Integrative
Medicine

Integrative Medicine

THIRD EDITION

David Rakel, MD
Associate Professor of Family Medicine
Director and Founder
University of Wisconsin Integrative Medicine
University of Wisconsin School of Medicine and Public Health
Madison, Wisconsin

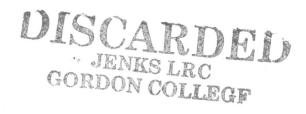
ELSEVIER
SAUNDERS

ELSEVIER
SAUNDERS

1600 John F. Kennedy Blvd.
Ste 1800
Philadelphia, PA 19103-2899

INTEGRATIVE MEDICINE ISBN: 978-1-4377-1793-8

Notices

Knowledge and best practice in this field are constantly changing. As new research and experience broaden our understanding, changes in research methods, professional practices, or medical treatment may become necessary.

Practitioners and researchers must always rely on their own experience and knowledge in evaluating and using any information, methods, compounds, or experiments described herein. In using such information or methods they should be mindful of their own safety and the safety of others, including parties for whom they have a professional responsibility.

With respect to any drug or pharmaceutical products identified, readers are advised to check the most current information provided (i) on procedures featured or (ii) by the manufacturer of each product to be administered to verify the recommended dose or formula, the method and duration of administration, and contraindications. It is the responsibility of practitioners, relying on their own experience and knowledge of their patients, to make diagnoses, to determine dosages and the best treatment for each individual patient, and to take all appropriate safety precautions.

To the fullest extent of the law, neither the Publisher nor the authors, contributors, or editors assume any liability for any injury and/or damage to persons or property as a matter of products liability, negligence, or otherwise or from any use or operation of any methods, products, instructions, or ideas contained in the material herein.

Library of Congress Cataloging-in-Publication Data

Integrative medicine / [edited by] David Rakel. – 3rd ed.
 p. ; cm.
 Includes bibliographical references.
 ISBN 978-1-4377-1793-8 (hardcover : alk. paper)
 I. Rakel, David.
 [DNLM: 1. Integrative Medicine–methods. 2. Complementary Therapies–methods. 3. Preventive Medicine–methods. 4. Primary Health Care–methods. WB 113]
 616—dc23

2012009514

Senior Content Strategist: Kate Dimock
Content Development Specialist: Julie Mirra
Publishing Services Manager: Anne Altepeter
Senior Project Manager: Doug Turner
Designer: Steve Stave

Printed in the United States of America
Last digit is the print number: 9 8 7 6 5 4 3

For my wife, Denise

Contributors

Robert Abel, Jr., MD
Delaware Ophthalmology Consultants
Wilmington, Delaware;
Former Clinical Professor of Ophthalmology
Thomas Jefferson University School of Medicine
Philadelphia, Pennsylvania

Ather Ali, ND, MPH
Assistant Director
Integrative Medicine, Prevention Research Center;
Associate Research Scientist, Pediatrics
Yale University School of Medicine
New Haven, Connecticut

Patricia Ammon, MD
Ridgway, Colorado

Bruce Barrett, MD, PhD
Associate Professor
Department of Family Medicine
University of Wisconsin School of Medicine and
    Public Health
Madison, Wisconsin

Iris R. Bell, MD, PhD
Department of Family and Community Medicine
The University of Arizona College of Medicine
Tucson, Arizona

Paul E. Bergquist, MD
Clinician
Family Practice and Complementary Medicine Clinic
Vernon Memorial Hospital Clinics
Medical Director
Vernon Memorial Hospital Home Health and Hospice
    Program
Viroqua, Wisconsin;
Medical Director
Sannes Skogdalen Nursing Home
Soldiers Grove, Wisconsin

Apple A. Bodemer, MD
Assistant Professor
Department of Dermatology
University of Wisconsin
Madison, Wisconsin

Robert Alan Bonakdar, MD
Director of Pain Management
Scripps Center for Integrative Medicine
Assistant Clinical Professor
Department of Family and Preventative Medicine
University of California, San Diego School of Medicine
La Jolla, California

Jennifer M. Capra, OMS-IV
College of Osteopathic Medicine
Kansas City University of Medicine and Biosciences
Kansas City, Missouri

Remy R. Coeytaux, MD, PhD
Associate Professor
Department of Community and Family Medicine
Duke Clinical Research Institute
Durham, North Carolina

Stephen M. Dahmer, MD
Attending Family Physician
Continuum Center for Health and Healing
New York, New York

Douglas E. Dandurand, PhD, MDiv
Spiritual Facilitator
Allina Center for Healthcare Innovation
The Penny George Institute for Health and Healing
Minneapolis, Minnesota

Alan M. Dattner, MD
CEO, HolisticDermatology.com
President, HealthDataLink.com
Director, Integrative Medicine and Dermatology
New York and New Rochelle, New York

Brian Degenhardt, DO
Associate Research Professor
Kirksville College of Osteopathic Medicine
A. T. Still University
Director
A. T. Still Research Institute
Kirksville, Missouri;
Co-Medical Director
Ridgway Integrative Medicine
Ridgway, Colorado

Ankit D. Desai, PharmD
Clinical Pharmacist
Harper University Hospital
Detroit, Michigan

Gautam J. Desai, DO
Associate Professor
Department of Family Medicine
College of Osteopathic Medicine
Kansas City University of Medicine and Biosciences
Kansas City, Missouri

Stephen Devries, MD
Preventive Cardiologist
Associate Professor of Medicine
Division of Cardiology
Northwestern University
Chicago, Illinois

Dennis J. Dowling, DO
Private Practice
Osteopathic Manipulative Medicine Associates
Syosset, New York;
Director of Osteopathic Manipulative Services
Physical Medicine and Rehabilitation Department
Nassau University Medical Center
East Meadow, New York;
Director of Osteopathic Manipulative Medicine
Clinical Skills Testing Center
National Board of Osteopathic Medical Examiners
Conshohocken, Pennsylvania

Jeffery Dusek, PhD
Research Director
Integrative Health and Medicine Research Center
Allina Center for Healthcare Innovation
The Penny George Institute for Health and Healing
Minneapolis, Minnesota

Connie J. Earl, DO
Integrative Medicine Fellow
UCSF Santa Rosa Family Medicine Residency
Santa Rosa, California

Brian Earley, DO
Assistant Professor
Department of Family Medicine
University of Wisconsin School of Medicine and
    Public Health
Madison, Wisconsin

Joseph Eichenseher, MD, MAT
Petaluma Health Center
Petaluma, California;
Adjunct Faculty
Touro University
Vallejo, California

Ann C. Figurski, DO
Family Medicine Physician
Healdsburg Family Practice
Sutter Medical Group of the Redwoods
Healdsburg, California

Luke Fortney, MD
Assistant Professor
Integrative Medicine Program
Department of Family Medicine
University of Wisconsin School of Medicine and
    Public Health
Madison, Wisconsin

Louise Gagné, MD
Clinical Assistant Professor
Department of Community Health and Epidemiology
University of Saskatchewan
Saskatoon, Saskatchewan, Canada

Leo Galland, MD
Director
Foundation for Integrative Medicine
New York, New York

Paula Gardiner, MD, MPH
Assistant Professor
Department of Family Medicine
Boston Medical Center
Boston, Massachusetts

Andrea Gordon, MD
Director of Integrative Medicine
Tufts University Family Medicine Residency Program
Cambridge Health Alliance
Malden, Massachusetts

Jeff Grassmann, DO
Integrative Medicine and Family Practice
Martin's Point Health Care
Portland, Maine

Russell H. Greenfield, MD
Director
Greenfield Integrative Healthcare, PLLC
Charlotte, North Carolina;
Clinical Assistant Professor of Medicine
University of North Carolina–Chapel Hill School of
    Medicine
Chapel Hill, North Carolina

Steven Gurgevich, PhD
Clinical Assistant Professor of Medicine
University of Arizona College of Medicine
Arizona Center for Integrative Medicine
Faculty, Fellow and Approved Consultant
The American Society of Clinical Hypnosis
Private Practice
Behavioral Medicine, Ltd.
Tucson, Arizona

Fasih A. Hameed, MD
Director of Integrative Medicine
Petaluma Health Center
Petaluma, California;
Assistant Clinical Professor
UCSF Santa Rosa Family Medicine Residency
Santa Rosa, California

Patrick J. Hanaway, MD
Chief Medical Officer
Genova Diagnostics
Asheville, North Carolina

James Harvie, PEng
Executive Director
Institute for a Sustainable Future
Duluth, Minnesota

Michael T. Hernke, PhD
Research Fellow
Department of Operations and Information Management
School of Business
University of Wisconsin
Madison, Wisconsin

Michael J. Hewitt, PhD
Research Director for Exercise Science
Department of Exercise Physiology
Canyon Ranch Health Resort
Tucson, Arizona

Ravi S. Hirekatur, MD
Clinical Assistant Professor
Department of Family Medicine
University of Wisconsin Urgent Care
University of Wisconsin Medical School
Madison, Wisconsin

Randy J. Horwitz, MD, PhD
Medical Director
Arizona Center for Integrative Medicine;
Assistant Professor of Medicine
University of Arizona College of Medicine
Tucson, Arizona

Corene Humphreys, ND
Director
Nutritional Medicine Ltd
Medical Research Consultant
Faculty Wellpark College of Natural Therapies
Auckland, New Zealand

Robert S. Ivker, DO
Co-Founder and Former President
American Board of Integrative Holistic Medicine
Medical Director
Fully Alive Medicine
Boulder, Colorado

Julia Jernberg, MD
Clinical Assistant Professor of Medicine
Department of Internal Medicine
Section of Geriatrics, General Medicine, and Palliative
    Medicine
University of Arizona College of Medicine
Tucson, Arizona;
Clinical Assistant Professor of Medicine
Department of Internal Medicine
University of Wisconsin Hospitals and Clinics
Madison, Wisconsin

Wayne Jonas, MD
Associate Professor of Family Medicine
Uniformed Services University of Health Sciences
President and Chief Executive Officer
Samueli Institute
Alexandria, Virginia

Amanda J. Kaufman, MD
Assistant Professor
Department of Family Medicine
University of Michigan
Ann Arbor, Michigan

Kathi J. Kemper, MD, MPH
Caryl J. Guth Chair for Complementary and Integrative
    Medicine
Professor of Social Science/Health Policy and Pediatrics
Wake Forest University School of Medicine
Winston-Salem, North Carolina

Dharma Singh Khalsa, MD
Founding President and Medical Director
Alzheimer's Research and Prevention Foundation
Tucson, Arizona

Sarah K. Khan, RD, MPH, PhD
Adjunct Professor
University of Wisconsin School of Medicine and
    Public Health
Founder and Director
Institute of Food, Healing, and Culture
Madison, Wisconsin

David Kiefer, MD
Clinical Assistant Professor of Medicine
Arizona Center for Integrative Medicine
University of Arizona
Tucson, Arizona;
Research Fellow
Department of Family Medicine
University of Wisconsin School of Medicine and
    Public Health
Madison, Wisconsin

Benjamin Kligler, MD, MPH
Vice Chair and Research Director
Beth Israel Department of Integrative Medicine
Continuum Center for Health and Healing
New York, New York

Wendy Kohatsu, MD
Assistant Professor of Family Medicine
Oregon Health & Science University
Portland, Oregon;
Visiting Assistant Professor
University of Arizona College of Medicine
Tucson, Arizona

Greta J. Kuphal, MD
Clinical Assistant Professor
University of Wisconsin Integrative Medicine
Department of Family Medicine
University of Wisconsin School of Medicine and
    Public Health
Madison, Wisconsin

Roberta A. Lee, MD
Vice Chair
Department of Integrative Medicine
Beth Israel Medical Center
New York, New York

David M. Lessens, MD, MPH
Integrative Medicine Fellow
University of Wisconsin Integrative Medicine
Department of Family Medicine
University of Wisconsin School of Medicine and
    Public Health
Madison, Wisconsin

Edward (Lev) Linkner, MD
Founding Member
American Board of Integrative Holistic Medicine
Clinical Associate Professor
Department of Family Medicine
University of Michigan Medical School
Faculty, Department of Family Practice
St. Joseph Mercy Hospital
Private Practice
Ann Arbor, Michigan

Yue Man Onna Lo, MD
Family Physician
Asian Health Services
Oakland, California

Amy B. Locke, MD
Assistant Professor
Integrative Medicine Wellness Center
Department of Family Medicine
University of Michigan Medical School
Ann Arbor, Michigan

Erica A. Lovett, MD
Integrative Family Medicine Physician and Faculty
Central Maine Medical Center Family Medicine
    Residency
Portland, Maine;
Clinical Assistant Professor of Family Medicine
Boston University
Boston, Massachusetts;
Associate Faculty
University of New England College of Osteopathic
    Medicine
Biddeford, Maine

Tieraona Low Dog, MD
Fellowship Director
Arizona Center for Integrative Medicine
Clinical Associate Professor of Medicine
University of Arizona Health Sciences
Tucson, Arizona

Michael Lumpkin, PhD
Chair
Department of Physiology and Biophysics
Georgetown University
Washington, District of Columbia

Junelle H. Lupiani, RD
Registered Dietician and Nutrition Expert
Miraval Spa and Resorts
Tucson, Arizona

Victoria Maizes, MD
Executive Director
Arizona Center for Integrative Medicine
Professor of Clinical Medicine, Family Medicine,
    and Public Health
University of Arizona
Tucson, Arizona

Geeta Maker-Clark, MD
Integrative Family Physician
NorthShore University HealthSystem
Evanston, Illinois

D. Jill Mallory, MD
Physician
Wildwood Family Clinic
Madison, Wisconsin

John Douglas Mann, MD
Professor of Neurology
Department of Neurology
University of North Carolina
Chapel Hill, North Carolina

Lucille R. Marchand, MD, BSN
Professor
Family Medicine
University of Wisconsin School of Medicine and
    Public Health
Medical Director
St. Mary's Hospital Palliative Care Inpatient Service
Clinical Director
Integrative Oncology Services
University of Wisconsin Carbone Cancer Center
Madison, Wisconsin

John D. Mark, MD
Clinical Professor of Pediatrics
Pediatric Pulmonary Medicine
Stanford University School of Medicine
Palo Alto, California

Patrick B. Massey, MD, PhD
Medical Director
Complementary and Alternative Medicine
Alexian Brothers Hospital Network
Elk Grove Village, Illinois

Patrick E. McBride, MD, MPH
Professor
Departments of Medicine and Family Medicine
Co-Director
Preventive Cardiology Program
Associate Dean for Students
University of Wisconsin School of Medicine and
    Public Health
Madison, Wisconsin

Mark W. McClure, MD
Associated Urologists of North Carolina
Raleigh, North Carolina

Leslie Mendoza Temple, MD
Clinical Assistant Professor of Family Medicine
University of Chicago Pritzker School of Medicine
Medical Director
Integrative Medicine Program
NorthShore University HealthSystem
Glenview, Illinois

Michelle J. Mertz, MD
Family Medicine Resident
UCSF Santa Rosa Family Medicine Residency
Santa Rosa, California

Aaron J. Michelfelder, MD
Professor of Family Medicine and Bioethics and
    Health Policy
Loyola University Chicago Stritch School of Medicine
Family Physician, Medical Acupuncturist, and Integrative
    Medicine Physician
Loyola University Health System
Maywood, Illinois

Daniel Muller, MD, PhD
Associate Professor of Medicine and Rheumatology
University of Wisconsin School of Medicine and Public Health
Madison, Wisconsin

Matthew P. Mumber, MD
Department Chair
Radiation Oncology
Co-Director
Harbin Clinic Integrative Oncology Program
Co-Director
Harbin MD Ambassador Program
Harbin Clinic
Rome, Georgia

Harmon Myers, DO
Preceptor
Program in Integrative Medicine
University of Arizona College of Medicine
Tucson, Arizona

Richard Nahas, MD
Assistant Professor
Department of Family Medicine
University of Ottawa
Medical Director
Seekers Centre for Integrative Medicine
Ottawa, Ontario, Canada

Rubin Naiman, PhD
Clinical Assistant Professor of Medicine
Arizona Center for Integrative Medicine
University of Arizona
Tucson, Arizona

Wadie I. Najm, MD, MSEd
Clinical Professor
Department of Family Medicine
Susan Samueli Center of Integrative Medicine
University of California, Irvine
Irvine, California

Sanford C. Newmark, MD
Head, Pediatric Integrative Neurodevelopmental Clinic
Osher Center for Integrative Medicine
University of California, San Francisco
San Francisco, California

James P. Nicolai, MD
Medical Director
Andrew Weil, MD, Integrative Wellness Program
Miraval Spa and Resorts
Tucson, Arizona

Brian Olshansky, MD
Professor of Medicine
Department of Internal Medicine
University of Iowa Hospitals and Clinics
Iowa City, Iowa

Sunil T. Pai, MD
President and Medical Director
Sanjevani LLC
Integrative Medicine Health and Lifestyle Center
Sanjevani Nutraceuticals/Cosmeceuticals LLC
Sante Fe, New Mexico

Danna Park, MD
Medical Director
Integrative Healthcare Program
Mission Hospitals System
Asheville, North Carolina

Adam I. Perlman, MD, MPH
Executive Director
Duke Integrative Medicine
Associate Professor
Division of General Internal Medicine
Duke University
Durham, North Carolina

Surya Pierce, MD
Integrative Family Physician
Little Axe Clinic
Absentee Shawnee Tribe
Norman, Oklahoma

Judy Platt, MD
Director of Maternity Care
Tufts University Family Medicine Residency Program
Cambridge Health Alliance
Malden, Massachusetts

Gregory A. Plotnikoff, MD, MTS
Senior Consultant
Allina Center for Healthcare Innovation;
Integrative Medicine Physician
The Penny George Institute for Health and Healing
Minneapolis, Minnesota

Rian J. Podein, MD
Family Physician
Mayo Clinic Health System
Lake City, Minnesota

David Rabago, MD
Assistant Professor
Department of Family Medicine
University of Wisconsin School of Medicine and
    Public Health
Madison, Wisconsin

David Rakel, MD
Associate Professor of Family Medicine
Founder and Director
University of Wisconsin Integrative Medicine
University of Wisconsin School of Medicine and
    Public Health
Madison, Wisconsin

Gayle Reed, PhD, RN
Owner
Forgiveness Recovery LLC
Madison, Wisconsin

Robert Rhode, PhD
Clinical Psychologist and Adjunct Lecturer
Department of Psychiatry
Arizona Health Sciences Center
Tucson, Arizona;
Clinical Assistant Professor
Applied Behavioral Health Policy Division
Arizona State University
Tempe, Arizona

J. Adam Rindfleisch, MD, MPhil
Associate Professor
University of Wisconsin Integrative Medicine
Fellowship Director
Department of Family Medicine
University of Wisconsin School of Medicine and
    Public Health
Madison, Wisconsin

Melinda Ring, MD
Medical Director
Northwestern Integrative Medicine;
Assistant Professor of Clinical Medicine
Feinberg School of Medicine
Northwestern University
Chicago, Illinois

Lawrence D. Rosen, MD
Founder
The Whole Child Center
Oradell, New Jersey;
Clinical Assistant Professor
University of Medicine and Dentistry of New Jersey
Newark, New Jersey

Lisa Rosenberger, ND, LAc
Research Fellow, Integrative Medicine
Prevention Research Center
Yale University School of Medicine
New Haven, Connecticut

Martin L. Rossman, MD
Clinical Associate Professor
Department of Medicine
School of Medicine
University of California, San Francisco
San Francisco, California;
Director
Collaborative Medicine Center
Founder
The Healing Mind, Inc.
Greenbrae, California;
Co-Founder
Academy for Guided Imagery
Malibu, California

Robert B. Saper, MD, MPH
Director of Integrative Medicine
Department of Family Medicine
Boston Medical Center
Associate Professor
Boston University School of Medicine
Boston, Massachusetts

Craig Schneider, MD
Director of Integrative Medicine
Department of Family Medicine
Maine Medical Center
Portland, Maine;
Assistant Clinical Professor
Tufts University School of Medicine
Boston, Massachusetts

Howard Schubiner, MD
Department of Internal Medicine
Providence Hospital
Southfield, Michigan;
Clinical Professor
Wayne State University School of Medicine
Detroit, Michigan

Nancy J. Selfridge, MD
Associate Professor
Department of Integrated Medical Education
Ross University School of Medicine
Commonwealth of Dominica, West Indies

Tanmeet Sethi, MD
Faculty Physician
Director of Integrative Medicine Curriculum
Swedish Cherry Hill Family Medicine Residency
Clinical Associate Professor
University of Washington
Seattle, Washington

Howard Silverman, MD
Associate Dean for Information Resources and Educational
    Technology
Clinical Professor
Departments of Family and Community Medicine
The University of Arizona College of Medicine, Phoenix
Clinical Professor of Biomedical Informatics
Arizona State University
Phoenix, Arizona

Adam D. Simmons, MD
Assistant Professor of Neurology
University of Connecticut School of Medicine
Farmington, Connecticut

Coleen Smith, DO
Founder
Johnson City Osteopathic Medicine
Johnson City, Tennessee

Pamela W. Smith, MD, MPH
Co-Director
Master's Program in Medical Sciences
University of South Florida College of Medicine
Tampa, Florida

Tina M. St. John, MD
Owner and Principal
St. John Health Communications and Consulting
Vancouver, Washington

Alicia Stanton, MD
Physician
Enfield, Connecticut

Joel M. Stevans, DC
Postdoctoral Fellow
Department of Physical Therapy
University of Pittsburgh
Pittsburgh, Pennsylvania

Larry Stoler, PhD, MSSA
Clinical Psychologist and Medical Qigong
WholeHealth Chicago
Chicago, Illinois

Nancy L. Sudak, MD
Executive Director
American Board of Integrative Holistic Medicine
Duluth, Minnesota

Jacob Teitelbaum, MD
Medical Director
Fibromyalgia and Fatigue Centers
Chronicity (Nationally)
Annapolis, Maryland

Gail Underbakke, RD, MS
Nutrition Course Director
University of Wisconsin School of Medicine and
    Public Health
Nutrition Coordinator
Preventive Cardiology Program
University of Wisconsin Hospital and Clinics
Madison, Wisconsin

Malynn L. Utzinger-Wheeler, MD, MA
Integrative Medicine Private Practice
Greenwich, Connecticut, and Manhattan, New York

Donald Warne, MD, MPH
Director
Master of Public Health Program
North Dakota State University
Fargo, North Dakota

Allan Warshowsky, MD
Private Practice
Rye, New York

Andrew Weil, MD
Director
Arizona Center for Integrative Medicine
Clinical Professor of Medicine
Professor of Public Health
University of Arizona
Tucson, Arizona

Joy A. Weydert, MD
Associate Professor of Pediatrics and Integrative Medicine
Department of Pediatrics
University of Kansas Medical Center
Kansas City, Kansas

Myrtle Wilhite, MD
Medical Director
A Woman's Touch Sexuality Resource Center
Madison, Wisconsin

Ted Wissink, MD
Integrative Medicine and Family Medicine
Department of Family Medicine
Maine Medical Center
Portland, Maine

Andrew J. Wolf, MEd
Exercise Physiologist
Miraval Spa and Resorts
Tucson, Arizona

Jimmy Wu, MD
Family Practice Post-Graduate Year 3
Santa Rosa Family Practice Residency Program
Santa Rosa, California

Sean H. Zager, MD
Integrative Medicine Fellow and Clinical Lecturer
Department of Family Medicine
University of Michigan
Ann Arbor, Michigan

Aleksandra Zgierska, MD, PhD
Assistant Professor
Department of Family Medicine
University of Wisconsin School of Medicine and
    Public Health
Madison, Wisconsin

Foreword

With the publication of the revised and expanded third edition, *Integrative Medicine* has become an established textbook in this new and rapidly growing field of clinical medicine. As I wrote in the foreword to the second edition:

> David Rakel and I and our growing number of colleagues feel strongly that integrative medicine is the way of the future. Not only is it the kind of medicine that most of our patients want, it is the kind that more and more physicians want to practice, because it restores the core values of the profession that have so eroded in the era of managed care. We also believe that it offers hope for rescuing a health care system on the verge of collapse. The reason is that integrative medicine can save money by bringing lower-cost treatments into the mainstream while preserving outcomes (or even improving them). At some point, we believe, we will be able to drop the word *integrative*. This will just be good medicine.

Most needed now are outcomes studies to document the effectiveness and cost-effectiveness of integrative versus conventional treatments for common health conditions. It is not so easy to design and conduct such studies, which are expensive and require large enough study populations to generate meaningful data. Clinical outcomes studies are not within the mission of the National Institutes of Health, and few researchers are trained to work with the complex and individualized treatments that practitioners of integrative medicine (IM) use. But demonstrating that IM works and saves money is the only way to change policies of reimbursement that are now the main impediment to taking IM mainstream.

The Arizona Center for Integrative Medicine will soon have graduated 1000 physicians from its intensive fellowship training and has been successful in making IM training a required, accredited part of residency training in family medicine. We are now expanding Integrative Medicine in Residency to pediatrics and internal medicine. As more and more clinicians learn IM, there is greater need for reliable, evidence-based treatment guidelines. I believe that *Integrative Medicine* answers that need.

This new edition includes more conditions (some of which are multiple sclerosis, Parkinson disease, insomnia, Lyme disease, polycystic overian syndrome, and erectile dysfunction), as well as discussions of the healing encounter, human energetic therapies, and other topics of relevance to IM practice. As in previous editions, there is strong emphasis on prevention and a visual icon to help readers evaluate evidence for both the benefits and risks of treatments.

David Rakel is committed to keeping this text current and informed by the best available research data. He has made the new edition even better and more useful than the last.

Andrew Weil, MD
Director, Arizona Center for Integrative Medicine
Clinical Professor of Medicine
Professor of Public Health
University of Arizona
Tucson, Arizona
July 2011

Preface

I am excited to present the third edition of *Integrative Medicine*. This text is focused on empowering the clinician to practice an integrative approach using therapies that address all aspects of health to facilitate healing.

We have worked hard to make this edition more efficient so the clinician can access evidence-based information quickly without having to sift through a lot of text. We have reduced the page count while increasing the density of content. There are 114 chapters with 37 new authors and 12 new chapters that include topics such as Lyme disease, polycystic ovarian syndrome, insomnia, and hormone replacement in men and women.

The text is divided into three parts. Part 1, "Integrative Medicine," is an overview of the field of integrative medicine and focuses on the philosophy of integrative medicine, how to create optimal healing environments, and key ingredients of the healing encounter. Part 2, "Integrative Approach to Disease," is the core of the text and discusses integrative approaches to treating disorders that range from insomnia to diabetes to various forms of cancer. Part 3, "Tools for Your Practice," includes practical, how-to information on common integrative therapeutic interventions.

The text format makes the information easy to find. Each disease-focused chapter concludes with a Therapeutic Review section that summarizes an integrative approach. Evidence-versus-harm icons provide the clinician a quick and efficient way to assess the level of evidence compared with the level of the potential harm for recommended therapies. Potential for harm has been an important missing factor in evidence-based rating scales (see "Using the Evidence-Versus-Harm Grading Icons" following the preface). Each chapter also has a Prevention Prescription, which summarizes key factors that will help prevent the disease being discussed and its recurrence. The text can also be accessed electronically.

Integrative medicine offers a path to improve the value of heatlh care by lowering cost and improving quality as health and healing become our primary objectives. I hope that this text proves to be a useful tool as you partner with your patients to find health within the complexity of life. Thank you for engaging in this work.

David Rakel, MD

Using the Evidence-Versus-Harm Grading Icons

In the busy practice of medicine, being able to access information quickly and efficiently is important for obtaining the highest quality data in the shortest period of time in the effort to enhance care.

The Strength of Recommendation Taxonomy (SORT)[1] rating for evidence has been an excellent step in this direction. The A, B, and C ratings give us a quick and simple way to judge the quality of evidence for a particular intervention. There are limitations to making decisions based only on the evidence. One limitation is the absence of the potential harm of the evidence. Even if the evidence may be grade A, the potential harm of that intervention may negate its effect.

An example is the Randomized Aldactone Evaluation Study (RALES) published in the *New England Journal of Medicine* in 1999.[2] This study showed that spironolactone significantly improved outcomes in patients with severe heart failure. A follow-up article published in the same journal in 2004[3] showed that after the publication of this study, the number of prescriptions written for spironolactone significantly increased in Ontario, Canada, from 34 per 1000 patients in 1994 to 149 per 1000 patients in 2001. Thus the Canadian physicians were practicing evidence-based medicine, and their prescribing habits resonated with this. The follow-up study also noted that despite this evidence-based practice, there was a significant increase in the number of hospital admission and in the death rate related to hyperkalemia when spironolactone and ACE inhibitors were used together. In fact, when the investigators took into account the number of deaths related to hyperkalemia, there was no decrease in the number of admissions or the death rate for congestive heart failure patients after the publication of RALES. The initial benefit of improving outcomes in congestive heart failure with spironolactone seen in the original study was not evident in the application of the evidence in the clinical setting. The potential harm of the evidence was not taken into account, and this drug may have caused more harm than good.

Adding a rating for potential harm will enhance the rating of the evidence for the clinician but is by no means a final guiding rule. Decision making goes beyond the evidence and the harm and is grounded in the much broader insights obtained through relationship-centered care. It is only a tool that we hope will make the clinician's life a little easier in recommending specific therapeutic interventions.

Grading the Evidence

The authors of this text used the SORT criteria for grading the evidence for the therapies that are recommended in the Therapeutic Review sections of the chapters. A simplified summary follows:

Grade A	Based on consistent, good-quality, patient-oriented evidence (e.g., systematic review or meta-analysis showing benefit, Cochrane Review with clear recommendation, high-quality patient-oriented randomized controlled trial). Example: Acupuncture for nausea and vomiting.
Grade B	Based on inconsistent or limited-quality patient-oriented evidence. Example: Ginger for osteoarthritis.
Grade C	Based on consensus, usual practice, opinion, disease-oriented evidence (e.g., study showing a reduction in blood sugar but no studies in humans to show a benefit to those with diabetes).

Grading the Potential Harm

Unlike grading for evidence, there is no unified, acceptable grading system for harm. In grading the three levels of harm, we used the following grading scale:

Grade 3 (most harm)	This therapy has the potential to result in death or permanent disability. Example: Major surgery under general anesthesia or carcinogenic effects of the botanical *Aristolochia* (birthwort).
Grade 2 (moderate harm)	This therapy has the potential to cause reversible side effects or interact in a negative way with other therapies. Example: Pharmaceutical or neutraceutical side effects.
Grade 1 (least harm)	This therapy poses little, if any, risk of harm. Examples: Eating more vegetables, increasing exercise, elimination diets, encouraging social connection.

The resulting icons incorporate a weighing of the evidence versus the potential harm. If the evidence is strong (A) with the least potential harm (1), the arrow will point up. If the evidence is weak (C) with the most potential harm (3), the arrow will point down.

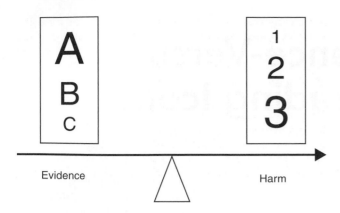

Evidence ——————————△—————————— Harm

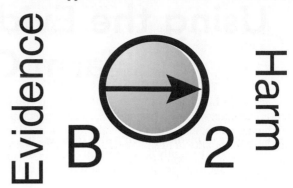

- Zinc supplementation for infectious diarrhea (B,2)

Examples:

Clinical Recommendation

- Exercise for diabetes management (A,1)

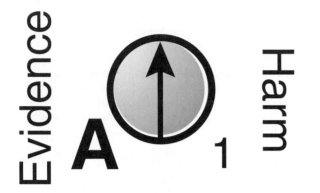

- Hypnosis for irritable bowel syndrome (B,1)

- Astragalus root for infectious hepatitis (C,2)

- *Aristolochia* (birthwort) to support immunity (C,3)

Rating Options	Arrow	Icon
(A,1)	↑	A⊕₁
(A,2) (B,1)	↗	A⊕₂ B⊕₁
(A,3) (B,2) (C,1)	→	A⊕₃ B⊕₂ C⊕₁
(B,3) (C,2)	↘	B⊕₂ C⊕₂
(C,3)	↓	C⊕₃

Strengths of Evidence-Versus-Harm Grading

- Gives quick access to the balance of available evidence and potential harm for a given therapy.

- Works best for therapeutic interventions for chronic disease compared with acute or emergency treatments.

- Gives more credibility to therapies that have little potential harm. For example, we know that encouraging social support, reducing stress, and enhancing spiritual connection are beneficial for quality of life and health, but the evidence may not be strong. The potential harm will always be low, giving the benefit a more positive outlook.

- Helps us honor our primary goal, which is to "first, do no harm." This rating scale allows us to include this important fact in medical decision making. This is very important, seeing that adverse drug reactions from medical therapy have been found to be the sixth leading cause of hospital deaths in the United States.[4]

Limitations of Evidence-Versus-Harm Grading

- Is used only for those therapies proved to have a positive benefit. There may be good evidence showing that a therapy does not work. If this was the case, the therapy was not included in the Therapeutic Review.

- Does not reward the potentially life-saving interventions that are risky and have little available evidence showing benefit. For example, there has not been a meta-analysis showing that emergency repair of a dissecting aortic aneurysm has therapeutic benefit. The potential harm of this therapy is high (Grade 3). On the evidence-versus-harm scale, this therapy would have an arrow pointing toward the negative side, but without the therapy the patient would likely die.

- Those therapies that have the most potential for economic gain often have the most evidence. For example, there are more resources to do high-quality research for a potentially profitable pharmaceutical that can be patented than for a whole food or plant that cannot. Therapies such as pharmaceuticals will have a higher quality of evidence in general when compared with botanicals, mind-body therapy, and spiritual connection.

- This rating scale can be reductionistic. It is much easier to complete high-quality research based on our scientific model on a physical process, drug, or supplement. It is harder to show an enhanced quality of life or a reduction in suffering from reducing social isolation, for example.

Summary

This model includes potential harm along with the strength of the evidence. The arrows will give a quick reference for potential benefit when the evidence and harm are weighted against each other. For example, strong (heavy) evidence with little (light) potential harm will result in an arrow pointing up. This will be most helpful for recommendations for chronic disease. Unlike acute life-threatening conditions that often need more aggressive intervention with higher potential risk, chronic disease is often managed using lifestyle choices that will be supported by this model.

References

1. Ebell MH, Siwek J, Weiss BD, et al. Strength of recommendation taxonomy (SORT): a patient-centered approach to grading evidence in the medical literature. *Am Fam Physician*. 2004;69:548–556.
2. Pitt B, Zannad F, Remme WJ, et al. The effect of spironolactone on morbidity and mortality in patients with severe heart failure. Randomized Aldactone Evaluation Study Investigators. *N Engl J Med*. 1999;341:709–717.
3. Juurlink DN, Mamdani MM, Lee DS, et al. Rates of hyperkalemia after publication of the randomized aldactone evaluation study. *N Engl J Med*. 2004;351:543–551.
4. Lazarou J, Pomeranz BH, Corey PN. Incidence of adverse drug reactions in hospitalized patients. *JAMA*. 1998;279:1200–1205.

Acknowledgments

This text would not have been possible without the talents of a passionate group of people. I would like to thank my colleagues at Elsevier—Kate Dimock, Julie Mirra, Doug Turner, and Kate Crowley—for their support, advice, and hard work. I am very appreciative of the more than 100 authors who took time from their personal lives and families to write this text. I am thankful to the faculty and staff at the University of Wisconsin Department of Family Medicine, UW Health Hospitals and Clinics, and the Program in Integrative Medicine for their support and friendship. I am grateful to my colleagues at the Arizona Center for Integrative Medicine, the Consortium of Academic Health Centers for Integrative Medicine (CAHCIM), and the American Board of Integrative Holistic Medicine (ABIHM) for contributing to this text and helping define a new model for health care delivery. It is an honor to be able to work with such a talented and caring group of people. I would also like to thank the students, residents, and fellows from the University of Wisconsin and across the country for all that they have taught me and encouraged me to think about and explore. And finally, I am thankful to my wife, Denise, and children, Justin, Sarah, and Lucas, for their love and presence.

Contents

Part One Integrative Medicine

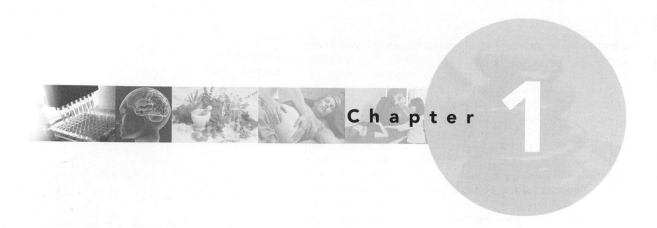

Chapter 1

Philosophy of Integrative Medicine

David Rakel, MD, and Andrew Weil, MD

A Brief History of Integrative Medicine

> When religion was strong and medicine weak, men mistook magic for medicine;
>
> Now, when science is strong and religion weak, men mistake medicine for magic.
>
> *Thomas Szasz, The Second Sin*

The philosophy of integrative medicine is not new. It has been talked about for ages across many disciplines. It has simply been overlooked as the pendulum of accepted medical care swings from one extreme to the other. We are currently experiencing the beginning of a shift toward recognizing the benefits of combining the external, physical, and technologic successes of curing with the internal, nonphysical exploration of healing.

Long before magnetic resonance imaging and computed tomographic scanners existed, Aristotle (384-322 BC) was able simply to experience, observe, and reflect on the human condition. He was one of the first holistic physicians who believed that every person was a combination of both physical and spiritual properties with no separation between mind and body. It was not until the 1600s that a spiritual mathematician became worried that prevailing scientific materialistic thought would reduce the conscious mind to something that could be manipulated and controlled. René Descartes (1596-1650), respecting the great unknown, did his best to separate the mind and the body to protect the spirit from science. He believed that mind and spirit should be the focus of the church, thus leaving science to dissect the physical body. This philosophy led to the "Cartesian split" of mind-body duality.

Shortly afterward, John Locke (1632-1704) and David Hume (1711-1776) influenced the reductionistic movement that shaped our science and medical system. The idea was that if we could reduce natural phenomena to greater simplicity, we could understand the larger whole. So to learn about a clock, all we need to do is study its parts. Reductionism facilitated great discoveries that helped humans gain control over their environment. Despite this progress, physicians had few tools to treat disease effectively. In the early twentieth century, applied science started to transform medicine through the development of medical technologies. In 1910, the Flexner report[1] was written and had a significant impact on the development of allopathic academic institutions. They came to emphasize the triad that prevails today: research, education, and clinical practice. Reductionism and the scientific method produced the knowledge that encouraged the growth of these institutions.

The scientific model led to greater understanding of the pathophysiologic basis of disease and the development of tools to help combat its influence. Subspecialization of medical care facilitated the application of the new information. We now have practitioners who focus on the pieces and a society that appreciates their abilities to fix problems. Unfortunately, this approach does not work well for chronic disease that involves more than just a single part. In fact, all body organs are interconnected, so that simply repairing a part without addressing the underlying causes for its failure provides only temporary relief and a false sense of security.

More Technology, Less Communication

The tremendous success of medical science of the twentieth century was not without cost. Total health care expenditures reached $2.5 trillion in 2009, an amount that was 17.6% of the Gross Domestic Product (GDP) and translates to $8086 per U.S. resident. The health care market grows when more attention is focused on parts that can be treated with drugs or procedures. In just 6 years (2003 to 2009), drug spending in the United States rose 39% from $180 billion to $250 billion.[2] Financial rewards increase when we have more subtypes of disease to which treatments can be matched. The system encourages patients to believe that tools are the answer to their physical woes and discourages them from paying attention to the interplay of mind, community, and spirit. Technology is the golden calf in this scenario. We have become dependent on it, and overuse has widened the barrier of communication between patient and provider. The old tools of the trade—rapport, gestalt, intuition, and laying on of hands—were used less and less as powerful drugs and high-tech interventions became available.

To help curtail costs, managed care and capitation were born. These new models reduced excessive costs and further eroded the patient-provider relationship by placing increased time demands on physicians that did not involve patient care. Physician and patient unrest followed. Physicians are unhappy in part because of loss of autonomy in practicing medicine. Patients are unhappy in part because they believe they are not receiving the attention they need. Most upset are patients with chronic medical conditions whose diseases do not respond well to the treatments of specialized medicine. This comes at a time when the incidence of chronic and degenerative diseases is at an all-time high. Diseases such as heart disease, diabetes, irritable bowel syndrome, chronic fatigue, and chronic pain syndromes are quite common. They require evaluation and treatment of much more than any one organ. The public has started to realize the limitations of Western medicine and wants more attention paid to health and healing of the whole person, especially when someone has no "part" to be fixed.

Public Interest Influences Change

The deterioration of the patient-provider relationship, the overuse of technology, and the inability of the medical system to treat chronic disease adequately has contributed to rising interest in complementary and alternative medicine (CAM). The public has sent its message with their feet and their pocketbooks. In fact, more visits were made to CAM providers in the early 1990s than to all primary care medical physicians, and patients paid for these visits out of pocket, with an estimated expenditure of $13 billion.[3] This trend continued throughout the 1990s; 42% of the public used alternative therapies, and expenditures increased to $27 billion from 1990 to 1997.[4] Patients are also demanding less aggressive forms of therapy, and they are especially leery of the toxicity of pharmaceutical drugs. Adverse drug reactions have become the sixth leading cause of death in hospitalized patients,[5] and in 1994, botanicals were the largest growth area in retail pharmacy.[6] Research shows that people find complementary approaches to be more aligned with "their own values, beliefs, and philosophical orientations toward health and life."[7] The public, before the medical establishment, realized that health and healing involved more than pills and surgery. Less invasive, more traditional treatments such as nutrition, botanicals, manipulation, meditation, massage, and others that were neglected during the explosion of medical science and technology were now being rediscovered with great enthusiasm (Fig. 1-1).

FIGURE 1-1
Integrative medicine pie chart.

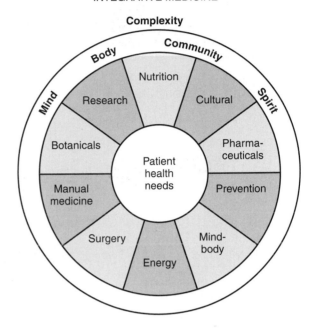

Medicine Gets the Message

The popularity of CAM therapies created a need for research in these areas. In 1993, an Office of Alternative Medicine was started within the National Institutes of Health (NIH). The initial budget was $2 million, a fraction of the $80 billion budget of the NIH. The office was later upgraded to the National Center for Complementary and Alternative Medicine (NCCAM), and the amount of money available for scholarly research kept pace with this growth. By 2010, the NCCAM budget grew to $127 million.[8] This allowed for needed research to explore ways in which these areas of medicine could enhance health care delivery. At first, researchers tried to use traditional methods to learn about CAM therapies. These methods were sufficient for studying some areas such as botanicals. The limitations of the reductionistic model became apparent, however, when it was applied to more dynamic systems of healing such as homeopathy, traditional Chinese medicine, and energy medicine. New methods were required to understand the multiple influences involved. Outcome studies with attention to quality of life were initiated. Research grants in "frontier medicine" were created to help learn about fields such as energy medicine, homeopathy, magnet therapy, and therapeutic prayer. Interest grew in learning how to combine the successes of the scientific model with the potential of CAM to improve the delivery of health care.

Academic Centers Respond

In 1997, one of the authors of this chapter, Andrew Weil, started the first fellowship program in integrative medicine at the University of Arizona. This 2-year clinical and research fellowship was created to train physicians in the science of health and healing and to teach more about therapies that

FIGURE 1-2
Adults and children who have used complementary and alternative medicine (CAM): United States, 2007. (From Barnes PM, Blook B, Nahin R. *Complementary and Alternative Medicine Use among Adults and Children: United States, 2007.* National health statistics report no. 12. Hyattsville, Md: National Center for Health Statistics; 2008.)

FIGURE 1-3
The 10 most commonly used complementary and alternative medicine (CAM) therapies among adults and a list of the most significant increases in therapies from 2002 to 2007. (From Barnes PM, Blook B, Nahin R. *Complementary and Alternative Medicine Use among Adults and Children: United States, 2007.* National health statistics report no. 12. Hyattsville, Md: National Center for Health Statistics; 2008.)

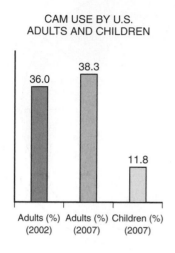

CAM USE BY U.S. ADULTS AND CHILDREN

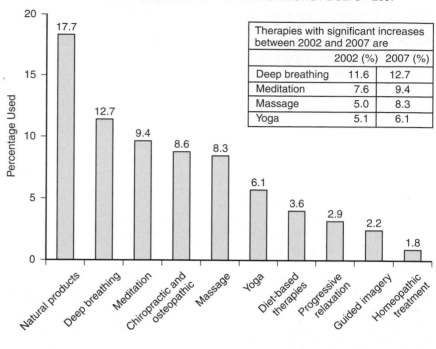

10 MOST COMMON CAM THERAPIES AMONG ADULTS—2007

Therapies with significant increases between 2002 and 2007 are	2002 (%)	2007 (%)
Deep breathing	11.6	12.7
Meditation	7.6	9.4
Massage	5.0	8.3
Yoga	5.1	6.1

were not part of Western medical practice. Other fellowship programs have been created since this time, as well as projects to incorporate integrative medicine into a 4-year family medicine residency training model. NIH-sponsored R-25 grants have been awarded to medical schools across the country to bring these concepts into medical school curriculums. The Consortium of Academic Health Centers for Integrative Medicine (CAHCIM) now comprises more than 45 medical schools across the United States and Canada, and it brings academic leaders together to transform health care through rigorous scientific studies, new models of clinical care, and innovative educational programs that integrate biomedicine, the complexity of humans, the intrinsic nature of healing, and the rich diversity of therapeutic systems.[9]

> Integrative medicine is defined as healing-oriented medicine that takes account of the whole person (body, mind, and spirit), including all aspects of lifestyle. It emphasizes the therapeutic relationship and makes use of all appropriate therapies, both conventional and alternative.

Complementary and Alternative Medicine Use Grows in the United States

Because of the popularity of CAM in the United States, the Institute of Medicine (IOM) published the results of a review of CAM in 2004 to create a better understanding of how it can best be translated into conventional medical practice. The IOM recommended that health profession schools incorporate sufficient information about CAM into the standard curriculum to enable licensed professionals to advise their patients competently about CAM.[10]

Data collected from National Health Interview Survey in 2002 by the Centers for Disease Control and Prevention's National Center for Health Statistics showed that 62% of U.S. adults used CAM within 12 months of being interviewed. When prayer was excluded as a CAM therapy, the percentage dropped to 36%.[11] This survey was repeated in 2007, during which the use of CAM rose slightly from 36% to 38.3%. The 2007 survey included children, in whom it showed 11.8% use of CAM therapy, most commonly for back/neck pain (6.7%) and colds (6.6%) (Fig. 1-2). The 10 most commonly used CAM therapies can be reviewed in Figure 1-3. The use of natural products was the most common at 17.7%. Pain conditions were the most common reason for CAM therapy in adults, and low back pain accounted for the highest CAM use, at 17.1% (Fig. 1-4).[12] A review also showed an increase in use of CAM in those who did not have access to conventional medical care, thus showing the importance of CAM as an option for the uninsured.[13] These data suggest that people value other ways of treating illness and that they want to be empowered to be active participants in their care. They also feel that CAM offers them more opportunity to tell their story and explore a more holistic view of their problem.[14]

DISEASES/CONDITIONS FOR WHICH CAM IS MOST
FREQUENTLY USED AMONG ADULTS—2007

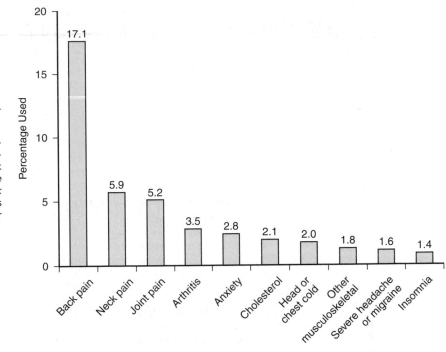

FIGURE 1-4
Diseases and conditions for which complementary and alternative medicine (CAM) is most frequently used in adults. (From Barnes PM, Blook B, Nahin R. *Complementary and Alternative Medicine Use among Adults and Children: United States, 2007.* National health statistics report no. 12. Hyattsville, Md: National Center for Health Statistics; 2008.)

Avoiding Complementary and Alternative Medicine Labels

With the growth of good scientific research regarding many CAM therapies, we are realizing that the labels once used to classify these therapies are no longer needed (Fig. 1-5). The use of the terms *complementary* and *alternative* serve only to detract from a therapy by making it sound second class. Therapies that are often labeled under the heading of CAM include nutrition and spirituality. Many would argue that a lack of attention to these important influences on health has resulted in an epidemic of obesity, diabetes, and substance abuse. Stress, which many CAM-labeled mind-body therapies address, was found to be the second leading risk factor for heart disease after smoking in one of the largest studies ever completed across multiple cultures.[15] CAM therapies are hardly of lesser significance than conventional therapies.

FIGURE 1-5
Evolution of titles in the field.

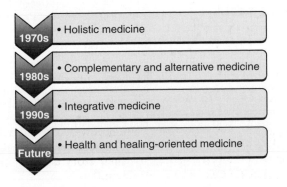

Labeling therapies as CAM also avoids the deeper issues that need to be addressed in health care delivery and promotes further fragmentation of care. Simply adding CAM therapies without changing our health care model is like increasing the number of specialists with no primary care infrastructure, an approach that increases cost and reduces the quality of care.[16] Having multiple providers treating the patient in many different ways prevents what is needed most in the restructuring of health delivery: a medical home that is founded in relationship-centered care.

The term *integrative medicine* stressed the importance of using the evidence to understand how best to integrate CAM therapies into our health care model and allowed us to understand better how they can be used to facilitate health and healing. This evolving understanding helped influence positive change in our health care system.

Changing the Medical Culture

In 2001, the IOM published a report on the overall state of U.S. health care. The IOM concluded that the U.S. health care system was so flawed it could not be fixed and an overhaul was required.[17] In 2006, a report from the American College of Physicians (ACP) stated that

> Primary care, the backbone of the nation's health care system, is at grave risk of collapse due to a dysfunctional financing and delivery system. Immediate and comprehensive reforms are required to replace systems that undermine and undervalue the relationship between patients and their personal physician.[18]

This crisis has led to proposals toward a restructuring of health care that resonate with the philosophy of integrative medicine. The family medicine community has joined the IOM and the ACP in creating their own proposal on a new model for care that promotes a relationship-centered medical home for the establishment of excellence in health creation in the outpatient setting. Principles of the medical home include the following:[19]

1. Access to care based on an ongoing relationship with a personal primary care clinician who is able to provide first contact and continuous and comprehensive care
2. Care provided by a physician-led team of professionals within the practice who collectively take responsibility for the ongoing needs of patients
3. Care based on a whole-person orientation in which the practice team takes responsibility for either providing care that encompasses all patient needs or arranging for the care to be done by other qualified professionals
4. Care coordinated or integrated across all elements of the complex health care system and the patient's community
5. Care facilitated by the use of office practice systems such as registries, information technology, health information exchange, and other systems to ensure that patients receive the indicated care when and where they need and want it in a culturally and linguistically appropriate manner
6. A reimbursement structure that supports and encourages this model of care

A similar set of goals was stated by the IOM in their proposal for a new health system for the twenty-first century (Table 1-1).

TABLE 1-1. Simple Rules for the Twenty-First Century Health Care System

OLD RULE	NEW RULE
Care is based primarily on visits.	Care is based on continuous healing relationships.
Professional autonomy drives variability.	Care is customized according to patient's needs and values.
Professionals control care.	Patient is the source of control.
Information is a record.	Knowledge is shared, and information flows freely.
Decision making is based on training and experience.	Decision making is evidence based.
"Do no harm" is an individual responsibility.	Safety is a system priority.
Secrecy is necessary.	Transparency is necessary.
The system reacts to needs.	Needs are anticipated.
Cost reduction is sought.	Waste is continuously decreased.
Preference is given to professional roles rather than the system.	Cooperation among clinicians is a priority.

From Institute of Medicine, Committee on Quality of Health Care in America. *Crossing the Quality Chasm: A New Health System for the 21st Century.* Washington, D.C.: National Academy Press; 2001.

In 2009, the Bravewell Collaborative sponsored a summit on Integrative Medicine and the Health of the Public at the Institute of Medicine in Washington, D.C. The goal of this conference was to share the science in the field and the potential for ways in which it can improve the health care of the nation. It succeeded in opening up dialogue among clinicians, administrators, and politicians to bring awareness of how the field could bring balance to a health care system that is weighted heavily toward disease management. A report of the meeting is available online.[20]

The field of integrative medicine was created not to fragment the medical culture further by devising another silo of care but to encourage the incorporation of heath and healing into the larger medical model. The culture of health care delivery is changing to adopt this philosophy, and the integration of nontraditional healing modalities will make this goal more successful.

> It is important to see the benefits and limitations of our current allopathic system and realize that science alone will not meet all the complex needs of our patients.[21]

Integrative Medicine

Integrative medicine is healing oriented and emphasizes the centrality of the physician-patient relationship. It focuses on the least invasive, least toxic, and least costly methods to help facilitate health by integrating both allopathic and complementary therapies. These therapies are recommended based on an understanding of the physical, emotional, psychological, and spiritual aspects of the individual (Table 1-2).

> The goal of integrative medicine is to facilitate health within complex systems, from the individual to the communities and environment in which all things live.

Health and Healing-Oriented Medicine

"Health" comes from the Old English word *Hal,* which means wholeness, soundness, or spiritual wellness. Health is defined by the World Health Organization (WHO) as "a state of complete physical, mental, and social well-being

TABLE 1-2. Defining Integrative Medicine

- Emphasizes relationship-centered care
- Integrates conventional and complementary methods for treatment and prevention
- Involves removing barriers that may activate the body's innate healing response
- Uses natural, less invasive interventions before costly, invasive ones when possible
- Engages mind, body, spirit, and community to facilitate healing
- Maintains that healing is always possible, even when curing is not

and not merely the absence of disease or infirmity."[22] Cure, on the other hand, refers to doing something (e.g., giving drugs or performing surgery) that alleviates a troublesome condition or disease. Healing does not equal curing. We can cure a condition such as hypertension with a pharmaceutical product without healing the patient. Healing would facilitate changes that reduce stress, improve diet, promote exercise, and increase the person's sense of community. In doing this, we help improve the balance of health of the body that may result in the ability to discontinue a pharmaceutical agent and thereby reduce the need for the cure.

An example of this can be seen in Figure 1-6. Here we have two trees, A and B. Tree A is obviously in a better state of health than tree B. This is likely because of its ability to be in balance with its environment. If a branch breaks on tree A, we can feel comfortable that if we mend the branch, it will likely heal well, or even heal itself. If a branch breaks on tree B and we mend it, the branch not going to heal because the tree is not in a state of health. The point here is that our focus in medicine has been on fixing the branch while neglecting the health of the tree. If we give more attention to helping tree B find health either by removing barriers that are blocking its own ability to heal or by improving areas of deficiency, the branch will heal

itself—we will not need to spend as much time and money fixing the parts.

Integrative medicine is about changing the focus in medicine to one of health and healing rather than disease. This involves understanding the influences of mind, spirit, and community, as well as the body. It entails developing insight into the patient's culture, beliefs, and lifestyle that will help the provider understand how best to trigger the necessary changes in behavior that will result in improved health and thus bring more value to health care delivery.

> Cure and fix when able, but if we ignore healing, the cure will likely not last or will give way to another disease that may not have a cure.

Increasing Value Through Integrative Medicine

Achieving high value for patients and incentivizing practitioners to foster health will become the overarching goal of health reimbursement in the future. Value is defined by the health outcomes achieved per dollar spent. It depends on results, not just inputs, and should be measured by the ways we can improve the quality of patients' lives, not by the number of patients seen in a day. This will require a reimbursement model that rewards team-based care that transcends the one-on-one office visit and allows multiple avenues for patient communication and education among an interdisciplinary team of professionals.

Integrative medicine can increase value and lower costs through two of its foundational values: (1) by shifting the emphasis of health care to health promotion, disease prevention, and enhanced resiliency through attention to lifestyle behaviors; and (2) by bringing low-tech, less expensive interventions into the mainstream that preserve or improve health outcomes. This approach requires that these professionals have time to recognize the complexity of someone's life, and it cannot be done without a sound commitment to the practitioner-patient relationship.

Relationship-Centered Care

> It is much more important to know what sort of patient has a disease than what sort of disease a patient has.
> *Sir William Osler*

Observing practitioners of various trades such as biomedicine, manual medicine, Chinese medicine, and herbal medicine helps us realize that some practitioners have better results with their chosen trade. Those with more success are able to develop rapport, understanding, and empathy that help them facilitate healing with their therapy. The relationship fosters healing not only by allowing the practitioner to gain insight into the patient's situation but also by building the patient's trust and confidence in the provider. This trust acts as a tool to activate the patient's natural healing response and supports whatever technique the provider uses, whether it is acupuncture, botanicals, pharmaceuticals, or surgery.

FIGURE 1-6
Healthy (**A**) and sickly (**B**) trees. It is important to see the benefits and limitation of our current allopathic system and to realize that science alone will not meet all the complex needs of our patients.[21]

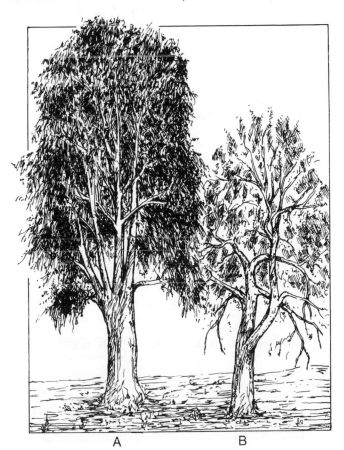

A   B

The evidence behind the benefits of relationship-centered care is solid, particularly with regard to reducing health care costs. This approach to care has been found to reduce expenditures on diagnostic tests,[23] reduce hospital admissions,[24] and lower total health care costs.[25,26]

Developing a holistic understanding and relationship with patients allows the practitioner to guide them toward health more efficiently. The integrative clinician can point the way toward health while realizing that the patient will have to do the work to get there. This attitude does a great deal to remove pressure and guilt from providers who have been trained to think of themselves as failures when they cannot fix problems. In fact, relationship-centered care is a necessity when dealing with the many chronic conditions that do not have simple cures. Success is now defined as helping the patient find an inner peace that results in a better quality of life, whether the problem can be fixed or not (see Chapter 3, The Healing Encounter).

Prevention

Integrative medicine encourages more time and effort on disease prevention instead of waiting to treat disease once it manifests. Chronic disease now accounts for much of our health care cost and also causes significant morbidity and mortality. The incidence of heart disease, diabetes, and cancer could be significantly reduced through better lifestyle choices. Instead, these diseases are occurring in epidemic proportions. The system needs a reallocation of resources. Unfortunately, this is a large ship to turn. In the meantime, integrative practitioners can use their broad understanding of the patient to make recommendations that will lead to disease prevention and slow or reverse disease progression.

Integration

Integrative medicine involves using the best possible treatments from both CAM and allopathic medicine based on the patient's individual needs and condition. This selection should be based on good science and neither rejects conventional medicine nor uncritically accepts alternative practices. It integrates successes from both worlds and is tailored to the patient's needs, by using the safest, least invasive most cost-effective approach while incorporating a holistic understanding of the individual.

CAM is not synonymous with integrative medicine. CAM is a collection of therapies, many of which have a similar holistic philosophy. Unfortunately, the Western system views these therapies as tools that are simply added on to the current model, one that attempts to understand healing by studying the tools in the tool box. David Reilly said it well in an editorial in *Clinical Evidence:*

> We are the artists hoping to emulate Michelangelo's David only by studying the chisels that made it. Meantime, our statue is alive and struggling to get out of the stone.[27]

Integration involves a larger mission that calls for a restoration of the focus on health and healing based on the provider-patient relationship.

Five Questions to Consider Before Prescribing a Therapy

The integrative medicine practitioner uses relationship-centered care to develop insight into the most effective therapy for the patient's needs. Before prescribing a specific therapy, the practitioner should consider the following five questions:

1. **Does the therapy result in symptom resolution or symptom suppression?**

   Our initial goal should always be the resolution of the symptom, to enable us to use fewer external influences to maintain health. This often requires that we explore the mind and spiritual aspects of a symptom. A symptom is our body asking for some type of change. If we simply suppress the symptom without understanding what it may need to go away, it will likely recur or arise in another part of the body. A good example of this is the use of proton pump inhibitors (omeprazole [Prilosec], lansoprazole [Prevacid], rabeprazole [Aciphex]) for epigastric pain. These are excellent medications to help suppress symptoms or heal ulcers. If we overrely on this technology, however, it prevents us from exploring the symptom further. It may keep us from listening to the patient's story in which the use of metaphor may give us further insight into the mind-body influences on health. A person with epigastric pain may say that his or her job is "eating me up inside." If we do not deal with this stress, the body will not truly heal even though the symptom is suppressed. This can lead to long-term use of a medication that can result in a change of the natural environment of the body. Long-term suppression of acid production can lead to the following: an increased risk of pneumonia[28]; malabsorption of B vitamins, calcium, magnesium, and iron[29]; a higher prevalence of *Clostridium difficile* colitis[30]; and fractures of the hip[31,32] and spine.[33]

   To foster symptom resolution, we need to explore both the external and internal reasons for its expression (Fig. 1-7). An external therapy (medications, acupuncture, surgery, body work) will not have lasting benefit unless it is coupled with an internal exploration of why the symptom is there (emotions, stress, meaning, and purpose). The physical and nonphysical are inseparable, and if we do not address both, it will be difficult for the symptom to resolve. When we have explored both and found no underlying internal source, then it is appropriate to suppress the symptom with our tools to reduce suffering and improve quality of life.

FIGURE 1-7
Dynamic interplay between the physical and nonphysical influences on health and disease.

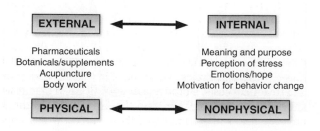

2. **What is the evidence?**

The scientific model allows us to understand which therapies have the most intrinsic value. Once we have reviewed the evidence, we can combine it with the "art of medicine" to stack the deck further in favor of a positive response. Unfortunately, the amount of evidence we have to rely on is limited. Out of 2404 treatments reviewed in medical care, 15% were found to be beneficial and 47% were not adequately tested.[34]

It is quite expensive to do good research, and the therapies that have the best quality of evidence are often those therapies that have the greatest potential for economic gain. Unfortunately, little economic incentive exists to promote therapies that result in healing in our current health care model. You will not see representatives from the wood and paper industry promoting the use of pencils and paper to support the health benefits of journaling on asthma and rheumatoid arthritis despite the evidence showing benefit.[35] The responsibility falls to the academic institutions and the government to provide funding to research all potential therapies despite their lack of economic rewards.

3. **What is the potential harm?**

It can be dangerous if we look at the evidence only for the potential benefit of a therapy without looking at the evidence for potential harm. In the 1950s, evidence showed that diethylstilbestrol prevented miscarriages, but the potential harm to the unborn fetus was not taken into consideration until after many lives were affected. For supraventricular tachycardia, evidence indicated that flecainide improved the rhythm on the electrocardiogram, but not until later did further research find the drug to increase mortality.[36] The integrative medicine practitioner uses the least harmful, least invasive therapy before using more invasive therapies. It is important that we continue to research not only the potential benefits but also the potential harm of the therapies we prescribe. Because of the potential risk of the external influences on health, we should encourage lifestyle habits with the least potential risk (whole food nutrition, stress reduction, exercise, spiritual connection) so that fewer high-risk interventions are needed, thereby resulting in the least potential risk of harm. For this reason, this text includes an icon that weighs the evidence of benefit against the evidence of harm to help guide the clinician.

4. **What is the cost?**

One of the first duties of the physician is to educate the masses not to take medicine.

Sir William Osler

Despite spending more on health care delivery than any nation in the world by almost 47%, the United States ranks fifteenth in quality when compared with the top 25 industrialized countries according to the 2000 WHO report. Despite this high cost, in 2006 the United States ranked thirty-ninth for infant mortality, forty-third for adult female mortality, forty-second for adult male mortality, and thirty-sixth for life expectancy.[37] Success of the higher-ranked countries comes from a strong primary care infrastructure[38] and healthier lifestyle habits. White and Ernst[39] showed that those primary care providers who provided a range of CAM therapies had a reduced number of referrals and treatment costs. Unfortunately, not all CAM therapists are primary care providers, and the use of CAM without the direction and continuity of these clinicians will only fragment care further and increase costs. The key is to incorporate this integrative philosophy into medical education so that primary care is enhanced and CAM therapies can be used to enable the provider to facilitate health.

CAM therapies are generally low tech and low cost and reduce the need for more expensive interventions. Users of CAM report that their use of prescription drugs and conventional therapies decreases.[40] When CAM was combined with biomedicine, one study showed a reduction of pharmaceutical use by 51.8%, a decrease in outpatient surgeries and procedures use by 43.2%, and a reduction of hospital admissions by 43%.[41]

Much economic incentive exists for physicians in the United States to do the fixing and little for them to do the lifestyle education that would reduce the need for expensive pills and procedures. Ornish et al[42] showed how coronary heart disease can be reversed by incorporating lifestyle changes including nutrition, exercise, stress management, group psychosocial support, and smoking cessation. This is an excellent example of how an integrative approach can result not only in self-healing but also in great savings in morbidity, mortality, and the money needed to treat them. The implementation of integrative medicine has the potential to result in tremendous cost savings, improved efficiency, and quality of care.

5. **Does the therapy match the patient's culture and belief system?**

In our conventional medical system, we have traditionally pulled patients into our paradigm of thought and have told them what they need. This method is often necessary for acute illness, but for chronic conditions that have no "right" answer, we will be more effective if we offer treatment plans that best match patients' belief systems. In this way, we can activate the internal healing response, a process that we know as the placebo effect. Instead of brushing this off as a nuisance, the talented clinician will use it to enhance healing. Becoming able to integrate methods of healing from various cultures will further enable the clinician to match the therapy to the individual. The art of medicine may lie in the clinician's ability to activate this response without deception. We should give patients what they need before we give them what we know. It is nice when we have knowledge about what our patients need, but this often requires collaborative treatments with an integrative team of providers who work toward a common goal of health for the patient.

Reducing Suffering

The secret of the care of the patient is in caring for the patient.

Francis Peabody, MD

Good caring and a weak medicine can give a better outcome than poor caring and a strong medicine.

Unknown

At the core of the delivery of health and healing is our ability to relieve suffering. This is not something that we learn in a book but requires that we explore our own suffering before we can understand how to help others with theirs. We are our own first patient, and part of our continuing education requires a recurring exploration of our inner self so we can understand what it means to be truly present without judgment.

> The integrative medicine practitioner is not afraid to turn toward suffering in the care of another. As each addresses what is real, the authenticity of the truth draws both toward healing.

In learning this, it is helpful to understand how suffering influences the severity of pain and our quality of life. Pain and suffering are intricately connected but are not the same. Pain is a normal bodily reaction; suffering is not. Pain helps protect us against further harm; suffering is an opportunity to learn. Suffering influences how our body perceives pain—"the more I suffer, the more pain I experience" (Fig. 1-8). Our job is to reduce suffering so we can distill the pain to the most physiologic reason for its presence. In treating someone's suffering, we can often make pain more tolerable. In recognizing the severity of suffering, we can often avoid long-term medications that are used to suppress the symptom. It is often through our listening and our presence that we are best able to treat suffering. When no "right" answer or "drug cure" exists, it is our human compassion, connection, and unconditional positive regard that always works, even when our tools do not. This is the most important part of our work and is the reason that we heal in the process of helping others do the same.

The Future

The information age will continue to increase the number of data on the variety of therapies available but will only complicate how we apply them. Informed patients will be looking for competent providers who can help them navigate the myriad therapeutic options, particularly for those conditions for which conventional approaches are not effective. These patients will demand scientifically trained providers who are knowledgeable about the body's innate healing mechanisms and who understand the role of lifestyle factors in creating health, including nutrition and the appropriate use

FIGURE 1-8
Suffering's effect on the same source of pain. Treating suffering will help reduce the severity of pain and improve the quality of life and should be at the core of our work in integrative medicine.

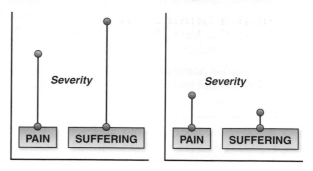

of supplements, herbs, and other forms of treatment from osteopathic manipulation to Chinese and Ayurvedic practices. They will be seeking providers who can understand their unique interplay of mind, body, and spirit to help them better understand what is needed to create their own balance of health. This will require a restructuring of medical training that will involve more research and education on how the body heals and how the process can be facilitated.

Conclusion

The philosophy of health based on a balance of mind, body, and spirit is not new or unique to integrative medicine. This understanding has been around since the time of Aristotle. What we call it is not important, but the underlying concepts are. It is time that the pendulum swings back to the middle, where technology is used in the context of healing and physicians acknowledge the complexity of mind and body as a whole. Integrative medicine can provide the balance needed to create the best possible medicine for both the physician and patient. We will know that we are near this balance when we can drop the term integrative. Integrative medicine of today will then simply be the good medicine of the future.

THERAPEUTIC REVIEW

- ### Integrative Medicine

  - Emphasizes relationship-centered care

  - Develops an understanding of the patient's culture and beliefs to help facilitate the healing response

  - Focuses on the unique characteristics of the individual person based on the interaction of mind, body, spirit, and community

  - Regards the patient as an active partner who takes personal responsibility for health

  - Focuses on prevention and maintenance of health with attention to lifestyle choices, including

    nutrition, exercise, stress management, and emotional well-being

  - Encourages providers to explore their own balance of health that will allow them better to facilitate this change in their patients

  - Requires providers to act as educators, role models, and mentors to their patients

  - Uses natural, less invasive interventions before costly, invasive ones when possible

  - Recognizes that we are part of a larger ecosystem that requires our efforts in sustaining its health so we can continue to be a part of it

  - Uses an evidence-based approach from multiple sources of information to integrate the best therapy for the patient, be it conventional or complementary

- Searches for and removes barriers that may be blocking the body's innate healing response
- Sees compassion as always helpful, even when other therapies are not
- Focuses on the research and understanding of the process of health and healing (salutogenesis) and how to reproduce it
- Accepts that health and healing are unique to the individual and may differ for two people with the same disease

- Works collaboratively with the patient and a team of interdisciplinary providers to improve the delivery of care
- Maintains that healing is always possible, even when curing is not
- Agrees that the job of the physician is to cure sometimes, heal often, support always—*Hippocrates*

KEY WEB RESOURCES

Consortium of Academic Health Centers for Integrative Medicine (CAHCIM). http://www.imconsortium.org.	This organization strives to advance the principles and practices of integrative health care within academic institutions. Its members include more than 45 academic health centers in North America.
Bravewell Collaborative. http://www.bravewell.org.	This is a community of leading philanthropists who work together to transform our health care system and improve the health of the U.S. public through the advancement of integrative medicine. The Web site has many resources that help guide the advancement of the field.
American Board of Integrative Holistic Medicine. http://integrativeholisticdoctors.org/.	This board offers continuing medicinal education and credentialing toward becoming a diplomate.
University of Arizona Center for Integrative Medicine. http://integrativemedicine.arizona.edu/.	This center offers education and fellowship training in integrative medicine for physicians, family nurse practitioners, and physician's assistants.
University of Wisconsin Integrative Medicine Program. http://fammed.wisc.edu/integrative.	This program offers patient handouts and educational material for integrative approaches to common medical conditions. It focuses on bringing integrative medicine into primary care delivery models.
National Center for Complementary and Alternative Medicine. http://nccam.nih.gov/.	This branch of the National Institutes of Health focuses on complementary and alternative medicine (CAM) research. It includes literature reviews and education on CAM and common conditions for which CAM is used.

References

References are available online at expertconsult.com.

Chapter 2

Creating Optimal Healing Environments

David Rakel, MD, and Wayne Jonas, MD

Many health practitioners who go into primary care want to both treat and heal, to care for the whole person, to be patient advocates, to apply the best science, and to serve the suffering. In short, we seek to be healers.

However, we often find in medical school and in our practice that the skills needed to be healers and the environment needed to execute those skills are not taught, available, or funded. We know, for example, the factors that increase the risk of disease, but we wait until illness arrives. We understand that relationships, a positive attitude, and behavioral skills form the foundation for compliance and self-care, prevention, and well-being, but we find ourselves without the time to develop them. We see the search for meaning in patients' eyes when they suffer from a serious illness, and yet our science cannot help them find the coherence they seek. For optimal healing to take place, we need to be proactive in creating an environment where these things can happen.

With every medical recommendation is a dynamic environment in which care is delivered. This environment consists of both physical and nonphysical elements. It often includes a synergy among factors that can either promote or hinder the healing process. Our goal is to describe foundational characteristics of an optimal healing environment (OHE) so that any therapy that is prescribed within this space (shown as a container in Fig. 2-1) will be more successful.

Creating an Environment That Enhances the Person's Ability to Heal

A growing amount of research shows how an environment based in positive intention, wholeness, and relationship-centered care can enhance the healing process independent of the treatment used, be it drugs or acupuncture needles.[1,2]

Optimal Healing Environments

We define an OHE as an environment in which the social, psychological, spiritual, physical, and behavioral components of health care are oriented toward support and stimulation of innate healing capacities and the achievement of wholeness. It is an expansion of Engel's biopsychosocial model, which created a foundation for understanding the dynamic influences of health.[3] These components include at least six domains, in addition to the physical and organizational structures that support them, which are summarized in Table 2-1.[4–28] The six core domains of an OHE are the following:

1. Development of intention and awareness
2. Experience of wholeness
3. Relationship-centered care
4. Health promotion with self-care and lifestyle skills
5. Collaborative treatment
6. Spiritual connection

Intention and Awareness

Intention can have an influence on motivation for change, understanding, and compliance.[9] Being fully present with positive intention for another human is perceived by those we are with and enhances the healing effects of the encounter.[9] It is difficult to connect truly with intention until we have explored our own inner nature. Patient care starts with ourselves. As this connection grows, our ability to sit fully with another suffering human will be enhanced, and appreciation in our work will grow. This growth brings forward foundations in healing that include positive expectation, hope, faith, and unconditional positive regard.[4,29]

FIGURE 2-1
Schematic showing that the therapy we prescribe comes from within
a container of influences that can enhance its effectiveness.

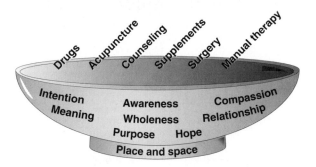

Optimal Healing Environments

Healing can be defined as the dynamic process of
recovery, repair, reintegration, and renewal that increases
resilience, coherence, and wholeness. Healing is an
emergent, transformative process of the whole person—
physical, mental, social, spiritual, and environmental.
It is a unique personal and communal process and
experience that may or may not involve curing.[2]

Wholeness

Health is a result of a dynamic balance of biopsychosocial
and spiritual influences. To facilitate healing, it is necessary to develop insight into how these factors are expressed
in each unique individual. The holistic model requires that
mind, body, emotions, and spirit are explored to understand
best how to facilitate positive change so the person can heal
most effectively.[11]

Relationship-Centered Care

Relationship is the bond that removes isolation and fear. It
enhances insight, understanding, and sense of control. When
two people develop trust, significant benefit results by enhancing social connection and by fostering communication,
empathy, and compassion. Through relationship, unhealthy
emotions are released and optimism and positive expectation are born.[13,15] Patient-oriented, relationship-centered
care has been found to improve efficiency of care by reducing the need for medical tests and referrals.[30]

Health Promotion

Empowering the individual to learn how best to take care of
himself or herself so both the provider and the patient are active
participants in the healing process is a key ingredient. All healing is self-healing, and we, as integrative medicine practitioners, are at our best when we are able to facilitate individuals
to care for themselves most successfully. This approach often
includes nutrition, physical activity, lifestyle choices, and management of stress and anxiety. These factors can have epigenetic influences on the expression of a healthy phenotype.[18,19]
Grounded in relationship and continuity of care, primary care
practitioners are in a unique position to influence healthy lifestyle changes before the onset of chronic disease.

Collaborative Treatment

The provider who has developed a relationship and an understanding of the individual's story will then use the most effective tools possible to facilitate health, be they conventional or
complementary. This integrative approach begins with less
invasive measures before costly invasive ones are needed, when
possible. It often involves working with a team of providers
who are able to offer practices that help the body heal. It combines the best of technology, when needed, but is grounded in
humanism and compassionate care so the least harmful, most
effective approach is implemented to influence health.[23-25]

Spiritual Connection

Spirituality is a journey toward, or experience of, connection
with sources of ultimate meaning, as defined by each individual. Spirituality includes connection with oneself, with
others, with nature, and with a higher power.[31] If we providers can help patients work toward facilitating awareness of
these connections, spirituality will enhance a sense of purpose for living, reduce suffering, buffer stress, and optimize
self-healing (see Chapter 110, Taking a Spiritual History).
Spirituality also is one of the most effective tools in helping
change unhealthy behavior (see Chapter 99, Motivational
Interviewing Techniques).[32]

Healing Spaces

The six key elements just discussed are enhanced by the
physical structure in which they are provided. Nature, color,
light, fresh air, music, fine arts, and architecture should be
used to create external influences that support the health and
well-being of those who enter the space.

Healing Places

Leadership and teamwork are essential to the delivery of
OHEs. If employees do not respect and communicate with
one another and feel safe to deal with conflict and empowered to contribute toward improvement, these deficiencies
will be experienced by patients and will therefore inhibit
healing. A culture of healing starts with modeling self-care
and core values by the leaders and then flows into the mission, vision, planning, and behavior of health care teams.

Creating an Optimal Healing Environment in the Clinical Setting

How can we bring the components of an OHE into a busy practice? Although transforming a practice into a healing environment may seem like a daunting task, or one with little practical
value, experience and evidence indicate that attention to simple and inexpensive details often gradually moves the focus of
care from cure only to one filled with healing activity.[33]

The practitioner can develop healing-oriented sessions
within the clinical space without having to go through major
renovations. The primary care practitioner already has the
foundational tools needed to create an OHE. The nonphysical intention is much more important than the physical
space. Healing can occur anywhere, whether it is in an
$8 million healing center or in an underfunded inner city
clinic for the homeless (Table 2-2).

TABLE 2-1. Optimal Healing Environments: Key Components and Skills and Tools to Create Them

COMPONENT	SKILLS	TOOLS
Intention and awareness[4]	Familiarity with cross-cultural medicine and how to maximize therapeutic effect for patients within various cultural and religious traditions[5,6] Awareness of placebo literature and how to help the body self-heal[7,8] Use of intention in one's own practice[9] Personal participation and guidance of others in mindfulness practices	Take a mindfulness course. Take a retreat to define your own spiritual connection and develop awareness, to manage this appropriately with others (see Chapter 98, Recommending Meditation).
Wholeness[10]	Attitude of unconditional acceptance of those seeking care Ability to guide others toward understanding the body's energetic as a mechanism for healing and growth Personal participation in or ability to guide others in personal growth enhancements[10] Philosophy of holism and patient-centered care[11,12] Interviewing practices that focus on all aspects of the patient Ability to create a healing team that has an underlying holistic approach	Study and follow some of the following resources: Engel's biopsychosocial model[3] Ken Wilber's *A Brief History of Everything** Information from the American Holistic Medical Association (AHMA) Regular personal mind-body practices
Healing relationships[13]	Skills in relationship-centered care, empathy, and rapport building[14,15] Understanding how patients relate to their surrounding communities[16] Skill with involving family[17] or other members of the support system in patient care Ability to guide support groups and help patients help each other	Make friends and see how it makes you feel. Look at your medical career as a privilege to be able to make a living taking care of your friends who are also your patients.
Health promotion	Personal experience with living a healthy lifestyle and helping others do the same; skill in helping others take personal responsibility in their care[18,19] Solid background in preventive care and familiarity with principles of nutrition,[20] exercise,[21] stress management,[22] and addictions Ability to educate patients and other providers effectively through information technology, clinic-run education sessions, and so forth	Develop your own health plan. Expand your knowledge base of lifestyle choices and health (nutrition, exercise, mind-body, spiritual connection). Take the American Board of Integrative Holistic Medicine (ABIHM) review course.
Collaborative treatment[23,24]	Skill in integrative approaches to practice[25] Familiarity with the variety of modalities available and when or where they are most useful[26] Understanding the safety of various modalities Ability to draw together and contribute to a diverse group of providers who can work together to create an optimal healing environment Ability to facilitate positive team dynamics and resolve conflicts Knowledge of the treatments available within the community Skill in use of scientific literature, such as Cochrane collaboration (www.cochrane.de) in making evidence-based treatment decisions	Develop relationships with a community of providers whom you trust and with whom you will enjoy working. Obtain therapies first hand from your colleagues. This is a great way to learn about the therapy, the art of the practitioner, and its potential benefits.
Spiritual connection	Incorporation of some of the following questions in your history taking: What gives your life meaning? If life were perfect and resources were limitless, what would it look like for you? How do you want to leave your mark on this world? Who do you want to become?	Become familiar with spiritual assessment tools such as FICA, HOPE, SPIRIT, LET GO (see Chapter 110, Taking a Spiritual History). Explore and define your own spiritual connection. Be careful not to project your beliefs onto others inappropriately.
Healing spaces[27,28]	Skill with using architecture, the arts, sensory stimulation, and ambience to maximize healing Hiring an interior decorator to modify your clinic	Visit spaces that make you feel good and incorporate key elements into your clinical space.

*Wilber K. *A Brief History of Everything*. Halifax, Nova Scotia, Canada: Shambhala; 2001.

TABLE 2-2. Optimal Healing Environment

OHE INGREDIENTS	Description of Sample Case Study	
	OHE PRESENT	**OHE ABSENT**
General case description	Mike is a 42-year-old man with low back pain for 8 weeks. He has no history of acute injury, no radicular symptoms, and no improvement despite chiropractic manipulation and over-the-counter NSAIDs.	Mike is a 42-year-old man with low back pain for 8 weeks. He has no history of acute injury, no radicular symptoms, and no improvement despite chiropractic manipulation and over-the-counter NSAIDs.
Relationship-centered care	Mike goes to see Dr. Smith because he knows and trusts her. She helped him through his divorce several years ago.	Mike has no primary care provider. He goes to a local health care clinic close to his home and sees whichever physician is available at the time he visits.
Healing space	Mike likes Dr. Smith's office. It is warm and welcoming and makes him feel at ease, safe, and comfortable.	The clinic is cold and uninviting. You can hear traffic noises from the busy street as you hear the paging system overhead telling the physician that the patient is ready in Room 3.
Self-care	Dr. Smith seems to "walk the talk." Mike sees her jogging around town at lunch, and she never seems "stressed out" like so many other physicians.	Dr. Jones seems rushed and stressed by the demands of all the patients backed up in the waiting room. She appears to be overweight, pale, and fatigued.
Intention and awareness	What Mike likes best about his physician is that she seems totally present when she sees him. He feels like he is the most important thing on her mind during his visits.	Mike feels sorry for the overworked physician and wants to give her information in an efficient manner so that she can do her job quickly. She remains standing, offers little eye contact, and seems distracted by the many demands on her time. Mike feels disconnected.
Holism	Dr. Smith does a full physical examination that shows muscle spasm in the right quadratus lumborum muscle group but no other concerning signs. Mike feels comfortable telling Dr. Smith about the loss of his job a few months back. She educates him about how the body can sympathize and experience symptoms when the mind is under stress.	Dr. Jones focuses on Mike's back pain and asks directed questions related to his discomfort. Time does not allow for questions beyond Mike's physical symptoms. The examination shows muscle spasm in the right quadratus lumborum muscle group, but no other concerning signs are noted.
Collaborative care	Dr. Smith refers Mike for counseling to develop further insight into how his life situation can influence his health. He will also see a massage therapist to loosen up his muscle spasm.	Dr. Jones is concerned about the length of Mike's symptoms without resolution. She orders an MRI scan and refers Mike to an orthopedic surgeon for further evaluation. She educates Mike about the potential benefits of an epidural block.
Lifestyle	Dr. Smith sees that Mike has gained 18 lb in the last year and discusses the need for him to start a gradual exercise program and work on getting back to his ideal body weight. She also recommends a book that discusses the relationship between back pain and stress.	Mike is given a prescription for hydrocodone and a patient education handout on low back pain exercises. He is told that if nothing helps, he may be a candidate for long-term opioid pain management.
Spiritual connection	Dr. Smith knows that Mike has a love of photography and the outdoors. Many of his photographs can be found around town in local shops. She encourages Mike to take this opportunity to direct his career to fulfill those things that he loves to do.	Mike leaves hopeful that the medication will reduce his pain and discomfort.
Compare and Contrast	**OHE Present**	**OHE Absent**
Outcome	Dr. Smith encourages the development of personal insight into how Mike's life situation is influencing his health. He understands what Mike can do to help this situation resolve.	With Dr. Jones' approach, the lack of a holistic view and of relationship-centered care result in a focus on the physical symptom without encouraging the patient's insight.
Goal	The initial goal is symptom resolution.	The initial goal is symptom suppression.

Continued

TABLE 2-2. Optimal Healing Environment—cont'd

Compare and Contrast	OHE Present	OHE Absent
Symptom management	This recruits internal resources to facilitate health and healing.	This relies on external influences for symptom management.
Use of resources	The use of resources is reduced.	The use of resources increases.
Cost	The long-term cost is low.	The long-term cost is high.
"Side effects"	Most side effects are potentially positive (e.g., joy in a new hobby, insight into behavior, increased well-being, and reduced risk factors).	Most side effects are potentially negative (e.g., nausea from hydrocodone, potential drug addiction, and possible surgery).

MRI, magnetic resonance imaging; NSAIDs, nonsteroidal antiinflammatory drugs; OHE, optimal healing environment.

Foundations of a Healing Encounter

To understand the intrinsic value of a therapeutic modality, the scientific model requires that we isolate it from the environment in which it is prescribed. The investigation is also blinded so that the belief systems of the patient and the prescriber do not influence the results. This is important for research but unrealistic when we look at the more complicated environment in which health care is delivered. In fact, the environment in which the prescribed therapy is given may be more effective than the therapy itself.[34]

In the early 1990s, Frank and Frank[35] described four ingredients that were present in a healing encounter:
1. An emotionally charged relationship with a helping person
2. A healing setting (an expected place to go for healing)
3. An explanation for the symptoms that resulted in a sense of control and understanding
4. A ritual, procedure, or plan that involves active participation of both parties that each believes will restore the person to a state of health (a mutual belief followed by an action to overcome the problem)

When one of the chapter authors, David Rakel, was in practice in rural Idaho, he believed that his most successful drug was a selective serotonin reuptake inhibitor. In retrospect, however, the fulfillment of these four criteria may have played the major role in patient improvement. If we look at a case of what happens before we put someone who is depressed on a medication, we can better understand this.

A depressed gentleman whose life is in chaos comes to see you, his physician, with whom he has a relationship based on trust and a holistic understanding of who he is. The patient has come to a healing setting (medical clinic), where he has the expectation that he will receive help. You give him a logical explanation for his symptoms ("a reduction in the level of serotonin") that offers a sense of control and understanding. Both you and the patient agree on a prescribed therapy that you both believe will restore health. You then write down the "answer" on a prescription pad and hand it to him, which then completes the healing ceremony.

When this ritual was performed in a study of St. John's wort, sertraline (Zoloft), and placebo for major depression, it was not the plant or the pill that had the greatest effect, but the ritual (placebo) 8 weeks after initiating therapy.[36] A meta-analysis and review of data submitted to the U.S. Food and Drug Administration for drug treatment of depression also found little difference between the medication and the placebo for mild to moderate depression; both had beneficial effects[37,38] (see Chapter 3, The Healing Encounter).

During the early development of family medicine, this process was known as the art of medicine and was held to be a rare feature of the specialty. With the rise and dominance of pharmaceuticals and evidence-based medicine, it became known as the placebo effect and was not supported in medical care. Subsequently, accumulating evidence on the importance of the healing context and encounter resulted in a reinterpretation as the creation of an OHE.[39] In this chapter, we describe those elements and how they can be systematically brought into clinical practice.

The Practitioner's Influence on Healing

Psychotherapy is a good area to explore the ways in which the therapeutic interaction influences healing because it has few external physical tools such as drugs and surgery. When researchers looked at factors that influenced positive health change in psychotherapy, the factor in the therapist's control that influenced healing the most (30%) was the establishment of a therapeutic relationship in which the patient felt a sense of trust and rapport.[40] A study looking at the "most effective" psychotherapists found that those patients receiving counseling from therapists most talented in developing trusting relationships were much more likely to respond positively to medications than were those patients seeing less effective therapists.[41]

In fact, when psychiatrists rated high in relationship and rapport treated depressed patients with placebo, they had better outcomes than did psychiatrists who were rated lower and who used active drug.[42] Thus, the practitioner, rather than the pill, had the largest impact on outcome.

The quality of the clinician-patient interaction influences outcomes. Studies looking at practitioners' effects on the severity and duration of the common cold and irritable bowel syndrome showed significant enhancement of the therapeutic effect when the treatment was given through an "enhanced" or "augmented" clinical visit in which the clinician took time to create a connection that was perceived as empathetic.[43,44]

In treating one of the most common conditions encountered in primary care—diabetes—high ratings of physician empathy by diabetic patients correlated with better outcomes in diabetes management.[45] The nonspecific healing

FIGURE 2-2
Influences on the healing process.

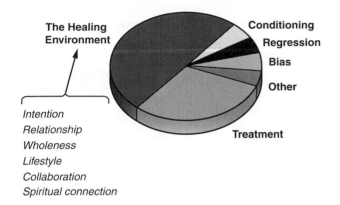

Contributions to the Healing Process

The Healing
Environment

Conditioning

Regression

Bias

Other

Treatment

Intention
Relationship
Wholeness
Lifestyle
Collaboration
Spiritual connection

influences found within the clinical encounter create intention toward health that should be the foundation of the medical home (Fig. 2-2).[46]

> Creating an optimal healing environment will bring more joy to your work. It will allow you to connect with those key elements that attracted you to health care, and in doing so you will find more meaning and purpose.

The Medical Home

The term medical comes from the Latin word *medērī*, which means "to heal." Unfortunately, this word has been shaped by our culture to be perceived as a medicine or an external treatment that is given to the patient. The healing power of the medical home comes from the healing intention of a team of professionals who understand that both inner and outer environments are necessary for health (Table 2-3). One of the most important ingredients is the social connection with a team of people who can support positive lifestyle behaviors while also diagnosing and managing disease. The positive behaviors have been found to have the most significant impact on longevity and the reversal of chronic disease if the disorder is caught early. Behaviors such as avoidance of smoking, weight management, improved nutrition, adequate physical activity, sufficient sleep, and avoidance of substance abuse can reduce the incidence of premature death by 40%[46] and extend life by 14 years.[47] To create this positive change, the medical home environment must empower individuals to do this for themselves. Empowerment requires a self-reflective process that results in a choice to act in a new way. The importance of this approach is exemplified in the care of diabetes, in which 98% of the care is patient directed.[48] Empowerment for behavior change is best facilitated through trusting relationships in which the clinician and the health care team recognize the unique needs of the individual and help create a supportive path toward health. It also honors the unique skills of the team to foster this growth.

Health Teams

New models of care are being defined to improve value and access and reduce cost in the United States. The practitioners of integrative medicine will be leaders in this movement because its philosophy places health creation as its highest priority. Both integrative medicine and conventional medicine will need to create teams of professionals based on the health needs of the community they serve, however, not simply a potpourri of professionals working independently in proximity. For example, if 30% of a community suffers from obesity, metabolic syndrome, and diabetes, the strategic medical home will recruit professionals best suited to address this need. This team may include nutritionists, exercise physiologists, spiritual guides, psychologists, health coaches, and physicians. These team members need adequate communication so that services of each are used when the patient will benefit most. When professionals from varied disciplines come together, shared knowledge allows for insight from different perspectives that can stimulate an "ah ha!" moment in which new ideas allow them to transcend old models of care. When this happens, an interdisciplinary team becomes a transdisciplinary team, and new models of delivery are defined.[49] Multifaceted team-based interventions in primary care are more effective in influencing positive lifestyle behaviors than is isolated specialty care[50-52] (Table 2-4).

TABLE 2-3. Optimal Healing Environments

INNER ENVIRONMENT TO THE OUTER ENVIRONMENT						
Healing intention	Personal wholeness	Healing relationships	Healing organizations	Healthy lifestyles	Integrative collaborative medicine	Healing spaces
Expectation	Mind	Compassion	Leadership	Diet	Person oriented	Nature
Hope	Body	Empathy	Mission	Movement	Conventional	Light
Understanding	Spirit	Social support	Culture	Relaxation	Complementary	Color
Belief	Family	Communication	Teamwork	Addictions	Culturally appropriate	Architecture
	Community					
Enhanced awareness expectancy	Enhanced personal integration	Enhanced caring communication	Enhanced delivery process	Enhanced healthy habits	Enhanced medical care	Enhanced healing structure

Modified from Jones WB, Chez RA. Toward optimal healing environments in health care. *J Altern Complement Med.* 2004;10(suppl 1):51–56.

TABLE 2-4. Defining Disciplinary Teams

TERM	DEFINITION
Multidisciplinary team	**Additive.** "Comprising more than two professionals from different health care disciplines who work with the same patient, set of patients, or clinical condition, but provide care independently of each other" (interdisciplinary team building). For example, a patient may have visits with both a primary care practitioner (PCP) and a physical therapist (PT). Although the PCP may view clinical notes or a report from the PT, the two disciplines usually do not interact.
Interdisciplinary team	**Interactive.** "Dedicated to the ongoing and integrated care of one patient, set of patients, or clinical condition" (interdisciplinary team building). Team members develop collegial relationships with shared goals and joint decision making. They interact, support, as well as question each other's opinions, and negotiate to develop health strategies based on the needs of the individual.
Transdisciplinary team	**Holistic.** Professionals learn from each other and in the process transcend traditional disciplinary boundaries that may result in the emergence of new knowledge. Often, the greater the difference between professions (epistemologic distance, e.g. engineering and humanities), the more likely insight will develop toward the creation of a new way to solve a problem.

From Rakel DP, Jonas W. The patient-centered medical home. In: Rakel R, Rakel D, eds. *Textbook of Family Medicine*. 8th ed. Philadelphia: Saunders; 2011; data from Choi BC, Pak AW. Multidisciplinarity, interdisciplinarity, and transdisciplinarity in health research, services, education and policy: 3. Discipline, inter-discipline distance, and selection of discipline.*Clin Invest Med.* 2008; 31:E41–E48.

Environment's Influence on Genetic Expression

The goal of an integrative medicine health-oriented team is to work together to create OHEs. Environments can have an influence on the genome of the living beings that live within them. The scientific evidence of this epigenetic influence is exploding and gives power and hope to the individual to make positive lifestyle choices by attending to and changing their environment (Fig 2-3).

Animal studies showed that genetically identical agouti mice bred to develop obesity and diabetes could have this expression suppressed when the mothers were fed methyl-donating foods (genestein) before they gave birth.[53] An Amish community assessed to see whether carriers of the *FTO* obesity gene would become overweight found that carriers who averaged 18,000 steps a day remained at a normal weight. Their lifestyle habits trumped their genetic risk.[54]

Telomers are the protective DNA-protein complexes at the end of the chromosomes that promote stability. Loss in their length has been associated with increased risk of

FIGURE 2-3

Depicted is a balance representing the person's unique genetic constitution and the direction into which his or her decisions will poise the organism's well-being, determined by the presence of nutrients, ailments, or pollutants. A nutrient can be understood as any element that nourishes the body and mind.

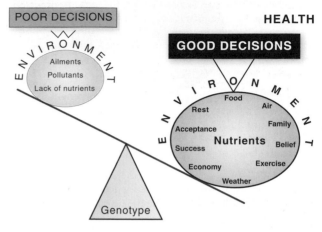

disease and premature mortality. Telomere shortening is counteracted by the enzyme telomerase, and more of this is beneficial. Ornish et al[55,56] looked at telomerase levels in 30 men with prostate cancer. After 3 months of healthy lifestyle changes, including moderate exercise, a low-fat plant-based diet, and social support, the telomerase levels rose,[55] and oncogene expression was inhibited.[56] Exercise alone can increase telomerase activity[57] and brain volume.[58] Stress can decrease telomerase levels,[59] whereas practicing the relaxation response can have a positive influence on genetic expression.[60] Although these behaviors are powerful, they are not the sole dictator of outcomes. The body-mind is complex and mysterious. The clinician should be careful not to instill guilt regarding lifestyle habits when cancer or heart disease is diagnosed. Instead, the clinician should reassure the patient that, even when disease progresses, improved well-being and function are more likely if he or she continues or adopts healthy behaviors.

Health as a Continuum

The continuum of health starts with ourselves, is supported by others, is influenced by lifestyle choices, and is shaped by our inner and outer environments. This continuum recognizes the importance of the interconnectedness of all things. Health is not found in isolated parts but throughout the whole. Being an integrative medicine practitioner means recognizing the dynamic and complex ecosystem in which we live and working to support its health. In doing so, we occasionally pause to witness the mystery of how nature continuously strives for balance despite the odds we have created for it.

I would rather live in a world where my life is surrounded by mystery than live in a world so small that my mind could comprehend it.

Harry Emerson Fosdick

Several years ago, a primary care clinic in England introduced a spiritual healer into its practice. This was done quietly, without advertisement. Patients who had refractory, chronic illnesses, who were high health care users, and who were taking multiple drugs were offered 12 sessions with the healer. Health care use costs, symptoms, and well-being were measured before and after the study period. Almost all patients got better: health care visits decreased; patients improved in their energy and well-being; and although the diseases were not actually cured, suffering was relieved. Costs were reduced by $2000 per patient per year. Most interesting, however, was the change this approach had on the physicians in the practice. When the investigators examined what the healer did during sessions, the procedures were simple. The healer spent a long time listening intently to the patients and hearing what their concerns were about the illness, linking it up with family events, and challenging patients to perceive their connectivity beyond themselves, to imagine a future that was better and improved. The healer then spent time doing some bioenergy work, holding her hands over the patient in the traditional laying-on-of-hands manner. The physicians in the clinic soon realized that many of these same behaviors were similar to things they had been taught to value in medical school but had not often been able to incorporate into their own practice. These physicians then found themselves spending a few more moments with patients and asking them about social and family issues that earlier they would have glossed over or ignored, getting and giving feedback about the meaning of a person's illness, and listening and responding in a warmer fashion. In other words, the physicians realized that they, too, could become healers in the classic sense of the term.[61]

KEY WEB RESOURCES

Samueli Institute. http://www.siib.org/research/research-home/optimal-healing.html

The Samueli Institute has sponsored research in the development of optimal healing environments. This site contains research papers and resources on the topic.

References

References are available online at expertconsult.com.

Chapter 3

The Healing Encounter

David Rakel, MD, and Luke Fortney, MD

To find health should be the object of the doctor. Anyone can find disease.

T. Still, MD

To write prescriptions is easy, but to come to an understanding of people is hard.

Franz Kafka

What kind of doctor do I need to be for this patient today?

Michael Balint

Medical encounters in the recent past have been dominated by the 15-minute office visit that focuses on a symptom or disease state. This is a pathogenic encounter focusing on the genesis or creation of disease. The healing encounter requires a different goal of salutogenesis that focuses on the creation of health.[1] The clinician's intent is to develop an understanding of what the person needs to self-heal and to help the person find a balance in which he or she can interact smoothly with the environment. This chapter focuses on how the clinician can most efficiently allow this process to unfold. At its deepest beauty, this healing process is not one sided, but one in which both the patient and the clinician are transformed. The result is the most rewarding aspect of the profession.

Salutogenesis (the creation of health) is the opposite of pathogenesis (the creation of suffering or disease). The goal of the healing encounter is to facilitate the creation of health that transcends the physical and results in less suffering and an overall improved quality of life.

Practitioner Versus Pill

The mind often attributes healing to external influences outside of ourselves such as from drugs, herbs, or an acupuncture needle. These specific variables are often the most thoroughly studied and are thought to have the most benefit, partly because they are physical treatments that can be quantified. The gold standard in medical research, the double-blind placebo-controlled trial, focuses on removing the nonspecific variables that can often be more powerful than the pill or procedure being studied. These nonspecific variables include aspects of care that are difficult to quantify. They may include trust, empathy, a sense of control, and compassion, which are key ingredients of the healing encounter. These nonspecific variables have been found to enhance the effects of acupuncture for irritable bowel syndrome,[2] shorten the duration of the common cold,[3] trump antidepressants for mild to moderate depression,[4-6] and improve clinical outcomes in patients with diabetes.[7] The nonspecific effects that have been most thoroughly studied in influencing healing in the clinical encounter can be summarized through the PEECE mnemonic: P, positive prognosis; E, empathy; E, empowerment; C, connection; and E, education.[8] Many of these healing influences are cultivated in the process of mindfulness.

Mindfulness in Your Practice

Mindfulness is a way of being in the present moment, on purpose, non-judgmentally.

Jon Kabat-Zinn[9]

When we sit with a patient, the mind will naturally wander and be distracted. Without intentional redirection of the attention back to the patient, however, we lose the opportunity to understand the person sitting across from us. When we are not present and anchored in the moment, we can slip into seeing patients not as who they truly are but as we project them to be. Medical training conditions us to label patients with disease. As we become more adept at recognizing the disease states within people, however, our perception of each other changes to honor the label and not the individual.

In an observational study from 1973, eight *sane* people presented to eight different psychiatric hospitals in California with the complaint of, "*I am hearing thuds.*" After being admitted, these people behaved in a normal and healthy way. The researchers wanted to see what diagnoses they would be given and how long they would remain in the hospital. All eight were given the diagnosis of schizophrenia in remission, and the average length of stay was 19 days. One of the eight was in the hospital for 52 days.[10] The doctors and nurses were not able to see the *sane* patients for who they really were because of their disease-focused conditioned thinking. Recognizing disease patterns is an important part of a clinician's everyday work. If we are not aware and do not recognize the habitual nature of these snap judgments, however, we risk being stuck in these conditioned perspectives and may not recognize arising moments and situations when it is appropriate to step out of these perspectives. The people who questioned the appropriateness of the eight *sane* patients' admissions to the psychiatric hospital were not the doctors or nurses but their fellow inpatients—those with whom the sane people developed relationships through meals, group therapy, and daily activities. Through close relationships the other inpatients were able to see the individuals as they truly were.

Self-Reflection

The healing encounter requires that the practitioner be aware of and recognize their own mind states that may or may not be helpful. Noticing personal bias can help minimize inappropriate judgments and projections. The mindful clinician will be able to meet patients where they are by recognizing their true needs. We will be more successful in helping others if we are able to recognize our own beliefs and then do our best to see the world through the lenses of our patients and their life perspectives (Fig. 3-1). Primary care clinicians trained in mindfulness report improved mood and sense of personal well-being, which, in turn, has a positive impact on patient care.[11,12] To be of service to a person in need is difficult if the clinician is suffering more than the patient. As the saying goes, "you can't give what you don't have."

FIGURE 3-1
Seeing from the patient's perspective.

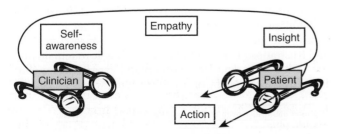

There is nothing like a difficult patient to show us ourselves.

William Carlos Williams

Most people do not listen with the intent to understand; they listen with the intent to reply. They're either speaking or preparing to speak. They're filtering everything through their own paradigms, reading their autobiography into other people's lives.

Stephen Covey

> A study of psychotherapists in training found that the patients taken care of by those therapists who practiced mindfulness had better outcomes, including greater symptom reduction, than did the patients of therapists who did not practice mindfulness. The personal practice of clinicians may influence the outcomes of the patients in their care.[12]

Empathy

Empathy is defined as a cognitive attribute that involves an understanding of experiences, concerns, and perspectives of the patient, combined with the capacity to communicate this understanding.[13] Empathy is a foundational ingredient of the healing encounter. It asks that we initially set aside what we know, feel what patients are communicating, and then communicate this back to them so that they know they were heard. Patients often do not remember what you tell them, but they remember how you made them feel. We feel first through empathy, and then we take action second, based on the information obtained through mindful listening that is combined with medical knowledge and training. We must listen and feel first, however. It is not surprising that empathy significantly declines through medical school and residency as learners focus more on increasing their knowledge at the expense of emotional health and awareness.[14] The combination of this empathetic insight with knowledge best serves the authentic needs of the patient to experience healing. Both are important and necessary.

Insight and Intuition

Insight requires empathy and is the process by which information is gained that allows clinicians to understand how best to serve the health needs of the patient. Intuition is a unique human ability. It is the process of taking a variety of different unrelated bits of information and arriving at a logical conclusion. The more information we have to work with, the more accurate the intuition. If a patient is seen as a disease or an organ system, the clinician will often start with what he or she knows, and the information obtained through listening and feeling will not be incorporated into the patient's care. This is why ongoing relationship-centered care is so important: it can enhance the accuracy of our intuition and insight. A clinician who has known a patient for 10 years is likely to have more accurate insight and intuition based on the many bits of information (analytical and emotional) assimilated over time. This insight results in action that guides the patient most efficiently to health (Fig. 3-2).

FIGURE 3-2
The dynamic process of facilitating health and healing. (From Rakel DP. The healing power of relationship-centered care. In: Rakel DP, Faass N, eds. *Complementary Medicine in Clinical Practice.* Boston: Jones & Bartlett; 2006.)

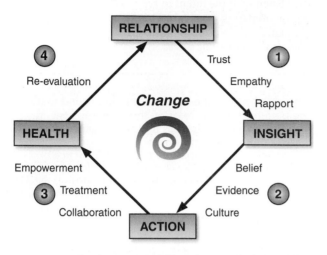

Functional magnetic resonance imaging research has shown a strong coupling between speakers' and listeners' brains that vanishes when communication is poor. In good communication, the listener can anticipate what is going to be communicated before speech is produced, thus leading to greater understanding of the information conveyed.[15]

Action

The Buddhists have the following saying: "action without wisdom is dangerous, and wisdom without action is useless." The healing encounter requires a collaborative action that both the clinician and patient believe will bring health. If we do not take a mindful stance to listen before moving to action, we may not serve the needs of the patient and even potentially cause harm. When we recommend a therapy that the patient does not follow through with, the clinician may blame the patient for being noncompliant. In actuality, the clinician should share the blame for not taking the time to understand the patient's concerns and make a recommendation that would better match the need. Noncompliance represents two people working toward different goals. The healing encounter involves a process that must unfold before action can be of service and the patient goals can be met. To simplify, we summarize this process into the three Ps of a healing encounter: pause, presence, and proceed.

The 3 Ps: Pause, Presence, and Proceed

Pause

Before entering the clinical examination room, take a moment to pause, take a deep breath, and allow yourself to direct your attention to the patient in the room. Use the threshold of the examination room doorway to remind you to drop into the

FIGURE 3-3
The four As of the healing encounter.

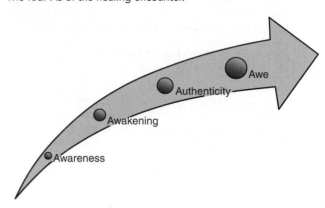

sensations of your own breathing, so that you may be more present with the patient. A threshold is a metaphor for a transition to a new understanding or awareness that the clinician and patient find together. Taking advantage of the opportunity to pause, drop in, and be present can help us center and be more attentive to the patient.*

 More information on this topic can be found online at expertconsult.com.

Presence

Intentionally directing the attention to the physical sensations of breathing or feeling the feet making contact with the floor helps ground and center the mind. Taking two to three deep breaths into the lower abdomen just beneath the umbilicus is a good start (see Chapter 89, Breathing Exercises). In martial arts, this area is called the *hara*, and bringing awareness to this area of the body allows the settled mind to respond more appropriately to the changing needs of each moment. According to Eastern practices, life energy flows from the hara (see Chapter 112, Human Energetic Therapies). A suggestion to "practice in your practice" involves using your computer log-in as an opportunity to drop in and check in with your own body as you prepare to work with a patient. When the mind and body show up in the same place at the same time, the clinician is better equipped to engage the patient. The computerized or paper chart does not need to be a barrier between patient and provider.

Being present and alert moment by moment can awaken us to mystery and awe in an authentic way (Fig. 3-3). When we pause and become present with what is really happening, we are more likely to recognize what is beautiful in each moment, such as in seeing a flower or a living cell. The same holds true with suffering. Even though suffering is associated with pain and discomfort, the more we explore and lean into it, the more we come to understand and learn from it. The mindful encounter brings two people together in the fullness of life including suffering, joy, peace, unrest, creativity, and frustration. The mindful clinician is able to remain present with a wide range of emotions and experiences without being overwhelmed by or overidentifying with suffering.

*For more information on this topic, go to http://www.fammed.wisc.edu/mindfulness/pip.

Patients are able to feel whether you are truly present and listening. If they sense that you are compassionate and attentive, they will feel more comfortable and will often share important information and amazing stories. Creating this space results in more meaningful conversation that engenders understanding. In telling their stories, patients are able to reflect on the cause of their symptoms. This insight can be empowering and help motivate the patient to make changes. The clinician's empathy provides comfort and reduces the feeling of isolation that patients with chronic illness often have. Mindful listening may be our most effective therapeutic tool.[16] As the saying goes, "you were given two ears and one mouth to be used in that proportion."

Proceed

In pausing, being present, and listening to the patient, insight arises. This insight allows a plan to be created that both the clinician and patient believe will be of benefit. The plan increases the sense of control that patients feel in taking action that helps them move from disease to wellness. The health plan should recognize both physical and nonphysical factors that the patient can use to manage symptoms and prevent illness in the future. Helpful questions that can bring an understanding to this process are reviewed in Box 3-1.

The health plan may have one recommendation or several, based on the needs of the patient. For example, if a patient has had recurring headaches and diarrhea ever since his or her divorce, the health plan may only involve one recommendation, such as working toward self-care and forgiveness (see Chapter 97, Healing Through Forgiveness). If another patient wants to prevent a recurrence of breast cancer, however, the health plan may include recommendations on stress reduction, nutrition, spiritual connection, improving sleep, and the use of medications and supplements.

Before computerized medical records, the "answer" to the patient's problem was often conveyed as a quick fix on the prescription pad. The practice of integrative medicine recognizes that health is defined by much more than a medication, but the power of the prescription ritual should not be lost (see Chapter 114, Creating Ceremony and Ritual in the Medical Encounter). This ritual transfers knowledge and a sense of control that gives confidence that something may

help the patient transcend suffering. The clinician's recommendations, based on the insight that arises from the healing encounter, should be summarized in writing and given to the patient at the conclusion of the visit.

> Healing is not something easily reproduced or taught. Often, the best we can do is create an environment where it can unfold, grow, and teach us.

Creating Salutogenesis-Oriented Sessions

A healing encounter can be created in a brief, 5-minute interaction or during an hour-long discussion. To serve the complexity of health and healing most effectively, however, practitioners need to protect time in their schedules to create the ceremony for a healing ritual, the salutogenesis-oriented session (SOS)[17] (see Chapter 114, Creating Ceremony and Ritual in the Medical Encounter).

Recipe for a Salutogenesis-Oriented Session

Any health care clinic can create an SOS that stacks the deck in favor of the healing encounter. The following subsections describe key ingredients that will help create a healing environment for this approach to unfold and be sustainable.

Protect Time in Your Schedule

Carve out time in your work week to schedule an SOS. Some practitioners may schedule these as they would a yearly physical; others may protect a half-day a week focused only on these sessions. Many integrative medicine consultative clinics work in this way. Each session should be scheduled for at least 45 minutes.

Create Space

Consider redecorating an existing examination room to give the feeling that you are in a special and comforting place. Incorporate more soft colors and fabric, and limit sterile and cold medical paraphernalia. If you are unable to do this, simply bring in an element of nature such as a flower, plant, or water fountain.

Create Patient Expectations

Let the patient know that these sessions are intended to allow time for exploring deeper issues that may help you understand how best to facilitate salutogenesis. A typical scenario for creating expectation may be something like the following:

We have ruled out a physical cause for your headaches, and no evidence indicates a tumor. We do not have time scheduled today, but I would like you to come back on a Wednesday morning when I have set aside time for a session that will allow us more time to explore other aspects of life that can have a significant impact on physical health. I want to understand more clearly what may be going on in your life that may be influencing the amount of pain, fatigue, and sleep problems you have been experiencing. Often, in these sessions, we find common underlying causes that may help us get at the root of many of your symptoms.

Offer Support

Relationship-centered care is based on trust and support. An SOS can result in the emergence of past traumas or events that must be supported and further processed. Often, we may need to collaborate with a psychologist colleague to help understand how we can help patients heal from these events. We should not create an environment in which this information comes out and then not offer support and guidance on how to process it. This represents abandonment and turns an SOS into a pathogenesis-oriented session. Collaborative care allows healing to occur within a team that can support it.

Code Appropriately

We need to make sure that our time is appropriately coded so these sessions can be incorporated into clinical care as an important factor. The hope is that the medical system will eventually recognize the cost-saving potential of an SOS. As we explore the root of how the body self-heals, we will need fewer costly interventions. As the cost of disease-focused care escalates, this approach will gain more acceptance.

You need 40 minutes of face-to-face time to bill a "99204" (new patient) or a "99215" (established patient). Be sure to document the amount of time spent and include that "greater than 50% of time was spent counseling and/or coordinating care." This needs to be included if you are billing for time spent with the patient. If you document only total time and not the percentage of time spent counseling and coordinating care, then you must document the required components of the history, examination, and medical decision making.

For integrative medicine consultations, the code is "99244" for a 60-minute appointment and "99245" for an 80-minute appointment. Be sure to document the practitioner who referred the patient for consultation.

Conclusion

Pausing to be present before proceeding toward a plan for health is a simple task that, if practiced, can help two people efficiently find a healing path within a dynamic and complex ecosystem. Ideally, the visit itself is healing even before something is prescribed. Communication between clinician and patient gives the patient perspective and support that encourages both parties to pause, learn from symptoms, and proceed toward a better place, together.

The meeting of two personalities is like the contact of two chemical substances; if there is any reaction, both are transformed.

Carl Jung

KEY WEB RESOURCES

University of Wisconsin Integrative Medicine Program. http://www.fammed.wisc.edu/mindfulness.

This Web site includes instructions, exercises, videos, and audio-files to help the clinician bring mindfulness into the clinical encounter. It complements this chapter.

References

References are available online at expertconsult.com.

Part Two Integrative Approach to Disease

Section I Affective Disorders

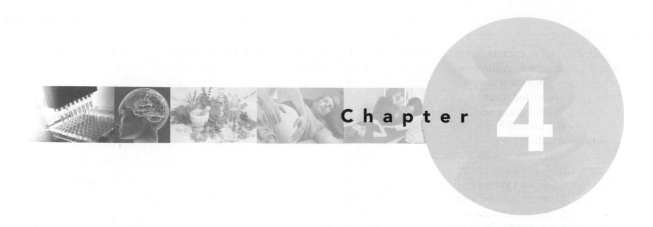

Depression

Craig Schneider, MD, and Erica A. Lovett, MD

Centers for Disease Control and Prevention surveys indicate that nearly 1 in 10 residents of the United States who is 18 years old or older has a depressive disorder.[1] In fact, depression is one of the chronic conditions for which alternative therapies are most frequently used.[2] This is not surprising considering that pharmaceutical antidepressant medications are not as effective as once believed for many patients with less severe forms of depression.[3] Many people seen in primary care settings do not meet the diagnostic criteria for many of the well-known depressive disorders set forth in the fourth edition of the *Diagnostic and Statistical Manual of Mental Disorders* (DSM-IV) but rather fall under the DSM-IV category "depressive disorder not otherwise specified (NOS)." The Patient Health Questionnaire (PHQ)-9 (see Key Web Resources, later) is a simple, brief, and well-validated instrument for diagnosing depression and a reliable and responsible measure of treatment outcomes in the primary care setting.[4]

Pathophysiology

The pathophysiology of depression is not fully understood. The stress-diathesis model of illness emphasizes that significant emotional, social, and environmental antecedents such as the loss of a family member or a romantic or professional disappointment, as well as genetic and acquired vulnerabilities, are clearly involved. Significant stressors appear to be more frequently involved with initial episodes. In recurrent depression, vulnerability appears to increase as episodes become less and less related to stress and more autonomous in a process known as kindling.[5,6] With repeated episodes of illness (kindling), central nervous system dysfunction increases, as manifested by hypercortisolemia, decreased slow-wave (restful) sleep, and increased rapid eye movement (arousing) sleep and disruption of neuroplasticity.[7] The biochemical impact of depression may be stored in neurons through changes in the activity of gene transcription factors and neuronal growth factors.[8] The common final pathway is the biochemical imbalance of biogenic amines or neurotransmitters (e.g., serotonin, norepinephrine, gamma-aminobutyric acid [GABA], and dopamine) and their relationships with their respective receptors in the brain. Potential effects on neurotransmitters include impaired synthesis, increased breakdown, and increased pump uptake, with consequent alterations in neurotransmitter levels. Successful pharmaceutical approaches to treating depression involve correction of these altered neurotransmitter levels and of neurotransmitter receptor interactions.

Integrative Therapy

Exercise as Medicine

More than 1000 trials examined the relationship between exercise and depression, and most of these studies demonstrated an inverse relationship between them.[9,10] Physical activity may also prevent the initial onset of depression.[11,12]

Regularly performed exercise is as effective an antidepressant as psychotherapy or pharmaceutical approaches.[9,13–17] Well-designed studies also support that exercise combined with pharmacologic treatment is superior to either alone, but exercise appears to be superior in maintaining therapeutic benefit and preventing recurrence of depression.[18–22] A Cochrane Review, however, demonstrated conflicting results and no statistically significant effect of exercise on depression.[23] The Cochrane Review results may be explained by the inability to blind properly for the active intervention of exercise.[24] The additional benefits that may be attained by patients who exercise, including increased self-esteem, increased level of fitness, and reduced risk of relapse, make exercise an ideal intervention for patients suffering from depression.

Both aerobic and anaerobic activities are effective.[15,19,24,25] Regardless of the type of exercise, the total energy expenditure appears more important than the number of times a week a person exercises, and high-energy exercises are superior to low-energy exercises.

Exactly why exercise relieves or prevents depression is not understood. Although exercise may increase levels of serotonin, norepinephrine, and endorphins, its benefits have been reported even when naloxone is administered to block endorphins. Exercise may also increase nerve cell growth in the area of brain that modulates mood, similar to pharmaceuticals.[26,27]

Exercise is inexpensive, has proven benefits beyond the treatment of depression, has a low occurrence of side effects, and is available to everyone. The appropriate exercise prescription depends on the specific patient's health, motivation, level of fitness, and interests (see Chapter 88, Writing an Exercise Prescription). For more seriously depressed patients and those with significant psychomotor retardation, the exercise regimen should be started as adjunctive therapy.

> Write an exercise prescription for all patients; tailor the type of exercise to something the patient enjoys, whether aerobic or anaerobic.

Nutrition

Caffeine and Simple Sugars

Cross-national epidemiologic studies suggest a correlation between sugar intake and rates of major depressive disorders.[28] Examination of the diets of people suffering from depression reveals increased consumption of sucrose compared with the general population.[29] A small cohort trial found that eliminating refined sucrose and caffeine from the diets of people experiencing unexplained depression resulted in improvements by 1 week, and symptoms worsened when patients were challenged with these substances but not with placebo.[30] Regular high-level caffeine consumption (750 mg daily) appears to be associated with depression.[31] A large epidemiologic study in Finland, however, demonstrated an inverse relationship between daily tea drinking and the risk of being depressed.[32]

Dietary Patterns

A large cross-sectional study of women consuming traditional diets (vegetables, fruit, beef, lamb, fish, and whole grains) in Australia found a 35% reduced likelihood of major depression or dysthymia compared with women consuming a Western-style diet (more fried, refined, and processed foods), after adjusting for potential confounders (age, socioeconomic status, education, physical activity, alcohol, smoking, and total energy intake).[33] Populations with high adherence to a Mediterranean dietary pattern ensuring adequate intake of omega-3 fatty acids (from fish), monounsaturated fatty acids (from olive oil), and natural folate and other B vitamins (from legumes, fruit and nuts, and vegetables) demonstrate significant reductions in depression risk as well.[34]

Alcohol

A systematic review confirmed that alcohol-related problems are more common in depressed individuals than in the general population and are associated with worse outcomes.[35] Although consumption of alcohol transiently increases the turnover of serotonin, the long-term result is diminished levels of serotonin and catecholamines.[36] Because of the safety, potential health benefits in other areas, and low cost of this intervention, discontinuation of alcohol consumption is warranted.

> Recommend that patients adhere to a traditional or Mediterranean dietary pattern and limit sugar, caffeine, and alcohol consumption.

Omega-3 Fatty Acids

Epidemiologic data suggest that a deficiency of omega-3 fatty acids or an imbalance in the ratio of omega-6 and omega-3 fatty acids correlates positively with increased rates of depression,[37] and this is not explained by known confounders such as inflammation and atherosclerosis.[38] Because dietary polyunsaturated fatty acids and cholesterol are the major determinants of membrane fluidity in synaptic membranes involved in the synthesis, binding, and uptake of neurotransmitters, investigators have hypothesized that alterations may lead to abnormalities contributing to increased rates of depression.[39] Although the current evidence does not support using omega-3 fatty acids as monotherapy to treat depression,[40] small, well-designed studies support the use of omega-3 fatty acids as adjuncts to conventional antidepressant therapy.[41,42] Preliminary evidence also suggests that children with depression and women with depression during pregnancy may benefit from supplementation with omega-3 fatty acids.[43,44]

The effective dose of omega-3 fatty acids for treating depression is not yet known. A dose-ranging study suggested that 1 g daily may be superior to 2 or 4 g daily.[45] Consumption of two or three servings each week of smaller cold-water fish (herring, mackerel, wild salmon, sardine) is comparable. Omega-3 fatty acids also support cardiovascular health and are generally safe. One caveat to consider is the issue of heavy metal and pesticide contamination of available seafood and supplemental fatty acids. Larger fish and farmed fish may bioconcentrate toxins, including mercury and polychlorinated biphenyls. Most studies suggest that eicosapentaenoic acid (EPA) or combinations of docosahexaenoic acid (DHA) and EPA are more helpful than DHA alone. Vegetarian alternatives to consider include flaxseed oil or ground flaxseed meal (2 tablespoons daily) and a small handful of walnuts each day, but these substances have not been studied in depression (see Chapter 86, The Antiinflammatory [Omega-3] Diet).

> Docosahexaenoic acid is generally more structural (important for brain and retina development), and eicosapentaenoic acid is generally more functional (improves communication across cell membranes).

Dietary Supplements

Vitamin D

A large Dutch cohort study of people aged 65 years and older demonstrated an inverse relationship among vitamin D levels, depression status, and depression severity even after adjusting for potential confounders. We do not yet know whether low vitamin D status in patients with depression is a cause or an effect.[46] Supplementing vitamin D is safe and inexpensive, however, and emerging evidence suggests that it may play a role in preventing multiple problems including falls in older persons, cardiovascular disease, and colon cancer.[47-49]

B Vitamins

Folic acid and vitamin B_{12} are intimately linked with the synthesis of S-adenosylmethionine (SAMe), and each functions as a methyl donor, carrying and donating methyl molecules to a variety of brain chemicals, including neurotransmitters. Although large-scale clinical studies are lacking, a trial of a B-complex vitamin is advisable, particularly for older patients, in whom B_{12} deficiency is common, and for persons with suboptimal diets. Vitamin B_6 is essential in the manufacture of serotonin, and vitamin B_6 levels have been found to be low in many depressed patients, particularly in premenopausal women taking oral contraceptive pills or replacement estrogen.[21,37,50]

■ Dosage
Vitamin B complex 100, one tablet daily (contains approximately 100 mg each of the major B vitamins).

Folic Acid

Up to one third of depressed adults have borderline or low folate levels. A subgroup of depressed patients with folate deficiency and impaired methylation and monoamine neurotransmitter metabolism has been identified.[51] In fact, depression is the most common symptom of folate deficiency.[52] Patients with low levels of folate also appear to respond more poorly to therapy with selective serotonin reuptake inhibitors (SSRIs).[52] Limited evidence from a Cochrane Review suggested that the addition of folate to conventional antidepressant therapy is beneficial.[53] Folate is used as an adjunctive treatment.[54]

Folate may also have other health benefits (i.e., prevention of neural tube defects and reduction of elevated homocysteine). It makes sense to supplement with vitamin B_{12} concomitantly to avoid masking a deficiency.

■ Dosage
400 mcg to 1 mg daily (although doses of 5 to 20 mg daily have been used in studies).

■ Precautions
High doses of folic acid have been reported to cause altered sleep patterns, vivid dreaming, irritability, exacerbation of seizure frequency, gastrointestinal disturbances, and a bitter taste in the mouth, and concerns have emerged about possible increased risk of some cancers.

S-Adenosylmethionine

SAMe (Fig. 4-1) is the major methyl donor in the body and is involved in the metabolism of norepinephrine, dopamine, and serotonin. Its synthesis is impaired in depression, and supplementation results in increased brain monoamine levels, enhanced binding of neurotransmitters to receptors, and increased brain cell membrane fluidity. Although larger trials are warranted, multiple open and randomized

FIGURE 4-1
S-Adenosylmethionine (SAMe) metabolism. SAMe may cause hypomania or mania in patients with bipolar disease and should be avoided in this population. ATP, adenosine triphosphate; CH₃, methyl group.

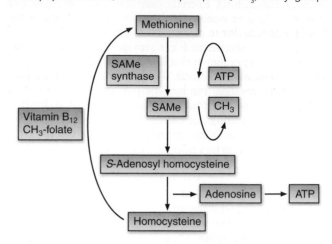

controlled trials (RCTs) suggest that SAMe is an effective natural antidepressant. An RCT comparing SAMe (1600 mg orally, daily) with imipramine (150 mg orally, daily) over 6 weeks demonstrated equivalent efficacy and superior tolerability of SAMe.[55] Another small double-blind placebo-controlled trial of SSRI nonresponders with major depression compared adjunctive SAMe (800 mg orally, twice daily) with placebo and found SAMe significantly more likely to lead to remission.[56] An Agency for Healthcare Research and Quality evidence report and technology assessment in 2002 found SAMe to be superior to placebo and comparable to conventional antidepressants, based on available evidence. SAMe is generally well tolerated and has a more rapid onset of action than that of standard pharmaceutical antidepressants.[57] Because of this characteristic, some clinicians start SAMe concurrently with another dietary supplement or pharmaceutical approach to therapy of depression that has been more thoroughly studied and then taper the dose of SAMe to zero as the other antidepressant begins to take effect. The most stable and bioavailable oral form appears to be 1,4-butane-disulfonate (Actimet), which is stable for up to 2 years at room temperature. SAMe is relatively free of side effects and does not have known cardiac, anticholinergic, or orthostatic effects. Larger clinical trials comparing SAMe with placebo and standard of care will help elucidate its role in treating depression.

■ Dosage
Initial treatment of depression may require 1600 mg daily given in equal doses, followed by a maintenance dosage of 200 mg twice daily. We recommend starting with 200 mg once or twice daily, to minimize any gastrointestinal side effects, and then titrating upward to effect over 1 to 2 weeks. In treating SSRI nonresponders, 800 mg orally twice daily may be used.

■ Precautions
High dosages can cause nausea, vomiting, flatulence, and diarrhea. Avoid giving the second dose close to bedtime because it can cause insomnia.

Hydroxytryptophan

Hydroxytryptophan (5-HTP) is the intermediate in the metabolism of tryptophan to serotonin. Open trials and RCTs have suggested that 5-HTP is as effective as standard antidepressants.[58,59] A Cochrane Review found only 2 of 108 trials of sufficient quality for inclusion, but in these trials, 5-HTP was superior to placebo.[60] Tryptophan itself appeared promising as a treatment for insomnia and depression but was removed from the market (although it is available again) when a contaminated batch was linked to an outbreak of eosinophilia myalgia syndrome in people with abnormal activation of the kynurenin pathway. Although 5-HTP is not metabolized along this pathway, case reports link 5-HTP to an illness resembling eosinophilia myalgia syndrome. The suspected culprit is a family of contaminants known as peak X that is commonly found in commercially available 5-HTP.[61] Because uncertainty surrounding 5-HTP remains, it seems advisable to avoid recommending its use pending further information. Case reports of seizures in Down syndrome and of dermatomyositis in conjunction with the use of carbidopa have appeared in the literature. Use with other serotonin agonists is not recommended, to avoid serotonin syndrome.

■ Dosage

100 to 200 mg three times daily, enteric-coated 5-HTP, 20 minutes before meals.

Botanicals

St. John's Wort (Hypericum perforatum)

The exact mechanism of action of St. John's wort (SJW) remains unknown, but this botanical affects serotonin, dopamine, norepinephrine, and GABA reuptake inhibition and also in vitro monoamine oxidase inhibition and L-glutamate.[55] SJW also appears to inhibit interleukin-6 and increase cortisol production, which may result in an additional indirect antidepressant effect.[62] Clinical effects are probably the result of a combined contribution of multiple mechanisms, each individually too weak to account for the action.[63] SJW has been a licensed prescription medication in Germany since 1984, and nearly twice the number of prescriptions are written for it as for all other antidepressants in that country. Two large U.S. trials found that SJW was not effective for treating severe major depression.[64] The most recent Cochrane Reviews examined the findings of 29 trials (almost 5500 patients) comparing SJW with placebo or standard antidepressants and concluded that available evidence suggests that SJW is superior to placebo and is as effective as conventional antidepressants and better tolerated.[65] Large-scale postmarketing surveillance studies of SJW extracts (14,245 patients) recorded rates of adverse effects 10-fold lower than for conventional antidepressants.[66]

■ Indication

SWJ is indicated for mild to moderate depression.

■ Dosage

SJW, 900 mg daily given in three equal doses, has been used most frequently in clinical trials. Choose a product standardized to a minimum of 2% to 5% hyperforin or 0.3% hypericin

such as those used in clinical trials. Examples include Lichtwer LI 160 found in Kira; Lichtwer LI 160 WS, the hyperforin stabilized version of LI 160 found in Quanterra Emotional Balance; ZE 117, containing 0.2% hypericin in Remotiv. Once clinical improvement has been obtained, consider twice-daily dosing. Up to 2 months may be required before full effects are noted.

■ Precautions

Although side effects are fewer than with current pharmacologic antidepressants, they can include gastrointestinal upset, allergic reaction, fatigue, dry mouth, restlessness, constipation, sexual side effects, and possibly increased risk of cataracts.

> St. John's wort can activate the cytochrome P-450 3A4 detoxification system in the liver and thereby reduce the serum levels of drugs metabolized by this pathway. Caution should be used in patients receiving antiretroviral, warfarin, cyclosporine, and oral contraceptive therapy.

Ginkgo biloba

Ginkgo, the most prescribed botanical in Europe, is considered "safe and effective" by the German Commission E for treatment of cerebral insufficiency. It also has been found to be useful in treating older patients with depression related to organic brain dysfunction. Small double-blinded placebo-controlled trials support the effectiveness of giving ginkgo to older adults (51 to 78 years of age) with depression unresponsive to standard drug treatment.[67,68] Larger, well-designed prospective trials are warranted, but ginkgo is generally well tolerated.

■ Indication

Ginkgo is given as an adjunctive agent for treatment-resistant depression in patients older than 50 years of age.

■ Dosage

The recommended regimen is 40 to 80 mg three times daily of an extract standardized to 24% ginkgo flavonglycosides and 6% terpenoids. Many patients respond within 2 to 3 weeks, but it may take up to 3 months for full effects to be noted.

■ Precautions

Rare cases of mild gastrointestinal upset, headache, and allergic skin reactions have been reported. Ginkgo has an antiplatelet effect, so caution should be taken when prescribing this to patients taking anticoagulants.

Mind-Body Therapy

Antidepressants and psychotherapy are first-line treatments for depression according to the American Psychiatric Association (APA); even so, only 60% of those treated will have a clinically significant response, and many others may have residual symptoms.[69] Many patients turn to a mind-body approach as another tool to improve their health. Additionally, the use of multiple treatment methods may end up being the best approach for preventing relapse and treating current depressive episodes.

The mind-body approach is common for those suffering from depression. One fourth of patients have tried some type of mind-body therapy,[27,70] and two thirds of those who tried a mind-body approach found it beneficial.[27]

With an understanding that no single mind-body exercise will treat all individuals or one individual completely, a pilot study by Little and Kligler demonstrated a positive response using a variety of mind-body techniques including psychoeducation, lifestyle modification, meditation, and mind-body skills training.[71] A larger study is pending. Another small study demonstrated that depressed pregnant patients treated with interpersonal psychotherapy and massage therapy (MT) improved more compared with those who had only psychotherapy.[72] One benefit of MT was that the patients also participated in more of their psychotherapy sessions.

Psychotherapy and Meditation
Depression-specific psychotherapies are designed to provide acute, time-limited interventions. They are present oriented and pragmatic, focusing on depression and issues considered relevant to both its onset and its perpetuation.[73] According to the APA, psychotherapy is a reasonable first-line or combination approach to all levels of depression, whether mild, moderate, or severe.[74] Primary care physicians can provide limited, supportive psychotherapy at frequent visits necessary to monitor the effectiveness of medications.[75] In fact, generic counseling appears to be preferred by patients over antidepressant drugs and is as effective, although slower in onset for treating mild to moderate depressive illness.[76]

Cognitive Therapy
Cognitive therapy is the most-studied psychotherapeutic approach to major depression. The physician or the therapist assists the patient in replacing negative patterns of thinking with a more positive, realistic approach. Multiple studies have demonstrated the equivalency of this modality to rigorous antidepressant medication regimens.[73] One controlled trial demonstrated that monthly cognitive therapy was as effective as antidepressant medications were for prophylaxis against recurrence over 6 months, but not all studies support this.

■ Mindfulness-Based Cognitive Therapy
A specific type of cognitive therapy that includes meditation is called mindfulness-based cognitive therapy (MBCT). This specific method has been successful for treating depression in a variety of patient populations from those with chronic pain or different types of cancer to patients with congestive heart failure or myocardial infarctions.[77] Several initial studies also demonstrated that MBCT can decrease recurrence of depression.[78-80] One study followed depressed patients through their acute treatment with pharmaceutical antidepressant medication and into remission and maintenance care. Once in remission, subjects were randomized into continued preventive strategies of medication, MBCT, or placebo. Patients with

an unstable remission ("periodic symptom flurries") during the acute phase of improvement had a significantly and equally reduced risk for subsequent relapse when they were in the continued medication or MBCT groups. Patients who were stable during the acute phase of remission did not benefit more from the active preventive interventions.[81] Mindfulness may be a critical component in patients with depression. Interpersonal therapy and problem-solving therapy have also been successful.[73,82]

Other Mind-Body Therapies
■ Yoga
Yoga is a specific form of exercise that combines poses, breath work, and meditation. Several studies, including one RCT, examined the effect of 4 to 6 weeks of yoga classes lasting 45 to 60 minutes per session; the results showed a positive trend toward supporting yoga as a therapeutic treatment for patients suffering mild to moderate depression.[27,83,84] At this point, distinguishing among the different types of yoga is not possible, although initial studies using Hatha and Vinyasa yoga both appeared promising.[83,85]

■ Other Traditional Healing Techniques
Although well-designed clinical studies investigating the role of meditation, hypnosis, and imagery in the treatment of depression have been limited, centuries of experience in traditional healing systems (e.g., Ayurvedic, Tibetan) support this kind of therapeutic approach. In our experience, these mind-body techniques are often extremely useful therapeutic adjuncts that appear to enhance the efficacy of other treatments. Emerging data suggest that relaxation therapy appears promising.[86] Evidence has also shown the effectiveness of prayer as an adjunct to other therapy for depression.[87] We recommend that interested patients explore one of these approaches (see Chapter 92, Prescribing Relaxation Techniques).

Acupuncture
Acupuncture has been used for centuries in Asia for the treatment of virtually all known disease states. The exact mechanism of action is unknown, but human and animal studies have demonstrated that the stimulation of certain acupuncture points can alter neurotransmitter levels.[88] The United Nations World Health Organization recognized acupuncture as effective in treating mild to moderate depression. Case series indicate that acupuncture is promising for treating depression; this finding is supported by several uncontrolled and controlled studies. Some trials detected an additive benefit of combining acupuncture with medications for treating depression. Reviews of available RCTs of acupuncture for depression (including translations of relevant Chinese language studies) found general trends suggesting that acupuncture is as effective as antidepressants in the limited studies available for comparison. Placebo acupuncture tends to perform as well as true acupuncture, however, so it remains unclear whether condition-specific needling has a precise effect on depression. Because of the limitations of these studies (small sample sizes, imprecise enrollment criteria, problems with randomization and blinding, brief duration of study, and

lack of follow-up), evidence supporting acupuncture for depression remains inconclusive pending further study, and the Cochrane Reviews investigators concluded that evidence was insufficient to recommend acupuncture for depression.[89,90]

Serious adverse effects of acupuncture have been reported but are rare. One prospective survey of more than 34,000 treatments (for all conditions) by traditional acupuncturists in Britain revealed no serious adverse events over a 1-month period.[91] Another review of 12 prospective studies surveying more than a million treatments concluded that the risk of a serious adverse event with acupuncture is estimated to be 0.05 per 10,000 treatments.[92]

Phototherapy

Phototherapy is commonly used for patients with seasonal affective disorder, but it may also be useful as an adjunctive modality with pharmacotherapy in both unipolar and bipolar depression.[93] Two meta-analyses supported at least modest benefit of bright light phototherapy when compared with placebo for nonseasonal depression.[94,95] The APA guidelines for the treatment of major depressive disorder consider bright light therapy a low-risk and low-cost option.[96] Consider recommending 30 to 60 minutes of bright, white (full-spectrum, 10,000 Lux) light daily from special bulbs, lamps, or light boxes.

Pharmaceuticals

Antidepressants are believed to work by inhibiting the degradation and reuptake of neurotransmitters important in regulating psychological and neurovegetative function (i.e., serotonin, norepinephrine, dopamine) and thus increasing neurotransmitter availability at the synaptic level. Newer theories suggest that pharmaceuticals may also mediate intracellular signaling systems that affect neurotrophic factors vital to the functioning of neuronal systems involved in mood regulation. Attempts to determine the most cost-effective approach to treating depression are limited by the quality of these evaluations, but SSRIs and newer antidepressants such as venlafaxine, mirtazapine, and nefazodone consistently are superior to tricyclic antidepressants (TCAs).[97] Studies of antidepressant medications increasingly are questioned because of the potential bias owing to unblinding, given that side effects of the drugs (as opposed to inert placebos) may reveal the identity of the true medication to participants or investigators. Trials using an "active" placebo that mimics some of the side effects of antidepressants to counteract this potential bias suggest that differences between antidepressants and active placebos are small.[98]

Selective Serotonin Reuptake Inhibitors and Mixed Reuptake Blockers

The APA continues to recommend the use of an SSRI as first-line treatment for all levels of depression: mild, moderate, and severe.[74] Recommendations for secondary steps include switching or augmenting current therapy (pharmacotherapy or psychotherapy) and depend on the initial treatment choice. *Maintenance therapy* is defined as continuation of the initial treatment to prevent recurrence of depression.

Safety in overdose and side effect profiles for SSRIs and mixed reuptake blockers are greatly improved over those for cyclic antidepressants and monoamine oxidase inhibitors. Even so, 50% of patients discontinue their medication in the first 4 months after treatment initiation, and two thirds of these patients report a side effect as the reason for stopping treatment.[99] Be aware that concern is emerging over the long-term effects of SSRIs, including uncommon but serious neurologic sequelae of seizures and extrapyramidal symptoms,[100] as well as worsening of long-term outcomes despite effective short-term control.[101] The Food and Drug Administration (FDA) has mandated a black box warning on SSRIs regarding the risk of increasing suicidality in children and adolescents. This risk appears to occur within the first 2 weeks of initiating therapy, and whether this risk exists for adults is unclear.[99]

■ Dosage
See Table 4-1.

■ Precautions
Nausea, cramping, agitation, insomnia, headache, decreased libido, delayed ejaculation, erectile dysfunction, and anorgasmia have been reported in patients taking SSRIs.[99] Gastrointestinal side effects are more pronounced with sertraline but may be minimized by taking the drug with food and water. Fluoxetine is generally the most activating. Paroxetine has mild anticholinergic properties, including nausea and possibly weight gain. Venlafaxine has side effects similar to those of the other SSRIs but may cause serious hypertension over time. Although venlafaxine and paroxetine may have an increased risk of nausea, this can be reduced by using the extended-release forms.[99] Citalopram and escitalopram have the fewest side effects and the least impact on the cytochrome P-450 enzyme system. Duloxetine appears to play a role in mediating chronic pain and appears effective in older patients.[102] Rare side effects of SSRIs may include increased risk of gastrointestinal bleeding when these drugs are used with nonsteroidal antiinflammatory drugs, but more research is needed.[99] Other rare side effects include cardiac conduction abnormalities with venlafaxine and liver enzyme abnormalities with duloxetine.[99]

Tricyclic Antidepressants
TCAs have significant side effects (anticholinergic effects, weight gain, and cardiac dysrhythmias) and can be lethal in overdoses as small as an average 10-day supply.

Heterocyclic Antidepressants
Heterocyclic antidepressants are much safer than TCAs in overdose, and they have side effect profiles that make them useful in specific clinical circumstances. Several studies demonstrated that heterocyclic antidepressants are equally effective compared with SSRIs.[103] Amoxapine is useful in treating psychotic depression. Trazodone is highly sedating and is useful in low doses (25 to 50 mg nightly) when it is taken in combination with SSRIs to induce sleep. Bupropion is highly stimulating and may be a good option for patients wishing to discontinue smoking tobacco; it also has decreased fatigue and somnolence, but it is associated with seizures in underweight people. Nefazodone has anxiolytic properties and

TABLE 4-1. Drug and Supplement Dosages Used in Depression Treatment

DRUG/SUPPLEMENT	INITIAL DOSE (mg[†])	RANGE (mg/day[†])	FREQUENCY
Vitamin B complex 100	1 tablet	—	Daily
Folic acid	400 mcg	400–800 mcg	Daily
Fish oil	1,000	1000–6000	Daily
SAMe (1,4-butane-disulfonate)	200	200–800	bid
Hydroxytryptophan (enteric coated)	100	100–200	tid
St. John's wort (standardized to 5% hyperforin)*	300	900–1200	tid
Ginkgo biloba extract (standardized to 24% ginkgo flavonglycosides and 6% terpenoids)	40	60–240	tid
Selective Serotonin Reuptake Inhibitors and Mixed Reuptake Blockers			
Fluoxetine	20	20–80	Daily (AM)[‡]
Sertraline	50	50–200	Daily
Paroxetine	20	20–50	Daily (AM)
Paroxetine, extended release	12.5	25–62.5	Daily
Fluvoxamine	50	50–300	Daily (at bedtime)[§]
Citalopram	20	20–60	Daily
Escitalopram	10	10–20	Daily
Serotonin Norepinephrine Reuptake Inhibitors			
Venlafaxine, immediate release	37.5	75–375	bid
Venlafaxine, extended release	37.5	75–225	Daily (at bedtime)
Desvenlafaxine	50	50	
Duloxetine	40–60	60–120	Divided daily-bid
Dopamine Norepinephrine Reuptake Inhibitor			
Bupropion, immediate release	150	300–450	tid[ǁ]
Bupropion, sustained release	150	300–400	bid
Bupropion, extended release	150	300–450	Daily
Heterocyclic Antidepressants/Serotonin Modulators			
Nefazodone	200	200–600	bid
Norepinephrine Serotonin Modulator, Alpha 2 Antagonist			
Mirtazapine	15	15–45	Daily (at bedtime)

bid, twice daily; SAMe, *S*-adenosylmethionine; tid, three times daily.
*Cytochrome P-450 3A4 and drug pump P-glycoprotein induction by St. John's wort requires that care be taken when prescribing this botanical in the setting of other drugs metabolized along these pathways. Perhaps the most clinically relevant interactions occur with cyclosporine (lowering serum cyclosporine concentration) and with other antidepressants, particularly the selective serotonin reuptake inhibitors (SSRIs; serotonin syndrome), antiretroviral therapy (reducing the concentration of protease inhibitors in patients infected with human immunodeficiency virus), and warfarin-type anticoagulants (increasing anticoagulation). Concern exists that St. John's wort may interfere with the efficacy of oral contraceptives. Avoid the use of St. John's wort concurrently with SSRIs; also avoid its use in pregnancy and lactation. High doses may predispose patients to photodermatitis.
[†]Unless otherwise indicated.
[‡]Maximum range is 20 to 80 mg.
[§]Doses greater than 100 mg should be divided dose, with the greater dose given at bedtime.
[ǁ]Initial dose: 100 mg bid for 3 days; then 100 mg tid.

may be useful in patients who develop anxiety and insomnia while taking SSRIs. Nefazodone and bupropion also tend to have fewer sexual side effects compared with the SSRIs and serotonin norepinephrine reuptake inhibitors. Nefazodone and bupropion have the least likelihood of causing weight gain compared with SSRIs, whereas mirtazapine increases appetite and tends to cause weight gain. Mirtazapine also increases fatigue and somnolence, which may be desirable in some cases.[99]

Rare side effects that need further investigation in heterocyclic antidepressants include the following: seizures and atopic reactions with bupropion; thrombocytopenia, neutropenia, and bone marrow suppression with mirtazapine; and hepatotoxicity, cardiac conduction problems, and priapism with trazodone.

Electroconvulsive Therapy

Electroconvulsive therapy (ECT) reportedly is effective in achieving remission in 70% to 90% of patients with depression within 7 to 14 days in clinical trials (although it is less effective in community settings).[104] Generally, ECT is reserved for suicidal, psychotic, or catatonic patients; it is also helpful in patients refractory to other treatment modalities. ECT should be used with caution in patients with recent myocardial infarction, cardiac arrhythmia, or intracranial space-occupying lesions. Transient postictal confusion and anterograde and retrograde memory impairment are expected.[96]

■ Dosage
ECT, which requires referral to an experienced treatment center, generally involves sessions three times a week for up to 4 weeks, until symptoms abate.

Therapies to Consider for Depression

Estrogen Replacement Therapy
No abnormality of ovarian hormones has been identified that distinguishes women with depression from those without depression during the menopause transition.[105] However, estrogen replacement was demonstrated to reduce symptoms in perimenopausal and postmenopausal women with depression in some small studies, and discontinuation of hormone replacement therapy (HRT) appears to be associated with the rapid recurrence of depression in some women with a history of depression.[106] An RCT comparing HRT (estradiol valerate 2 mg, dienogest 2 mg) with placebo suggested that in women with mild to moderate depression in the setting of postmenopausal syndrome, HRT clearly and clinically relevantly reduced symptom severity by the Hamilton Rating Scale for Depression HAM-D at 24 weeks.[107] Studies assessing the relationship between hormone status and depression are inconsistent, and this remains an active area of research. Practitioners should consider recommending HRT after weighing the risks and benefits.

Transcranial Magnetic Stimulation
Transcranial magnetic stimulation uses a magnetic coil close to the scalp to generate rapidly alternating magnetic fields to produce electrical stimulation of superficial cortical neurons. It requires no general anesthesia and has minimal side effects. This technique was cleared by the FDA in 2008 for use in patients with major depressive disorder who have not responded adequately to at least one antidepressant trial. It is currently being studied as an alternative to ECT, but it has not consistently demonstrated superiority to ECT or sham.[108]

Aromatherapy
Aromatherapy, which is the use of essential oils most often topically combined with MT or as inhaled vapors, has roots in ancient healing traditions. Several small studies demonstrated the impact of aroma on mood. One small open pilot trial found that adjunctive aromatherapy allowed for reductions in dose of antidepressants compared with usual therapy. This nonrandomized trial included patients using various types and doses of antidepressants.[109] Short-term but not persistent benefits were found for aromatherapy MT with citrus oil in patients with cancer who were dealing with depression.[110] Aromatherapy may be promising as a gentle adjunctive therapy, but larger, well-designed trials are necessary before conclusions can be drawn.

Music Therapy
In music therapy, patients actively perform or listen to music to promote health and healing. This is an active area of research, but most trials are small and lack appropriate control for attention of professionals. In addition, concurrent interventions that are not music specific (e.g., guided imagery and relaxation) make conclusions difficult to draw. Numerous trials of music therapy, largely in an older population, suggested potential antidepressant benefits when this modality was added to usual care, and a dose effect appeared to occur with increased response as treatment continued.[111] However, a Cochrane Review identified only five trials meeting inclusion criteria and concluded that although music therapy is well tolerated by people with depression and appears to be associated with improvements in mood, the small number and low quality of studies preclude clear determination of effectiveness until better studies are conducted.[112] The risks of music therapy are low, and although proof of benefits will require more thorough study, interested patients so inclined should not be discouraged.

Massage
Several studies reported the benefits of MT for improving mood in healthy and ill individuals, but MT has not been studied extensively for the treatment of depression. Small randomized trials have suggested that the addition of MT to psychotherapy in pregnant women with depression may be more helpful than psychotherapy alone[113] and that MT by the woman's partner is superior to standard treatment.[114] However, the most recent systematic review continues to point to a lack of evidence for MT in the treatment of depression.[115] When performed by a qualified therapist, MT can be a safe and pleasant experience and may be considered appropriate adjunctive therapy for depressed individuals who are so inclined.

PREVENTION PRESCRIPTION

The following steps are recommended for prevention of depressive symptoms:

- Remove exacerbating factors.
- Review current medications and supplements that could be contributing to depression, and consider decreasing dosages or discontinuing drugs that are suspect if they are not vital to the patient's well-being.
- Recommend a whole foods/low–processed foods diet such as the Mediterranean or antiinflammatory style eating plan, low in refined sugar (sucrose), caffeine, and alcohol. Encourage a diet rich in omega-3 fatty acids. Recommend two or three servings of cold-water fish (salmon, herring, mackerel, sardines) each week and 2 tablespoons of ground flaxseed or flaxseed oil daily.
- Consider recommending vitamin D$_3$ 1000 units daily.
- Consider recommending a B-complex vitamin daily.
- Prescribe physical activity. Encourage daily aerobic (e.g., walking, jogging, cycling) or anaerobic (weight-lifting) exercise. Explore options, and help patients select activities they feel are enjoyable. Emphasize starting slowly and setting realistic short-term goals. Gradually increase to an ideal exercise prescription (see Chapter 88, Writing an Exercise Prescription).
- Foster an increase in a sense of community and investment in meaningful relationships to reduce social isolation.

THERAPEUTIC REVIEW

▥ Lifestyle

- Suggest regular practice of aerobic or anaerobic exercises most days of the week.

- Encourage activities that will increase social connection and enhance meaningful relationships.

▥ Nutrition

- Eliminate caffeine and simple sugars from the diet.

- Consume a Mediterranean-style or whole foods (low–processed foods) diet.

▥ Dietary Supplements and Botanicals

- Vitamins: Augment conventional antidepressant medication with vitamin B complex and 400 mcg to 1 mg of additional folic acid daily.

- St. John's wort: Take 900 mg daily in three equal doses. Choose a product standardized to a minimum of 2% to 5% hyperforin or 0.3% hypericin. Examples include Kira, Quanterra Emotional Balance, Remotiv, or Movana. If no improvement is seen after 4 to 6 weeks, consider switching to SAMe or a pharmaceutical antidepressant. Concurrent psychotherapy is recommended, if this approach is acceptable to the patient.

- S-Adenosylmethionine (SAMe): Start at 200 mg once or twice daily to minimize gastrointestinal side effects; then titrate upward to effect over 1 to 2 weeks. Initial treatment of depression may require 1600 mg daily given in two equal doses, followed by a maintenance dose of 200 mg twice daily.

- If recommending a pharmaceutical antidepressant, consider using SAMe initially (because of its rapid onset of action) along with it to minimize the latency period. SAMe may be withdrawn after 4 to 6 weeks.

- If SAMe is given without a pharmaceutical antidepressant, consider switching to another agent if no resolution of symptoms is noted after 2 weeks. Choose a product containing 1,4-butane-disulfonate (Actimet), which is stable for up to 2 years at room temperature. Concurrent psychotherapy is recommended, if this approach is acceptable to the patient.

- Fish oil: Take 1 g daily. If this dose is not effective, consider titrating up to 6 g of omega-3 fatty acids. In the case of an intake higher than 3 g per day, caution must be used because antiplatelet effects are more likely. Choose a product that has been tested for pesticides and heavy metal residues and keep refrigerated.

▥ Psychotherapy

The combination of supportive psychotherapy with antidepressant supplements or pharmacotherapy is generally recommended. Primary care physicians can provide limited psychotherapy at frequent visits to monitor lifestyle modifications, dietary supplements, or drug therapy. Alternatively, referral for cognitive or interpersonal therapy is recommended.

▥ Pharmaceuticals

If no improvement is obtained with the use of lifestyle modification measures and dietary supplements (or if the patient has severe depression), discontinue the supplements, and start a pharmaceutical antidepressant. All currently approved antidepressant drugs are equally effective and have similar latency periods.[47] Choice of a selective serotonin reuptake inhibitor, mixed reuptake blocker, or heterocyclic antidepressant should be guided by matching the most appropriate side effect profile to each patient's symptoms. Continue treatment for at least 6 months after improvement, and consider full-dosage maintenance if the patient has a history of recurrent depression ([moderate to severe depression] or [mild depression]). If only a partial response has occurred at 6 weeks, either change the class of antidepressant medication or continue the antidepressant and consider adding lithium carbonate, 300 mg three times a day (necessitates experience in monitoring serum levels), or liothyronine sodium (Cytomel), 25 to 50 mcg.

▓ Phototherapy

Suggest phototherapy with 30 to 60 minutes of bright, white (full-spectrum, 10,000 Lux) light daily from special bulbs, lamps, or light boxes.*

▓ Referral

Consider referral to a psychiatrist if the patient remains refractory to treatment, is suicidal or psychotic, or requires psychiatric hospitalization or electroconvulsive therapy or transcranial magnetic stimulation.

*Information and therapeutic lights are widely available, including from the following manufacturers: BioBrite, Inc., 1-800-621-LITE (1-800-621-5483), www.biobrite.com; and SunBox Company, 1-800-548-3968, www.sunboxco.com

KEY WEB RESOURCES

American Psychiatric Association. http://www.psychiatryonline.com/pracGuide/pracGuideTopic_7.aspx	American Psychiatric Association Guidelines for Treatment of Major Depression
http://www.depression-primarycare.org/clinicians/toolkits/materials/forms/phq9/	The PHQ-9 questionnaire, a useful tool to diagnose and monitor depression treatment.
http://www.consumerlab.com	Independent testing of dietary supplements
http://naturaldatabase.therapeuticresearch.com	Evidence-based resources on dietary supplements

References

References are available online at expertconsult.com.

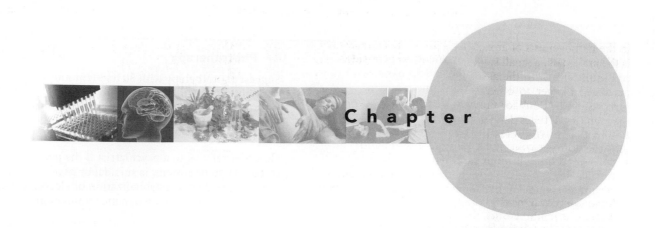

Chapter 5

Anxiety

Roberta A. Lee, MD

Anxiety disorders are one of the most commonly encountered medical conditions in primary care. According to the National Institute of Mental Health, the 1-year prevalence rate is 18.1% of the population, or 40 million people. Underdiagnosis is common; the average patient with an anxiety disorder consults 10 health care professionals before a definitive diagnosis is made.[1] Furthermore, patients who carry the diagnosis use primary care services three times as often as other patients.[2] In the past, when underdiagnosis was more common, patients received elaborate medical workups, but the definitive diagnosis remained elusive. These patients became categorized as the "worried well." Nevertheless, because anxiety can be masked in numerous psychosomatic ways, practitioners must maintain a high index of suspicion for this disorder.

Anxiety disorders encompass a wide variety of subtypes, the most common being generalized anxiety disorder (GAD), obsessive-compulsive disorder (OCD), panic disorder, phobias, and posttraumatic stress disorder (PTSD). All are marked by irrational, involuntary thoughts. One of the most defining diagnostic elements of anxiety disorders is the disruption of daily life by overt distress. Frequently, patients have a significant reduction in the ability to carry out routine tasks, whether social, personal, or professional.[3] In this chapter, the focus is on an integrative approach to the management of GAD, as defined in the fourth edition of the *Diagnostic and Statistical Manual of Mental Disorders* (DSM-IV). In primary care practice, the prevalence of GAD can be as high as 10% to 15%.[2]

Definition and Diagnostic Criteria

GAD involves unremitting, excessive worry involving a variety of issues. These concerns may be related to family, health, money, or work. Once the initial concern subsides, another quickly takes its place. The practitioner observes over time that the concerns seem pervasive and repetitive. Additionally, the distress seems out of proportion to the actual life circumstance.

To meet the DSM-IV criteria for GAD, intense worrying must occur on a majority of days during a period of at least 6 continuous months.[3] In addition, three of the following signs and symptoms must be present: easy fatigability, difficulty concentrating, irritability, muscle tension, restlessness, and sleep disturbance. Patients usually present with physical complaints and fail to recognize the stress-related origin. The most frequent signs and symptoms are diaphoresis, headache, and trembling.[4] GAD can have psychological manifestations as well. Patients often report impaired memory or a diminished ability to concentrate or take directions, and they frequently make statements such as "I can't seem to stop thinking of. . . ."

Comorbid Conditions

Approximately 40% of people with GAD have no comorbid conditions, but many develop another disorder as time evolves.[5] In fact, concurrent or coexistent organic or psychiatric disease is the rule rather than the exception in patients with GAD.[5] For example, panic disorder is common among persons who have irritable bowel syndrome; a shared brain-gut mechanism incorporating a serotonin link has been theorized.[6] Psychiatric overlap is common. Anxiety disorders and depression frequently coincide—either can trigger the other. In the case of coexisting depression, especially of significant severity, treatment of the depression is the primary objective. Subsequent visits will reveal whether the anxiety is relieved simply by addressing depression. Many persons coping with anxiety use alcohol or drugs to mask their distress. Approximately 30% of people with panic disorder abuse alcohol, and use of drugs occurs in 17%.[1]

Pathophysiology

The pathophysiology of GAD is multifactorial and remains incompletely understood. Studies in animals and humans have attempted to pinpoint body structure and systems involved in the pathogenesis of anxiety. One that has been identified is the amygdala, a small structure deep inside the brain that communicates with the autonomic nervous system to relay perceived danger to other centers of the brain, which, in turn, ready the body for the perceived danger. Furthermore, the memory of these dangers stored in the amygdala appears to be indelible, thus creating a pathophysiologic phenomenon that may progress to GAD.

> Although the pathophysiology of generalized anxiety disorder is multifactorial, the amygdala in the brain appears to be a focus for stressful memories that stimulate the autonomic nervous system when the body and mind perceive danger.

Other contributing factors may lie in the realm of cognitive phenomena. Research is currently under way to evaluate exposure to stress early in life and subsequent development of GAD.[7]

In PTSD, a subtype of anxiety, studies have identified low cortisol levels (and high levels of corticotropin-releasing factor) and an overabundance of norepinephrine and epinephrine as contributing factors.[8]

Finally, genetic factors are thought to be another influence. Studies indicate genetic concordance with certain genetic loci that produce functional serotonin polymorphisms.[9]

Ruling Out Organic Disease

The symptoms of anxiety disorders can resemble those of a variety of medical conditions, and a full medical workup is in order if the possibility of disease exists (Table 5-1).

Integrative Therapy

Exercise

Numerous studies assessing the effects of both short-term and long-term exercise on anxiety exist. The bulk of these studies measured the effects of exercise by the presence of signs and symptoms of elevated anxiety, rather than by using a diagnostic system such as that of the DSM.[10] Nonetheless, the results of most studies generally showed a reduction in symptoms with increased physical activity.

Aerobic exercise programs seem to have produced a larger effect than obtained with weight training and flexibility regimens, although all appear effective for improvement in mood.[10,11] The length of physical activity also seems important. In one study, programs exceeding 12 minutes for a minimum of 10 weeks were needed to achieve significant anxiety reduction.[12] The beneficial effect appeared to be maximal at 40 minutes per session.[10] Furthermore, the benefits seem to be lasting. In one study assessing the long-term effects of aerobic exercise, participants evaluated at 1-year follow-up examination were found to maintain the psychological benefits initially recorded. Their exercise routines over the 12-month follow-up were either the same as those in the original study design or less intensive.[13]

TABLE 5-1. Medical Conditions Often Associated With Symptoms of Anxiety	
SYSTEM	**SPECIFIC DISORDER**
Cardiovascular	Acute myocardial infarction Angina pectoris Arrhythmias Congestive heart failure Hypertension Ischemic heart disease Mitral valve prolapse
Endocrine	Carcinoid syndrome Cushing's disease Hyperthyroidism Hypothyroidism Hypoglycemia Parathyroid disease Pheochromocytoma Porphyria Electrolyte imbalance
Gastrointestinal	Irritable bowel syndrome
Gynecologic	Menopause Premenstrual syndrome
Hematologic	Anemia Chronic immune diseases
Neurologic	Brain tumor Delirium Encephalopathy Epilepsy Parkinson disease Seizure disorder Vertigo Transient ischemic attack
Respiratory	Asthma Chronic obstructive pulmonary disease Pulmonary embolism Dyspnea Pulmonary edema

The exact reason for the improvement of mood with exercise is not completely known. However, increased physical activity has been correlated with changes in brain levels of monoamines—norepinephrine, dopamine, and serotonin—that may account for improved mood.[14] The endorphin hypothesis is another explanation for the beneficial effects of exercise on mood. Many studies have demonstrated significant endorphin secretion with increased exercise, with beneficial effects on state of mind. However, blockade of endorphin elevation with antagonists such as naloxone during exercise does not correlate with decreased mental health benefits.[14] Some investigators have argued that the latter finding reflects flaws in methodologic design.

> Both the length of the exercise session and the duration of the physical activity program seem important in maximizing the beneficial effect of exercise on anxiety reduction.

No matter what the hypothesis, the involvement of each patient in active recovery may confer a sense of independence leading to increased self-confidence. In turn, the patient's ability to cope with challenging life events is increased. This process is consistent with the integrative philosophy of healing. Furthermore, paucity of side effects, low cost, and general availability all make exercise a crucial component of integrative management.

The level of exertion and the specific exercise prescription should be determined by the patient's level of fitness, interests in specific physical activities, and health concerns (see Chapter 88, Writing an Exercise Prescription).

Nutrition

Caffeine

On average, U.S. residents consume 1 or 2 cups of coffee a day, which represents approximately 150 to 300 mg of caffeine. Although most people can handle this amount with no effect on mood, some experience increased anxiety. People who are prone to feeling stress have reported that they experience increased anxiety from even these small amounts. With long-term use, caffeine has been linked with anxiety as well as depression. Discontinuation is warranted.[15]

Alcohol

With long-term use, alcohol has been found to diminish levels of serotonin and catecholamine. Discontinuation of alcohol consumption is therefore warranted.[16]

Omega-3 Fatty Acids

Epidemiologic data suggest that an omega-3 fatty acid deficiency or imbalance between the ratio of omega-6 and omega-3 fatty acids in the diet correlates with increased anxiety and depression. Investigators clearly documented in animal studies that levels of polyunsaturated fats and cholesterol metabolism influence neuronal tissue synthesis, membrane fluidity, and serotonin metabolism.[17] Primarily indirect evidence, particularly in depression, suggests that correction of the ratio of omega-6 to omega-3 consumption may improve mood. Given the evidence concerning neuronal tissue synthesis and serotonin metabolism, increased supplementation with omega-3 fatty acids seems beneficial.[18] Recommending consumption of cold water fish (sardines, mackerel, tuna, salmon, herring) at least two or three times a week or flaxseed oil (1000 to 2000 mg) or freshly ground flaxseed (2 tablespoons daily) or as a supplement seems reasonable (see Chapter 86, The Antiinflammatory Diet).

Supplements

B Vitamins

A deficiency of a variety of nutrients can alter brain function and therefore lead to anxiety. Deficiency of certain vitamins, including the B vitamins, has been linked with mood disorders. The B vitamins, including B_6 (pyridoxine) and B_{12}, are linked with the synthesis of S-adenosylmethionine (SAMe), which carries and donates methyl molecules to many chemicals in the brain including neurotransmitters. Vitamin B_6 is essential for the production of serotonin and has been linked with improvement in various mood disorders including anxiety when it is used as a supplement.[19] Although large-scale clinical studies are lacking, a trial of a B-complex supplement seems advisable, especially in older persons and in persons taking medications that may deplete this vitamin (e.g., oral contraceptives or replacement estrogen [Premarin].[20])

■ Dosage

The dose is a B-complex vitamin.

Folic Acid

Studies have shown that folic acid supplementation is helpful in persons who are depressed (see the section on folic acid use in Chapter 4, Depression). Patients with low levels of folic acid also have been reported to respond less well to selective serotonin reuptake inhibitors (SSRIs).[21] Serum vitamin B_{12} levels should be checked if folic acid supplementation is used, especially if megaloblastic anemia is noted in laboratory tests, because vitamin B_{12} deficiency can be masked by folic acid supplementation.

■ Dosage

The recommended dose of folic acid for supplementation is 400 to 800 mcg per day.

■ Precautions

High doses of folic acid have been reported to cause altered sleep patterns, exacerbation of seizure frequency, gastrointestinal disturbances, and a bitter taste in the mouth.

5-Hydroxytryptophan

5-Hydroxytryptophan (5-HTP) is an amino acid precursor used in the formation of serotonin. 5-HTP has been used as an oral supplement alternative to boost serotonin.[22] It has been shown in studies to improve depression, but only preliminary evidence is available suggesting that 5-HTP also may improve anxiety. L-Tryptophan, another amino acid found to improve mood, is converted to 5-HTP and then to serotonin. 5-HTP readily crosses the blood-brain barrier. The metabolism of 5-HTP by monoamine oxidase and aldehyde dehydrogenase forms 5-indoleacetic acid, which is excreted in the urine.

■ Dosage

For anxiety or depression, the dose is 150 to 300 mg daily.

■ Precautions

Anyone using conventional medications for depression or anxiety, particularly those agents that boost serotonin, should discuss the use of 5-HTP with his or her health care practitioner before initiating supplementation, to avoid excessively elevated levels of serotonin. 5-HTP can cause gastrointestinal side effects such as nausea, belching, and heartburn.

■ Caution

Some concern exists that 5-HTP, like L-tryptophan, can cause a condition known as eosinophilia myalgia syndrome. The suspected culprit is a group of contaminants identified from the peak X family. However, current evidence is insufficient to suggest that this element is consistently responsible. Case reports have been sporadic.[23]

Pharmaceuticals

Conventional options for initial therapy in GAD are based on various factors and drug side effect profiles. Depression frequently coexists with GAD, so antidepressants are often considered.

None of the SSRIs has a formal indication for the treatment of GAD, although some agents have been approved for panic disorder, social phobia, and PTSD. Because less cardiotoxicity is associated with SSRIs than with tricyclic antidepressants, an SSRI may be a better choice for patients with heart disease. Other conventional options for treatment of GAD involve the use of multiple receptor agents. Venlafaxine (Effexor) is the only serotonin norepinephrine reuptake inhibitor approved for GAD. The use of tricyclic antidepressants has always been a consideration, but the difficulty in using these medications is that they can have anticholinergic and cardiovascular side effects, as well as a more pronounced sedative effect. Most experts recommend a trial of at least 4 to 6 weeks to determine efficacy.

For short-term treatment of GAD, the use of anxiolytics, especially benzodiazepines, has always been a consideration. However, the risk of abuse and habituation has made most primary care practitioners cautious about prescribing these medications. The nonbenzodiazepine anxiolytic buspirone (BuSpar) may be a conventional alternative lacking the problematic issue of drug dependence and excessive sedation.

▪ Dosage
See Table 5-2.

Botanicals

Kava (Piper methysticum)
In the realm of botanical pharmaceuticals, kava has become known as a botanical option for the treatment of GAD in the United States and Europe. It is derived from the pulverized lateral roots of a subspecies of a pepper plant, *Piper methysticum*, and is indigenous to many Pacific Island cultures. In Europe, kava is recognized by health authorities as a relatively safe remedy for anxiety.[24] Seven small clinical trials evaluated the efficacy of kava in GAD.[25] In all trials, kava was found to be superior to placebo in the symptomatic treatment of GAD.

The constituents considered to be most pharmacologically active are the kava lactones, which have a chemical structure similar to that of myristicin, found in nutmeg.[26] These lactone structures are present in the highest concentration in the lateral roots and are lipophilic. Of the 15 isolated kava lactone structures, 6 are concentrated maximally in the root and vary depending on the variety of *Piper methysticum*.[27] The mechanism of action of kava in GAD has not been completely elucidated, although the action seems similar to that of benzodiazepines. Results of studies in rats and cats are conflicting, however.

Benzodiazepines exert their actions by binding to the gamma-aminobutyric acid (GABA) site and benzodiazepine receptors in the brain; animal studies analyzing kava's anxiolytic action, however, show mixed and minor effects at both sites. Other studies indicate that kava constituents produce anxiolytic effects by altering the limbic system, especially at the amygdala and hippocampus.[28] Other documented uses of kava have been as a muscle relaxant, an anticonvulsant, an anesthetic, and an antiinflammatory agent.

▪ Indication
Mild to moderate GAD.

TABLE 5-2. Supplement and Drug Recommendations for Treatment of Anxiety

DRUG/SUPPLEMENT	INITIAL DOSE (RANGE)	FREQUENCY
Vitamin B complex 100	1 tablet	Daily
Folic acid	400–800 mcg	Daily
Kava	50–70 mg (of kava lactones)	tid
Valerian root	150–300 mg every AM and 300–600 mg at bedtime	
5-Hydroxytryptophan	150–300 mg	Daily
Selective Serotonin Reuptake Inhibitors and Mixed Reuptake Blockers		
Fluoxetine (Prozac)	10–20 mg (10–80)	Daily
Fluvoxamine (Luvox)	50 mg (50–300)	Daily
Paroxetine (Paxil)	10 mg (10–60)	Daily
Sertraline (Zoloft)	50 mg (50–200)	Daily
Escitalopram (Lexapro)	10 mg (10–20 mg)	Daily
Citalopram (Celexa)	20 mg (20–40 mg)	Daily
Others		
Venlafaxine (Effexor)	75 mg (37.5–75 mg)	bid
Nefazodone (Serzone)	200 mg (100–300 mg)	bid
Bupropion (Wellbutrin)	100 mg (50–125 mg)	bid
Azapirones		
Buspirone (BuSpar)	5 mg (15–30 mg)	bid

bid, twice daily; tid, three times daily.

Dosage

Kava is taken for anxiety at a dose of 50 to 70 mg (of the purified extract, kava lactones) three times daily or kava dried root 2 to 4 g boiled as a decoction three times daily.

Precautions

Anecdotal reports have noted excessive sedation when kava is combined with other sedative medications.[29] Extrapyramidal side effects were reported in four patients using two different preparations of kava. Kava thus should be avoided in patients with Parkinson syndrome.[30] The effects diminished once the extract was discontinued. In patients taking high doses from heavy kava consumption, a yellow, ichthyosiform condition of the skin known as kava dermopathy has been observed. This condition is reversible with discontinuation of the kava.[31] The overdose potential appears to be low. In many cases, the rash, ataxia, redness of the eyes, visual accommodation difficulties, and yellowing of the skin reported in the literature from Australia and the Pacific region emerged after ingestion of up to 13 liters per day, equivalent to 300 to 400 g of dried root per week. This amount represents a dose 100 times that of the recommended therapeutic dose.[32]

Caution

Data are insufficient to determine teratogenicity; for this reason, it is wise to avoid use of kava during pregnancy. Kava is present in the milk of lactating mothers; therefore, use is discouraged during breast-feeding.[33] The use of kava should be avoided with other sedative medications.

Kava has been reported to cause idiopathic hepatotoxic hepatitis. To date, all case reports (a total of 31) have been in patients from Europe who used concentrated extracts manufactured in Germany or Switzerland. The exact cause of the effects is under investigation. Kava should not be used in individuals who have liver problems, nor should it be used concomitantly in patients who are taking multiple medications that are metabolized in the liver or in individuals who drink alcohol on a daily basis.[34] Liver tests should be routinely performed in individuals who use kava on a daily basis, and patients should be counseled on the signs and symptoms of hepatotoxicity (jaundice, malaise, and nausea). Furthermore, kava should be discontinued from daily use after approximately 4 months.

Valerian (Valeriana officinalis)

Valerian is another botanical alternative for the treatment of GAD. The clinical efficacy of valerian has been evaluated mostly for treating sleep disturbances; fewer clinical studies assessing its use in anxiety are available. Nevertheless, valerian has been used in Europe for more than a thousand years as a tranquilizer and calmative.[35] The use of valerian in combination with either passionflower (Passiflora incarnata) or St. John's wort (Hypericum perforatum) for anxiety has been studied in small clinical trials. One study evaluated valerian root in combination with passionflower (100 mg of valerian root with 6.5 mg of passionflower extract) compared with chlorpromazine hydrochloride (Thorazine) (40 mg daily) over a period of 16 weeks. In this study, 20 patients were randomly assigned to the two treatment groups after being identified as suffering from irritation, unrest, depression, and insomnia. Electroencephalographic changes in both groups consistent with relaxation were comparable; two psychological scales measuring these qualities demonstrated

scores consistent with reduction in anxiety.[36] Another study evaluated anxiety in 100 anxious persons receiving either a combination of 50 mg of valerian root plus 90 to 100 mg of standardized St. John's wort for 14 days or 2 mg of diazepam (Valium) twice daily in the first week and up to 2 capsules twice daily in the second week. The results showed reduction of anxiety in the phytomedicine treatment group to levels in healthy persons. Patients in the diazepam treatment group still had significant anxiety scores.[37]

Indication

Mild to moderate anxiety.

Dosage

For adults with anxiety, a dose of 150 to 300 mg in the morning and another dose of 300 to 600 mg in the evening, using a standardized product containing 0.1% valerenic acid, can be taken. Combinations with lemon balm and hops (Humulus lupulus) may be considered. These additions are based on herbal tradition and empirical medicine; no clinical trials demonstrating efficacy are available.[38,39]

> Contrary to common belief, valerian is not suitable for acute treatment of anxiety or insomnia. A beneficial effect may take several weeks.

Precautions

Valerian root is not suitable for the treatment of acute insomnia or nervousness because it takes several weeks before a beneficial effect is obtained. An alternative that gives a more rapid response should be taken when valerian root is initiated.[13] Products with Indian and Mexican valerian should be avoided owing to the mutagenic risk associated with their high concentrations of valpotriates and baldrinals (up to 8%).[38] Adverse effects are rare with products that do not contain valpotriates. Occasional reports have noted headache and gastrointestinal complaints.

Mind-Body Therapy

Psychotherapy

Psychotherapy has been shown to be effective as a therapeutic option in the treatment of GAD with or without medical intervention. Two clinically proven forms are used frequently: behavioral therapy and cognitive-behavioral therapy. Behavioral therapy focuses on changing the specific unwanted actions by using several techniques to stop the undesired behavior. In addition, both behavioral therapy and cognitive-behavioral therapy help patients to understand and change their thinking patterns so that they can react differently to their anxiety.

Relaxation Techniques

Relaxation training, stress reduction techniques, and breath work are of proven benefit. In fact, imaginal exposure is used as a tactic for repeated exposure to induce anxiety (in a gradual way). Patients learn through repeated exposure to cope with and manage their anxiety, rather than to eliminate it. Relaxation training paired with this interceptive therapy is useful. I often encounter patients who admit to their anxiety and are willing to confront and learn to cope with it but lack the ability to relax completely. Depending on their preferences, I help them choose a relaxation technique that reinforces a sense of calm. Therapies that can be used for this purpose are massage, sound therapy, aromatherapy, guided interactive imagery, and hypnosis. Because many patients have somatic sensations that accompany their anxiety, a complementary therapy that imparts a "remembrance" of a deeply relaxed state (see Chapter 93, Relaxation Techniques) should also be reinforced on a more somatic-kinesthetic level.

Therapies to Consider

Traditional medical systems such as acupuncture and Ayurvedic medicine can provide other options for the treatment of anxiety.[41,42] Several small trials assessing relaxation in an anxiety state showed reduction of anxiety in a psychologically normal patient population through the use of auricular acupuncture.[41-43] Although the mechanisms are not well elucidated, these systems may somehow interface favorably to balance the autonomic nervous system.

PREVENTION PRESCRIPTION

- Maximize nutrition to include foods rich in omega 3-fatty acids, B vitamins, and folic acid.
- Follow a regular exercise routine (even walking and tracking use with a pedometer).
- Institute a daily mind-body exercise program to enhance the relaxation response.
- Keep a journal; take a "feeling inventory," and enhance self-awareness.
- Limit your use of personal digital assistants, cellphones, and BlackBerry devices. Do not access these devices during meals and special times with family and friends. Turn to "off" at 10 AM and "on" at 6 to 7 AM, and do not recharge these devices right next to your bed!
- Get enough sleep to feel refreshed.

THERAPEUTIC REVIEW

The following four steps are recommended for initial management of patients with generalized anxiety disorder (GAD).

1. Remove exacerbating factors. Review current medications and supplements that could contribute to anxiety (especially botanical supplements such as ephedra and over-the-counter preparations that are stimulants). Supplements that are unnecessary should be discontinued.

2. Screen for diseases that mimic anxiety. Screening should be performed for underlying medical conditions that produce anxiety, for instance, hyperthyroidism or a withdrawal syndrome.

3. Improve nutrition. Nutritional support such as with omega-3 fatty acid supplementation (two to three servings of cold water fish per week, or flaxseed oil 2 tablespoons a day or 1000 mg of flaxseed oil in a capsule) is recommended. In addition, caffeine and alcohol consumption should be avoided. $A\textcircled{\uparrow}_1$

4. Institute physical activity. Physical activity (aerobic or anaerobic) at least 5 days out of 7 should be encouraged. To ensure long-term compliance, an activity that is enjoyable to the patient is important. Furthermore, adherence to a regular exercise regimen and setting realistic short-term goals may need emphasis. Increases in exercise level and intensity should be gradual (see Chapter 88, Writing an Exercise Prescription). $A\textcircled{\uparrow}_1$

■ Supplements

- Vitamin B_6 included in a vitamin B 100 complex preparation with the addition of folic acid (400 mcg daily) should be considered. $B\textcircled{\nearrow}_1$

- Vitamin B_6  $A\textcircled{\nearrow}_2$
- Folic acid $B\textcircled{\rightarrow}_2$

- 5-Hydroxytryptophan (150 to 300 mg daily) could be considered as a serotonin boosting alternative, but close monitoring should be undertaken to screen for eosinophilia myalgia syndrome. $C\textcircled{\downarrow}_3$

■ Botanicals

- Kava, 50 to 70 mg three times a day (of the purified kava lactones), can be given. Choose a standardized product with either a 30% or a 50% to 55% kava lactone concentration.

- If no improvement is observed over 4 to 6 weeks, consider valerian or a valerian combination or a pharmaceutical anxiolytic (use for at least 6 weeks before evaluating efficacy). $B\textcircled{\rightarrow}_2$

- Concurrent psychotherapy is highly recommended if this approach is acceptable to the patient.

■ Mind-Body Therapy

- Psychotherapy: The combination of psychotherapy in conjunction with supplements, botanicals, or a pharmaceutical anxiolytic or antidepressant is highly recommended, especially in GAD. An integrative therapeutic approach is associated with higher success rates in cases of severe anxiety. Often, psychotherapy can provide the patient with skills for coping with anxiety, as opposed to extinguishing the symptoms. Primary care physicians can monitor lifestyle modification, dietary and supplement interventions, and drug therapy. However, referral to a psychotherapist is advised. $A\textcircled{\uparrow}_1$

- Relaxation training: Educate the patient in relaxation techniques that will empower him or her to bring anxiety symptoms under control when needed.

Continued

Traditional Medical Systems

- Use of traditional medicine systems (TMSs) is problematic in that TMSs have historically been used to provide primary care for a variety of medical ailments (including anxiety). As an allopathic physician, I generally designate the use of TMSs as an adjunctive modality. However, for those patients who have strong feelings about the use of singular botanical preparations (mostly as being insufficient for treatment) or whose medical conditions appear mild, I am more than willing to be a medical partner and consider the use of a TMS (e.g., Chinese medicine or Ayurvedic medicine) as a primary therapeutic option, as long as the well-being of the patient is not in jeopardy.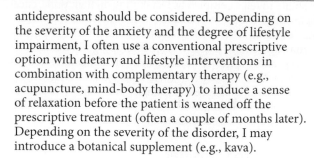

Pharmaceuticals

- If no improvement is obtained with lifestyle measures, dietary measures, and supplement interventions in conjunction with botanical supplements, use of a pharmaceutical anxiolytic or antidepressant should be considered. Depending on the severity of the anxiety and the degree of lifestyle impairment, I often use a conventional prescriptive option with dietary and lifestyle interventions in combination with complementary therapy (e.g., acupuncture, mind-body therapy) to induce a sense of relaxation before the patient is weaned off the prescriptive treatment (often a couple of months later). Depending on the severity of the disorder, I may introduce a botanical supplement (e.g., kava).

- Obviously, different clinical responses will be obtained with the various anxiolytics (and selective serotonin reuptake inhibitors). Optimal management may require a change of medication, depending on the patient's symptoms. For long-term therapy, I refrain from the use of benzodiazepines because tolerance can be problematic.

- Consider referral to a psychiatrist if the patient remains refractory to treatment, is suicidal or psychotic, or requires psychiatric stabilization in a hospital unit.

KEY WEB RESOURCES

Benson-Henry Institute for Mind Body Medicine. http://www.massgeneral.org/bhi/.

The Institute was founded in 1988 as a nonprofit scientific and educational organization building on the work of Herbert Benson at Harvard Medical School on the relaxation response. The Web site covers research, education, training programs, clinical programs, books, videotapes, audiotapes, and more.

Mind and Life Institute. www.MindandLife.com.

The Institute is dedicated to creating dialogue and collaboration in research at the highest possible level between modern science and the great living contemplative traditions, especially Buddhism. The Web site describes conferences and events, research initiatives, publications, and the work of the Dalai Lama.

Mindfulness-Based Stress Reduction (MBSR). www.umassmed.edu/cfm.

The Center for Mindfulness at the University of Massachusetts sponsors the MBSR program. The Web site covers clinical care, education, research, training, a bibliography, and more.

Continuum Center for Health and Healing: Preparing for Surgery/Learning Mind/Body Techniques. http://www.preparingforyoursurgery.org/.

This free online course teaches stress management techniques that are easy to learn and simple to practice. These techniques can help manage fear, worry, and anxiety and can help promote faster healing with less pain or discomfort. These same relaxation practices can be used whenever one feels stress building up in daily life.

Shambhala. www.shambhala.org/.

This worldwide network of meditation centers was founded by Chogyam Trungpa Rinpoche, a Tibetan Buddhist master of the Shambhala and Buddhist teachings. The Web site is a guide to Shambhala centers internationally and their activities, books and recordings, and essays on mindfulness meditation.

Transcendental Meditation (TM) Program. www.tm.org/.

The official U.S. Web site of the TM program, the Web site covers a description of the program, the scientific research on TM, news articles and books, places to study, and an explanation of the uses of TM to enhance function and treat a variety of conditions.

Wildmind Buddhist Meditation. www.wildmind.org/.

This Web site provides a wealth of information on Buddhist practices, including guided meditations in RealAudio format and online meditation courses led by an experienced instructor.

References

References are available online at expertconsult.com.

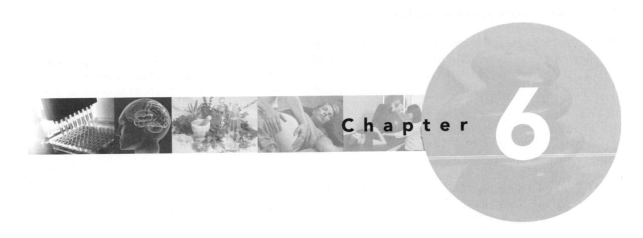

Attention Deficit Hyperactivity Disorder

Kathi J. Kemper, MD, MPH

Pathophysiology, Definitions, and Epidemiology

In the 1930s, hyperactivity, impulsivity, learning disability, and distractibility in childhood were described as "minimal brain damage" or "minimal brain dysfunction." This label was modified in the 1950s to "hyperactive child syndrome" and in 1968 to "hyperkinetic reaction of childhood." More recently, investigators have recognized that for nearly 66% of patients, the core symptoms of impulsivity and distractibility characteristic of attention deficit hyperactivity disorder (ADHD) persist into adulthood.

One of the most commonly diagnosed and costly mental health problems in the United States, ADHD is diagnosed in 3% to 10% (depending on age and gender) of school-age children. It is diagnosed more commonly in boys than girls (3:1 ratio); the peak age of diagnosis is between 8 and 10 years old. The drugs used to treat ADHD, such as methylphenidate (Concerta), atomoxetine (Strattera), and a combination of amphetamine and dextroamphetamine (Adderall), are three of the top five (ranked by spending) for children younger than 18 years in the United States. The prevalence of ADHD in adults is estimated at 2.5%. Unlike an acute bacterial infection, ADHD is a chronic condition requiring ongoing management.

The classic image is that of an energetic boy who talks a lot, interrupts others, acts as if driven by a motor, fidgets and squirms, has a messy room, acts impulsively, has trouble following rules, and often breaks or loses things; he is often admonished to sit still, pay attention, and clean up his room. The quiet girl who daydreams and is inattentive in class has a second classic type of ADHD (ADHD without hyperactivity). The diagnosis is based on consistent perceptions of a particular pattern of behavior:

- Early onset (by age 7 years)

- Persistence (at least 6 months)

- Pervasive (present in at least two settings) pattern of distractibility and impulsivity (at least 6 symptoms of each), with or without hyperactivity, that

  - Disrupts age-appropriate academic, social, or occupational functioning

Knowledge of normal child development is essential to making the diagnosis because normal behavior for a 2 year old includes impulsivity and a short attention span that would be abnormal in an 8 year old.

Most clinicians use behavioral checklists such as the Vanderbilt Parent and Teacher Rating Scales to make the diagnosis and monitor progress. No laboratory or imaging study exists to confirm the diagnosis, although clinicians often use laboratory or neuropsychological tests to rule out contributory problems such as hearing or vision problems, anemia, hypothyroidism, absence seizures, reading or math learning disabilities, and short-term memory impairment.

Common comorbidities include oppositional defiant disorder and conduct disorders (30% to 50%), mood or anxiety disorders (15% to 30%), learning disabilities (20% to 25%), sleep problems, and tic disorders such as Tourette syndrome.[1,2] Strengths often include creativity, imagination, sociability, and flexible attention, interest in the environment, energy, vitality, enthusiasm, adaptability, confidence, exuberance, spontaneity, and desire to please others.[3] A strengths-based, specific behavioral goal-oriented approach to management is popular.

Consequences of persistent, poorly treated ADHD include the following: an increased risk of injuries; increased cost of medical care; an increased risk of addiction to tobacco, alcohol, and illicit drugs; an increased risk of incarceration; and a diminished ability to maintain employment or relationships.[4,5]

Although a single pathophysiologic pathway has not been determined, genetic associations, multiple environmental agents, and psychosocial characteristics (e.g., poverty, stressed parents and households, families with mental health or substance abuse challenges, difficulty setting limits, disorganized routines) affect the risk of developing or being labeled with ADHD. Genes showing significant associations with ADHD include *DRD4, DRD5, DAT, DBH, 5-HTT, HTR1B,* and *SNAP-25*. Other risk factors for ADHD include male gender, maternal tobacco use during pregnancy or early childhood, intrauterine growth retardation, excessive exposure to television, and exposure to certain pesticides.[6–8] Of the 358 industrial chemicals, pesticides, and pollutants found in studies of the umbilical cord blood of infants in the United States, more than 200 are known to be toxic to the brain. Multiple brain regions, including the prefrontal cortex, frontostriatal networks, and cerebellum, and neurotransmitters, particularly dopamine and norepinephrine, appear to be involved in ADHD deficits.[9–12]

In summary, ADHD is a common clinical diagnosis in both children and increasingly in adults, and it has multiple genetic, environmental, and psychosocial contributions to dysfunction from several neurotransmitter systems and regions of the brain.

Integrative Therapy

Integrative therapy focuses on the goals of the patient and family in the context of values, culture, and community. Goals for treating ADHD may include improvements in the ability to focus or pay attention and in following directions, greater persistence in the presence of difficulty, improved ability to delay gratification, more consistent anticipation of consequences, improving grades, better organizational skills, better short-term memory, greater neatness, less procrastination, improved social relationships, greater obedience, better sleep, and fewer injuries, among other goals. Each of these goals requires a complex interaction of specific skills and resources.

Requirements for learning to manage attention are as follows:
1. Motivation (it is easier to pay attention to things that interest us)
2. The ability to *perceive* sensory data such as sounds (as words) and symbols (written words or gestures) accurately and to *process* these data into meaningful information
3. *Tuning out of irrelevant* sensory information (e.g., ignoring music or conversation in the background while reading a book) while being *flexibly responsive* to changing priorities (a fire by a smoke detector, a cry for help, or ringing telephone)
4. *Monitoring* of one's own attention ("Oh, was I listening to the music instead of focusing on the words? How many times have I read this sentence?")
5. *Redirection* of attention (let us get back to the book.)

In addition to managing attention, learning to *follow directions* also requires certain abilities:
1. Understanding the meaning of the request
2. Recognizing the tools and skills needed to complete it
3. Assessing the availability of these tools and skills
4. Using available resources and asking for help when needed
5. Monitoring performance

The choice of specific therapies depends to some extent on an individual's specific goals, but general mental and physical health can always be supported by appropriate attention to the fundamentals: *healthy habits in a healthy habitat.* Four fundamental healthy habits have been identified: exercise, balanced with optimal sleep; nutrition and avoidance of toxins in the diet; management of stress and emotions; and establishment of healthy communication and supportive, rewarding social relationships. A healthy habitat includes the physical and psychosocial environment (Fig. 6-1).

Exercise

A minimum of 30 to 60 minutes of aerobic activity daily is necessary for general physical and mental health.[13] A 2009 study in children with developmental coordination disorder found that regularly playing table tennis was helpful both for their coordination and for their ability to sustain focus.[14] Exercise outdoors in nature is even better than exercise in a gym or urban setting.[15] Exercise increases brain-derived neurotrophic factor levels and enhances neurogenesis, thus promoting overall cognitive function, including attention and memory, which are both required for academic achievement.[16,17] Cerebellar dysfunction has been implicated in ADHD.[18] This has led to growing interest in activities that build balance and coordination such as yoga, juggling, cross-midline exercises, the Interactive Metronome method, and Brain Gym. Quiet, mindful exercises such as tai chi and yoga encourage focus on the body as it moves and can thereby improve the ability to focus and to be more deliberate and less impulsive.[19] Martial arts training promotes discipline. Dr. David Katz of Yale University in Connecticut recommends the ABCs—Activity Bursts in the Classroom (or Corporation).[20]

> A minimum of 30 to 60 minutes of aerobic activity daily is needed for mental and physical health.

Safety

Impulsive, distracted people are prone to injuries. Encourage appropriate use of bike and ski helmets, as well as protective padding for skateboarding. Encourage enrollment in organized sports or lessons with small classes with close supervision and low student-teacher ratios (karate, tae kwon do, tai chi, or yoga) to help develop better body awareness and self-discipline. Counsel the patient to avoid overuse injuries.

Sleep

Sleep deprivation impairs focus, organizational skills, diligence, and self-discipline during boring tasks. Inadequate sleep and poor sleep quality impair attention and judgment, increase fidgeting, lower performance, and lead to more mistakes, automobile collisions, and injuries. Although many patients with ADHD report sleep problems even before starting treatment, stimulant medications can contribute to insomnia. Improved sleep may lead to improvements in daytime focus on behavior. Clinicians should inquire routinely about sleep and recommend sleep hygiene measures

FIGURE 6-1
Healthy habits in a healthy habitat.

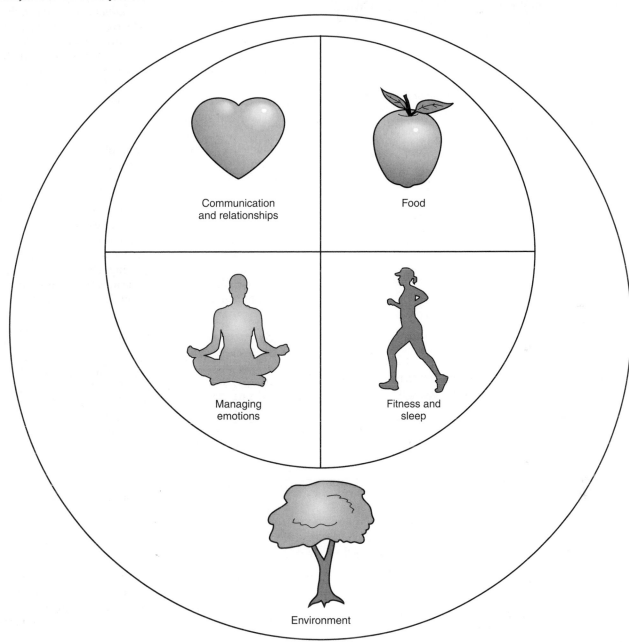

Nutrition

Although its weight is less than 5% of the body's total, the brain uses approximately 20% of the body's energy supply. To function well, it needs a steady supply of high-quality fuel (Table 6-1). This means regular meals supplying optimal amounts of essential fatty acids for cell membranes, of the amino acids used to make neurotransmitters, and of the vitamin and mineral cofactors necessary for their production and metabolism, as well as a steady supply of glucose for energy needs. Optimally, these nutrients are ingested in the diet, but for those who do not eat well, supplements may be useful.

Omega-3 Fatty Acids

Low levels of omega-3 fatty acids are linked to ADHD and behavioral problems in both adults and children.[21,22] Supplementing with fish oils (which are rich sources of omega-3 fatty acids) can alleviate ADHD symptoms and decrease depression, anger, anxiety, impulsivity, and aggression; it can also improve academic achievement.[23–29] Although flaxseed, walnuts, and green leafy vegetables contain the omega-3 fatty acid

(e.g., cool, quiet, dark room; comfortable bedding; avoidance of television in the bedroom or exercise late in the day; routine bedtime) to promote optimal sleep.

TABLE 6-1. Dietary Essentials for Optimal Attention

DIETARY ESSENTIALS	FOODS SOURCES
Amino acids	Soy, tofu, beans, lentils Seeds and nuts Milk, cheese, eggs Fish, fowl, meat
Essential fatty acids (omega-3 fatty acids: EPA, DHA and linolenic acid)	Fish (tuna, salmon, sardines, and mackerel) Flax seeds, walnuts Dark green leafy vegetables Animals that have eaten omega-3–rich diets (e.g., eggs from chickens fed flaxseed; pasture-raised and grass finished beef; lamb; bison; wild game)
B vitamins, including folate and B_{12}	Beans, lentils, nuts and seeds Leafy green vegetables, asparagus Oranges and other citrus fruits and juices Whole grains Yeast (e.g., brewer's), dairy, eggs, meat, poultry, fish and shellfish
Minerals: iron, magnesium, zinc	Peas, beans, lentils, peanuts, peanut butter Leafy green vegetables: spinach, avocado Raisins Whole grains, brown rice, wheat bran and germ Nuts: almonds, cashews Dairy, eggs Meat, fish, poultry, oysters

DHA, docosahexaenoic acid; EPA, eicosapentaenoic acid.

linolenic acid, humans convert only 5% to 10% of linolenic acid to the useful *eicosapentaenoic acid* (EPA) and *docosahexaenoic acid* (DHA). Encourage patients either to eat sardines, salmon, or mackerel twice weekly or consume 1 to 2 tablespoons of flaxseeds daily or to consider a supplement containing between 500 and 2000 mg of combined EPA and DHA.

Amino Acids

Two small studies suggested that *carnitine* supplements can help improve attention and behavior in children and adults with ADHD, particularly the inattentive type.[30,31] Additional studies are desirable to determine optimal dosing, frequency, and duration, particularly for patients with varying intake of foods rich in amino acids.

Minerals

Iron deficiency interferes with memory, concentration, behavior, and both physical and mental performance, and correcting deficiencies (indicated by low ferritin levels) can improve attention and restlessness.[32-36] *Magnesium* supplements have helped children with ADHD who are excitable, easily stressed, or worriers, as well as those who also suffer from constipation.[37] *Zinc* supplements can improve behavior for those who are deficient in zinc.[38,39] The best dietary sources of essential minerals are plants and animals raised on mineral-rich soils.

Vitamins

The B vitamins serve as essential cofactors in the production of neurotransmitters. Many children who avoid leafy green vegetables consume insufficient amounts of folate. Those who are strict vegans may benefit from vitamin B_{12} supplements. For picky eaters or those who eat poor-quality diets, multivitamin and mineral supplementation may be helpful, but megadoses are not useful and may have side effects.[40]

Water

Dehydration can impair attention and mood.[41] In a small study of first graders, ingestion of some water before taking a test led to better attention and greater happiness.[42]

Sugar

At least a dozen double-blind studies have shown that sugar does not cause hyperactivity. However, eating simple sugars can cause blood sugar swings that impair mental and emotional stability. It is preferable to consume calories from complex carbohydrates such as whole grains rather than simple sugars.[43] Furthermore, many sweet processed food products also contain artificial colors and preservatives that can contribute to behavior problems.

Feingold Diet, Artificial Colors, Flavors, and Preservatives

The Feingold diet does not ban sugar, but it does eliminate salicylates (at least initially; it slowly reintroduces fruits containing them), several synthetic food additives, and certain synthetic sweeteners:

- Artificial colors (petroleum-based certified FD&C and D&C colors)
- Artificial flavors
- BHA, BHT, TBHQ (preservatives)
- The artificial sweeteners Aspartame (now called Truvia), Neotame, and Alitame

Artificial food colors significantly worsen hyperactivity for many people.[44] The Center for Science in the Public Interest (CSPI) has called on the U.S. Food and Drug Administration (FDA) to ban dyes linked to hyperactivity and behavior problems. The colorings the CSPI would like to see banned are as follows:

- Blues 1 and 2
- Green 3
- Orange 8
- Reds 3 and 40
- Yellows 5 and 6

In studies of children with ADHD who received the Feingold diet, 73% had improved behavior.[45,46] Studies involving more than 1800 children showed significant improvements in the children's hyperactive behavior on a diet free of benzoate preservatives and artificial colors and flavors.[47,48] Some families find whole foods diets free of artificial colors, flavors, and preservatives difficult to follow. When families focus on healthy foods, use supplements wisely, and avoid exposure to artificial ingredients and environmental toxins, however, they often see remarkable improvements in mood, attention, and behavior. Some patients have been able to reduce their reliance on stimulant medications.

Coffee and Other Caffeine-Containing Foods

Caffeine improves attention better than placebos, but it is not as potent as prescription medications.[49–52] Some families find caffeine a useful substitute for stimulant medications. In addition to caffeine, green tea also contains the amino acid theanine, which leads to a feeling of calm that can counteract the jitteriness some people experience with coffee.[53] Coffee and tea contain variable amounts of caffeine, depending on growing conditions and preparation techniques. Side effects include insomnia, jitteriness, anxiety, palpitations, panic attacks, and dehydration. Coffee can be addictive; withdrawal symptoms include headaches and feeling irritable, sleepy, depressed, anxious, or fatigued. Withdrawal symptoms can occur with as little as 1 to 2 cups daily. Caffeinated sodas or energy drinks often contain artificial flavors, colors, and preservatives and are not as good a choice as coffee or tea. Caffeine should not be used as a substitute for regularly getting a good night's sleep.

Food Sensitivities

Approximately 6% to 10% of children have allergies or sensitivities to foods. In addition to classic allergies, many people are lactose intolerant, and approximately 1% of people are sensitive to gluten. The most common food sensitivities are to wheat, corn, soy, milk products, eggs, tree nuts, shellfish, citrus, and peanuts. If sensitivities are suspected, encourage families to keep a careful *food diary*. In some cases, blood testing, skin testing, biopsies (for gluten sensitivity), and elimination diets may be useful. However, because many reactions are not true allergies, allergy test results may be negative even if a food is problematic. Some studies support the use of few foods or oligoantigenic diets to improve symptoms in more than half the children with ADHD.[54] An elimination diet typically removes all the foods and artificial ingredients that commonly cause problems for at least 2 weeks and then slowly reintroduces one at a time every 3 to 4 days. Recommend nutritional counseling to avoid deficiencies if families pursue this option.

Organic or Not?

Produce with the highest levels of pesticide contamination includes apples, bell peppers, celery, cherries, imported grapes, nectarines and peaches, pears, potatoes, raspberries, spinach, and strawberries. Organic crops contain lower levels of pesticides and other agrochemical residues than do nonorganic crops.[55] Children who eat organic produce have lower levels of these toxic pesticide chemicals than do children who eat nonorganic produce.[56] As historical farming practices waned, mineral levels in fruits, vegetables, meat, and milk fell up to 76% between 1940 and 1991.[57] Organic crops contain significantly more minerals and antioxidants than do crops raised with petroleum-derived (so-called conventional) fertilizers.[58,59] Milk from cows that graze on grass (botanically diverse pasture) has higher levels of the essential omega-3 fatty acids than does milk from cows that eat grain such as corn.[60,61]

TABLE 6-2. Stress Management Strategies

Common Sense

Gratitude. Develop the habit of listing three things you are grateful for before meals or bed.

Count on it. Count to 10 before reacting.

Identify your early warning signs: tight muscles, faster breathing, red face, clenched hands, and tight jaw.

Know yourself. Plan activities based on whether you are a morning person or a night owl and a visual or auditory learner.

Plan ahead. Being organized and consistent reduces stress.

Reflect. Develop the daily practice of reflecting on what went well and what could be improved.

Rehearse. Anticipate difficult situations and rehearse or role play before the situation.

Formal Practices, Often Learned With a Teacher or Trainer

Sitting meditation (concentration or mindfulness types)

Moving meditation (e.g., yoga, tai chi, qi gong)

Other Practices, Often Best Learned with Professional Coaching

Biofeedback

Autogenic training, guided imagery

Managing Stress and Emotional Self-Regulation

Learning to manage stress is an important lifelong skill. Major pediatric stressors include divorce, moving, parental loss of a job or loss of a house, serious health challenges, war, neighborhood violence, parental addiction or depression, and loss of a loved one. Stress interferes with concentration and self-discipline. Numerous successful strategies for managing stress are available. Some are common sense, and some require training and practice or professional counseling.

Common Sense Stress Management

Common sense strategies include preventive strategies such as practicing gratitude (counting blessings) and in-the-moment strategies such as taking a deep breath and counting to 10. Learning to understand one's own triggers, strengths, and weaknesses is also helpful to plan proactively how to manage stressful situations such as tests, running late, and losing something. Night owls may want to save perplexing problems until later in the day, whereas morning people (larks) may want to get up earlier to tackle challenging tasks. Reflecting on the day's events after the heat of the moment can also identify unskillful patterns and create opportunities for meeting challenges. Similarly, rehearsing an anticipated event can help decrease the stress of the actual experience (Table 6-2).

Meditation

Meditation improves attention, creativity, and mental clarity and reduces errors, aggressiveness, anxiety, and depression, particularly in the presence of stress or distractions. Meditation leads to calm coherence with more focused electroencephalographic (EEG) patterns.[62,63] Regular meditation practice changes cortical blood flow and increases the size of areas dealing with attention, focus, planning, emotional self-regulation, and mood.[64-69]

Just as many kinds of sports improve physical fitness, many kinds of meditation improve attention and reduce stress reactivity. Just as some kinds of sports involve rackets, bats, or balls, meditation can be done with eyes open or closed, while sitting still or moving, in silence or not, while visualizing or not, and alone or in groups. *Concentration-based* meditation practices involve focusing on a word, sound, object, idea, emotion (e.g., gratitude) or movement; when other thoughts, sensations, or emotions arise, they are gently placed aside, and the mind returns to its object of concentration. Students who practiced concentration-types of meditation had fewer problems with absenteeism and suspension for behavioral problems,[70] less distractibility and better creativity,[71] and better cognitive function and grades.[72,73] *Mindfulness* meditation is the moment-to-moment practice of nonjudgmental awareness of sensations, thoughts, emotions, and experiences; when the mind wanders to past or future concerns, it is also gently returned to the present. Studies in school settings show that mindfulness-based meditation training can improve attention, emotions, and behavior; students have fewer fights and better grades.[74-80] For hyperactive patients, moving meditation such as yoga, tai chi, or qi gong may be a better fit than sitting meditation.[19,81] Regular practice reduces test anxiety and improves academic achievement. Those who practice the most reap the greatest rewards.[82]

The need for formal training and the intensity, duration, and frequency of practice vary. Some clinicians undertake specific training and certification to provide specific kinds of meditation training (e.g., mindfulness-based stress reduction, mindfulness-based cognitive-behavioral therapy, or dialectical behavior therapy). Nevertheless, because of the absence of consistent state or national certification for mind-body training, it is prudent to ask about a provider's training and experience. As with other clinicians, look for those who are welcoming, warm, and empathetic and who show genuine interest in people, not just in their favorite techniques. The most effective teachers and trainers offer steadfast acceptance and positive regard. They create an atmosphere of safety and trust while fostering independence and acknowledging students' strengths and capacities.

Just as national guidelines recommend 30 to 60 minutes daily of physical exercise to maintain physical health, recommendations for meditation practice typically range from just a few minutes for young children to 10 minutes twice daily for school-age children to 40 to 60 minutes daily for older adolescents and adults.

Biofeedback
EEG biofeedback (neurofeedback) can significantly improve behavior, attention, and intelligence quotient (IQ) scores.[83-91] In fact, neurofeedback is as effective as standard therapies, even for children with Asperger's syndrome and those with mental retardation.[88,92-96] Most studies provided at least 20 EEG biofeedback training sessions with a professional trainer. EEG biofeedback training develops a skill. Unlike medications, whose effects stop when the pills stop, EEG biofeedback training benefits can be expected to persist if the skill is mastered and practice continues.

Typical costs range from $75 to $200 per session; insurance reimbursement for neurofeedback varies. Most professionals who offer EEG biofeedback are psychologists, however, and as such their professional services may be covered by insurance. Patients should check their insurance policies and ask clinicians to assess their unique situations.

> Electroencephalographic frequencies correlated with levels of alertness and processing:
> - Beta wave (>14 Hz) = Active processing
> - Alpha wave (8–13 Hz) = Active alert
> - Theta wave (4–7 Hz) = Transitional state (associated with meditation, relaxation, imagery, and hypnosis

Professional Counseling
Large studies suggest that, at least in the short term, the most effective treatment for children with ADHD is an integrated strategy including both behavioral therapy and stimulant medication.[97] Cognitive-behavioral therapy can be particularly useful in helping patients learn to question assumptions and thoughts underlying negative emotions. Given all the negative feedback patients with ADHD have received about their behavior and academic performance, it is not surprising that they have internalized many of these messages. Negative self-labels are sometimes projected onto others, thus leading to blaming and oppositional behavior. By recognizing, questioning, and transforming negative self-talk, one can build confidence and problem-solving capacities. Professional counseling may be particularly helpful for those who have coexisting conditions such as anxiety or depression or for families whose parents were not fortunate enough to have good role models for effective parenting skills. Psychological or neuropsychological testing and advice help identify and treat children with specific learning disabilities. For adults with ADHD, "metacognitive" therapy can help teach skills such as time management, organization, and planning. This training promotes significant improvements in daily living skills and job performance.[98]

Professional counseling takes a little longer to show a benefit than does medication. However, the skills learned in behavioral therapy can persist for years after the therapy officially ends.[99] Although it may appear to be more expensive in the short term, behavioral therapy can be an excellent cost-effective investment.

Social Relationships
Social support is useful for most families managing chronic conditions such as ADHD. National support groups usually have local chapters with ongoing support and local resources:

All Kinds of Minds (AKOM) is a nonprofit organization that aims to help individuals with learning differences achieve success in school and in life. Their Internet site has toolkits and other resources for parents, schools, and health professionals.

Children and Adults with Attention Deficit Hyperactivity Disorder (CHADD) is a national nonprofit organization that works to improve the lives of those affected by ADHD through education, advocacy, and support. Their home page offers links to local chapters, as well as international activities.

The National Federation of Families of Children's Mental Health is a parent-run organization to support families caring for children and youth with emotional, behavioral, or mental disorders. The Web site provides links to publications, research, and state chapters.

Learning Disabilities Association of America (LDA) was founded in 1963 to support people with learning disabilities and their families, teachers, and health professionals. It sponsors an annual conference. The Web site provides resources, legislative updates, and links to state chapters.

Mental Health America, formerly known as the National Mental Health Association, is the national's oldest and largest community-based network dedicated to promoting mental health, preventing mental disorders, and achieving victory over mental illness through advocacy, education, research, and delivering programs and services. The organization strongly supported the Mental Health Parity law that became effective in 2010 and continues to provide updates, action alerts, and advocacy to ensure effective implementation. The Web site provides links to local affiliates and a wealth of advocacy information.

Alliance With Schools

Clinicians should help teachers and school administrators recognize the child's unique gifts and challenges. Families should schedule regular meetings with their child's teachers to monitor progress and advocate for seating arrangements that put the child near the front of the classroom. Encourage families to advocate for the child to receive the public services to which he or she is legally entitled. According to the 1999 addendum to the U.S. Individuals with Disability Education Act (IDEA), children and youth whose disabilities adversely affect their educational performance should receive special services or accommodations that address their problem (e.g., ADHD) and its effects. Section 504 of the U.S. Vocational Rehabilitation Act prohibits discrimination against any person with a disability. Under Section 504, students may receive services such as a smaller class size, tutoring, modification of homework assignments, help with organizing, and other assistance.

If the patient has not received sufficient services or accommodation within 6 months of asking the teacher or principal, write to the school district's director or chairperson for special educational services. The letter should specifically request an evaluation for specific learning disabilities and a functional assessment to determine how the disabilities are affecting the child's classroom performance. These evaluations are required to develop an Individual Educational Plan (IEP) or a 504 Accommodation Plan. Middle school and high school students diagnosed with ADHD are also entitled to these evaluations and, if appropriate, an IEP or accommodation plans. With an IEP, the child may qualify for extra help, special classes, extra time for tests or projects, an extra set of books for home study, permission to take notes on a computer keyboard rather than by hand, extra breaks in the day, fewer classes, and other accommodations. Support teachers and administrators who offer creative, effective strategies to promote children's strengths.

Encourage parents to try other activities that explore the child's interests, talents, and possible life-long passions or vocations. When choosing activities, consider the adult-child ratio. Music, art, tutoring, and individual language lessons may offer more individual attention than soccer leagues. Look for consistency. A class that meets every Tuesday is easier to schedule and attend than a sports team that has inconsistent practice and game schedules requiring frequent changes in the family driving routine.

Environment

Increasing time in nature may help soothe irritable children and adults, allow room for exploratory and creative play, and build on innate strengths and skills. Encourage families to reduce electronic screen time to less than 2 hours daily. Ask, advise, and assist families in reducing or eliminating exposure to tobacco smoke and adults who model using alcohol and illicit drugs as primary stress management strategies. Remind families to use proper safety equipment (e.g., seat belts, helmets). Reduce the use of pesticides at home and in schools. Consider using music as a way of reinforcing positive behavior, a learning strategy (songs with rhymes to assist in memorization), and a way to influence the environment subtly to cue wake up times and bedtimes. Encourage families to use calendars and posted schedules to promote structure and predictability for the day, week, and month (Table 6-3).

Additional Therapies

Botanicals and Other Dietary Supplements

Melatonin

Melatonin does not improve daytime symptoms of ADHD, but it can help improve sleep, particularly for shift workers and those with delayed sleep phase syndrome.[100-103] The typical adult dose of melatonin is 0.3 to 5 mg 1 hour before the desired bedtime. Melatonin is not a substitute for a healthy sleep routine. One study followed children with ADHD who had started taking melatonin as part of a clinical trial on sleep; nearly 4 years later, more than two thirds of these children were still using melatonin because it was helpful and had no serious side effects.[104]

TABLE 6-3. Environmental Dos and Don'ts

Do

Spend more time in nature.

Be more mindful of use of music to calm, focus, and reinforce behavior.

Use clocks, calendars, and lists to organize time.

Post schedules, chore charts, and other tools to organize activities and expectations.

Use proper safety equipment (e.g., bike helmets and seat belts).

Don't

Spend more than 2 hours in front of electronic devices daily.

Spend time around tobacco smoke.

Model the use of alcohol or drugs as skillful stress management strategies.

Calming Herbs

Historically, some herbs have been used to promote calm and decrease agitation, but none can replace a healthy lifestyle. Calming herbs, such as chamomile, hops, kava, lavender, lemon balm, passionflower, and valerian, may promote sleep, but they are not usually helpful for calming daytime hyperactivity, inattentiveness, or impulsivity.[105]

Other Herbs

Coffee and tea containing caffeine are natural stimulants. Green tea also contains theanine, which can be calming, thereby offsetting some of the unpleasant side effects of caffeine.[106-108] Caffeine helps enhance attention and promote positive cognitive performance in both children and adults.[109-112] To minimize the risk of insomnia from caffeine, caffeinated beverages should not be consumed within 6 hours of planned bedtime. No controlled trials are available to show significant benefits for other commonly used stimulant herbs such as ginseng for ADHD. A pilot study from Italy indicated that ginkgo may help improve ADD symptoms.[113] A Canadian product (AD-fX) that combines ginseng and ginkgo benefitted patients with ADHD or dyslexia in one manufacturer-sponsored study.[114] Similarly, pycnogenol or European pine bark extract was significantly better than placebo in improving concentration and decreasing hyperactivity in children in several European studies funded in part by pycnogenol producers.[115-117] Neither evening primrose oil (which contains gamma-linoleic acid [GLA]) nor St. John's wort supplements have proved any more useful than placebo for ADHD. Variations in the quality of herbal products and the paucity of effectiveness research mean that routine recommendations for these products should await further study and standardization of products (Table 6-4).

TABLE 6-4. Herbs as Additional Therapy

Calming Herbs

Tea: chamomile, hops, lemon balm, passionflower

Valerian: tincture, glycerite, or capsule

Aromatherapy: chamomile, lavender

Avoid kava because of concerns about hepatotoxicity

Stimulant Herbs

Coffee

Tea: black and green

Ginseng or ginseng/ginkgo combination

Other Herbs

Pycnogenol (pine bark extract, also known as OPC): benefits shown in small, industry-funded studies

Evening primrose oil: ineffective in a randomized controlled trial

St. John's wort: ineffective in a randomized controlled trial

Pharmaceuticals

In the United States, stimulant medications combined with behavioral therapy comprise first-line treatment for youth, although the long-term effectiveness of this therapy is unclear.[118,119] The British National Institute for Health and Clinical Excellence (NICE) guidelines for treating ADHD recommend stimulant medications as a first-line therapy for adults with ADHD, but only for children with severe symptoms, not mild or moderate ADHD.[120] Initially, stimulants (which are classified as controlled substances) benefit approximately two thirds of patients. Stimulant medications do not generally improve oppositional or defiant behaviors or overall quality of life, however, and their adverse effects on appetite, sleep, and growth require ongoing monitoring. Research conducted by scientists without conflicts of interest (unlike previous studies, in which investigators sometimes received payments from pharmaceutical companies) showed that stimulants were little better than placebo.[121]

> The National Institute of Clinical Excellence (NICE) recommends stimulant medications only for children with severe symptoms, not for children with mild to moderate ADHD.

Stimulant medications include short-acting (3 to 6 hours), medium-acting (4 to 8 hours) and long-acting (more than 8 hours) methylphenidate (Ritalin and Methylin) and amphetamines (Adderall, Dexedrine, Dextrostat, and Vyvanse). Related compounds include dexmethylphenidate (Focalin) and extended-release methylphenidate and amphetamine (Adderall, Metadate, and Concerta). A patch medication (Daytrana) provides controlled release of methylphenidate. Like coffee, most stimulants start working within approximately 20 minutes. Short-, medium-, and long-acting medications are available (Table 6-5).

Nonstimulant medications used to treat ADHD include atomoxetine (Strattera), modafinil (Provigil), clonidine (Catapres), guanfacine (Tenex and extended-release Intuniv), bupropion (Wellbutrin), and other antihypertensive, antidepressant, and antiseizure medications. Atomoxetine is the most commonly prescribed nonstimulant medication for ADHD. It is much better than placebo for improving the ability to focus, to be organized, and to regulate attention and emotions, as well as enhancing short-term memory in adults.[122] Atomoxetine has also been beneficial for children with ADHD, but side effects such as sleepiness and decreased appetite limit its appeal.[123] Many of the other medications are prescribed off label, that is, they have not been approved by the FDA for treatment of ADHD.

In addition to not working for some people, medications have several problems:

1. Side effects. The most common side effects of stimulant medications are decreased appetite, poor growth, and insomnia. Less common side effects include nausea, headaches, stomachaches, sweating, jitteriness, tics, dizziness, a racing heart, and, paradoxically, drowsiness. Of greater concern, stimulant use is linked to psychosis, hallucinations, heart arrhythmias, and sudden death.[124,125]
2. Failure to work when they are not taken. Medications are not a cure for ADHD. When a dose is missed, the

TABLE 6-5. Short-, Medium-, and Long-Acting Stimulant Medications for Attention Deficit Hyperactivity Disorder

SHORT (3–6 hr)	MEDIUM (4–8 hr)	LONG (> 8 hr)
Ritalin (methylphenidate) 5, 10, 20 mg bid or tid	Ritalin LA (methylphenidate long acting) 20, 30, 40 mg daily	Concerta (methylphenidate) 18, 36, 54 mg daily
Methylin (methylphenidate) 5, 10, 20 mg bid or tid	Ritalin SR (methylphenidate sustained release) 20 mg daily to bid	Focalin XR (dexmethylphenidate extended release) 5, 10, 20 mg daily
Focalin (dexmethylphenidate) 2.5 mg, 5, 10 mg bid	Metadate CD (methylphenidate extended release) 10, 20, 30, 40, 50, 60 mg daily	Daytrana (methylphenidate patch) 10, 15, 20, 30 mg daily
Metadate ER (methylphenidate extended release) 10–20 mg daily to bid	Methylin ER (methylphenidate extended release) 10, 20 mg daily to bid	Adderall XR (amphetamine/dexamphetamine extended release) 5, 10, 15, 20, 25, 30 mg daily
Adderall (amphetamine/dexamphetamine) 10, 20, 30 mg daily to bid		Vyvanse (lisdexamfetamine) 20, 30, 40, 50 mg daily

bid, twice daily; tid, three times daily.

medication cannot work. If someone stops taking it, it stops working. More than half the patients with ADHD stop taking stimulant medication without being advised to do so by their physician.[126,127]

3. Reliance on medications. Patients may rely on these agents instead of making healthy changes in lifestyle and environment.

4. Long-term costs. Continuous dependence on medications is costly for individuals and society. Stimulant use has increased from 0.6% of children less than 19 years old in 1987 to 3.4% in 2003. In terms of overall costs of medications, of the top five drugs prescribed for children, three were medications for ADHD.

5. Long-term effects. The effects of long-term medication use or of the concurrent use of multiple medications are unknown. Although stimulant medications have been used for decades, no long-term studies have evaluated the developmental impact of using these medications daily for 30 years. Short-term use has been evaluated for one drug at a time, but the impact of taking multiple medications simultaneously is unknown.

6. Misuse, diversion and abuse. As the number of prescriptions for stimulant medications has grown, so has the number of reports that these drugs are being diverted or sold to people who do not have ADHD. A 2009 study reported a 76% increase in the number of calls to Poison Control Centers related to adolescent abuse of prescription ADHD medications.[128]

Given these concerns about medications, many pediatricians do not write prescriptions for stimulant medications without first conducting N-of-1 trials to determine the short-term benefits and risks for individual patients. Such trials can be repeated annually to assess the ongoing need for medications.

Massage, Chiropractic, and Other Biomechanical Therapies

Scientific studies support the regular use of massage for improving ADHD symptoms.[129–131] Massage affects blood flow and neurotransmitters that influence focus and clarity.[132,133] Massage also reduces stress,

improves mood, decreases pain, and alleviates anxiety, all of which can improve concentration, deliberation, and self-discipline.[132,134–136] Even a 15-minute chair massage can improve speed and accuracy on standard tests.[137] Additional studies would be useful to help determine the best type of massage, the duration and frequency of treatments, and whether massage provided by friends or family members is as helpful as care from a licensed professional.

Massage is safe when common sense precautions are used, such as avoiding massage over rashes, infections, bruises, or burns. Do not force massage therapy on someone who has suffered physical or sexual abuse or who is very shy. Respect adolescents' desires for privacy. In the United States, massage therapists are licensed or certified as health professionals in 40 states; elsewhere, cities or counties license them. Licensed professionals in the United States can be identified through the American Massage Therapy Association's Locator Service.

PREVENTION PRESCRIPTION

■ Advise pregnant women to stop smoking and avoid drinking alcohol.

■ Advise parents not to smoke around their children and to limit exposure to television and pesticides.

■ Encourage families to live a healthy lifestyle focusing on the following: a whole foods diet that limits intake of artificial colors, flavors, sweeteners, and preservatives and foods that cause sensitivity reactions and that avoids deficiencies of essential omega-3 fatty acids, amino acids, vitamins and minerals; daily physical activity, preferably outdoors in natural surroundings; adequate sleep; effective stress and emotional self-management; strength-based communication skills and participation in supportive community networks; and a safe, structured, well-organized environment.

THERAPEUTIC REVIEW

■ Accurate Diagnosis

- Use standard rating scales such as the Vanderbilt Parent and Teacher Rating Scales to assess ADHD symptoms and response to interventions.

- Rule out medical and neuropsychological conditions that impair attention and self-discipline such as hypothyroidism, vision, hearing, and specific learning deficits. Consider requesting a neuropsychological examination to assess IQ and learning difficulties.

■ Encouraging Healthy Habits in a Healthy Habitat

- Dietary

  - Assess diet and correct nutritional deficiencies with a better diet or dietary supplements.

  - Encourage patients to maintain a steady blood glucose level by eating regular meals with foods having a low glycemic index. Foods containing artificial colors, sweeteners, flavors, and preservatives should be avoided, as should foods with a heavy burden of pesticides.

  - Instruct patients to avoid dehydration.

  - Consider recommending coffee or tea as mild dietary stimulants and monitoring for insomnia and other common side effects.

- Sleep and activity

  - Promote adequate sleep with sleep hygiene. Consider melatonin (0.3 to 3 mg an hour before bed) or sedative herbal remedies (a cup of chamomile tea or lavender aromatherapy) as a first-line approach to improving sleep.

  - Encourage vigorous daily activity, at least 30 minutes daily of activity vigorous enough to break a sweat or make it difficult to talk and move at the same time.

- Stress management and emotional self-management skills

  - Assess stress management and emotional self-management skills.

- Counsel families about stress management.

- Consider referral for meditation training, including moving meditation practices such as yoga and tai chi. Consider referral for effective counseling and cognitive-behavioral therapy.

- Social support

  - Refer families to support networks of other families such as Children and Adults with Attention Deficit Hyperactivity Disorder (CHADD).

  - Encourage positive family communication, focusing on goals rather than problems. Help families view overall long-term goals in terms of short-term achievable objectives. Help families learn to make specific, measurable, achievable, relevant, time-specific (SMART) plans, including ways to celebrate success.

  - Consider referring families for additional support for parenting and discipline skills, as well as time management and organizational skill development.

- Healthy environment

  - Advocate for appropriate testing and learning accommodations at school.

- Referral for additional professional assistance

  - Consider referral to a psychologist for neurofeedback.

  - Consider a referral for massage therapy.

- Pharmaceutical management

  - Remember that 65% of people do respond to stimulant medication, at least initially.

  - Consider recommending an N-of-1 trial of a stimulant medication, comparing a low dose (e.g., 5 mg methylphenidate twice daily) with a middle dose (10 mg twice daily) with placebo for 1 week each.

  - If patient notes improvement, consider switching to a longer-acting medication to reduce the number of pills or doses required daily.

- Monitor and support families with regular follow-up every 3 to 4 months.

KEY WEB RESOURCES

Rating Scales
Vanderbilt Teacher Rating Scale. http://www.brightfutures.org/mentalhealth/pdf/professionals/bridges/adhd.pdf.
Vanderbilt Parent Rating Scale. http://www.vanderbiltchildrens.org/uploads/documents/DIAGNOSTIC_PARENT_RATING_SCALE(1).pdf.

Activity
U.S. Centers for Disease Control and Prevention. http://www.cdc.gov/healthyyouth/physicalactivity/.
ABC for Fitness. Activity bursts in the classroom. http://www.davidkatzmd.com/abcforfitness.aspx.

Diet
Feingold diet. www.feingold.org.
Nutrition information from the Center for Science in the Public Interest. http://www.cspinet.org/.
Food pesticide levels from Environmental Working Group. http://www.foodnews.org/.

Support Groups
All Kinds of Minds (AKOM). www.allkindsofminds.org.
Children and Adults with Attention Deficit Hyperactivity Disorder (CHADD). www.chadd.org.

The National Federation for Families of Children's Mental Health. www.ffcmh.org.
Learning Disabilities Association of America (LDA). www.ldanatl.org.
Mental Health America. www.nmha.org.

Environment
Collaborative on Health and the Environment. www.healthandenvironment.org/.
National Environmental Education Foundation's Children and Nature Initiative. www.neefusa.org/health/children_nature.htm.
Pesticide information from Environmental Working Group. www.ewg.org/chemindex.
U.S. Department of Education information on attention deficit hyperactivity disorder and schools. http://www2.ed.gov/rschstat/research/pubs/adhd/adhd-identifying.html.

Biofeedback
Association for Applied Psychophysiology and Biofeedback. www.aapb.org.

Massage
American Massage Therapy Association. www.amtamassage.org.

References

References are available online at expertconsult.com.

Autism Spectrum Disorder

Sanford C. Newmark, MD

Autism is a neurodevelopmental disorder characterized by deficits in social interaction and language development and a restricted or stereotypical pattern of interests and activities. Formerly a relatively rare condition well out of the public eye, autism has increased in prevalence more than 10-fold since 1990, from an estimated prevalence of approximately 5 to 6 per 10,000 children to 110 per 10,000 according to the most recent estimate by the Centers for Disease Control and Prevention.[1] As a comparison, this disorder is now more than 5 times more prevalent than Down syndrome, which has a prevalence of approximately 20 per 10,000 (Fig. 7-1). No scientific agreement exists on the cause of this rapid increase in prevalence, often referred to as an "epidemic" in the media. The three most likely possibilities are the following:

1. A true increase in the prevalence of the disorder has occurred.
2. Case finding is increased because of heightened awareness of the disorder on the part of the public and medical and other professionals.
3. The definition of autism has been loosened so that more children are being included.

To complicate matters still further, other diagnostic categories such as autism spectrum disorder, pervasive developmental disorder, and Asperger syndrome have been added to the mix, including children with some features of autism but who do not meet strict criteria. Even so, the Brick Township, New Jersey study separated autism from autism spectrum disorder and Asperger syndrome and still recorded a prevalence of 40 per 10,000 for autism itself.[2] A study in Minnesota, in which autism was separated from these other categories, gave a striking picture of the rapidity of the increase in the prevalence of this disorder.[3]

Regressive autism refers to children who have normal development until the age of 1 to 2 years, after which they lose language, social interaction, and other developmental milestones. This type of autism has mainly caused the widespread public concern over the influence of the measles-mumps-rubella (MMR) and mercury-containing vaccines on the development of autism. However, the available studies indicate that regressive autism accounts for only 30% to 40% of autism cases.[4, 5]

The origin of this disorder is basically unknown. Investigators currently believe that autism is a genetically based disorder requiring some environmental trigger to manifest. This belief is supported by the 90% concordance rate in identical twins, as opposed to the 30% concordance rate in fraternal twins. The siblings of an affected patient also have a much higher risk of autism. Many gene loci have been associated with autism, but no single gene or even group of genes has been shown to have a large impact contribution to this order.[6] The genetic aspect of this disorder likely consists of simultaneous genetic variations in multiple genes. In addition, even in the previously mentioned identical twins, when one twin has classic autism, the other twin has only a 60% incidence of also having classic autism. This finding emphasizes the role of environmental influence. From a conventional medical point of view, investigators have had little discussion of possible environmental factors that may trigger the expression of this disease. However, as discussed in greater detail later in this chapter, integrative physicians have examined the role of toxin exposure (especially including mercury), nutritional factors, infectious disease, and autoimmunity as contributing factors.

Pathophysiology

The pathophysiology of autism is not completely defined, but the use of functional magnetic resonance imaging and other imaging techniques has advanced our knowledge significantly. We do know that children with autism exhibit increased brain growth in the first year of life compared with neurologically normal children, followed by a period of decreasing growth rate. Investigators have theorized that this rapid growth is characterized by disjointed and disorderly growth resulting in abnormal neuronal connections. Intriguing neuropathologic evidence indicates that these

FIGURE 7-1
Number of children classified as having an autism spectrum disorder (ASD) special educational disability in Minnesota from 1981 to 1982 through 2001 to 2002.

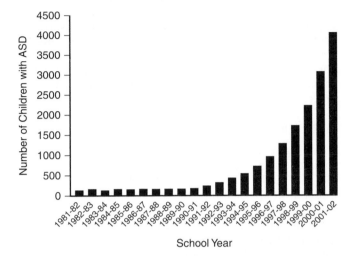

> Rather than thinking of autism as a brain disorder that has systemic effects, autism can be thought of as a systemic disorder that affects the brain.

abnormalities are associated with inflammation, thus raising the possibility that autism is, to some extent, a chronic inflammatory process. Patients have abnormalities of both gray and white matter. Evidence indicates that autism is, to a large degree, a problem of underconnectivity of cortical systems, especially interhemispheric communication, essentially a decreased ability of parts or systems of the brain to communicate with each other. This impairment results in difficulty with complex, higher-order functions, such as language and social skills. Autistic patients tend to have increased parietal and occipital activation, which is consistent with their greater reliance on visual-spatial as opposed to verbal skills. This feature also explains why autistic patients may have extremely high skills in areas not requiring this type of connectivity, such as mathematical calculation. Magnetic resonance imaging studies have shown abnormalities in the size of the cerebellum, amygdala, caudate, and various other parts of the brain, but the findings are not sufficiently reproducible to draw any definitive etiologic conclusions.[7]

Biomedical Approach

Some physicians and researchers have taken an alternative, or what is commonly referred to as a biomedical, approach to autism. The basis of this approach is that autism is a genetically based syndrome triggered by certain fetal, neonatal, and early childhood stimuli and that this syndrome results in a variety of nutritional, gastrointestinal, metabolic, and autoimmune abnormalities. Further, some of these abnormalities can be treated, and this treatment can improve the core symptoms of autism. Rather than thinking of autism as a brain disorder that has systemic effects, autism can be thought of a systemic disorder that affects the brain.[8]

Biomedical practitioners, including myself, have seen remarkable response to these treatments in some children with autism. The next sections discuss the strong evidence for the systemic nature of autism and the evidence for treatment efficacy.

Gastrointestinal System

One of the most common problems seen in children with autism is the wide variety of both gastrointestinal symptoms and clear gastrointestinal disease. The incidence of gastrointestinal problems in children with autism varies by study but seems to be in the range of 30% to 40%. Symptomatically, the most common reports are of chronic constipation or diarrhea and chronic abdominal pain; gastrointestinal disease is common and widespread. One study of children with autism and gastrointestinal symptoms showed that 69.4% of subjects had reflux esophagitis, 42% had chronic gastritis, and 67% had chronic duodenitis.[9] Because many of these children are nonverbal and cannot express gastrointestinal discomfort, many autistic children with these conditions may react to pain by exhibiting behaviors such as self-stimulation and temper tantrums that are not obviously referable to the gastrointestinal system.

Several studies have demonstrated definite disease of the small and large intestine. Torrente et al[10] performed biopsies on 25 children with autism and found duodenitis in almost all the children. These investigators described increased lymphocytic proliferation in both the epithelium and the lamina propria. This proliferation was associated with immunoglobulin G (IgG) and complement C1q deposition on the epithelial surface, indicating a possible autoimmune cause of the duodenitis. Horvath and Perman[11] also documented significant disaccharidase deficiencies in a population of children with autism and gastrointestinal symptoms.

> The gut–immune system interface is an area of opportunity in developing a better understanding of how to treat autism most effectively.

Dysbiosis

Dysbiosis, or abnormalities of gastrointestinal microflora, is also thought to be a common problem. Rosseneu et al[12] analyzed 80 children with autism and gastrointestinal symptoms and found that 61% had growth of abnormal aerobic gram-negative endotoxin-producing bacteria. The endotoxin produced by these aerobic gram-negative bacteria could cause ongoing bowel damage; 55% had overgrowth of *Staphylococcus aureus,* and 95% had overgrowth of pathogenic *Escherichia coli.* No abnormal amounts of yeast were noted in this study. In a fascinating pilot study, 11 of these children were treated with a nonabsorbable antibiotic. Not only did the abnormal flora disappear, but also both gastrointestinal symptoms and autistic behaviors decreased significantly. This study did not have a control group, and unfortunately, after 2 months the abnormal bacteria returned to pretreatment levels.[12] In another study,[13] vancomycin treatment of children with regressive autism and diarrhea resulted in decreased autistic behaviors, as measured by blinded observers.

Yeast

An overgrowth of yeast is widely believed to be part of dysbiosis and responsible for many gastrointestinal and behavioral symptoms of autism. Many children are therefore treated with antifungal agents as part of their "bowel detoxification" protocol. Very little research evidence for this yeast overgrowth exists, however. As mentioned earlier, Rosseneu's study failed to identify any yeast among the abnormal bacteria, and no good controlled studies have evaluated yeast overgrowth in autism. Some research has shown the presence of urine organic acids suggestive of yeast overgrowth in children with autism, but the significance of these byproducts is unclear. Antifungals such as nystatin, fluconazole, and ketoconazole are widely used, with much anecdotal evidence of positive results, but no controlled studies.

Intestinal Permeability

Yet another gastrointestinal abnormality commonly attributed to children with autism is "leaky gut," or increased intestinal permeability. Although this issue is ignored by most conventional practitioners, studies have shown it to be a pervasive problem. In a study by D'Eufemia et al,[14] examination of 21 autistic children with no known intestinal disorders confirmed increased intestinal permeability in 43%, as opposed to 0% of controls. In addition, Horvath and Perman[15] examined 25 children with autism and gastrointestinal symptoms by using lactulose-mannitol testing and found that 76% of these children had altered intestinal permeability. Finally, in 2010, de Magistris et al[16] found increased intestinal permeability in 36.7% of autistic patients and in 21.2% of their relatives, as compared with 4.8% of neurologically normal subjects.

Food Sensitivities

Food sensitivities or allergies are also thought to play an important role in the pathophysiology of autism. The evidence for this connection is indirect but suggestive. In one study, 36 children with autism were compared with healthy controls and were found to have significantly higher levels of IgA, IgG, and IgM and antigen-specific antibodies for specific food proteins such as lactoglobulin, casein, and beta-lactoglobulin compared with controls.[17] Two studies by Jyonouchi et al[18] showed that children with autism had higher intestinal levels of inflammatory cytokines directed against specific dietary proteins than did controls. In 2002, as previously noted, Torrente et al[10] showed increased lymphocyte proliferation and epithelial IgG deposition in the small intestine of children with autism, a finding suggesting an autoimmune process.

Some researchers believe that gluten and casein pass through a leaky gut barrier and form gluteomorphins and caseomorphins, which then have important central nervous system effects. Research in this area has been inconsistent, however. These putative food protein sensitivities do not manifest as immediate hypersensitivity on standard skin testing or IgE radioallergosorbent testing (RAST). This finding leads investigators to question whether children with autism have true food allergies or food sensitivities that are not IgE mediated.

In summary, available evidence suggests that significant percentages of children with autism have gastrointestinal abnormalities, including gastroesophageal reflux, duodenitis, ileitis, colitis, dysbiosis, increased intestinal permeability, and immune reactions to specific dietary proteins. Whether one or more of these conditions is primary and others are secondary is not clear. For example, does food sensitivity or dysbiosis cause increased intestinal permeability and inflammation, or does the increased permeability cause the food sensitivity? Similarly, is dysbiosis primary, leading to chronic damage to gut epithelia, or is it secondary to other pathologic processes?

Autoimmunity

Some studies suggest that autoimmune abnormalities are common in children with autism. Some of these abnormalities can be directly linked to the central nervous system. Connolly et al[19] examined the sera of children with autism for antibrain antibodies. IgG antibrain antibodies were present in the sera of 27% of children and in only 2% of controls. IgM antibodies were present in 36% of the sera of autistic children and in 0% of controls.

Another study looked at the prevalence of antibodies to various brain structures in 68 autistic children and 30 controls.[20] Forty-nine percent of autistic children had serum antibodies to the caudate nucleus, as opposed to 0% of controls. Antibodies to the cerebral cortex and cerebellum were 18% and 9%, respectively, again with 0% of controls having these antibodies. The reason that autistic children have the abnormal presence of antibodies to the brain and central nervous system is certainly not clear, nor is it known whether these antibodies cause neurologic problems or are merely a byproduct of central nervous system damage caused by other factors. However, these studies do suggest a possible role for autoimmunity in the origin of the neurologic abnormalities found in autism.

An epidemiologic study supported the importance of autoimmunity in autism.[21] Three groups of 101 families were examined. The first set of families had a child with autism, the second had a child with a classic autoimmune disease, and the third were healthy families, without autoimmune disease or autism. Families were then evaluated to find the number of first- or second-degree relatives with an autoimmune disorder. The surprising results were that autistic families had 1.87 relatives with autoimmune disorders. Thus, a family containing an autistic child was significantly ($P = .03$) more likely to have another relative with an autoimmune disorder than a family already containing a child with an autoimmune disorder.

Mitochondrial Abnormalities

One of the more fascinating aspects of autism research is the discovery that children with autism have a higher percentage of mitochondrial abnormalities than do other children. This finding was confirmed in several studies. In one study, Olivieri measured plasma lactate in 69 patients with autism. Fourteen patients, or 20%, had elevated plasma lactate; 11 of these patients underwent muscle biopsy, and 5 showed definite mitochondrial respiratory chain abnormalities. Thus, a total of 5 of 69, or 7.2% of autistic patients, had mitochondrial disease.[22] A 2011 review and meta-analysis estimated that the incidence of mitochondrial abnormalities is at least 5%, orders of magnitude higher than the general population.[23] Children with autism also demonstrated abnormalities in lactic acid, pyruvate, and carnitine levels compared with the general population.

Metabolic Disorders

Some studies demonstrated abnormalities in the metabolic functioning of children with autism, with defects in areas such as glutathione synthesis, sulfation deficits, and folate metabolism. For instance, a study reported in the *American Journal of Clinical Nutrition* demonstrated that relative to the control children, the children with autism had significantly lower baseline plasma concentrations of methionine, S-adenosylmethionine (SAMe), homocysteine, cystathionine, cysteine, and total glutathione and significantly higher concentrations of S-adenosylhomocysteine (SAH), adenosine, and oxidized glutathione.[24] This metabolic profile is consistent with impaired capacity for methylation (significantly lower ratio of SAMe to SAH) and increased oxidative stress.

In another study, activities of erythrocyte superoxide dismutase and erythrocyte and plasma glutathione peroxidase in autistic children were significantly lower than in neurologically normal children.[25] These results indicate that autistic children have low levels of activity of blood antioxidant enzyme systems.

An excellent review article by McGinnis[26] documented certain positive markers of oxidative stress in children with autism. Among other factors, he cited indirect markers for greater oxidative stress such as the following: (1) lower endogenous antioxidant enzymes and glutathione; (2) lower antioxidant nutrients; (3) higher organic toxins and heavy metals; (4) higher xanthine oxidase and cytokines; and (5) higher production of nitric oxide, a toxic free radical.

Heavy Metal Toxicity

Many clinicians and families involved in the alternative treatment of autism believe that increased body levels of heavy metals, especially mercury, are an important part of the pathophysiology of autism. This belief is related to the assumption that the thimerosal (ethylmercury) contained in, and later withdrawn from, infant immunizations, is a major factor in the autism "epidemic." Because children with autism are clearly not exposed to more mercury or other heavy metals than are other children, investigators have postulated that these children have impaired abilities to detoxify or excrete mercury and other heavy metals. This impairment is thought to result from the various methylation, sulfation, and antioxidant deficiencies discussed previously.

Little evidence supports the hypothesis that mercury is related to the development of autism. One of the problems in discussing heavy metal toxicity is that no simple tests are available for determining body levels of heavy metals. Blood tests for mercury are not useful because mercury remains in the tissues and not in the circulation. Hair analysis has been used, but whether low or high results correlate adequately with body levels is not clear. In conventional medicine, mercury toxicity is measured by giving a dose of a chelating agent, such as edetate disodium (EDTA) or dimercaptosuccinic acid (DMSA) and then measuring urine mercury levels. No published study exists in which this procedure has been done in autistic children. One study by Ip et al[27] compared blood and hair levels of autistic children with those of controls and found no significant differences; however, the investigators did not examine urine levels after chelation.

In another study, Holmes et al[28] compared the levels of mercury in the hair obtained during the first haircut of a set of babies with and without autism. These investigators found that hair mercury levels were significantly lower in autistic children than in controls, even though the exposure to mercury was the same or higher than that of controls. Because hair mercury level is a result of excretion of mercury, the investigators postulated that the toxic effect of mercury in autistic children could be caused by impaired excretion. In this article, hair mercury levels in controls were directly correlated with the number of mercury amalgams and with fish consumption in the mothers of these children, but no such correlation was noted in the autistic group.

If mercury is believed to be a cause of autism in some children, then why would these presumably neurologically normal children have impaired excretion resulting in higher than normal mercury levels? It would have to be postulated that the metabolic defects leading to impaired excretion were already present, perhaps on a genetic basis. This would explain why children genetically at risk for autism would react to mercury in a different way from nonautistic children to the same total mercury exposure. This hypothesis is plausible, but it has not yet been adequately investigated.

Finally, Bradstreet et al[29] performed a retrospective analysis of 221 children and 18 controls who had been treated with three doses of DMSA. Heavy metal concentrations in the urine were then analyzed. In this study, urinary concentrations of mercury were significantly higher in 221 autistic children than in the 18 controls. Moreover, vaccinated children showed a significantly higher urine mercury concentration than unvaccinated controls. No correlation was found between autism and urinary concentrations of lead or cadmium. The findings of this study implied that autistic children have significantly higher body burdens of mercury than controls, but the study had at least two significant limitations. First, it was a retrospective study with nonrandom selection of controls. Second, the imbalance between the number of cases and the control group was quite large.

In summary, although mercury is clearly a potent neurotoxin, especially in the developing brain, the idea that mercury exposure is a significant cause of autism is at this point largely unproven. To prove this association, a large study using postchelation urinary heavy metal levels in autistic children as compared with controls would be necessary.

> Although it is clear that mercury is a potent neurotoxin, especially in the developing brain, the idea that mercury exposure is a significant cause of autism is at this point largely unproven.

Role of Thimerosal in Immunizations in the Causation of Autism

The role of thimerosal in autism is a topic of great controversy, and entire book chapters could be written about it. This issue has caused a remarkable rift between the scientific mainstream and the "autism community" that seems to be completely impenetrable. This discussion is an attempt to describe the issue as succinctly as possible. First, even though mercury is a potent neurotoxin, it was used as a preservative in childhood vaccines until 1999. At that time, a review conducted by the U.S. Food and Drug Administration discovered that with the increased number of vaccines given in infancy, the amount of thimerosal, which is ethylmercury, received by infants in the first 6 months of life could exceed the U.S. Environmental Protection Agency guidelines for safe amounts of methylmercury. (The distinction between ethylmercury and methylmercury is important because safety standards are based on methylmercury.) Despite claims that thimerosal posed no danger or showed no evidence of harm, thimerosal was then withdrawn from all infant vaccines except the influenza vaccine. The autism community, however, aware of the huge increases in the diagnosis of autism, made the obvious connection and asserted that autism could in large part be caused by the thimerosal in childhood vaccines. This connection was supported by two analyses by Geier and Geier,[30,31] who claimed to link thimerosal-containing vaccines with autism through analyses of reports for the Vaccine Adverse Event Reporting System (VAERS) and through comparison of thimerosal vaccine rates and special education enrollment of children with autism. The authorities criticized reports on methodologic grounds, especially noting that VAERS is a passive reporting system and not suited to this type of analysis. Since then, several epidemiologic studies have failed to find a connection between thimerosal in vaccines and the incidence of autism, but opponents have refused to accept their statistics and have become suspicious of any report coming from government or medical "authorities."

Evidence that thimerosal in vaccines is responsible for a rise in autism is insufficient. The amount of mercury in vaccines since 2000 has been miniscule, yet we have not yet seen a corresponding drop in new cases of autism. Arguing that thimerosal was a major contributor to the so-called autism epidemic would be difficult without postulating that some "new" factor was causing the continued high incidence, now that thimerosal is no longer a factor.

This is not to say that environmental mercury or other toxins could not have a significant impact on the development of autism. A small study showed 287 environmental pollutants in the umbilical cord blood of newborn infants,[32] including mercury and a wide variety of organic and inorganic contaminants, such as polychlorinated biphenyls. Before their first breath, infants are already accumulating significant levels of mercury and other environmental toxins. Also true is that no levels of mercury exposure in the fetal brain are known to be "safe."

A study in Texas[33] showed a direct correlation between the incidence of autism and the amount of mercury expelled from industrial pollution. In fact, for each 1000 lb of environmentally released mercury, the investigators noted a 43% increase in the rate of special education services and a 61% increase in the rate of autism. Of course, this is a correlation only and does not prove causation, but it is nevertheless extremely concerning, especially as environmental mercury pollution continues to rise.

> Low levels of environmental toxins can affect neurologic development in animal models. Although evidence is not yet available for a strong relationship with autism, the precautionary principle should be implemented and practiced.

Measles-Mumps-Rubella Vaccine and Autism

Because regressive autism occurs between the first and second year of life, which is when the MMR vaccine is usually given, many parents have suspected this live vaccine as a cause of autism in their children. This concept was reinforced when research by Dr. Andrew Wakefield asserted the presence of small bowel disease in children with autism that is often associated with the presence of the measles virus. This study, however, was retracted by the *Lancet* after very serious allegations of irregularities in the research.[34]

What is the evidence? Several epidemiologic studies have failed to find any link between measles immunization and autism.[35-37] Therefore, on a population-wide basis, I believe it is clear that the MMR vaccine is not a significant contributor to the increased incidence of autism. Also true, however, is that epidemiologic studies would have a difficult time teasing out a small subpopulation of genetically predisposed children who were susceptible to an autoimmune reaction to the measles virus. Therefore, the possibility certainly exists that the MMR vaccine is the triggering event for autism in a small subset of individual patients. One study did show increased levels of measles antibody in immunized children with autism versus controls, a finding indicating a possible hyperimmune response to measles in children with autism.[38]

On a personal level, I have met some parents who ascribed their child's development of regressive autism to the MMR vaccine, even if the regression occurred months after an uneventful vaccine reaction. These associations do not seem credible. However, I have also met a few parents whose neurologically normal child received the MMR vaccine, had a severe physical reaction, including mental status changes, and immediately began losing milestones. These reports are more difficult to dismiss, although coincidence is always possible.

> No good evidence supports the potential relationship between the measles-mumps-rubella vaccine and the development of autism.

Nutritional Deficiencies

One tenet of the biomedical approach is that nutritional deficiencies are widespread and important in autism. These deficiencies are thought to be mainly linked to poor digestion and absorption of nutrients resulting from the aforementioned gastrointestinal problems, as well as abnormalities in the metabolic processing of nutrients. The evidence for these nutritional deficiencies, however, is somewhat uneven and rarely complete.

The beginning of the biomedical approach to the treatment of autism occurred when Bernard Rimland et al[39-41] began using supplements of vitamin B_6 in the early 1970s. These investigators reported controlled and uncontrolled studies of the effect of vitamin B_6 and magnesium on autistic symptoms, all of which were positive. However, many of these reports were not published in peer-reviewed journals, and they did not have a rigorous study design. In 2002, a Cochrane Review found only two articles of sufficient quality to analyze.[42] One was inconclusive, and the other showed no effect. A pilot study by Adams and Holloway[43] that evaluated the impact of a multivitamin and mineral study in a controlled double-blind fashion on a small group of children found statistically significant differences in sleep and gastrointestinal symptoms but not in the core symptoms of autism. The levels of vitamin B_6 were much higher in autistic children than in controls. This finding is postulated as reflecting the relatively poor conversion of pyridoxal to pyridoxal-5-phosphate, the enzymatically active form of the vitamin. This would explain why children with autism may need increased intake of vitamin B_6. A larger controlled study is currently under way.

Although no peer-reviewed studies have documented inadequate levels of vitamin C in children with autism, one study did show positive effects of up to 8 g/day of vitamin C in institutionalized autistic children.[44] This was a placebo-controlled double-blind crossover study, and total autism evaluation scores improved significantly in the treated group and worsened in the group going from vitamin C to placebo.

Omega-3 Fatty Acid Deficiency

A study by Vancassel et al[45] looked at levels of omega-3 fatty acids and other polyunsaturated fatty acids in the serum of children with autism compared with controls. Those children who had autism had 23% lower levels of omega-3 fatty acids in their plasma than did controls. They also had 20% lower levels of polyunsaturated fatty acids. This finding is in addition to two studies in the related diagnosis of attention deficit hyperactivity disorder (ADHD) that clearly showed lower levels of omega-3 fatty acids in both erythrocytes and serum in children with ADHD as compared with controls. The reason for this finding is unclear. Because no reason exists to assume that children with autism have different levels of omega-3 intake than control children, autistic children may have differences in how they use and metabolize these fats. This question is significant in that omega-3 fatty acids are a common supplement used in the integrative treatment of autism.

Integrative Therapy

Mind-Body Therapy

Conventional Behavioral Approaches

Intensive behavioral therapy is another common treatment for children with autism. With this therapy, direct behavioral intervention by trained facilitators occurs in home and school settings from 20 to 40 hours a week. Specific methods are used, such as Lovaas, Floortime, and applied behavior analysis. Intervention is directed at increasing appropriate social and language behavior while decreasing self-stimulatory activities. Overall, reasonable evidence indicates the effectiveness of this modality. A 2003 review in the *Canadian Journal of Psychiatry* concluded that "delivering interventions for more than 20 hours weekly that are individualized, well planned, and target language development and other areas of skill development significantly increases children's developmental rates, especially in language, compared with no or minimal treatment."[46]

Speech Therapy

Speech therapy is almost universally recommended to deal with the language deficits of children with autism. Most clinicians and parents, including myself, believe speech therapy to be helpful and effective in most children with autism. Very little convincing research supports the efficacy of speech therapy for autism, however. Although some showed specific areas of language improvement, all these involved a small number of subjects, and none of the studies were randomized or controlled. Considering the almost universal use of speech therapy in the treatment of autism, this is an area with surprisingly inadequate research.

Occupational Therapy

Occupational therapy is also commonly recommended for children with autism. As with speech therapy, anecdotal reports note improvement, but no convincing research evidence of efficacy exists.

▪ Precautions

In general, the effectiveness of the therapy is highly practitioner dependent. Practitioners should find the excellent therapists in their area. The usefulness of the conventional behavioral approaches must be evaluated on an ongoing basis. Families have limits in both time and money in what they can do.

Alternative Behavioral Approaches

Another modality commonly employed with children with autism is sensory integration therapy. Children with autism clearly have significant sensory issues. They often do not enjoy touching, can be upset by noisy environments, and exhibit other sensory difficulties. To modify these deficits, sensory integration therapy is often recommended. This therapy usually involves a variety of sensory stimuli administered under controlled conditions. As with the other therapies discussed earlier, only anecdotal evidence indicates effectiveness. Small noncontrolled studies have been conducted, but any evidence of efficacy is preliminary at best.

A second behavioral modality is auditory integration therapy. This technique is based on the idea that hypersensitivity to certain sounds can cause behavioral and emotional difficulties in autistic children. Essentially, auditory integration therapy attempts to reprogram and "integrate" the auditory system by sending randomized sound frequencies through earphones worn by the autistic child. This is usually done in 20- to 30-minute sessions over a period of 10 days or so. Many anecdotal reports of efficacy exist, but studies so far are uncontrolled and limited to very small numbers, so any positive evidence must be judged as preliminary. Finally, a few small studies have indicated that music therapy may be beneficial for autism.

Nutrition

Dietary Interventions

The most common alternative or biomedical intervention employed with autistic children is the gluten-free, casein-free (GFCF) diet. This diet is based on the previously discussed theory that food sensitivities, especially to gluten and casein, can produce not only gastrointestinal symptoms but, in association with gut inflammation and increased gut permeability (leaky gut), can lead to many of the neurologic manifestations of autism. In general, parents are advised strictly to avoid all foods containing gluten or casein for a period of at least 60 days and sometimes several months.

The anecdotal evidence for efficacy is abundant. In various support groups, chat groups, and other situations bringing together parents of children with autism, the GFCF diet is often described as promoting significant and positive changes in gastrointestinal symptoms, language, socialization, and other autistic behaviors.

Two controlled studies concerning the efficacy of the GFCF diet in the treatment of autism showed positive results. In the first study, by Knivsberg et al,[47] 10 matched pairs of children with autism were randomized to a GFCF diet or a placebo control for 1 full year. Autistic behaviors were then evaluated by blinded observers using the DIPAB, a Danish instrument for measuring autistic traits. After the intervention, the diet group had a mean DIPAB rating of 5.60, significantly ($P = .001$) better than the control group rating of 11.20. Specifically, social contact increased in 10 of 15 of the treated children, whereas ritualistic behaviors in that group decreased in 8 of 11 children. In the second study, by Lucarelli et al,[17] autistic children were found to have decreased behavioral symptoms after 8 weeks on an elimination diet. A third double-blind study in 2006, with 15 children, showed no statistically significant differences between groups.[48]

The GFCF diet can be extremely stressful to maintain. Autistic children tend to be picky eaters, and using this diet often removes some of their main foodstuffs. The diet can also cause a financial hardship, because many of the GFCF substitutes can be significantly more expensive. The potential for nutritional deficiencies exists if the diet is not supervised by a dietitian or physician. Both protein and calcium intake should be watched, as well as overall caloric intake.

With willing families and adequate supervision, these concerns are minor and easily manageable. I believe it is important, however, to make no other changes when instituting the diet, so that any improvements will be clearly the result of the diet itself and not related to other factors. Too often, the GFCF diet is started in conjunction with several nutritional supplements and other interventions, thus making it difficult to know whether behavioral or other improvements can be clearly attributed to the diet.

If gluten and other proteins can cause gastrointestinal disease and other manifestations of autism, what about other dietary proteins? The answer is that no reason exists that other foods cannot cause problems, and anecdotal reports abound of children with autism who react to a variety of food proteins, as well as certain preservatives and artificial colors and flavors. No controlled trials support these observations, however. Deciding how to determine whether a child is sensitive to these foods is interesting. As with gluten and casein, results of IgE skin tests and RAST testing are mostly negative. Many practitioners use RAST testing specific for IgG or IgG-4, tests that are usually obtained from alternative laboratories that are not covered by insurance and are less strictly regulated. These IgG tests are thought to reflect delayed-type food allergy, but the actual evidence linking IgG results to clinical allergy is scant. Moreover, problems with the reliability and accuracy of some of these laboratories have been reported. Another alternative is single or multiple food elimination diets, in which one or more groups of foods are removed for a period and behavior is observed. These diets can be very illuminating, but they depend on subjective impressions of the observer (see Chapter 84, Food Intolerance and Elimination Diet).

Another dietary intervention is known as the specific carbohydrate diet, made popular by Elaine Gottschall in *Breaking the Vicious Cycle*. This diet, which eliminates almost all carbohydrates and sugars except monosaccharides, was originally intended for patients with inflammatory bowel disease, celiac disease, and other gastrointestinal problems. The diet has been used by families of children with autism, however, and many have claimed positive results. It is even stricter than the GFCF diet, and essentially no scientific evidence exists of its efficacy in autism. Finally low-phenol and low-oxalate diets have some anecdotal success, again without any substantiating research.

■ Dosage (Length of Trial)

Most practitioners believe that at least 60 days on a GFCF diet is necessary to evaluate its efficacy fully. Some practitioners recommend at least 6 months.

■ Precautions

Make sure that caloric intake is adequate, including protein, fat, and carbohydrate. Depending on the diet, calcium or a multivitamin supplementation may be indicated. Monitor the child's weight.

Pearls for Instituting a Gluten-Free Diet for Autism

1. Make sure that no other interventions are being started simultaneously.
2. Discuss carefully the need for strict adherence during the trial period.
3. Discuss the reading of labels and locations where gluten-free, casein-free products can be obtained.
4. I also recommend eliminating artificial colors and flavors.
5. Use a supportive nutritionist whenever feasible.
6. Do not substitute large amounts of soy for casein. Soy is also a significant player in childhood food allergies.
7. Following this diet is *hard*. Parents need support and guidance.

Omega-3 Essential Fatty Acids

Many nutritional supplements are used in the treatment of autism, including omega-3 fatty acids, probiotics, zinc, vitamin B_6, and other multivitamin and mineral supplements.

Omega-3 fatty acids, as discussed previously, have been shown to be decreased in the serum of children with autism. (Other studies, have shown similar deficiencies in children with ADHD.) Therefore, these supplements are widely used in the treatment of autism. In one pilot study by Patrick and Salik,[49] 18 children were given an omega-3 fatty acid supplement (247 mg of omega-3 and 40 mg of omega-6) for 3 months. The language skills of these children were measured at baseline and after the 3-month trial. The investigators found a highly significant increase in language skills over a wide variety of measures. A literature review rated the overall evidence for the efficacy of omega-3 fatty acids in autism as insufficient to draw conclusions.[50] This review noted that only one small randomized controlled study has been done, and this showed a trend toward improvement in hyperactivity and stereotypy that did not reach statistical signficance.[50]

Another study of relevance concerned the use of omega-3 fatty acids in developmental coordination disorder.[51] This is not part of the autistic spectrum but is relevant because children with this disorder can have elements of learning disabilities, ADHD, and autism. In this double-blind controlled trial, 117 children were given either an omega-3 supplement or placebo for 3 months. Although no coordination improvement was found, the treated children made startling gains in reading, spelling, and mathematical skills compared with the placebo group. As an example, the average reading scores in the treatment group advanced 9.5 months in 3 months, as opposed to an increase of 3.5 months in the placebo group ($P = .004$). No clearly accepted guidelines exist for the dosage of omega-3 fatty acids in autism, or the ideal ratio of docosahexaenoic acid (DHA) and eicosapentaenoic acid (EPA), the crucial omega-3 fatty acids.

■ Dosage

Dosage is an area of uncertainty. I usually begin with 15 mg/lb of omega-3 fatty acids. Some studies have used 1.5 g of omega-3 fatty acids for children 5 to 14 years of age.

■ Precautions

Too high a dose, or sometimes even low doses, can trigger hyperactivity in a small subset of children.

Experiential Pearls for Using Omega-3 Fatty Acids in Autism

1. I tend to use a fairly balanced dose of docosahexaenoic acid and eicosapentaenoic acid for a total dose of 15 mg/lb.
2. I use Nordic Naturals, Carlson Laboratories, or Genova Diagnostics products. These manufacturers have a good variety of products, including reasonable-tasting liquids and chewable capsules. However, the chewable capsules can become expensive for older or larger children.
3. Start slowly and move up the dose. Hyperactivity is an occasional side effect and disappears when the dose is lowered.
4. I like to start omega-3 fatty acids, multivitamins, zinc, and probiotics at the same time. This approach may be less scientific, but synergy may exist among some of these products.

Probiotics

Probiotics are used frequently in the biomedical treatment of autism. As discussed previously, many children with autism have abnormal gut flora, as well as increased intestinal permeability. It seems reasonable to treat this problem with probiotic therapy. Unfortunately, treatment with antibiotics seems to result in only temporary changes in bowel flora, thus leading to the conclusion that ongoing use of probiotics may be necessary to ensure normal bowel flora. In addition, despite the widespread use of probiotics and anecdotal reports of their efficacy, no well-designed studies have been conducted on the impact of probiotic use in the treatment of autism.

An interesting problem in the use of probiotics is that many different strains of beneficial bacteria exist. Controlled studies using probiotics in other areas of medicine tend to use single strains such as *Lactobacillus* GG (Culturelle). However, many of the commonly available probiotics used in the treatment of autism contain 1 billion or more colony-forming units of *Lactobacillus acidophilus, Lactobacillus bulgaricus, Bifidobacterium* of various species, and others. Because many of these strains of beneficial bacteria are commonly present in the colon, it would seem to make sense to use a product that includes them, but scientific evidence concerning this choice is absent. The correct dosage of probiotics is equally unclear (see Chapter 102, Prescribing Probiotics).

■ Dosage

Dosage varies greatly, depending on the type of preparation.

■ Precautions

Start slowly and gradually increase the dose; otherwise, diarrhea may occur.

Zinc

Zinc is the most widely recommended single mineral used in the treatment of autism. Much of this is related to research by Dr. William Walsh of the Pfeiffer Institute (Warrenville, Ill),[52] who found that copper-to-zinc ratios were increased in more than 85% of children with autism. He also found that a dysfunction of metallothionein, a protein involved in the regulation of these and other metals, was present in 99% of 503 autistic children. Unfortunately, this research was published by the Pfeiffer Institute only and not in a peer-reviewed journal. However, given the possibility of reduced zinc levels or increased copper-to-zinc levels in autistic children, many clinicians include increased zinc as part of autism therapy. However, no controlled studies have been conducted to indicate the efficacy of zinc in the treatment of autism. Some related evidence is available in the case of ADHD; two studies showed that children with ADHD tend to be deficient in zinc, and two studies showed improvement in these children when they were given zinc supplementation.

■ Dosage

20 to 25 mg/day.

■ Precautions

Zinc can inhibit the absorption of copper, thus leading to deficiency.

Carnosine

Carnosine is an antioxidant and may affect neurotransmitter function. It is one of the few metabolic supplements for which at least reasonable research evidence is available. One study showed carnosine levels in autistic children to be significantly lower than in controls. A double-blind placebo-controlled study by Chez et al[53] showed that autistic children had significant benefits from carnosine supplementation compared with placebo.

▪ Dosage

The study by Chez et al[53] used 400 mg twice daily in 3- to 12-year-old children.

▪ Precautions

Watch for hyperactivity or excitability.

Other Supplements

Many different metabolic and nutritional supplements have been used for the treatment of autism. These include trimethylglycine, dimethylglycine, glutathione, dipeptidases, digestive enzymes, methylcobalamin (methyl vitamin B_{12}), phosphatidylcholine, and others. All of these are recommended based on various metabolic and nutritional defects discussed earlier, and many come with glowing anecdotal reports of efficacy. None has been subject to any type of controlled study, so it is difficult to know which, if any, of these supplements are worth recommending. Methyl vitamin B_{12} injections, given every 3 days, are probably the most widely used of these therapies, and in my experience they elicit the most positive responses from parents. Some families have stated that methyl vitamin B_{12} was the most clearly effective of the entire range of biomedical interventions. The only double-blind study of methyl vitamin B_{12}, with 30 children, did not show any difference between experimental and control groups in either autistic symptoms or glutathione status, however.[54]

Hyperbaric Oxygen

One of the more interesting newer treatments for autism is the use of hyperbaric oxygen. Long used in deep sea diving, wound healing, and more recently cerebral palsy, hyperbaric oxygen use in autism is based on the finding that autism has been associated with hypoperfusion to various areas of the brain in several studies. Whether this association is primary or secondary to abnormal neurologic development is unknown. After a few case reports and unblinded studies, Rossignol[55] performed a randomized placebo-controlled trial with 62 children with autism. Subjects received either 40 sessions of either hyperbaric treatment or a placebo that involved being in a hyperbaric chamber with normal pressures and oxygen. The experimental group had statistically significant improvement in a range of autistic symptoms compared with controls.

Given early positive evidence and the knowledge that hyperbaric oxygen is a fairly safe procedure, practitioners are tempted to recommend it as a therapy. However, it is very expensive (usually at least $4000 dollars) for a set of 40 treatments and obviously time consuming. So far, no research is available on the permanence of any gains made with hyperbaric therapy.

Treating Mitochondrial Disorders

No direct research has specifically concerned the treatment of children with autism and mitochondrial disorders, outside of normal recommendations for mitochondrial issues. Clinically, many biomedical practitioners recommend testing of lactate, pyruvate, or carnitine levels to determine which children may be at increased risk. Treatment for children with elevated levels, with or without muscle biopsy confirmation, may consist of antioxidants such as coenzyme Q10, B vitamins, carnitine, and other antioxidants. Carnitine is known to be important in mitochondrial function, and antioxidants may decrease the oxidative stress associated with mitochondrial dysfunction. The somewhat speculative nature of this treatment may be reasonably countered by the high level of safety of these particular supplements.

Pharmaceuticals

Investigators generally believe that conventional psychotropic medication does not affect the core symptoms of autism but may help related comorbid behaviors that may be problematic. The main classes of drugs used are the following:
1. Mood-stabilizing medication, especially more recently the atypical antipsychotics such as risperidone (Risperdal), for explosive behavior and mood stabilization
2. Selective serotonin reuptake inhibitors (SSRIs) for anxiety, agitation, and depression
3. The psychostimulants such as methylphenidate (Ritalin) and combined amphetamine and dextroamphetamine (Adderall) for comorbid hyperactivity, lack of focus, and decreased attention span

Risperidone

Risperidone has had several good controlled trials and seems to be effective for the treatment of explosivity and irritability in children with autism, at least in the short term. In 2002, the results of a multisite trial of risperidone for the treatment of irritability, aggression, and explosiveness in autism showed a positive response in 56% of respondents as compared with 14% of the placebo group.[56] Increased appetite, fatigue, drowsiness, dizziness, and drooling were more common in the risperidone group than in the placebo group, however. The average weight gain in 8 weeks was 2.8 kg. Of the positive responders, two thirds still had a positive response after 6 months, a finding indicating that approximately 36% of the original group maintained improvement for 6 months. A follow-up study by these same investigators showed continued effectiveness without significant dose increases and a return to baseline when the risperidone was withdrawn.[57]

Although many integrative physicians would prefer not to use psychotropic medicines as first-line therapy in autism, one can imagine the difficulty of dealing with an explosive and noncommunicative adult-sized teenager to see how this type of treatment may have an important place.

▪ Dosage
0.5 to 4 mg orally daily.

▪ Precautions
Watch for tardive dyskinesia, anxiety, gastrointestinal disturbances, skin sensitivity, weight gain, and diabetes.

Selective Serotonin Reuptake Inhibitors

Theoretical reasons exist to believe the serotonin inhibitors could be effective in autism. First, some studies have established abnormalities of serotonin metabolism in children with autism. Second, the repetitive behaviors seen in autism have similarities to those seen in obsessive-compulsive disorder, which can be treated with SSRIs. A placebo-controlled trial by Hollander et al,[58] who used an 8-week course of low-dose fluoxetine (Prozac) (average 10 mg/day), showed significant improvement in repetitive behaviors compared with placebo but did not demonstrate any significant improvement in the Clinical Global Impressions score or global effectiveness.[58] The rate of adverse effects was no higher in the treatment than in the placebo group. This finding contrasted with an earlier study in which a 50-mg dose of fluoxetine was effective in only 1 of 18 subjects and caused significant adverse effects.[59] A Cochrane Review of SSRIs for autism stated that these drugs had no evidence of efficacy, could cause harm, and could not be recommended.[60]

■ Dosage

Dosage varies with the specific SSRI. Fluoxetine should be started at 5 mg and advanced slowly if necessary.

■ Precautions

Given the paucity of evidence, especially longer term, use SSRIs cautiously. Watch for decreased alertness, irritability, and dysphoria.

Psychostimulants

Although psychostimulants have been quite widely used in autism, the literature on their effectiveness is limited. Some studies, however, demonstrated a positive effect on those children with autism and hyperactivity symptoms. One double-blind study did show positive changes in some aspects of social interaction and self-regulation.[61] However, stimulants are associated with a significant incidence of negative side effects in children with autism, and in one study the drugs caused a variety of adverse effects, such as agitation, dysphoria, and irritability, in more than half of the subjects.[62] Clinically, however, some children with autism have hyperactivity and lack of ability to focus so severe that a careful trial of these medications is warranted.

■ Dosage

Dosage varies depending on the specific medication, beginning at low doses and working up slowly. Long- or short-acting preparations can be used (e.g., amphetamine plus dextroamphetamine [Adderall] 5 mg to 10 mg, one in AM, one in early PM).

■ Precautions

Watch for hypertension, weight loss, growth suppression, and insomnia if the drugs are given too close to bedtime.

Therapies to Consider

Complementary therapies such as homeopathy, craniosacral therapy, Reiki and other energy medicine modalities, and traditional Chinese medicine all may have a place in the integrative approach to autism. Scattered anecdotal reports of efficacy exist, but no research evidence. Certainly, any of these approaches would be safe for most children with autism.

PREVENTION PRESCRIPTION

No definitive means exist to prevent autism. Some reasonable possibilities are the following:
- Have pregnant women avoid any unnecessary mercury intake. This would involve not eating certain fish and not having dental work done on amalgam fillings while pregnant.
- Encourage mothers to eat foods rich in omega-3 fatty acids during pregnancy and breast-feeding. If bottle-feeding, infants should use the omega-3–enriched formulas.
- Consider probiotics during pregnancy and infancy.
- If immunizations are a concern, the family could consider having fewer immunizations at once and separating immunizations when possible.
- Avoid exposure of pregnant mothers and infants to toxic household products of any kind.
- Avoid pesticide exposure wherever possible

 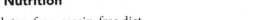

THERAPEUTIC REVIEW

■ Nutrition

- Gluten-free, casein-free diet
- See Chapter 84, Food Intolerance and Elimination Diet

■ Supplements

- Omega-3 fatty acids: 15 mg/lb total eicosapentaenoic acid and docosahexaenoic acid to start
- See Chapter 86, The Antiinflammatory Diet
- Probiotics: 1 to 10 billion colonies daily (one or two capsules)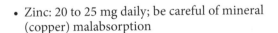

- Zinc: 20 to 25 mg daily; be careful of mineral (copper) malabsorption

■ Mind-Body Therapy

- Intensive behavioral therapy (Lovaas, applied behavior analysis, Floortime)
- Sensory integration therapy
- Auditory integration therapy

■ Other Therapy

- Speech therapy (for language development)
- Occupational therapy (for manual tasks and motor skill development)

KEY WEB RESOURCES

Talk about Curing Autism. www.TACAnow.org.	This very good Web site contains information about both conventional and biomedical treatment for autism, as well as various types of support for families who have a child with autism.
http://www.talkaboutcuringautism.org/tag/gfcf/.	This useful Web site, associated with Talk about Curing Autism, has information about the gluten-free, casein-free diet.
Autism Research Institute. www.autism.com.	This Web site provides information about research on and application of the biomedical approach. It also notes DAN (Defeat Autism Now) Conferences, which are appropriate for both practitioners and parents.
MIND (Medical Investigation of Neurodevelopmental Disorders) Institute at the University of California, Davis. www.ucdmc.ucdavis.edu/mindinstitute/.	This institute is at the forefront of research into childhood neurodevelopmental diseases. At this Web site, physicians can find good information and parents can find research studies for which their child may be eligible.

References

References are available online at expertconsult.com.

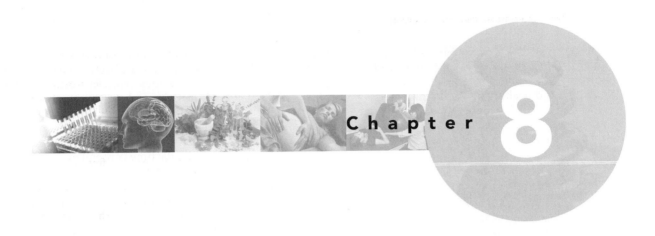

Chapter 8

Insomnia

Rubin Naiman, PhD

Insomnia is pervasive, associated with a broad range of illnesses, and presents a significant medical, social, and economic burden. Largely undiagnosed and untreated despite the existence of effective interventions, insomnia has been described as "unremitting, disabling, costly, pervasive, and pernicious."[1] Because it is strongly linked to lifestyle and body-mind dynamics and is resistant to conventional medical treatment, insomnia deserves much greater consideration from integrative medicine researchers and practitioners. In fact, a National Health Interview Survey reported that 1.6 million adults already use complementary and alternative medicine (CAM) to treat insomnia.[2]

The National Institutes of Health reports that 60 million adults in the United States struggle with insomnia annually.[3] Depending on definition, the prevalence of insomnia among adults ranges from 10% to 30% and increases with age and female gender, as well as with a broad range of medical and psychiatric comorbidities.[4]

Most patients with insomnia are at increased risk for comorbid medical disorders, including chronic pain, cardiovascular disease, cancer, neurologic and gastrointestinal disorders[5,6] obesity,[7] and diabetes.[8-10] Sleep loss has been associated with insulin dysregulation[9,10] disruptions of cortisol rhythms,[11,12] and immune function and inflammatory markers.[13-16]

Psychiatric illness, especially depression or anxiety,[17] is the most common comorbidity linked to insomnia.[18,19] Approximately 40% of adults with insomnia have a psychiatric illness—most commonly depression.[18,19] Persistent insomnia significantly raises the risk of clinical depression, anxiety disorders, and substance abuse.[20,21] The traditional presumption that insomnia is secondary to psychiatric illness has been challenged by several findings that suggest insomnia more often precedes and is likely a significant risk factor for mood disorders.[22-25]

Although psychiatric illness,[18] medical disorders,[26] and shift work[27] significantly increase the risk for insomnia, they are not causal but precipitating factors in patients already predisposed to the disorder.[28] Certain primary sleep and circadian rhythm disorders such as restless legs syndrome,[29] periodic limb movement disorders, delayed sleep phase, and sleep-related breathing disorders are also frequently associated with insomnia.[30]

Insomnia is associated with significant impairment in quality of life,[31-33] increased risk for accidents,[34] and decrements in work productivity.[35] The economic burden of insomnia has been estimated to be as high as $107 billion annually.[36]

Although conventional sleep medicine has clearly made advances in understanding and evaluating sleep and sleep disorders, one can argue that it lags in terms of developing effective treatment and prevention strategies for insomnia. Despite their serious limitations, hypnotic agents remain the primary focus of conventional insomnia treatment. Advances in cognitive-behavioral therapy for insomnia (CBT-I) challenge the conventional emphasis on medication and are associated with a growing chasm between conventional and behavioral sleep medicine. Among the most significant limitations of conventional approaches to insomnia is a widespread tendency to "treat the chart" that offers remarkably limited regard for subjective experiences of the patient. Among other consequences, this approach is associated with an unfortunate disregard for the role of rapid eye movement (REM) sleep and dreaming.

Because insomnia is so common and sleep is so vital a factor in general health, concern about the screening, evaluation, and treatment of insomnia should to be integral to primary health care. Along with nutrition, exercise, and stress management, sleep is clearly one of the four cornerstones of health. Because healthy sleep is associated with a broad range of biologic, psychological, behavioral, environmental, and lifestyle factors, the practitioner must approach insomnia from a comprehensive perspective.

Beyond bringing the best of conventional and CAM approaches together, integrative medicine takes the following approach to understanding and managing insomnia: (1) it restores the place of subjectivity, as is evident in CBT-I; (2) it emphasizes the restoration of sleep health, as opposed to suppression of symptoms; (3) it acknowledges the important social and relational context of sleep; (4) it acknowledges the important role of natural rhythmic processes in life and health; and (5) it strongly emphasizes the role of lifestyle. An integrated approach to insomnia also calls for sensitive personalization of treatment based on a thorough evaluation.

Definitions

Insomnia disorder refers to difficulties with initiating or maintaining sleep, as well as nonrestorative sleep that is associated with excessive sleepiness or fatigue and with functional decrements for at least 4 weeks. Primary insomnia is not attributable to medical or psychiatric causes, whereas secondary insomnia has historically been viewed as a symptom of a primary disorder that would resolve with its treatment.[28] A National Institutes of Health (NIH) State of the Science Conference[5] recommended that secondary insomnia be considered *comorbid insomnia,* to encourage its direct treatment. Insomnia is frequently comorbid with other conditions, most commonly primary sleep disorders (Box 8-1), chronic pain syndromes, and psychiatric disorders, especially depression and substance abuse.

Etiology

The etiology of insomnia is commonly understood in terms of a "3 P" model,[37,38] consisting of predisposing, precipitating, and perpetuating factors. Predisposing factors comprise a broad range of biomedical, psychological, and lifestyle factors that increase the risk for developing insomnia. These include the following: (1) dependence on substances such as alcohol, caffeine, nicotine, and other drugs; (2) the long-term use of stimulant, sedating, or circadian rhythm–disrupting medications; (3) illnesses associated with nocturnal pain or discomfort; (4) primary sleep disorders such as restless legs syndrome, periodic limb movements in sleep, gastroesophageal reflux disease, and obstructive sleep apnea; and (5) circadian rhythm disorders associated with shift work, jet lag, and advanced or delayed sleep-phase syndromes.

Precipitating factors in insomnia commonly include stress associated with family, occupation, or health challenges. These factors are usually negative challenges such as divorce, death of a loved one, or illness, but they can also involve stress associated with positive events such as the birth of the child or retirement.[37,38]

Perpetuating factors in insomnia are a range of behaviors that are intended to manage or compensate for insomnia but inadvertently exacerbate it. Examples include the following: (1) excessive waking time spent in bed; (2) an irregular sleep-wake schedule including napping and dozing; (3) excessive use of caffeine, alcohol, and other drugs; and (4) anxiety associated with attempts at controlling sleep, as well as the daytime consequences of sleeplessness. Dependence, habituation, and rebound effects associated with sedative-hypnotics, ironically, appear to be major perpetuating factors in insomnia.

Spending excessive time in bed in attempts to sleep or compensate for lost sleep results in conditioned insomnia, a negative association of the bed with wakefulness.

> Conditioned insomnia is measured in terms of *sleep efficiency,* the ratio of total time spent asleep to the amount of time spent in bed. Sleep efficiency lower than 85% is considered problematic.[37,38]

Additional biomedical factors that can predispose to, precipitate, or perpetuate insomnia include iatrogenic influences of extended hospitalizations, as well as a broad range of medications that interfere with sleep such as analgesics, benzodiazepines, antidepressants, and anticholinergic medications. Beta blockers, calcium channel blockers, diuretics, and other medications may also suppress melatonin (MT) and interfere with sleep. Box 8-2 provides a more extensive listing of medications that can interfere with sleep.

Ordinary room light exposure before bedtime suppresses MT onset and duration in humans,[39] and it potentially disrupts circadian rhythms and sleep. Other sleep environmental

---

BOX 8-1. Comorbid Primary Sleep Disorders

- Restless legs syndrome (RLS)
- Periodic limb movements in sleep (PLMS)
- Gastroesophageal reflux disease (GERD)
- Sleep-phase disorders
- Narcolepsy
- Obstructive sleep apnea (OSA)
- Nocturia

BOX 8-2. Medications That Can Interfere With Deep or Rapid Eye Movement Sleep

- Alcohol
- Antiarrhythmics
- Anticonvulsants
- Antihistamines
- Appetite suppressants
- Benzodiazepines
- Bronchodilators
- Caffeine
- Carbidopa/levodopa
- Corticosteroids
- Diuretics
- Decongestants
- Estrogen
- Lipophilic beta blockers
- Monoamine oxidase inhibitors
- Nicotine
- Pseudoephedrine
- Selective serotonin reuptake inhibitors
- Sedatives
- Statins
- Sympathomimetics
- Tetrahydrozoline
- Thyroid hormones
- Tricyclic antidepressants

factors such as sound, temperature, and air and bedding quality also appear to predispose to, precipitate, or perpetuate insomnia, although these factors have not received the research attention they warrant.

Pathophysiology

The most compelling pathophysiologic model for insomnia suggests a strong association with chronic cognitive-emotional hyperarousal, which may be a premorbid characteristic of the disorder.[40-42] Compared with controls, patients with insomnia have elevated heart rates,[43,44] increased body and brain metabolic rates,[45,46] elevated core body temperature,[47] increased beta and gamma electroencephalographic features, and neuroendocrine dysregulation including elevated nighttime cortisol and decreased serum MT.[48-51] Insomnia has also been linked to nocturnal sympathetic activation and overactivation of the hypothalamic-pituitary-adrenal axis.[52,53]

> Chronic cognitive-emotional hyperarousal associated with elevated metabolic rate, sympathetic overactivation, and chronic inflammation is a common substrate of insomnia.

Insomnia appears to be bidirectionally associated with chronic inflammation. A single night of sleep deprivation in human subjects can alter cellular immune responses[54] and increase levels of inflammatory markers.[55-58] In contrast, inflammatory conditions have been shown to disrupt sleep by increasing pain, anxiety, and depression.[59,60] Chronic inflammation is fundamentally a process of immune system overactivation, which can be viewed as another expression of hyperarousal.

Sleepiness and sleep propensity appear to be strongly influenced by circadian core body temperature rhythms. Specific types of insomnia have been linked to specific patterns of body temperature rhythm disruption. Sleep onset difficulties have been associated with a delayed circadian temperature rhythm, early morning awakenings with an advanced circadian temperature rhythm, sleep maintenance insomnia with a nocturnally elevated core body temperature, and mixed insomnia with a 24-hour elevation of core body temperature, consistent with the hyperarousal model.[61]

Hyperarousal can be further elucidated by the widely accepted dual-process model of sleep regulation,[62] which views sleep in terms of a dynamic interaction between homeostatic and circadian processes. As the homeostatic sleep drive gradually increases through the waking day, the circadian pacemaker exerts an equal but opposite force to maintain alertness. The potential for sleep normally occurs with the nightly, rhythmic release of circadian alertness.

Although patients with insomnia are generally less sleepy during the day than normal sleepers, they appear to be significantly more fatigued (a construct independent of sleepiness).[63,64] Fatigue is very strongly associated with major depression.[65] Theoretically, fatigue, which draws one toward rest, and hyperarousal, which draws one toward activity, can result in a state of chronic isometric tension that characterizes the insomnia-depression complex. Suspended in a limbic zone between fatigue and hyperarousal, both a healthy descent into sleep and a passionate ascension into waking are inhibited.[66]

Anecdotal evidence strongly suggests that modern lifestyles are associated with widespread suppression of REM sleep. Excessive alcohol consumption, many sleep medications, and most psychiatric medications suppress REM sleep. Sleep maintenance insomnia, obstructive sleep apnea, and dream avoidance can further limit REM sleep and dreaming.[67]

Some human and animal studies confirmed that the selective deprivation of REM sleep results in its rebound in the form of reduced REM latency and disrupted deep sleep. The most common pattern of depression-related insomnia includes damaged REM sleep, most prominently reduced REM latency.[68] Could the classic psychodynamic notion that depression is "a loss of one's dreams" possibly have a literal underpinning?

> Hyperarousal may be understood as circadian alertness (wakefulness) that has gone awry and overrides both normal sleep drive and the excessive daytime sleepiness one would expect with chronic insomnia.

Evaluating Insomnia

The scope of the insomnia evaluation should be comprehensive, including any and all biomedical, psychological, and environmental factors potentially affecting sleep. Box 8-3 provides a list of essential clinical interview and history topics.

> Subjective measures, including the clinical interview and history, are the most critical components of the evaluation of insomnia.

The adage that as important as knowing which disease the patient has is knowing which patient has the disease is most pertinent here. It is critical to elicit each patient's personal sleep *and dream* story. Evidence from the study of bad

---

BOX 8-3. Clinical Interview and History

1. The presenting complaint
2. The sleep-wake routine
3. Daytime functioning and symptoms
4. Sleep conditions and routines
5. Previous treatment effects
6. Other sleep disorder symptoms
7. Comorbid medical conditions
8. Psychiatric conditions and stressors
9. Medication and substance use
10. Relevant family history

Adapted from Mai E, Buysse DJ. Insomnia: prevalence, impact, pathogenesis, differential diagnosis, and evaluation. *Sleep Med Clin.* 2008;3:167–174.

dreams and nightmares suggests that patients may respond to these dreams with sleep avoidant behaviors.[68] Eliciting the patient's basic posture toward sleep and dreams is a critical component of the insomnia evaluation. In addition to providing essential diagnostic information, doing so can engage the patient more deeply, strengthen the therapeutic alliance, and improve treatment adherence. The patient's story should be complemented with information gathered through personalized sleep logs or diaries, which should be recorded over a period of 1 to 2 weeks. Sleep logs and diaries (see Key Web Resources) provide data about sleep patterns, habits, and daytime effects, as well as related cognitive, affective, and behavior patterns. Interviewing available bed partners may also be helpful, to corroborate information about snoring and movement disorders.

Self-Report Scales

Self-report scales can be a useful adjunct to the interview for the general measurement of insomnia and specific assessment of sleepiness, fatigue, and hyperarousal. Self-report scales can be helpful in both the initial evaluation and treatment outcome measurements. The available empirically supported insomnia rating scales include the Pittsburgh Insomnia Rating Scale,[69] the Athens Insomnia Scale,[70] and the Bergen Insomnia Scale.[71] The Epworth Sleepiness Scale[72] is a brief, public domain questionnaire that provides an effective measure of current sleepiness (see Key Web Resources). Although the Epworth Sleepiness Scale is helpful as a screening device, it does not provide useful discriminative information for insomnia, although it may have value in screening for comorbid sleep apnea, narcolepsy, or other sleep disorders. Also in popular use, the Stanford Sleepiness Scale[73] offers sensitivity to patterns of daytime wakefulness. Finally, the Insomnia Severity Index[74] is a self-report scale that assesses insomnia type, severity, and impact on daily life.

Objective Measures

Polysomnography (PSG), as its name implies, measures multiple sleep parameters including indices of respiration, electroencephalography, and movement and muscle tone. Widely considered the gold standard of sleep evaluation, PSG is not, however, routinely indicated for insomnia because it provides little information useful for diagnosis or treatment.

PSG may be necessary to rule out periodic limb movements in sleep, obstructive sleep apnea, or other conditions underlying persistent insomnia.[75] With advances in remote monitoring technologies, home-based PSG is on the increase. Other home use devices such as actigraphy allow for longitudinal studies that can reveal useful information about circadian rhythms and other sleep parameters.[5]

Integrative Therapy

"The best cure for insomnia," said W.C. Fields, "is sleep." A common temptation among both patients and practitioners is to oversimplify the causes and treatment of insomnia. As suggested earlier, treatment of insomnia calls for lifestyle change. Promoting general health with proper nutrition, exercise, and psychological well-being provides an essential backdrop to the comprehensive integrative treatment of

insomnia. No magic bullets exist. Treatment usually requires a comprehensive, multicomponent approach that addresses all 3 P factors contributing to the noise of hyperarousal, including comorbid medical and psychiatric conditions. Ongoing monitoring and evaluation using subjective reports, as well as the Epworth Sleepiness Scale and the Fatigue Severity Scale , should be an integral part of treatment.

> If there is a secret to a good night's sleep, it is a good day's waking.

From the patient's perspective, interventions for insomnia can be classified in terms of two basic approaches: *taking something to sleep* and *letting go of something to sleep*. Patients who struggle with insomnia are inclined to consume sleeping medication, alcohol, warm milk, herbal teas, MT, botanicals, nutraceuticals, a wide range of comfort foods, and more. The fundamental belief underlying this approach is that insomnia results from *insufficient sleepiness* that can be ramped up with sleep-promoting ingestibles.

Sleep Promotion: Principles of Taking Something to Sleep

That good general health practices, including adequate exercise, good nutrition, and effective stress management, would promote healthy sleep is a safe assumption. When challenged by insomnia, conventional and CAM approaches offer an array of options for *taking something to sleep*.

Situations certainly exist (e.g., personal or medical crises) for which taking something to sleep may be indicated. Short-term use of a safe alternative will minimize the risk of dependence and of erosion of sleep self-efficacy. With the possible exception of MT, which regulates circadian rhythms, both conventional and alternative sleep aids do little to address the underlying noise of hyperarousal.

> Most chronic insomnia results not from insufficient sleepiness, but from excessive wakefulness. *Letting go of something to sleep* refers to an approach concerned with reducing the noise of this excessive wakefulness.

Pharmaceuticals

Epidemiologic studies suggest that over-the-counter antihistamines, alcohol, and prescription medications are the most common treatments used by patients with insomnia. Data suggesting that sedative-hypnotics can be effective in ameliorating insomnia raise serious questions about pharmaceutical industry influence and bias. At best, positive outcomes found are negligible, and harmful side effects are substantial.[76]

Box 8-4 provides a list of the most common U.S. Food and Drug Administration–approved and off-label medications used to treat insomnia. Long-term use of most of these medications is associated with serious side effects (Box 8-5). Studies raised concerns that the use of hypnotic agents may increase the risk of cancer.[77,78] Additional findings revealed a 10% to 15% increase in mortality among occasional users of sleeping pills and a 25% increase in mortality among nightly users of these drugs.[79]

BOX 8-4. Common Medications for Insomnia

Over-the-Counter Agents
- Diphenhydramine
- Doxylamine
- Benzodiazepines
- Estazolam
- Flurazepam
- Quazepam
- Temazepam
- Triazolam

Nonbenzodiazepine Hypnotics
- Eszopiclone
- Zaleplon
- Zolpidem
- Melatonin Receptor Agonists
- Ramelteon

Antidepressants (Tricyclic or Tetracyclic Antidepressants)
- Amitriptyline
- Doxepin
- Trazodone
- Mirtazapine

Other Agents
- Clonidine
- Gabapentin
- Quetiapine
- Sodium oxybate (gamma-hydroxybutyric acid sodium salt [GHB])

BOX 8-5. Common Side Effects of Sedative-Hypnotics

- Dependence
- Tolerance
- Damaged sleep architecture
- Diminished deep sleep
- Rapid eye movement suppression
- Parasomnias
- Anterograde amnesia
- Morning hangover
- Undermined self-efficacy
- Rebound insomnia with discontinuation
- Increased risk of falls
- Cognitive impairment
- Symptom suppression
- Increased mortality

In the end, most sleep medications do little more than temporarily suppress the neurophysiologic symptoms of hyperarousal—and they do so with risk.

Despite these concerns, an unprecedented surge has occurred in the use of sleeping medications since 2000.[80] In addition are growing concerns about substantial increases in related polypharmaceutical practices.[81] Why is this the case? This approach is driven by two faulty presumptions: (1) the common belief that insomnia is primarily the result of insufficient sleepiness, rather than excessive noise; and (2) a culture-wide, naive conceptualization of healthy sleep that equates it with a knockout.

Supplements

Numerous botanical sleep aids have been in use around the globe for centuries. In contrast to conventional sleep medications, CAM sleep aids, including botanical medicines as well as nutraceuticals, provide less of a knockout and more of a gentle assist to sleep with significantly fewer adverse effects. Although L-tryptophan and 5-hydroxytryptophan (5-HTP), precursors to serotonin and MT, are widely used, reports about the effectiveness of these agents in treating insomnia are mixed. Kava has empirical support for use with insomnia, but findings have raised serious questions about its safety.[82] More rigorous research into such alternatives has been hindered by limited financial incentives, conventional sleep medicine biases, and the natural complexity of many botanicals. Of the many alternatives to conventional sleep medications available, MT, valerian, and hops, reviewed in greater detail, are in common use and are generally regarded as safe.

Melatonin

Synthesized from tryptophan via 5-HTP and serotonin, MT is a neurohormone found in most living organisms. MT production is normally inhibited during the day by exposure to the blue wavelength of light and is disinhibited by dim light and darkness.[83] In addition to regulating circadian rhythms, MT mediates sleep and dreaming, decreases nocturnal body temperature, and has antiinflammatory, immune-modulating, and free-radical scavenging effects.[84] The suppression of endogenous MT through overexposure to light at night,[85–87] in advancing age,[88] and by common substances and medications (e.g., caffeine, nicotine, alcohol, beta blockers, diuretics, calcium channel blockers, and over-the-counter analgesics[89]) may be a factor in insomnia, depression, and cancer. A growing number of animal, human, and population studies suggest that MT may have oncostatic properties.[90,91] Tetrahydrocannabinol (THC) has been shown to cause a 400-fold increase in endogenous MT.[92] Other findings suggest that high doses of MT may actually disrupt sleep.[93] Anecdotal reports suggest that MT may heighten awareness of dreams. Doses as high as 50 mg can dramatically increase REM sleep and dreams. Certain psychoactive drugs, including cannabis and lysergic acid diethylamide(LSD), increase MT synthesis and may emulate MT activity in the waking state as a "waking dream."[94] Although an Agency for Healthcare Research and Quality report suggested that MT had limited effectiveness in treating insomnia,[95] a more recent meta-analysis of the effects of exogenous MT confirmed its beneficial effects on sleep onset latency, total sleep time, and sleep efficiency.[96]

■ Preparations

MT is available in oral, sublingual, and transdermal immediate or sustained-release formulations. Sublingual MT can avoid first-pass liver metabolism, thereby likely resulting in more reliable serum levels. Given its short half-life (approximately 0.5 to 2 hours) sustained-release forms are more likely to maintain effective levels throughout the sleep period.

■ Dosage
The dose is 0.3 to 0.5 mg for adults.[96]

■ Precautions
MT generally has a good safety profile. One meta-analysis found adverse effects uncommon and more likely with high doses.[97,98]

Valerian Root (Valeriana officinalis)
Valerian is a sedating botanical with purported anxiolytic and hypnotic properties. In contrast to prescription sedative-hypnotics, valerian does not impair psychomotor or cognitive performance.[99,100] One review concluded that valerian was safe but did not have significant effects on sleep.[101] A second study concluded that valerian appeared effective for mild to moderate insomnia.[102] Valerian is nonaddictive, resulting in no withdrawal symptoms on discontinuation. Valerian may sometimes require weeks of nightly use before producing an effect.[103]

■ Preparation
Valerian is available as whole powdered root and an aqueous or ethanolic extract standardized to 0.8% valerenic acids. High-quality products have an unpleasant odor, which confirms potency.

■ Dosage
For adults: 300 to 900 mg standardized extract of 0.8% valerenic acid or as a tea of 2 to 3 g of dried root steeped for 10 to 15 minutes and taken 30 to 120 minutes before bedtime for 2 to 4 weeks to assess effectiveness.

■ Precautions
Valerian has a good safety profile.[101] Possible herb-drug interactions can increase sedation or alter drug metabolism. Caution should be exercised during pregnancy or in patients with a history of liver disease.

Hops (Humulus lupulus)
Hops refers to the flower clusters atop the *Humulus lupulus*. Best known for its use in beer, hops has also been used in traditional preparations to treat a broad range of conditions, including insomnia. The German Commission E Monographs listed hops as an approved remedy for insomnia.[103] More recent findings showed a modest hypnotic effect for a valerian-hops combination for treating adult insomnia.[104] Hops is believed to have antispasmodic properties that can help reduce muscle tension and promote relaxation.[105] Additional evidence suggests that hops may be beneficial in alleviating hot flashes and other menopausal symptoms.[106]

■ Dosage
Prescribe 5:1 ethanolic extract, one-half to one dropper full, 30 to 60 minutes before bedtime.

■ Precautions
Although no evidence indicates toxicity in medicinal dosages, avoiding the use of hops in pregnancy may be advisable.

Noise Reduction Approach to Insomnia
The breadth of an integrative approach to insomnia treatment can overwhelm patients. Too often, the misguided temptation is to reduce sophisticated integrated strategies that support a shift in consciousness and lifestyle to a simple sleep hygiene checklist. The Noise Reduction Approach for Insomnia (NRAI)[107] provides a comprehensive and face valid framework for patients by organizing complex and numerous etiologic and therapeutic recommendations into an understandable and manageable system. More specifically, the NRAI uses a body, mind, and bed framework in which body refers to biomedical factors, mind refers to psychological factors, and bed refers to sleep environmental factors.

The NRAI conceptualizes healthy sleep in terms of a *sleepiness-to-noise ratio*, in which *sleepiness* refers to the propensity to sleep and *noise* refers to any kind of stimulation that interferes with sleep. Noise is used to denote the subjective experience of hyperarousal. Both sleepiness and noise can derive from body, mind, or bed factors. Insomnia can result from insufficient sleepiness caused by daytime sleep or dozing, inadequate activity, sedating medications, and circadian rhythm disorders. For the most part, however, insomnia results from excessive noise.

Noise resulting from body, mind, or bed factors is cumulative. For example, the stimulating effects of ordinary work stress or of 2 cups of coffee or minor reflux alone may not interfere with sleep, but their cumulative effect could well reach a threshold that does. Insomnia occurs when a person's noise levels exceed his or her sleepiness, whereas sleep occurs when noise levels fall to less than the threshold of sleepiness. Because the propensity to sleep is our natural default, the NRAI is less concerned with promoting sleepiness and more concerned with the identification and management of factors that produce noise.

Reducing Body Noise
The essential focus of body noise reduction is decreasing physiologic manifestations of hyperarousal. In addition to the importance of promoting basic health through exercise, nutrition, and stress management mentioned earlier, reducing body noise involves attending to a range of biomedical and lifestyle factors that commonly disrupt sleep. Box 8-6 summarizes the main components of reducing body noise.

Simultaneously addressing all comorbid disorders is essential. This is especially true for depression, primary sleep disorders, and disorders characterized by pain and discomfort. The reasonable assumption is that doing so may have a synergistic effect. For example, reducing pain will obviously improve sleep, but improving deep and REM sleep can raise pain thresholds by 60% and 200%, respectively.[108]

BOX 8-6. Reducing Body Noise

- Manage all comorbid conditions, especially other sleep disorders, depression, and chronic pain.
- Manage the sleep side effects of medications.
- Manage alcohol and caffeine use.
- Manage symptoms of women's health issues (e.g., premenstrual dysphoric disorder, menopause).

Managing the sleep disruptive side effects of medications (see Box 8-2) discussed earlier will help reduce body noise, as will managing caffeine and alcohol. Although considerable individual variation exists, the half-life of caffeine is approximately 5 hours and can range from 2 hours for tobacco smokers to more than 10 hours for women who are pregnant or using oral contraceptives. Consuming two 8-ounce cups of drip coffee within an hour of morning awakening will leave approximately 35 mg of caffeine, the amount found in a cola drink, in one's system near bedtime. "Energy drinks," which contain 2 to 500 mg of caffeine per serving, have soared in popularity. Because the depressant effects of alcohol can facilitate sleep onset, it is widely used as a sleep aid. Insomnia increases the risk of relapse in patients recovering from alcoholism.[109] Alcohol, especially if consumed without food or near bedtime, commonly compromises sleep quality and results in arousals early in the night.

Common women's health concerns, including premenstrual syndrome and premenstrual dysphoric disorder,[110] pregnancy,[111] and menopause,[112] are strongly linked to insomnia. These conditions and any associated insomnia are most effectively addressed independently. Additionally, MT may be helpful in managing premenstrual syndrome and premenstrual dysphoric disorder,[113,114] possibly through regulating rhythmic features of the disorder. Menopausal symptoms, particularly hot flashes, are commonly blamed for repeated awakenings. Disrupted sleep, however, is not an inevitable consequence of hot flashes.[115]

> Menopausal symptoms likely function as precipitating factors of insomnia for women who were previously predisposed to it.

Reducing Mind Noise
The essential focus of mind noise reduction is decreasing psychological and behavioral expressions of hyperarousal. This approach is largely centered on the CBT-I set of strategies. CBT-I combines cognitive restructuring, which addresses insomnia-related dysfunctional thoughts and beliefs, with behavioral interventions including sleep hygiene education, stimulus control therapy (SCT), sleep restriction therapy (SRT), and relaxation practices. CBT-I also addresses common maladaptive coping reactions to insomnia that function as perpetuating factors. In addition to the treatment of individuals, CBT-I can be used in group settings, as well as through automated and Web-based formats. Box 8-7 provides a list of mind noise reduction therapies. This list primarily contains CBT-I components, but it is expanded to include dream health, which is not typically addressed in conventional treatment.

Compelling evidence indicates the effectiveness of CBT-I for primary insomnia,[5,116,117] and support for CBT-I in comorbid insomnia is growing.[22] CBT-I was shown to be at least as effective as prescription medications in the short-term treatment of chronic insomnia, with beneficial effects that extended well beyond the completion of treatment and no evidence of adverse effects.[118] Patients with insomnia who were treated with CBT-I experienced greater increases in deep sleep and decreases in wake time than those treated with zopiclone (Canadian hypnotic similar to eszopiclone). These benefits were still present at a 6-month follow-up, in contrast to patients treated with zopiclone, who showed no ongoing benefits of treatment.[119] CBT-I alone was also found to be no less effective than CBT-I paired with zolpidem.[120] CBT-I has also been shown to enhance depression outcomes for patients with comorbid insomnia.[121]

Sleep Hygiene
Sleep hygiene refers to a list of various behavioral and environmental recommendations that promote healthy sleep.[122] These can include most of the suggestions reviewed earlier, such as managing substances, regulating one's sleep-wake schedule, obtaining exercise, and creating an environment conducive to sleep. Sleep hygiene has not been demonstrated effective as a stand-alone intervention, although most sleep specialists believe that it can be an effective aid to a multicomponent treatment approach.

Cognitive Restructuring
Cognitive restructuring techniques systematically review, reconsider, and replace thoughts and beliefs that trigger sleep disruptive anxiety and rumination. Box 8-8 provides examples of common dysfunctional thoughts about sleep. These thoughts are dysfunctional because they distort the truth, set up unrealistic expectations, and inevitably trigger anxiety. For example, the belief that "I can and must get myself to sleep" is nearly ubiquitous among patients with insomnia. Because it implies that falling asleep is under one's conscious control, this belief leads to excessive sleep effort, which then backfires by increasing arousal. Similarly, the common belief that "I should always sleep through the night" sets the stage for a reflexive reaction of frustration, disappointment, and even self-recrimination with wakefulness after sleep onset. In reality, what wakes one up is not necessarily what keeps one awake. Frequently, our strong reaction to the awakening, which is based on a dysfunctional belief, is the real problem. Similar cycles of disappointment, frustration, arousal, and anxiety can ensue from comparable dysfunctional thoughts and beliefs, and their effects can be cumulative.

BOX 8-7. Mind Noise Reduction (Cognitive-Behavioral Therapy for Insomnia)

- Sleep hygiene education
- Cognitive restructuring
- Stimulus control therapy
- Sleep restriction therapy
- Relaxation practices
- Restoring dream health

BOX 8-8. Dysfunctional Thoughts About Sleep

- I should sleep at least 8 hours every night.
- I should fall asleep quickly.
- I should always sleep through the night.
- I can and must get myself to sleep.
- I should just rest in bed if I cannot sleep.
- I will have a terrible day if I do not sleep well.

BOX 8-9. Stimulus Control Therapy Instructions

1. Get into bed with the intention to sleep only when sleepy.
2. Use the bed and bedroom only for sleep and sexual activity.
3. Do not watch the clock.
4. If awake after approximately 15 minutes, leave the bedroom, engage in restful activity, and return to bed when sleepy. Repeat as needed.
5. Keep a fixed morning rising time irrespective of the amount of sleep obtained.
6. Avoid napping until nighttime sleep is normal.

■ Stimulus Control and Sleep Restriction Therapies

Both SCT and SRT are effective behavioral interventions for managing conditioned insomnia and reducing sleep efficiency.[123,124] Both approaches systematically minimize the amount of waking time spent in bed in an effort to increase sleep efficiency. SCT does so through self-monitoring and staying out of bed when sleepless. Box 8-9 provides basic SCT instructions.

SRT requires patients to limit the amount of time in bed to their average total sleep time established at baseline. Time in bed is then gradually increased as sleep efficiency improves. The administration of SRT is challenging to both patients and clinicians and should be used only by professionals trained in this intervention. Both SCT and SRT may be contraindicated in patients with sleep apnea, mania, epilepsy, and parasomnias and those at risk of falling.

■ Relaxation Practices

Relaxation practices, which have been included under the rubric of CBT-I, are useful in reducing sympathetic tone, decreasing mind noise, and familiarizing patients with the waking state of rest that serves as a transition to sleep. A myriad of effective techniques are available (Box 8-10), and they should be matched to patients' interests and personalities. Breathing exercises are among the easiest and most portable practices.[125] Early research combining mindfulness meditation and CBT-I showed a reduction of sleep-related arousals.[126]

■ Restoring Dream Health

In contrast to conventional approaches, integrative therapies for insomnia are concerned with the restoration of dream health. From antiquity through recent times, dreams have

---

BOX 8-10. Relaxation Practices

- Breathing exercises
- Mindfulness meditation
- Progressive muscular relaxation
- Gentle yoga/yoga nidra
- Self-hypnosis
- Guided imagery
- Biofeedback and neurofeedback
- Transcranial stimulation

BOX 8-11. Promoting Healthy Dreaming

- Identify and manage dream thieves.
- Arise slowly in the morning to enhance recall.
- Journal or talk about dreams.
- Join a dream circle or support group.
- Note dreamlike aspects of waking life.

---

been revered as rich sources of psychological insight, healing, and spirituality. Healthy REM sleep and dreaming are critical to the consolidation of procedural memory, as well as to the processing of emotion.[127]

Trying to promote healthy sleep without considering dreams is like trying to promote healthy nutrition without regard for the taste of food.

Given the frequency of bad dreams and the common belief that high-quality sleep is devoid of dreaming, it is not surprising when patients with insomnia state that they would prefer not to dream at all. Dream avoidance, evident in Hamlet's classic remark, "To sleep perchance to dream...," is clearly seen in patients with frequent nightmares and can result in sleep avoidance and arousals.[68]

Box 8-11 offers recommendations for promoting healthy dreaming. Simply asking patients whether they have dream recall can be an essential first step in sensitizing them to the importance of dreaming. In addition to avoiding dream thieves—REM-suppressant drugs, substances, and activities—it may be useful intentionally to recall and attend to one's dreams.[128] Because we usually awaken from dreams, arising slowly in the morning with a receptive attitude can improve recall. Bridging dream experiences to waking life through journaling, discussion, and noting the "waking dream," dreamlike aspects of ordinary waking life, can also be helpful.

Reducing Bed Noise

Although the sleep environment can have a critical impact on sleep, it has not yet received the attention it warrants. Recognizing the bedroom as not only a physical location, but also a temporal and psychological space, the goals of bed noise reduction include (1) minimizing the toxic burden of the physical environment, (2) regulating circadian rhythms through entrainment with light and darkness, and (3) creating a sense of sanctuary that is free of ordinary waking life stimulation.

■ A Healthy Sleep Environment

Sensitivities or allergies to bedroom irritants or toxins can be pronounced or subtle. Awareness is increasing, as reflected in the growth of the natural mattress industry, of the importance of an environmentally friendly and toxin-free bedroom. In addition to recommendations to keep the bedroom quiet and cool (no hotter than 68 °F), compelling arguments have been made on behalf of "green" (organic) beds and bedding and clean bedroom air.[128,129] Box 8-12 lists common sources of bedroom toxicity that should be evaluated and addressed to improve sleep. Bedroom air quality can be improved with

BOX 8-12. Common Sources of Bedroom Toxicity

- Pesticide-laden fabrics in bed and bedding
- Synthetic materials in mattresses and pillows
- Outgassing from furnishings, floors, walls, or carpeting
- Polluted indoor air
- Electromagnetic fields

BOX 8-13. Regulating Circadian Rhythms

- Use phototherapy, with timed exposure to light and darkness.
- Maintain a regular sleep-wake pattern.
- Simulate dusk by dimming the lights or using blue blocker technology 1 to 2 hours before sleep.
- Supplement with melatonin.
- Sleep in total darkness.

BOX 8-14. Creating a Sense of Sanctuary

- Establish the bedroom as a stress-free and work-free zone.
- Limit exposure to stressful imagery from books, television, and radio.
- Conceal ready access to clocks.
- Establish a sense of personal safety.
- Maintain peace with your sleep partner.

high-efficiency particulate air (HEPA) filtration systems as well as with varieties of ordinary houseplants. Because electromagnetic fields can suppress endogenous MT,[130] it is advisable to clear them from the sleep area.

Regulation of Circadian Rhythms

Time can be conceptualized in two distinct ways. Ordinary waking life is structured by linear or clock time. Human biology, however, including sleep-wake cycles, operates on cyclic time, most evident in circadian rhythms. Nature's darkness may invite us to sleep, whereas culture, with its vast array of evening distractions, encourages us to stay awake.[70]

> Sleep disorders, in part, are chronic skirmishes between nature and culture—between linear and cyclic time.

A factor that regulates circadian rhythms is called a Zeitgeber (from the German: "time giver"). Such factors include temporal patterns of feeding, exercise, and socialization, although the most potent ones are exposure to light and darkness. Bright light signals the start of morning, whereas dim light or darkness conveys a sense of night to the brain's circadian pacemaker. Sleep-phase disorders, most commonly advanced or delayed sleep-phase syndromes, are frequent predisposing factors in the origin of insomnia. These disorders are usually treated by systematically manipulating exposure to light and darkness to restructure the position of the patient's sleep phase within the circadian cycle.

Regulating circadian rhythms (Box 8-13) is a critical component of treating insomnia. Maintaining a regular sleep-wake pattern 7 days per week is essential to promoting a healthy sleep rhythm. Bright light exposure for approximately 30 to 45 minutes shortly after morning arising is a most potent Zeitgeber,[131] as well as a potential antidepressant.[132] When natural light is not an option, light boxes that provide comparable lux levels are commercially available. Exposure to higher lux levels of natural light throughout the waking day may also reduce daytime sleepiness.[133]

Given the relentless demands of daily living, dusk simulation practices—dimming lights for 2 to 3 hours before bedtime—are particularly challenging. Dim light diminishes the blue wavelength of light prominent in natural daylight, artificial lighting, and computer and television screens. The blue wavelength of light has been shown to signal the brain to suppress MT production, thus delaying the start of the sleep phase.[134] Newer blue light filtration technology in the form of goggles and light bulbs can provide illumination without

suppressing MT (see Key Web Resources) and can minimize the negative impact of reading or watching television.

> Because even small amounts of light can trickle across closed eyelids and suppress melatonin, sleeping in total darkness or with a sleep mask is ideal.

Creating a Sense of Sanctuary

For many who struggle with insomnia, the bedroom is a place of work, entertainment, and other associations that may be antagonistic to sleep. Reimagining the bedroom as a sanctuary (Box 8-14), a place of retreat from the world of waking, is helpful. To do so, the bedroom should be a work-free, stress-free, and clock-free zone. Exposure to stressful imagery from reading material, television, or radio should be avoided. Clock watching is a common compulsion among patients with insomnia and serves only to exacerbate sleeplessness by tethering them to the waking world of linear time. Establishing a deep sense of personal or psychological safety in the bedroom is also important. For some patients, this may mean installing a security system, whereas for others it may mean keeping a religious icon on the bed stand.

The percentage of couples sleeping apart, largely as a result of sleep disorders, has increased dramatically and now stands at 23%.[135] Sleeping apart is associated with negative effects on the relationship.[136] Addressing sleep symptoms (e.g., snoring or periodic limb movements in sleep) that may provoke one's sleep partner is helpful. Differing sleep environment preferences can also be negotiated. Creating a sense of sanctuary in the bedroom encourages an essential shift from waking to *night consciousness*.[70]

> Fundamentally, insomnia is associated with inadvertently smuggling waking consciousness into the world of night and sleep.

Behavioral Sleep Medicine Specialists

Although some components of CBT-I can be implemented by patients on their own, this complex therapy generally requires levels of specialized training. The stepped care model for CBT-I recommends a hierarchy of five increasing levels of interventions associated with clinician expertise and patients' needs (Fig. 8-1). Behavioral sleep medicine specialists, formally trained and certified in the use of CBT-I, are a small but steadily growing and key professional resource in this model (see Key Web Resources).

Spirituality

Sleep has historically been viewed as a deeply personal and even spiritual experience.[70] World sacred traditions have typically viewed dreaming as a portal to spirituality. Some traditions have established elaborate spiritual practices around sleep and dreams. One of the central themes found in spiritual perspectives of sleep is an emphasis on the need to let go or surrender to sleep. At their core, most CBT-I techniques reflect sensitivity to this central process of letting go. With this recognition, the place of a personal evening ritual in healing insomnia becomes evident. The many recommendations commonly offered the patient with insomnia can be best organized and implemented in the context of such ritual. Slowing down, dimming the lights, practicing relaxation techniques, journaling with a cup of soporific tea, and surrendering to sleep are much more than clinical recommendations. They are practices that will facilitate a shift not only in lifestyle, but also in consciousness.

PREVENTION PRESCRIPTION

Preventing insomnia by intentionally maintaining healthy sleep is considerably less daunting than treating it.
- Recognize the value and joy of sleep.
- Attend to and journal dreams.
- Engage in relaxation practices daily.
- Obtain adequate regular exercise.
- Obtain daily exposure to morning light.
- Limit the use of stimulants and sedatives.
- Maintain a regular sleep-wake schedule.
- Dim lights or use blue blocker tools 1 to 2 hours before sleep.
- Sleep in total darkness or use a sleep mask.
- Consider low-dose melatonin replacement therapy.

FIGURE 8-1
A stepped care model for cognitive-behavioral therapy for insomnia (CBT-I). This evidence-based model for CBT illustrates how patients may be allocated to resources. *Arrows* represent referral movements. BSM, behavioral sleep medicine. (From Espie CA. "Stepped care": a health technology solution for delivering cognitive behavioral therapy as a first line insomnia treatment. *Sleep.* 2009;32:1549–1558.)

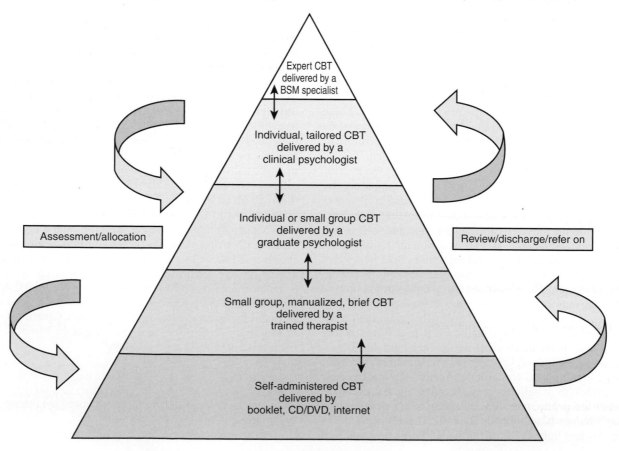

THERAPEUTIC REVIEW

■ Reduce Body Noise

- Directly address all comorbid conditions, especially primary sleep disorders, depression, chronic pain, and women's health issues. Evaluate and manage sleep side effects of all medications (see Box 8-2). Evaluate and manage alcohol, caffeine, and other stimulant use.   B / 1

- Melatonin: 0.3 to 0.5 mg at bedtime, especially if the patient may have an associated circadian rhythm disorder   A ↑ 1

- Avoid sedative-hypnotics , and use complementary and alternative medicine sleep aids as needed, preferably on a short-term (2- to 4-week) basis. Consider one or a combination of the following: A / 2

  - Valerian, for adults: 300 to 900 mg standardized extract of 0.8% valerenic acid or as a tea of 2 to 3 g of dried root steeped for 10 to 15 minutes and taken 30 to 120 minutes before bedtime for 2 to 4 weeks to assess effectiveness   B → 2

  - Hops: in a 5:1 ethanolic extract, ½ to 1 dropper full, 30 to 60 minutes before bedtime   C → 1

■ Reduce Mind Noise

- Encourage patients to select and engage in a daily relaxation practice. The 4-7-8 relaxing breath exercise (Box 8-15) is an easy and effective option.   A ↑ 1

- Use stimulus control therapy for sleep efficiency lower than 85%.   A ↑ 1

- Evaluate and discuss basic dysfunctional beliefs and thoughts about sleep. Refer the patient to a behavioral sleep medicine specialist for more elaborate cognitive restructuring therapy as needed.   A ↑ 1

BOX 8-15. 4:7:8 Relaxing Breath Exercise

1. Place the tip of your tongue against the ridge behind your front teeth and exhale completely through your mouth.
2. Inhale through your nose for a count of 4.
3. Hold your breath for a count of 7.
4. Exhale through your mouth with a swooshing sound to the count of 8.
5. Repeat this cycle three more times for a total of four breaths.
   The ratio of 4:7:8 is key, not the actual time spent on each breath cycle. Practice at least twice daily, beginning with no more than four breath cycles at one time for the first month and increasing to eight breath cycles afterward if desired. This exercise can be used to increase presleep relaxation and to facilitate sleep onset in bed.

- Encourage dream recall by limiting "dream thieves," and promote daily dream journaling and participation in dream support groups. Refer patients with chronic nightmares to a behavioral sleep specialist for image rehearsal therapy.   A ↑ 1

■ Reduce Bed Noise

- Recommend reduction of bedroom toxicity from beds, bedding, and furnishings, as well as air filtration with high-efficiency particulate air (HEPA) filters or houseplants. Encourage evaluation of and protection from electromagnetic fields.   C → 1

- Urge the patient to maintain a regular sleep-wake schedule, including on weekends. The patient should simulate dusk by dimming lights or using blue blocker technology (see Key Web Resources) 1 to 2 hours before sleep, and sleep in total darkness. Exposure to morning light is important.   B / 1

- Encourage patients to create a sense of sanctuary by establishing the bedroom as a stress-free and work-free zone, limiting exposure to stressful imagery and clocks, ensuring a sense of personal safety, and maintaining peace with bed partners.   C → 1

KEY WEB RESOURCES

American Academy of Sleep Medicine: http://www.aasmnet.org/	This Web site provides professional information and resources for sleep medicine.
Society of Behavioral Sleep Medicine: http://www.behavioralsleep.org/	This official Web site includes links to lists of certified behavioral sleep medicine specialists.
Epworth Sleepiness Scale: http://epworthsleepinessscale.com/	This official Web site provides an overview of and access to the Epworth Sleepiness Scale.
Fatigue Severity Scale: http://www.medscape.org/viewarticle/472869	This Medscape Web site provides information about fatigue and the Fatigue Severity Scale.
Sleep diary forms: http://www.sleepeducation.com/pdf/sleepdiary.pdf or http://sleep.buffalo.edu/sleepdiary.pdf	These documents assist patients in collecting and monitoring data essential for initial and ongoing evaluation.

The Dark Side of Sleeping Pills: http://www.darksideofsleepingpills. com/all.html

Dr. Daniel Kripke's complementary e-book discusses the risks of sedative-hypnotics.

Low Blue Lights: https://www.lowbluelights.com/index.asp

This commercial Web site provides information, research, and products related to blue light filtering technology.

SHUTi (Sleep Health Using the Internet): http://www.shuti.net/

This is an automated Web-based program of cognitive-behavioral therapy for insomnia that was developed by the University of Virginia.

Dr. R. Naiman: http://www.drnaiman.com/

This Web site promotes the development of integrative sleep medicine.

References

References are available online at expertconsult.com.

Section II Neurology

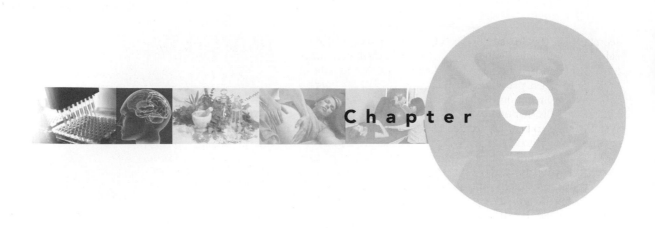

Chapter 9

Alzheimer Disease

Dharma Singh Khalsa, MD

Renowned gerontologist Ken Dychtwald, PhD,[1] has stated, "It's easy to overlook the remarkableness of aging." According to Dychtwald, throughout 99% of human history, the average life expectancy at birth was less than 18 years of age. In the past, people did not age; they died. Infectious diseases, accidents, violence, and other hazards often brought life to an early close. Until very recently, therefore, people were much more likely to die young than to live into old age.

Beginning in the last century, however, something unprecedented happened. Thanks to advances in sanitation, public health, food science, pharmacy, surgery, medicine, and, more recently, wellness-oriented lifestyles, the number of people in the United States who were more than 65 years old multiplied 11-fold during the twentieth century, from 3 million to 33 million. According to the U.S. Bureau of the Census, by the year 2035 some 70 million people—60 million of whom will be older baby boomers—will be 65 years old and older. Although we should applaud the increase in life span enjoyed by many people, a major problem is associated with it: with increasing longevity comes an increasing incidence of cognitive decline, dementia, and Alzheimer disease (AD).[2]

In 2009, 5.3 million people had AD in the United States. The costs were $148 billion a year, and more than 9.9 million people were unpaid caregivers. The 2010 report showed these figures to be increased to $172 billion in costs and 10.9 million unpaid caregivers. AD was the sixth leading cause of death in 2009, although more recently it was reported to be the seventh.

More telling however, is that AD is now the number one worry of aging baby boomers, thus surpassing cancer and heart disease. The integrative medical model is based on good science and good sense. Conventionalists, who focus narrowly on this gene or that neurotransmitter or a plaque or tangle, often overlook the fact that the brain is a flesh-and-blood organ. Because the brain is flesh and blood, like the heart, for example, it responds to health-promoting interventions such as improved blood flow, good nutrition, stress reduction, and exercise. An integrative approach brings surviving neurons to their optimal potential; therefore, using it can reverse many of the symptoms of AD and slow its progression.

Like many degenerative diseases associated with aging, memory loss spans a spectrum of signs, symptoms, causes, pathogenesis, and prognosis. Although the term memory loss does not imply a specific cause, it signifies a clinical syndrome characterized by the acquired loss of cognitive and emotional abilities that is severe enough to interfere with daily functioning and quality of life.

Pathophysiology

The term age-associated memory impairment was initially used to describe the minor memory difficulties that were previously believed to accompany the aging process. This impairment is now known to exist in patients as young as 50 years of age. An at-risk population with both subjective cognitive impairment (SCI) and mild cognitive impairment (MCI) that converts to AD at a rate of approximately 12% per year has been identified and is discussed later in the chapter.[3] Moreover, Lupien et al[4] noted a conversion to AD in subjects with cortisol-induced, stress-related memory loss. This chapter includes this emerging etiology for cognitive dysfunction in the discussion on chronic stress. Neuroscientists now agree that memory loss is a disease that begins to attack the brain 30 to 40 years before symptoms appear. Snowden et al[5] showed that nuns who displayed linguistic difficulties in their 20s had a higher incidence of AD later in life. Using positron emission tomographic scans, Reimen et al[6] noted that patients can have lesions consistent with severe cognitive decline years before symptoms are seen. It is becoming increasingly clear that AD is an insidious process similar to other chronic diseases such as heart disease, and therefore AD has lifestyle management implications.

Plaques or Tangles?

For a century, scientists have wondered which of the brain lesions associated with AD are more important—the plaques that litter the empty spaces between nerve cells or the stringy tangles that erupt from within the cell. An enzyme called secretase on the surface of the brain cell makes a protein called beta amyloid. Patients with AD have too much amyloid, which forms the so-called plaques on the outside of brain cells. These plaques grow so dense that they trigger an inflammatory reaction from the brain's immune system that kills nerve cells. Among the powerful weapons the immune system brings to bear are oxygen free radicals, and this helps explain why antioxidants such as vitamin E are helpful.

A strong piece of evidence supporting the beta amyloid theory is that significant numbers of mice genetically engineered to develop plaques remained plaque free compared with controls after vaccination with a fragment of beta amyloid. Researchers then vaccinated 1-year-old mice whose brains were riddled with plaques. These mice became plaque free. Unfortunately, this vaccine has not been successful in tests on humans.

The second major school of thought among neuroscientists concerns tau, a molecule that acts much like the ties on a railroad track. Tau assembles microtubules that support the structure of the nerve cell. Chemical changes in the nerve cell cause the tau molecules to change shape so that they no longer hold the microtubule in place. The "railroad ties" begin to twist and tangle, causing neuronal cell death.

Many questions remain. Are the plaques and tangles seen in AD causative or simply tombstones? Does some still unknown biochemical event precede the formation of plaques and tangles and cause the inflammatory death knell? AD, no less than heart disease, certainly has multiple causes. As in aging itself, risk factors affect the development of AD. This means that lifestyle choices, especially relating to stress management, are critically important.

Risk Factors for Memory Loss

Hard Risk Factors

- *Increased age:* This is the most important risk factor. Ten percent of persons 65 years old develop AD. The incidence at age 85 years is as high as 50%.

- *Family history:* The risk of developing AD is increased threefold to fourfold if a first-degree relative has the disease.

- *Genetic factors:* Individuals with two *APOE4* genes on chromosome 19 are at least eight times more likely to develop AD. Gatz et al[7] noted that the *APOE4* gene exerts its maximal effect on people in their 60s and is a strong predictor of AD. The *APOE4* gene is also a strong predictor for heart disease. More recently, investigators have revealed that people with two *APOE4* genes begin developing cognitive decline perhaps as early as in their 20s.

- *Head injury:* AD risk doubles in patients who have suffered traumatic brain injuries early in life. Moderate head injury increases the risk of AD by two to three times, whereas severe head injury more than quadruples the risk of dementia.

- *Gender:* Because women have longer life spans than men, they have a higher incidence of AD. Lower estrogen levels may also play an important role in AD.[8]

- *Educational level:* The risk of developing AD decreases with the number of years of formal education. This finding highlights research suggesting that mental activity throughout life is neuroprotective.[9]

Warning signs of AD are shown in Table 9-1.

TABLE 9-1. Warning Signs of Alzheimer Disease

- Recent memory loss that affects job skill
- Difficulty performing familiar tasks
- Problems with language
- Disorientation to time and space
- Poor or decreased judgment
- Problems with abstract thinking
- Misplacement of important objects
- Changes in mood or behavior
- Changes in personality
- Loss of initiative

Lifestyle Risk Factors
Subjective Cognitive Impairment

Many specialists treating neurologic diseases once thought that complaints of benign senescent forgetfulness were insignificant because this condition had no potential to progress to true AD. However, a newer study revealed that, over a 7-year period, healthy adults who reported having the feeling that their memory was not functioning as well as it should progressed to MCI and AD at a higher rate than did those without SCI.[10]

In the study, researchers found that SCI in older persons without manifestation of symptoms is a common condition with a largely unclear prognosis. Patients were followed over a sufficient period by using conversion to MCI or to dementia to clarify SCI prognosis and determine whether the prognosis of patients with SCI would differ from that of demographically matched healthy subjects with no cognitive impairment (NCI).[10]

A consecutive series of healthy subjects, 40 years old or older, presenting with NCI or SCI to a brain aging and dementia research center during a 14-year interval, was studied and followed up during an 18-year observation window. The study population (60 NCI, 200 SCI, 60% female) had a mean age of 67.2 ± 9.1 years, was well educated (mean, 15.5 ± 2.7 years), and was cognitively normal based on scores of the Mini-Mental State Examination (MMSE 29.1 ± 1.2).[10]

In this study, 213 subjects were followed up over a mean period of 6.8 ± 3.4 years, and subjects had a mean of 2.9 ± 1.6 follow-up visits. Seven NCI (14.9%) and 90 SCI (54.2%) subjects had a decline in their cognitive function. Of NCI decliners, 5 declined to MCI, and 2 to probable AD. Of the 90 SCI decliners, 71 declined to MCI, and 19 to AD. Controlling for baseline demographic variables and follow-up time, SCI subjects had a higher likelihood of decline and declined more rapidly. The study also showed that mean time to decline was 3.5 years longer for NCI than for SCI subjects.[10]

Crucially, these results suggested that SCI in subjects with normal cognition was a possible indication of future decline in most subjects during a 7-year follow-up interval. Relevance for community populations and prevention studies in this at-risk population should be explored further.

Mild Cognitive Impairment

MCI is characterized primarily by recent memory loss. This is the transitional state from normal aging to SCI and dementia. People with MCI are at an increased risk of developing AD, at a rate of 12% to 15% per year. Symptoms of

MCI are distinguished from normal aging by recent memory loss. For example, people with MCI suffer frequently from forgetfulness and may visibly have difficulty learning new information and recalling previously learned information. The primary distinction between people with MCI and those with AD appears to be in the areas of cognition outside of memory. Unlike people with AD, those with MCI are able to function normally in daily activities requiring other cognitive abilities such as thinking, understanding, and decision making.[11]

■ Stress and the Brain

Stress is represented by a bell-shaped curve, with demand on the horizontal axis and performance on the vertical axis. As depicted on the graph, when a person's ability to perform is exceeded by the demand, stress ensues. At some point, however, a person's ability to perform is exceeded by the demand placed on him or her. That is when the chronic stress reaction comes into play, with the release of cortisol from the adrenal glands. Cortisol then flows throughout the bloodstream and has been shown to kill brain cells in the memory center of the brain, known as the hippocampus. Cortisol also suppresses immune system function.

Cortisol produces memory dysfunction by the following means:

1. Preventing the uptake of glucose by the hippocampus
2. Inhibiting synaptic transmission
3. Causing neuron injury and cellular death.[12]

For those skeptical about this notion, one simply has to look at the title of the book written by eminent brain researcher Professor Robert Sapolsky from Stanford University: *Stress, the Aging Brain, and the Mechanisms of Neuron Death*.[13] Beyond that, McEwen and Sapolsky, in their landmark article "Stress and Cognitive Function,"[14] also showed evidence suggesting that the glucocorticoid cortisol has a direct effect on synaptic plasticity and dendritic structures. Additionally, according to McEwen and Sapolsky, prolonged exposure to stress leads to loss of neurons, particularly in the hippocampus. Moreover, Stein-Behrins and Sapolsky, in their landmark article, "Stress, Glucocorticoids, and Aging,"[12] revealed that illness and aging are a time of decreased ability to handle stress.

As one reaches beyond the age of 46 up to more than 55 years, the amount of cortisol in the blood during chronic stress becomes elevated and drops more slowly. Part of the reason for this is that cortisol kills the same brain cells in the hippocampus that are responsible for the negative feedback loop in shutting off the release of cortisol from the adrenal glands in the first place. The mechanism of which Sapolsky wrote has been delineated in that the neurotoxic excitatory amino acid glutamate is usually taken up by the glial cells. With chronic stress, however, excess cortisol blocks this uptake by the glial cells in the synaptic cleft. High levels of free glutamate in the synapse therefore activate the N-methyl-D-aspartate (NMDA) receptors and cause an influx of calcium into the postsynaptic neuron. In addition, glutamate activation of the NMDA receptor blocks calcium efflux out of the postsynaptic neuron.[15] This excessive synaptic neuron calcium leads to free radical damage, inflammation, and cell death. Lupien et al[4] revealed that hippocampal volume was inversely related to cortisol levels in the serum.

Other work has revealed the effects of cortisol and stress on the development of dementia. For example, Crow et al[16] showed that greater reactivity to stress predicted a higher risk of dementia in individuals who reported a high incidence of work-related stress. The risk was not the work-related stress itself, but how the individual reacted to that stress. This 30-year longitudinal study included more than 2000 people. In addition, Newcomer et al[17] showed decreased memory performance in healthy humans who were injected with stress levels of cortisol intravenously. Wilson et al[18] revealed that unbalanced stress doubled the risk of AD. Moreover, Peavy et al[19] unveiled that stress produced more reactivity and higher levels of cortisol, with subsequent worse effects on memory function in older individuals who were *ApoE4* positive and therefore at greater risk for the development of AD.

More recently, work by Choi et al[20] at the University of California, Los Angeles (UCLA) School of Medicine revealed a reduction in telomerase activity in human T lymphocytes exposed to cortisol. This finding is significant because reduction in telomerase activity means that the telomeres in the DNA shortened precipitously, and shortened telomeres thereby accelerate aging and illness. This finding is especially important because the work of Lukens et al[21] showed that telomere length in peripheral blood was diminished in individuals with AD.

To summarize, chronic, unbalanced stress causes excessive cortisol release from the adrenal gland into the bloodstream. This cortisol then travels to the hippocampus, where it causes brain cell death and shuts off the inhibition of production of further cortisol from the adrenal gland. This excess of cortisol not only causes inflammation and hippocampal neuronal cell death, but also has an accelerated aging effect by decreasing telomere length in the stressed individual. Shortened telomeres may lead to accelerated aging, inflammation, cardiovascular disease, cancer, and AD.

Diagnosis

1. Patient history: Family history is important because of the correlation between AD in patients and their first-degree relatives. A personal history of illnesses, especially cardiovascular disease, and metabolic disorders such as diabetes mellitus is also useful. Other areas of concern include medication usage and a history of head trauma. In general, the diagnosis of MCI can be made if an individual has a memory complaint and an abnormal memory for his or her age and education. Moreover, the person demonstrates normal activities of daily living and a normal level of general cognitive function. The patient with MCI is not demented.
2. Cognitive assessment: I have found the MMSE to be valuable in an office setting. This test offers a relatively rapid and reliable means of assessing cognitive function, memory, and visual-spatial skills (Fig. 9-1). Individuals with low levels of education, however, tend to do more poorly on the test, independent of any effects of cognitive function. Moreover, the test is less sensitive in individuals with higher educational levels; they may have a normal score on the MMSE yet have early signs of dementia. Repeated MMSE testing offers a good means of tracking disease progression and monitoring the effects of treatment.

FIGURE 9-1
Mini-Mental State Examination.

One point for each answer.

1. Orientation

	Correct	Incorrect
What is the year we are in?	1	0
What season is it?	1	0
What is today's date?	1	0
What day of the week is today?	1	0
What month are we in?	1	0
What state are we in?	1	0
What country are we in?	1	0
What town are we in?	1	0
Can you tell me the name of this place?	1	0
What floor of the building are we on?	1	0

Subtotal Correct. [ ]

2. Registration

Ask the patient if you may test his/her memory. Then say the names of 3 unrelated objects, clearly and slowly, about one second for each. After you have said all 3, ask him/her to repeat them. This first repetition determines his/her score (0-3), but keep saying them until he/she can repeat all 3, up to 6 trials. If he/she does not eventually learn all 3, recall cannot be meaningfully tested.

Score   [0] [1] [2] [3]

3. Attention and Calculation

Ask the patient to begin with 100 and count backwards by 7. Stop after 5 subtractions (93, 86, 79, 72, 65). Score the total number of correct answers.
If the patient cannot perform this task, ask him/her to spell the word world backwards. The score is the number of letters in correct order (e.g., dlrow = 5, dlorw = 3)

Score   [0] [1] [2] [3] [4]

4. Recall

Ask the patient if he/she can recall the 3 words you previously asked him/her to remember. Score 0-3.

Score   [0] [1] [2] [3]

5. Naming
a. Show the patient a wrist watch and ask him/her what it is.
b. Repeat for a pencil.

Score   [0] [1] [2]

6. Repetition
Ask the patient to repeat this sentence after you—"No If's, And's, or But's."

Score   [0] [1]

7. 3-Stage Command
Have the patient follow this command—"Take a paper in your hand, fold it in half, and put it on the floor."

Score   [0] [1] [2] [3]

8. Reacting
On a blank piece of paper print the sentence "Close your eyes" in letters large enough for the patient to see clearly. Ask him/her to read it and do what it says. Score 1 point only if he/she actually closes his/her eyes.

Score   [0] [1]

9. Writing
Give the patient a blank piece of paper and ask him/her to write a sentence for you. Do not dictate a sentence; it is to be written spontaneously. It must contain a subject and a verb and be sensible. Correct grammar and punctuation are not necessary.

Score   [0] [1]

10. Copying
On a clean piece of paper, draw intersecting pentagons, each side about one inch, and ask him/her to copy it exactly as it is. All 10 angles must be present and 2 must intersect to score 1 point. Tremor and rotation are ignored.

Score   [0] [1]

Total Score [ ]

Total Possible Score = 30
Score suggesting dementia ≤ 23

* Using a cut-off score of 23, the MMSE has a sensitivity of 87% and a specificity of 82%.

3. Physical examination and laboratory tests: The physical examination and standard neurologic evaluation may reveal evidence of a stroke. Focal findings of hemiparesis, sensory loss, cranial nerve deficits, and ataxia are not consistent with a diagnosis of AD. Conventional laboratory testing should include a complete blood count, electrolyte and metabolic panels, a thyroid function test, vitamin B_{12} levels, and tests for syphilis and human immunodeficiency virus. Beyond that, the integrative medical practitioner also tests for certain hormone levels. Measuring dehydroepiandrosterone (DHEA) has proved clinically useful. In my experience, patients with AD have markedly low levels of DHEA. I also measure levels of free testosterone in men and estrogen in women. Although full hormone replacement therapy is not a regular part of my work, I do order an insulin-like growth factor-I level. Urinalysis, electrocardiogram, chest radiograph, and determination of folate levels are no longer recommended. Low folic acid levels, however, are a risk factor for the development of AD.

4. Neuroimaging: The Alzheimer's Association neuroimaging initiative has gained a large amount of support. The time to use neuroimaging is somewhat controversial, but I have found this modality useful in identifying lesions such as hippocampal and cerebral atrophy that are consistent with AD. I believe that neuroimaging can help in determining the stage of dementia and the patient's prognosis. Some experts suggest computed tomography or magnetic resonance imaging for all patients with suspected AD. Others consider positron emission tomography more

useful when the diagnosis is uncertain, and it can be used to identify a declining metabolic rate in the parietal-temporal lobe that is characteristic of AD.

5. Genetic testing: Determining *APOE4* gene status can contribute to diagnostic accuracy in patients who already have a clinical diagnosis of AD. This testing is most commonly used in academic medicine. Current controversy revolves around the routine use of genetic testing to offer information to people interested in knowing their genetic potential for developing AD. The concern is what can be offered to people who are *APOE4* positive. Some believe that nothing can be done. I disagree. My two decades of clinical experience has led me to believe that AD can be delayed or prevented and its progression slowed.

Integrative Therapy

A true integrative medical model combines evidence from therapies based on nutrition, stress reduction, exercise, and pharmaceuticals into a total synergistic program. Gould et al[22] showed that this type of program can reverse coronary artery disease, and I have had compelling success in my own practice involving patients with AD.

At this juncture, a large difference of opinion exists between the conventionalist who prescribes only a cholinesterase inhibitor such as donepezil (Aricept) and rarely vitamin E in the treatment of MCI or AD and the more forward-thinking clinician who practices integrative medicine. The integrative medicine practitioner understands, by virtue of experience and knowledge, that much can be done in patients with SCI, MCI, and AD to slow the progression and, in many cases, reverse the symptoms. What follows is an organized and scientific approach to the treatment of cognitive decline.

Lifestyle Factors

Physical Exercise

Aerobic conditioning has been shown to improve some aspects of mental function by 20% to 30%. Smith and Fredlund[23] demonstrated that physical exercise has a retardant effect on the development of AD. In a retrospective analysis of subjects aged 40 to 60 years, those with a regular exercise program did not develop AD as frequently as those who followed no exercise program. Exercise increases cerebral blood flow and the production of nerve growth factors. A more recent study on this topic by Jedrziewski et al[24] revealed results from the National Long-Term Care Study that provided evidence supporting an exercise-related lowering of risk for cognitive decline. In this 10-year study, the amount of exercise was inversely associated with the onset of cognitive impairment.[24]

Cognitive Exercise

Based on research by Diamond et al,[25] an integrative medical program that includes cognitive stimulation such as headline discussion, crossword puzzles, music, or art could help to maintain cognitive ability. Mental training increases dendritic sprouting and enhances central nervous system plasticity.[26] In addition to inducing positive medical benefits, cognitive exercise allows patients and their spouses to spend quality time together. In my view, computerized cognitive training is neither necessary nor cost effective.

Nutrition

The key points in nutrition are to reduce dietary fat and cholesterol, add omega-3–rich foods such as salmon and tuna, and lower caloric consumption.

Some studies have shown that a diet restricted in calories and consisting of 15% to 20% fat can help prevent and treat AD. This approach extends the life expectancy of animals and enhances health and cognitive ability of humans. U.S. citizens, who consume a high-calorie, high-fat diet, have a much higher incidence of AD than people living in countries where a relatively low-fat diet is eaten. High-fat and high-calorie intake leads to oxidative stress, which contributes to the onset and progression of cognitive decline.

Researchers at New York University's Nathan Kline Institute put transgenic mice on high-fat diets and then observed an increase in the rate at which beta amyloid built up in their brains. Cholesterol-lowering medication slowed the rate of plaque formation.[27,28] The studies using statins to prevent dementia, however, have been equivocal.

The dietary consumption of fish—especially salmon and tuna, which contain docosahexaenoic acid (DHA), an omega-3, long-chain, polyunsaturated fatty acid—is considered beneficial to cognitive health. Although supplementation with DHA was not found to reduce functional decline in AD in a large randomized trial,[29] a study by Yurko-Mauro et al,[30] published in *Alzheimer's and Dementia* in 2010, did, in fact, show beneficial effects of DHA on cognition in age-related cognitive decline.

In my consultation practice, the nutritionist works to create a 15% to 20% fat diet based on patient preferences. This has proved beneficial.[31-33]

Results of the Biosphere II experiment on caloric restriction and reduced fat showed reductions in triglyceride and cholesterol levels, which are important in the treatment of AD.[34]

Mind-Body Therapy

Stress-relieving techniques such as meditation have been shown to reduce cortisol levels and enhance cognitive function in patients with MCI and AD.[35] Moreover, I have seen that an innovative mind-body exercise called kirtan kriya (KK) activates the posterior cingulate gyrus, the first area to decline in patients with AD.[36]

Meditation

Because of the effects of chronic, unbalanced stress and cortisol secretion on memory, it is beneficial to suppress elevated glucocorticoid levels or normalize their release. Given that age increases the vulnerability to stress and cortisol-induced hippocampal damage, stress-relieving meditation is highly recommended for patients of all ages to reduce cortisol and limit the loss of hippocampal neurons.

Meditation has consistently been found to decrease cortisol levels and promote normalization of adaptive mechanisms.[37] Practitioners of meditation also display lower levels of lipid peroxidase, a marker of free radical production, and higher levels of the hormone DHEA, which is considered important for optimal brain function. Wallace[38] reviewed studies that noted the positive health benefits of meditation on cognition. In a landmark study in older adults, investigators found that meditators had a greater life expectancy than nonmeditators[39] (see Chapter 98, Recommending Meditation).

▦ Physiology of Meditation

The most significant physiologic change induced by meditation is a drop in oxygen consumption (MVO_2). This effect was described by Herbert Benson in the late 1960s.[40] As seen in the graph in Figure 9-2, Benson showed that when one elicits the relaxation response, MVO_2 drops approximately 14% over the control or waking state. This finding is in contrast to sleep, in which MVO_2 has been shown to decrease 10% after 5 or 6 hours. To summarize, when one elicits the

relaxation response or practices basic meditation for as little as 10 or 20 minutes, MVO_2 drops by as much as 14%.

At least 11 forms of basic meditation are recognized:
1. The relaxation response
2. Transcendental meditation
3. Mindfulness or Zen Buddhist meditation
4. Many types of yoga
5. Autogenic training
6. Progressive muscle relaxation
7. Affirmations
8. Visualization
9. Listening to music
10. Receiving a therapeutic massage, which is a passive activity in which the relaxation response is induced
11. Prayer, when the requirements previously described are followed

FIGURE 9-2
Before (**A**) and after (**B**) kirtan kriya. **C**, The key physiologic effect of the antistress response. (**A** and **B**, From Khalsa D, Amen D, Hanks C, et al. Cerebral blood flow changes during chanting meditation. *Nucl Med Commun.* 2009;30:956–961; **C**, from Benson H. *The Relaxation Response.* New York: HarperTorch; 1976.)

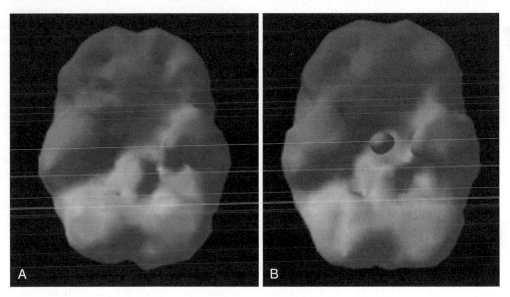

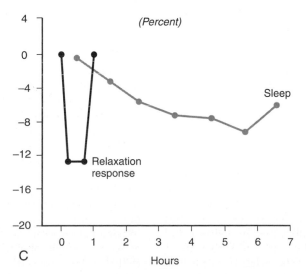

Moreover, at least 13 different physiologic effects of basic meditation have been observed[41]:

1. Decrease in pulse and increased heart rate variability
2. Decrease in respiratory rate
3. Decrease in blood pressure
4. Decrease in total peripheral resistance
5. Decrease in MVO_2
6. Decrease in stress hormones epinephrine and norepinephrine
7. Decrease in cortisol
8. Decrease in lactic acid, signifying a decrease in anxiety levels
9. Decrease in lipid peroxidase, which reveals a decrease in free radical formation
10. An increase in the hormone DHEA
11. Increase in the sleep and antiaging hormone melatonin
12. Enhanced immune system function
13. Reduction in inflammatory molecules

Even the most basic form of the relaxation response or meditation has a very high benefit at a very low cost. Generally, it has no side effects. However, sometimes people do become frustrated when they struggle to meditate. Very rarely, people have had idiosyncratic reactions, such as uncomfortable out of body experiences.

Almost 300 articles have been published on the many benefits of the regular elicitation of the relaxation response and various forms of meditation, going all the way back to the late 1960s. Although many of these studies were not well executed, the overwhelming data showed beneficial effects.

With regard to the prevention of AD and maximizing cognitive function in aging baby boomers, blood pressure regulation is critically important. Benson et al[42] demonstrated that the relaxation response decreased blood pressure in pharmacologically treated hypertensive patients. The hypometabolic state elicited by the response seems to represent an integrated hypothalamic mechanism. Benson et al[43] also showed that the relaxation response helped patients decrease the number of premature ventricular contractions, a finding demonstrating a salubrious effect on stable ischemic heart disease. In a similar study, Peters and Benson[44] showed that daily relaxation response breaks in a working population had a positive effect on self-reported measures of well-being after 12 weeks. This finding is highly significant because telomeres, as mentioned previously, are found to be shortened in patients with AD. As discussed later, self-reported measures of well-being either decreased the rate of shortening of telomeres or, in fact, lengthened them. This information may have profound significance for enhancing cognitive function as people age.

Kirtan Kriya

Specific brain exercises called kriyas are derived from the science of Kundalini yoga as taught by Yogi Bhajan. They combine breathing, finger movements, and regenerating sound currents. The practice of these exercises serves a dual purpose because they induce a meditative state and stimulate the central nervous system. Kriyas have been clinically shown to be useful in increasing global brain energy. Positron emission tomography scans demonstrate that these types of exercises enhance regional cerebral blood flow, oxygen delivery, and glucose use. Beyond that, research at Harvard University in Cambridge, Massachusetts, proved that what I call medical meditation, based on kriyas, is quite specific in increasing activity to the hippocampus compared with basic meditation. Moreover, this same research group is studying the effect of meditation on cortisol levels and grades in school-age children.[45]

In advanced meditative work, these five attributes—breath, posture or position, mantra or sound, fingertips or mudras, and focus of concentration—may be different, depending on the meditation that is chosen for a specific effect. Advanced meditations, such as KK, are therefore prescriptive or medical meditations. I described this in detail in the book *Meditation as Medicine* in 2001.[46]

Method of Kirtan Kriya

This exercise is called Kirtan Kriya and involves the chanting of the primal sounds. Say each of these words repeatedly, in order: Saa Taa Naa Maa. The "a" in these words is pronounced as a soft a, or ah. Repeat this mantra while sitting with your spine straight and your mental energy focused on the area of your brow, or forebrain. Yogis believe that this stimulates your pituitary. You can find this spot by rolling your eyes to the top, or root, of your nose. The mudras, or finger positions, are important in this kriya. On Saa, touch the index fingers of each hand to your thumbs. On Taa, touch your middle fingers to your thumbs. On Naa, touch your ring fingers to your thumbs. On Maa, touch your little fingers to your thumbs. For 2 minutes, chant in your normal voice. For the next 2 minutes, chant in a whisper. For the middle 4 minutes, chant silently, while still touching the fingertips. Then reverse the order, whispering for 2 minutes and chanting the mantra out loud for the last 2 minutes. The total time is 12 minutes. At the end, inhale deeply, stretch your hands above your head, and then bring them down in a sweeping motion as you exhale.

KK is thought to operate by several mechanisms. According to Yogi Bhajan, PhD, Master of Kundalini and White Tantric Yoga, the use of the tongue in KK during the chanting, or saying of the sounds, stimulates the 84 acupuncture meridian points on the roof of the mouth in a certain permutation and combination that sends a signal to the hypothalamus, as well as to the brain itself.

How this works on a chemical level is theoretical, but I postulate that practicing KK may rejuvenate the brain synapses by increasing important brain chemicals such as acetylcholine. This concept needs further evaluation. What we do know, however, is that meditation does increase levels of dopamine, serotonin, and melatonin.

What is not theoretical is the map of the brain, known as the homunculus, shown in *Gray's Anatomy*, as well as Penfield and Rasmussen's *The Cerebral Cortex of Man: A Clinical Study of Localization of Function*. The fingertips, hands, lips, tongue, and other aspects of vocalization are highly represented in the motor and sensory areas of the brain. Therefore, when the practitioner uses the fingertips in conjunction with the sound, specific areas in the brain, as seen on single photon emission computed tomography (SPECT) scans, are activated.

In a SPECT study published in *Nuclear Medicine Communications*, my colleagues and I[36] showed particular cerebral blood flow changes during the practice of KK. Perhaps most significantly, as seen in Figure 9-3, the frontal lobes of the brain showed increased cerebral blood flow, as did the whole brain itself. Beyond that, the posterior cingulate gyrus was activated. This finding is significant because the posterior cingulate gyrus is one of the first areas that demonstrate decreased activity on a scan when one develops AD.

One could therefore postulate that if an individual practiced KK meditation on a consistent basis, and activated the posterior cingulate gyrus, that person could decrease the risk of developing cognitive decline or even frank AD. This is also important because we know that AD may take as long as 20 to 40 years to develop.

In a follow-up to that study, Newberg et al[47] described positive effects of KK on cognitive function and cerebral blood flow in subjects with memory loss. In this preliminary study involving 15 experimental subjects and 5 subjects in a control group who listened to music, the participants in the experimental group kept a practice log revealing a high degree of compliance. When they returned to the university study area after 8 weeks of practice, the participants were scanned in the baseline state and after the meditation. They also had their neuropsychological tests repeated. The testing revealed a significant improvement in scores on tests of verbal fluency, animal naming, and attention. These neuropsychological tests tap into executive functioning skills.

Subjectively, the study subjects also reported improvement in their overall memory functioning. Given the findings of Reisberg et al about SCI,[10] this may be significant, because individuals with SCI were at higher risk for progression to MCI and later AD.

Of greatest significance is that this was the first study to explore meditation in people diagnosed with memory impairment. Also noteworthy, KK was revealed to have a positive effect in enhancing cerebral blood flow and improving cognitive functioning.

As can be seen in the scans in Figures 9-3, 9-4, and 9-5, a difference was evident in activation in the frontal lobe, posterior cingulate gyrus, and anterior cingulate gyrus, both the

FIGURE 9-3
Enhanced cerebral blood flow in the frontal lobe.

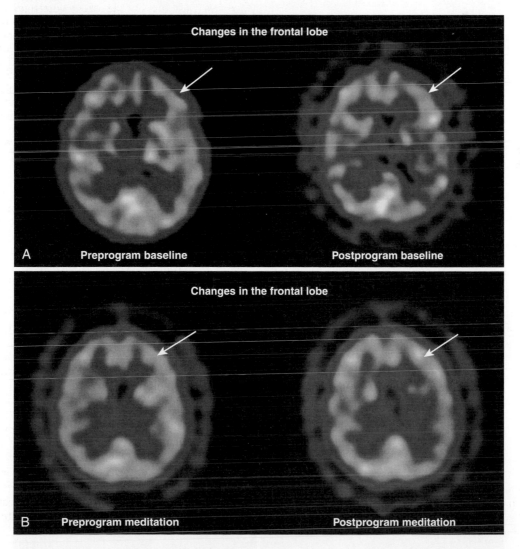

FIGURE 9-4
Enhanced cerebral blood flow in the posterior cingulate gyrus.

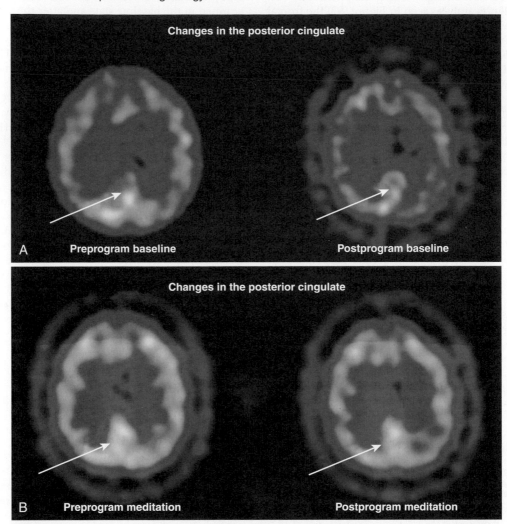

FIGURE 9-5
Enhanced cerebral blood flow in the anterior (Ant) cingulate gyrus. PFC, prefrontal cortex.

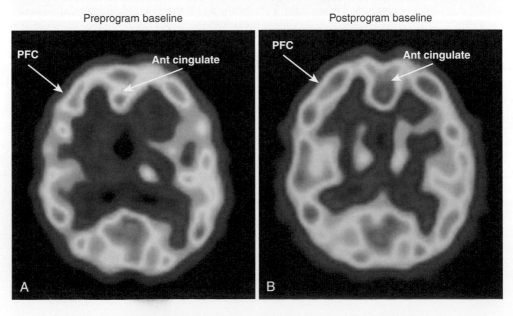

first time the subjects practiced the meditation and, more prominently, after 8 weeks of meditating only 12 minutes a day. MacLullich et al[48] showed that a smaller anterior cingulate cortex is associated with impaired hypothalamic-pituitary-adrenal axis regulation in healthy older men. In my view, enhancing activity and size of the anterior cingulate gyrus could improve hypothalamic-pituitary-adrenal axis function and normalize the stress response so that not as much cortisol bathes the hippocampus.

■ Kirtan Kriya, Telomeres, and Prevention of Alzheimer Disease

Telomeres are the cap on the DNA. When they shorten, a person ages, and when they elongate, a person is healthier and longer lived. Shortened telomeres have been associated with cancer, heart disease, and AD.

Although Dusek, Benson, and their colleagues[49] showed that stress reduction through meditation and yoga actually improved a person's genetic response to stress, Ornish et al[50] also revealed that improved diet, meditation, and other integrative medical interventions could actually turn off the disease-promoting process in men with prostate cancer. This work by Ornish et al, published in *The Lancet Oncology*, also showed increased telomerase activity with these comprehensive changes.[51]

The enzyme telomerase decreases the rate at which telomeres are shortened, and perhaps increases their length, which is an indicator of enhanced health and longevity. According to Ornish et al,[51] the telomeres increased 29% with meditation as part of this lifestyle program. Other aspects of the stress management program included, yoga, breathing, and imagery.

In July 2009, at the Conference of the International Society of Psycho-Neuro Immunology, Jacobs et al[52] presented work from the Samantha Meditation Project. This work showed that subjects taken to a retreat center who practiced mindfulness meditation for 5 hours a day for 3 months increased their psychological well-being, as well as their telomere length.

The following six facets of psychological well-being were thought to play a significant part in the enhanced telomere length:
1. Self-confidence
2. Self-acceptance
3. Personal growth
4. Purpose and meaning
5. Positive relationships
6. Sense of independence

Our preliminary research showed that KK meditation also appears to improve several aspects of psychological well-being. Noteworthy is that the amount of time necessary was only 12 minutes a day for 8 weeks, rather than 5 hours a day for 3 months. In a second study with Wang et al,[53] we also revealed that KK decreased stress, increased spiritual connection, and improved psychological well-being. In a study at UCLA, investigators revealed a positive relationship among KK, cognitive enhancement, well-being, and telomerase activation. This study had 44 subjects, 39 of whom completed the study (23 meditated, and 16 listened to relaxation tapes for 25 minutes a day for 8 weeks). Both groups demonstrated improvement in depression and anxiety, resilience, and perceived burden. The KK group improved significantly more compared with the relaxation tape group on measures of perceived support, physical suffering, energy,

emotional well-being, and cognitive tests of memory and executive function. A subgroup also showed improvement in inflammatory processes.

Supplements

The following brain-specific nutrients play a part in the prevention and treatment of AD: B-vitamins; vitamin E in the form of mixed tocopherols; phosphatidylserine (PS), with an intake of up to 300 mg/day; coenzyme Q10 (ubiquinone), up to 100 mg/day; ginkgo (*Ginkgo biloba*), at a dose up to 240 mg/day; and the omega-3 fatty acid DHA, at 1500 mg/day. Other nutrients that hold promise are huperzine A, at 100 to 200 mg/day, and vinpocetine, at 2.5 to 10 mg/day.

B Vitamins

The B-complex vitamins are critical for neurotransmitter control and carbohydrate energy metabolism. Niacin itself (vitamin B_3) has been shown to have memory-improving benefits.[54] Folate reduces homocysteine, high levels of which have been implicated in heart disease and AD. A high intake of folate was found to be associated with a reduced risk of AD in the Baltimore Longitudinal Study of Aging.[55] An integrative brain program should also contain adequate antioxidants and vitamin C in the diet, as well as through supplementation.[56]

Vitamin E

Vitamin E, at a dose of 2000 units/day, has been shown to slow the progression of midstage AD primarily because it protects cell membranes from oxidative damage.[57] Combining vitamin E, at 1000 units daily, with donepezil (Aricept), at 5 mg daily, may help slow cognitive decline in AD.[58] Vitamin E does not appear to have a significant effect in preventing the progression from MCI to AD, however.[59] Moreover, the Baltimore Longitudinal Study of Aging did not show that dietary sources or supplemental vitamin E reduced the risk of AD.[55]

Phosphatidylserine

PS is a negatively charged phospholipid that is almost exclusively located in cell membranes. It has a set of unique physiologic properties that are important to neuronal functions, including stimulation of neurotransmitter release, activation of ion transport mechanisms, and augmentation in glucose and cyclic adenosine monophosphate levels in the brain. In the aging brain, a decline in these functions is associated with memory impairment and deficits in cognitive abilities.

PS has been the subject of 23 studies, 12 of which were double-blind trials. The findings indicate that PS improves short-term memory, mood, concentration, and activities of daily living.[60] Although early research used bovine PS, concern over possible slow viral infection prompted the search for an alternative, plant source. A novel PS product made by enzymatic conversion of soy lecithin has been developed and has been shown to be beneficial in patients with memory loss, including those with AD.[61] In my experience, PS is highly effective, especially at improving the recall of names and objects, both of which are symptoms of AD. For some reason, conventionalists have decided not to include PS in their armamentarium against AD.

Dosage
The dose is 100 to 300 mg/day.

Precautions
None are known.

Coenzyme Q10
Coenzyme Q10, a powerful neuroprotective agent, works as a dynamic antioxidant. It is present throughout the brain cell membrane and mitochondria, where it is involved in the production of high-energy phosphate compounds.[62]

Dosage
The dose is 100 mg/day.

Precautions
Coenzyme Q10 can lead to gastritis, loss of appetite, nausea, and diarrhea when taken in doses greater than 300 mg/day. It can also elevate serum aminotransferase levels.

Botanicals

Ginkgo biloba Extract
Although *Ginkgo biloba* enjoys a continuous, old stellar reputation for effectiveness among practitioners and patients alike, a more recent spate of controversial articles has reported negative outcomes.[63–65] In my view, these negative reports are flawed because the subject population was older, and most people who take ginkgo, especially for prevention, fall into younger groups. I personally still do employ ginkgo in my practice, and my patients benefit from it.

Ginkgo increases microvascular circulation, scavenges free radicals, and helps improve concentration and short-term memory in patients with SCI, MCI, and AD. A 52-week, randomized, double-blind, placebo-controlled, parallel-group, multicenter study showed modest but significant improvements in 309 patients with mild to severe AD or multiinfarct dementia. These changes were equal to those induced by drugs with a higher side effect profile and were of a sufficient magnitude to be recognized by the patients' caregivers.[66]

Dosage
The dose is up to 240 mg/day.

Precautions
Reports in the medical and lay media have emphasized the need to exercise caution when combining vitamin E and ginkgo, especially in patients taking anticoagulants. In patients taking warfarin (Coumadin), for example, I measure the appropriate coagulation parameters and perhaps lower the dose of all the compounds. I believe it is a disservice to the patient with MCI or AD, however, automatically to withhold compounds with a proven benefit in fighting AD because of a purely theoretical concern. If the patient is not taking warfarin, I do not believe that the patient is in danger of excessive bleeding; in my clinical experience I have not seen it, nor have I heard of it from any practitioner of integrative medicine.

Huperzine A
Huperzine A is a natural anticholinesterase inhibitor derived from Chinese club moss. Many studies, most of which were done in China, showed that huperzine A surpassed donepezil in reversing memory deficits in aging animals. Huperzine's activity is also reportedly long lasting. What makes huperzine attractive is its apparent lack of serious side effects and low toxicity.

Dosage
I use 50 mg once or twice daily, depending on the severity of symptoms.

Precautions
Huperzine A can cause nausea, sweating, blurred vision, and fasciculations, but less often than prescription anticholinesterase inhibitors.

Vinpocetine
Vinpocetine, a nutrient derived from the periwinkle plant, has been shown to increase cerebral blood flow and enhance neuronal metabolism. A Cochrane Review reported evidence of beneficial effects on cognitive function, but most of the studies reviewed were of short duration.[67]

Dosage
I find the dose of 2.5 to 5 mg twice daily to be less stimulating and hence more effective than higher doses recommended by others.

Precautions
Gastrointestinal distress, dry mouth, low blood pressure, and rash are rare. Vinpocetine should be avoided in pregnancy.

Pharmaceuticals

Acetylcholinesterase Inhibitors
Currently, five drugs are approved by the U.S. Food and Drug Administration to treat early AD. These are acetylcholinesterase inhibitors, which increase the level of the neurotransmitter acetylcholine. Acetylcholine is critically important for memory formation and retrieval.

The first, tacrine (Cognex), was minimally effective and had poor patient compliance because of its side effects; it is no longer used. The second, donepezil (Aricept), is moderately effective in improving short-term memory in patients with early AD. Neither drug has any effect on the progression of the disease. Rivastigmine (Exelon) is slightly more effective than the others and has the best side effect profile of the available cholinesterase-inhibiting drugs.[68]

The other drugs are galantamine (Razadyne), which affects neurotransmitter function, and memantine (Namenda), which inhibits the toxic compound glutamate. Memantine has been shown to be effective in the moderate to later stages of AD.

Hormones
DHEA and pregnenolone, both neurospecific hormones and precursors to estrogen, are also useful. An animal study demonstrated that DHEA affected excitability in the hippocampus, thereby enhancing memory function at doses of 50 mg/day. Another study showed that DHEA enhanced

acetylcholine release from hippocampal neurons in the rat brain. DHEA levels have been shown to be consistently low in patients with AD.[69] Alternatively, an article by Grimley et al in 2006,[70] which reviewed four studies on DHEA supplementation while showing epidemiologic evidence that DHEA may protect against heart disease and AD risk factors, nevertheless concluded that little support exists for a beneficial effect of DHEA in prevention or treatment of AD. Individual integrative medical practitioners must decide whether DHEA is useful in their practice. I do prescribe it.

Pregnenolone has been the subject of research in both animals and humans. This hormone has been found to be a powerful memory enhancer. One study demonstrated improved memory with pregnenolone use in older adults.[71]

Estrogen deficiency in postmenopausal women is a factor in the development of AD. Observational studies indicated that estrogen replacement delays the expression of AD by 40% to 70%, enhances hippocampal plasticity, and increases nerve growth factor. Estrogen has antioxidant properties that protect the neuron from oxidative stress. Estrogen also enhances glucose transport in neuronal tissue, which may be impaired in AD. Finally, estrogen stimulates the production of several neurotransmitters whose deficiency characterizes AD.[72]

The hormone melatonin is a reasonable alternative to benzodiazepines in patients with AD for sleep. Melatonin restores circadian rhythm and may help prevent wandering.

Dosage
A good starting dose for melatonin is 1 to 3 mg at bedtime.

Spirituality

Beyond reported improvements in memory, concentration, learning ability, and activities of daily living, patients enrolled in an integrative medical program for cognitive enhancement also note positive changes in what can be described as personal awareness. This awareness sometimes appears as a sense of increased self-knowledge or what many people call spirituality and leads to a feeling of connectedness. Some patients report that this spiritual connection leads to a profound level of wisdom: the combination of age, intelligence, and experience. This wisdom, or maturity, brings greater life satisfaction. These changes are consistent with the work of Benson, Larson, and Matthews, who established that an integrative medical program, including mind-body interactions, enhances spirituality.[73] Spirituality was expressed as experiencing the close presence of a higher power. Furthermore, spirituality, faith, belief, and religion are now well known to be associated with fewer medical symptoms and better outcomes when medical interventions are needed. A preliminary study presented by Dr. Yaku Kaufmann at the 2005 American Academy of Neurology meeting demonstrated that patients with AD who lived a rewarding spiritual lifestyle had slower progression of their illness. This lifestyle was defined as being connected with a spiritual presence in the life, whether it took the shape of a family member, close friend, support network, meditation, yoga, or prayer. I have seen this in my patients as well.

As the population ages, cognitive decline, including SMI, MCI, and AD, is expected to rise. An integrative medical program can have a powerful impact on these diseases.

PREVENTION PRESCRIPTION

- Recommend a low-fat diet (15% to 20%). Most of the fat should be rich in omega-3 fatty acids (see Chapter 86, The Antiinflammatory Diet).
- Encourage stress management. Meditation, deep breathing, prayer, and various other relaxation techniques are shown to lower cortisol levels, improve memory, and lower blood pressure.
- Exercise. Physical, mental and mind-body exercises all are essential for a healthy body and a healthy mind.
- Consider measuring hormone levels (dehydroepiandrosterone, estrogen, pregnenolone) and replace hormones to keep at optimal levels.

THERAPEUTIC REVIEW

Nutrition
- Recommend a diet containing 15% to 20% fat based on patients' preferences. Include organic fruits and vegetables, and fish or seeds rich in omega-3 fatty acids, such as salmon or flaxseed oil.

Supplements
- Vitamin E: 2000 units/day
- *Ginkgo biloba:* 240 mg/day
- Phosphatidylserine: 100 to 300 mg/day

- Fish oil (docosahexaenoic acid [DHA] and eicosapentaenoic acid): 500 to 1000 mg/day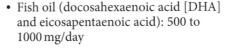
- Huperzine A: 50 to 100 mcg/day
- Vinpocetine: 2.5 to 10 mg/day
- Coenzyme Q10: 100 to 300 mg/day

Be aware of the rare possibility of increased clotting time in patients taking maximum doses of ginkgo, vitamin E, and DHA, especially with warfarin and aspirin.

Mind-Body Therapy
- Control stress: Perform daily morning meditation for at least 12–20 minutes.

 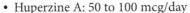

Continued

- Exercise: Physical, mental, and mind-body exercise should be part of the integrative prescription.

Pharmaceuticals

- Deprenyl, 5 mg twice daily, slows progression.

- Rivastigmine is the most effective acetylcholinesterase inhibitor available. Start with 2.5 mg twice daily and work up per package insert.

- Memantine is usually started with 5 mg in the morning for 2 weeks and then is often increased to a maximum of 40 mg/day slowly over a 2-week period.

Caution: Do not use deprenyl with antidepressant medication because fatal reactions can occur. Deprenyl can be used in conjunction with anticholinesterase drugs.

Hormone Replacement Therapy

- Dehydroepiandrosterone (DHEA): 25 to 100 mg/day, depending on blood level

- Pregnenolone: 10 to 100 mg/day

- Melatonin (for sleep): 3 mg/day at bedtime. A proper dose allows a complete night's sleep without morning grogginess.

When using DHEA in men, measure and follow the prostate-specific antigen level. If it is elevated, do not use DHEA. Also consider using saw palmetto with DHEA.

KEY WEB RESOURCES

Alzheimer's Research & Prevention Foundation. www.alzheimers-prevention.org.	This Web site provides education on holistic and preventive medicine.
Alzheimer's Foundation of America. www.alzfdn.org.	This resource has information on local and national awareness events such as Free Memory Screening Day.
Alzheimer's Association. www.alz.org.	The focus is on caregiver support and education on the latest medical developments.
Alzheimer's Disease Education and Referral Center. www.nia.nih.gov/alzheimers.	This government-sponsored education site gives an overview of all the scientific research and has in-depth referral center.

References

References are available online at expertconsult.com.

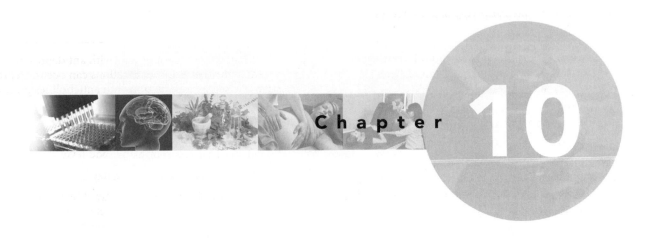

Chapter 10

Headache

John Douglas Mann, MD, and Remy R. Coeytaux, MD, PhD

Headache is one of the most common complaints that brings a patient to the attention of health care providers.[1] Ninety percent of all headaches are either migraine, with or without aura, tension-type headache (TTH), or a mixture of the two. Sixteen percent of women and 6% of men suffer from migraine.[2] The remaining 10% of headaches seen by caregivers are secondary to disorders of the tissues of the head and neck including the cervical spine, sinuses, temporomandibular joints, dental structures, soft tissue trauma and posttraumatic conditions, with primary tumors, infection, and metastatic cancers constituting a small fraction of possible causes.

"Red flag" symptoms of life-threatening disorders include the following: early morning headaches that awaken the patient, a suggestion of increased intracranial pressure; visual dimming or double vision; headaches that are increasing in frequency or severity over weeks to months; headaches made significantly worse by postural changes; explosive onset of new, severe head pain; and headaches associated with mental status changes, focal motor or sensory deficits, syncope, seizures, fever, or stiff neck. Headaches in the setting of systemic illness, weight loss, human immunodeficiency virus infection, or known malignant disease clearly require thorough investigation. Findings on examination that prompt further diagnostic workup include focal neurologic signs, evidence of head or neck trauma, temporal artery tenderness, papilledema, stiff neck, fever, and physical evidence of local or systemic infection or malignant disease.

The emphasis in this chapter is on complementary and conventional therapies that are effective in the treatment of the primary headaches, migraine and TTH.

MIGRAINE

Pathophysiology

Characteristics typical of migraine include subacute onset of throbbing head pain (unilateral or bilateral) associated with nausea and vomiting, photophobia, or sonophobia.

Headaches are heralded by visual or other painless premonitory symptoms in approximately 20% of those with migraine. The duration is usually more than 6 hours, and headaches may last several days with fluctuating intensity. Precipitating factors can include menses, specific foods, stress or letdown following stress, changes in the weather, infection, fatigue, and bright sunlight.

Although the origin of the pain of migraine is not fully understood, evidence points to a role for potent vasodilators such as substance P and calcitonin gene–related peptide, released by peripheral nerve endings of cranial nerve V on blood vessels in the scalp and meninges.[3] This process leads to sterile inflammation and edema of blood vessels, with increased sensitivity to mechanical stimulation that causes pain. Glutamate, nitric oxide, and vanilloid receptors are also implicated in migraine. Translation of this information to therapy is very active. For instance, calcitonin gene–related peptide receptor antagonists are currently in phase I and II clinical trials.[4] In the periphery, release of serotonin by platelets in the early stages seems to increase pain and prolong the headache. Centrally, the presence of a "headache generator" in the midbrain and pons is supported by findings from positron emission tomographic studies obtained during migraine attacks. Genetic influences are evident in most patients, who have one or more family members experiencing migraine. Although the individual attacks of migraine are often stereotypical, variation is not uncommon, and comorbid TTH is frequent.

Patients with migraine often suffer from tension-type headache and other forms of headache. A carefully recorded history of headache symptom characteristics helps establish criteria that lead to diagnoses and helps to highlight distinctions that guide specific therapies.

The following sections describe complementary approaches that are potentially useful for integration with conventional therapies in the treatment of migraine

TABLE 10-1. Summary of Migraine Therapies

TYPES OF THERAPY	SPECIFIC EXAMPLES/COMMENTS
Preventive	
Lifestyle	Sleep hygiene, exercise, stress management
Nutrition	Elimination of "food triggers," consideration of food allergy, maintenance of good hydration
Supplements	Magnesium, riboflavin, coenzyme Q10, omega-3 fatty acids, alpha-lipoic acid
Botanicals	Feverfew, petasites, melatonin, and valerian root (sleep); ginger root (nausea)
Pharmaceuticals	Tricyclic antidepressants, beta blockers, calcium channel blockers, anticonvulsants, NSAIDs, botulinum toxin; reduction of the risk of analgesic rebound headache by addressing analgesic polypharmacy
Mind-Body Techniques	
Biofeedback	Motivation required to practice and use as a life skill
Relaxation	Progressive muscle relaxation, focused breathing exercises, guided imagery
Cognitive-behavior therapy	Modification of maladaptive thoughts and reactions to feelings and sensations
Neurolinguistic programming	Alteration of the subjective experience of pain and modification of expectations
Self-hypnosis	Use for both headache prevention and pain control
Mindfulness meditation	Improvements in mood, coping, blood pressure, muscle tone, pain control, and pain perception
Body work	Craniosacral therapy and chiropractic
Bioenergetics	Effectiveness in both preventing and treating migraine
Abortive and Acute	
Pharmaceuticals	NSAIDS, ergot alkaloids, isometheptene, intranasal lidocaine, triptans, valproate, magnesium, narcotics, antiemetics (ginger)
Chiropractic, massage	Use especially for headaches associated with neck discomfort
Acupuncture	Use for severe acute attacks

NSAIDs, nonsteroidal antiinflammatory drugs.

(Table 10-1). Conventional approaches rely heavily on pharmaceutical interventions to prevent or abort headaches, and these agents are usually prescribed with analgesics and antiemetics. Although these measures by themselves are effective in the management of symptoms, they are often expensive, have significant side effects, and fail to address the underlying physical, psychological, and energetic issues that lead to headache. Patients with headache currently use a variety of alternative and complementary therapies,[5] many of which are reviewed in this chapter.

Integrative Therapy

Lifestyle

Effective management of migraine requires a careful assessment of lifestyle issues relating to sleep, nutrition, exercise, stress management, and relationships. Regularizing mealtimes, developing an exercise routine, and correcting poor sleep can significantly reduce the frequency of migraine. Sleep hygiene guidelines are readily available, easy to implement, and often lead to a decrease in both duration and frequency of migraine.[6] A 30-minute exercise program three times per week at aerobic levels has beneficial effects on headache intensity and variable effects on frequency.[7,8]

Nutrition

Dietary choices clearly influence migraine, and exploration of diet is an important therapeutic avenue for improving migraine outcomes.[9] Dietary triggers are found in 8% to 20% of patients with migraine.[10] Patients usually know which foods they need to avoid. Red wines, dark beers, aged cheeses, some nuts, onions, chocolate, aspartame, and processed meats containing nitrates such as hot dogs and pepperoni are common offenders. Caffeine withdrawal can temporarily exacerbate migraine or TTHs, whereas caffeine taken during a migraine can reduce pain in some patients, possibly because of its vasoconstrictive effects on scalp and meningeal vessels. Caffeine excess (more than 5 cups of coffee per day) can contribute to maintaining chronic daily headache. Raising the possibility of dietary triggers with patients is important because these triggers sometimes go unnoticed. Specific mechanisms may include direct effects of ingested substances on neuronal elements governing headache (e.g., tyramine in cheeses and wine) or allergic responses to foods such as wheat or dairy products. Diets containing large quantities of omega-6 fatty acids are usually proinflammatory and are likely to aggravate migraine and chronic TTH.

Supplements

Magnesium

Levels of ionized tissue magnesium are often low in patients with migraine, especially in those with menstrual migraine.[11-13] Oral supplementation with magnesium has been shown to be beneficial in preventing different types of migraine.[14-17] The mechanisms leading to improvement with magnesium supplementation may include reduction in cerebral cortical neuronal excitability or alteration in magnesium-dependent, circadian regulatory mechanisms that are frequently disturbed in migraine.[18-20] One study showed that oral magnesium dicitrate, 600 mg, given once a day, significantly reduced the frequency of migraine compared with placebo.[6,21] In another study, oral administration of 360 mg of pyrrolidine carboxylic acid magnesium daily for 2 months was associated with greater pain relief than was placebo in women with menstrual migraine.[22] Patients with menstrual migraine should continue magnesium for at least 3 months to determine effectiveness because beneficial effects may be delayed for several cycles.

Preventive benefit can be achieved with oral potassium magnesium aspartate (500 to 1000 mg/day at bedtime). Magnesium oxide is more readily available and cheaper than other forms, but it is poorly absorbed, especially when combined with calcium, zinc, or iron. Magnesium may cause diarrhea, particularly in those with irritable bowel syndrome, a common comorbid condition. For acute treatment of migraine, 2 g in 100 mL of saline given intravenously over 30 minutes appears to be effective and safe in an outpatient setting.[23-25] Magnesium can be used safely for both prevention and acute therapy of migraine during pregnancy.

◼ Dosage
For prevention: potassium magnesium aspartate, 500 to 1000 mg at bedtime

◼ Precautions
Magnesium may cause diarrhea; consider magnesium gluconate as an alternate form.

Riboflavin (Vitamin B₂)
Patients with migraine have been shown to have reduced phosphorylation potential in brain and muscle, a finding suggesting a mitochondrial defect in electron transport.[26] Riboflavin is a precursor for two coenzymes involved in electron transfer for redox reactions. One hypothesis for the mechanism of action of riboflavin is that it improves mitochondrial energy reserves without changing neuronal excitability.[27] Several clinical studies of riboflavin as a supplement in migraineurs noted significant preventive effects.[28,29] Riboflavin may have synergistic preventive effects when it is used concurrently with a beta blocker.[27] No head-to-head studies have compared riboflavin with other preventive measures. Results in children with migraine are mixed.[30,31]

◼ Dosage
Give 200 mg twice daily with meals.

◼ Precautions
Riboflavin is well tolerated and does not influence the metabolism of other agents. Patients may notice that their urine turns an intense yellow with daily use. Riboflavin is safe in pregnancy.

Coenzyme Q10
The rationale for studying coenzyme Q10 relates to lower phosphorylation potentials found in patients with a variety of chronic disorders including migraine.[32] The findings of an open-label trial showing reduction in headache frequency at 3 months with daily doses of 150 mg of coenzyme Q10 were confirmed in a double-blind, placebo-controlled, randomized trial (RCT) in 42 patients with migraine.[33,34] Oral coenzyme Q10, 100 mg three times a day, resulted in a reduction in attack frequency of 47.6% compared with 14.4% in the control subjects at 3 months. Headache days were also significantly reduced. As with riboflavin, no change in headache intensity or duration was noted once a headache occurred. No major recent studies have been conducted.

◼ Dosage
Prescribe 150 to 300 mg/day; minimum 3-month trial, based on the research of Sandor et al.[34]

◼ Precautions
Coenzyme Q10 is well tolerated, with rare gastrointestinal side effects. It is relatively expensive and safe in pregnancy.

Fish Oil
Rationale for the use of omega-3 fatty acids in migraine includes their antiinflammatory properties, vascular relaxation effects, and inhibition of serotonin release from platelets. Reports include a crossover randomized trial in 27 adolescents with migraine, comparing daily omega-3 fatty acids with an olive oil control over 2 months. Both olive oil and omega-3 fatty acid were associated with a striking reduction in headache frequency compared with baseline and washout frequencies.[35] Results of a larger study in 96 adults with migraine were negative.[36] The dosing ranges studied were 2 to 6 g/day. Side effects included nausea and symptoms of gastric reflux. Fish oil is safe during pregnancy.

Alpha-Lipoic Acid
The rationale for use of alpha-lipoic acid in migraine is similar to that for riboflavin and coenzyme Q10, in that it is a mitochondrial cofactor directly involved in energy production while additionally being a potent antioxidant. One high-quality study found that daily use for 3 months was associated with reduced frequency of migraine and a significant decrease in headache severity and headache days.[37]

◼ Dosage
The dose 200 mg three times a day.

◼ Precautions
None are reported. It is safe in pregnancy.

> Daily use of a compound containing 400 mg of riboflavin, 300 mg of magnesium, and 100 mg of feverfew has been shown to be effective in reducing the frequency of migraine in adults.[38]

Botanicals

Feverfew (Tanacetum parthenium Leaf)
Johnson et al[39] reported a significant increase in migraine severity and frequency when feverfew was stopped in a small group of migraineurs who were taking it for prevention. In one well-designed study, a 70% reduction in headache frequency and severity was shown in 270 patients with

migraine.[40] Variations in the standardization of the dried leaf constituents confound replication studies of this herb. A reproducibly manufactured extract of feverfew showed preventive efficacy in a double-blind RCT.[41] No long-term studies documenting safety and no head-to-head trials with other preventive medications have been conducted. The mechanism of action of feverfew in migraine may be related to its inhibiting effects on platelet aggregation and inflammatory promoters such as serotonin and prostaglandins or possibly its effect in dampening vascular reactivity to amine regulators of blood flow.

Dosage

Oral administration of up to 125 mg/day of the dried leaf standardized to a minimum of 0.2% parthenolide. Beneficial effects may take weeks to develop.

Precautions

Aphthous ulcers and gastrointestinal irritation develop in 5% to 15% of users. Abrupt cessation of feverfew occasionally results in agitation and increased headache. Feverfew is not recommended during pregnancy because it prolongs of bleeding times.

Butterbur (Petasites hybridus *Root*)

In a large, three-arm, dose-finding RCT of a standardized extract of the root of this perennial shrub, investigators found that migraine attack frequency was reduced by almost 50%. Of patients taking the highest dose, 68% had a 50% or greater reduction in headache frequency.[42] This effect continued for at least 4 months. One smaller study showed similar results,[43] and another study in 108 children and adolescents with migraine also had positive results.[44] One study that compared butterbur root extract with both music therapy and placebo in the prevention of migraine in children had mixed findings; butterbur demonstrated efficacy compared with placebo in long-term follow-up but not in short-term follow-up.[45]

A systematic review of the published literature on the effectiveness of *Petasites hybridus* revealed that higher-dose extracts (150 mg) were associated with a lower frequency of migraine attacks after 3 to 4 months, compared with a lower dose and placebo.[46] The extract is commonly standardized to 15% of the marker molecule (petasins), and known carcinogens are removed. Drug-herb interactions have not been studied.

Dosage

Start with 50 mg three times a day for a month, then 50 mg twice a day.

Precautions

The effects of butterbur in pregnancy are unknown. Excessive belching is a side effect.

Supplements for Sleep

Sleep management is a major therapeutic strategy in helping patients gain control over their headaches. Melatonin and valerian root can be used on a temporary basis to improve sleep.

Melatonin

Melatonin is used in management of migraine to improve sleep and circadian rhythms. Sleep maintenance, as opposed to sleep induction, is improved with melatonin. Melatonin is recommended nightly for 4 to 6 weeks and then is tapered. During that period, a sleep hygiene program can be put into place to reduce the need for the supplement. Melatonin has few side effects. Leone et al[47] demonstrated that a daily intake of 10 mg of melatonin for 14 days significantly reduced cluster headache frequency. Other investigators have shown beneficial effects of melatonin in migraine and other types of headache, including for migraine prevention in children[48-50] However, a more recent double-blind placebo-controlled crossover study comparing extended-release melatonin at a dose of 2 mg 1 hour before bedtime did not demonstrate improvement in migraine frequency compared with placebo.[51]

Dosage

Usual dose is 2 to 12 mg. Start at 2 mg and titrate up every 4 days as needed for sleep. Lower doses are needed if taken each evening for weeks. Higher doses (more than 15 mg) are needed to induce sleep acutely over several days (jet lag).

Precautions

Fatigue, drowsiness, dizziness, abdominal cramps, and irritability are all possible.

Valerian (Valeriana officinalis *Root*)

When taken at night for sleep, valerian rarely results in residual drowsiness on awakening. Valerian is nonaddictive and useful as an anxiolytic when it is given during the daytime (up to 250 mg three times per day). It generally does not impair psychomotor or cognitive performance.[52] The mechanism of action includes stimulation of central nervous system gamma-aminobutyric acid (GABA) receptors along with enhanced release, and inhibition of reuptake, of GABA. In clinical trials, including use for sleep and anxiety, valerian has been judged safe.[52-55] Gastrointestinal irritation is the most common side effect (15%).

Dosage

Prescribe 100 to 300 mg of the extract, standardized to 0.8% valerenate at bedtime or 250 mg every 6 hours for anxiety.

Precautions

Valerian has an extremely unpleasant smell that may aggravate nausea during migraine. It may cause worsening of TTH if taken regularly for more than 3 months. Valerian should not be used during pregnancy.

> Magnesium aspartate, in contrast to magnesium oxide, is easily absorbed and rarely causes diarrhea when used for migraine prevention. Avoid giving either preparation at the same time as calcium, zinc, or iron. Dose: 500 to 1000 mg each night.

Pharmaceuticals

The integration of conventional and complementary approaches in the treatment of headache has no inherent difficulty. Conventional pharmacologic therapy includes the use of preventive and abortive medications. The pharmaceutical approaches discussed here are those with the greatest evidence of efficacy and clinical usefulness.[56-60]

Preventive Pharmaceutical Therapies

Application of preventive pharmacologic therapies in practice is typically organized around classes of medications, including tricyclic antidepressants, selective serotonin reuptake inhibitors, beta blockers, calcium channel blockers, anticonvulsants, and other miscellaneous agents. The goals are reduction in headache frequency and severity, improved function, and increased responsiveness to abortive and analgesic agents.

The decision to start preventive therapy is based on (1) headache frequency of more than two per month or more than 3 days per month lost to headache, (2) willingness of the patient to take a medication or supplement daily for at least 3 months, and (3) ability to keep a headache diary. Medications for prevention are administered according to the half-life and according to a schedule that minimizes side effects. Effectiveness is best measured by having the patient keep a headache diary, noting headache frequency and intensity, as well as significant life events such as stressful circumstances, menses, vacations, and major changes. Patients may respond to any of several beta blockers (e.g., propranolol, atenolol, metoprolol, or timolol), thus making the choice of an agent highly individualized. One cannot predict who will respond to a given agent in advance, although the history of a family member who achieved effective prevention with a given agent may guide initial choices. Comorbid depression, a history of active asthma, and thyroid disease limits the use of beta blockers, whereas obesity limits the use of tricyclic antidepressants and valproate.

Medications and supplements are prescribed one at a time and are tapered up to a maximum dose or until satisfactory benefit is realized at lower doses. Most drugs are started at less than half the predicted maximum dose. Often, patients achieve satisfactory results at doses much lower than the maximum, particularly with the tricyclic antidepressants. Conversely, verapamil usually must be given at doses of at least 320 mg/day for benefit to occur. Magnesium, vitamin B_2, coenzyme Q10, and daily aspirin mix well with conventional preventive agents.

Once improvement is achieved, the medication combination is continued for 3 to 6 months, with periodic gradual reductions in one or more agents to determine the minimum effective dose. Effective preventive agents allow time for patients to work on lifestyle issues including management of stress, sleep, nutrition, and exercise, as well as time to develop life skills such as relaxation, biofeedback, and self-hypnosis. Preventive agents are also chosen to facilitate treatment of comorbid depression and sleep dysfunction. As patients improve, diaries that focus attention on pain are discontinued.

Tricyclic Antidepressants

Amitriptyline, in doses of up to 150 mg at bedtime, starting as low as 10 mg, is effective for prevention. A few patients do well on very low doses such as 10 mg at night. Other useful medications in this group include nortriptyline, up to 100 mg at bedtime. Sleep is often improved, which reduces migraine frequency. Dry mouth, morning drowsiness, and constipation are significant side effects.

Beta Blockers

Medications in this class that have been shown to be effective for migraine include propranolol, nadolol, timolol, atenolol, and metoprolol. Long-acting formulations have not been formally studied. Side effects include fatigue, depression, insomnia, dizziness, and nausea. Rebound headaches may occur if beta blockers are withdrawn suddenly. Dosing regimens for propranolol for migraine prevention range between 80 and 240 mg/day in two or three divided doses.

Calcium Channel Blockers

Calcium channel blockers shown to be effective include verapamil, nimodipine, flunarizine, and nifedipine. Delayed onset (weeks) of effectiveness is typical, and side effects such as abdominal pain, bloating, weight gain, constipation, and even headache are not uncommon. A typical dose of verapamil is 180 to 360 mg once daily.

Anticonvulsants

The major members of this group prescribed for migraine are sodium valproate, gabapentin (Neurontin), topiramate (Topamax), zonisamide (Zonegran), and levetiracetam (Keppra).[57,58] A typical adult dose of sodium valproate for prevention is 1500 mg/day, with a starting dose of 250 mg twice daily. Side effects include weight gain, alopecia, tremor, and nausea. Sodium valproate is available in 125-, 250-, 500-mg and sustained-release formulations. Topiramate is the most consistently effective of the four most commonly used drugs in this class, but cognitive side effects and nausea can be limiting. Levetiracetam and zonisamide have the fewest side effects.

Nonsteroidal Antiinflammatory Drugs

Trends toward reduction in migraine frequency have been seen with daily use of aspirin, naproxen, ketoprofen, and tolfenamic acid. Gastric side effects are common, and patient compliance is poor. Dosages include the following: naproxen, 500 mg twice daily; aspirin, 350 to 975 mg/day; and ketoprofen, 150 mg/day. These drugs are not safe in pregnancy.

Abortive Pharmaceutical Therapies

The following are descriptions of medications that, when taken early in the course of migraine, can abort further development of the headache.

Nonsteroidal Antiinflammatory Drugs

Ibuprofen (800 mg) and naproxen sodium (200 to 400 mg) can block headache progression when they are given during the first few hours when the headache is building. Ibuprofen in liquid form (200 to 400 mg) is recommended when nausea occurs early in the headache. Individual variation in responsiveness to nonsteroidal antiinflammatory drugs (NSAIDs) is high so that it is worth trying several different agents in this class early in headache.

Ergot Alkaloids

Now largely supplanted by the triptans, ergot alkaloids can be useful in patients who cannot tolerate other abortive methods. A typical dose is ergotamine tartrate, 1 mg orally or 2 mg sublingually, or dihydroergotamine (DHE-45), 2 mg subcutaneously (self-injection) every 4 hours for up to three doses. A nasal inhalational form is also available.

Isometheptene

Isometheptene (Midrin) has a low side effect profile and modest cost. It is a weak vasoconstrictor of scalp vessels. The dose is two or three capsules at the start of a headache, then one every 45 minutes for three more doses as needed within 24 hours.

Intranasal Lidocaine

Intranasal lidocaine is effective for all forms of migraine and is particularly useful when it is given during an aura and when nausea and vomiting are prominent early in the headache. Lidocaine (4% liquid) is applied with a dropper, 0.25 to 0.50 mL up each nostril with the patient supine and the head hyperextended. Side effects include a transient burning sensation in the nose and numbness in the throat. Repeat dosing can be hourly for 4 to 6 hours.

Triptans (5-Hydroxytryptamine Receptor 1B/1D Agonists)

The triptans, on average, are the most effective agents available for aborting migraine.[61-65] They act by blocking the release of inflammatory cytokines from the distal nerve endings of the trigeminal system onto scalp and meningeal vessels, as well as by their vasoconstrictive effects on scalp vessels. Multiple products are available by prescription, including tablet or melt forms, self-injection kits, and nasal sprays. The efficacy of a single dose is 60% to 80% for pain and nausea relief, with a 25% to 30% recurrence rate necessitating a second dose. The choice of triptan depends on the patient's response, the side effect profile, and the preferred route of administration. Long-acting forms, including naratriptan (Amerge) and frovatriptan (Frova), can be effective when recurrence rates are noted with the more rapidly acting triptans. Oral melt formulations and nasal sprays are useful when nausea is prominent early in the headache.

Usual dosing is at 2-hour intervals if necessary for a maximum of three doses in 24 hours.

Sumatriptan (Imitrex): 25-, 50-, 100-mg tablets, 20-mg nasal spray, and injection kits of 6 and 4 mg/0.5 mL
Naratriptan (Amerge): 1- or 2.5-mg tablets
Rizatriptan (Maxalt): 5- or 10-mg tablets or melt tablets
Zolmitriptan (Zomig): 2.5- or 5-mg tablets or melt tablets
Almotriptan (Axert): 12.5-mg tablets
Frovatriptan (Frova): 2.5-mg tablets
Eletriptan (Relpax): 40-mg tablets

Triptans are contraindicated in pregnancy, cardiovascular disease, complex migraine, and poorly controlled hypertension. Cost is a major factor. Rebound headache can occur with daily use. Side effects include transient pressure sensations in the chest, neck, and head. These drugs are ineffective in TTH but occasionally effective in cluster headache. Insurance coverage varies widely.

Botulinum Toxin

Botulinum toxin has been found to prevent migraine when it is injected in small quantities at multiple sites into the muscles of the forehead, temples, and posterior neck, as well as the trapezius muscle.[66-68] Effects last an average of 2 to 4 months. That botulinum toxin has also been reported to be effective in TTH suggests a common pathophysiology.[69] The U.S. Food and Drug Administration has approved botulinum toxin for treatment of chronic daily headache (more than 15 headache days per month). Side effects can include transient weakness of injected muscles. Dosing is 100 to 200 units total, injected with a 27-gauge needle over 15 to 25 sites (approximately 2 to 10 units per site).

Mind-Body Techniques

Biofeedback

Biofeedback can provide significant benefit for patients with migraine and TTH without major side effects. Thermal biofeedback, in which patients learn to increase the temperature of their hands through guided imagery and relaxation, is a commonly employed technique. The combination of thermal biofeedback and relaxation training has been shown to improve migraine symptoms significantly.[70] Meta-analysis of 25 controlled studies revealed that biofeedback is comparable to preventive pharmacotherapy.[71] Another meta-analysis of five studies revealed a 37% improvement in headache symptoms associated with thermal biofeedback.[72] A systematic review of 94 studies concluded that biofeedback was effective for both migraine and TTH.[73] Biofeedback, however, did not appear to provide additional benefit in a study involving 64 patients randomized to relaxation training or relaxation training plus biofeedback.[74]

No criteria are available for predicting benefit from biofeedback, and training requires a significant time commitment (10 to 15 hour-long sessions in addition to home practice). Pharmacotherapy combined with biofeedback may have variable results. This is an important point because vascular reactivity (a major target in biofeedback training) may be modified by medications used for headache prevention (e.g., beta blockers), thus potentially limiting the effects of training. Conversely, biofeedback could be favorably synergistic with magnesium or topirimate.[75] Biofeedback is indicated for patients intolerant to medications, those oriented toward self-efficacy in pain management, and in pregnancy, and it is especially suited to patients willing to practice the techniques regularly.

Relaxation

The category of relaxation includes progressive muscular relaxation, focused breathing exercises, and guided imagery. Holroyd and Penzien[71] reported that these techniques are as effective as biofeedback. Treatment effects were enhanced by beta blockers and other preventive agents, thus making integration both feasible and effective. Some patients are able to identify the early stages of a headache in time to deploy focused relaxation or guided imagery to abort the full development of pain. D'Souza et al[76] demonstrated that relaxation training improved headache frequency and disability associated with migraines among college students, compared with written emotional disclosure or a neutral writing group control. These techniques can be taught in groups and then practiced individually using audiotapes. Relaxation appeals to those with an internal locus of control and above-average motivation (see Chapter 93, Relaxation Techniques).

Cognitive-Behavioral Therapy

Cognitive-behavioral therapy is a stress management approach designed to help patients identify maladaptive thought patterns (e.g., self-blame, hopelessness, helplessness, worthlessness, and catastrophizing), as well as emotional states such as anger and anxiety, that can precipitate and amplify headache. Acknowledgment of present-moment and historical emotional states, shifting of habitual thought patterns, and modification of physiologic responses are the key steps in this approach. This type of therapy has been shown to be effective alone or in combination with other behavioral therapies for headache.[77] Combining cognitive-behavioral and biofeedback therapies is effective.

Neurolinguistic Programming

Neurolinguistic programming[78,79] relies on the following: establishing excellent rapport between provider and patient; developing an agreed-on, positively stated, and well-formed set of therapeutic goals; and skillfully applying a set of linguistic techniques that provide the patient with tools to deal with pain. Therapeutic approaches include reframing the meaning of headache, shifting the sensory coding of the pain, practicing dissociation techniques, modifying expectations, accessing coping resources, and anchoring effective resource states during and between episodes of pain. Patients respond favorably to the highly specific methods for pain management that are not medication based, are easily learned, and are readily applicable.

Hypnosis

Hypnosis has been shown to reduce the number of headache days and to decrease headache intensity among patients with chronic TTH.[80] For abortive therapy, hypnosis is useful in helping patients identify the early stages of migraine so that they can initiate relaxation or self-hypnosis routines. Patient motivation and regular practice are vital components of this strategy. Self-hypnosis can also be useful in resetting expectations about future successes with treatment, reducing rumination about past and future, and modifying patterns of negative thought (see Chapter 92, Self-Hypnosis Techniques).

Mindfulness Meditation

Meditation has been shown to have positive effects on mood, cardiac function, blood pressure, and muscle tone when it is practiced regularly. Effects are believed to be mediated by the development of nonjudgmental awareness of feelings, thoughts, and sensations, combined with a sense of gratitude while optimizing sympathetic and parasympathetic nervous system balance. Group instruction is based on the work of Jon Kabat-Zinn et al,[81,82] and this technique is taught as an 8-week course, including 2 to 3 hours of formal training each week, combined with daily practice of at least half an hour of meditation. Patients report improved sleep and less anticipatory anxiety relating to headache, as well as reduction in headache intensity.[83] Home practice is important in maintaining benefits.[84,85]

Biomechanical Techniques

Physical Therapy

Physical therapy alone does not appear to be effective in the treatment of migraine, but it can be useful as an adjunct to biofeedback and relaxation training when patients have significant reactive muscle tension in the upper body with limitation of head and neck movement.[70]

Chiropractic and Craniosacral Therapy

One published RCT of chiropractic spinal manipulative therapy for migraine revealed improvement in frequency, duration, disability, and medication use compared with a control group.[86] Another study revealed moderate improvement of symptoms among patients with migraine who received either chiropractic manipulation or mobilization (compared with medical care only). Chiropractic may serve as adjunctive therapy when guided by patient reports of significant neck discomfort during and between headaches. It may be especially useful when combined with biofeedback. Cost analysis has been favorable, and studies have supported its use in migraine, cervicogenic headache, and intractable headache during pregnancy, but not for TTH.[87-89]

Craniosacral therapy, derived from osteopathic theory and practice, is a gentle manipulative approach that is effective for both migraine and TTH.[90,91] Beneficial effects of four to six treatments can be long lasting.

Bioenergetics

Acupuncture

Findings from a systematic review and meta-analysis of acupuncture for migraine prophylaxis, involving 22 trials with 4419 participants, suggest that acupuncture is more effective than routine care only, but not more effective than sham acupuncture. Acupuncture was found to be associated with slightly better outcomes and fewer adverse effects than prophylactic drug treatment.[92] A systematic review and meta-analysis of acupuncture for the management of chronic headache (including chronic migraine) concluded that acupuncture is superior to sham acupuncture and medication therapy in decreasing headache intensity and frequency and in improving response rate to treatment.[93] In sum, current evidence clearly suggests that acupuncture is effective as an adjunct to usual care in the treatment of migraine, but the degree to which placebo effects contribute to this efficacy is unknown.

Homeopathy

One study of homeopathy in a group of 98 patients with mixed headaches found a 20% overall improvement rate, which was stable at 1 year. Half the patients continued homeopathic treatments with or without conventional therapy. The investigators concluded that the patients who had the most improvement suffered from both TTH and migraine and had an average disease history of 25 years.[94] Other reports are of poor quality or are inconclusive.[95] Side effects of homeopathic remedies are usually minimal, and any positive effects make integrative efforts worthwhile (see Chapter 111, Therapeutic Homeopathy).

PREVENTION PRESCRIPTION: MIGRAINE

- Identify and avoid environmental factors that consistently lead to headache (e.g., allergens, fluorescent lights, loud noises, fumes, and dust).
- Implement a sleep hygiene program, using a prebedtime routine that signals a time leading to restorative sleep. Avoid excessive sleep as well as inadequate sleep.
- Eliminate foods that lower the threshold for migraine (e.g., chocolate, aged and yellow cheeses, caffeine, red wine, dark beer, shellfish, and meats processed with nitrates).
- Water and fluid intake should be a minimum of 40 to 60 oz per day for an adult.
- Maintain an exercise program: aerobic level activity, for a minimum of 30 minutes, three times a week.
- Regularize meals, sleep, exercise, and use of medications for prevention.
- Keep a diary documenting headache frequency and intensity, response to medications, association with major life changes, stress, and changes in physiologic states, such as menses, pregnancy and illness. Share diary information with caregivers.

THERAPEUTIC REVIEW: MIGRAINE

Migraine Prevention

Lifestyle

- Regular meals and sleep, sleep hygiene, aerobic exercise three times a week, headache calendar, stress management, avoidance of environmental triggers $A\;^{①}_{1}$

- Consideration of discontinuation of hormonal birth control method if menstrual migraine is evident or the history suggests cause and effect

Nutrition

- Elimination of food triggers: wine, aged cheese, cashews, chocolate, processed meats, caffeine $A\;^{①}_{1}$

Biochemical Supplements

- Magnesium aspartate: 500 to 1000 mg nightly $B\;^{→}_{2}$
- Riboflavin: 200 mg twice daily $B\;^{↗}_{1}$
- Coenzyme Q10: 150 mg daily $B\;^{↗}_{1}$

Botanicals

- Feverfew: 125 mg up to three times daily $B\;^{→}_{2}$
- Butterbur (Petasites hybridus): 50 mg three times daily $A\;^{①}_{1}$
- For sleep: valerian root extract: 100 to 300 mg nightly; melatonin: 6 to 10 mg nightly $B\;^{→}_{2}$

Pharmaceuticals

- Aspirin: 325 mg daily $C\;^{↘}_{2}$
- Amitriptyline: 10 to 150 mg nightly $A\;^{↗}_{2}$
- Propranolol: 60 to 180 mg daily $A\;^{↗}_{2}$

- Gabapentin: 300 to 600 four times daily $C\;^{↘}_{2}$
- Topiramate: 100 to 200 mg nightly $A\;^{↗}_{2}$
- Verapamil: 180 to 480 mg daily $B\;^{→}_{2}$
- Valproate: 500 mg three times daily $A\;^{↗}_{2}$
- Botulinum toxin: subcutaneous 100 units every 3 months $B\;^{↗}_{1}$

Mind-Body Therapy

- Biofeedback: 10 sessions $A\;^{①}_{1}$
- Cognitive behavioral therapy $A\;^{①}_{1}$
- Hypnosis $B\;^{↗}_{1}$
- Mindfulness meditation: 8-week course $B\;^{↗}_{1}$

Biomechanical Techniques

Consider in cases where muscle tension in the jaw, neck, or shoulder is prominent:

- Chiropractic $C\;^{↘}_{2}$
- Craniosacral therapy $C\;^{→}_{1}$
- Massage $C\;^{→}_{1}$

Bioenergetics

- Acupuncture: six to eight sessions over 8 weeks, repeated as needed $A\;^{①}_{1}$

Acute Migraine Treatment

Use of specific abortive measures depending on efficacy, cost, side effects, and ease of administration; use of narcotics and antiemetics not covered

Lifestyle

- Darkened, quiet environment, maintenance of hydration, meals if possible, sleep

Biochemical Supplements and Herbals

- Magnesium sulfate: 2 g IV in 100 mL saline over 30 minutes
- Ginger tea for nausea: 8 oz every 3 hours
- Aromatherapy (peppermint)

Pharmaceuticals

- Naproxen sodium: 250 to 500 mg every 4 hours
- Ibuprofen liquid: 200 to 400 mg every 2 hours
- Lidocaine 4% liquid: 0.25 mL in each nostril every 1 hour
- Isometheptene (Midrin): two tablets at onset, then one tablet every 45 minutes × three
- Triptans: many available; dosing routines identical: initial dose at the onset of head pain, followed no sooner than 2 hr by a second dose if necessary; limit: three doses in 24 hr

- Valproate: 1 g IV over 1 hour
- DHE-45: 1.5 mg IV over 30 minutes preceded by promethazine (Phenergan) 20 mg IV

Mind-Body Therapy

- Self-hypnosis training
- Practiced biofeedback routine
- Relaxation

Biomechanical Techniques

- Craniosacral therapy
- Massage, slow stretch

Bioenergetics

- Acupuncture
- Reiki

IV, intravenously.

TENSION-TYPE HEADACHE

TTH may exist in a spectrum with migraine, as shown by positive responses to antimigraine agents in some patients, with or without coexisting migraine. History and physical examination suggest intermittent muscle traction of pain-sensitive tendons and connective tissues of the head and neck. Pain is typically bilateral, nonthrobbing, and bandlike, with trigger points at the base of the skull, the temples, the masseters, and the forehead. The pain is typically slow in onset and intermittent, with little or no nausea or sensory sensitivity. Positive responses to NSAIDs suggest that inflammatory and myofascial influences dominate, with modest secondary contributions from vascular structures.

Certain pericranial conditions (e.g., brain tumor and central nervous system infection) can manifest with features of TTH and little else. It is rare for a vascular headache pattern to be the presenting complaint for such conditions. Warning symptoms and signs that suggest the need for head imaging and other studies are reviewed in the first section of this chapter.

Integrative Therapy

An integrated treatment approach to TTH has considerable overlap with migraine treatment. Lifestyle issues surrounding stress, sleep, exercise, and diet are central to effective management, and all need to be reviewed carefully for both the work and home environments. Individuals with baseline TTH may develop conditions that abruptly amplify the pain. Examples include sinus and dental infections, head trauma, refractive errors, glaucoma, cervical disk disease, depression, and occult hypertension.

A thorough physical examination may lead to discovery of tender areas and trigger points in the head, the neck, or the shoulders that promote or sustain head pain. Observation of the patient while he or she is sitting, walking, and lying down can provide useful clues to musculoskeletal imbalances. Examination of temporomandibular joints is important in all patients because daytime clenching, nocturnal bruxism, and joint disease all can contribute to the pain of TTH.

Patient education in ergonomics, posture, and breathing is often useful in treating TTH. Mind-body approaches are equally effective in migraine and TTH and are usefully integrated with conventional therapies. The effectiveness of biofeedback, stress management, guided imagery, and self-hypnosis is documented in TTH.[96] Time-contingent and limited use of analgesics is needed to avoid analgesic rebound headache.

Chronic daily headache is often caused by excessive use of medications, including prescription and over-the-counter analgesics, decongestants, sleep aids, and even caffeine. Integrating nonpharmacologic approaches early in treatment, aimed at eliminating polypharmacy, can help prevent or reverse difficult-to-treat chronic analgesic rebound headache.

A combination of sleep hygiene and regularization of daily schedules is effective in reducing pain in motivated and compliant patients. The botanicals for sleep described previously for migraine can be equally effective for those with tension-type headache (TTH). Patients should be strongly encouraged to reduce consumption of sugar, caffeine, and red meat, along with increasing omega-3 fatty acids to reduce sympathetic nervous system activity and to enhance production of antiinflammatory prostaglandins (see Chapter 86, The Antiinflammatory Diet). Detoxification from unneeded drugs is part of effective TTH management. One often overlooked area is dehydration. Poorly hydrated muscles tend to cramp and contract painfully.

Pharmaceuticals have a limited role because of the risk of rebound headache and because they tend to reduce motivation to attend to needed lifestyle adjustments. NSAIDs should be medium to long acting and strictly limited to less than 20 doses per week. Muscle relaxants provide limited short-term benefit and tend to lead to psychological dependence and rebound headache. Triptans are rarely effective in TTH.

When TTH occurs daily or almost daily without evidence of an underlying organic condition, analgesic rebound headache is likely, especially when patients take more than a total of 20 doses of analgesics (NSAIDS and opiates), decongestants, muscle relaxants, and caffeine per week. Caffeine consumption, when more than three drinks a day, should be tapered slowly over 2 to 3 weeks, along with short-acting analgesics. Pain is managed with patient education, biofeedback, relaxation, slow-stretch exercises, massage, heat, long-acting NSAIDs, and low-dose tricyclic antidepressants given at night (10 to 50 mg amitriptyline, or equivalent).

Chiropractic

A few older studies investigated chiropractic or osteopathic manipulation in TTH. Hoyt et al[97] reported a 50% reduction in headache severity after a single 10-minute cervical manipulation session. In posttraumatic headache, patients had a 57% reduction in pain intensity and a 64% reduction in analgesic use over a 2-week period after two cervical spine manipulation treatments, compared with treatment with ice packs.[98] Another group found no difference between chiropractic manipulation and daily amitriptyline at the end of a 6-week course of treatment in patients with chronic TTH. However, patients who received chiropractic manipulation had fewer headaches on follow-up 6 weeks after the end of treatment.[99] Finally, an RCT comparing soft tissue therapy plus spinal manipulation with soft tissue therapy plus placebo laser treatment for episodic TTH did not show a statistical difference in outcomes between the two arms of the trial.[100] Credible more recent studies are lacking.

Acupuncture

A three-arm RCT involving 270 patients with TTH demonstrated that a course of up to 12 acupuncture treatments over 8 weeks was associated with significantly improved clinical outcomes compared with no acupuncture, but not when compared with a sham acupuncture comparison group.[101]

A systematic review and meta-analysis of acupuncture for the treatment of TTH included 11 trials with 2317 participants. Wide variability in comparison groups complicates interpretation of the findings among the trials collectively. The two large trials that included a no-treatment control demonstrated statistically significant and clinically relevant benefit associated with acupuncture. A meta-analysis with data from five trials that compared acupuncture with a sham acupuncture control demonstrated small but statistically significant benefits for treatment response and other clinical outcomes. The authors of the systematic review concluded "that acupuncture could be a valuable nonpharmacologic tool in patients with frequent episodic or chronic tension-type headaches."[102] Although further research is needed to differentiate placebo effects from purely physiologic responses to needling, available evidence suggests that patients with TTH may benefit from a course of acupuncture.

PREVENTION PRESCRIPTION: TENSION-TYPE HEADACHE

- Notice physiologic reactions to stressful situations in the home and the workplace, especially muscle contraction in the neck and shoulders, breathing patterns, chest sensations, and gastrointestinal responses such as nausea, pain, and diarrhea.
- Develop a daily relaxation routine that focuses attention on posture and muscles of the head and neck.
- Maintain adequate sleep, regular aerobic exercise, and adequate hydration.
- Modify the diet to ensure regular consumption or supplementation of omega-3 fatty acids.
- Be alert to conditions that may contribute to, or intensify, muscular head pain, such as sinus or dental infection, jaw clenching, tooth grinding, head thrusting, anxiety, and depression.
- Be checked for hypertension at least twice a year.
- Consult a physician if symptoms of weakness, loss of sensation, poor coordination, difficulty with speech, fever, or syncope occur with TTH.

THERAPEUTIC REVIEW: TENSION-TYPE HEADACHE

Emphasis is placed on lifestyle and mind-body techniques and reduced reliance on medication.

■ Lifestyle

- Stress management, sleep hygiene, nutritional choices, ergonomic awareness, regular aerobic exercise

■ Nutrition

- Increased omega-3 fatty acid per diet or supplements; reduced sugar, caffeine, red meats, tobacco, and alcohol

■ Sleep and Exercise

- Sleep hygiene
- Aerobic exercise for 30 minutes, three times per week

■ Supplements and Herbals

- Melatonin: 6 to 10 mg nightly
- Valerian root: 100 to 300 mg nightly

■ Pharmaceuticals

- Time-contingent NSAIDs
- Limit total of NSAIDS, decongestants, and caffeine to less than 20 doses per week to prevent rebound headaches

■ Mind-Body Therapy

- Biofeedback and relaxation training
- Stress management, cognitive-behavioral therapy, and mindfulness meditation

■ Biomechanical Techniques

- Manipulative therapy, massage, and craniosacral therapy

■ Bioenergetics

- Acupuncture: 6 to 10 weekly sessions with follow-up as needed

NSAIDs, nonsteroidal antiinflammatory drugs.

KEY WEB RESOURCES

National Institutes of Health (NIH) National Center for Complementary and Alternative Medicine (NCCAM). http://nccam.nih.gov/health/acupuncture/acupuncture-for-pain.htm.

This Web site contains current practice guidelines, ongoing research, and research findings relating to acupuncture for pain, including headache. The NCCAM home page links to headache management using other complementary approaches.

NIH National Institute of Neurologic Disorders and Stroke (NINDS). http://www.ninds.nih.gov/disorders/migraine/migraine.htm.

This Web site contains diagnosis criteria, treatment information, and details of recently funded research on migraine headache and pain.

American Headache Society. http://www.achenet.org/education/patients/index.asp.

This Web site provides information for patient education and on research on headache.

National Headache Foundation. http://www.headaches.org/cms.

This Web site has information for patients with headache and professionals who treat headache.

National Headache Foundation Headache Diary. http://www.headaches.org/For_Professionals/Headache_Diary.

Migraine Disability Assessment Test (MIDAS). http://www.headaches.org/pdf/MIDAS.pdf.

References

References are available online at expertconsult.com.

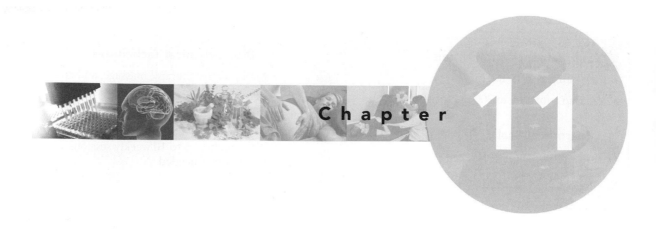

Chapter 11

Peripheral Neuropathy

Sunil T. Pai, MD

Pathophysiology

Peripheral neuropathy, or peripheral neuritis, is a common neurologic disorder resulting from damage to the peripheral nerves. It may be caused by diseases of the nerves or may be the result of systemic illnesses. It has various causes including toxic trauma (Table 11-1), certain prescription medications and chemotherapeutic agents (Table 11-2), and mechanical injury causing compression or entrapment, as with carpal tunnel syndrome (see Chapter 66, Carpal Tunnel Syndrome). Even simple pressure on superficial nerves, such as from prolonged use of crutches or sitting in the same position for too long, can lead to the disorder. Nutritional deficiencies can cause peripheral neuropathy, as seen in B-vitamin deficiency (i.e., from alcoholism, pernicious anemia, isoniazid-induced pyridoxine deficiency, malabsorption syndromes). Other causes include viral and bacterial infections and other infectious diseases (e.g., human immunodeficiency virus [HIV] infection, Lyme disease), autoimmune reactions (e.g., Guillain-Barré syndrome, chronic inflammatory demyelinating polyneuropathy, multifocal motor neuropathy), cancer (e.g., lymphoma, multiple myeloma), collagen-vascular disorders (e.g., systematic lupus erythematosus, rheumatoid arthritis, polyarteritis nodosa, Sjögren syndrome), endocrinopathies (e.g., hypothyroidism, acromegaly), and rare inherited genetic abnormalities (e.g., hereditary sensory neuropathy types I, II, III, and IV; Krabbe disease; Charcot-Marie-Tooth disease). Despite a thorough history and physical examination, the origin remains a mystery in approximately 50% of cases.[1]

One of the most common causes is diabetes; peripheral neuropathy is estimated to be present in approximately 40% to 60% of persons with diabetes of 25 years' duration.[2] Diabetic neuropathy is now thought to be the most common form of peripheral neuropathy that afflicts humans,[3] and the incidence increases significantly with age.[4] Although the exact pathophysiology of diabetic neuropathy has not yet been clearly identified, the origin is multifactorial. Persistent hyperglycemia and autoimmune and microvascular mechanisms are important factors.

Persistent hyperglycemia is the most common primary factor responsible for the development of diabetic neuropathy. Persistent hyperglycemia is thought to increase the activity of the polyol pathway, which results in the intraneural accumulation of fructose and sorbitol and thereby damages the nerves.[5] This form of hyperglycemia alone, however, cannot account for the development of nerve damage because diabetic neuropathy also occurs in patients with well-controlled disease, whereas other patients with poorly controlled disease have no evidence of neuropathy.[2]

In addition to accumulation of intraneural fructose and sorbitol, immunologic mechanisms have a role in the development of diabetic neuropathy. This damage is caused by antineural autoantibodies that circulate in the serum of some diabetic patients. Antiphospholipid antibodies may also be present and may contribute to nerve damage in combination with vascular abnormalities.[6]

Finally, endoneural vascular insufficiency resulting from decreased nitric oxide or impaired endothelial function, impaired sodium/potassium-adenosine triphosphatase (Na^+/K^+-ATPase) activity, and homocysteinemia has been found to be a primary cause of diabetic neuropathy.[6-9] Investigators have postulated that ischemia related to endoneural and epineural vascular changes causes nerve damage by thickening the blood vessel wall. Eventually, occlusion of the vessel may occur, leading to vascular permeability and compromise of endoneural blood flow (Fig. 11-1).

Other multifactorial mechanisms implicated in the development of diabetic neuropathy are body habitus, environmental factors (including alcohol, smoking, exposure to heavy metals), and genetic predisposition.

By these mechanisms, the sensory, autonomic, and motor nerves all may be affected, beginning with the distal lower extremities and spreading to involve the upper extremities as the diabetes continues.[3] Diabetic neuropathy usually manifests in a "stocking-and-glove" distribution, with sensory loss, dysesthesias, and painful paresthesias, most commonly in the lower

TABLE 11-1. Agents Causing Symptoms Associated With Toxic Neuropathy

Acrylamide (truncal ataxia)

Alcohol

Allyl chloride

Arsenic (sensory alterations, brown skin, Mees' lines)

Buckthorn toxin

Carbon disulfide

Cyanide

Dichlorophenoxyacetic acid

Dimethylaminopropionitrile (urinary complaints)

Biologic toxin in diphtheritic neuropathy (pharyngeal neuropathy)

Ethylene oxide

Germanium

Hexacarbon (n-hexane) (glue sniffing; occupational exposure to solvents, glue, or glue thinner)

Lead (wrist drop, abdominal colic)

Lucel-7 (cataracts)

Mercury

Methylbromide

Mold (in water-damaged buildings)

Nitrous oxide inhalation

Organophosphorus esters (triorthocresyl phosphate, leptophos, mipafox, trichlorphon) (cholinergic symptoms, neuropathy of delayed onset)

Polychlorinated biphenyls

Tetrachlorbiphenyl

Thallium (pain, alopecia, Mees' lines)

Trichloroethylene (trigeminal neuralgia)

Vacor

Modified from Wyngaarden JB, Smith LH Jr, Bennett JC, eds. *Cecil Textbook of Medicine*. 19th ed. Philadelphia: Saunders; 1992:2246.

TABLE 11-2. Pharmaceutical Agents Associated With Generalized Neuropathy

5-Azacytidine

5-Fluorouracil

Amiodarone

Antiretrovirals (didanosine [ddl], zalcitabine [ddC], stavudine [d4T])

Aurothioglucose

Chloramphenicol

Clioquinol

Cytarabine

Dapsone*

Disulfiram

Ethambutol

Ethionamide

Etoposide

Gemcitabine

Gold

Glutethimide

Hexamethylmelamine

Hydralazine

Ifosfamide

Isoniazid†

Metronidazole, misonidazole

Nitrofurantoin*

Penicillamine

Perhexiline

Phenytoin

Pyridoxine† (in excessive amounts)

Platinum† (cisplatin, oxaliplatin)

Sodium cyanate

Statins (3-hydroxy-3-methyl-glutaryl coenzyme A reductase inhibitors)

Stilbamidine

Suramin

Taxoids (paclitaxel, docetaxel)

Thalidomide†

Vinblastine

Vincristine

VM-26

Modified from Wyngaarden JB, Smith LH Jr, Bennett JC, eds. *Cecil Textbook of Medicine*. 19th ed. Philadelphia: Saunders; 1992:2247.
*Predominantly motor.
†Predominantly sensory.

extremities. Common symptoms include the following: tingling, prickling, or numbness; burning or freezing pain; sharp, stabbing, or electric pain; extreme sensitivity to touch; muscle weakness; and loss of balance and coordination.

Integrative Therapy

One survey showed that 43% of patients with peripheral neuropathy used complementary and alternative medicine (CAM) therapies. The most frequent were megavitamins

FIGURE 11-1
Pathophysiologic factors in diabetic neuropathy. ATPase, adenosine triphosphatase; K⁺, potassium; Na⁺, sodium. (From Head K. Peripheral neuropathy: pathological mechanisms and alternative therapies. *Altern Med Rev.* 2006;11:295.)

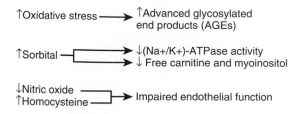

(35%), magnets (30%), acupuncture (30%), herbal remedies (22%), and chiropractic manipulation (21%). Twenty-seven percent thought their neuropathy improved with these approaches. The most common reason (32%) for using CAM was inadequate pain control. Almost half the patients did not consult a physician before starting CAM.[10]

Because diabetic neuropathy is the most common peripheral neuropathy encountered in clinical practice, and its symptoms consist primarily of pain, the management of neuropathy involves not only prevention and control of underlying disease—in this case, diabetes—but also alleviation of the painful symptoms that result.

Lifestyle

Nutrition and Exercise

Good diabetic control can be one of the best preventive measures for peripheral neuropathy and must not be underestimated or overlooked. The benefits of near normoglycemia on nerve function in the Diabetes Control and Complications Trial adequately demonstrated that strict glycemic control may reduce the incidence of diabetic neuropathy by up to 64%.[11]

In addition, multiple studies have shown that following a whole foods, low-fat, high-fiber, plant-based diet along with exercise alone can decrease type 1 diabetic medications by up to 40%[12] or eliminate them completely for type 2 diabetes.[13-16] Therefore, strong emphasis should be placed on patient education about lifestyle changes, including a whole foods, low-fat, high-fiber, plant-based diet. Reduction of medications will help reduce health care costs and potential risk of side effects.[17] Maintaining diabetic control and avoiding environmental toxins such as heavy metals, cigarettes, alcohol, and pollution are of the utmost importance. Healthy eating habits should be established (see Chapter 32, Diabetes), and body habitus can play an important role in control of glycemia. Regular exercise of walking for a minimum of 30 minutes three times a week should be implemented. An optimal regimen would be daily walks for 30 minutes to 1 hour as tolerated (see Chapter 88, Writing an Exercise Prescription).

Although evidence is inadequate to evaluate the effect of exercise on the functional ability in people with peripheral neuropathy,[18] some evidence indicates that strengthening exercises improve muscle strength in peripheral neuropathy. Most of the studies involved conventional exercises such as cycling, running, and walking. However, patients may be fearful that exercise may exacerbate their symptoms, as well as increase the possibility of injury.[18] Physical limitations of their current state of health can lead to decreased compliance, and thus proper guidance and support must be given.

Yoga

In randomized controlled trials, nonrandomized trials, and uncontrolled trials, yoga was shown to improve glucose tolerance and insulin insensitivity, reduce body mass index, reduce lipid concentrations, reduce blood pressure, decrease stress and anxiety, increase energy levels, improve well-being and self-esteem, and control fluctuations of blood glucose better than oral hypoglycemic agents alone.[19-25] Yoga was shown to be helpful in children, adolescents, and adults with diabetes,[26-30] and it increased nerve conduction velocity in those patients with neuropathy.[31] Benefits can be seen in as little as 9 to 10 days.

■ Frequency

Benefits of yoga can be seen with a minimum of two to three sessions per week for a duration of 30 to 90 minutes. Daily practice is the most beneficial. Yoga asanas including Suryanamskar, Tadasana, Konasana, Paschimottansana Ardhmatsyendrasana, Shavasana, Pavanmukthasana, Sarpasana, Trikonasana, Sukhasana, Padmasana, Pawanmuktasana, Bhujangasana, Vajrasana, Dhanurasana, Bhastrika, and Padmasana Pranayama are beneficial for diabetes mellitus.

■ Precautions

Some asanas (postures) are contraindicated in patients with severe heart disease and retinopathy. Heated yoga should be avoided. A certified yoga instructor experienced in working with patients with chronic diseases should be recommended.

Tai Chi

Studies show that as little as 6 weeks to 6 months of performing tai chi can improve performance (6-minute walk, leg strength, time up-and-go), enhance balance (greatest improvements with those with large sensory losses), improve plantar sensation, decrease glycated hemoglobin (HbA1c), and improve peripheral nerve conduction velocities.[32-36] Tai chi can be used as a safe and effective intervention for patients with peripheral neuropathy.

Movement therapies such as yoga and tai chi are usually gentler and less strenuous and, as such, may lead to better compliance. With proper instruction and supervision, these techniques may be valuable lifestyle behaviors to help patients who may not be able to exercise using conventional modalities (see Chapter 90, Prescribing Movement Therapies).

Mind-Body Therapy

Biofeedback

Biofeedback may be used to reduce stress and improve coping skills, which may aid in improving compliance, thereby promoting better glycemic control and reducing pain associated with diabetic neuropathy.[37-38] Biofeedback has been shown to reduce HbA1c directly and to increase blood flow in the extremities, which, in turn, decreases neuropathic pain, reduces stress levels, improves psychological health, and enhances quality of life.[39-43] The patient should be referred to a behavioral therapist or psychologist who teaches biofeedback techniques. Recommendation is for a minimum of six 1-hour biofeedback sessions at approximately 1-week intervals. Usually, treatments include sessions of guided imagery or relaxation techniques (see Chapter 95, Guided Imagery; Chapter 93, Relaxation Techniques). During these sessions, the patient wears a biofeedback device that indicates physiologic responses, such as electromyographic or electrodermal responses, and a vital sign monitor typically for blood pressure, pulse, or oxygen saturation. The monitoring enables patients to conceptualize how emotion, anxiety, stress, and pain can affect their physiologic status.

Once patients gain the ability to alter their physiologic state, they are taught to perform the relaxation biofeedback techniques at home with the use of a biofeedback home-use computer program[43] (e.g., emWave Desktop [Institute of HeartMath, Boulder Creek, Calif]), audio CDs, DVDs, or guided imagery exercises 10 to 20 minutes each day to attain the same result without the monitoring equipment (see Chapter 94, Enhancing Heart Rate Variability). Thus, biofeedback is a tool the patient can use to control certain physiologic parameters during times of stress or pain to help alleviate symptoms.

Bioenergetics

Infrared Therapy

The use of monochromatic near-infrared photo energy (MIRE) has been demonstrated to provide symptomatic reversal of peripheral neuropathy.[44,45] It provides a drug-free, noninvasive treatment for the consistent and predictable improvement of sensation in diabetic patients with peripheral neuropathy of the feet. Increasing foot sensitivity may substantially reduce the incidence of new foot wounds, and reversal of peripheral neuropathy is associated with a decrease in the absolute number of falls (78%), a reduced fear of falling (79%) and improved activities of daily living (72%).[46,47] Restoration of sensation, reduced pain, and improved balance in diabetic peripheral neuropathy was demonstrated in a double-blind, randomized, placebo-controlled study with MIRE.[48] This study used a medical device called the Anodyne Therapy System (ATS), which consists of therapy pads containing 60 near-infrared (890-nm) gallium aluminum arsenide diodes used three times a week for 40 minutes each visit.[48] In addition, a randomized clinical trial with photon stimulation reported significant improvements in pain quality, sensation, and quality of life outcomes for patients with severe peripheral neuropathy symptoms.[49] Photo stimulation is light emitted by light-emitting diode (LED) lights in the near-infrared wavelengths of 750 to 1500 nm.

Bioelectromagnetics

Static magnetic fields can penetrate up to 20 mm and appear to target the ectopic firing nociceptors in the epidermis and dermis. Although the exact mechanism of action is not well understood, investigators have speculated that magnets may lessen the sensation of pain by altering nerve C fiber firing frequency, possibly by stimulating K^+ internal rectifying channels to repolarize or hyperpolarize. A multicenter randomized, double-blind, placebo-controlled trial showed that subjects with diabetic peripheral neuropathy stage II or III who constantly wore static magnetic (450 G) shoe soles for 4 months showed statistically significant reductions in burning, numbness and tingling, and exercise-induced foot pain.[50] These results follow a previous study in which biomagnetic techniques were used in pain management. Positive outcomes were reported in 90% of patients suffering from diabetic neuropathy who used a magnetic footpad insole device (Magsteps [475 G], Nikku, Irvine, Calif) constantly for 4 months.[51] A systematic review of well-conducted controlled trials suggested that static magnetic fields are able to induce analgesia in all types of pain including neuropathy.[52] This included a double-blind, randomized controlled study that reported significant reductions in pain and increases in motor nerve conduction velocity by using frequency-modulated electromagnetic neural stimulation (FREMS).[53]

Acupuncture

Acupuncture and electroacupuncture have been found to be useful in neuropathic pain. Because beta endorphins have been found to be involved in the pathogenesis of both painful and painless neuropathy,[54] acupuncture may exert its well-known effect by stimulating the production of endorphins in the central nervous system.[55] Although acupuncture cannot be easily explained by known neurophysiologic mechanisms, several studies have examined the effect of acupuncture for the treatment of various types of peripheral neuropathy, including diabetic, HIV-associated, chemotherapy-induced, and neuropathy of mixed origin.[56] In randomized controlled studies, case series, and sham studies, acupuncture was shown to improve nerve conduction velocity, decrease numbness and pain (66% to 87%), and improve symptoms even more effectively than conventional medical treatment for peripheral neuropathy induced by chemotherapeutic drugs (66% versus 40%), especially for moderate and severe sensory nerve disorder.[57-63] In some cases (67%), patients were able to reduce or stop their pain medications.[64]

> Acupuncture has a positive effect on neuropathic pain and often results in the ability to reduce or stop pain medications.

Patients can receive six courses of classical acupuncture analgesia[65,66] to both lower limbs over a 10-week period. In addition to classical acupuncture, electroacupuncture in a small clinical pilot study of biweekly treatments for 4 weeks demonstrated a reduction of continuous pain from 32.9% to 15.9% and a decreased intensity of pain attacks from 59% to 44%.[67] Electroacupuncture may have a positive influence on nerve conduction velocity and may also relieve neuropathic pain.[65] Electroacupuncture is performed in two cycles of five sittings each (10 sessions) at 2-day intervals.

A more comprehensive mixture of body acupuncture and scalp acupuncture (with or without electrical stimulation) can improve outcomes clinically by using the following protocol. Scalp points: upper one fifth sensory area, foot motor and sensory area; ear points: ShenMen, sympathic, foot; body points: GB-40, GB-34, SP-10, SP-6, ST-44, LR-3, and Bafeng (extra point). Electrical stimulation can be used for the ear and body points at a frequency of 100 Hz at low intensity for 10 to 15 minutes for enhanced response.[68]

Before such therapies can be recommended, a constitutional evaluation by a practitioner trained in acupuncture should be considered because each modality is prescribed on the basis of the unique symptoms and physical characteristics of the patient. A comprehensive review of medical acupuncture and scalp acupuncture for physicians may be found in the various texts by Dr. Joseph Helms[69] and Dr. Jason Hao.[68]

Botanical Medicine

Diabetes, like most diseases, is considered to be partly the result of inflammatory responses, especially when pain is involved. Many herbs are used for diabetes (see Chapter 32, Diabetes Mellitus), but a few Ayurvedic herbs, such as curcumin, [70-90] *Boswellia,*[91-105] and ginger,[106-116] are used to treat the pain of diabetic neuropathy and the other complications and comorbidities associated with diabetes.

Curcumin

Curcumin is the active ingredient in turmeric. It is widely used as a spice and food colorant throughout India. For more than 4000 years, curcumin has been used in traditional Ayurvedic medicine to treat a wide variety of ailments. It is one of the most researched natural medicines to date, with more than 5000 studies published.

Curcumin has shown to be beneficial in treating many different inflammatory diseases. It reduces inflammation in more than 97 biologic mechanisms including c-reactive protein, cyclooxygenase-2, 5-lipoxygenase, interleukin (IL)-1beta, IL-6, IL-12, tumor necrosis factor-alpha, interferon-gamma, activator protein-1, nuclear factor-kappaB, macrophage inflammatory protein, matrix metalloproteinase, human leukocyte elastase, several types of protein kinases, adhesion molecules, and genes involved with inflammation.[81-85] In addition, curcumin has been shown to improve endothelial function[86,87] and reduce vascular inflammation[88,89] and down-regulate adipokines, including resistin, leptin, and monocyte chemotactic protein-1.[81] Curcumin also shows antinociceptive activity by attenuating diabetic neuropathic pain[90] and provides other benefits for diabetic complications in in vitro, animal, and human studies.[83] Therefore, curcumin can be used as a safe analgesic for neuropathic pain while assisting in reversal of insulin resistance, hyperglycemia, hyperlipidemia, and obesity, which is common in diabetic patients as well as in the general population.[81]

▮ Dosage

Dosing for curcumin C3 Complex: 500 to 1000 mg orally three times daily; or Bosmeric-SR (a sustained-release formulation that combines boswellia and ginger along with black pepper to enhance absorption), two caplets orally twice daily.*

▮ Precautions

Although curcumin is nontoxic to human subjects at high doses,[82] many curcumin supplements may contain contaminants such as lead and are not standardized to the curcuminoids that provide the health benefits. Curcumin C3 Complex is a patented form of curcumin that is standardized to 95% curcuminoids, including curcumin (70% to 80%), bidemethoxycurcumin (2.5% to 6.5%), and

demethoxycurcumin (15% to 25%). Curcumin C3 Complex has the most research in human studies at major hospitals and universities and thus is a safe and effective form to be recommended.

Geranium Oil (Pelargonium *spp.*)

A patented formulation of geranium oil, Neuragen PN, has been clinically studied. It contains a proprietary blend of five essential oils and six homeopathic ingredients. A multicenter double-blind crossover trial and a randomized, double-blind, placebo-controlled clinical trial showed a significant reduction in neuropathic pain in 93% of patients of the patients within 30 minutes of application of Neuragen PN. In addition to the immediate reduction of neuropathic pain, 70% to 80% had lasting relief up to 8 hours.[117,118] Geranium oil provides significant pain relief in as little as 5 minutes and lasts up to 8 hours. Therefore, geranium oil can be used as monotherapy or used in conjunction with other treatments for diabetic neuropathy for breakthrough pain or immediate pain relief.

▮ Dosage

Neuragen PN is highly concentrated, and thus one needs to apply one to two drops to the affected area, rub in, and allow to absorb. This can be applied several times a day but no more than five times daily. For efficient application to wider areas, or for extremely sensitive skin, it is recommended to dilute four or five drops in 1 tablespoon of carrier oil such as grapeseed oil or jojoba oil before application. Neuragen PN is now also available in a gel for easy application. Pain relief may be immediate but usually is noticed within 30 minutes. If relief is not experienced within the first application, repeat the application over a period of 3 days.

▮ Precautions

As with any essential oil, only a few drops are needed because they can irritate the skin. For patients with sensitive skin, it is best mixed with carrier oil first before direct application is attempted. Wash hands after use; avoid contact with eyes and open sores. Discontinue if rash occurs.

Evening Primrose Oil

Evening primrose oil (EPO) is extracted from the seeds of *Oenothera biennis.* EPO is a rich source of omega-6 essential fatty acids, primarily gamma-linolenic acid (GLA) and linoleic acid, both essential components of myelin and the neuronal cell membrane.[119] GLA has provided positive results in the treatment of experimental diabetes and may be more beneficial than docosahexaenoic acid (DHA) in preventing diabetic neuropathy.[120-122] GLA is converted to prostaglandin E_1 (PGE_1) preferentially over PGE_2. PGE_1 has antiinflammatory, antiplatelet, and vasodilating properties. In patients with diabetes, however, levels of PGE_1 are decreased and levels of PGE_2 and thromboxane are increased[132] and thus tend to promote inflammation, vasoconstriction, and platelet aggregation.[124] Supplementing the diet with GLA has been shown to augment the production of PGE_1 (by bypassing the blocked enzymatic step delta-6-desaturase) seen in patients with hyperglycemia.[125-127]

Two of three randomized controlled trials showed positive effects of GLA in diabetic neuropathy.[119] Two of the trials demonstrated, with GLA at 360 mg/day for 6 months and 480 mg/day for 1 year, statistically significant improvements in neuropathy scores, nerve conduction velocities, and action

---

*Editor's Note: Dr. Pai has financial interests to the company that produces Bosmeric-SR.

potentials. Therefore, EPO may be helpful for mild to moderate diabetic peripheral neuropathy.

■ Dosage
The dose is 360 mg/day of GLA from EPO (the most researched source of GLA, as opposed to borage oil or black currant oil), and it may be increased up to 480 mg/day. Obtain high-quality oil (preferably certified organic), packaged in light-resistant containers, refrigerated, and marked with a freshness date to avoid rancidity.

■ Precaution
EPO may increase the effectiveness of ceftazidime, chemotherapy agents, and cyclosporine and may interact with phenothiazines, thus causing an increase in seizures. Patients taking antiplatelet agents or anticoagulants should use EPO cautiously or not at all. Theoretically, the use of nonsteroidal antiinflammatory drugs (NSAIDs) may counteract the effect of EPO.

Supplements

Many supplements have been shown to be helpful for symptoms of diabetes (see Chapter 32, Diabetes) and specifically for peripheral neuropathy. Those supplements with the best results for peripheral neuropathy are discussed here.

Acetyl-L-carnitine
Acetyl-L-carnitine (ALC) is an acetylated form of L-carnitine, an amino acid responsible for transport of fatty acids into a cell's mitochondria. ALC is far superior to normal L-carnitine in terms of bioavailability in that it is absorbed by the gastrointestinal tract, enters cells, and crosses the blood-brain barrier more readily than does unacetylated carnitine.

Peripheral neuropathy is a common side effect of chemotherapy drugs belonging to platinum or taxane families. Animal studies showed the benefits of ALC as a specific protective agent when it was given concomitantly and also after treatment for chemotherapy-induced neuropathy after cisplatin, paclitaxel, and vincristine without showing any interference with the antitumor activity of the drugs.[128,129] Further studies in humans showed that ALC, given as a 1-g/day infusion over 1 to 2 hours for at least 10 days, improved chemotherapy-induced peripheral neuropathy in up to 73% of the patients.[130] Patients with chemotherapy-induced peripheral neuropathy treated with oral ALC (1 g three times a day) for 8 weeks showed sensory improvement (60%) and motor improvement (79%), and their total neuropathy scores that included neurophysiologic measures improved (92%), with symptomatic improvement persisting at median 13 months after treatment of ALC.[131] In addition to chemotherapy-induced peripheral neuropathy, multiple long-term (1-year) randomized, double-blind, placebo-controlled studies showed that ALC improves pain, nerve regeneration, and vibratory perception in patients with chronic diabetic neuropathy.[133,134] ALC appeared to work more effectively in patients with type 2 diabetes with a shorter duration of neuropathy than in patients with type 1 diabetes.[132]

■ Dosage
The recommended dose is 500 mg orally twice a day to 1000 mg orally three times a day. Better pain control is seen at the higher dose regimen.

■ Precautions
ALC may cause nausea, vomiting, diarrhea, headache, bladder irritation or infection, unusual body odor, stuffy nose, and rash. Other side effects associated with ALC include restlessness and difficulty sleeping.

Alpha-Lipoic Acid
Alpha-lipoic acid, also known as thiotic acid, is approved for clinical use in the management of diabetic neuropathy in Germany and has been used there extensively in medical practice since 1959.[134] Alpha-lipoic acid is a universal antioxidant, exerting direct (scavenges free radicals) and indirect (participates in the process of recycling other natural antioxidants, thereby increasing glutathione, vitamins C and E, and coenzyme Q10) antioxidant activity.[135-138] Alpha-lipoic acid chelates transition metal ions (e.g., iron and copper) and effectively mitigates toxicities associated with heavy metal poisoning.[139] Investigators have established that alpha-lipoic acid protects from lipid peroxidation and increases the activity of antioxidant enzymes—catalase and superoxide dismutase—in peripheral nerves. By decreasing oxidative stress, alpha-lipoic acid normalizes impaired endoneural blood flow and the impaired nerve conduction velocity.[140]

Several studies established the neurogenerative and neuroprotective effects of alpha-lipoic acid. The efficacy and safety of alpha-lipoic acid in peripheral and autonomic diabetic neuropathy were demonstrated in many randomized, double-blind, placebo-controlled trials.[141-145] A meta-analysis provided evidence that treatment with alpha-lipoic acid significantly improves both positive neuropathic symptoms and neuropathic deficits to a clinically meaningful degree in diabetic patients with symptomatic polyneuropathy.[146] Further studies showed the oral forms of alpha-lipoic acid to be effective on peripheral neuropathy.[147] Alpha-lipoic acid was shown effective for diabetic mononeuropathy of the cranial nerves, with full recovery of all the patients in the study.[148] The studies ranged from a minimum of 3 weeks to 2 years, and thus 3 weeks is likely to be the minimum amount of treatment time. Although greater improvements were seen with higher doses, so were adverse effects such as gastrointestinal upset and headaches.[146]

Most studies of alpha-lipoic acid used parenteral doses ranging from 600 to 1800 mg, which demonstrate more rapid response than oral doses of the same range, and found a continuous daily improvement in symptom scores beginning on the eighth day of treatment.[146] Unfortunately, the parenteral form of alpha-lipoic acid is not currently available as a prescribed therapy in the United States; only the oral form is available in various doses. In most studies, 600 mg seems to be the starting dose. To obtain similar results, patients should use high-quality products from manufacturers that source the alpha-lipoic acid from Europe (Germany or Italy).

■ Dosage
Alpha-lipoic acid is given orally at 600 to 1800 mg daily. Start with 600 mg daily, and increase up to 1800 mg daily in divided doses if needed.

■ Precautions
Although no evidence has indicated that alpha-lipoic acid affects glycemic control, case studies have shown improved glucose handling in diabetic patients.[139] As a precaution, patients predisposed to hypoglycemia, including those

receiving hypoglycemic agents, should have blood glucose levels monitored closely. In addition, because alpha-lipoic acid acts as a chelator, monitor for possible mineral deficiencies. Gastrointestinal upset may occur at higher doses. Rarely, this supplement may cause rash.

B Vitamins

■ Benfotiamine: Vitamin B_1

Benfotiamine, which is also known as *S*-benzoylthiamine-*O*-monophosphate, is a lipid-soluble derivative of vitamin B_1 (thiamine) and is absorbed up to 3.6 times more than water-soluble forms. Vitamin B_1 is associated with a 120-fold greater increase in the levels of metabolically active thiamine diphosphate. Its lipid solubility allows it to penetrate the nerves more readily. It has been found to give higher bioavailability of thiamine than its water-soluble counterparts.[149-151] Studies have shown benfotiamine to improve neuropathy scores significantly[152,153] and to increase nerve conduction velocity.[154-156] In a randomized, placebo-controlled, double-blind pilot study, investigators also demonstrated a pronounced effect on the decrease in pain[157] in conjunction with the earlier described benefits. Benfotiamine may also be beneficial in preventing diabetic nephropathy[158] and retinopathy.[159] Therapeutic benefits can be seen as early as 3 weeks, with the most significant improvement in patients taking the highest-dose benfotiamine.[160]

Dosage

The recommended dose of benfotiamine is 150 to 300 mg twice daily specifically for diabetic peripheral neuropathy.

■ Methylcobalamin: Vitamin B_{12}

Methylcobalamin is the active form of vitamin B_{12}. In a small double-blind, placebo-controlled trial of patients with type 1 and 2 diabetes with neuropathy, those given oral methylcobalamin at a dose of 500 mcg three times daily showed significant improvements of somatic and autonomic symptoms compared with placebo.[161] A review of several clinical trials of the use of methylcobalamin alone or combined with other B vitamins found overall symptomatic relief of neuropathy symptoms that was more pronounced than electrophysiologic findings.[162] Additionally, supplementation of 1500 mcg/day methylcobalamin for 2 months resulted in improved vibratory perception thresholds and heart rate variability (a sign of improvement in signs of autonomic neuropathy) in patients with diabetes.[163]

Dosage

The dose is 500 mcg three times daily or 1500 mcg daily of methylcobalamin or 5-adenosylcobalamin for best bioavailability and absorption. Most generic vitamins contain the cyanocobalamin, which may not be as effective or as beneficial.

B-Complex Multivitamin

Vitamins B_1 (thiamine), B_6 (pyridoxine), and B_{12} (cobalamin) play an important role in the pathogenesis of peripheral neuropathy in deficiency syndromes such as those resulting from alcoholism or pernicious anemia, from isoniazid-induced pyridoxine deficiency, and from malabsorption syndromes. If peripheral neuropathy is caused by deficiency syndromes, then use B-100 complex (a multivitamin that usually contains 25 to 100 mg of thiamine, riboflavin, niacin, pyridoxine, and pathothenic acid and also may include other vitamins such as folate) for ease of administration and intake of all B vitamins.

Dosage

B-complex multivitamin (B-100), one tablet once or twice daily is taken for peripheral neuropathy caused by deficiency syndromes. The B vitamins such as methylcobalamin and 5-adenosylcobalamin (vitamin B_{12}) and the 5-methyltetrahydrofolate (5-MTF) form of folate should be used in these formulas.

Precautions

Avoid excessive doses of vitamin B_6 (pyridoxine). Doses higher than 250 mg/day can cause reversible nerve damage.

> In prescribing B-complex vitamins, make sure that the patient is not already taking another vitamin supplement that may contain B vitamins. Vitamin B_3 (niacin) in doses greater than 300 mg/day may cause headache, nausea, skin tingling, and flushing. Vitamin B_6 in doses greater than 250 mg/day may cause reversible nerve damage.

Fish Oil: Omega-3 Fatty Acids

Similar to EPO (GLA), omega-3 fatty acids are also essential for healthy nerve cell membranes and blood flow.[164] Omega-3 fatty acids have been found to have neuroprotective effects against experimental diabetic neuropathy, to reduce proinflammatory cytokine production, and to benefit macrovascular and microvascular functioning in diabetics.[165-168] A clinical study of diabetic patients with neuropathy who consumed 1800 mg eicosapentaenoic acid (EPA) daily for 48 weeks reported significantly decreased cold and numb sensations, vibrational perception, and improved vibratory threshold in these patients. Circulation, measured in the dorsal is pedis artery, and lipid profiles also significantly improved.[169]

■ Dosage

Doses are EPA, 1000 to 2000 mg/day, and DHA, 500 to 1000 mg/day. The natural triglyceride form provides superior absorption and bioavailability up to 70% more than preparations with ethyl ester forms.[170] For patients who are vegetarian or allergic to fish, a plant-based form of EPA and DHA called NutraVege is available. It contains *Echium plantagineum* oil (stearidonic acid, a precursor of EPA) and algal DHA and GLA. High-potency fish oils should be used to obtain the clinical dose. They also should be independently tested for purity (e.g., no heavy metals), potency, and label claims. Sources that are sustainably harvested are preferred to preserve the ocean's ecosystem and reduce overfishing.

■ Precautions

Possible blood thinning effect may occur with higher doses. Patients taking anticoagulant medications should be closely monitored.

Pharmaceuticals

Capsaicin

Capsaicin, an extract of chili peppers, when applied topically, has been demonstrated to relieve neuropathic pain by affecting sensory fibers, especially C fibers,[171] and by depleting endogenous neurotransmitter stores associated with pain transmission, such as substance P, vasoactive intestinal peptide, cholecystokinin, and somatostatin.[172] Capsaicin does not reverse, stabilize, or lessen neuropathy but decreases the pain that occurs from it. The result can be a burning sensation with the first few weeks of use. Successive application, however, results in a dose-dependent degeneration and desensitization of afferent fibers blocking further action potential conduction.[171] Patients should be advised to continue use, if the pain is tolerable, for at least 4 to 6 weeks before full benefits are appreciated.

A Cochrane Database Systematic Review showed that capsaicin, either as repeated application of a low-dose (0.075%) cream or a single application of a high-dose (8%) patch, may provide a significant degree of pain relief to some patients with painful neuropathic conditions.[173] In addition, patients with postherpetic neuralgia and painful HIV-associated distal sensory polyneuropathy were studied in randomized, double-blind, multicenter trials using a high-concentration capsaicin dermal patch successfully for up to 1 year; this patch is now available by prescription.[174-176]

Dosage

Capsaicin cream is available over the counter (Capzacin HP, Zostrix HP). Various strengths range from 0.025% to 0.1%, although clinical studies use the 0.075% strength. The cream is applied to the affected area up to three or four times daily for at least 4 to 6 weeks. Clinical trials show that application must take place three or four times a day for improvement.[173] Using daily, twice daily, or on an as-needed basis is likely ineffective.

Capsaicin 8% patch (Qutenza) is by prescription only and is applied in a physician's office. The painful area is pretreated with anesthetic, and the patch is applied for 1 hour and then removed. One patch provides relief for up to 3 months. Follow insert directions for specific application procedure.

Precautions

Application with gloves is recommended. Wash hands immediately after application, and avoid contact with eyes or mucous membranes. Local skin irritation, which is often mild and transient but may lead to withdrawal, is common. Systemic adverse effects are rare.

Antidepressants

The Neuropathic Pain Special Interest Group of the International Association developed evidence-based guidelines for pharmacologic treatment of neuropathic pain using first-line treatment options including tricyclic antidepressants (TCAs), dual reuptake inhibitors of serotonin and norepinephrine, and calcium channel α_2-δ ligands.[177] The results of a systematic review defined clinical success as a 50% reduction in pain. Investigators found that TCAs were the most effective analgesics, followed by traditional anticonvulsants, and then the newer-generation anticonvulsants.[178] However, the review concluded that the efficacy of most of these pharmacologic treatments is limited, because for any particular drug, only 30% of patients treated will experience analgesia.[49] With these low analgesic response rates and the risk of side effects, the use of integrative therapies and dietary supplements is therefore recommended as a trial of benefit before treatment with pharmaceuticals.

Tricyclic Antidepressants

TCAs such as amitriptyline (Elavil, Endep), nortriptyline (Aventyl, Pamelor), and desipramine (Norpramin) have been commonly used as the mainstays in the palliation of pain secondary to diabetic neuropathy.[179] Many placebo-controlled, randomized controlled trials found TCAs to be efficacious for several different types of neuropathy.[180] TCAs work by increasing the postsynaptic concentration of norepinephrine. Because the inhibitory pathways in the spinal cord use norepinephrine as a neurotransmitter, TCAs are believed to increase the inhibitory influence on nociceptive transmitting neurons.[181] The selective serotonin reuptake inhibitors (SSRIs) such as fluoxetine and paroxetine have also been used; although they are better tolerated than the TCAs, they have little or no efficacy in relieving pain.[182-184]

Dosage

To minimize side effects and encourage compliance, start therapy with amitriptyline or nortriptyline at a dose of 10 mg at bedtime. Titrate this dose upward to 25 mg at bedtime as side effects allow, in 10-mg to 25-mg increments. Even at lower doses, patients generally report rapid improvement in sleeping and begin to experience some pain relief in 10 to 14 days. If no relief of pain is obtained with increased doses (usual range, 50 to 300 mg/day), the addition of gabapentin (Neurontin) alone or in combination with nerve blocks with local anesthetics is recommended.[185] The slow onset of action of TCAs and their potential side effects often require a gradual dose buildup (6 to 8 weeks) before maximum efficacy and tolerance are achieved.

Precautions

Significant anticholinergic side effects, including dry mouth, constipation, sedation, and urinary retention, are common. TCAs are contraindicated in patients who have significant ischemic heart disease, and these drugs may also cause arrhythmias and orthostatic hypotension (thus should be avoided in older persons because of the risk of falling). Limit doses to less than 100 mg/day when possible. Screening electrocardiography for patients older than 40 years is recommended. These agents are not to be used with monoamine oxidase inhibitors (MAOIs).

Serotonin Norepinephrine Reuptake Inhibitors

- Venlafaxine (Effexor)

- Duloxetine (Cymbalta)

Although both drugs have been used traditionally as antidepressants, studies on venlafaxine and duloxetine have demonstrated beneficial treatment for reduction of painful diabetic neuropathy with better tolerability and fewer side effects than TCAs.[186-190] Although these studies are positive and duloxetine has been granted U.S. Food and Drug Administration (FDA) approval for treatment of neuropathic pain, they were less than 12 weeks in duration, and thus the long-term efficacy and safety are unknown.

Dosage

For venlafaxine ER, the dose is 150 to 225 mg daily; start with 150 mg daily, and increase to 225 mg daily if a greater analgesic effect is needed. The maximum dose of duloxetine is 60 mg daily; start with 30 mg daily and increase to 60 mg daily if an increase in analgesic effect is needed. With both medications, higher doses increase the risk of side effects.

Precautions

Nausea, dyspepsia, somnolence, and insomnia are possible. Venlafaxine may cause cardiac rhythm changes. Duloxetine may decrease sodium, uric acid, chloride, gamma-glutamyltransferase, and alanine aminotransferase. It may also increase bicarbonate and alkaline phosphatase levels.

Anticonvulsants

- Gabapentin: First-line choice
- Pregabalin (Lyrica): First-line choice
- Phenytoin (Dilantin)
- Carbamazepine (Tegretol)

Phenytoin and carbamazepine have been used with varying degrees of success, either alone or in combination with antidepressants.[191] Gabapentin has been shown to be highly efficacious in the treatment of various painful neuropathic conditions, including postherpetic neuralgia and diabetic neuropathy.[192] Based on the reviewed randomized controlled trials, gabapentin shows good efficacy, a favorable side effect profile (especially when compared with phenytoin and carbamazepine), and few drug interactions; therefore, it may be a first-choice treatment in painful diabetic neuropathy, especially in older adults.[193,194] The precise mechanism of action of anticonvulsants that accounts for their analgesic efficacy is unknown. Anticonvulsants modulate both peripheral and central mechanisms through sodium channel antagonism, inhibition of excitatory transmission (e.g., *N*-methyl-D-aspartate receptor), or enhancement of gamma-aminobutyric acid–mediated inhibition.[195]

Pregabalin is a selective high-affinity ligand for the α_2-δ subunit of voltage-gated calcium channel,[196] which plays a role in pathologic changes believed to be associated with neuropathic pain in humans.[197,198] Double-blind, placebo-controlled trials showed that pregabalin is effective in the treatment of diabetic peripheral neuropathy and postherpetic neuralgia, and it produces significant improvement of various pain scores as well as reduced sleep interference.[199,200] The FDA has approved pregabalin for the management of neuropathic pain associated with diabetic peripheral neuropathy and postherpetic neuralgia. Pregabalin is structurally and mechanistically related to gabapentin but differs from gabapentin in exhibiting linear pharmacokinetics with increasing dose and low intersubject variability. These properties may make pregabalin easier to prescribe and could impart a more effective dose range with potentially fewer side effects. Although pregabalin has become a first-line agent in the treatment of diabetic peripheral neuropathy and postherpetic neuralgia, all studies were less than 13 weeks in duration, and thus the long-term durability of response and safety are unknown. Physicians should also consider the cost before prescribing this agent.

■ Gabapentin
Dosage

A single bedtime dose of 300 mg of gabapentin for 2 nights can be followed by 300 mg given twice daily for an additional 2 days. If the patient tolerates this twice-daily regimen, the dose can be increased to 300 mg three times a day. Additional titration upward can be carried out in 300-mg increments as side effects allow. Total daily doses greater than 3600 mg are not currently recommended.[185] A possible combination with 10 to 25 mg of TCAs (see earlier) can be added for patients with sleep disturbance.

Precautions

The most serious concern with gabapentin is leukopenia. This drug can also cause somnolence, dizziness, ataxia, and fatigue. Taper dose over 7 days or longer to discontinue.

■ Pregabalin (Lyrica)
Dosage

Pregabalin is taken at 50 to 150 mg daily, divided into two or three doses. After an initial daily dose of 150 mg, it should be titrated with patient's response and tolerability over 2 weeks to a maximum of 300 mg daily. Pregabalin dosage adjustment should be considered in case of renal impairment.[201]

Precautions

The most common side effects are dizziness, somnolence, headache, dry mouth, and peripheral edema.

Analgesics

Simple analgesics such as acetaminophen, aspirin, naproxen, and ibuprofen may be used in conjunction with anticonvulsants and antidepressants, but the response is very poor. Caution must be taken because many of these NSAIDs received black box warnings and can cause fatal cardiac and gastrointestinal events. Do not exceed the recommended daily dose because of the risk of renal and hepatic toxicity, particularly in diabetic patients.

Narcotic analgesics also are suboptimal agents for pain control. Owing to their significant central nervous system and gastrointestinal side effects, coupled with problems of tolerance, dependence, and addiction, these agents should rarely be used, if ever. If a narcotic analgesic is considered, the analgesic tramadol (Ultram), which binds weakly to opioid receptors, may provide some symptomatic relief.

Dosage

Tramadol, 50 to 100 mg, is taken every 6 hours as needed for pain; the maximum dose is 400 mg per day.

> Caution should be used with the combination of tramadol, antidepressants, and anticonvulsants, owing to increased seizure risk.

Biomechanical Modalities
Electrical Stimulation

Electrical stimulation modalities such as transcutaneous electrical nerve stimulation (TENS)[202] and application of spinal cord stimulators[203] have been used successfully to alleviate the pain and discomfort associated with peripheral neuropathy. TENS portable units that generate a biphasic, exponentially decaying wave form (pulse width 4 msec, 25 to 35 V, more than 2 Hz) should be used for 30 minutes daily for 4 weeks. A study showed that percutaneous electrical nerve stimulation

(PENS), in addition to decreasing pain, improves patients' capacity for physical activity, sense of well-being, and quality of sleep while reducing the need for oral nonopioid analgesic medication.[204] PENS is similar to electroacupuncture in that electrical stimulation is given by disposable acupuncture-type needles. It differs in that it is delivered along the peripheral nerves innervating the region of neuropathic pain, rather than being delivered at acupuncture points or along meridians. Although use of alternating low and high frequencies of 15 and 30 Hz at 30-minute intervals three times a week is recommended, the patient should be evaluated by a health care professional familiar with electrical stimulation techniques for adjustment of frequencies and time intervals as tolerated.

Neural Blockade

Local anesthetic peripheral and sympathetic blocks provide useful diagnostic information but tend to confer only temporary therapeutic benefit in patients with peripheral neuropathy.[205]

Surgery

Entrapment neuropathies such as carpal tunnel syndrome may be relieved by surgical decompression (see Chapter 66, Carpal Tunnel Syndrome). In addition, compression or entrapment from cancers may be addressed by removal of the tumor directly.

Therapies to Consider

Physiologic Regulating Medicine: Biotherapeutics.

Physiologic Regulating Medicine (PRM) is a safe and effective approach to treatment of neuropathic pain that has been used in Europe for many years and is gaining awareness in the United States. The GUNA Method (Guna, Whitehall, Pa) represents the most cutting-edge integration of conventional and homeopathic medicines. The GUNA Method includes the most up-to-date knowledge about homeopathy, homotoxicology, psychoneuroendocrine immunology, and nutrition.

PRM adds a new therapeutic concept to classical homeopathy by restoring physiology through communicating molecules such as hormones, neuropeptides, interleukins, and growth factors prepared in homeopathic dilutions at the same physiologic concentration as the biologic milieu. The unique homeopathic preparation method of dilution-dynamization or sequential kinetic activation makes these communicating molecules even more effective and provides a biofeedback mechanism capable of restoring the body's homeostatic balance.

Treatment is given through oral therapies (drops) as well as injectables specific for neural pain that includes classical homeopathic ingredients, beta endorphins, anti-interleukins 1α and 1β, and neurotrophin, all given in specific acupuncture and trigger points by using a mesodermal technique. These molecular microdoses are capable of reactivating the appropriate biologic immune response that work in synergistic coordination to reverse inflammatory processes and their resultant physiologic effects.[206] No known side effects have been reported with use, and thus PRM can be used along with the other recommendations in this chapter.

PREVENTION PRESCRIPTION

- Eat a whole foods, low-fat, high-fiber, plant-based diet.
- Avoid environmental toxins such as heavy metals, cigarette smoke, alcohol, pesticides, and herbicides.
- Prevent adult-onset diabetes by maintaining ideal weight and staying physically fit and active.
- If possible, avoid specific toxins (see Table 11-1) and pharmaceutical agents known to cause neuropathy (see Table 11-2).
- Avoid doses of vitamin B_6 (pyridoxine) greater than 250 mg/day.
- If taking the chemotherapeutic medications cisplatin, paclitaxel (Taxol), or vincristine, consider acetyl-L-carnitine, 1 g three times daily for 8 weeks.

THERAPEUTIC REVIEW

Lifestyle and Nutrition

- Daily exercise of walking at least 30 minutes per day three times per week should be implemented. If walking is not possible because of painful peripheral neuropathy, gentler forms of exercise such as yoga or tai chi three times a week for 30 to 90 minutes are therapeutic. A whole foods, low-fat, high-fiber, plant-based diet with strict glycemic control should be strongly advised. Environmental and other toxins such as heavy metals, cigarette smoke, alcohol, and pollution should be avoided.

Mind-Body Therapy

- Biofeedback: Recommendation is for at least six 1-hr biofeedback sessions at approximately 1-week intervals. Thereafter, relaxation biofeedback techniques can be performed at home with the use of biofeedback home-use programs (e.g., emWave Desktop or emWave [Institute of HeartMath]), audio CDs, or guided imagery exercises (for 10 to 20 minutes each day).

Bioenergetics

- Infrared: Monochromatic near-infrared photo energy (MIRE), that is, the Anodyne Therapy System (ATS), which consists of therapy pads containing 60 near-infrared (890 nm) gallium aluminum arsenide diodes used three times a week for 40 minutes each

Continued

visit. Four treatments of photostimulation using light-emitting diodes (LEDs) at wavelengths between 750 and 1500 nm may be beneficial.

- Bioelectromagnetics: Magnetic footpad insole devices (i.e., Magstep) with a range of 450 to 475 G steep field gradient can be worn for up to 24 hours of direct contact, and for up to 4 months, to obtain symptomatic relief.

- Acupuncture: Scalp points: upper one fifth sensory area, foot motor and sensory area; ear points: ShenMen, sympatic, foot; body points: GB-40, GB-34, SP-10, SP-6, ST-44, LR-3, and Bafeng (extra point). Electrical stimulation can be used for the ear and body points at a frequency of 100 Hz at low intensity for 10 to 15 minutes for enhanced response. Patients can receive 2 treatments per week for 10 weeks.

- Electroacupuncture: This treatment can be performed in two cycles of five sittings each (10 sessions) at 2-day intervals.

Botanicals

- *Curcumin longa, Boswellia serrata,* and ginger (e.g., Bosmeric-SR, two caplets twice daily) or Curcumin C3 Complex: 1000 mg three times daily.

- Geranium oil (*Pelargonium* spp.): For topical pain relief, apply a few drops (i.e., Neuragen PN) to the affected area several times a day.

- Evening primrose oil (EPO; *Oenothera biennis*): 360 mg orally daily of GLA from EPO. The dose may be increased up to 480 mg orally daily.

Supplements

- Acetyl-ʟ-carnitine (ALC): 500 mg orally twice daily to 1000 mg orally three times daily. ALC is used for both chemotherapy-induced and diabetic peripheral neuropathy.

- Alpha-lipoic acid: 600 to 1800 mg orally daily; start with 600 mg orally daily and increase up to 1800 mg orally daily in divided doses if needed.

- Benfotiamine: Lipid-soluble vitamin B$_1$, 150 to 300 mg twice daily specifically for diabetic peripheral neuropathy.

- Methylcobalamin or 5-adenosylcobalamin: Better-absorbed vitamin B$_{12}$, 500 mcg three times daily or 1500 mcg daily.

- B-complex multivitamin (B-100): One tablet once or twice daily for peripheral neuropathy caused by deficiency syndromes.

- Fish oil (omega-3 fatty acids): Eicosapentaenoic acid (EPA), 1000 to 2000 mg/day, and docosahexaenoic acid (DHA), 500 to

1000 mg/day or a vegetarian plant-based option (i.e., NutraVege).

Pharmaceuticals

For topical relief:

- Capsaicin cream 0.075%: Apply to the affected area up to three or four times daily for at least 4 to 6 weeks.

- Capsaicin patch (8%): One patch to area for 1 hour (after preanesthetic applied) and then removed. It is applied in a doctor's office under supervision.

For acute pain management, consider:

- Analgesics: Nonsteroidal antiinflammatory drugs (NSAIDs) as usually prescribed for pain, as well as narcotics. All should be used very cautiously due to black box warnings.

For chronic pain management:

- Antidepressants

  - Amitriptyline or nortriptyline: 10 mg orally nightly; titrate the dose upward to 25 mg orally nightly as side effects allow (usual range: 50 to 300 mg/day).

- Anticonvulsants

  - Gabapentin (first-line choice): 300 mg orally nightly for 2 days, then 300 mg orally twice daily for 2 days; can be increased to 300 mg orally three times daily as tolerated, with increases in 300-mg increments as side effects allow; maximum daily dose, 3600 mg.

  - Pregabalin: 50 mg three times daily. After an initial daily dose of 150 mg, it should be titrated with the patient's response and tolerability over 2 weeks to a maximum of 300 mg daily.

Biomechanical Therapy

- Transcutaneous electrical nerve stimulation (TENS): Use of a TENS portable unit for 30 minutes daily for 4 weeks is recommended.

- Percutaneous electrical nerve stimulation (PENS): This modality can be used three times a week; stimulation is delivered along the peripheral nerves innervating the region of neuropathic pain.

- Neural blockade: This provides only temporary therapeutic benefit.

- Surgery: Surgical decompression may relieve symptoms in carpal tunnel syndrome; with neuronal entrapment from cancer, removal of the tumor itself may also be helpful.

KEY WEB RESOURCES

National Institute of Neurological Disorders and Stroke. www.ninds.nih.gov/disorders/peripheralneuropathy/peripheralneuropathy.htm.

This page has information about organizations that support neuropathic conditions, as well as up-to-date clinical trials.

MedlinePlus, National Library of Medicine. http://www.nlm.nih.gov/medlineplus/ency/article/000593.htm.

Simplified information is provided for patients about neuropathy and its associated conditions with definitions.

WebMD. www.webmd.com/brain/understanding-peripheral-neuropathy-basics.

This page on understanding peripheral neuropathy contains the basics for patients.

Neuropathy Association. http://www.neuropathy.org/site/PageServer.

This patient source describes neuropathic treatment centers and support groups.

References

References are available online at expertconsult.com.

Chapter 12

Multiple Sclerosis

Surya Pierce, MD, and Patricia Ammon, MD

Pathophysiology

Multiple sclerosis (MS) is the most common cause of chronic neurologic disability in young adults, with a prevalence varying by geographic region from 1 to 2.5 per 1000.[1]

Although the origin and exact mechanisms remain uncertain, MS is a complex disorder characterized by axonal injury, inflammation, and demyelination. This demyelination impairs the transmission of nerve impulses and results in fatigue, weakness, numbness, locomotor difficulty, pain, loss of vision, and other health problems. MS is generally viewed as an autoimmune disorder that transpires when internal antibodies mistakenly direct their "attack" against the body's own nerve cells.

Research suggests that MS is more correctly thought of as one end of a spectrum of central nervous system (CNS) disorders resulting from a byproduct of the malfunctioning of a physiologic immune response whose purpose is protective. According to this view, all individuals are endowed with the potential ability to evoke an autoimmune response to CNS injuries (viral, bacterial, toxin, or direct injury). The inherent ability to control this response so that its beneficial effect will be expressed is limited and is correlated with the individual's inherent ability to resist autoimmune disease induction.[2]

Because of the wide variability of the disease presentation and of the development of treatment protocols, investigators have found it useful to categorize patients with MS into the following four groups[3]:
1. Relapsing-remitting (RR) disease occurs at onset in 80% of cases and is characterized by acute attacks followed by remissions with a steady baseline between attacks.
2. In 50% to 80% of patients with RR disease, progressive deterioration with less marked attacks occurs within 10 years of onset; the disease in these patients is called secondary progressive phase MS (SP-MS).
3. Primary progressive MS (PP-MS) occurs in 10% to 15% of patients and is characterized by progressive deterioration from the outset without superimposed relapses.

4. Approximately 6% of patients with PP-MS also experience relapses in parallel with their disease progression and are said to have progressive-relapsing MS (PR-MS).

Etiology

The search for the cause of MS is made difficult by the marked variation in disease expression. It is not clear whether MS is one disease with variable symptoms or whether the different subtypes represent unique causes.[4] At present, four major theories of the cause of MS are recognized: immunologic, environmental, infectious agent, and genetic factors.

Immunologic Factors

The theory that MS is an organ-specific autoimmune disease is, although unproven, widely accepted. Antibodies against antigens located on the surface of the myelin sheath cause demyelination either directly or by complement-mediated processes. Investigators have suggested that priming of myelin-reactive T cells occurs as part of the disease process in MS. Primed T cells reactive to myelin antigens may develop a phenotype making them more resistant to regulatory processes. The concept that autoantigens can drive B-cell clonal expansion and contribute to autoimmunity has been demonstrated in other autoimmune diseases. A role of B cells in the recovery from inflammatory demyelination has also been hypothesized.[5]

Environmental Factors

Several decades of research have documented that the incidence of MS increases with increasing distance from the Equator. Possible explanations for this finding include genetic predisposition in population groups, dietary factors, and levels of the active form of vitamin D. Evidence indicates that the timing of the exposure to an environmental agent plays a role, with exposure before puberty predisposing a person to develop MS later in life.[6] The dietary influence on MS was first reported by Swank et al in 1952.[7] Dr. Swank noted that people living in colder climates tend to consume diets higher in fat compared with those living in more tropical regions, and this dietary difference was linked to a higher incidence of MS in colder regions.[7]

The relationship between mercury from dental fillings and MS is one of extreme controversy; some studies concluded a clear relationship between mercury and MS,[8] and other studies showed a relationship between the extent of dental caries and MS but no association between MS and the number of fillings.[9] At present, mercury toxicity and MS have too many similarities to be ignored.

The possible connection between viral vaccines and MS is another area of controversy. Although it appears that immunity to tetanus is protective against the development of MS,[10] even stronger evidence indicates that hepatitis B vaccination can induce autoimmune demyelinating diseases.[11]

Exposure to cigarette smoke has been demonstrated to be a clear risk factor for developing MS, as well as increasing the severity of illness.[12,13] These findings suggest the possibility of environmental toxins or pollutants in the pathogenesis of MS.

Infectious Agents

At least 16 different infectious agents have been implicated as causes of MS; however, none has been definitely associated with the disease. At present, three agents are receiving the most attention: human herpesvirus-6, *Chlamydia pneumoniae,* and Epstein-Barr virus.

Genetic Factors

Although most cases of MS are sporadic, susceptibility to MS is substantially affected by genetic factors. For example, clear associations exist between certain subtypes of the major histocompatibility human leukocyte antigen (HLA)-DRB1 gene and susceptibility and disease course in MS.[14] However, the aggregate contribution of germline genetic variants to the disease expression of a given patient with MS may be modest. This concept is highlighted by observations that the clinical expression of MS may be quite different between monozygotic twin siblings who both have the disease; it is therefore likely that several postgermline events influence the clinical expression of MS.[15]

Diagnosis

The hallmark for the clinical diagnosis of MS is neurologic dysfunction that is disseminated in space and time. Objective evaluation includes magnetic resonance imaging (MRI), evaluation of cerebrospinal fluid, and evoked potential tests (measuring the electrical activity of the brain in response to stimulation of sensory nerve pathways). The pathologic hallmark of MS is the presence of demyelinated plaques involving the periventricular white matter, optic nerves, brainstem, and cerebellum or spinal cord white matter (Figs. 12-1 and 12-2).

Integrative Therapy

Lifestyle

Smoking Cessation

As previously mentioned, tobacco smoke exposure is a risk factor for developing MS and is associated with a worse prognosis. Smokers with MS should be offered appropriate counseling and support measures to quit.

FIGURE 12-1
Multiple sclerosis. **A,** T2-weighted magnetic resonance imaging (MRI) scan of the brain demonstrates multiple lesions located in the white matter characteristic of multiple sclerosis *(arrow).* **B,** T1-weighted MRI scan of the spine indicates a demyelinating plaque of multiple sclerosis in the midcervical region *(arrow).* (From Johnson MV. Demyelinating disorders of the CNS. In: Kliegman RM, Behrman RE, Jenson HB, eds. *Nelson Textbook of Pediatrics.* 18th ed. Philadelphia: Elsevier; 2007.)

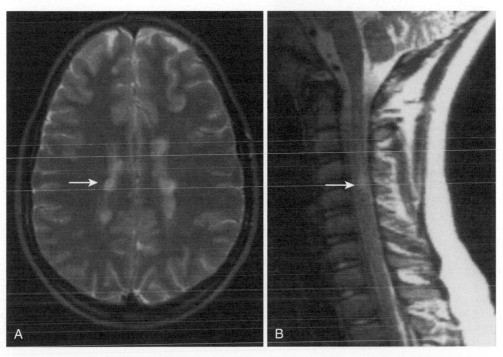

FIGURE 12-2

Changes in magnetic resonance imaging (MRI) scans with duration of disease. **A, B,** and **C,** Comparison of three scans from patients with different disease duration, indicating the appearance of atrophy and ventricular dilatation with time. **D,** As brain atrophy appears, it is common to observe that the number of gadolinium-enhancing lesions declines. (From Lublin FD, Miller AE. Multiple sclerosis and other inflammatory demyelinating diseases of the central nervous system. In: Bradley WG, Daroff RB, Fenichel GM, Jankovic J, eds. *Neurology in Clinical Practice.* 5th ed. Munich: Butterworth-Heinemann; 2008.)

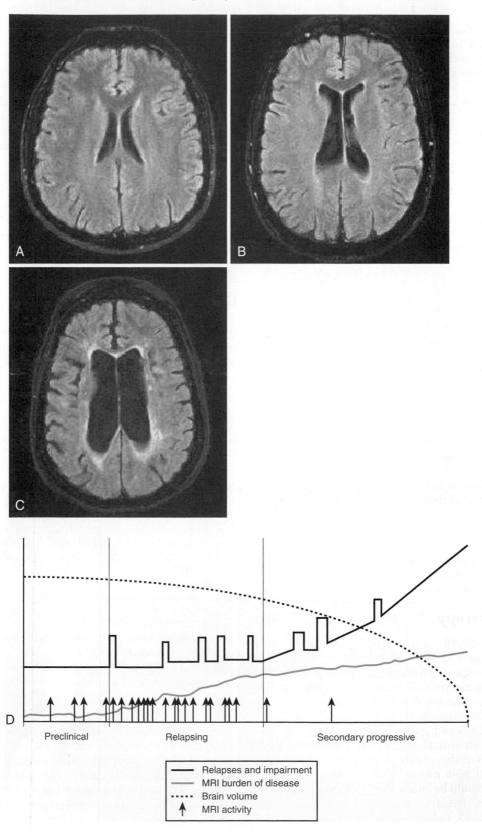

In addition to affecting risks of other diseases, tobacco smoking is probably the most important disease-specific modifiable risk factor for patients with multiple sclerosis who smoke.

Stress and coping should be addressed with each patient with multiple sclerosis and may affect both relapse frequency and disease progression.

Exercise

Although physical fitness and exercise have been associated with better function for patients with MS,[16–18] the exact role of exercise in treating MS remains uncertain, likely because of the variability of the disease. The main question is which patients will benefit from which types of exercise. Accordingly, this is an active area of research.

A reasonable approach is to recommend exercise programs designed to activate working muscles but avoid overload that results in conduction block. Before recommendations are made, physical activity patterns and physical effects of MS should be assessed in individual patients.[19] Research shows that for people with MS, exercise capacity is reduced in response to a single bout of continuous exercise to maximal effort; however, minimally impaired people with MS often exhibit cardiorespiratory responses similar to those of healthy individuals during discontinuous exercise.[20]

Aquatic and other body weight–supported activities are generally considered the most appropriate form of exercise for the population with MS. Water can provide adequate support for patients with gait and balance problems, by allowing movement that may be difficult to achieve with full weight bearing. Modified yoga classes may also provide benefit to patients with MS (see Mind-Body Therapy, later).

Sunshine

Sunlight has been postulated as having a protective effect in the development of MS, which has a clear increase in incidence in extreme latitudes. Furthermore, exposure to sunlight is associated with improved vitamin D levels, decreased relapse rate, and lower mortality in MS.[21] Whether the association of sunlight is entirely attributable to vitamin D is unclear.

Alcohol

Minimal research suggests a dose-related association between modest alcohol consumption and decreased disability for patients with MS.[22] Further research is needed.

Mind-Body Therapy

Psychosocial Factors

Depression is common in MS, and death by suicide occurs seven times more frequently than in the general population. Combining counseling with body work therapies can be highly effective in countering this depression.

Psychological stress has been clearly identified as a trigger for relapses of MS and possibly contributes to disease progression.[23–25] Furthermore, coping styles may effect susceptibility to the harmful effects of stress in MS.[26] Given the relatively modifiable nature of life stress and coping, patients with MS should be encouraged to learn some form of stress reduction, stress management, or coping techniques (see Chapter 93, Relaxation Techniques).

Yoga

Yoga techniques have been shown to improve circulation, balance, the ability to relax, flexibility, and eyesight and to reduce muscle tension—all features typically affected by MS.[27] A yoga class modified specifically to the needs of patients with MS and performed similarly to a modified exercise class in improving fatigue for patients with MS.[28] In the absence of a yoga class for MS, an individualized yoga program developed closely with a qualified yoga teacher or therapist is likely to produce similar benefits.

Mindfulness

Mindfulness-based stress reduction is a mind-training approach that has been successfully applied for coping with difficult life circumstances and illness (see Chapter 98, Recommending Meditation). An 8-week mindfulness-based intervention demonstrated significant improvement in measures of nonphysical quality of life, depression, fatigue, and anxiety compared with usual care in patients with MS.[29] This benefit persisted for 6 months after the intervention.

Nutrition

The following are nutritional and dietary recommendations for patients with MS that generally target inflammation:

- Increase intake of foods rich in omega-3 essential fatty acids: cold-water fish, nuts, seeds, and dark green leafy vegetables.[30] These foods reduce inflammation by their effect on prostaglandins and leukotrienes (see Chapter 86, The Antiinflammatory Diet). If patients find it more convenient to take supplements of these essential fatty acids, suggest a docosahexanoic acid (DHA) dose of 400 to 600 mg/day and a gamma-linolenic acid (GLA) dose of 240 to 320 mg/day.

- Consume less than 5% of energy from saturated fat. This approximates to 10 g of saturated fat per day. Dietary saturated fat and cholesterol trigger the arachidonic acid cascade and increase the production of proinflammatory leukotrienes.[31]

- Consume less than 1% of energy from trans fat. This is approximately 2 g/day. This is done by avoiding processed or packaged foods. Avoiding trans fats altogether is possible because trans fat occurs infrequently in nature. Trans fat may be even more vulnerable to oxidation, and thus an inflammatory reaction, than saturated fat.

- Consider a reduced-gluten or gluten-free diet. Case reports have noted gluten sensitivity manifesting as optic neuritis,[32] and other studies have shown an increase in some proteins from the gut in patients with MS and immunoglobulin G against gliadin and gluten.[33] Considering the difficulty of instituting a gluten-free diet, a reasonable course would be to conduct simple laboratory testing for tissue transglutaminase and gliadin antibodies in the patient newly diagnosed with MS.

Supplements

Vitamin D

The role of vitamin D in decreasing the incidence of MS and in alleviating the symptoms has been thoroughly evaluated.[34] Vitamin D was shown to prevent the development of experimental allergic encephalomyelitis—an MS-like disease—completely in a mouse model.[35] The dose of vitamin D is variable, depending on the patient's exposure to sunlight. Doses up to 4000 units a day have been used without toxicity for up to 6 months. A general guideline is to recommend 2000 units/day from April through October and 4000 units/day from November through March.

▪ Dosage

Usual dose is 800 to 4000 units/day. Titrate for a serum level near 40 ng/mL.

▪ Precautions

Watch for symptoms of hypercalcemia such as weakness, fatigue, sleepiness, headache, and loss of appetite.

> For dark-skinned individuals and those living farthest from the Equator, be sure to monitor 25-hydroxyvitamin D levels and supplement to keep the level near 40 to 50 ng/mL.

Calcium

Calcium supplementation has been found to be synergistic with vitamin D for suppressing experimental allergic encephalomyelitis in mice.[36]

▪ Dosage

Give calcium 800 to 1200 mg/day in divided doses. Take with vitamin D.

Alpha-Lipoic Acid

Alpha-lipoic acid is rapidly absorbed from the gut, crosses the blood-brain barrier, and has powerful antioxidant activity. It not only augments the function of vitamins C, E, and glutathione,[37] but also raises the body's level of glutathione.[38]

▪ Dosage

The dose is 600 to 1200 mg/day.

▪ Precautions

Nausea, vomiting, and rash are possible.

Glutathione

Endogenous glutathione provides the primary cellular defense against free radicals. Glutathione functions both as an antioxidant (in the form of glutathione peroxidase) and as a detoxifying agent for many xenobiotics.[39] The most effective way of raising intracellular levels of glutathione is by intravenous infusion.

▪ Dosage

The dose is 600 to 800 mg intravenously diluted in 10 to 20 mL sterile water and infused over 15 to 20 minutes two or three times a week.

▪ Precautions

Rapid infusion of glutathione can provoke respiratory distress, coughing, rhinorrhea, and vertigo.

N-Acetylcysteine

N-Acetylcysteine taken orally raises glutathione levels. Nausea and vomiting are common with doses higher than 2 g/day.

▪ Dosage

Prescribe 1 g twice daily.

▪ Precautions

It can cause nausea, vomiting, and diarrhea, and it has an unpleasant odor.

Magnesium

Magnesium is required for adequate levels of metabolized vitamin D products to be maintained in circulation. At 800 mg/day, magnesium also has a mild effect on the muscle spasticity often associated with MS.

▪ Dosage

The dose is 600 to 1200 mg/day.

▪ Precautions

Individual tolerances for magnesium are variable. Advise patients to decrease the dose if diarrhea develops.

B-Complex Vitamins

The B vitamins have been shown to aid in cognitive function, act as antioxidants, and decrease the production of inflammatory cytokines.

▪ Dosage

Varies by preparation.

Vitamin B_{12}

Deficiency of vitamin B_{12} and errors in vitamin B_{12} metabolism are known to cause demyelination of the CNS.[40] High doses of vitamin B_{12} given intramuscularly have been shown to improve brainstem nerve function in chronic, progressive MS.[41] Teaching patients self-injection of vitamin B_{12} can be a cost-effective way of improving overall well-being.

▪ Dosage

Oral doses are 1000 to 2000 mcg/day in the form of methylcobalamin. Intramuscular doses of hydroxycobalamin are 1000 mcg/day for 5 days, then twice weekly for 4 weeks, and then twice monthly.

Botanicals

Ashwagandha (Withania somnifera)

Ashwagandha is an Ayurvedic herb (see the discussion of Ayurveda later), also known as winter cherry, that is sometimes called Indian ginseng in reference to its rejuvenating and tonic effects on the nervous system. Ashwagandha's antiinflammatory, antioxidant, anxiolytic, and antidepressant activities all make this herb an important supplement for patients with MS.[42,43]

Dosage
Give 1 to 6 g of the whole herb in powdered form two or three times a day.

Precautions
Some Ayurvedic herbs have been found to have high levels of contaminants such as lead. By knowing the supplier's source of the herb, you can be sure your patient is not taking a contaminated product.

Ginkgo biloba
Ginkgo, in addition to its antioxidant effects, also enhances neurotransmission.[44]

Dosage
The dose is 120 to 240 mg/day.

Marijuana (Cannabis sativa)
Numerous case reports and randomized controlled trials support the use of smoked marijuana, cannabis extracts, and synthetic cannabinoids for MS-related symptoms, especially spasm and tremor.[45–47] Potential legal issues and unwanted side effects must be considered. This is an active area of research.

Dosage
The dose varies considerably with the potency of the whole herb. Consider products standardized to 2.5 to 30 mg delta-9 tetrahydrocannabinol or equivalent daily in divided doses.

Hormones

Estriol
Most patients with MS who become pregnant experience a significant decrease in symptoms. Research has shown that estriol causes an immune shift from T-helper 1 to T-helper 2 cells. Studies have documented a reduction in symptoms and a decrease in gadolinium-enhancing lesions on MRI in women and men with MS who are treated with estriol[47,48] (see Chapter 34, Hormone Replacement in Men, and Chapter 35, Hormone Replacement Therapy in Women).

Dosage
Prescribe 4 mg twice daily. Estriol is available only through compounding pharmacies at this time.

Precautions
Although estriol is considered a "weak" estrogen compared with estradiol, it remains a hormone with the same potential risks, albeit lower, as any hormone treatment. When prescribing estriol to nonmenstruating women with an intact uterus, adding small amounts of progesterone (25 to 50 mg/day) is prudent.

Testosterone
Much like estriol's protective role in women, testosterone has been found to ameliorate MS symptoms in male and female patients.[49] Laboratory measurement of testosterone before treatment is important to determine optimal dosing, and monitoring levels periodically is important to decrease the potential for side effects.

Dosage
Use micronized testosterone from compounding pharmacies.

- For men: 10 to 30 mg/day
- For women: 2 to 5 mg/day

Precautions
Because testosterone can influence prostate physiology, use only after a complete evaluation of prostate function, and continue to monitor men for signs and symptoms of prostatic hypertrophy or prostatic carcinoma.

Dehydroepiandrosterone
Dehydroepiandrosterone (DHEA) serves as a metabolic intermediate in the pathway for synthesis of testosterone, estrone, and estradiol. It also affects lipogenesis, substrate cycling, peroxisome proliferation, mitochondrial respiration, protein synthesis, and thyroid hormone function.[50] Although the evidence for benefit from DHEA in lupus is stronger, researchers in MS have clinically associated low DHEA levels with MS relapses.

Dosage
- Men: 10 to 30 mg/day
- Women: 5 to 15 mg/day

Precautions
DHEA is a hormone that can have potential untoward effects in an individual patient. Monitor the patient and serum levels carefully while prescribing this substance.

Pharmaceuticals

Corticosteroids
Evidence indicates that the administration of corticosteroids improves symptoms of and disability from acute MS relapses.[51] High-dose regimens have become the mainstay of the approach to relapse. Evidence indicates that oral therapy can have the same results as intravenous therapy,[52] although intravenous therapy is generally indicated for acute optic neuritis. Whether corticosteroids affect the overall degree of recovery or the long-term course of the disease is unclear.[51] Plasma exchange is indicated for patients with severe attacks refractory to high-dose corticosteroids.

Dosage
Methylprednisolone, 1 g/day intravenously or (equivalent oral regimen); prednisone, 1250 mg orally daily for 3 to 5 days. Low-dose oral dosage regimens vary; the most common regimen is prednisone 60 mg orally once a day for 5 days, then 40 mg orally for 5 days, then 20 mg for 5 days, then 10 mg for 5 days, and finally 5 mg for 5 days.

Precautions
Side effects include congestive heart failure, hypertension, psychosis, osteoporosis, peptic ulcer with possible perforation, immune suppression with increased susceptibility to infection, and decreased carbohydrate tolerance. Gastric side effects are substantially increased with the oral route of administration. High-dose corticosteroids may be associated

with defects in long-term memory,[53] possibly through affecting memory consolidation[54] and disruption of sleep architecture.[55] A further concern is that use of high-dose corticosteroids outside of a relapse may actually contribute to progression of disability in some patients.[56]

Interferon Beta

Interferon beta-1b (Betaseron) and interferon beta-1a (Avonex, Rebif) were originally thought to increase the resistance of tissues, including those of the CNS, against viral infections. Currently, no data suggest that viral inhibition underlies the effects of interferon beta on MS in any way.[57] The precise mechanism of action of these drugs is not known. Clearly, the effect of interferon beta on disease progression is only modest, and some studies showed no benefit compared with placebo.[58] Long-term benefit (beyond 2 years) is also uncertain.

▪ Dosage

Interferon beta-1b comes as a powder that must be mixed with saline solution immediately before injection and given subcutaneously every other day. The cost is approximately $10,000 per year. Interferon beta-1a preparations are injected intramuscularly once a week (Avonex) or three times per week (Rebif).

▪ Precautions

Injection site reaction, headache, fever, flulike symptoms, pain, diarrhea, constipation, lymphocytopenia, elevation of liver enzymes, myalgias, depression, and anxiety may occur.

Glatiramer Acetate

Glatiramer acetate (Copaxone) is a synthetic copolymer of the most prevalent amino acids in myelin basic protein. The drug is thought to work by mimicking myelin basic protein and thus redirecting inflammatory cells to the drug instead of the myelin. Again, the effects of glatiramer acetate on disease progression are only modest.

▪ Dosage

The dose is 20 mg subcutaneously daily.

▪ Precautions

Glatiramer is well tolerated by most patients. Local injection site reaction is the most prominent adverse reaction.

Mitoxantrone

Mitoxantrone (Novantrone) is an antineoplastic agent that is used predominantly with secondary progressive phase MS.

▪ Dosage

Individualized.

▪ Precautions

Cardiotoxic effects are the major limitation associated with using this agent.

Natalizumab

Natalizumab is a selective adhesion molecule inhibitor used for the treatment of relapsing forms of MS. It was withdrawn from the market shortly after U.S. Food and Drug Administration approval because of the development of progressive multifocal leukoencephalopathy in two patients. This drug is being reintroduced for MS therapy on a selective, controlled basis.

Corticosteroids and immunomodulatory drugs have proven efficacy for treating multiple sclerosis, but they also have potentially serious side effects. The high financial cost of immunomodulatory drugs should also be considered when making recommendations.

Therapies to Consider

Traditional Healing Systems

▪ Traditional Chinese Medicine

Traditional Chinese medicine (TCM) is a codified ancient healing system with a holistic approach that employs therapies such as acupuncture, herbs, and behavioral recommendations. It generally views MS as representing a heterogeneous group of causes and disease processes. From a TCM perspective, patients with MS often exhibit the signs of spleen deficiency with dampness blocking the channels or liver or kidney deficiency. In the hands of an experienced practitioner familiar with MS, TCM can be a safe and effective modality. Additionally, separate aspects of TCM such as acupuncture are often used for MS-related symptoms. Use of acupuncture has been reported in up to 35% of patients with MS.[59] As with TCM, acupuncture is safe and possibly effective for MS when it is performed by a qualified practitioner.

▪ Ayurveda

Ayurveda is among the oldest existing healing traditions. In explaining disease and healing processes, it relies on the interplay of the three *doshas,* or cardinal humors: *vata* (formed of ether and air), *pita* (formed of fire and water), and *kapha* (formed of earth and water). The Ayurvedic description of MS is analogous to that of biomedicine: an excess of pita (inflammation) burns up the kapha (myelin) and results in an excess of vata (weakness, fatigue).[60] Ayurvedic treatments for MS often target the reduction of pita (inflammation) and the replenishing of the kapha (myelin) with medicinal oils, diet, herbs, and lifestyle changes.

PREVENTION (OF RELAPSE) PRESCRIPTION

- Eliminate tobacco smoke.
- Practice some form of stress reduction technique regularly.
- Exercise moderately and consistently; do not exercise to the point of fatigue.
- Ensure adequate rest and sleep.
- Get adequate sunlight or at least 800 units of vitamin D daily.
- Consume less than 10 g of saturated fat a day.
- Eliminate trans fat.
- Increase foods rich in omega-3 fats.
- Supplement with docosahexanoic acid at 400 to 600 mg/day.
- Supplement with gamma-linolenic acid at 240 to 320 mg/day.
- Reduce or eliminate gluten from the diet.

THERAPEUTIC REVIEW

Lifestyle

- Smoking cessation
- Aquatic exercise
- Moderate alcohol intake
- Regular sunshine

Mind-Body Therapy/Stress Reduction Techniques

- Yoga
- Mindfulness meditation

Nutrition

- Limit saturated fat to less than 10 g/day.
- Eliminate trans fats.
- Increase foods rich in omega-3 fatty acids, or take supplements of docosahexanoic acid, 400 to 600 mg daily, and gamma-linolenic acid, 240 to 320 mg daily.
- Reduce or eliminate gluten.

Supplements

- Vitamin D: 2000 units daily if deficient (keep serum level near 40 ng/mL)
- Calcium: 800 mg daily
- Glutathione: 600 to 800 mg intravenously two or three times weekly
- N-Acetylcysteine: 1 g twice daily
- Alpha-lipoic acid: 600 to 1200 mg daily
- Magnesium: 600 to 1200 mg daily
- B-complex vitamins: doses vary by preparation

- Vitamin B$_{12}$ oral dose: 1000 to 2000 mg daily OR
- Vitamin B$_{12}$ intramuscular injection: 1000 mcg twice a month

Botanicals

- *Ginkgo biloba:* 120 to 240 mg daily
- Ashwagandha: 1 to 6 g two to three times daily
- Medical marijuana: 2.5 to 30 mg of delta-9 tetrahydrocannabinol daily in divided doses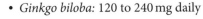

Hormones

- Estriol: 4 mg twice daily topically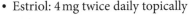
- Testosterone: men, 10 to 30 mg daily; women, 2 to 5 mg daily
- Dehydroepiandrosterone: men, 10 to 30 mg daily; women, 5 to 15 mg daily

Pharmaceuticals for Acute Attacks

- Corticosteroids: methylprednisolone (Solu-Medrol), 1000 mg daily for 3 to 5 days, or prednisone, 1250 mg orally daily for 3 to 5 days with no taper

Pharmaceuticals for Relapsing-Remitting Disease

- Interferon beta: Avenox, 30 mcg intramuscularly every week; or Rebif, 44 mcg by subcutaneous injection three times weekly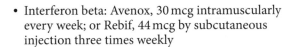
- Glatiramer acetate (Copaxone): 20 mg by subcutaneous injection once daily
- Natalizumab (Tysabri): 300 mg intravenously every 28 days

Pharmaceuticals for Secondary Progressive Multiple Sclerosis

- Mitoxantrone (Novantrone): 12 mg/m^2 intravenously once every 3 months

KEY WEB RESOURCES

Multiple Sclerosis Foundation. http://www.msfocus.org/default.aspx.

This not-for-profit organization seeks to provide "a comprehensive approach to helping people with MS maintain their health and well-being" through programming and education. The Web site provides a wide variety of information including disease basics, support group contacts, articles on complementary and alternative medicine therapies, online forums, and links for health professionals.

National Multiple Sclerosis Society. http://www.nationalmssociety.org.

The Society's mission is to "mobilize people and resources to drive research for a cure and to address the challenges of everyone affected by MS." The Web site features updates on fundraisers and research, a multimedia library, and advocacy and research-oriented resources.

References

References are available online at expertconsult.com.

Chapter 13

Parkinson Disease

Adam D. Simmons, MD

Pathophysiology

Clinical Signs and Symptoms

Parkinson disease is a progressive neurodegenerative disorder. People with Parkinson disease often exhibit a characteristic tremor, a shuffling gait, and a masked facial expression. However, the effects of Parkinson disease are much more widespread.

Preclinical Stage

Parkinson disease likely starts many years before it is first recognized by either physicians or patients. The early symptoms are subtle and nonspecific. Usually, Parkinson disease progresses slowly, but the rate of progression is highly variable. In retrospect, many people can point to early signs that may have existed years before they first suspected they had Parkinson disease. The most common of these early symptoms are constipation and a decreased sense of both smell and taste. Sleep difficulties such as rapid eye movement (REM) sleep behavior disorder and restless legs syndrome may also predate motor symptoms by many years. Family members may have noted a decrease in the range of facial expression, a softness and flatness in the voice, and a more passive personality. Some people diagnosed with Parkinson disease are found to have suffered from late-onset depression for several years before diagnosis.

Early Symptoms

Although the cardinal features of Parkinson disease are described as resting tremor, rigidity, bradykinesia, akinesia, postural instability, flexed posture, and "freezing" episodes, these do not all manifest at once. Early motor signs may be subtle and nonspecific. Often they are recognized only in retrospect. A decrease in arm swing or stride length on one side while walking can lead to pain in the shoulder, upper back, low back, or hip. Decreased fine motor coordination can cause difficulty with buttons and clasps. Thus, getting dressed in the morning may become a slower process.

Additional movements may slow and decrease in amplitude. For example, handwriting often becomes smaller and more difficult to read. When tremors first appear, they often are intermittent and most obvious during stressful situations.

As the disease progresses, physical signs become more obvious. Tremor often is more constant. However, it may be absent altogether in some people, especially older ones. Parkinsonian tremor usually is present only at rest. Some people learn to control the tremor by keeping their hands active. As walking becomes more difficult, people with Parkinson disease tend to become more sedentary. Difficulty with initiating movement, in combination with worsening balance, can make arising from soft chairs and car seats an arduous process. As the disease advances, akinesia (lack of movement) and bradykinesia (slowness of movement) continue to become more prominent. Posture may become more stooped. People with Parkinson disease may attribute these signs to weakness or stiffness of their limbs and body.

Nonmotor Symptoms

In addition to the better-known motor symptoms of Parkinson disease, people with this disorder experience a wide range of nonmotor symptoms. Sometimes these symptoms can be even more disabling than the motor symptoms. The nonmotor symptoms of Parkinson disease can be categorized broadly as psychiatric, autonomic, sleep-related, and sensory symptoms (Table 13-1).

Advanced Disease

Unfortunately, some symptoms of advanced Parkinson disease are not responsive to any of the currently available medications or surgery. Motor freezing, or episodes when people feel that their feet are "glued to the floor," can be difficult to treat with medications. However, specially modified canes and walkers, which use a laser to project a red line for patients to step over, can be useful for breaking these episodes. Other strategies include walking to a rhythm, such as a marching song. Safety modifications in the home such as grab bars in the bathroom and kitchen can help prevent falls

TABLE 13-1. Nonmotor Symptoms in Parkinson Disease

Psychiatric	Depression Anxiety Apathy Dementia Hallucinations Impulse control disorders
Autonomic	Constipation Orthostasis (lightheadedness on standing) Excessive sweating Urinary incontinence
Sleep Disorders	Insomnia REM sleep behavior disorder Restless legs syndrome Excessive daytime sleepiness Fatigue
Sensory	Impaired sense of smell and taste Blurred vision Numbness and tingling Pain

REM, rapid eye movement.

and extend a patient's independence. As fine motor skills diminish, switching to garments without buttons and shoes with Velcro or elastic laces can help with getting dressed. People who have low voice volume may be helped by the Lee Silverman Voice Therapy (LSVT) program.[1]

Prevalence

Parkinson disease is one of the most common neurodegenerative disorders. It is estimated to affect 500,000 people in the United States.[2] Parkinson's disease typically begins after the age of 50, and its prevalence increases with age. The lifetime risk of developing this disorder is 2% for men and 1.3% for women.[3]

Risk Factors

Epidemiologic studies have investigated factors that increase the risk of developing Parkinson disease. By design, such studies cannot identify definitive causes. Although Parkinson disease generally is more common in industrialized societies, it is found with greater frequency in rural areas[4] and increases with exposure to pesticides,[5] heavy metals,[6] and drinking well water.[7]

Large doses of the pesticide rotenone cause a parkinsonian syndrome in laboratory rats that is used experimentally as a model for studying Parkinson disease.[8] Ironically, rotenone is allowed in organic farming practices, although typical exposure rates have not been shown to cause Parkinson disease.

Trichloroethylene (TCE) is a degreaser used to clean metal in factories, as a dry cleaning solvent, and in some household cleaning agents. Results of a study of twins showed that occupational exposure to TCE increased the risk of Parkinson disease fivefold.[9]

Increasing exposures to cigarettes and coffee are correlated with a lower risk of developing Parkinson disease.[6] It is not clear whether these agents are protective or whether early changes in the dopamine-mediated reward systems in the brains of people destined to develop Parkinson disease make them less susceptible to the addictive qualities of nicotine and caffeine. Smoking and coffee drinking certainly are not recommended as preventive measures.

A large, prospective population-based study in Rotterdam, The Netherlands, found that a higher dietary intake of omega-3 fatty acids was associated with a decreased risk of Parkinson disease.[10] The effect was entirely the result of intake of plant-based alpha-linolenic acid, rather than fish oils. Even if it is not preventive, fish oil may still have value for patients with Parkinson disease. A separate double-blind, placebo-controlled study of patients with Parkinson disease and major depression found improved mood symptoms in patients taking fish oil, with or without antidepressants.[11] Additionally, fish oil supplements were shown to reduce the risk of sudden cardiac death in otherwise healthy men in the Physician's Health Study.[12]

Nutrition Suggestions for People With Parkinson Disease
- Eat foods high in fiber to lessen constipation.
- Foods high in omega-3 fatty acids may be beneficial.
- Eat colorful fruits and vegetables for dietary sources of antioxidants.

Pathogenesis

The underlying cause of Parkinson disease remains elusive. The variety in the constellation of symptoms and in the rate of progression suggests that Parkinson disease is a collection of similar disorders rather than a single entity. A single etiology therefore is unlikely to emerge. The variety of epidemiologic risk factors suggests multiple competing factors including genetics and toxic exposures. The balance of these factors determines whether an individual will go on to develop Parkinson disease.

Lewy Bodies
The hallmark pathologic features of Parkinson disease are the death of dopaminergic neurons in the brainstem and the presence of intraneuronal inclusions called Lewy bodies. Lewy bodies contain multiple constituents. However, research has focused on aggregations of the protein alpha-synuclein bound to the intracellular chaperone protein ubiquitin[13] (Fig. 13-1).

Braak Hypothesis
A German pathologist, Hideo Braak, and his colleagues, conducted an extensive and detailed study of the progression of Lewy body pathology in Parkinson disease.[14,15] They demonstrated that the pathology of Parkinson disease begins not in the motor centers of the brain but in the lower brainstem. It spreads up to involve the dopaminergic neurons of the substantia nigra pars compacta only later in its course. This evolution and Braak's proposed staging system support the concept of a preclinical stage of Parkinson disease. The study also suggested that Parkinson disease is not simply a disease of dopamine deficiency. Other neurotransmitters, including the serotonergic, histaminergic, and noradrenergic systems, are affected as well. These other neurotransmitters are involved in the etiology of many of the nonmotor symptoms of Parkinson disease.

FIGURE 13-1
A combination of a pale body *(arrow)* and a small Lewy body *(arrowhead)* in melanized projection cells of the substantia nigra. (From Braak H, Del Tredici K, Rüb U, et al. Staging of brain pathology related to sporadic Parkinson's disease. *Neurobiol Aging.* 2003;24:197–211.)

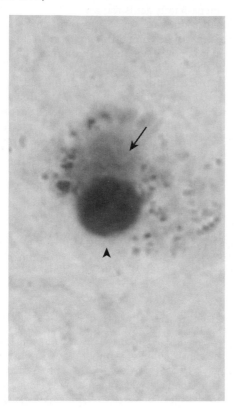

Mitochondrial Hypothesis

One recurring theme in theories on the etiology of Parkinson disease is dysfunction of the mitochondria. Evidence indicates damage to mitochondrial complex I in people with Parkinson disease.[16] Impaired energy metabolism in the mitochondria of dopaminergic neurons may lead to production of reactive oxygen species.[17] The resulting oxidative damage to cell proteins, lipids, and DNA eventually can cause cell death.[18]

Alpha-Synuclein

Alpha-synuclein has been implicated in the pathogenesis of Parkinson disease, although the mechanism still is uncertain. Alpha-synuclein can be found bound to ubiquitin within Lewy bodies in areas of the brain affected by Parkinson disease.[13] However, unbound alpha-synuclein may be more harmful to neurons.[19] In conjunction with dopamine, alpha-synuclein enhances a neuron's susceptibility to death from oxidative stress.[20,21] Studies have also suggested that misfolded alpha-synuclein can spread from cell to cell, analogously to how the prion proteins spread in Creutzfeldt-Jacob ("mad cow") disease.[22,23]

Integrative Therapy

An integrative approach to treating Parkinson disease should start with optimizing general health through exercise and diet. Some people choose to take supplements for their potential neuroprotective benefits, whereas others prefer to wait for definitive studies. As Parkinson disease progresses, pharmaceuticals are eventually needed to help control motor symptoms. A thorough discussion of the integrative treatment of the nonmotor symptoms of Parkinson disease would be very lengthy and is beyond the scope of this chapter. However, addressing patients' nonmotor symptoms may be even more important to improving quality of life than treating their motor symptoms.

Exercise and Movement

Aerobic Exercise

Aerobic exercise has a multitude of benefits for people with or without Parkinson disease. A systematic review including multiple exercise modalities found significant benefit for people with Parkinson disease.[24] Improvements were found in physical functioning, health-related quality of life, strength, balance, and gait speed. Data from animal studies suggested that aerobic exercise also may be neuroprotective and slow the progression of Parkinson disease.[25,26] Furthermore, exercise is helpful in reducing depression and anxiety,[27] both very common issues in Parkinson disease. The forms of exercise that have been studied range widely from treadmill exercise,[28] to playing games on a Nintendo Wii,[29] to dancing the tango.[30] No clear evidence favors one form of exercise over another. Therefore, choosing an exercise program that is enjoyable enough to be continued is the best strategy.

Tai Chi

Tai chi is a martial art that started in ancient China as a means of self-defense. However, over time people began to use it primarily for health purposes. Tai chi emphasizes the cultivation of internal energy, *qi,* through the meditative properties of paying close attention to the details of its movements. Many different styles of tai chi are practiced, but all involve slow, relaxed, graceful movements. Each movement flows into the next. The body is in constant motion, and posture is important. Individuals practicing tai chi also must concentrate and put aside distracting thoughts. They must breathe in a deep and relaxed but focused manner. In the Chinese community, people commonly practice tai chi in nearby parks—often in early morning before going to work.[31]

Tai chi has been shown to reduce the risk of falls in an older population without Parkinson disease.[32] Although large controlled studies on Tai chi in Parkinson disease are lacking,[33] some preliminary reports on its efficacy have been published. One randomized clinical trial found tai chi to be effective in the prevention of falls.[34] Another pilot study showed promising improvements in balance and mobility, but it concluded that larger and longer studies were needed.[35] An additional study showed no objective benefit on gait or balance after 16 weeks of tai chi training, although the participants subjectively reported improvement.[36] Therefore, although overwhelming evidence of its efficacy is not yet available, tai chi certainly is safe, and it shows promise as potentially effective in helping people with Parkinson disease.

Benefits of Exercise in Parkinson Disease
Aerobic exercise has multiple benefits including:
- Increasing energy levels
- Decreasing depression and anxiety
- Potentially slowing disease progression
- Tai chi and yoga can help maintain and improve balance.

Supplements

Coenzyme Q10

Coenzyme Q10 (CoQ10), or ubiquinone, is the electron receptor in mitochondrial complexes I and II. Its level is significantly reduced in the mitochondria of people with early Parkinson disease.[37] In animal studies, oral supplementation was shown to increase CoQ10 levels in brain mitochondria.[38] Oral CoQ10 was also shown to reduce the loss of dopaminergic neurons in an animal model of Parkinson disease.[39] One randomized controlled trial in people with Parkinson disease showed a statistically significant slowing of the decline in a clinical rating scale (Unified Parkinson's Disease Rating Scale) at the highest dose of 1200 mg of CoQ10 with 1200 units of vitamin E.[40] The trend was for the 300-mg and 600-mg doses to provide some benefit; however, the 300-mg dose was slightly better than the 600-mg dose. A second trial using 1200 and 2400 mg along with 1200 units of vitamin E is now under way.[41]

■ Dosage
The dose is 1200 mg in three or four divided doses daily.

■ Precautions
CoQ10 is well tolerated with few side effects. No significant long-term safety data are available at these doses.

Glutathione

Glutathione is a potent, naturally occurring intracellular antioxidant. Its levels are significantly reduced in the substantia nigra of people with early Parkinson disease.[42] Glutathione was tried as a twice-daily intravenous infusion in one small open-label study.[43] A more recent double-blinded study using intravenous infusions three times a week showed a positive trend early, but the condition worsened after the treatments stopped.[44] Currently, not enough evidence is available to support the use of glutathione.

N-Acetylcysteine

Although some evidence indicates that glutathione can be transported actively across the blood-brain barrier, this agent cannot cross passively or in large volume.[45] Therefore, endogenous production is likely the primary source of brain glutathione stores. N-acetylcysteine is a precursor to glutathione that is able to cross the blood-brain barrier.[46] It may therefore be a more effective way of increasing intraneuronal glutathione. In animal studies, N-acetylcysteine was shown to increase glutathione in the brain.[47] It was also shown to protect against cell death in animal models of Parkinson disease.[48] Although it smells like rotten eggs, N-acetylcysteine can be well tolerated in people.[49]

■ Dosage
The dose is 1200 mg per day, generally divided into 600 mg twice daily.

■ Precautions
Frequent side effects include nausea, vomiting, and diarrhea.[50]

Vitamin D

Vitamin D is a secosteroid hormone that has modulating effects on immune and neural cells in addition to its classical actions on calcium and bone metabolism.[51] This vitamin can be consumed in the diet, as well as manufactured in the skin with exposure to sunlight. Vitamin D deficiency is markedly more common in people with Parkinson disease.[52,53] Additionally, in a dose-dependent fashion, one study linked vitamin D deficiency with a greater risk of developing Parkinson disease. People with serum 25-hydroxyvitamin D concentrations greater than 20 ng/mL had a 65% lower risk than did people with levels lower than 10 ng/mL.[54] Vitamin D was also demonstrated to be neuroprotective in animal models of Parkinson disease.[55,56] Administration of 1,25-dihydroxyvitamin D_3 was shown to increase glial cell line–derived neurotrophic factor (GDNF) mRNA and protein levels in the striatum of rats.[57] GDNF shows promise as a neuroprotective agent in animal models of Parkinson disease.[58,59]

■ Dosage
Consider supplementing with vitamin D_3 to keep serum levels between 30 and 80 ng/mL. A general rule of thumb is that 1000 units a day of vitamin D_3 will increase the serum level by 8 to 10 ng/mL.

Vitamin E

Vitamin E (tocopherol) has been looked at in one of the longest studies on neuroprotection. Ten-year follow-up data from the Deprenyl and Tocopherol Antioxidative Therapy for Parkinson's Disease (DATATOP) study found no evidence that 2000 units of vitamin E could slow the progression of Parkinson disease.[60] Additionally, 14-year data from the Nurses' Health Study did not find any reduction in the risk of developing Parkinson disease associated with taking vitamin E supplementation. However, eating nuts, which are high in vitamin E, did significantly reduce the risk of developing Parkinson disease. Nut consumption may have served as a marker for a healthier diet.[61]

Vitamin B₆ (Pyridoxine)
Vitamin B_6 can increase the peripheral conversion of levodopa to dopamine and should therefore be avoided in people taking carbidopa/levodopa. The decarboxylase inhibitor carbidopa should prevent this effect, but it may not at high doses of vitamin B_6.[62]

Creatine

Creatine is a supplement often used to improve athletic performance and increase muscle mass. Creatine is obtained both through diet and synthesis in the body.[63] It is found primarily in skeletal muscles. However, creatine crosses the blood-brain barrier easily and subsequently is converted into phosphocreatine. Phosphocreatine can serve as an energy buffer, decreasing the demand for mitochondrial adenosine triphosphate (ATP) production by donating its phosphate group.[18] In animal models of neurodegenerative diseases, creatine was shown to protect neurons from oxidative damage and death.[64] Because of this theoretical promise, creatine was included in a group of trials designed for rapid identification of agents that warrant further study in neuroprotective trials. In a small, 12-month trial, creatine was found to slow the progression of Parkinson disease marginally.[65] Additionally, no safety issues were identified. However, the same percentage of subjects in the creatine and placebo groups had progressed to require pharmaceutical treatment of their Parkinson disease symptoms.[66] A much longer, 5-year-long study with 1720 subjects now is under way, although the results will not be known until at least 2015.[67]

Dosage
Prescribe 5 g orally twice per day.

Precautions
Creatine supplementation has been documented as being associated with a weight gain of approximately 1 to 2 kg from water retention. Anecdotal reports have also noted gastrointestinal distress, renal dysfunction, muscle cramps, and hepatic dysfunction.[68]

Cytidine Diphosphate–Choline
Cytidine diphosphate (CDP)–choline, or citicoline, is an intermediate in the synthesis of phospholipids, which are essential components in the assembly and repair of cell and mitochondrial membranes. Therefore, CDP-choline may have neuroprotective qualities as well as therapeutic effects in Parkinson disease.[69,70] Several studies investigated CDP-choline as a supplement to levodopa. Investigators found that CDP-choline allowed for a reduction of the levodopa dose by up to 50% without any reduction in symptom control.[69] CDP-choline may enhance dopaminergic therapy in Parkinson disease through multiple mechanisms. It decreases reuptake of dopamine and thereby increases levels at the synapse. Additionally, it activates tyrosine hydroxylase and leads to greater dopamine production.[71]

Dosage
The dose is 500 to 1200 mg orally per day.

Precautions
CDP-choline can worsen levodopa side effects and lead to increased dyskinesias. A reduction in levodopa dosing may be warranted if CDP-choline is added.

Botanicals

Green Tea (Epigallocatechin Gallate)
Epidemiologic studies suggested that drinking three cups of tea per day can decrease the risk of developing Parkinson disease by 28%. Although other caffeinated beverages such as coffee are also linked with a reduced risk of Parkinson disease,[6] evidence indicates that other constituents of green tea may account for at least some of the beneficial effects.[72] In addition to caffeine, green tea contains multiple polyphenols, catechins, and flavonols.[73] The potent antioxidant epigallocatechin gallate (EGCG) is the most thoroughly studied. Moreover, green tea may be helpful in Parkinson disease not only as an antioxidant but also as an inhibitor of both apoptosis and toxic alpha-synuclein fibrils.[74-76]

Dosage
Recommended dose is three cups per day.

Precautions
Green tea can be a strong diuretic.

Curcumin
Curcumin is a phenolic compound with antiinflammatory properties that is found in the spice turmeric. Turmeric is used commonly in Indian and Asian foods, especially in curries. Curcumin has been used also for centuries in the Ayurvedic medical tradition in India. Curcumin has been shown to be a potent antioxidant that can attenuate loss of glutathione in cultured dopaminergic cells.[77] It was also shown to reduce cell loss in an animal model of Parkinson disease.[78] Additionally, curcumin protected against apoptosis in a cultured dopaminergic cell line.[79] The aggregation of alpha-synuclein and toxic misfolded variants was reduced.[80]

Dosage
Studies in people with Parkinson disease have not yet been done. However, typical doses of curcumin for other conditions range from 450 mg of curcumin capsules to 3 g of turmeric root daily in divided doses.[81] As an alternative to taking curcumin capsules, people may incorporate more turmeric into their diet.

Precautions
Curcumin may cause mild stomach upset at high doses of several grams.

Mucuna pruriens (Cowhage)
Mucuna pruriens (velvet bean or cowhage) is a leguminous plant that has been used for centuries in Ayurvedic medicine for the treatment of Parkinson disease. Mucuna pruriens contains levodopa as well as two components of the mitochondrial electron transport chain, CoQ10 and reduced nicotinamide adenine dinucleotide (NADH).[82] In a single-dose, randomized controlled trial, a Mucuna seed powder formulation was as effective as levodopa in reducing Parkinsonian symptoms.[83] This formulation had a quicker onset and caused less dyskinesia than levodopa. An open-label study of another formulation in 60 patients over 12 weeks suggested that HP-200 was well tolerated and helped alleviate parkinsonian symptoms.[84] Currently, neither formulation is available commercially.

Acupuncture

Acupuncture is the insertion of fine needles into specific points along energy pathways called meridians. Acupuncture traditionally is part of the whole medical system of traditional Chinese medicine. Few studies have been conducted on the effects of acupuncture in people with Parkinson disease. Two meta-analyses of the current literature suggested that evidence is not sufficient to support or refute the use of acupuncture in Parkinson disease.[85,86] Both reviews concluded that larger randomized controlled trials were warranted, especially because some studies with design flaws did show promising results. For Parkinson disease, acupuncture may be especially useful in the treatment of some nonmotor symptoms or associated symptoms such as back and joint pains. One open-label study of acupuncture in 20 patients with Parkinson disease showed statistically significant improvements in sleep.[87] Additionally, 85% of patients reported subjective improvement in at least one individual symptom. Another pilot study showed positive trends toward decreased nausea, improved sleep, greater ease of activities of daily living, and improved quality of life.[88]

Pharmaceuticals

Levodopa
Levodopa remains the gold-standard therapeutic agent in Parkinson disease. It is an amino acid that easily crosses the blood-brain barrier, where it is converted into dopamine to increase the neuronal supply. Levodopa is combined with a DOPA decarboxylase inhibitor (carbidopa in the United States or benserazide in Europe) to prevent conversion in the peripheral bloodstream. Levodopa remains the most effective treatment for most of the motor symptoms of Parkinson disease, with the possible exception of tremor. The use of this agent often is delayed to reduce the risk of developing fidgety movements, known as dyskinesias, as a side effect. Levodopa is delayed frequently in the mistaken belief that early treatment will shorten the number of years that it will be effective.

Dosage
Carbidopa/levodopa 25/100 three times a day in early disease. As Parkinson disease progresses, people may take up to 2 g of levodopa per day in doses divided as frequently as every 2 hours.

Precautions
Levodopa can cause lightheadedness, fatigue, nausea, confusion, hallucinations, dyskinesias, and lower extremity edema. However, in comparison with the dopamine agonists, levodopa tends to cause less severe side effects for proportionately greater benefit.

Dopamine Agonists
Ropinirole and pramipexole are the two primary dopamine agonists used in the United States. They have very similar efficacy and are extremely effective for treating primarily the motor symptoms of Parkinson disease. These medications act as a replacement for the brain's decreased dopamine levels by directly stimulating dopamine receptors. They often are used in early Parkinson disease to delay the introduction of levodopa and reduce the risk of developing dyskinesias.[89] Extended-release formulations of both ropinirole and pramipexole are available.

Dosage
Ropinirole: Start at 0.25 mg three times a day (maximum, 24 mg per day). Pramipexole: start at 0.125 mg three times a day (maximum, 4.5 mg per day).

Precautions
Both dopamine agonists have a similar range of side effects. The most common side effects are sleepiness, fatigue, nausea, and lower extremity swelling. Some people have fallen asleep while driving without first feeling sleepy.[90] Dopamine agonists also can increase obsessive and compulsive behaviors.[91] Rarely, serious problems (i.e., gambling, sexual obsessions) can occur. Milder impulse control problems are common.

Rasagiline
Rasagiline is a highly selective monoamine oxidase type B (MAO-B) inhibitor. It slows the endogenous breakdown of dopamine and its precursor, levodopa. Unlike rasagiline's older cousin, selegiline, no amphetamines are produced during its degradation in the body. This difference is significant because amphetamines are thought to be neurotoxic. Rasagiline can be used as a stand-alone treatment in early Parkinson disease although its symptomatic effect is rather mild. In later disease, rasagiline can extend the length of action of levodopa and reduce "off" time.

Studies have suggested that rasagiline may be neuroprotective through antiapoptotic effects. In one study using a delayed start design, rasagiline slowed the progression of clinical symptoms of Parkinson disease.[92,93]

Dosage
Prescribe 1 mg orally, once per day.

Precautions
Rasagiline usually is very well tolerated with few side effects. However, it rarely can cause a dangerous excess of serotonin when it is taken in conjunction with antidepressant medications. Symptoms of serotonin syndrome include flushing, sweating, tremors, diarrhea, and elevated blood pressure. In addition, rasagiline also should not be taken with medications containing dextromethorphan.

Catechol-O-Methyltransferase Inhibitors
Entacapone and tolcapone both inhibit the degradation of dopamine and levodopa by blocking the enzyme catechol-O-methyltransferase (COMT). Entacapone is used much more frequently because tolcapone has been associated with rare cases of liver failure. In patients taking tolcapone, hepatic enzymes must be monitored carefully. Entacapone can increase the length of action of levodopa when the two agents are taken concurrently. However, entacapone has no effect on its own. It is also available as a combination pill with carbidopa/levodopa.

Dosage
The dose is 200 mg taken with each dose of carbidopa/levodopa (maximum, 1600 mg per day [eight doses]).

Precautions
Entacapone can potentiate the side effects of levodopa including dyskinesia, lightheadedness, confusion, and hallucinations. People should be warned that entacapone can turn the urine dark orange or dark yellow.

Amantadine
Amantadine is an antiviral medication used to treat and prevent influenza infections. It was serendipitously found to reduce Parkinson disease motor symptoms when it was given prophylactically in a nursing home. This drug can be used as a stand-alone treatment or in conjunction with rasagiline for early symptoms, including tremor.[94,95] Later in the course of the disease, it can be used to reduce dyskinesias, fidgety movements that are a side effect of levodopa.

Dosage
Give 100 mg two to three times a day.

Precautions
Amantadine can cause confusion and hallucinations, especially in older patients. Fatigue, lower extremity edema, a lacy rash (livido reticularis), and lightheadedness are other common side effects.

Zonisamide

Zonisamide is an antiepileptic medication that has been found to be effective in Parkinson disease as well. It has specific efficacy for reducing tremor. Zonisamide may work by several mechanisms. It has been found to stimulate dopamine synthesis and also may directly inhibit the basal ganglia's indirect pathway through delta opioid receptors.[96] Zonisamide was shown to reduce neuronal and astroglial cell loss in animal models of Parkinson disease.[97,98]

■ Dosage

The dose is 25 to 100 mg per day as one dose or divided into two doses.

■ Precautions

Because kidney stones can occur in up to 1% to 2% of people taking zonisamide,[99] people taking this drug should be advised to keep well hydrated. Other side effects include weight loss, dry mouth, fatigue, and nausea.

Anticholinergic Medications

Anticholinergic medications rarely are used as a primary treatment for Parkinson disease given the high incidence of side effects such as hallucinations, confusion, drowsiness, dry mouth, urinary retention, and blurry vision. However, trihexyphenidyl can be very effective for treating tremor that is refractory to other medications.

■ Dosage

Trihexyphenidyl dose may be titrated up from 1 mg once or twice daily to three times daily and then up to a maximum of 15 mg total per day as clinically indicated.

Surgery

Deep Brain Stimulation Surgery

Deep brain stimulation surgery for Parkinson disease involves the placement of a permanent electrode into the basal ganglia for continuous high-frequency electrical stimulation. Deep brain stimulation is considered when patients still are responsive to levodopa yet the effects of the drug wear off too quickly. Some surgical candidates may seem to cycle rapidly from feeling "frozen" to being wildly dyskinetic without spending much time in a comfortable state. Other people may be considered for surgery if they cannot tolerate a high enough dose of levodopa because of side effects. In a study of 255 patients who fit these criteria, deep brain stimulation surgery was shown to be more effective than optimal medical management.[100] This study found that people who received deep brain stimulation were more likely to experience clinically significant improvement in motor function (71% versus 32%). On average, they gained 4.6 hours of time with good motor function per day. However, serious adverse events were more common with deep brain stimulation. In another study, significant improvements in motor function were seen 4 years after surgery.[101]

Mind-Body Therapy

Depression and anxiety are extremely common in Parkinson disease. Approximately 20% to 40% of surveyed patients report these conditions.[102,103] Depression in Parkinson disease frequently can go unrecognized, in part because of the significant overlap of outward manifestations.[104] In Parkinson disease, depression may decrease quality of life even more than motor symptoms.[105] It is important to screen for these disorders and then to initiate counseling and other treatments as needed.

Increased stress levels have been observed to exacerbate the symptoms of Parkinson disease temporarily. Although no significant evidence exists for or against their use, mindfulness-based stress reduction programs may be considered. Other mind-body exercises such as yoga and qi gong should be considered as well.

PREVENTION PRESCRIPTION

For Parkinson disease, risk reduction rather than prevention is the goal.
- Engage in regular aerobic exercise.
- Drink three cups of tea per day, preferably green tea.
- Maintain a diet high in antioxidants and omega-3 fatty acids.
- Eat a handful (not a canful) of nuts daily (rich in vitamin E and in B vitamins).
- Reduce exposure to pesticides. Wash all fruits and vegetables carefully, including those that are grown organically.
- Reduce exposure to heavy metals. Test and filter well water as appropriate.
- Reduce exposure to industrial solvents and dry cleaning.

THERAPEUTIC REVIEW

Given here is a summary of the therapeutic options for Parkinson disease. Because Parkinson disease can have such a variety of manifestations and symptoms, the ladder approach will not always work. However, for mild motor symptoms, it may be useful to consider. Because this disease is chronic and progressive, most patients eventually will need to use strategies from multiple rungs of the ladder.

Removal of Exacerbating Factors

• If other medical conditions allow, stop all medications that can induce parkinsonism. These medications include neuroleptics such as haloperidol, risperidone (Risperdal), and perphenazine, as well as metoclopramide and prochlorperazine. More rarely, lithium, valproate, amlodipine, and amiodarone lead to parkinsonism. Reduce exposures to pesticides. Have well water tested annually for heavy metals and pesticides. Remedy any abnormalities.

Mind-Body Therapy

• Facilitate optimism. The placebo effect is very strong in Parkinson disease.

Exercise

• Encourage regular aerobic exercise.

• Consider tai chi for stress management and improving balance.

Nutrition

• A high-fiber diet can help with constipation.

• Encourage foods rich in omega-3 fatty acids such as salmon, walnuts, pumpkin seeds, and flax seeds.

• Use turmeric when cooking.

• Drink three cups of tea per day, preferably green tea.

Neuroprotection

• Coenzyme Q10: 400 mg three times daily

• Creatine: 5 g twice daily

• N-acetylcysteine: 600 mg twice daily

• Rasagiline: 1 mg daily

Therapeutic Supplements

• CDP-choline: 500 to 1200 mg daily

• If the patient is taking carbidopa/levodopa, reduce its dose by 30% to 50% when CDP-choline is prescribed.

Acupuncture

• Acupuncture may help with the nonmotor and pain symptoms of Parkinson disease.

Pharmaceuticals

The general strategy is to start with a monoamine oxidase B inhibitor (as long as it is not contraindicated) and then try either amantadine or a dopamine agonist. In patients with mild cognitive impairment, consider starting with carbidopa/levodopa.

• Rasagiline: 1 mg daily

• Amantadine: 100 mg two to three times daily

• Dopamine agonists

  • Ropinirole: Start with 0.25 mg three times daily and titrate up to a maximum of 24 mg per day.

  • Pramipexole: Start with 0.125 mg three times daily and titrate up to a maximum of 4.5 mg per day.

  • Carbidopa/levodopa IR: Slowly titrate up from 25/100 mg ½ tablet three times daily. Stop at lowest effective dose. May increase up to 1 g of levodopa (i.e., one 25/250 mg tablet four times daily) as necessary. May divide into more frequent but smaller doses.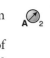

• For tremor-predominant Parkinson disease, start with

  • Zonisamide: 25 to 100 mg daily

  • Trihexyphenidyl: Titrate up from 1 mg once or twice daily and then three times daily (maximum of 15 mg per day).

• If carbidopa/levodopa wears off early, consider adding

  • Rasagiline: 1 mg daily (if not already being used)

  • Entacapone: 200 mg with each dose of carbidopa/levodopa up to eight doses per day

• If dyskinesias develop and are causing the patient problems, try decreasing the dose of carbidopa/levodopa or divide it into smaller but more frequent doses. If these modifications are not possible, consider adding

• Amantadine: 100 mg two to three times daily

Surgery

• Consider deep brain stimulation surgery targeting either the subthalamic nucleus or the globus pallidus internus for patients who respond to levodopa yet have severe motor fluctuations with rapid wearing off or dyskinesias.

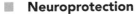
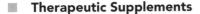

KEY WEB RESOURCES

Worldwide Education and Awareness for Movement Disorders. http://wemove.org.	Information on Parkinson disease for patients
American Parkinson Disease Association. http://www.apdaparkinson.org.	Local and national Parkinson disease events
Michael J. Fox Foundation for Parkinson's Research. http://www.michaeljfox.org.	News about current Parkinson disease research
Environmental Working Group's 2011 Shopper's Guide to Pesticides in Produce. http://www.foodnews.org/walletguide.php.	List of the most and least contaminated crops
U.S. Environmental Protection Agency Ground Water and Drinking Water. http://www.epa.gov/safewater.	Information on water testing, filtering, and safety
ActiveForever laser light. http://www.activeforever.com/p-630-u-step-walker-laser-light-for-parkinsons-freezing.aspx.	Laser light to attach to a walker to help with freezing episodes (provides a red line for patients to step over)
LSVT Global. http://www.lsvtglobal.com.	Lee Silverman's voice training program for improving speech in Parkinson disease

References

References are available online at expertconsult.com.

Section III Infectious Disease

Chapter 14

Otitis Media

Lawrence D. Rosen, MD

Pathophysiology

Otitis media (OM) literally means "inflammation of the middle ear" and is commonly known as an "ear infection." Fluid, either sterile or containing infective pathogens, develops behind the tympanic membrane (TM), with drainage impeded by a congested eustachian tube (Fig. 14–1). In children, the eustachian tube is small and at times tortuous, leading to increased susceptibility to OM. The National Institutes of Health[1] delineates OM into three categories: acute OM (AOM), OM with effusion (OME) and chronic OM with effusion (chronic serous OM, or CSOM). AOM is the most frequently diagnosed subtype, typically following upper respiratory congestion and causing acute inflammatory symptoms such as pain and fever. Earache may be caused by inflammation of the TM and by distention of the TM by pressure from fluid trapped behind the TM. OME may persist asymptomatically for some time following AOM, but it may also be associated with recurrent AOM episodes, as well as chronic inflammatory changes. This state of persistent fluid presence behind the TM, known as CSOM, may be associated with auditory and speech impairment.[2] Most cases of AOM are preceded by upper respiratory tract inflammation and congestion. Common triggers include viral (influenza, adenovirus) and bacterial pathogens (nontypeable *Haemophilus influenzae, Streptococcus pneumoniae, Moraxella catarrhalis*),[3] atopy (allergic rhinitis and cow's milk allergy),[4,5] exposure to prenatal and postnatal tobacco smoke,[6] and exposure to air pollution.[7]

Conventional Therapy

Although widely debated, the use of antibiotics for AOM is currently the standard of care for children younger than 2 years old and for many older children and adults as well, even though up to 80% of cases resolve spontaneously.[3] Great concern exists about the appropriate use of antibiotics for the condition in an age when we are witnessing increasing rates of microbial resistance to antiinfectives.[8] Furthermore, antibiotic use is associated with an increased rate of adverse effects, including diarrhea and allergic reactions. AOM is most frequently diagnosed in young children (ages 6 to 15 months), and more frequent use of antibiotics in early childhood is now linked to increased incidence of atopic disease such as asthma.[9] A "wait-and-see" approach is now increasingly prescribed, using symptomatic relief measures instead of initial antibiotic treatment; the documented decrease in antibiotic usage has not been associated with a corresponding increase in adverse sequelae.[10]

> A "wait-and-see" approach is now increasingly prescribed, using symptomatic relief measures instead of initial antibiotic treatment.

Conventional prevention recommendations include advocating for universal childhood administration of influenza and pneumococcal vaccines. Evidence supporting this policy is inconclusive. Some studies have demonstrated a decrease in episodes of AOM and OME in vaccinated versus unvaccinated groups,[11] whereas others have not.[12] In the case of pneumococcal immunization, concerns have been raised regarding the emergence of new, nonvaccine strains and antibiotic-resistant pneumococcal subtypes despite the reduction in vaccine strains associated with OM.[13,14] The conventional management of CSOM includes a wait-and-see approach, and if fluid persists for some length of time (more than 3 months), myringotomy and pressure-equalizing tube placement is advised.[2] CSOM is the most common reason for elective surgery in children (other than circumcision) in the United States.[15] Even this approach, however, is under scrutiny with regard to when and whether the benefits outweigh the risks.[16]

Concern about the safety and efficacy of conventional approaches has led more practitioners to develop an interest in integrating complementary and alternative medicine (CAM) therapies for the prevention and treatment

FIGURE 14-1
The ear. The Eustachian tube in children is small.

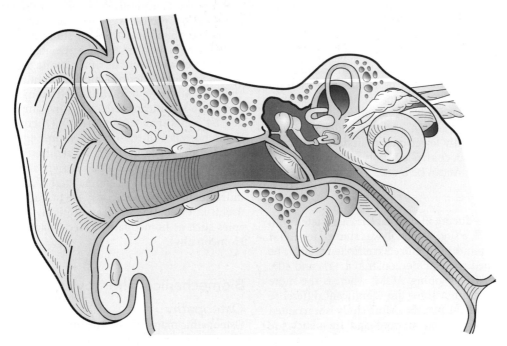

of OM. Additionally, many patients use over-the-counter remedies for management of symptoms—pain, fever, and congestion—associated with OM. The use of these products in infants and young children is strongly discouraged by the U.S. Food and Drug Administration because of concerns about lack of efficacy and potential for harm.[17] Therefore, safe and effective alternatives for symptom management are desirable.

Integrative Therapy

In integrative care, the primary goal is prevention of OM, and the secondary goal is the use of natural methods for symptom management to optimize children's inherent healing mechanisms. Effective preventive measures include breast-feeding[18,19] and avoiding environmental triggers such as second-hand smoke and air pollution.[20,21]

> Effective preventive measures include breast-feeding and avoiding environmental triggers such as second-hand smoke and air pollution.

Regarding symptom management, patients can be educated to view OM-associated symptoms such as fever and congestion as the body's way of fighting infection. Natural viral infections theoretically allow for natural immune system development. Of course, one must consider the degree of symptoms and the possibility of overwhelming bacterial infection requiring the use of pharmaceutical agents, including antibiotics. Commonly used CAM therapies for OM management include biologically based therapies (botanical and nutritional), homeopathy, and manipulative and body-based methods.

Botanicals

Combination Herbal Extract Ear Drops

Botanically based naturopathic topical ear drops were shown to be effective and safe in prospective randomized and controlled trials.[22,23] The specific product tested included the following extracts: garlic oil *(Allium sativum)*, mullein flower *(Verbascum thapsus)*, calendula flower, St. John's wort *(Hypericum perfoliatum)*, lavender, and vitamin E, in an olive oil base. These components have antiviral, antibacterial, antifungal, and anti-inflammatory properties. This topical botanical combination was as effective for AOM pain relief as prescription anesthetic ear drops with or without concurrent antibiotic use. No significant adverse effects were reported in these two trials.

■ Dosage
The product used in this study is from Israel and may be difficult to find in the United States. A similar product, *Ear Drops Children's Formula* by Gaia Herbs (Brevard, NC) is available. It also contains goldenseal and lobelia but does not include calendula.

Larch Arabinogalactan

Larch arabinogalactans, polysaccharides made from the bark of the larch tree and consisting of galactan backbones with side-chains of galactose and arabinose sugars, were linked in one report to decreased frequency and severity of pediatric AOM.[24] Larch arabinogalactan is a source of dietary fiber and also serves as a prebiotic, or substrate for growth of probiotic organisms. Whether its immune stimulating effects result from this mechanism or from others is unclear.

■ Dosage
One teaspoon of larch arabinogalactan powder in juice or water two to three times a day until symptoms have resolved.

■ Precautions
It can cause gas or bloating similar to fiber.

Nutrition

Cod Liver Oil
Cod liver oil, which contains omega-3 essentially fatty acids as well as vitamins A and D, was studied in combination with selenium (an antioxidant mineral) in a small pilot trial for prevention of AOM.[25] Eight children, serving as their own historical controls, received this combination of nutritional supplements for one "OM season" and were noted to receive antibiotics for significantly fewer days than during the previous OM season. Larger, controlled trials are needed before general recommendations can be made.

Xylitol
Based on success in reducing mouth bacteria associated with dental cavities, xylitol, a sugar alcohol, was studied for AOM prevention in four blind randomized controlled trials. The two earliest published trials[26,27] demonstrated 41% and 40% reductions in risk of developing AOM, whereas the more recent two trials[28,29] did not show any significant difference in AOM prevention versus placebo. More study is warranted to determine whether dosing amount and frequency are related to the success of xylitol in preventing AOM episodes. Xylitol has few noted adverse effects, mainly diarrhea and mild abdominal pain in a minority of children studied. It can be found commercially in chewing gum preparations.

Probiotics
Probiotics have been studied for both prevention and treatment of OM and OM-associated upper respiratory infections. A Finnish trial in 571 children 1 to 6 years old who were in child care centers compared prevention with *Lactobacillus* GG–containing milk versus milk that did not contain probiotic, three times per day, 5 days per week for 7 months.[30] Children who drank the probiotic milk were absent 1 less day from child care over the study period. This finding was statistically although not clinically significant. A follow-up study by the same research group compared a daily probiotic blend with placebo for 24 weeks in 306 AOM-prone children 10 months to 6 years old.[31] Probiotic treatment did not reduce the occurrence of AOM episodes. Finally, a Swedish study examined the efficacy of a probiotic nasal spray for prevention of AOM in 108 children 6 months to 6 years old.[32] This complex study design also included treatment with prophylactic antibiotics at various intervals and compared the study group with a placebo control group. During the study period, significantly more children in the probiotic study group had no AOM recurrences and normal middle ear examinations than did the placebo group. Reported adverse effects did not differ significantly between groups (see Chapter 102, Prescribing Probiotics).

■ Dosage
The foregoing study included two strains of *Streptococcus sanguis,* two strains of *Streptococcus mitis,* and one strain of *Streptococcus oralis* in equal proportions. The mixture corresponded to a suspension of 5×10^8 colony-forming units per milliliter. Dosing was three puffs into each nostril twice a day for 10 days.

Homeopathy
Table 111–6 in Chapter 111 suggests homeopathic remedies for OM. Five published studies evaluated the efficacy of homeopathic remedies for treatment of AOM in children.[3] Overall, despite limitations in study design, findings suggested a reduction in AOM-associated symptoms such as pain, as well as a decrease in antibiotic use and AOM recurrences. In the one double-blind randomized controlled trial, children receiving individualized homeopathic remedies had more significant reductions in symptoms (pain) at 24 and 64 hours than did controls.[33] Of course, extrapolating the importance of these positive findings of individualized treatments to a larger, generalized pediatric population is difficult. However, this study design did take into account the actual practice of homeopathy, which is based on individualizing remedies. N-of-1 study designs may be useful in evaluating efficacy of highly individualized therapies such as homeopathy[34] (see Chapter 111, Therapeutic Homeopathy).

Biomechanical Therapy

Osteopathy
Osteopathic manipulative treatment was studied in two published trials for preventing recurrent OM, with the goal of decreasing the need for surgical intervention for CSOM and recurrent AOM. Degenhardt and Kuchera[35] treated eight children with recurrent AOM in an uncontrolled pilot study. Patients received weekly osteopathic manipulative treatment for 3 weeks; intervention was performed in a complementary manner, concurrently with traditional medical management. Five children had no recurrence of symptoms, and only one child required myringotomy and tube placement surgery at 1-year follow-up.

Mills et al[36] performed a prospective, controlled trial of osteopathic manipulative treatment in 57 children with recurrent AOM. The control group received routine pediatric care, and the intervention group received osteopathic manipulative treatment plus routine care for 9 visits over the 6-month study period. Children receiving osteopathic manipulative treatment had significantly fewer episodes of AOM, surgical procedures, and "surgery-free months." No adverse reactions were reported.

> Children receiving osteopathic manipulative treatment have significantly fewer episodes of acute otitis media, surgical procedures, and "surgery-free months."

Chiropractic
Chiropractic treatments have been anecdotally reported to reduce recurrence of AOM and the need for surgical tympanostomies and pressure-equalizing tube placements for CSOM. Published trials to date were uncontrolled nonrandomized cohort studies.[37-39] All trials reported improvement during the treatment course. Given the typical course of AOM to resolve spontaneously, however, studying the efficacy and safety of chiropractic in a randomized controlled trial would be instructive.

Pharmaceuticals

Conventional pharmaceutical treatment for AOM historically has relied on antibiotics that target the most common bacterial pathogens such as *Streptococcus pneumoniae*, *Haemophilus influenzae*, and *Moraxella catarrhalis*. First-line treatment is typically amoxicillin, at a dose of 50 mg/kg divided twice daily, with second-line therapy including amoxicillin-clavulanic acid (Augmentin or generic), second-generation cephalosporins (cefdinir compliance is typically excellent given good palatability and ease of administration with a 5-day dosing option), or azithromycin (also convenient, given once daily for 5 days).

Surgery (Myringotomy With Tympanostomy Tube Placement)

Myringotomy with placement of tympanostomy tubes is the preferred surgical procedure for CSOM under certain conditions. Guidelines for circumstances when the procedure is warranted have changed over time. The most recent, relevant American Academy of Pediatrics policy was published in 2004.[2] This policy notes that the need for surgery depends on "hearing status, associated symptoms, the child's developmental risk, and the anticipated chance of timely spontaneous resolution of the effusion." Specifically, "candidates for surgery include children with OME lasting 4 months or longer with persistent hearing loss or other signs and symptoms, recurrent or persistent OME in children at risk regardless of hearing status, and OME and structural damage to the tympanic membrane or middle ear." Most important, the authors of the policy wisely counsel that "ultimately, the recommendation for surgery must be individualized based on consensus between the primary care physician, otolaryngologist, and parent or caregiver that a particular child would benefit from intervention."

PREVENTION PRESCRIPTION

- Limit exposure of children to environmental tobacco smoke and air pollution.
- Encourage exclusive breast-feeding for the first 4 to 6 months of life.
- Recommend a diet high in nutritious foods such as fresh fruits and vegetables, whole grains, and hormone- and antibiotic-free proteins.
- Advise those with clinical signs and symptoms of allergy and inflammation to avoid cow's milk, and identify all food allergies and eliminate consumption of offending foods.
- Avoid unnecessary antibiotic exposures.
- Consider preventive use of cod liver oil given once daily with dosing based on omega-3 fatty acids as appropriate for age and weight, xylitol at 10 g/day divided five times per day, and prebiotics or probiotics given once daily at a dose typically exceeding 5 billion colony-forming units of live probiotics.

THERAPEUTIC REVIEW

Environmental

- Remove potential allergens and triggers of upper respiratory inflammation (tobacco smoke, cow's milk protein). B/1

Botanicals

- Naturopathic/botanical ear drops: Instill 2 drops in affected ear(s) every 4 hours as needed for pain. B/2

Homeopathy

- Use individualized homeopathic remedies for symptoms associated with acute otitis media (see Table 111-6 in Chapter 111, Therapeutic Homeopathy). C/2

Manipulative and Body-Based Methods

- Consider a trial of osteopathic or chiropractic treatment, especially for patients with otitis media with chronic effusion who are at high risk for surgical intervention. C/2

Pharmaceuticals

- Use antibiotics judiciously in children less than 6 months of age and in all patients with significant systemic symptoms (fever, irritability) affecting daily functioning. A/2
- Use ibuprofen or acetaminophen judiciously for pain relief. B/2

Surgery

- Myringotomy tubes. B/2

KEY WEB RESOURCES

American Academy of Pediatrics (AAP) Section on Complementary and Integrative Medicine. http://www.aap.org/sections/CHIM

National Center for Complementary and Alternative Medicine (NCCAM). *Complementary and Alternative Medicine Use and Children.* http://nccam.nih.gov/health/children

Pediatric Complementary and Alternative Medicine Research and Education (PedCAM) Network. http://www.pedcam.ca

References

References are available at expertconsult.com.

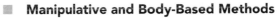

Chronic Sinusitis

Robert S. Ivker, DO

Pathophysiology

Prevalence

Since 1981, chronic sinusitis has been the most common chronic disease in the United States. It is currently the most common respiratory condition in the world. According to the National Center for Health Statistics (a division of the Centers for Disease Control and Prevention [CDC]), approximately 40 million residents of the United States of all age groups suffer from this ailment.[1] Chronic sinusitis affects nearly 15% of the population or 1 out of every 7 people. Twenty-two percent of all women between the ages of 45 and 64 years have chronic sinusitis (15% of men in this age group have it), an incidence approximately equal to that of hypertension. Sinusitis is second only to arthritis among the most common chronic diseases for women in this age group. In men in this age group, sinusitis ranks fourth, behind hypertension, hearing impairment, and arthritis. It was the primary reason for nearly 12 million physician office visits in 1995,[2,3] and more than 200,000 sinus surgical procedures were performed in 1994,[4] (the current estimate is approximately 300,000). Medical costs for diagnosing and treating this condition are estimated to be greater than $10 billion annually.

When sinusitis is considered together with allergic rhinitis (the fourth most common chronic condition), asthma, and chronic bronchitis (the eighth and ninth most common conditions, respectively), respiratory disease resulting from these ailments affects more than 90 million people—nearly 1 out of every 3 U.S. residents—and thus constitutes our first environmental epidemic. In the 1960s, not 1 of these 4 conditions was among the top 10 chronic health problems.

Etiology

The modern-day plague of *air pollution* is insidiously destroying the respiratory tract of those breathing polluted air. According to the Environmental Protection Agency (EPA), 60% of U.S. residents currently live in areas where the air quality makes breathing a risk to their health. A 1993 study performed by the EPA and Boston's Harvard School of Public Health reported that 50,000 to 60,000 deaths a year are caused by particulate air pollution.[5] A subsequent study in 1995 bolstered the earlier findings while concluding that people who live in highly polluted cities die earlier (approximately 10 years sooner, a 15% decrease in life expectancy) than if they had been breathing healthier air. In addition to particulates, other components of toxic air include carbon monoxide, ozone, sulfur dioxide, nitrogen dioxide, hydrocarbons, and lead.

The nose and sinuses are lined by the respiratory epithelium. By virtue of the histologic and physiologic characteristics of its outermost lining, the *ciliated mucous membrane* or *mucosa,* the nose and sinuses serve as the body's *air filter, humidifier,* and *temperature regulator,* as well as *protector of the lungs.* This continuous mucous membrane that extends from just inside the nostrils to the alveolar sacs in the lungs is a connected porous protective shield for the body's air portal. The respiratory epithelial mucosa serves as a vital component of the immune system and acts as the first line of defense against bacteria, viruses, pollen, animal dander, cigarette smoke, dust, chemicals, automobile exhaust, and other potentially harmful air pollutants. The bulk of its job of filtration, humidification, and temperature regulation occurs in the nose and in the four pairs of paranasal sinuses (maxillary, ethmoid, frontal, and sphenoid) comprising the entrance and vestibule of the respiratory tract.

Although the human body is a self-healing organism, this self-rejuvenating process typically requires a period of rest and recovery. The primary challenge preventing healing of the respiratory mucosa is that we breathe continuously approximately 20,000 times per day. When the air that we breathe is polluted and dry, as indoor air tends to be, especially during the winter months, the mucous membrane can easily become mildly inflamed from the chronic irritation, in addition to one or more of the etiologic factors listed later. Without the opportunity for rest and recovery, this situation often leads to *chronic inflammation,* the underlying pathophysiologic process of chronic sinusitis. A chronically inflamed mucosa is weak and therefore more vulnerable to cold viruses, the most common trigger for sinus infections. It can also become hyperreactive and more sensitive to a wide variety of allergens, foods, and chemicals.

Nothing is more important to optimal physical well-being than the quality of the air breathed and the ability to breathe it. Pollutant-laden air often has far less than the optimal 20% oxygen or negative ion content (3000 to 6000 ions/cm³), thus adding to its effect as a chronic irritant in creating inflamed and hypersensitive mucous membranes. Chronically inflamed mucosa often results in increased mucus secretion (rhinorrhea and postnasal drip), head and nasal congestion with some degree of obstruction of the ostia, headaches, and nasal allergy.

Risk Factors for Acute and Chronic Sinusitis

- Infections: The common cold causes inflammation and ciliostasis. Candidiasis, yeast overgrowth, or fungal sinusitis can cause severe respiratory and systemic inflammation.

- Environment (air pollution, both indoor and outdoor, and pollen)

- Lifestyle (diet, cigarettes, and other sources of smoke)

- Allergies: Half of chronic sinusitis sufferers have allergies to pollen or food.

- Food sensitivities

- Emotional stress, especially repressed anger and grief (unshed tears)

- Dry air: Air with less than 30% relative humidity occurs in an arid or semiarid climate and is also the result of forced-air heating systems, air conditioning (especially in cars), oxygen therapy, and wind.

- Cold air: The ideal temperature is higher than 65°F.

- Occupational hazards: Those at highest risk include automobile mechanics, construction workers (especially carpenters), painters, beauticians, firemen, and airport and airline personnel.

- Gastroesophageal reflux disease

- Dental infection: Infection in the upper teeth can spread to the maxillary sinuses.

- Malformations (polyps, cysts, deviated septum)

Fungal Sinusitis

Since the early 1990s, I have treated the patients who have presented with the most severe and challenging cases of chronic sinusitis by using an antifungal regimen. A landmark Mayo Clinic (Rochester, Minn) study,[6] published in September 1999, reported that an immune system response to fungus rather than to bacterial infection is the cause of most cases of chronic sinusitis. The investigators reached this conclusion after studying 210 patients with chronic sinusitis and finding 40 different kinds of fungus, including *Candida*, in the mucus of 96%. In a control group of normal, healthy volunteers, very similar organisms were found. The investigators concluded that the immune system response to these fungi in patients with chronic sinusitis is markedly different from that in healthy people and that this unusual immune reaction is responsible for the chronic inflammation, pain, and swelling of the mucous membranes associated with sinusitis. These investigators called the condition "allergic fungal sinusitis." However, the investigators failed to speculate on the possible impact of previous multiple courses of broad-spectrum antibiotics on the immune response to the fungal organisms in these patients. The resultant profound disruption of the normal bacterial flora of the mucosa likely contributed to the immune response observed. This issue was not addressed, however, and this study concluded simply by stating that "We must begin looking at chronic sinusitis as more than simply a bacteriological and/or anatomical problem, but as a dysfunction of the immune system mediated by a fungus."

Between October 1999 and February 2000, my colleagues and I[7] conducted a study with 10 patients of an allergist-immunologist who were symptomatic despite aggressive conventional treatment for their chronic sinusitis. (Four of the patients also had asthma.) The study consisted of 5 group sessions with follow-up evaluations at 1-year and again at 7.5 years. Dr. William Crook's *Candida* Questionnaire and Score Sheet (Fig. 15-1) was used as part of the baseline measurement, and all 10 patients scored in the "probably yeast-connected" category or higher. They were treated with the Sinus Survival Program (currently called the Respiratory Healing Program; discussed later), in addition to fluconazole. Statistically significant improvement was measured 1 month following the introduction of fluconazole and again at the end of the 5-month study. Although asthma outcomes were not measured, 3 of the 4 asthmatic patients also reported a marked improvement in their asthma, and they were able to reduce the dose or stop using their inhalers. In both the 1-year and 7.5-year follow-up assessments, improvements in sinusitis symptoms and quality of life were either maintained or enhanced in all participants. This is the only published long-term study of a nonsurgical treatment for chronic sinusitis and the only long-term study of the treatment of fungal sinusitis.

> An allergic inflammatory response to fungal organisms is an important etiologic factor in chronic sinusitis.

The Common Cold and Sinitus

 Information on this topic can be found online at expertconsult .com

Symptoms and Diagnosis

Chronic sinusitis is defined as persistent or recurrent episodes of infection or inflammation of one or more sinus cavities, episodes that produce most or all of the following symptoms and signs: headache, facial pain, head congestion, purulent postnasal drainage or rhinorrhea, and fatigue.[9] I now recognize that purulent mucus does not always mean infection, but it does always indicate some degree of inflammation. Although most otolaryngologists rely on the computed tomography scan for a definitive diagnosis of sinusitis, in a primary care setting I have found that a good history and physical examination to detect the presence of most or all of the defining signs and symptoms can provide a reliable diagnosis of acute sinusitis. In my experience, the patients who are most debilitated by chronic sinusitis have some degree of fungal sinusitis. Unfortunately, even in 2010, no consistently

FIGURE 15-1
Candida Questionnaire and Score Sheet. (From Crook W. *The Yeast Connection: A Medical Breakthrough*, 3rd ed. Jackson, TN: Professional Books; 1986.)

Candida Questionnaire and Score Sheet

This questionnaire is designed for adults and the scoring system isn't appropriate for children. It lists factors in your medical history that promote the growth of *Candida albicans* (Section A), and symptoms commonly found in individuals with yeast-connected illness (sections B and C).

For each "Yes" answer in Section A, circle the point score in the box at the end of the section. Then move on to sections B and C and score as directed. Filling out and scoring the questionnaire should help you and your doctor evaluate the possible role of candida in contributing to your health problems. Yet, it will not provide an automatic "Yes" or "No" answer.

SECTION A: HISTORY POINT SCORE:

(1) Have you taken tetracyclines (Sumycin, Panmycin, Vibramycin, Minocin, etc.) or other antibiotics for acne for one month or longer? 25

(2) Have you, at any time in your life, taken other "broad spectrum" antibiotics* for respiratory, urinary, or other infections for 2 months or longer or in shorter courses 4 or more times in a 1-year period? 20

(3) Have you taken a broad spectrum antibiotic* — even in a single course? 6

(4) Have you, at any time in your life, been bothered by persistent prostatitis, vaginitis, or other problems affecting your reproductive organs? 25

(5) Have you been pregnant
2 or more times? 5
1 time? 3

(6) Have you taken birth control pills
For more than 2 years? 15
For 6 months to 2 years? 8

(7) Have you taken prednisone, Decadron or other cortisone-type drugs, by injection or inhalation:
For more than 2 weeks? 15
For 2 weeks or less? 6

(8) Does exposure to perfumes, insecticides, fabric shop odors and other chemicals provoke:
Moderate to severe symptoms? 20
Mild symptoms? 5

(9) Are your symptoms worse on damp, muggy days or in moldy places? 20

(10) Have you had athlete's foot, ringworm, jock itch or other chronic fungus infections of the skin or nails? Have such infections been:
Severe or persistent? 20
Mild to moderate? 10

(11) Do you crave sugar? 10

(12) Do you crave breads? 10

(13) Do you crave alcoholic beverages? 10

(14) Does tobacco smoke really bother you? 10

TOTAL SCORE, SECTION A:

* Including ampicillin, amoxicillin, Augmentin, Keflex, Ceclor, Bactrim, Septra, Levaquin, Zithromax, and many others. Such antibiotics kill off "good germs" while they are killing off those which cause infection.

SECTION B: MAJOR SYMPTOMS

For each of your symptoms, enter the appropriate figure in the point score column:
Not at all 0 points
Occasional or mild 3 points
Frequent and/or moderately severe 6 points
Severe and/or disabling 9 points
Add total score and record it in the box at the end of this section.

POINT SCORE:

(1) Fatique or lethargy
(2) Feeling of being "drained"
(3) Poor memory or concentration
(4) Feeling "spacey" or "unreal"
(5) Depression
(6) Numbness, burning, or tingling
(7) Muscle aches
(8) Muscle weakness or paralysis
(9) Pain and/or swelling in joints
(10) Abnominal pain
(11) Constipation
(12) Diarrhea
(13) Bloating
(14) Troublesome vaginal discharge
(15) Persistent vaginal burning or itching
(16) Prostatitis
(17) Impotence

(18) Loss of sexual desire
(19) Endometriosis or infertility
(20) Cramps and/or other menstrual irregularities
(21) Premenstrual tension
(22) Spots in front of the eyes
(23) Erratic vision

TOTAL SCORE, SECTION B:

SECTION C: OTHER SYMPTOMS
For each of your symptoms, enter the appropriate figure in the point score column:
Not at all 0 points
Occasional or mild 1 point
Frequent and/or moderately severe 2 points
Severe and/or disabling 3 points
Add total score and record it in the box at the end of this section.

POINT SCORE:

(1) Drowsiness
(2) Irritability or jitteriness
(3) Incoordination
(4) Inability to concentrate
(5) Frequent mood swings
(6) Headache
(7) Dizziness/loss of balance
(8) Pressure above ears, feeling of head swelling and tingling
(9) Itching
(10) Other rashes
(11) Heartburn
(12) Indigestion
(13) Belching and intestinal gas
(14) Mucus in stools
(15) Hemorrhoids
(16) Dry mouth
(17) Rash or blisters in mouth
(18) Bad breath
(19) Joint swelling or arthritis
(20) Nasal congestion or discharge
(21) Postnasal drip
(22) Nasal itching
(23) Sore or dry throat
(24) Cough
(25) Pain or tightness in chest
(26) Wheezing or shortness of breath
(27) Urinary urgency or frequency
(28) Burning on urination
(29) Failing vision
(30) Burning or tearing of eyes
(31) Recurrent infections or fluid in ears
(32) Ear pain or deafness

TOTAL SCORE, SECTION C:

TOTAL SCORE, SECTION A:

TOTAL SCORE, SECTION B:

GRAND SCORE:
The Grand Total Score will help you and your doctor decide if your health problems are yeast-connected. Scores in women will run higher as 7 items in the questionnaire apply exclusively to women, while only 2 apply exclusively to men.

IF YOUR SCORE IS: SYMPTOMS ARE:

180 (women)
140 (men)   almost certainly yeast-connected

120 (women)
80 (men)   probably yeast-connected

60 (women)
40 (men)   possibly yeast-connected

Less than
60 (women)
40 (men)   probably not yeast-connected

reliable laboratory tests are available to make this diagnosis definitively. I have relied on the patient's history, Dr. William Crook's *Candida* Questionnaire and Score Sheet (see Fig. 15-1), and the therapeutic response to antifungal treatment to confirm the diagnosis of fungal sinusitis.

Integrative Therapy: Respiratory Healing Program

Although antibiotics have been the mainstay of conventional medical treatment for chronic sinusitis, often followed by sinus surgery if the problem has not resolved, these therapeutic modalities increasingly offer only temporary relief and fail to resolve or cure the problem of chronic sinusitis. In a study of 161 children with acute sinusitis, researchers concluded that "antimicrobial treatment offered *no benefit* in overall symptom resolution, duration of symptoms, recovery to usual functional status, days missed from school or child care, or relapse and recurrence of sinus symptoms."[10] For the growing numbers of patients who have failed to respond to repeated courses of broad-spectrum antibiotics and surgery, for postoperative patients, and for the growing numbers of people who elect not to have (or are not candidates for) surgery or to take antibiotics, the Respiratory Healing Program has consistently produced successful outcomes.

The *goal* of this integrative holistic treatment program for chronic sinusitis is to address the primary cause (inflammation) by healing the chronically inflamed mucous membrane. Although this is a relatively complex problem with multiple risk factors contributing to chronic inflammation, what makes this approach so effective is that each of these factors is either mitigated or eliminated.

Components of the Respiratory Healing Program for Chronic Sinusitis

1. Treating and preventing sinus infections and colds
2. Practicing nasal hygiene: spraying, steaming, and irrigating
3. Eating a healthy, antiinflammatory, and hypoallergenic diet in combination with antiinflammatory and antioxidant vitamins and supplements
4. Improving indoor air quality
5. Treating yeast overgrowth or fungal sinusitis
6. Detoxification
7. Strengthening and restoring balance to the immune system
8. Healing the issues in the tissues: mental, emotional, spiritual, and social health factors

If the patient closely adheres to the first seven components listed here, he or she will usually experience significant improvement in 1 to 2 months, regardless of how many years the patient has suffered with chronic sinusitis. Depending on the patient—the severity of the condition, the level of commitment, and my sense of the patient's capability—I'll typically introduce all but the last two components at the first session, followed a month later by measures to strengthen immunity. The third and fourth sessions, 2 and 3 months into the program, are focused on mental and emotional health and on spiritual and social health, respectively.

The keys to curing chronic and fungal sinusitis are becoming a highly skilled practitioner in the *art of preventive medicine* (specifically preventing sinus infections) and making a commitment to *healing one's life.* My more than 3 decades of experience in treating extremely challenging cases of chronic sinusitis have made it apparent that mental, emotional, social, and spiritual factors have a profound impact on the degree of inflammation and immune dysfunction. Specifically, repressed anger may be the single most significant cause (see Chapter 100 Emotional Awareness for Pain). To have the greatest therapeutic benefit, the recommendations that follow should be practiced on a daily basis and incorporated into one's lifestyle. From the foregoing published study and from statistics I have derived from patient questionnaires since 1990, more than 90% of patients who make at least a 3-month commitment (and three to four office visits) to the Respiratory Healing Program experience, at a minimum, a significant improvement, and in most cases, chronic sinusitis is cured.

Integrative Therapy: Treating and Preventing Sinus Infections and Colds*

Natural "Antibiotics"

Garlic

Allimed or Allimax (both are 100% pure allicin, the active ingredient in garlic) is my first choice because studies have shown it to be highly effective as an *antibacterial,*[11,12] *antiviral* (kills cold viruses),[13] and *antifungal.*[14] In my practice, it has been consistently effective in treating and preventing sinus infections and colds. However, it needs to be taken in therapeutic doses. Allimed (450 mg/capsule) and Allimax (180 mg/capsule) are both available in liquid form for children.

■ Dosage

For treating a sinus infection: Allimed, two capsules three times daily for 10 days; Allimax, five capsules three times daily for 10 days. For treating colds and preventing sinus infections: at the first sign of a cold, Allimed, two capsules (or Allimax, five capsules) three times daily for 2 to 3 days; then if symptoms have subsided, one capsule (or Allimax, two capsules) twice daily for 2 to 3 days.

Echinacea and Elderberry

The commercial formulation EchinOsha with Elderberry contains two antiviral herbs, *Echinacea*[15] and elderberry[16] (also effective for the influenza virus), as well as osha root, which helps to strengthen the immune system. This preparation is contraindicated during pregnancy and in patients with autoimmune disease.

■ Dosage

EchinOsha, for treating colds and flu: 1 to 2 teaspoons every 2 to 4 hours for as long as symptoms are present. Or *Echinacea* extract, 2 dropperfuls four to five times a day.

*Editor's Note: Dr. Ivker has financial ties to some of these products, which are sold through his Web site.

Yin Chiao

This antiviral Chinese herb is available in health food stores.

■ Dosage

For treating colds: three to five tablets or capsules (300 to 500 mg each) four or five times a day in the first 48 hours.

Grapefruit Seed Extract

In capsule or liquid form, grapefruit seed extract, which is antifungal and antiviral, is available in health food stores.

■ Dosage

The dose is 250 mg three times daily or 10 drops in water three times daily (the liquid has an unpleasant taste).

Nasal Sprays

Sinus Survival Spray

This saline nasal spray contains aloe, calendula, and yarrow leaf (antiinflammatory herbs), in addition to grapefruit seed extract (Table 15-1).

■ Dosage

One to two sprays in each nostril every 1 to 2 hours during infection; apply a dab of peppermint oil to the *outside* of the nostrils following each application. Use for both treatment and prevention on a daily basis.

Nasal Rescue (Ionic Silver Spray)

This is highly effective in killing bacteria, viruses, and fungi. It contains ionic silver.

■ Dosage

One spray in each nostril every 15 to 20 minutes for maximum effectiveness; apply a dab of peppermint oil to the outside of the nostrils following each application. Use only for treating infection.

Nasal Hygiene (see Table 15-1)

Steam Inhaler

This acts as a decongestant[17,18] and mucolytic. Add a highly medicinal eucalyptus oil, peppermint oil, and tea tree oil to the steam. Use three to four times a day for at least 15 to 20 minutes if treating an infection and once or twice daily preventively and for treating chronic inflammation.

Irrigation

Perform three to four times a day for treating a sinus infection, immediately following use of the steam inhaler.[19,20] A pulsatile irrigator is the most effective irrigating device and the only one that has been shown to remove the biofilm. Irrigation is one of the best methods for quickly eliminating (and preventing, once or twice daily) sinus infections, as well as for treating chronic and fungal sinusitis (see Chapter 109, Sinus Irrigation).

Antiinflammatory and Antioxidant Vitamins and Supplements

Vitamin C

A regimen of 3000 to 5000 mg three times a day with meals is followed, for the antiinflammatory and antioxidant effects. Use this high dosage until symptoms subside, and then reduce the dose to 2000 mg three times a day. Vitamin C is

TABLE 15-1. Physical and Environmental Health Components of Sinus Survival Program

MEASURE	PREVENTIVE MAINTENANCE	TREATMENT
Sleep	7–9 hr; no alarm clock	8–10+ hr/day
Negative ions or air cleaner	Continuous operation; use ions especially with air conditioning	Continuous operation
Room humidifier, warm mist	Use during dry conditions, especially in winter if heat is on and in summer if air conditioner is on	Continuous operation
Saline nasal spray	Use daily, especially with dirty or dry air	Use daily every 2–3 hr
Steam inhaler	Use as needed with dirty or dry air	Use two to four times/day; add eucalyptus oil
Nasal irrigation	Use as needed with dirty or dry air	Use daily, two to four times/day, after steam
Water, filtered	Drink ½ oz/lb body weight; with exercise, drink 2–3 oz/lb	½–⅓ oz/lb of body weight
Diet	Emphasize fresh fruit and vegetables, whole grains, fiber; limit sugar, dairy, caffeine, and alcohol	No sugar, dairy, alcohol
Exercise, preferably aerobic	Minimum of 20–30 min three to five times/wk; avoid outdoors with high pollution or pollen levels and extremely cold temperatures	No aerobic; moderate walking allowed; avoid outdoors with high pollution or pollen levels and cold temperatures

Modified from Ivker RS. *Sinus Survival: The Holistic Medical Treatment for Sinusitis, Allergies, and Cold.* 4th ed. New York: Tarcher/Putnam; 2000.

most effective if it is taken in the form of Ester C or a mineral ascorbate (for better absorption and gastrointestinal tolerance), rather than as ascorbic acid. If diarrhea occurs, then the dose should be reduced.[21-26]

Vitamin D₃

The dose is 100,000 units daily for the first 3 days of a sinus infection. Vitamin D_3 is a potent immune strengthener and can safely be taken at 5000 to 10,000 units daily on an ongoing basis. Studies have revealed that most illnesses are accompanied by a deficiency in vitamin D.[27-31]

Grape Seed Extract

Patients should take 300 mg in the morning on an empty stomach. Grape seed is a powerful antioxidant, antiinflammatory, and antihistamine.[32-34]

Fish Oil

Eicosapentaenoic acid 1000 to 3000 mg/docosahexaenoic acid 500 to 900 mg per day. This is an omega 3/omega-6 combination. Fish oil is a potent natural antiinflammatory.[35-37]

Sinupret Plus

One tablet three times daily. This herbal combination serves as a highly effective natural antiinflammatory for the mucous membrane of the upper respiratory tract.

Sleep

Nine to 10 or more hours for treating sinus infections; 7 to 9 hours for prevention. Adequate sleep is perhaps the most effective and convenient and least expensive way to strengthen the immune system.

Diet

Patients should eat mostly organic vegetables and fruits, nongluten grains (brown rice, quinoa, millet, buckwheat, amaranth), fiber, and protein; they should *avoid* sugar, dairy, wheat, other carbohydrates (especially gluten grains), caffeine, and alcohol. Sugar weakens immunity; wheat, dairy, and gluten grains are most common causes of food allergy (often a trigger of sinus infections).

Patients should also drink filtered water, at least ½ oz/lb of body weight (e.g., 160 lb = 80 oz/day). For colds, patients should drink lots of warm or hot liquids; ginger root or peppermint tea is recommended, possibly including ginger, honey, lemon, cayenne, cinnamon, and a teaspoon of brandy.

Emotional Factors

Treat the emotional cause. Most sinus infections are triggered by repressed anger or unshed tears. I recommend the safe release of anger, as well as reflecting on whether the patient is feeling grief or some sense of loss. The feeling of grief or loss is typically not as obvious as the anger, but it is probably there, just a bit deeper. Journaling is another excellent method for releasing either or both of these painful emotions (see Chapter 96, Journaling for Health).

Improving Indoor Air Quality

Ideal air quality is rated by clarity (freedom from pollutants), humidity (between 35% and 55%), temperature (between 65°F and 85°F), oxygen content (21% of total volume and 100% saturation), and negative ion content (3000 to 6000 .001 micron ions/cm³). Air that is clean, moist, warm, oxygen rich, and high in negative ions is healing to the mucous membrane (see Table 15-1). To create optimal indoor air I recommend the following:

- A negative ion generator[38-40]: used as an air cleaner and placed in the rooms in which patients spend the bulk of their time, especially the bedroom and office
- Furnace filter: an electrostatic or a pleated filter (e.g., Filtrete by 3M)
- Air duct and furnace cleaning
- Carpet cleaning
- Use of a humidifier: a warm mist room unit, especially during the winter months
- Plants, especially those that can remove formaldehyde (Boston fern, chrysanthemums, striped *Dracaena*, dwarf date palm) and carbon monoxide (spider plant)

Treating Yeast Overgrowth and Fungal Sinusitis

Most severe and unresponsive (to conventional treatment) cases of chronic sinusitis require anti-*Candida* antifungal treatment. Although very similar in its holistic scope, the comprehensive treatment program for fungal sinusitis or yeast overgrowth and candidiasis is more challenging than the regimen for simple chronic sinusitis (i.e., without a significant degree of *Candida* overgrowth), chiefly because of the restrictive *Candida*-control diet. The treatment program depends on how sick the patient is, which can be reliably determined through the patient's medical history and Dr. Crook's *Candida* Questionnaire and Score Sheet (see Fig. 15-1). If yeast symptoms are confined to the gastrointestinal tract or vagina, the program is shorter and simpler than if the yeast toxins have spread throughout the body and are causing recurrent sinus infections along with inflammation in other parts of the body (e.g., myalgia, arthralgia, mental "fog," or severe fatigue). In the case of systemic inflammation, which is most often the situation in patients with severe chronic sinusitis, curing the condition can take from 6 months to 1 year.

The treatment program for fungal sinusitis consists of four components. I recommend integrating all four of the following components simultaneously for the best possible outcomes:

1. Reduce the overgrowth of *Candida*.
2. Eliminate the fuel for the growth of *Candida* organisms through diet. Starve them!
3. Restore normal bacterial flora in the bowel.
4. Strengthen the immune system.

Reducing the Yeast Overgrowth

Until recently, I relied heavily on the prescription antifungal fluconazole (Diflucan) to kill *Candida*. The dosage I prescribe is 200 mg daily for 6 weeks, followed by 200 mg every other day for 3 weeks. Although this drug works well, it often results in a *die-off*, or Herxheimer reaction, which usually occurs during the first 2 weeks of treatment and typically lasts for 2 days to 1 week. The medication is so effective in killing yeast that as the organisms die, they release a "flood" of toxins into the bloodstream that can cause fatigue, headaches, congestion, increased mucus drainage, nausea, loose stools, flulike aches and pains, and any other symptom (usually resulting from inflammation) that yeast toxins are known to produce. Distilled water, both drunk and used as an enema, vitamin C, and ibuprofen can all help to relieve these die-off symptoms.

Although for a short time patients may possibly feel worse than they did before they started taking the drug, they may also choose to look at the "regression" resulting from die-off as a confirmation of the diagnosis of *Candida* overgrowth, as well as a hopeful sign that they are eliminating yeast and will be feeling much better very soon. Following die-off, most patients experience a level of health significantly greater than they had before treating the *Candida* overgrowth.

Prescription drugs, however, rarely provide the entire solution. In addition to antifungal supplements and probiotics, patients must also be prepared to adhere strictly to the dietary recommendations.

In 2004, I discovered antifungal supplements, Allimax and Allimed, that are nearly as effective as fluconazole, although not as fast acting as the drug. These supplements have no harmful side effects (antifungal drugs have a minimal risk of liver toxicity), and the die-off reaction is usually less severe. Allimed contains the same 100% pure allicin, called allipure, as Allimax, but each capsule is 450 mg, rather than the 180-mg capsules of Allimax. Allimed is available only through practitioners and is slightly less costly than Allimax, although it is still expensive. Allimed has become my first choice for mild to moderate candidiasis; in patients with severe cases, I use it in conjunction with fluconazole. These supplements also work well in treating sinus infections, as noted earlier, because they are highly effective antibacterial agents.

Other antifungal supplements that I have had success with include the following:

- Candex or Candisol: This supplement contains an enzyme that destroys the cell wall of *Candida* organisms and reduces die-off symptoms. It is especially helpful in patients who have both sinusitis and asthma. Not infrequently, the die-off symptoms worsen asthma and make breathing more difficult. This supplement is well tolerated and is a consistent component of the *Candida* treatment program. Candex is readily available in most health food stores; Candisol, which has a higher strength of the active ingredient, is available only through practitioners.

- Flora-Balance or Latero-Flora: This unique strain of bacteria, *Bacillus laterosporus B.O.D.*, is available in some health food stores as Flora-Balance or through physicians as Latero-Flora. It has been tested extensively and found to be highly effective for gastrointestinal dysfunction, food sensitivities, and candidiasis.

- Grapefruit seed extract: In liquid or capsule form, this supplement is also available in nearly all health food stores.

- CandiBactin-AR (Metagenics, San Clemente, Calif): This supplement is a combination of essential oils from the mint family, especially red thyme oil and oregano oil. Although I have not had much experience with it personally, I do know several practitioners who have had success using it. I am also aware of successful treatment of candidiasis with just oregano oil.

I take an aggressive approach to treating fungal sinusitis and usually use several of the foregoing products in combination (but not all of them together), along with either fluconazole or Allimed.

Numerous products available in health food stores can help to eliminate *Candida*. Most contain caprylic acid, garlic, pau d'arco, plant tannins, grapefruit seed extract, oregano oil, and other herbs that act directly on *Candida* or indirectly by strengthening the immune system. Although most of these products do not work as quickly as the regimen I have recommended here, I have observed that patients find it helpful to *rotate* antifungal supplements and not continue using the same one longer than approximately 2 months.

Eliminating the Fuel for Candida Through Diet

While at the same time strengthening the immune system, diet is the foundation of any antifungal treatment program. Because every individual has a unique body chemistry, no two *Candida*-control diets will be exactly the same. Moreover, every physician who treats candidiasis and fungal sinusitis has somewhat different dietary recommendations. However, most people with yeast overgrowth are far more susceptible to food allergies, and the following basic principles apply to almost anyone who opts for a *Candida*-control, hypoallergenic, and antiinflammatory diet:

- The diet consists primarily of protein and fresh organic vegetables and a limited amount of complex carbohydrates and fat-containing foods, along with a small amount of fresh fruit.

- Sugar and concentrated sweets are always avoided.

- The minimum time frame for maintaining the diet is 3 to 6 months, although the diet can be less restrictive the longer it is followed.

- The best practice is to rotate the acceptable foods and not eat a particular food more than once every 3 or 4 days. This is especially true for grains.

- Changing one's diet can be a challenge. The more involved the patient is in the process—planning, shopping, and cooking—the easier and more rewarding it will be.

For the first 21 days, avoid starch and high-sugar foods, including fruit. Also avoid yeast and mold foods (see later).

■ Foods to Include at the Onset of the Diet

- Vegetables: should be eaten freely; 50% to 60% of total diet; raw or lightly steamed; organic and clean (wash well); vegetables with high water content and low starch preferable

- Green leafy: all lettuce, spinach, parsley, cabbage, kale, collard greens, watercress, beet greens, mustard greens, bok choy, sprouts
- Other low-starch vegetables: celery, zucchini, summer squash, crookneck squash, green beans, broccoli, cauliflower, brussels sprouts, radish, bell pepper (green, red, yellow), asparagus, cucumber, tomato, onion, leek, garlic, kohlrabi
- Moderately low starch: carrot, beet, rutabaga, turnip, parsnip, eggplant, artichoke, avocado, water chestnuts, peas (green, snow peas), okra

- Protein: emphasis at breakfast and lunch with no less than 60 g per day; antibiotic-free and hormone-free meats; fresh deep-water ocean fish; raw organic seeds and nuts; acceptable proteins: fish, canned fish (salmon and tuna, no more than twice per week), turkey, ground turkey, chicken, lamb, wild game, Cornish hens, eggs (two to four per week), and seeds and nuts (almonds, cashews, pecans, filberts, pine nuts, Brazil nuts, walnuts, pistachios, sunflower seeds, sesame seeds [raw or dry roasted], pumpkin seeds)
- Complex carbohydrates: starchy vegetables, legumes (introduced after the first 21 days), and whole grains; only enough consumed to maintain energy (ideally, one serving a day or less); restriction varied according to food allergy, which can be determined with food rotation
  - Starchy vegetables: new and red potatoes, sweet potatoes, yams, winter squash (acorn, butternut), pumpkin
  - Legumes: lentils, split peas, black-eyed peas, beans (kidney, garbanzo, black, navy, pinto, lima, adzuki)
  - Nongluten grains: brown rice, millet, quinoa, buckwheat, and amaranth, sprouted or cooked, organic and clean; available in bulk at health food stores; grains rotated every 4 days; tasty as breakfast cereals, in salads and soups, and in casseroles and stir-fry; stored away from light and heat in airtight containers; other whole grains (with gluten) that should be eaten in only limited amounts: barley, spelt, wild rice, corn, oats, cornmeal, bulgur, couscous
- Flaxseed oil: 1 to 2 tablespoons daily; used on grains or vegetables or as a salad dressing, *not* heated or used for cooking; kept refrigerated and away from light; other acceptable oils (cold-pressed): extra virgin olive oil, canola, walnut, macadamia nut, used within 6 weeks of opening

Foods to Include After 21 Days

- Fruits: Fruits are introduced into the diet slowly, one serving per day until the patient is sure they do not make symptoms worse. One starts with melons, berries (blueberries, raspberries, huckleberries, blackberries), lemon, and grapefruit (only after the first 21 days of the diet) and then chooses from among most other fresh fruits, all of which are generally sweeter than the first group. These include apple, pear, peach, orange, nectarine, apricot, cherry, and pineapple. Fruit juices should be very diluted, at least 1:1 with water. Freshly squeezed is best. Full-strength fruit juices, canned fruit juices, and all dried fruits are avoided.

- Yeast- and mold-containing foods: These are allowable only if the patient is not allergic. However, I would introduce them very gradually (no more than one particular food every 3 to 4 days) and not before at least 3 weeks into the diet. These foods include the following: fermented dairy products such as yogurt, kefir, buttermilk, low-fat cottage cheese, and sour cream; fermented foods such as tofu, tempeh, miso, and soy sauce; and raw almond butter and raw sesame tahini.

Foods to Avoid

- *Refined sugar and sugar-containing foods:* cakes, cookies, candy, doughnuts, pastries, ice cream, pudding, soft drinks, pies; anything containing sucrose (table sugar), fructose, maltose, lactose, glucose, dextrose, corn sweetener, corn syrup, sorbitol, or mannitol; honey; molasses; maple syrup; date sugar; barley malt; rice syrup; NutraSweet; and saccharine; table salt (often contains sugar; sea salt preferred)
- *To diminish sugar cravings:* chromium picolinate, 200 mcg twice daily; biotin, 500 to 1000 mcg twice daily; and a yeast-free B-vitamin complex, 50 mg twice daily, only if the patient is not already taking a comprehensive multivitamin; craving also eliminated by 4 days without any sugar
- *Milk and dairy products:* all cheeses (unsweetened soy milk and butter allowed, but not in excess)
- Bread and other yeast-raised baked items, including cakes, cookies, and crackers; whole grain cereals; pastas; tortillas; waffles; and muffins
- Beef and pork
- *Mushrooms:* all types
- Rye and wheat (avoided for first 3 weeks)
- Grapes, plums, bananas, dried fruit, canned fruit, and canned vegetables
- Alcoholic beverages
- *Caffeine:* both tea and coffee (herbal tea and green tea allowed)
- White or refined flour products, packaged or processed and refined foods
- Fried foods, fast foods, sausage, and hot dogs
- Vinegar, mustard, ketchup, sauerkraut, olives, and pickles (raw apple cider vinegar allowed)
- Margarine, preservatives (e.g., in frozen vegetables)
- Refined and hydrogenated oils
- Leftovers (can be frozen for later)
- Rice milk (high carbohydrate content)

This diet is meant to be a guide. The responses to it will vary greatly depending on the severity of the candidiasis, food allergies, and the type of medication (if any) the patient is taking to eliminate *Candida*. Most people who closely adhere to it will experience a significant improvement within 1 month. If the diet is followed for 3 to 4 weeks in addition to taking medication or antifungal supplements and the patient reports no improvement, however, then I would recommend going back to the basic vegetable (low-starch) and protein diet and being highly suspicious of food allergy or leaky gut syndrome. The offending food is often something that is eaten every day and for which the patient has developed a craving. If new foods are reintroduced very gradually, every 3 to 4 days, then the offending food should be easily detected from the symptoms that arise after eating it.

Initially many patients complain, "There's nothing to eat on this diet." Losing 8 to 10 lb during the first month is not unusual. Many different nutritious and tasty choices are available, however, and the weight loss will subside after the first month unless your patient is significantly overweight. A key factor in successfully maintaining the diet lies in finding desirable recipes. *Candida*-control diet cookbooks are relatively easy to locate in most health food stores.

This *Candida*-control, hypoallergenic, and antiinflammatory diet is essentially the same diet I recommend to all my patients with chronic sinusitis, although it need not be quite as restrictive if fungal sinusitis is not a significant factor.

> My basic dietary recommendations are to avoid milk and dairy products, sugar, wheat, caffeine, and alcohol,[41-46] as well as to increase intake of fresh organic vegetables and fruits, whole grains, fiber, and protein.

Restoring Normal Bowel Bacterial Flora

The best way to restore normal bacterial flora in the bowel is through the administration of probiotics, specifically containing *Lactobacillus acidophilus* and *Bifidobacterium bifidum* (see Chapter 102, Prescribing Probiotics). Patients should start taking a probiotic supplement at the very beginning of the treatment program for fungal sinusitis. The beneficial bacteria cannot grow back fully until the yeast overgrowth in the bowel has been greatly diminished. The intestinal bacteria can be restored through a multitude of *Lactobacillus acidophilus* and *Bifidobacterium bifidum* products available in health food stores.

Many yogurt products do not contain a high amount of viable organisms by the time they reach the consumer. This is especially true of highly processed yogurt products and those with many additional ingredients. People who are sensitive to dairy products, as well as those with chronic respiratory disease, should not use yogurt as a consistent source of beneficial bacteria because the milk protein may contribute to inflammation of the mucous membrane. Brands of yogurt that have added sweeteners should be avoided.

Strengthening the Immune System

Immune strengthening is a vital aspect of treating *Candida* overgrowth and fungal sinusitis. The three steps described previously can all contribute in varying degrees to a stronger immune system.

Both regular aerobic exercise[47] and, especially, adequate sleep, in addition to the recommendations for strengthening mental, emotional, social, and spiritual health (see later), can have a profound impact on creating a strong immune system. The combined effect of these aspects of the Respiratory Healing Program can potentially have a far greater effect on immune function than can any single supplement or food.

The improvement in chronic sinusitis can become evident within 2 to 3 weeks of beginning the *Candida* treatment program, but a period lasting 3 months to 1 year (the most severe cases can take this long) is usually required to complete the healing process. Practitioners should strongly recommend that patients maintain a healthy diet without reverting back to excess sugar and alcohol or an excess of any food.

Detoxification

In conjunction with treating *Candida* overgrowth (especially because these organisms are releasing massive amounts of toxins as they die), a detoxification process should be initiated (see Chapter 104, Detoxification). Options for detoxification include the following:

Water
Patients are advised to drink lots of water (filtered or distilled), at least half an ounce per pound of body weight.

UltraInflamX-360
The core medical food drink UltraInflamX-360 (Metagenics, San Clemente, Calif) *reduces inflammation and promotes accelerated detoxification.* This highly researched nutraceutical contains patented, proprietary ingredients. Published research is available in the literature,[48-50] and clinical trials originated from the Functional Medicine Research Center in Gig Harbor, Washington. I recommend a 3-month course of UltraInflamX-360, with the following regimen:

- First week: one scoop twice daily
- Second and third weeks: two scoops twice daily
- Following the third week, for 3 days only, no food eaten, and two scoops taken four to five times per day
- Fourth, fifth, and sixth weeks: two scoops twice daily
- Seventh, eighth, and ninth weeks: two scoops once daily
- Tenth, eleventh, and twelfth weeks: one scoop daily

Natural Cellular Defense
Natural Cellular Defense (NCD, Waiora, Boca Raton, Fla) is a detoxifier, alkalinizer, and immune strengthener. It is composed of a mineral (clinoptilolite zeolite), micronized and purified by a patented process, and suspended in sterile water. The supplement is approved by the Food and Drug Administration as generally recognized as safe (GRAS). NCD removes heavy metals, dioxins, and petrochemical and other environmental toxins. As an alkalinizer (raises digestive pH), NCD assists immune function by eliminating many bacteria and viruses in the gastrointestinal tract, as well as *Candida* (they thrive in a more acidic environment).

Colon Hydrotherapy
I recommend *colonic treatments* as a rapid method of removing excess *Candida* from the bowel and mitigating die-off effects. Much more effective than an enema, colon

hydrotherapy is best done on a weekly basis (twice during the first week) for 6 weeks, in conjunction with taking an antifungal drug. The hydrotherapy can help cleanse the bowel of *Candida,* toxins, and dead yeast organisms while assisting the inflamed lining of the bowel to begin the healing process. Colonic treatments can also significantly enhance the detoxification process by stimulating the liver to release toxins (the liver is the primary detoxification organ in the body) while also helping to flush the small bowel with all the water that the body is absorbing through the colon (large bowel). These treatments need to be performed by trained colon hydrotherapists, who are usually found in most cities by calling the office of a naturopath or chiropractor.

Far-Infrared Sauna

Although I have had no experience either personally or with patients who have used a far-infrared (FIR) sauna, numerous reports and references[51-53] on its efficacy for detoxification have been published. Several FIR sauna devices are portable, convenient, and economical and can be used in the privacy of the patient's home.

The primary advantage of the FIR sauna is that a conventional sauna heats the air in the chamber to a very high temperature, which, in turn, heats the body. The FIR sauna works differently. Neither oxygen nor nitrogen molecules in the air can block the FIR wave, thus allowing the FIR wave to penetrate the body to a depth of approximately 2 inches, without hurting the skin by the hot air.

Mind-Body Therapy

Mental and Emotional Health Recommendations

Most sufferers of chronic sinusitis have repeatedly heard the message "You're going to have to live with it" from their physicians, or they have come to this conclusion themselves. This belief often adds to already existing feelings of anger, sadness, fear, and possibly hopelessness. Essential mental and emotional components of the Respiratory Healing Program include the following: modifying beliefs and attitudes through *affirmations* and *visualizations*; creating a *goal list* and an *ideal life vision* (developing clarity about personal and professional objectives); learning to express painful emotions, especially through the *safe release of anger, journaling,* and finding more *humor, optimism,* and *play* in life.

Physical problems with the nose and sinuses bioenergetically correspond to mental and emotional issues associated with self-evaluation, truth, intellectual abilities, openness to the ideas of others, the ability to learn from experience, emotional intelligence (the ability to identify, experience, and express feelings), and feelings of adequacy. These issues are all associated with the sixth ("third eye") chakra in Ayurvedic medicine. I have found most patients with chronic sinusitis to be high achievers, perfectionists who set very high standards of performance for themselves and who tend to be unforgiving of themselves and others for making mistakes. The repressed anger felt by most sinus sufferers is often self-directed. Assisting the patient to a heightened sense of awareness of these possible contributing factors can help to begin the process of healing.

■ Mental and Emotional Health Practices

- Affirmations
- Visualizations[54]
- Goal or ideal vision list

These first three items should be practiced daily for 10 to 20 minutes. Affirmations are most effective when written, recited, and visualized.

- Anger release (safely): punching (a punching bag, sofa, or pillow), screaming, or stamping while simultaneously exhaling the "shhhh" sound; highly therapeutic for chronic sinusitis
- Journaling[55]
- Optimism
- Humor
- Biofeedback
- Psychotherapy: cognitive therapy and family therapy
- Play
- Energy medicine modalities: healing touch, Reiki, qi gong, or craniosacral therapy

Spirituality

Spiritual and Social Health Recommendations

Integrative holistic medicine is based on the belief that *unconditional love is life's most powerful healer.* Its corollary, *the perceived loss of love is our greatest health risk,* is also the spiritual cause of chronic sinusitis and all disease. Healing the spirit is by far the most powerfully therapeutic component of the Respiratory Healing Program. Spiritual health is simply learning to love ourselves in body, mind, and spirit. The first step in the Respiratory Healing Program is to love and nurture the sinuses (i.e., to heal the chronically inflamed mucous membrane). To heal the self spiritually involves connecting to a higher power (God, Spirit, or whatever term one is comfortable with) in a personal way and becoming attuned to this energy. By engaging in this spiritual healing process, individuals experience a profound reduction in feelings of fear and a greater capacity for unconditional love of self and of others. They also heighten their sense of soul awareness and are better able to identify special talents and gifts. This awareness helps them to fulfill their life's purpose while fully experiencing the power of the present moment. The spiritual practices I recommend most are *prayer, meditation,*[56] *gratitude,* and *spending time in nature.*

Relationship with others is the crucible that most strongly determines the spiritual health of each person. Optimal *social health* consists of a strong positive connection to others in community and family and intimacy with one or more people. It is often much easier to feel a connection with Spirit during moments of solitude than it is to express that connection through interactions with others. At the same time, relationships offer the greatest opportunities for spiritual growth and for learning how to receive and impart unconditional love. *True spiritual health is a balance between the autonomy of the self and intimacy with others.*

On the basis of a growing number of relationship studies, researchers have concluded that social isolation is statistically just as dangerous as smoking, high blood pressure, high cholesterol, obesity, or lack of exercise. Another study has shown that marital conflict can weaken immunity.[57]

The primary opportunities available to each person for improving social health include *forgiveness, friendships, selfless acts and altruism, support groups,*[58] and especially *marriage, committed relationships,* and *parenting.* Practicing forgiveness is particularly challenging for and most helpful to the typical patient with chronic sinusitis. Much of the patient's anger, which often precipitates a sinus infection,

is ultimately self-directed for making mistakes. In learning to forgive themselves, such patients are able to expand their capacity to forgive others and thereby heighten intimacy in their relationships (see Chapter 97, Forgiveness).

> The three primary components of the Respiratory Healing Program for treating, preventing, and curing chronic sinusitis are as follows: stop infection, reduce or eliminate inflammation of the mucous membrane, and strengthen immunity.

PREVENTIVE PRESCRIPTION

- Become more *aware* of the quality and quantity of the air you are breathing, water you are drinking, the food you are eating, the exercise and sleep you are getting, and, most importantly, the stress you are experiencing, especially *anger* with yourself or others.
- Pay more *attention* to how each of the foregoing factors affects the condition of your sinuses.
- Once you have learned what factors contribute most to the way your sinuses feel, then determine which of the recommendations in the earlier Integrative Therapy section are consistently effective in improving the way you feel. The *daily practices* that are most helpful to nearly every sinus sufferer are adequate sleep and water intake, elimination of dairy products and a significant reduction in sugar intake, use of a saline or aloe nasal spray, inhalation of medicinal eucalyptus oil, nasal irrigation (any method), journaling, anger processing, and a spiritual or meditative practice.
- *Repeat* to yourself several times a day:
  - I am always doing the best I can. There are no mistakes, only lessons.
  - Everything is happening at just the right time.
  - I love and approve of myself.
- Remember that you are a unique individual with a different set of needs, desires, beliefs, and gifts than anyone else. As you heighten your level of *self-awareness,* you will be much better able to care for yourself, heal your life, and potentially cure your chronic sinusitis.

THERAPEUTIC REVIEW

Lifestyle

- Sleep: Adequate good-quality sleep can help improve immune function.

- Use a negative ion generator as an air cleaner in the bedroom and office.

- Saline nasal spray: Use daily every 2 to 3 hours. Saline sprays containing aloe vera and grapefruit seed extract are most helpful.

- Steam inhaler: Use this device for 15 to 20 minutes two or three times daily.

- Medicinal eucalyptus oil: This can be added to the steam for optimal benefit or inhaled from a tissue.

- Nasal irrigation: Use one of several methods for nasal irrigation, although a pulsatile irrigator is most effective. Perform two to three times daily. This modality is best performed following steam inhalation therapy.

- Exercise: Engage in regular aerobic exercise three to five times per week for at least 20 to 30 minutes.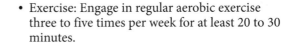

Nutrition

- Avoid milk and dairy products, sugar, wheat, caffeine, and alcohol.

- Increase intake of fresh organic vegetables and fruits, whole grains, fiber, and protein.

- Increase water intake (filtered or distilled) to at least ½ oz/lb of body weight.

- If candidiasis is suspected (e.g., history of multiple antibiotics), strict adherence to a *Candida*-control diet is recommended. This diet avoids yeast-containing foods such as breads and foods that promote yeast growth such as refined sugars, processed foods, cheeses, peanuts, vinegar, and alcoholic beverages.

Supplements

- Vitamin C: 1000 to 2000 mg three times daily

- Vitamin D₃: 5000 to 10,000 units daily

Continued

- Grape seed extract: 100 to 300 mg daily in the morning on an empty stomach $\quad$ B 1

- Selenium: 100 to 200 mcg daily $\quad$ B 2

- Essential fatty acids: 2 tablespoons/day of flaxseed oil and 3 to 4 g docosahexaenoic acid/eicosapentaenoic acid daily $\quad$ B 1

■ Botanicals

- Garlic as 100% pure allicin (Allimed or Allimax): 450 mg daily preventively or 900 mg three times per day for treating a sinus infection or fungal sinusitis $\quad$ B 2

- Echinacea: 2 dropperfuls four to five times per day daily for treating a sinus infection $\quad$ B 2

- Grapefruit seed extract: 250 mg twice daily for treating a sinus infection or fungal sinusitis $\quad$ C 2

■ Pharmaceuticals, Surgery, and *Candida* or Fungal Sinusitis Treatment

- Fluconazole or other antifungal drugs, if the history and symptoms indicate *Candida* or yeast overgrowth and fungal sinusitis $\quad$ B 2

- *Candida*-control diet $\quad$ C 1

- Antifungal supplements $\quad$ C 1

- Probiotics containing *Lactobacillus acidophilus* and *Bifidobacterium bifidus* $\quad$ B 1

- Surgery (polypectomy), usually indicated for nasal polyps $\quad$ A 3

■ Mind-Body Therapy

- Affirmations, visualizations, goals or ideal life vision list, practiced daily for 10 to 20 minutes $\quad$ C 1

- Anger release (safely) $\quad$ C 1

- Journaling $\quad$ B 1

- Biofeedback $\quad$ B 1

- Psychotherapy $\quad$ B 1

- Energy medicine modalities: healing touch, Reiki, qi gong, or craniosacral therapy $\quad$ C 1

■ Spirituality

- Prayer, meditation $\quad$ B 1

- Gratitude, intuition, spiritual practices: observing a weekly Sabbath; fasting; practices around earth, air, fire, and water $\quad$ C 1

- Forgiveness, communication exercises: shared vision, attentive listening $\quad$ B 1

- Support groups $\quad$ A 1

KEY WEB RESOURCES

Respiratory Healer Network. www.respiratoryhealer.com.

This Web site, with which I am affiliated, offers on-line respiratory healing training for practitioners.

Sinus Survival. www.sinussurvival.com.

This Web site, with which I am affiliated, provides products and educational resources for patients engaged in implementing the Respiratory Healing Program.

References

References are available at expertconsult.com.

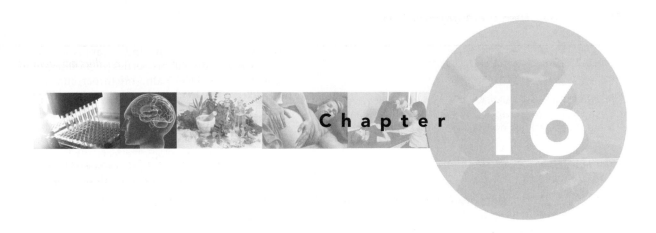

Chapter 16

Viral Upper Respiratory Infection

Bruce Barrett, MD, PhD

Viral infection of the upper respiratory tract causes the common cold, humanity's most frequent illness.[1-4] Acute viral respiratory infections are often categorized as being caused by influenza, the most serious of the viruses, or all others.[5-7] Noninfluenza upper respiratory infection (URI), or common cold, accounts for more than 25 million doctor visits and 40 million lost days of school and work each year in the United States alone.[8] Total annual economic costs are estimated at approximately $40 billion in the United States, thus making noninfluenza URI the seventh most expensive illness.[9] Although colds are often considered a nuisance rather than a major public health threat, even rhinovirus, the least pathogenic of the common cold viruses, causes death among older and immunocompromised patients.[10-12] On average, children experience four to six symptomatic colds per year, along with several asymptomatic infections. Day care attendance is a reported risk factor.[13,14] For adults, the average is two to three symptomatic colds per year and perhaps one or two asymptomatic infections.[15-17] Some people are especially prone to colds; others get them infrequently.[18] We do not really know why. Despite numerous investigations, both biologic and psychosocial determinants of susceptibility are poorly understood.[19-27]

Pathophysiology

As an experienced *illness*, the common cold is characterized by nasal congestion and drainage, sneezing, sore or scratchy throat, cough, and general malaise.[28-30] Cough may or may not be present and tends to occur later in the disease. The cough sometimes lasts for weeks after other symptoms have resolved. The severity of symptoms varies markedly, from barely noticeable to truly debilitating.[31] Although true fever is not typical, feelings of feverishness and chilliness are common.[32]

As an infectious *disease*, viral URI is characterized by replication of viruses in oral, nasal, and upper respiratory epithelium,[33] as well as by activation of local and systemic immune responses.[34-36] Viral replication within epithelial cells triggers cytokine-mediated local inflammatory reactions and recruitment of white blood cells. Parasympathetic neural pathways activate and coordinate local responses. Blood vessels dilate and capillaries leak, causing edematous tissue swelling in the nasal passages.[37] Mucous glands are activated, leading to copious discharge in some people. Inflammatory changes in the respiratory epithelium persist for days or weeks after viral shedding subsides. Nevertheless, viruses are sometimes cultured from occasional hosts weeks after the initial infection. Activation of inflammatory mechanisms leading to bronchial constriction makes viral URI the most frequent cause of asthma exacerbation.[38]

Rhinovirus is the single most common etiologic agent, but it accounts for less than half of all URIs.[39-41] Other viruses include adenovirus, coronavirus, enterovirus, influenza virus, parainfluenza virus, and respiratory syncytial virus.[4,42] Metapneumovirus,[43,44] and then bocavirus,[45-47] were more recently discovered. Others as yet undiscovered may exist, given that even the best research laboratories fail to identify an etiologic agent in up to one fourth of people with obvious colds. A few bacteria, such as *Streptococcus* and *Haemophilus influenzae*, may cause illnesses with symptoms similar to those of the common cold.

Respiratory viruses follow seasonal patterns. Influenza and respiratory syncytial virus infection occur only during the winter months. Rhinovirus URIs tend to occur in the fall and spring. Adenovirus appears year round. Parainfluenza miniepidemics are episodic. Outbreaks of atypical agents, such as the pertussis bacteria *(Bordetella pertussis)*, may further complicate the picture.

Integrative Therapy

No effective cure exists for the common cold. Even the best positive trials report only modest symptomatic benefit and little or no duration benefit.

Exercise

Although moderate regular exercise protects against infection, excess activity such as running a marathon increases the risk of infection temporarily.[48-50]

Nutrition

Chicken Soup

Hot chicken soup is the epitome of traditional cold remedies and could no doubt be supported by many personal testimonies. Chicken soup as a cold remedy is also somewhat supported by at least two human studies, one reporting inhibited neutrophil chemotaxis[51] and the other suggesting increased nasal mucus velocity and decreased nasal airflow resistance.[52] No randomized controlled trials (RCTs) using patient-oriented outcomes are available. Use of soup made from free-range chickens and substantial quantities of wholesome organic vegetables can be cautiously supported.

Hot Toddy

I have been impressed by the number of people, including several physicians, who have come up after a lecture to tell me that their favorite cold remedy was some form of hot alcoholic beverage, such as a "hot toddy" or hot buttered rum. Although to my knowledge no trials have tested any of these remedies, testimonies of symptomatic benefit should not be totally disregarded. At a societal level, the inverse relationship between moderate regular consumption of alcoholic beverages and the number and severity of colds is well known.[22] Those who consume one or two drinks daily have fewer and less severe colds than both those who drink heavily and those who drink not at all. One study found this relationship to be most pronounced for red wine.[53] Personally, I like to add a bit of rum to a cup of hot orange juice as a nighttime cold remedy. However, this would be contraindicated in patients with alcohol use disorders, in children, in pregnant women, and in anyone needing to use a motor vehicle or operate hazardous machinery.

Healthful exercise, nutritious diet, positive attitude, and healthy relationships are important.

Botanicals

Plants have long been used for medicinal purposes.[54-57] Those used for upper respiratory tract infections are discussed here.

Andrographis: Andrographis paniculata (also Known as Justicia paniculata)

Andrographis is indigenous to Asia, with traditional use most prominent in India. Of 28 *Andrographis* species, *Andrographis paniculata* is most commonly used. According to Ayurvedic tradition, andrographis is attributed many important medicinal properties, including use for constipation, digestion, fever, pain, sore throat, and snake bite, as well as to clean the blood. In the West, andrographis is most commonly used as common cold treatment or preventive.

Various laboratories have reported antimicrobial,[58] antihyperglyemic,[59,60] antiinflammatory,[61] immunomodulatory,[62,63] and psychopharmacologic[64] effects attributable to andrographolide, flavonoids,[65] and other phytochemical constituents. At least 8 RCTs have been conducted, with more than 1000 subjects, to test various andrographis derivatives in URIs, including pharyngitis.[66-73] Systematic reviews by Coon and Ernst[74] and Poolsup et al[75] concluded the following:

> Collectively, the data suggest that *A. paniculata* is superior to placebo in alleviating the subjective symptoms of uncomplicated upper respiratory tract infection. There is also preliminary evidence of a preventative effect. *A. paniculata* may be a safe and efficacious treatment for the relief of symptoms of uncomplicated upper respiratory tract infection; more research is warranted.[74]

> Current evidence suggests that *A. paniculata* extract alone or in combination with *A. senticosus* extract may be more effective than placebo and may be an appropriate alternative treatment of uncomplicated acute upper respiratory tract infection.[75]

The most recent trial was not included in those reviews, but it also reported positive results.[76] Based on published evidence, and with no indications of serious safety concerns, for adults seeking relief from URI symptoms to try andrographis-based cold remedies seems reasonable. Evidence is not sufficient to favor one product over another, any specific dosing regimen, or any particular standardization procedure for phytochemical content. For pregnant women and children, it seems prudent to recommend against use because of the paucity of data from these populations and because of the possible risk of harm.

◼ Dosage and Standardization

Most clinical trials used products standardized to 4% andrographolide. One reasonable dose regimen would be a 300-mg tablet, four times daily, for the first few days of a cold.

◼ Precautions

This herb is generally well tolerated. It can, however, cause gastrointestinal distress, urticaria, fatigue, and headache. In high doses, it may cause transient elevation of liver enzymes.

Several trials support the use of *Andrographis*. This is one to watch.

Astragalus: Astragalus membranaceus; Astragalus mongholicus

Astragalus is an important medicinal plant in traditional Chinese medicine.[77] Although dozens, if not hundreds, of reported uses are recognized, astragalus extracts are commonly used for both treatment and prevention of the common cold.[78] Even though some antiviral activity has been reported, immunomodulation is the purported mechanism of action. Indeed, several studies have reported immunoactivity from astragalus, from enhanced immunoglobulin production to restoration of lost T-cell activity.[79-83] Astragalus root contains astragaloside, flavonoids, and saponins, which are thought to be involved in various hypothesized mechanisms of action. Unfortunately, because no human URI trials have been conducted, no clear recommendations can be made for or against use for treatment or prevention of common cold.

▪ Dosage
The dose is 4 to 7 g (up to a maximum of 28 g) daily.

▪ Precautions
Astragalus is generally well tolerated. Immune suppression can occur with doses greater than 28 g daily.

Chamomile: Matricaria chamomilla; Matricaria recutita *(German chamomile);* Chamaemelum nobile *(Roman chamomile)*
Chamomile has been used widely as botanical remedy for centuries for a variety of purposes, including dysmenorrhea, gingivitis, hemorrhoids, infantile colic, indigestion, insomnia, nausea, and vaginitis, as well as topically for numerous skin conditions.[84] In the United States, chamomile is most often used as calmative or sedative and for irritable bowel syndrome. However, chamomile is also used for acute respiratory infection, hence it merits inclusion in this discussion. As a remedy for the common cold, chamomile can be taken as herbal tea (i.e., chamomile tea), or the flowering tops can be boiled and the vapors inhaled. One trial testing inhaled vapors from boiling chamomile reported benefit, but the study was of insufficient quality to make firm conclusions.[85]

▪ Dosage
Although this practice has no good supporting evidence, a cup or two of chamomile tea as supportive treatment for the common cold is certainly safe, and it may be beneficial.

▪ Precautions
Even though no dose-dependent adverse reactions to chamomile are known, allergic sensitivities, including several cases of anaphylaxis, have been reported.[86]

Echinacea: Echinacea angustifolia; Echinacea purpurea; Echinacea pallida
All dozen species from the genus *Echinacea* are indigenous to North America. Native peoples discovered dozens of medicinal uses for this plant and later transferred their knowledge to European settlers.[87] In the 1920s, echinacea was introduced into Germany, where it has been popular ever since. Today, in North America, Europe, and elsewhere, echinacea extracts are widely used, especially for prevention and treatment of the common cold.[88] A considerable body of research exists regarding these uses, including 20 randomized trials with more than 3000 participants, as well as dozens of in vitro and animal studies.[89-91] Although some consensus exists that echinacea extracts display immunologic activities such as macrophage activation and cytokine expression,[92-99]

investigators disagree about which of many echinacea-derived phytochemicals are involved. Various alkylamides, glycoproteins, polysaccharides and caffeic, cichoric, and caftaric acids are all implicated. Differing extracts from all three species and from various plant parts have shown immunoactivity in laboratory models. No head-to-head, dose-finding, or viral load outcome studies have been reported.

Double-blind RCTs testing echinacea extracts for prevention and treatment of the common cold were initially positive, and several European trials reported positive results.[100-107] More recent trials, including several in North America, reported mixed results, with the higher-quality trials finding no benefit.[108-112] I myself have directed two trials. Results of the first were flatly negative,[113] but results of the second trended in positive directions.[114] A trial using *Echinacea angustifolia* extracts in an induced cold rhinovirus inoculation study found little or no effect.[115] However, when all three rhinovirus inoculation studies are considered together, the results look more favorable.[116] In general, systematic reviews tend to be positive.[117-123] One negative review argued that the positive trial results could have reflected inadvertent unblinding with either placebo effect or participant reporting bias that contributed to false-positive results.[124] The possibility also exists that studies with negative results went unreported. A comprehensive safety review noted some reported allergic reactions but suggested no dose-dependent adverse effects or major drug interaction concerns.[125]

Given that echinacea extracts appear safe and that most published trial results remain positive, cautious support of echinacea use for adults, especially those with favorable personal experiences and positive expectations, seems reasonable. My opinion is that echinacea use in children should be discouraged because the only pediatric RCT found no positive effects but did report a slight increase in rash among patients randomized to echinacea.[126] Although a modest case control study found no adverse effects in pregnancy,[127] I caution against this use because the theoretical risks are substantive.

▪ Dosage and Standardization
Trials with positive results have used differing formulations, with preparations made from leaf and flower of *Echinacea purpurea* used most widely. However, preliminary evidence suggests that alkylamides from roots of *E. purpurea* and *E. angustifolia* may have the best bioavailability and immunoactivity.[128-130] Although no consensus on standardization criteria exists, most experts do agree that echinacea extracts should be used as early as possible in the course of a cold, with multiple doses per day for the first few days of symptoms.

> Actually, more evidence is available on echinacea and vitamin C than on any single conventional therapy. Unfortunately, for every positive trial result, a negative one has been reported.

Elderberry: Sambucus nigra
Preliminary research suggested that elderberry extracts may have antiinflammatory and antiviral antiinfluenza properties.[131,132] One Norwegian RCT of 60 volunteers suggested a potential symptom reduction benefit in influenza-like

illness.[133] With only one small limited trial and no good safety data, elderberry extract is probably not ready for widespread use.

▪ Dosage
Elderberry fluid extract, 15 mL (1 tablespoon) four times daily, or elderberry extract lozenges (175 mg four times daily), should be taken within the first 48 hours of symptoms.

Garlic: Allium sativum
Garlic is very widely used as a food and flavoring. Medicinally, garlic has dozens, if not hundreds, of reported uses. The most prominent of these is moderation of cholesterol and other lipids, for which modest beneficial activity has been reasonably established.[134-136] Use for prevention or treatment of the common cold is fairly widespread but less well researched.

Although in vitro studies have reported antibacterial and antiviral effects, only one relevant human trial has been conducted. Josling[137] reported a trial in which 146 participants were randomized to daily garlic or placebo capsule for 12 weeks. Dramatic between-group differences were observed, with 65 colds in the placebo group and 24 in the garlic group ($P < .001$). The average cold duration was 5.0 days among those taking placebo compared with 1.5 days among those taking garlic ($P < .05$). Although the study was reported as a double-blind trial, proof of blinding was not provided. The active treatment was "an allicin-containing garlic supplement" dosed at "one capsule daily." No further information on extraction methods, phytochemical composition, or amount of garlic was provided. Nevertheless, tentative support of garlic use may be reasonable because the risk of side effects is low, cardiovascular benefits are likely, and garlic is tasty.

▪ Dosage
Fresh garlic should be used in cooking as much and as often as palatable while keeping in mind positive expectations about cardiovascular and cold prevention benefits.

Ginseng: Panax ginseng, Panax quinquefolium
Asian (*Panax ginseng*) and American (*Panax quinquefolium*) ginseng are used for many different purposes. The genus name *Panax* chosen by Linnaeus, in fact, derives from the same root word as Panacea, the Greek goddess of healing. The most widespread medical theory supporting the use of ginseng derives from traditional Chinese medicine.[138] Ginseng is thought to have "adaptogenic" attributes, which bring balance, homeostasis, and healing.[139-141] Evidence for effectiveness of a *P. ginseng* extract in preventing the common cold comes from an Italian trial of 227 people followed for 12 weeks.[142] A series of Canadian studies of a polysaccharide-rich *P. quinquefolium* extract reported immunomodulatory changes.[143,144] An RCT of 198 older nursing home residents reported reductions in both cold and flu episodes.[145] A second preventive trial using the same formulation among 323 subjects reported a statistically significant 13% difference in incidence in cold and flu episodes during 4 months of observation.[146] The proprietary formula used in this series of research has been approved for use in Canada. In the United States, for prevention-minded people to use small doses of ginseng extracts regularly during cold and flu season seems reasonable, but because evidence is preliminary and safety has not been established, use of ginseng in pregnancy and in children is not advised.

▪ Dosage
For prevention during times of high risk, take 100 mg daily. For acute infection, consider 100 mg twice daily for 9 days.

▪ Precautions
Ginseng is generally well tolerated. The most common side effect is insomnia. It can also cause tachycardia, palpitations, and hypertension.

Goldenseal: Hydrastis canadensis
Goldenseal is among the top-selling botanicals in the United States. In addition to cold remedies, *Hydrastis* extracts are found in treatments for allergy and in digestive aids, feminine cleansing products, mouthwash, shampoo, skin lotion, and laxatives.[84] Goldenseal accompanies echinacea in many cold therapies. However, currently no RCTs have evaluated goldenseal either alone or in combination with echinacea. The phytochemical constituent berberine is pharmacologically active and in overdose can cause significant toxicity, including cardiac arrhythmia and death.[147] Goldenseal is contraindicated in pregnancy and lactation. Berberine-rich extracts are included in many traditional Chinese medications. The demand for goldenseal has led to overharvesting and to the substitution of other plants containing berberine or similar compounds. Given these considerations, I do not recommend goldenseal to prevent or treat the common cold.

Peppermint: Mentha piperita
Peppermint and other members of the mint family are widely used for various medicinal purposes, including coughs and colds, as well as for several gastrointestinal purposes. For treating colds, mint teas and infusions are taken internally; mint oils are applied topically. Peppermint oil is composed primarily of menthol, menthone, and menthyl acetate. Menthol especially has been extracted and included in various topical cold remedies classified as "menthol rubs." Although neither mint teas nor menthol rubs have been subjected to rigorous RCTs for the common cold, both applications seem reasonable from the perspectives of cost, risk, and potential benefit, at least for adults. More concentrated preparations such as peppermint oil should not be applied to the mucosa of infants or young children because direct inflammatory toxicity can result. Bronchospasm, tongue swelling, and even respiratory arrest have been rarely reported.[147,148]

Umckaloabo: Pelargonium sidoides
Various preparations of the South African umckaloabo plant have been used for centuries, following ethnobotanical tradition.[149-151] Three RCTs in adults ($N = 746$) and three RCTs in children ($N = 819$) yielded inconsistent yet generally positive findings.[152-154] Although no dose-dependent adverse effects are known, one published report suggested that allergic reactions may be a relatively frequent problem.[155] Scientific interest in *Pelargonium* is relatively recent, and conclusions to date are tentative, yet this seems a reasonable choice for adults looking for a natural treatment for cough, cold, or bronchitis.

▪ Dosage
EPs 7630 is an 11% aqueous ethanolic extract in which 100 g of finished product corresponds to 8 g of extracted plant material. This was the formulation used in the clinical trials,

but it may be difficult to find in the United States. The following dosage was used in clinical trials (although I do not support the use of this product in children):

Children younger than 6 years old: 10 drops three times daily
Children 6 to 12 years old: 20 drops three times daily
Those older than 12 years: 30 drops three times daily

A 1× homeopathic formulation is produced by Nature's Way (Lehi, Utah) called *Umcka ColdCare*. The dose is 1 mL of the tincture three to five times a day for those older than 12 years.

■ Precautions

Umckaloabo appears to be safe.

Nutritional Supplements

Vitamin C: Ascorbic acid

The use of vitamin C for prevention and treatment of the common cold became widespread after twice Nobel laureate Linus Pauling promoted his belief in this therapy in the 1950s and 1960s.[156] By the early 1970s, three major trials conducted in Toronto by T.W. Anderson et al[157-159] supported some preventive effectiveness. Over the next few decades, more than 30 trials including more than 12,000 participants were reported.[160] Approximately half of these trials reported positive results, far more than would be expected by chance, but not enough to convince the more skeptical scientists. Although no clear consensus exists to explain why some trials found benefit and others did not, tentatively concluding some preventive effectiveness seems reasonable, as noted by a Cochrane Systematic Review: "The consistent and statistically significant small benefits on duration and severity for those using regular vitamin C prophylaxis indicates that vitamin C plays some role in respiratory defense mechanisms."[161]

■ Dosage

The evidence supports modest preventive effectiveness for doses of 200 to 500 mg daily. Benefits of larger doses for prevention—or for treatment of new-onset colds—are supported by some trials and systematic reviews,[162] but not by others.[163] Given the generally accepted safety of ascorbic acid at doses up to several grams per day over short periods, cautious support of its use seems reasonable, especially among those with positive experiences and expectations. (Very high doses, such as the 10 g per day that Linus Pauling was reportedly taking up to his death at age 93 in 1994, have not been tested in trials and hence cannot be supported.) Regular intake of vitamin C–rich foods and juices can be enthusiastically supported because greater intake of fresh fruits and vegetables has no known risks and has been associated with many health benefits in dozens of large observational studies.

■ Precautions

Large doses of vitamin C can cause diarrhea, gastrointestinal distress, nausea, and heartburn.

Zinc

In some ways, the story of zinc for colds is similar to that of vitamin C. Reportedly, the physician George Eby noticed the rapid recovery from URI in a child hospitalized and given zinc for unrelated reasons. This observation was followed by an RCT in 1984 that reported positive results (but had several methodologic flaws).[164] Since then, at least 10 trials with more than 1000 participants have been conducted

using various zinc preparations.[165-169] As with vitamin C, only approximately half the studies had positive results, without clear indications of the reason for this disparity. Because most zinc preparations have a distinctive taste, adequate blinding may be an issue, as more skeptical experts have argued.[168,170]

Some concerns also exist over adverse effects, such as unpleasant taste and nausea. Although zinc is an essential mineral, with many known protective effects when it is ingested in foods in appropriate doses,[171,172] the use of relatively high doses during acute illness may or may not carry some risks. Advocates recommend frequent dosing (every 2 to 3 hours) for the first 2 or 3 days of a cold, a dosing regimen that some patients will not find convenient. More recently, nasal zinc preparations have been devised, and three out of four RCTs reported benefits.[170,173-175] Issues of specific preparation, dosing, and blinding complicate interpretation of study results. Nasal irritation is common, and loss of sense of smell has been reported.[176] Large, well-designed trials are needed before the benefits of oral or intranasal zinc for the common cold can be said to be proven. My personal recommendation is to support the use of oral or zinc preparations tentatively among those who have experienced benefit or express positive feelings about the treatment, but not to recommend the use of these preparations in children, in women, or in men who have not yet tried it.[177] The U.S. Food and Drug Administration (FDA) has collected more than 100 reports of loss of sense of smell for people using nasal zinc. Zicam has been withdrawn from the market. I recommend that nasal zinc not be used.

■ Dosage

Zinc gluconate, 9 to 24 mg of elemental zinc, is taken every 2 hours while symptomatic.

■ Precautions

Zinc can inhibit the absorption of other minerals (copper), and nasal formulations have been associated with loss of smell.

> Of a dozen trials of zinc, half the results are positive and half are negative.

Probiotics

Probiotics are live bacteria that are thought to support healthy gastrointestinal function. Several trials demonstrated benefit for antibiotic-associated diarrhea,[178] and others suggested benefit for irritable bowel syndrome and a few other conditions.[179-183] Reasonably strong preliminary evidence indicates that probiotics may also prevent or ameliorate URI illness. This evidence comes from several trials testing efficacy for preventing cold and flu illness episodes.[184-190] One RCT was of older persons,[187] and two involved children.[186,189] One of these studies was aimed at preventing diarrhea illness, but instead it provided some evidence of cold and flu prevention.[189]

■ Dosage

In children, prevention of URI was found with a milk product containing *Lactobacillus rhamnosus* and *Lactobacillus* GG (in one study) and *Lactobacillus acidophilus* and *Bifidobacterium animalis* (in another). The dose is 5 to 10 billion colony-forming units (CFUs) twice daily.

Precautions

Probiotics should be avoided in persons who have compromised immunity.

Nasal Irrigation and Humidification

Nasal Saline

What could be more healthful and therapeutic than a mild saltwater rinse of the nasal cavities? Although saline nasal lavage is a long-standing tradition in many cultures, only fairly recently has Western biomedicine begun to integrate this practice. Several trials with positive results were conducted in people with allergic rhinitis and chronic sinus symptoms, including one trial at the University of Wisconsin Department of Family Medicine in Madison, Wisconsin.[191]

To my knowledge only two RCTs of nasal saline in people with the common cold have been conducted. Adam et al[192] randomized 140 people to 1 of 3 groups: hypertonic saline, normal tonic saline, or no treatment (two squirts per nostril, three times per day.) No significant differences among the groups were found in terms of duration or severity of symptoms. Diamond et al[193] reported a trial in which 955 participants were randomized to 1 of 3 doses of nasal ipratropium, to the "placebo" saline vehicle, or to no treatment at all. The nasal saline vehicle yielded greater benefit compared with no treatment than did any of the ipratropium doses when compared with each other or with saline.

Dosage

I suggest a mild salt water solution made with warm tap water and just enough salt to make it taste like tears (a half teaspoon of salt in 6 oz of warm water). To instill the solution, the head and neck should be nearly horizontal, with one ear down, and the nose should be positioned over a sink or basin. Using a neti pot (small tea pot) or a bulb syringe, gently pour the saline into the higher nostril. The soothing, cleaning fluids will run through the nasal cavity, coming to the other nostril and to the throat. Spit out any fluids from the mouth, and gently blow the nose with a handkerchief or tissue. Repeat the process with the other ear down. I suggest treatment twice daily for the first few days of a cold (see Chapter 109, Sinus Irrigation).

Hot Moist Air

One widespread traditional cold remedy involves the inhalation of hot moist air, often with a botanical or other additive. As noted earlier, the benefits of inhalation of vapors from chamomile tea were reported in one clinical trial.[85] At least two RCTs suggested significant benefit of nasal inhalation of unadulterated hot moist air.[194,195] However, two subsequent trials found no benefit.[196,197] Although recommending humidification when the air is dry and perhaps advocating the inhalation of hot moist air for those who find it comforting seem reasonable, water boils at 100 °C, and inhalation of vapors near this temperature may cause significant thermal damage. Be careful.

Dosage

Some patients find it beneficial to add a handful of chamomile flowers or 5 to 10 drops of eucalyptus essential oil to the water. Place the head under a towel, and inhale the steaming vapors for 10 to 15 minutes. Repeat as needed.

Mind-Body Therapy

Placebo, Meaning, and Mind-Body Effects

Since 2000, I have read the reports of hundreds of trials and dozens of systematic reviews of common cold research and have become increasingly convinced of the importance of mind-body effects, otherwise described as placebo or meaning effects.[198-202] Positive thinking, suggestion, expectancy, and belief in the therapeutic value of a given remedy can be powerful healing forces. Although regular exercise, balanced nutrition, and tobacco cessation are clearly associated with fewer and less severe illness episodes, so too are positive mental health attributes such as a favorable psychological profile and healthful social relationships. Psychological predispositions, especially sociability and a positive emotional style, are predictive of both symptomatic and physiologic outcomes. For the integrative clinician, this means that understanding an individual's belief system may be a crucial part of the therapeutic encounter. If a patient already believes in a safe therapy, reinforcing that belief may enhance the therapeutic response. If a patient is wary of a remedy mentioned, do not press the issue. Remember that reassurance, empathy, empowerment, and positive prognosis can all be usefully employed in the clinical encounter.

> Belief in a therapy—positive expectation—should usually be supported rather than discounted.

Psychosocial Influences

As in virtually all illness, the common cold involves both psychological and physiologic elements and is influenced by social factors. Stress, both acute and chronic, increases risk. In a series of groundbreaking studies, Cohen et al showed that certain psychosocial variables predicted whether volunteers would become infected when they were exposed to rhinovirus. Childhood socioeconomic status,[203] number and quality of social relationships,[204] acute and chronic stress,[205-207] and negative emotion[208,209] measured before rhinovirus inoculation all predicted subsequent infection and viral shedding, as well as severity and duration of cold symptoms. Work by other investigators confirmed these findings.[210-215] Together, these observations suggest that maintenance of psychological and social health (positive attitude, healthy relationships) may be as important as maintenance of physical health (exercise, nutrition, hand washing, smoke avoidance) for preventing colds and moderating symptoms.

Conventional Therapies

Antihistamines

Drugs blocking the effects of histamine have been sold as cold remedies for more than a century, but they have been subjected to less in terms of rigorous RCT research than alternatives such as vitamin C, zinc, and echinacea. Nevertheless, some reasonable evidence indicates modest benefit, in terms of reduction of nasal drainage, for first-generation antihistamines such as diphenhydramine, clemastine fumarate, or chlorpheniramine.[216-219] These effects appear to result more from anticholinergic mechanisms than from antihistamine effects, however, and second-generation "nonsedating" antihistamines do not seem to provide benefit.[220] For adults who do not mind the potential sedating or membrane-drying effects, or for patients with an allergic response, a first-generation antihistamine may be a reasonable choice. For children, in whom no positive evidence of benefit in colds exists whatsoever, antihistamines should be reserved for allergic rather than infectious rhinitis.

Decongestants

The oral decongestant pseudoephedrine was tested in several clinical trials and appears to have minor benefit in terms of reduction of nasal congestion and drainage.[221-224] Side effects including anxiety, dizziness, insomnia, and palpitations are fairly common. More worrisome is the potential for elevated blood pressure and cardiac arrhythmia. Phenylpropanolamine, for decades a popular over-the-counter decongestant, was taken off the market after studies suggested increased mortality, especially in older persons.[225]

The topical intranasal decongestant oxymetazoline was shown to decrease nasal airway resistance, as well as mucus production and drainage.[226-229] Intranasal phenylephrine has been less extensively studied but likely has similar effects. Unfortunately, these proven benefits come at the risk of nasal membrane dryness, discomfort, or nosebleed. These drugs should be used for no more than 4 days because rebound nasal congestion can occur.

> Conventional treatments such as antihistamines, decongestants, and cough remedies may help slightly with some symptoms, but they do tend to have side effects.

Cough Suppressants

Dextromethorphan, the active ingredient in cough remedies designated with "DM," is widely used as an over-the-counter cough suppressant. Codeine and, to a lesser extent, hydrocodone are prescribed for cough. Presumably, these drugs work through similar opioid-mediated mechanisms and as such have side effects including sedation, constipation, and, potentially, respiratory suppression. Although most patients and clinicians agree that these remedies work, considerable debate exists over effect size and mechanism of action, given that little appropriate evidence is available.[230-232] The best systematic review of cough remedies for children and adults concludes: "There is no good evidence for or against the effectiveness of OTC medicines in acute cough."[233] Benzonatate (Tessalon Perles) is licensed as a prescription antitussive, but it appears to have been given this indication without any good evidence.

Analgesics and Antipyretics

There is little doubt that acetaminophen and nonsteroidal antiinflammatory drugs (NSAIDs) such as aspirin, ibuprofen, and naproxen are effective for pain and fever, which may accompany common cold. However, some suggestion also exists that viral shedding may be prolonged.[234,235] Although the limited use of NSAIDs for pain reduction is eminently reasonable, the widespread use of NSAIDs for general common cold symptoms is not justified. Evidence of benefit is marginal, and many thousands of people die each year from NSAID-attributable gastrointestinal hemorrhage and congestive heart failure.[236-238]

Anticholinergics

Ipratropium nasal spray was tested in several high-quality RCTs for amelioration of symptoms of infectious and allergic rhinitis.[239,240] These trials, including a dose-response trial of 955 patients with community-acquired common cold,[193] suggested a definite benefit in terms of reduced nasal congestion and drainage. Common side effects of these drugs include headache, uncomfortable nasal dryness, and nosebleed.

Combination Formulas

The multibillion dollar market in cold remedies is dominated by numerous products containing combination formulas. Loopholes in FDA regulations have allowed pharmaceutical companies to mix various decongestants, antihistamines, analgesics, and antitussives and then market them under a variety of brand names with exaggerated or false claims. Although some evidence of effectiveness from early trials exists for combining a decongestant with an antihistamine,[216] few, if any, of the currently marketed products have been tested in large, well-controlled RCTs. Personally, I recommend against using any combination cold formula, with a possible exception for patients who are convinced that a specific formula works for them. Perhaps most importantly, clinicians and parents should be made aware that no cold formula has ever been proved to work in children. For pain, acetaminophen (paracetamol) may be justified, but in my opinion, virtually nothing else is.

PREVENTION PRESCRIPTION

- Eat a nutritious diet with foods rich in vitamin C (fruits and vegetables) and zinc (meat, nuts, cereals, seafood, and pumpkin seeds).
- Do not smoke.
- Maintain regular exercise and movement, and be careful not to overstrain.
- Maintain supportive social relationships.
- Reduce exposure to people with colds.
- Reduce stressors, and foster positive emotions.
- Wash your hands frequently.
- Obtain an annual influenza vaccine.
- Vitamin C (200 to 500 mg daily), *Panax ginseng* (100 mg daily), and probiotics have some effectiveness for the prevention of colds and flu.

THERAPEUTIC REVIEW

The therapeutic options for the common cold are summarized here. None of these options are proved beyond reasonable doubt to be safe and effective. Nevertheless, they are all reasonable given the best current evidence of benefit and harm.

Botanicals

• Andrographis: 300 mg four times daily as soon as symptoms appear and continued for 3 to 4 days

• Echinacea: No one formulation appears to work better than another. Consider one of the following three to four times daily for the first 3 to 4 days of a cold:

  • 1 to 2 mL of extract in juice or water sublingually

  • 150 to 300 mg powdered extract

  • 1 to 5 mL of tincture (1:5 in ethanol)

• *Pelargonium*/umckaloabo: EPs 7630 is an 11% aqueous ethanolic extract in which 100 g of finished product corresponds to 8 g of extracted plant material. This was the formulation used in the clinical trials but may be difficult to find in the United States. Dosage used in clinical trials:

  • Those older than 12 years old: 30 drops three times daily

  • A 1 × homeopathic formulation is produced by Nature's Way called *Umcka ColdCare*. The dose is 1 mL of the tincture three to five times a day for those older than 12 years.

Nutritional Supplements

• Vitamin C: 500 to 1000 mg three times daily for the first 3 to 4 days of symptoms

• Zinc gluconate or acetate: 23-mg tablets every 2 hours while awake

Pharmaceuticals

• First-generation (sedating) antihistamines may decrease nasal congestion, but they may cause drowsiness.

  • Diphenhydramine: 25 to 50 mg every 6 hours

  • Clemastine: 1 to 2 mg two to three times daily as needed

  • Chlorpheniramine: 4 mg every 6 hours

• Intranasal decongestants appear to be effective in decreasing nasal congestion and drainage, but quite often they cause nasal dryness, irritation, or nosebleed, and, rarely, insomnia, palpitations, or elevated blood pressure.

  • Intranasal ipratropium appears to be effective in decreasing nasal congestion and drainage, but it may cause headache, nasal irritation, or nosebleed.

  • Nasal ipratropium 0.03%: two sprays in each nostril two to three times daily. It is also effective for nasal congestion.

Biomechanical Therapy

• Hot moist air: Consider adding 5 to 10 drops of eucalyptus oil or chamomile tea to the water, and inhale deeply for 10 to 15 minutes.

Nasal Irrigation

• Consider twice daily nasal irrigation with normal or hypertonic saline with a bulb syringe, nasal spray, or neti pot (see Chapter 109, Sinus Irrigation).

• Astragalus, chamomile, garlic, ginseng, peppermint, and chicken soup are all unproven but probably safe, supportive therapies.

KEY WEB RESOURCES

Department of Family Medicine, University of Wisconsin School of Medicine and Public Health. http://www.fammed.wisc.edu/research/past-projects/nasal-irrigation	Instructions on nasal irrigation available in English and Spanish
Integrative Medicine, Department of Family Medicine, University of Wisconsin School of Medicine and Public Health. http://www.fammed.wisc.edu/sites/default/files//webfm-uploads/documents/outreach/im/ss_andrographis.pdf	Monograph on *Andrographis*
Integrative Medicine, Department of Family Medicine, University of Wisconsin School of Medicine and Public Health. http://www.fammed.wisc.edu/sites/default/files//webfm-uploads/documents/outreach/im/ss_pelargonium.pdf	Monograph on *Pelargonium*
National Center for Complementary and Alternative Medicine, National Institutes of Health: http://nccam.nih.gov/news/newsletter/2010_february/coldnflu1.htm	Clinical information on the common cold

References

References are available at expertconsult.com.

HIV Disease and AIDS

Stephen M. Dahmer, MD, and Benjamin Kligler, MD, MPH

Pathophysiology

Acquired immunodeficiency syndrome (AIDS) is a potentially life-threatening disease caused by the human immunodeficiency virus (HIV). HIV infection in humans, considered pandemic by the World Health Organization (WHO), affects approximately 0.6% of the world's population. The virus, which is transmitted by sexual contact and contact with blood and certain other body fluids, attacks a class of T lymphocytes called CD4+ cells, macrophages, and dendritic cells and results in severe declines in both number and effective function of this arm of the immune system. The result is a dramatically weakened immune system with a host at risk for life-threatening opportunistic infections, including *Pneumocystis carinii* pneumonia (PCP), *Mycobacterium avium-intracellulare* sepsis, and cerebral toxoplasmosis, and Kaposi's sarcoma. Before the advent of effective antiretroviral medications, AIDS was a fairly progressive and almost universally fatal condition.

Currently, no vaccine or cure for HIV is publicly available. Since 1996, AIDS has been transformed into a serious but manageable chronic illness by the widespread use of antiretroviral medications (highly active antiretroviral therapy [HAART]). Many of the current challenges in the management of the HIV-positive patient in developed nations pertain to minimizing the possibility of developing viral resistance while maximizing quality of life by preventing or controlling the adverse effects associated with long-term use of antiretrovirals. In the developing world, where the HIV epidemic continues to spread, the cost of antiretroviral medications is prohibitive, and the number of deaths from AIDS continues to mount.

Integrative Therapy

People with HIV disease typically use alternative approaches for several reasons. First is to promote healthier functioning of the immune system; this approach can apply both to patients very early in the course of HIV infection who are not yet taking antiretroviral medications and to those with more advanced disease who are receiving conventional medications. Second is for a claimed antiviral effect of the therapy, as in the use of intravenous vitamin C infusions. Third is to treat an HIV-associated symptom or condition. Fourth is to mitigate one or more of the side effects of conventional antiretroviral medications, as in the use of glutamine supplements for protease inhibitor–associated diarrhea. Fifth is simply to improve their quality of life.

A 2008 review concluded that complementary and alternative medicine (CAM) use is more common among HIV-positive individuals who are men who have sex with men (MSM), nonminority, better educated, and less impoverished, and that the use of CAM is also associated with greater HIV-symptom severity and longer disease duration.[1] A study from New England confirmed that although the advent of effective pharmaceutical treatment for HIV has led to a decrease in the use of CAM, rates of use nevertheless remain high. In a cohort of HIV-positive adults ($N = 642$) followed semiannually in the Nutrition for Healthy Living (NFHL) study, between 1995 and 1999, HAART use increased from 0% to 70%, but ingested CAM decreased only from 71% to 52%.[2] The investigators concluded that most people with HIV at this point apparently feel that "CAM therapies complement, rather than replace, HAART [and that] physicians should routinely ask about ingested CAM therapy use in HIV-positive patients."[2]

Pharmaceuticals

Thirty medications have been approved by the U.S. government to fight HIV and AIDS, and many more are in development. These medications fall into several groups, or classes. The first category is the antiretrovirals, used for their specific activity against HIV. These agents are currently divided into three groups: (1) the nucleoside reverse transcriptase inhibitors, which include zidovudine (Retrovir), emtricitabine

(Emtriva), abacavir (Ziagen), didanosine (Hivid), stavudine (Zerit), and lamivudine (Epivir); (2) the protease inhibitors, which include indinavir (Crixivan), nelfinavir (Viracept), amprenavir (Agenerase), and numerous others; and (3) the nonnucleoside reverse transcriptase inhibitors, which include efavirenz (Sustiva) and nevirapine (Viramune), among others. Newer classes include entry inhibitors (including fusion inhibitors) such as enfuvirtide (Fuzeon), integrase inhibitors such as raltegravir (Isentress), and multiple-class combination drugs such as efavirenz + tenofovir + emtricitabine (Atripla). Currently, the most common approach is to use these agents in combinations of at least three drugs—usually two nucleoside reverse transcriptase inhibitors and either one protease inhibitor or one nonnucleoside reverse transcriptase inhibitor—to reduce the possibility of viral resistance. Research is looking at the possibility that antiviral medications should be withheld during the early stages of HIV infection to minimize the problems with long-term toxicity of these agents. Other investigators are examining the risk-to-benefit analysis of "drug holidays" (i.e., planned periods off medication to minimize toxicity).

The second category of pharmaceuticals, used less widely since the advent of effective antiretroviral medications, comprises the prophylactic agents used for prevention of specific HIV-related opportunistic infections. These drugs include trimethoprim-sulfamethoxazole (Septra, Bactrim) for PCP and toxoplasmosis prophylaxis and azithromycin and rifabutin for prophylaxis of *Mycobacterium avium* infection.

> Studies have shown that if CD4+ counts rise and remain higher than 250, prophylaxis for HIV-related opportunistic infections may be safely discontinued.

Nutrition

Early research in the 1980s showed that decreases in body weight, body mass index, and body fat percentage may be the first signs of declining nutritional status resulting from HIV disease and may begin even during the early asymptomatic phase of HIV infection. Many patients with HIV infection or AIDS experience HIV-associated wasting and lose body mass despite nutritional intake that should be adequate for their height and weight. In a study of nutritional status in 108 HIV-positive patients, some with and some without AIDS, body weight, serum cholesterol level, and CD4+ level progressively decreased over a 6-month period, and HIV-associated wasting persisted.[3] This study also found a significant relationship between low serum cholesterol—a marker for poor nutrition—and adverse patient outcome.

Nutrition counseling and intervention in the early stages of HIV disease constitute important components of a prevention-oriented treatment plan because these measures may help forestall adverse nutritional changes in HIV-positive patients. Although definitive data supporting specific nutritional recommendations are scarce, reasonable suggestions include the following: a diet high in omega-3 essential fatty acids such as flaxseed and fish oils; small, frequent meals to ensure intake of adequate calories and to reduce the likelihood of malabsorption; avoidance of simple sugars, which some studies show may inhibit immune function on a short-term basis; and avoidance of large amounts of alcohol and caffeine.

In 227 HIV-infected patients, adherence to a Mediterranean dietary pattern was favorably related to cardiovascular risk factors in patients with fat redistribution.[4]

Another purpose for which nutritional interventions are widely used is to address the problems with malabsorption experienced by many HIV-positive patients. Common recommendations include the use of *Lactobacillus*, *Bifidobacterium*, and other "friendly bacteria" to maintain proper balance of intestinal flora (see Chapter 102, Prescribing Probiotics); the use of a multivitamin supplement to prevent the development of subclinical vitamin deficiencies even in patients eating a well-balanced diet; and the use of glutamine supplements to promote the health of colonic mucosa. Although these recommendations have not yet been shown to affect the course of HIV disease progression, all are safe and reasonable to include in an integrative treatment plan.

Supplements

Multivitamins

Many clinicians have routinely recommended multivitamin supplementation for HIV-positive patients. A double-blind placebo-controlled study of multivitamin (vitamins B, C, and E) supplementation in 1078 HIV-positive pregnant women in Tanzania demonstrated that over a 6-year follow-up period, women taking multivitamins had significantly less progression to WHO stage 4 disease or died as compared with women given placebo (relative risk = 0.71).[5] Subjects in the multivitamin group also had significantly higher CD4+ and CD8+ cell counts and significantly lower viral loads. Adding vitamin A to this multivitamin regimen did not improve the outcomes and, in fact, reduced the benefit of multivitamin therapy on some of the outcome measures.

Vitamin A

Vitamin A supplementation has been extensively studied for ameliorating infection with HIV in adults and for possibly reducing the likelihood of vertical HIV transmission. An association between lower vitamin A levels, lower CD4+ counts, and higher risk of progression to AIDS was reported.[6] A study in African women demonstrated a connection between vitamin A deficiency and increased maternal-to-fetal transmission of HIV.[7] Other prospective trials, however, including one with 341 HIV-positive patients followed over 9 years, demonstrated no significant difference in risk of AIDS progression with vitamin A levels.[8] Trials of high-dose vitamin A supplementation also failed to show an effect on CD4+ or CD8+ counts, viral loads, lymphocyte responsiveness to mitogens, or progression of disease.[9] The association between vitamin A deficiency and increased vertical transmission of HIV initially reported in Kenya was not borne out in subsequent U.S. studies. The Women and Infants Transmission Study (WITS), a large prospective ongoing cohort study, found that vitamin A level does not correlate with increased risk of HIV vertical transmission in North America.[10] The investigators suggested that vitamin A supplementation in addition to prenatal vitamins is not necessary.

Vitamin B$_{12}$

Supplementation with a B-complex vitamin may be beneficial in HIV-infected patients. Lack of vitamin B$_{12}$ has been associated with peripheral neuropathy and myelopathy; a

9-year prospective cohort study in 310 patients found vitamin B_{12} levels to be an early and independent marker of HIV disease progression, and time to development of AIDS was found to be 4 years less on average in persons observed to have lower vitamin B_{12} levels.[11] Results of intervention trials using B_{12} supplementation have been equivocal. Nevertheless, vitamin B_{12} supplementation continues to be widely used in HIV disease.

Antioxidants: Vitamins C and E, Selenium, and Alpha-Lipoic Acid

Vitamins C and E both have been explored for a role in treatment of HIV disease, owing to their antioxidant properties. Other substances, including selenium and alpha-lipoic acid, are commonly used for the same purpose. In addition, vitamin C has been shown in vitro to inhibit viral replication at high doses.[12] On the basis of this finding, intravenous vitamin C has been widely used to achieve the high serum levels necessary for antiviral activity. No evidence supports this aggressive approach, although anecdotally it has not been proved to be as dangerous as was initially feared. The role of antioxidant supplements in general in HIV disease requires further study. A 2009 review of 19 studies showed that evidence to support standard selenium supplementation in patients with HIV is both limited and insufficient, yet although the available evidence for selenium supplementation is weak, its low toxicity and side effect profile seem to pose minimal risks, especially at low doses.[13] Vitamins E and C at more standard doses are safe and may decrease lipid peroxidation and enhance the immune system; however, conclusive evidence on the effects of these vitamins in HIV disease is still lacking.

Dosage
Vitamin E 400 units daily; vitamin C 500 to 2000 mg three times daily

N-Acetylcysteine

Because of the strong evidence that depletion of glutathione levels correlates with progression of HIV infection,[14] much interest has focused on use of the nutritional supplement N-acetylcysteine (NAC) as a means to replete intracellular glutathione levels. Despite its early promise, however, NAC has not been proved beneficial in the treatment of HIV disease. One randomized controlled trial[15] failed to show any influence of NAC on T-cell counts or disease progression. Despite the lack of evidence supporting its use, this supplement is commonly used.

Dosage
The dose is 600 to 1200 mg daily.

Precautions
No adverse effects of NAC supplementation have been reported.

L-Carnitine

L-Carnitine may be helpful in mitigating some of the adverse effects of antiretroviral medications, including peripheral neuropathy and dyslipidemia. Acetylcarnitine acts to facilitate transport of essential fatty acids across cell membranes and thus may have a role in normalizing intracellular lipid metabolism and regulating peripheral nerve function and regeneration. Decreased levels of carnitine have been found in HIV-positive people; in addition, patients with AIDS experiencing neuropathy with zidovudine or didanosine therapy had significantly lower levels of acetylcarnitine than did patients with AIDS but without neuropathy.[16] One open trial of oral acetyl-L-carnitine supplementation (1500 mg twice daily) for up to 33 months in 21 HIV-positive patients with established antiretroviral-induced neuropathy found an improvement in neuropathic grade in 76% of patients.[17] HIV RNA load and CD4+ and CD8+ cell counts were not altered.

An increased proliferation of peripheral blood mononuclear cells in vitro was noted after oral supplementation with L-carnitine; a significant decrease in triglyceride levels was also noted.[18]

Dosage
Give 2000 to 3000 mg orally daily for HIV-positive patients with peripheral neuropathy or high triglyceride levels.

Precautions
No significant adverse effects of or interactions with L-carnitine have been demonstrated to date; further study of this supplement is needed to substantiate the possible benefits.

L-Glutamine

L-Glutamine supplementation has been shown in animal models to speed proliferation of colonocytes. Glutamine deficiency is also hypothesized to play a role in the process of HIV-associated wasting.[19] Many patients taking protease inhibitors experience chronic diarrhea as a medication side effect. A randomized trial involving 35 HIV-positive men with protease inhibitor–induced diarrhea found that when added to a regimen of fiber and probiotic supplementation, L-glutamine (30 g/day) significantly decreased the frequency of diarrhea and the need for antidiarrheal medications.[20] Anecdotally, many patients find glutamine to be helpful in mitigating this side effect even at lower and more easily administered doses.

Dosage
Give 2000 mg daily in two or three divided doses, with the dose titrated upward as needed to 40 g daily.[21]

Calcium Carbonate

Several studies to date have shown that calcium carbonate supplementation can help reduce the frequency of protease inhibitor–associated diarrhea.[22,23] The dose typically used is 500 mg twice daily, although some clinicians report that a higher dose may be more effective. This treatment has no reported interactions or adverse effects.

Dosage
Usual dose is 500 mg twice daily.

Omega-3 Polyunsaturated Fatty Acids

Patients taking antiretroviral therapy are reported to have an increased risk of cardiovascular disease. One study randomized 51 patients in a placebo-controlled double-blind trial to receive either 2 capsules of Lovaza fish oil twice daily or 2 capsules of placebo. After 12 weeks, the omega-3 group noted slightly decreased plasma triglycerides and induced antiinflammatory effects by increasing formation of antiinflammatory leukotriene B_5.[24] Fifty-four persons with HIV and elevated serum triglycerides (higher than 150 mg/dL) were randomly assigned to a control group or an intervention group and given supplemental omega-3 fatty acids for 13 weeks. The investigators documented dramatically reduced serum triglycerides, decreased arachidonic acid in the phospholipid fraction, and reduced de novo lipogenesis associated with the metabolic syndrome in the intervention group.[25]

■ Dosage
Dose is 4 g/day of docosahexaenoic acid and eicosapentaenoic acid, the main essential fatty acids found in fish oil.

■ Precautions
High doses (more than 6 g) can increase free radical production and can have an antiplatelet effect.

Zinc
Adequate zinc is necessary for immune function, and zinc deficiency is estimated to occur in more than 50% of HIV-infected adults. A prospective randomized controlled clinical trial involving 231 HIV-infected adults with low plasma zinc levels revealed that zinc supplementation for 18 months reduced 4-fold the likelihood of immunologic failure while controlling for age, sex, food insecurity, baseline CD4+ cell count, viral load, and antiretroviral therapy (relative rate, 0.24; 95% confidence interval, 0.10 to 0.56).[26]

■ Dosage
The dose is 15 mg for men; 12 mg for women.

■ Precautions
High doses can inhibit the absorption of other minerals, most significantly copper.

Chromium
Chromium is an essential micronutrient, and deficiency has been reported to cause insulin resistance, hyperglycemia, and hyperlipidemia. A randomized double-blind placebo-controlled trial enrolled 52 HIV-positive subjects with elevated glucose, lipids, or evidence of body fat redistribution who also had insulin resistance. Chromium was tolerated without side effects and resulted in a significant decrease in the following: Homeostatic Model Assessment-Insulin Resistance (HOMA-IR, an insulin resistance indicator) (median [IQR]; pre, 4.09 [3.02 to 8.79]; post, 3.66 [2.40 to 5.46]; $P = .004$); insulin (pre, 102 [85 to 226]; post, 99 [59 to 131] pmol/L; $P = .003$); triglycerides, total body fat mass (mean ± SEM; pre, 17.3 ± 1.7; post, 16.3 ± 1.7 kg; $P = .002$), and trunk fat mass (pre, 23.8 ± 1.9; post, 22.7 ± 2.0%; $P = .008$).[27]

■ Dosage
The dose is 400 mcg/day chromium-nicotinate.

K-PAX Immune Support Formula
In 2006, a double-blind placebo-controlled randomized clinical trial of 40 HIV-infected patients showed that a broad-spectrum micronutrient supplement could produce a statistically significant 24% increase in the mean CD4+ cell count of individuals taking stable HAART ($P = .01$).[28]

The micronutrient supplement tested (K-PAX Immune Support Formula, Mill Valley, Calif) included 33 ingredients and was consumed twice daily with food. The supplement is currently paid for by the New York AIDS Drug Assistance Program. For ingredients of the immune support formula used in the research, see Table 17-1.

■ Dosage
Four capsules twice per day (for less than 120 lb) or eight capsules twice per day (for more than 120 lb).

Botanicals

Chinese Herbal Approaches
In the traditional practice of Chinese medicine, herbal formulas are typically individualized to suit a given patient's condition, rather than standardized as a treatment for a given "disease." In the United States, however, the use of standardized formulas for certain conditions has become quite popular. Early small randomized controlled trials of two such Chinese herbal formulas (Enhance and Clear Heat, formulated by Health Concerns in California) showed a trend (statistically nonsignificant) toward fewer symptoms in the treatment group than in the placebo group.[29] However, a more recent prospective placebo-controlled double-blind study of a different Chinese formula in 68 HIV-infected adults with CD4+ cell counts lower than 0.5×10^9/L found no significant differences between the intervention and placebo groups regarding viral loads, CD4+ counts, symptoms, or quality of life scores. No significant therapy-related toxicities were reported, although patients taking Chinese herbs reported significantly more gastrointestinal disturbances (79% versus 38%; $P = .003$) than those receiving placebo. The investigators concluded that this particular Chinese herbal formula was not effective when administered in a Western medicine setting.[30]

A study of 18 volunteers evaluated the safety and efficacy of CKBM-A01, a Chinese herbal medicine, and patient quality of life. Although CKBM-A01 appeared to be safe, it gave no significant improvement in quality of life in asymptomatic HIV-infected patients and no significant improvement in the treatment of HIV infection based on CD4+ cell counts and viral loads.[31] Well-controlled long-term follow-up studies of use of these Chinese herbal preparations are needed before Western practitioners can recommend them with confidence. Significant concerns remain regarding possible herb-drug interactions, given the large number of herbs in most Chinese formulas, especially in those patients concurrently taking conventional antiretroviral medications.

Milk Thistle
Milk thistle extract (silymarin) may help normalize liver function tests in patients taking antiretroviral therapies, especially if these patients are coinfected with hepatitis C. Numerous in vitro studies found that silymarin speeds regeneration of hepatocytes after chemical injury.[32] A significant improvement in liver function in patients with alcoholic hepatitis was noted after treatment with milk thistle extract.[33] At present, no firm evidence specifically links the hepatoprotective function of silymarin with liver damage from antiretrovirals. However, clinical experience suggests that milk thistle may be useful in this situation. Silymarin has no reported contraindications or adverse effects. Contrary to a widely held

TABLE 17-1. Immune Support Formula for HIV Infection Found in K-PAX Formulation

MICRONUTRIENT	TOTAL DAILY DOSAGE	MICRONUTRIENT	TOTAL DAILY DOSAGE
N-Acetyl cysteine (NAC)	1200 mg	Calcium	800 mg
Acetyl L-carnitine	1000 mg	Magnesium	400 mg
Alpha-lipoic acid	400 mg	Selenium	200 mcg
Beta-carotene	20,000 units	Iodine	150 mcg
Vitamin A	8,000 units	Zinc	30 mg
Vitamin C	1800 mg	Copper	2.0 mg
Vitamin B_1	60 mg	Boron	2.0 mg
Vitamin B_2	60 mg	Potassium	99 mg
Pantothenic acid	60 mg	Iron	18 mg
Niacinamide	60 mg	Manganese	10 mg
Inositol	60 mg	Biotin	50 mcg
Vitamin B_6	260 mg	Chromium	100 mcg
Vitamin B_{12}	2.5 mg	Molybdenum	300 mcg
Vitamin D	400 units	Choline	60 mg
Vitamin E	800 units	Bioflavonoid complex	300 mg
Folic acid	800 mcg	L-Glutamine Betaine HCL	100 mg 150 mg

From Kaiser J, Campa A, Ondercin JP, Leoung GS, Pless RF, Baum MK. Micronutrient supplementation increases CD4 count in HIV-infected individuals on highly active antiretroviral therapy: a prospective, double-blinded, placebo-controlled trial. *J Acquir Immune Defic Syndr.* 2006;42:523–528.

popular belief among patients with HIV disease and many practitioners, milk thistle has no documented antiviral effect either in HIV disease or in hepatitis C.

Dosage
The dose is 240 mg twice daily of standardized milk thistle (silymarin) extract.

Red Rice Yeast Extract
Hyperlipidemia is a common side effect of treatment with protease inhibitors. A standardized extract of Chinese red rice yeast can reduce cholesterol levels by up to 20% in certain patients. One randomized controlled trial showed a significant decrease in lipids with use of this supplement, with no significant toxicity.[34] Red rice yeast has not been tested specifically in protease inhibitor–related hyperlipidemia. No significant adverse effects have been reported to date in patients using this supplement (see Chapter 39, Dyslipidemias).

Dosage
The dose is 1200 mg orally twice daily.[35]

Precaution
Because this supplement can contain statin-like compounds, it is probably prudent to monitor liver function periodically in patients taking red rice yeast extract over the long term.

Herb-Supplement-Medication Interactions

An extremely active and important area of current research covers the questions of possible interactions among herbal medicines, supplements, and anti-HIV medications. In particular, herbs and supplements that induce elements of the cytochrome P-450 system have been found potentially to lead to lowered serum levels of protease inhibitors. St. John's wort, for example—an herb commonly recommended for depression—induces cytochrome P-450 activity and can lead to a decrease in indinavir levels of up to 57%; nevirapine levels can also be affected.[36] Garlic, commonly used for elevated cholesterol levels, can have similar effects through increased cytochrome P-450 activity.

Databases are now available that provide frequently updated information regarding known herb-drug and supplement-drug interactions, and practitioners caring for patients taking antiretrovirals should regularly consult these sites to provide informed counseling to patients regarding their concomitant use of herbs and supplements.

St. John's wort increases cytochrome P-450 activity and can reduce serum levels of medications metabolized by this system. It can decrease indinavir levels up to 57%.[28]

Mind-Body Therapy

Research in psychoneuroimmunology has clearly linked psychological stress to impaired immune function. Although a specific link between T-cell count or function and stress reduction in HIV disease has not been clearly established, one study did find a trend toward increased T-cell count in persons practicing a mind-body approach, and other studies found improvement in natural killer cell function and other immune parameters. Stress reduction approaches studied to date in HIV-positive patients include biofeedback, meditation, systematic relaxation, hypnosis, and cognitive-behavioral stress management training. A review of several mind-body applications from the literature follows.

Progressive Muscle Relaxation and Biofeedback

Ten HIV-positive men who were asymptomatic but had T-cell counts lower than 400 were enrolled in a randomized 10-week study in which the experimental group received a 1-hour training session twice weekly in progressive muscle relaxation and biofeedback-assisted relaxation.[35] The subjects were expected to practice the techniques daily. Follow-up at 1 month after the intervention was completed showed decreased anxiety and improved mood and self-esteem and increased T cell counts, as shown by the State Anxiety Inventory, the Profile of Mood States, the Self-Esteem Inventory, and a basic T-cell count. The extremely small sample size limits the generalizability of these findings, however.

The differing effects of guided imagery, progressive muscle relaxation, and no intervention were tested on 69 participants in an uncontrolled study over a span of 6 weeks.[38] Subjects were instructed in their particular intervention and then expected to continue daily practice for the duration of the study. The outcome showed improved quality of life scores for the guided imagery group but no change in the group practicing progressive muscle relaxation.

Mindfulness and Stress Reduction

Forty-eight HIV-1–infected adults were randomized to either an 8-week mindfulness-based stress reduction (MBSR) program or a 1-day control stress reduction education seminar. Findings provided an initial indication that mindfulness meditation training can buffer CD4+ T-lymphocyte declines in HIV-1–infected adults independent of antiretroviral medication use.[39]

A small nonrandomized study examined the effects of a structured, 8-week, MBSR program on perceived stress, mood, endocrine function, immunity, and functional health outcomes in HIV-positive adults. Although functional and quality of life outcomes were not significantly affected, natural killer cell activity and number increased significantly in the MBSR group compared with the comparison group.[40]

Another study of stress management training[41] focused on both CD4+ counts and quality of life measurements in 45 HIV-infected and AIDS patients (30 in the intervention group and 15 in the control group). This study found a lower mean stress level and a trend toward higher CD4+ counts in the intervention group. The intervention led to immediate increases in emotional well-being and perceived quality of life, but these outcomes were not sustained at a 6-month follow-up. The presence of illness-related intrusive thinking was higher in the control group at follow-up, whereas that of the intervention group actually decreased.

Further studies are needed to distinguish whether any one of the mind-body approaches is more effective than others in patients with HIV disease. Generally, these strategies are considered extremely safe. The one exception to this general rule is that patients with a history of psychosis or unstable behavior should avoid hypnosis and should undertake other deep relaxation approaches with caution because these practices may increase the risk of relapse in certain patients (see Chapter 93, Relaxation Techniques, and Chapter 98, Recommending Meditation).

Therapies to Consider

Acupuncture

Acupuncture has been widely used both to enhance immune function and general well-being in HIV-positive patients and to treat specific HIV- or medication-related symptoms. One randomized controlled trial that examined amitriptyline plus acupuncture found no benefit of standardized acupuncture over sham (placebo) acupuncture[42] in the treatment of HIV disease–related peripheral neuropathy. Methodologic challenges in studying acupuncture make it difficult to demonstrate a small positive effect of an acupuncture intervention. Specifically, to construct a valid placebo intervention (i.e., sham acupuncture) that does not in itself carry a therapeutic benefit beyond that of placebo is difficult. In addition, individualized strategies both for specific symptoms and for overall health may have higher efficacy than that of standardized treatment protocols more amenable to study in such trials; however, these individualized strategies are extremely difficult to study in blinded trials. Thus, a trial such as this one examining standardized acupuncture treatment versus individualized choice of points may fail to show efficacy because of the lesser efficacy of the standardized approach.

Many acupuncturists believe that for this modality to be effective in peripheral neuropathy, treatment must be initiated as soon as possible after the onset of symptoms. Perhaps future acupuncture trials in HIV disease should focus on efficacy in treating new-onset neuropathies.

Massage Therapy

Massage therapy has been shown to reduce anxiety levels. Massage therapy is proposed to have a positive impact on quality of life and immune function through stress mediation. The ability of massage to produce significant effects in the treatment of patients with HIV disease or AIDS in particular requires further study. A randomized trial of massage therapy in HIV-exposed neonates showed a significant benefit[43]; other evidence is all anecdotal. Although massage therapy has not been proved to affect CD4+ levels per se, evidence showed that daily massage in HIV-positive men improved natural killer cell function and increased CD8+ cell counts.[44] A Cochrane Systematic Review examined the safety and effectiveness of massage therapy on quality of life, pain, and immune system parameters. The investigators concluded that some evidence supports the use of massage therapy to improve quality of life for people living with HIV infection or AIDS, particularly in combination with other stress management modalities, and that massage therapy may have a positive effect on immunologic function.[45] The benefits in terms of mood and decreased anxiety and the lack of adverse effects make massage therapy a reasonable choice for the HIV-positive patient.

THERAPEUTIC REVIEW

If viral load exceeds 30,000, if CD4$^+$ counts fall to less than 500, or if patients are in any way symptomatic of HIV disease, good practice requires that they be offered combination antiretroviral medication as the mainstay of treatment. This approach does not preclude the use of integrative strategies as supportive adjuncts and to alleviate certain disease-related or medication-related symptoms.

■ Pharmaceuticals

- Consultation with a physician familiar with the rapidly changing range of medication options is recommended for proper choice of pharmaceutical approaches.

■ Nutrition

- Nutritional consultation early in the course of HIV infection should be recommended.
- Adequate calorie consumption and an emphasis on high intake of omega-3 essential fatty acids are important elements.
- Absorption issues should be considered as well.

■ Supplements

- Multivitamin daily, emphasizing vitamins B, C, and E and avoiding additional vitamin A

- L-Carnitine: 2000–3000 mg daily, especially in peripheral neuropathy or lipid disturbance
- L-Glutamine: 2000 mg daily, especially in chronic diarrhea or malabsorption syndromes
- Calcium carbonate supplementation: 500 mg twice daily for protease inhibitor–induced diarrhea

■ Botanicals

- Milk thistle extract: 240 mg twice daily, in patients with elevated values on liver function tests or coinfection with hepatitis C
- Red rice yeast: 1200 mg twice daily for hyperlipidemia
- Use of Chinese herbal formulas in patients not meeting criteria for pharmaceutical treatment
- High level of awareness among practitioners regarding possible interactions between herbal medicine, especially cytochrome P-450 inducers, and antiretroviral medications

■ Mind-Body Approaches

- Biofeedback, deep relaxation therapy, visualization, cognitive-behavioral stress reduction training, or another mind-body strategy

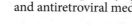
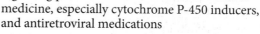

KEY WEB RESOURCES

- National HIV/AIDS Clinicians' Consultation Center. http://www.nccc.ucsf.edu/

  This University of California San Francisco/San Francisco General Hospital–based AIDS Education & Training Centers clinical resource for health care professionals includes toll-free numbers linking physicians to expert clinical advice on HIV/AIDS management and managing health care worker exposures to HIV and hepatitis B and C, as well as consultation on antiretroviral use in pregnancy, labor and delivery, and the postpartum period.

- The Body, a subsidiary of HealthCentral Network. http://www.thebody.com/index.html

  This community-oriented commercial Web site in English and Spanish has information on prevention and treatment, coverage of major HIV/AIDS conferences, online community discussion threads, and an extensive ask-the-experts feature.

- Johns Hopkins Medicine. http://hopkins-aids.edu/.

  A comprehensive HIV guide for clinicians is available from Johns Hopkins and requires signing up for an account (free).

  http://locator.aids.gov/

  This Web site links people to HIV testing, treatment, mental health and substance abuse services, housing, and other resources.

- National Institutes of Health HIV/AIDS Prevention & Service Provider Locator. www.aidsinfo.nih.gov

  This U.S. Department of Health and Human Services project offers the latest federally approved information on HIV/AIDS clinical research, treatment and prevention, and medical practice guidelines for people living with HIV/AIDS, their families and friends, health care providers, scientists, and researchers.

References

References are available online at expertconsult.com.

Chapter 18

Herpes Simplex Virus

Jeff Grassmann, DO, and Ted Wissink, MD

Pathophysiology

Herpes simplex is a viral disease caused by both herpes simplex virus type 1 (HSV-1) and herpes simplex virus type 2 (HSV-2). The infection is common in the United States and abroad and is usually categorized based on the site of infection, although both HSV-1 and HSV-2 can cause infections anywhere on the body. Oral herpes, generally caused by HSV-1, is the most common type and typically occurs on the lips. These lesions are frequently referred to as cold sores or fever blisters. HSV-1 primarily causes infections in the mouth, throat, face, eye, and central nervous system. Genital herpes, usually referred to simply as herpes, is the second most common form and is generally caused by HSV-2. HSV-2 primarily causes anogenital infections.

HSV is contracted only by direct contact with an active lesion or body fluid of an infected person.[1] To infect an individual, HSV travels through very small (even microscopic) breaks in the skin or mucous membranes in the mouth and genital area. The virus prefers areas where the skin is thin or moist. The clinical manifestations of primary (first episode) genital herpes are quite variable. The initial presentation tends to be more severe than recurrences, with painful genital ulcers, fevers, myalgias, tender inguinal lymphadenopathy, and headache.[2] The average incubation period is 4 days (range, 2 to 21 days). After initial infection, the virus moves to the sensory nerves, where it becomes latent until reactivated. Potential triggers for reactivation are discussed later in the chapter and are summarized in Table 18-1.

Herpes has no known cure. Once a person is infected, the immune system never removes HSV from the body. As a result of the primary infection, the body produces antibodies to the particular type of HSV and prevents another infection of that type at a different site of the body.[3] Therefore, people with immature or suppressed immune systems (e.g., newborns, transplant recipients, patients with human immunodeficiency virus infection) are more prone to recurrences and more severe complications of HSV infections. Many people infected with HSV-1 and HSV-2 show no physical symptoms, a condition known as subclinical herpes.

Asymptomatic HSV shedding occurs at some point in most people infected with herpes, and this may represent the most common form of HSV-1 and HSV-2 transmission.[3]

Many HSV-infected people experience recurrences, often within the first year of infection. A prodrome of symptoms including tingling, itching, and pain can occur and last from hours to days before lesions develop. Fewer lesions usually develop during recurrences, and these lesions are usually less painful and heal faster. Outbreaks tend to be episodic and occur an average of four to five times per year when patients are not using antiviral therapy.[3]

Integrative Therapy

Lifestyle

Condoms offer some protection against HSV-2 in both men and women; consistent condom users have a 30% lower risk of HSV-2 acquisition compared with those who never use condoms.[4]

The virus cannot pass through a latex condom, but condoms do not completely prevent skin contact. People with any symptoms of herpes should abstain from sexual activity with uninfected partners.

During an outbreak, practitioners often recommend that people clean the areas with warm water and then keep the active lesions as dry as possible after this. One way to help prevent spread of the virus is to dry the area with a hairdryer on a low or cool setting instead of using a towel.

All causes of HSV reactivation are unknown, but several triggers have been identified and are summarized in Table 18-1. Changes in the immune system the week before

TABLE 18-1. Potential Triggers That May Reactivate Herpes Simplex Virus

HSV-1
- Ultraviolet light
- Immunodeficiency
- Stress, depression, anxiety (chronic)
- Poor sleep
- Trauma to mucosa
- Cold, windy, or dry weather
- Hot food or biting lips
- Food allergy
- Fever

HSV-2
- Immunodeficiency
- Stress, depression, anxiety (chronic)
- Poor sleep
- Food allergy
- Trauma to genital mucosa
- Menses (usually 5–12 days before onset)

HSV, herpes simplex virus.

TABLE 18-2. Dietary Considerations in Herpes Simplex Viral Infection

Foods to Avoid (High Arginine Levels)
- Chocolate
- Peanuts
- Almonds
- Cashews
- Sunflower seeds
- Gelatin

Foods to Include (High Lysine Levels)
- Vegetables
- Beans
- Fish
- Turkey
- Chicken

and during menstruation can play a role in HSV-1 reactivation.[5] Concurrent infections such as viral upper respiratory infections or other febrile illnesses can cause outbreaks, and this association led to the common names cold sores and fever blisters.

Trauma Prevention

Local injury to the face, lips, eyes, or mouth can lead to reactivation. Exposure to wind, ultraviolet light, and sunlight are also well-known triggers. Preventing mucosal injury from chapping or sunburn is important in the prevention of outbreaks. Use of lip balm to prevent injury, and specifically the ingredient zinc sulfate (discussed later in the chapter), can help heal and prevent recurrent herpes infections.

Stress and Sleep

Sleep deprivation from poor sleep habits or lifestyle factors can increase a person's chance of herpes recurrence. Stress and uncontrolled anxiety can often lead to recurrences as well. These two factors should be addressed in patients with recurrent outbreaks of herpes.

Nutrition

Increased Lysine and Decreased Arginine

Generally, a well-balanced diet high in fruits and vegetables is recommended as healthy. Specifically for people infected with HSV, a diet avoiding foods high in arginine and including foods high in lysine is often recommended for reducing herpes outbreaks. Table 18-2 provides a list of foods high in lysine and arginine. Tissue culture studies have demonstrated a beneficial effect on viral replication when the amino acid ratio of arginine to lysine favors arginine. The opposite, elevation of lysine to arginine, suppresses viral replication and inhibits cytopathogenicity of HSV.[6] Results of clinical studies using this theory of avoiding arginine-rich foods have not been conclusively positive.

Lysine supplementation is reviewed later in the chapter. Lysine intake can be increased by increasing consumption of lysine-rich foods, such as legumes and animal proteins and reducing intake of lysine-poor foods such as grains and refined sugars. Emphasizing foods that are not processed or cooked in ways that limit available lysine (boiling or poaching preserves lysine, whereas grilling, broiling, or frying destroys it) also improves lysine nutritional status. Making these dietary changes may obviate the need for lysine supplementation in some cases.[7]

Refined Carbohydrates

Ingestion of large amounts of refined carbohydrates impairs certain parameters of immune function. In rats, the progressive addition of sucrose to the diet caused a dose-dependent reduction in the capacity to produce antibodies.[8] In healthy humans, acute ingestion of 75 g of glucose significantly depressed cell-mediated immune function after 30 and 60 minutes.[9] Although the relationship between refined carbohydrate intake and susceptibility to HSV has not been investigated, many patients notice that herpetic lesions recur when they eat too many sweets. In some cases, ingestion of even small amounts of refined sugar appears to trigger an exacerbation. Restriction of refined carbohydrate intake should therefore be considered on a case-by-case basis.

Food Allergies

Although the potential association between food allergy and recurrent HSV infection has not been studied, patients often report that outbreaks become less common after they identify and avoid specific foods. Repeated ingestion of allergenic foods could theoretically strain the immune system and potentially increase chances of HSV reactivation. Consider a trial of an elimination diet if food allergies are thought to play a role (see Chapter 84, Food Intolerance and Elimination Diet).

Supplements

Vitamin C

In early scientific studies in the 1930s, ascorbic acid was shown to inactivate a wide range of viruses in vitro, including HSV.[10] Oral and intravenous vitamin C, along with a vitamin C paste, was found to help alleviate HSV outbreaks in patients with acquired immunodeficiency syndrome (AIDS) in the 1980s. [11] In a small double-blind trial, patients with HSV outbreaks received 200 mg ascorbic acid and 200 mg water-soluble flavonoids (apparently from citrus) three times daily for 3 days or a placebo. The mean time until remission of symptoms was 57% shorter in the active treatment group than in the placebo group (4.2 versus 9.7 days; $P < .01$). Treatment was most effective when it was initiated during the prodromal stage. [12]

Thus, supplementation with vitamin C, with or without flavonoids, appears to be a worthwhile treatment for herpes simplex when supplementation is used early in an outbreak. Anecdotal evidence suggests that the antiviral effect of vitamin C is more pronounced at higher doses. For treatment of an acute episode, patients may consider increasing the daily consumption of vitamin C by eating fruits high in the vitamin and supplementing according to bowel tolerance for 5 to 10 days.

Zinc

Several studies have indicated that topical zinc preparations may be effective at shortening duration of outbreaks of HSV infection and preventing recurrence. One study of patients with frequent recurrences of HSV used a topical solution of 0.025% to 0.05% zinc sulfate. During an acute episode, zinc was applied daily until the lesions were gone. Treatment of healed lesions was continued once weekly for 1 month, then twice a month. During a follow-up period of 16 to 23 months, none of the patients experienced a recurrence of lesions. Results also showed that application of a 0.05% zinc sulfate solution, before and during sun exposure, at the site of previous HSV infections decreased relapses induced by sun exposure. [13]

Oral zinc seems to be helpful as well. Taking 23 mg zinc sulfate and 250 mg vitamin C, each twice daily for 6 weeks, appeared to reduce the duration and severity of HSV outbreaks during the supplementation period. [14]

▨ Dosage

Topical zinc sulfate 0.025% to 0.05% is applied daily for acute outbreaks. Oral zinc sulfate, 23 mg daily (with 250 mg of vitamin C) twice daily for 6 weeks, may reduce the duration and severity of outbreaks.

▨ Precautions

Long-term oral zinc supplementation may require a copper supplement to prevent zinc-induced copper deficiency. [15]

Lysine

A review of clinical trials showed that lysine supplements seem to be more effective for preventing a herpes outbreak than for reducing the severity and duration of an outbreak. [16] One such clinical trial included 114 patients (52 completed the trial) with recurrent orofacial herpes or genital herpes, or both. Patients were randomly assigned to receive, in double-blind fashion, 1 g lysine hydrochloride three times daily or placebo for 6 months. Among those who completed the trial, the proportion of patients who reported the treatment to be effective or very effective was 74% in the lysine group and 28% in the placebo group ($P < .01$). Lysine was significantly more effective than placebo in terms of frequency and severity of lesions and healing time. [17]

According to anecdotal reports, lysine supplementation accelerates the healing of acute herpes simplex outbreaks. Short-term administration of 1 to 3 g lysine daily has been found to reduce the duration of attacks, and higher doses are more effective than lower doses. [18] In a double-blind trial, however, administration of 1 g lysine at the first sign of infection, followed by 500 mg twice daily for a total treatment period of 5 days, had no significant effect on the healing rate. [19] Although anecdotal reports suggest that higher doses of lysine may be effective during acute outbreaks, no controlled trials have confirmed this.

▨ Dosage

For prevention, 1 g, three times daily for 6 months, is taken.

▨ Precautions

Gastrointestinal side effects such as diarrhea and abdominal pain have been reported with high doses (more than 10 g/day). A modest rise in low-density lipoprotein has been reported.

Topical Vitamin E

Topical application of vitamin E seems to relieve pain and aid in the healing of oral herpetic lesions (gingivostomatitis or herpetic cold sores). One study used topical cotton saturated with vitamin E oil (20,000 to 28,000 units/oz) placed over a dried lesion for 15 minutes. [20] In some cases, a single application was beneficial, but large or multiple lesions responded better when they were treated three times daily for 3 days. In another study, the content of a vitamin E capsule was applied to lesions every 4 hours. Prompt and sustained pain relief occurred, and the lesions healed more rapidly than expected. [21]

▨ Dosage

Empty the contents of a vitamin E capsule (*d*-alpha-tocopherol) onto a cotton stick and apply to crusted sores every 8 hours for 3 days.

Mind-Body Therapy

Antecedent stress has commonly been thought to instigate HSV outbreaks. However, this relationship has not always been clearly delineated in the literature. Some investigators have postulated that stress is induced by the recurrence itself and not causative. [22] In a 2009 review article, however, psychosocial stress was in fact shown to increase HSV recurrence significantly. [23] Further evidence for the link between stress and HSV recurrence was shown by a reduction in HSV-2 antibody titers in patients after cognitive-behavioral therapy. [24] Because high levels of circulating HSV antibodies have been correlated with HSV recurrence, this signifies a positive effect. Another interesting correlate has shown depressive symptoms to increase the rate of HSV recurrence. [25] Thus, it stands to reason that a focus on modalities to lower stress level and to treat depression when present would decrease the incidence of HSV outbreaks.

Relaxation Training

Relaxation exercises can be incorporated into a daily routine and also used to manage situational stress (see Chapter 93, Relaxation Techniques).

Meditation

Meditation can be an excellent way for patients to manage chronic stress. Encouraging the receptive patient to incorporate a meditative practice into daily life can have far-reaching health benefits (see Chapter 98, Recommending Meditation).

Botanicals

Lemon Balm

Lemon balm (*Melissa officinalis*), an herb from the mint family, is typically known for its calming properties. It is also a potent antiviral herb and has been used to treat herpes infections for many years. Studies have demonstrated its effect when used topically as a 1% cream or ointment of a 70:1 leaf extract applied two to four times a day. Topical application should be started with prodromal symptoms and continued for 2 to 3 days after the lesions have healed. One double-blind placebo-controlled study (*N* = 66) demonstrated significant improvement in discomfort, number of lesions, and size of lesions when compared with controls.[26]

Dosage

Lemon balm 1% cream or ointment of 70:1 extract applied to lesions two to four times daily from the start of symptoms to 2 to 3 days after healing.

Precautions

Lemon balm is likely safe and without long-term risk.

Siberian Ginseng

Siberian ginseng (*Eleutherococcus senticosus*) is an adaptogenic plant. Its root has been used to form a standardized extract containing 0.3% eleutheroside (Elagen). When taken orally, this extract was found to decrease frequency, duration, and severity of HSV-2 outbreaks.[27]

Dosage

Siberian ginseng extract standardized to contain eleutheroside E 0.3% is taken in a dose of 400 mg per day.

Precautions

Siberian ginseng can cause slight drowsiness, anxiety, irritability, melancholy, mastalgia, and uterine bleeding. These symptoms are often seen with doses higher than normal. It should be used with caution in patients with cardiovascular disease because hypertension, palpitations, and tachycardia can occur. Long-term use of Siberian ginseng has been associated with nerve inflammation and subsequent muscle spasm.

Rhubarb and Sage

A cream composed of 23 mg/g each of rhubarb (*Rheum officinale and Rheum palmatum*) and sage (*Salvia officinalis*) topically has been shown to be as effective as acyclovir cream.[28]

Dosage

Apply a cream containing 23 mg/g each of rhubarb and sage extracts every 2 to 4 hours while awake. Start treatment within 1 day of prodromal symptoms and continue for 7 days.

Precautions

Oral use of rhubarb may have significant side effects, but topical use appears to be safe. Rhubarb-containing products should not be used for longer than 8 days.

Propolis

Propolis is a resin-like substance collected by bees from a variety of plant structures. One study demonstrated the benefit of propolis in the treatment of HSV lesions with a 3% ointment applied four times a day.[29]

Dosage

An ointment of 3% propolis is applied to HSV lesions four times a day.

Precautions

Some allergic reactions have been reported with oral propolis use. Patients with bee allergies should also use caution with propolis. One case report noted acute renal failure in a patient using oral propolis who improved when propolis was stopped. Topical propolis may contain cosmetics that could induce eczematous contact dermatitis.

Sangre de Grado

Sangre de Grado is a tree indigenous to the Amazon of South America. Its resin contains SP-303, which has been used orally in the treatment of diarrhea. One study showed its benefit in reducing HSV lesions in the genital and perianal region in patients with AIDS. These patients used a standardized extract containing SP-303.[30,31]

Dosage

An ointment of 15% SP-303 (derived from Sangre de Grado) is applied topically to lesions three times a day for 21 days.

Precautions

SP-303 used topically can cause pain and burning.

Aloe Vera

Some data indicate that aloe vera 0.5% extract cream, applied topically three times a day, hastens healing time compared with aloe vera gel or placebo.[32]

Dosage

Aloe vera 0.5% extract cream is applied topically three times a day for 2 weeks.

Precautions

Topical aloe is generally well tolerated. Some burning, itching, or local dermatitis can be experienced.

Pharmaceuticals

Antivirals are the mainstay in conventional medicine for the treatment of primary and recurrent HSV infections. By inhibiting DNA polymerase in virally infected cells, these drugs work to interfere with viral replication. The greatest effects are seen when the drugs are prescribed within 48 to 72 hours of the initiation of symptoms from an outbreak. If a patient is experiencing new lesions after this time frame, however, initiation of an antiviral may still be warranted.

Studies demonstrated that the use of acyclovir can decrease the duration of lesions, fevers, and odynophagia, as well as reduce viral shedding compared with placebo.[33]

> Early treatment does not seem to decrease the risk for recurrent infection.[34]

Caution is advised in patients with renal disease because antiviral medications can worsen renal function, especially when these drugs are used with other nephrotoxic substances.

Primary Herpes Infection

Options include the following:
Acyclovir: 400 mg orally three times per day or 200 mg orally five times per day for 7 to 10 days[35]
Famciclovir: 500 mg orally three times daily for 7 to 10 days
Valacyclovir: 1000 mg orally twice daily for 7 to 10 days[36]

Famciclovir and valacyclovir offer less frequent dosing but are more expensive.

Recurrent Herpes Infection

Patients who experience minimal symptoms and infrequent recurrences may not need treatment at all. Those with more significant symptoms may benefit from antivirals when the drugs are started at the onset of prodrome symptoms (itching, burning, tingling).

Topical antiviral treatment has shown to have a modest benefit and may be helpful for certain patients. One study demonstrated a decrease in healing time, duration of pain, and viral shedding. [37] Topical options are as follows:
Acyclovir cream or ointment: applied six times a day for 7 days[38]
Penciclovir cream: applied every 2 hours while awake for 4 days[37]

Oral options include the following:
Acyclovir: 200 or 400 mg five times daily for 5 days [39]
Famciclovir: 750 mg twice daily for 1 day or 1500 mg as a single dose[40]
Valacyclovir: 2 g twice daily for 1 day[41,42]

Single-day dosing with famciclovir or valacyclovir can offer greater patient convenience and lower cost compared with 5 days of acyclovir.[42]

Pharmaceutical Prophylaxis

Prophylactic treatment should be prescribed on an individual basis and depends on the severity of symptoms with outbreaks or underlying conditions. In general, suppressive therapy is recommended if a patient has six or more recurrences per year. Practitioners should discontinue prophylactic antiviral medications once a year to see whether continuation is necessary.

Options include the following:
Acyclovir: 400 mg orally twice a day[43]
Valacyclovir: 500 mg orally once a day[44]

PREVENTION PRESCRIPTION

- Follow safe sexual practices, with the use of condoms and avoidance of oral sex if infectious status is unknown.
- Avoid contact with vesicular fluid to others or other body areas.
- Avoid trauma to the skin (physical trauma, rough intercourse, sunburns).
- Maintain a regular sleep-wake cycle with 8 hours of sleep daily.
- Avoid known food triggers.
- Eat lysine-rich food (vegetables, beans, fish, chicken, and turkey).
- Avoid excessive arginine-rich foods (chocolate, peanuts, almonds, cashews, sunflower seeds, and gelatin).
- Make lifestyle choices to reduce stress levels.
- Prevent and treat depression.
- Consider antiviral medications if outbreaks are frequent or you are immunosuppressed.

 ## THERAPEUTIC REVIEW

■ Acute Treatment

Supplements

- Zinc sulfate
  - Topical solution 0.025% to 0.05%: applied daily at the start of an outbreak, then once weekly for 1 month, then twice a month
  - Oral: 25 mg zinc added to 250 mg of vitamin C each twice a day for 6 weeks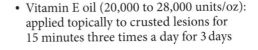
- Vitamin C: 200 to 250 mg three times a day for 3 days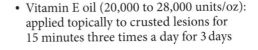
- Lysine: 1 g three times a day

- Vitamin E oil (20,000 to 28,000 units/oz): applied topically to crusted lesions for 15 minutes three times a day for 3 days

Botanicals

- Lemon balm 1% cream or ointment (70:1 extract): applied two to four times daily at onset of symptoms to 2 to 3 days after healing
- Siberian ginseng (eleutheroside E 0.3% standardized extract): 400 mg by mouth daily (higher doses and long-term use can lead to significant adverse effects)
- Rhubarb and sage extract cream containing 23 mg/g each: applied topically every 2 to 4 hours for 7 days

Continued

- Propolis 3% ointment: applied topically 4 times a day (use caution if patient has a bee allergy)

- Sangre de Grado (SP-303) 15% ointment: applied topically to lesions three times a day for 21 days

- Aloe vera 0.5% extract cream: applied topically three times a day for 2 weeks

Pharmaceuticals

- Primary infection

  - Acyclovir: 400 mg orally three times daily or 200 mg orally five times daily for 7 to 10 days

  - Famciclovir: 500 mg orally three times daily for 7 to 10 days

  - Valacyclovir: 1000 mg orally twice daily for 7 to 10 days

- Recurrent infection

  - Topical

  Acyclovir cream or ointment: applied 6 times a day for 7 days
  Penciclovir cream: applied every 2 hours while awake for 4 days

  - Oral

  Acyclovir: 200 to 400 mg five times daily for 5 days

  Famciclovir: 750 mg twice daily for 1 day or 1500 mg as single dose

  Valacyclovir: 2 g twice a day for 1 day

Prevention of Recurrences

Lifestyle

- Avoid trauma to genital and oral mucosa.

- Use sun protection.
- Encourage 8 hours of sleep each night.

Nutrition

- Encourage seven to eight servings of fruits and vegetables a day.
- Increase lysine-rich foods (see Table 18-2).
- Decrease arginine-rich foods (see Table 18-2).
- Consider an elimination diet.

Mind-Body Therapy

- Make lifestyle changes to reduce chronic stress, anxiety, and depression. Educate patients on techniques for relaxation such as breath work and meditation. Treat depression when present.

Supplements

- Zinc

  - Topical: 0.05% solution before and during sun exposure at the site of previous HSV infection

  - Oral: 25 mg twice a day (supplement with copper if long-term use)

- Lysine: 1 g three times a day

Botanicals

- Siberian ginseng (eleutheroside E 0.3% standardized extract): 400 mg a day (high doses and long-term use can lead to significant adverse effects)

Pharmaceuticals

- Acyclovir: 400 mg orally twice daily
- Valacyclovir: 500 mg orally once a day

References

References are available at expertconsult.com.

Chronic Hepatitis

Tina M. St. John, MD

Pathophysiology

Hepatitis is the Latin term for liver inflammation. It is characterized by hepatonecrosis and inflammatory cell infiltration. Viral and toxic agents are the most common causes of hepatitis. *Acute hepatitis* describes a process enduring less than 6 months. Hepatitis is deemed chronic when it is present for longer than 6 months. The ongoing inflammatory process may lead to fibrosis and eventually cirrhosis, with a concomitant increased risk of hepatocellular carcinoma.

Chronic hepatitis has various causes, in isolation or combination (Table 19-1). Most people with chronic hepatitis develop the disease gradually without an acute clinical illness or obvious symptoms. The condition is generally insidious and slowly progressive, declaring itself clinically only after cirrhosis develops with concomitant symptoms. Cases of chronic hepatitis diagnosed before the development of hepatic symptoms are often the result of incidental findings, especially unexpectedly elevated liver enzymes on routine biochemical panels.

The most common cause of chronic viral hepatitis in the United States is hepatitis C, accounting for approximately 50% to 75% of all cases.[1-3] Given its high prevalence and the associated implications for clinical practice, chronic hepatitis C (CHC) is the focus of this section. Integrative treatments aimed at controlling chronic hepatic inflammation and its sequelae, which underlie the pathologic process of CHC, are applicable to other conditions that share a similar pathophysiology.

The histologic hallmarks of hepatitis are hepatic necrosis and mononuclear infiltration (lymphocytes, macrophages, and plasma cells). These parameters are directly assessed with liver biopsy. Specimens are graded according to portal and lobular inflammatory activity and are staged based on the degree of fibrosis or the presence of cirrhosis. The hepatitis C virus (HCV) is hepatotropic but minimally cytopathic. A corollary of this observation is that HCV viral load does not affect the natural history of the disease in a given individual.[4,5] The detrimental effects of chronic HCV infection are predominantly a consequence of the associated chronic inflammatory process, which causes marked oxidative stress resulting from an overabundance of free radicals. In the presence of ongoing hepatonecrosis, connective tissue is laid down as the body attempts repair. An accumulation of extracellular connective tissue leads to fibrosis, which progresses predictably (Table 19-2). Cirrhosis is the final stage of the fibrotic process, characterized by diffuse hepatocyte damage, nodular regeneration, and aberrant architecture accompanied by impaired hepatocyte function and impeded portal blood flow.

Advanced fibrosis and cirrhosis are associated with increased risk for the development of hepatocellular carcinoma. Each year, 1% to 3% of people with HCV-related cirrhosis develop liver cancer.[6] The incidence of liver cancer in the United States tripled from 1975 to 2005, with the most significant increases occurring in black, white, and Hispanic men 50 to 59 years old.[7] Although 1-year, cause-specific survival for hepatocellular carcinoma increased from 25% to 47% from 1992 to 2004, more than half of all newly diagnosed patients succumb within the first 12 months after diagnosis.[7]

Liver biopsy remains the gold standard for making a histopathologic diagnosis of chronic hepatitis. Biochemical, serologic, and nucleic acid testing are the mainstays of etiologic diagnosis. Histologic information is particularly important for hepatitis C management decisions because fibrotic stage is often a key factor in such deliberations. Overall, approximately 5% to 25% of people with CHC develop cirrhosis over a period of 25 to 30 years.[8-10] Observational prospective studies and outcome modeling projections indicate that the risk of liver disease progression toward severe fibrosis or cirrhosis is minimal at 10 to 15 years in patients with persistently normal alanine aminotransferase (ALT) levels, approximately 5% to 10% in patients with elevated ALT and no fibrosis on initial liver biopsy, but greater than 30% to 40% in those with elevated ALT and portal fibrosis.[8,11]

A study of patients with newly diagnosed hepatitis C found that up to 20% of those patients with evidence of

TABLE 19-1. Common Causes of Chronic Hepatitis

ETIOLOGIC CATEGORY	SPECIFICS
Hepatitis viruses	Hepatitis C Hepatitis B (± hepatitis D)
Toxins and medications	Ethanol Methyldopa Isoniazid Nitrofurantoin Amiodarone
Autoimmune disease	Autoimmune hepatitis
Inborn metabolic disorders	Wilson disease Hemochromatosis Alpha$_1$-antitrypsin deficiency
Acquired metabolic disorders	Nonalcoholic steatohepatitis
Biliary diseases	Primary and secondary biliary cirrhosis Primary sclerosing cholangitis Biliary tree anomalies
Cryptogenic	—

TABLE 19-2. Stages of Liver Fibrosis

STAGE	CHARACTERISTICS
0	No fibrosis
1	Confined to enlarged portal zones
3	Architectural distortion (septal fibrosis, bridging) without obvious cirrhosis
4	Probable or definite cirrhosis

cirrhosis on liver biopsy were not suspected of having cirrhosis, based on clinical and laboratory findings.[12] Liver enzyme levels do not predictably correlate with liver histologic features. A 2006 study of 480 patients with CHC who had persistently normal ALT levels found that nearly two thirds of patients had evidence of portal fibrosis on liver biopsy, and roughly 1 in 10 patients had bridging fibrosis.[13] Laboratory panels that include multiple biologic markers of hepatic fibrosis, such as platelet count, hyaluronic acid, procollagen type 3 N-terminal peptide, and tissue inhibitor of matrix metalloproteinase-1, perform relatively well in predicting the presence or absence of advanced fibrosis or cirrhosis among patients with CHC who have no physical or other laboratory evidence of cirrhosis. These tests lack sensitivity and specificity with midrange fibrosis, however, and therefore cannot be used to track fibrosis progression.[6,14,15]

Although patients with clinical or laboratory evidence of frank cirrhosis can have an accurate diagnosis without liver biopsy, the reverse logic is untrue (i.e., cirrhosis cannot be ruled out based on clinical and laboratory assessments alone). In the absence of clinical evidence of cirrhosis, the only way to assess a patient's liver histologic features with a high degree of certainty is with liver biopsy. Histologic features other than

TABLE 19-3. Nonhistologic Factors Associated With Increased Risk of Development of Cirrhosis Among People With Chronic Hepatitis C

- Genotypic male
- Heavy alcohol consumption
- Coinfection with human immunodeficiency virus and/or hepatitis B virus
- Elevated serum alanine aminotransferase[160]
- Obesity[6]
- Age older than 35 yr at the time of initial infection

fibrotic stage (e.g., steatosis and iron accumulation) may also have predictive value for disease progression and response to interferon-based regimens.[16,17] Nonhistologic factors associated with accelerated disease progression and poor outcomes are shown in Table 19-3. Notably absent from this list are HCV genotype and viral load, factors that do not predict disease progression. Both these factors, however, correlate with the probability of response to interferon-based therapy.

Reducing Free Radicals

The primary care provider has an important role in promoting constitutional, hepatic, and immunologic health and wellness. The interplay of host and virologic factors that potentially influence CHC disease progression and may be affected by integrative interventions falls into two primary arenas: oxidative stress and immunologic function.[18-30] Chronic inflammation leads to an overabundance of oxygen-derived free radicals. The influence of free radicals in a given inflammatory reaction depends on the balance between the production and inactivation of these reactive metabolites.[18] To the extent that one can influence the balance favorably toward decreased oxidative stress, one can potentially limit or reduce damage caused by an overabundance of free radicals.

Enhancing Liver Detoxification

When considering therapy for chronic hepatitis, the practitioner should keep in mind the liver's detoxification function. The liver is the interface between the digestive tract and the rest of the body, and it orchestrates metabolic homeostasis. Blood delivered from the digestive tract is filtered and processed by the liver. Endogenous waste products and pollutant xenobiotics are detoxified and excreted into the bile. A two-phase detoxification process neutralizes and eliminates these chemicals. For optimal function of the hepatic detoxification system, the phases must be balanced and supported by adequate dietary intake to provide the necessary system elements. Phase I of the detoxification pathway is chemical neutralization, which is accomplished predominantly by the cytochrome P-450 system. This system is a versatile family of heme-derived enzymes that catalyze redox reactions on a wide variety of endogenous and exogenous substrates. When a chemical is neutralized by cytochrome P-450 enzymes, free radicals are produced, which can damage hepatocytes. Free radicals are removed by antioxidants in the liver; one of the most important is glutathione, which is also used in phase II of the detoxification process. High-level toxin exposure can deplete hepatic glutathione and thus hamper both phases of the detoxification process.

TABLE 19-4. Substances That Support Phase II Detoxification

DETOXIFICATION PATHWAY	REQUIRED NUTRIENTS
Glutathione conjugation	Dietary glutathione Vitamins B_2, B_6, and C N-Acetylcysteine Glycine, cysteine, glutamine, and methionine Zinc, copper, manganese, and selenium
Amino acid conjugation	Glycine, taurine, glutamine, arginine, and ornithine Magnesium
Methylation	S-Adenosylmethionine Vitamin B_{12} and folic acid Choline Molybdenum
Sulfation	Dietary sulfur-rich foods B vitamins Taurine, methionine, cysteine, and glutathione Zinc, copper, manganese, selenium, and molybdenum
Acetylation	Vitamins B_1, B_2, B_5 (pantothenic acid), and C Acetyl coenzyme A
Glucuronidation	Glucuronic acid and glutamine Magnesium Vitamins B_3 and B_6

Phase II of the detoxification process is elimination, which typically involves a conjugation reaction that renders the toxin water soluble and enables excretion of the toxin complex through bile or urine. The six phase II detoxification pathways are glutathione conjugation, amino acid conjugation, methylation, sulfation, acetylation, and glucuronidation.[31] Many experts consider glutathione conjugation to be the most important of these pathways. In summary, glutathione serves as both a potent antioxidant and an essential substrate for phase II detoxification. Table 19-4 lists substances needed to support the phase II detoxification pathways (see Chapter 104, Detoxification).

Patients with chronic hepatitis should be vaccinated against hepatitis A and B to decrease the risk of superinfection and acute fulminant hepatitis.

Integrative Therapy

The choice of therapeutic modalities used in an integrative approach to CHC management depends on numerous factors, including the patient's liver status, goals, and comorbid conditions. Regardless of the specific modalities chosen, the fundamental goals of integrative CHC management are to:
1. Decrease hepatic inflammation and thereby limit disease progression
2. Support and enhance hepatic detoxification capacity
3. Support healthy immune function
4. Decrease the risk of cirrhosis and hepatocellular carcinoma
5. Support and enhance quality of life

Pharmaceuticals

The National Institutes of Health Consensus Conference Statement on the Management of Hepatitis C[32] states that all patients with CHC are potential candidates for antiviral therapy. Current pharmacologic, state-of-the-art treatment for CHC is combination therapy with pegylated interferon alfa (peginterferon) and ribavirin. The American Association for the Study of Liver Diseases Practice Guideline on the Diagnosis, Management, and Treatment of Hepatitis C[6] recommends combination therapy for patients with bridging fibrosis or compensated cirrhosis on liver biopsy. The relative and absolute contraindications to interferon-based therapy are numerous, however, and include ongoing alcohol dependence, hepatic decompensation, and certain comorbid medical and neuropsychiatric conditions. Thus, many patients with CHC are ineligible for interferon-based treatment or fall outside this histologically defined group. Additionally, the side effect profiles of peginterferon and ribavirin are such that many patients decline or postpone aggressive pharmacologic therapy.

Deciding which patients should consider therapy with peginterferon plus ribavirin must be done on a case-by-case basis. Paradoxically, evidence indicates that patients with low-stage fibrosis are more likely to clear HCV in response to combination therapy compared with patients with advanced fibrosis or cirrhosis. Yet these are the same patients in whom the risk of progression to cirrhosis is lowest. Table 19-5 summarizes factors predictive of response to interferon-based therapy for CHC.

A challenge in pharmaceutical treatment is that patients who are most likely to respond to therapy are also least likely to progress to cirrhosis.

The decision to start therapy requires consideration of the patient's goals, liver status and likelihood of disease progression, comorbidities, and potential risks and benefits. Watchful waiting with supportive management, including periodic liver biopsy (every 4 to 5 years), is considered both safe and prudent for patients with minimal fibrosis on initial liver biopsy. At the other extreme, patients with decompensated hepatic cirrhosis are ineligible for interferon-based therapy and should be referred for liver transplant evaluation.

CHC is a highly variable disease. Although certain factors can be used to predict the most likely natural history of the disease, the clinical course in a given individual is inherently unpredictable. Accordingly, no clear consensus exists among gastroenterologists and hepatologists regarding absolute criteria for deciding which patients should be treated with interferon-based therapy. The challenge is to identify those patients for whom the formidable undertaking of interferon-based therapy is most likely to prove holistically healing. An overly aggressive or inappropriately passive approach can prove detrimental to a patient, depending on his or her circumstances.

TABLE 19-5. Factors Predictive of Viral Response to Interferon-Based Therapy for Hepatitis C Virus

FACTOR	ASSOCIATION WITH VIRAL RESPONSE
HCV genotype	Genotypes 2 and 3 significantly more responsive to peginterferon alfa plus ribavirin than genotypes 1 and 4*
HCV viral load	Probability of a viral response reduced by high pretreatment viral load (600,000 units/mL or more)[43]
Liver fibrosis stage	Fibrosis stage on liver biopsy inversely predictive of the likelihood of viral response; absence of bridging fibrosis or cirrhosis significantly positively predictive
Ethnicity	People of European or Asian ethnicity more likely to experience a viral response than are those of African or Hispanic ethnicity
Hepatic steatosis	Likelihood of a viral response adversely affected by the presence and severity of steatosis
Body mass index	Likelihood of a viral response negatively influenced by elevated body mass index
Insulin resistance	Probability of a viral response possibly reduced by insulin resistance
Age (among adults)	Overall, age inversely related to likelihood of a viral response

HCV, hepatitis C virus.
*In a study of more than 6000 patients with chronic hepatitis C in the United States, the genotype distribution was 73% genotype 1, 14% genotype 2, 8% genotype 3, 4% mixed genotype, and less than 1% for genotypes 4, 5, and 6.[162]
HCV genotype and viral load have predictive value with respect to the likelihood of response to interferon-based therapy. However, these factors are not predictive of liver fibrosis or disease progression.

Peginterferon Alfa

Interferons are a family of potent cytokines produced in response to viral infection and various other stimuli. Interferons are associated with complex antiviral, immunomodulatory, and antiproliferative actions. Interferon-stimulated genes inhibit viral replication and cell proliferation. Pegylation technology links interferon to the inactive, water-soluble polymer polyethylene glycol, which shields the molecules from proteolytic enzymes and prolongs the half-life of the drug. Two peginterferons have been approved by the U.S. Food and Drug Administration for the treatment of CHC: peginterferon alfa-2a (Pegasys) and peginterferon alfa-2b (Peg-Intron).

■ Dosage

Peginterferon alfa-2a dosing, in combination with ribavirin, for the treatment of CHC is 180 mcg/week subcutaneously. The recommended dose of peginterferon alfa-2b, administered in combination with ribavirin, is 1.5 mcg/kg/week subcutaneously.

■ Precautions

The most common side effects of peginterferons are flulike symptoms such as fatigue, lethargy, myalgia, and headache. Other potentially serious side effects include depression, anxiety, suicidal ideation, hypothyroidism, bone marrow suppression, and anorexia.

Ribavirin

Ribavirin is a guanosine analogue that has shown activity against a variety of RNA and DNA viruses in vitro and in vivo. Ribavirin alone has little in vivo effect against HCV. The combination of peginterferon alfa and ribavirin, however, has been definitively shown to lead to superior, durable response rates compared with monotherapy with either agent.[33,34] Four companies in the United States market ribavirin, which is administered orally twice daily.

■ Dosage

The dosage recommendation for ribavirin in combination with pegylated interferon depends on body weight, genotype, and whether peginterferon alfa-2a or alfa-2b is used. For HCV genotypes 1 and 4, the recommended dose of peginterferon alfa-2a is 1000 mg/day orally in two divided doses for patients weighing 75 kg or less and 1200 mg/day for those weighing more than 75 kg. If using peginterferon alfa-2b, the recommended dose of ribavirin is 800 mg/day for patients weighing less than 65 kg, 1000 mg/day for those weighing 65 to 85 kg, 1200 mg/day for those weighing 85 kg to 105 kg, and 1400 mg/day for patients weighing more than 105 kg. For HCV genotypes 2 and 3, the recommended dose of ribavirin with peginterferon alfa-2a or alfa-2b is 800 mg/day orally in two divided doses, regardless of body weight.

■ Precautions

Ribavirin is associated with two serious side effects: hemolytic anemia and birth defects. Other side effects of ribavirin include cough, dyspnea, insomnia, pruritus, rash, and anorexia.

Peginterferon plus Ribavirin Treatment and Response

The duration of combination peginterferon-based therapy for HCV varies by genotype. The standard duration of treatment is 48 weeks for HCV genotypes 1 and 4, and 24 weeks for genotypes 2 and 3.[6] Monitoring of HCV viral load after the initiation of therapy determines virologic response and may influence the duration of therapy. Early virologic response (EVR), a 100-fold or greater reduction in HCV viral load after the first 12 weeks of treatment, is predictive of sustained virologic response (SVR),[35,36] defined as undetectable HCV RNA 6 months after completion of therapy. In the absence of EVR, it is highly unlikely that continued antiviral treatment will successfully clear HCV. Treatment discontinuation is recommended in the absence of EVR.[6,33,37]

Rapid virologic response (RVR), defined as undetectable HCV using a molecular assay with a lower detection limit of 50 units/mL at week 4 of therapy, is highly predictive of SVR.[38,39] Among patients with RVR and difficulty tolerating treatment, consideration may be given to shortening the duration of therapy to 24 weeks for patients with HCV genotype 1, and to 12 to 16 weeks for those with genotypes 2 and 3, respectively.[39–42] Early discontinuation of treatment, however, increases the risk of relapse on completion of therapy.

SVR rates vary by HCV genotype. Approximately 80% of people with genotypes 2 and 3 who receive peginterferon plus ribavirin achieve SVR compared with roughly 50% of people with genotype 1.[33,37,43,44] Results of studies evaluating the long-term durability of SVR indicate that late relapse is rare and liver histology typically improves with time.[45,46] Among patients with marked pretreatment hepatic fibrosis, a low level of risk for the development of hepatocellular carcinoma persists, especially among those with preexisting cirrhosis.

> Hepatitis C genotypes 1 and 4 are associated with the poorest response to therapy.

Hepatitis A and B Vaccination

Anyone with documented chronic hepatitis who was not previously immunized and is without serologic evidence of immunity should be vaccinated for both hepatitis A and hepatitis B. Superinfection with a second hepatitis virus in a patient already chronically infected with another of the hepatitis viruses may cause acute fulminant disease. In the absence of an acute fulminant episode, new infection superimposed on preexisting chronic liver disease may accelerate disease progression and negatively affect prognosis.

Supplements

Glutathione

Glutathione is a potent antioxidant with many crucial functions, including detoxification and cytotoxic T lymphocyte (CTL) activation.[47] Most glutathione in the body is produced intracellularly in the liver from the amino acids cysteine, glutamate, and glycine. Glutathione levels are frequently below normal in people with alcoholic hepatitis and CHC.[48–50] One study found that patients with CHC who had the lowest glutathione levels had the highest viral loads and greater degrees of liver damage, compared with patients with the highest glutathione levels.[50]

The absorption of intact glutathione from dietary sources appears to be limited; glutathione is hydrolyzed by intestinal gamma-glutamyl transferase (GGT). Similarly, a study of oral glutathione supplementation found no increase in circulating levels.[51] Optimal glutathione levels are achieved by consuming a diet rich in foods with high levels of sulfur-containing amino acids (e.g., asparagus, avocados, broccoli, spinach, garlic, and unprocessed meats) and may be enhanced by nutritional supplements that promote glutathione production, such as vitamins C and E, N-acetylcysteine (NAC), selenium, silymarin, and curcumin.

> Glutathione is not absorbed well when taken orally. The best way to increase glutathione levels is to eat sulfur-containing foods (asparagus, avocados, broccoli, spinach, garlic) and supplement with nutrients that enhance production, including vitamin C, vitamin E, N-acetylcysteine, selenium, silymarin, and curcumin.

Vitamin C

Vitamin C is a powerful antioxidant and antiinflammatory agent, functions that may help limit the chronic inflammation and oxidative stress associated with CHC. In a 2008 study, investigators noted an inverse relationship between plasma vitamin C levels and aspartate aminotransferase (AST) among patients with CHC.[52] Evidence indicates that vitamin C also has in vivo immunomodulatory and anticarcinogenic functions. Finally, vitamin C has been found to preserve intracellular reduced glutathione concentrations and improve overall antioxidant protection capacity.[53]

■ Dosage

Vitamin C 200 to 250 mg twice daily (recommendations vary widely). The Institute of Medicine of the National Academies notes that the tolerable upper intake limit (UL) for vitamin C is 2000 mg/day.[54]

■ Precautions

Vitamin C modulates iron absorption and transport. High doses of vitamin C should be avoided by persons with hemochromatosis or other conditions with the potential for iron overload. High doses of vitamin C are also contraindicated in patients with a history of kidney stones or renal insufficiency. Excessive doses of vitamin C may result in bloating and diarrhea.

Vitamin E

Vitamin E is a fat-soluble antioxidant that also supports optimal glutathione levels. Research data on vitamin E in the setting of chronic hepatitis are mixed. A small study of patients with CHC found that nearly half of the participants taking 800 units daily experienced improvement of liver enzyme levels.[55] A separate study in which CHC patients took 945 units of vitamin E, 200 mcg of selenium, and 500 mg of vitamin C daily found no effect on serum ALT, HCV viral load, or oxidative markers after 6 months of treatment.[56] Some data indicate that vitamin E may have a role in interruption of the fibrotic process.[57,58]

■ Dosage

Dose is 400 International Units (IU)/day of d-alpha tocopherol.

■ Precautions

High doses of vitamin E may potentiate the effects of antithrombotic drugs (including aspirin), anticoagulants, and some herbs (e.g., garlic and ginkgo). Patients with vitamin K deficiencies (e.g., liver failure) should avoid high doses of vitamin E. The recommended UL for vitamin E is 1500 IU/day.

N-Acetylcysteine

NAC is a derivative of the amino acid L-cysteine. It is a reducing agent and an antioxidant. NAC is more stable than L-cysteine and may be better absorbed. Acetylcysteine (Mucomyst) is used therapeutically as an inhaled mucolytic and an oral antidote for acetaminophen poisoning. By increasing hepatic glutathione levels, NAC counters the marked depletion that characterizes acetaminophen poisoning. NAC is available over the counter as a dietary supplement, which is rapidly absorbed. It is a precursor in glutathione production and has been found to raise serum levels, although not as effectively as vitamin C.[59] Long-term safety of this product in otherwise healthy people is yet to be proved. One study found that doses greater than 1.2 g/day may have prooxidant effects.[60] The findings of studies examining the effects of NAC in people with CHC are conflicting; some studies show no benefit, and others report normalization of liver enzyme levels.[61-64] In animal models, NAC was found to relieve oxidative stress and dampen the hepatic inflammatory response associated with nonalcoholic steatohepatitis.[65,66] Because of the unestablished safety profile of NAC and because of its cost, support for optimal glutathione levels are best achieved using other supplements, such as vitamins C and E, silymarin, and selenium.

Dosage
NAC 800 mg/day

Precautions
Doses of NAC greater than 1.2 g/day may have prooxidant effects. Reported adverse reactions after oral administration include nausea, vomiting, diarrhea, headache, and rash. Renal stone formation has been reported, albeit rarely; patients taking NAC should be encouraged to drink six to eight glasses of water daily. Gastrointestinal symptoms may be reduced by taking NAC with meals.

Selenium

Selenium is an essential micronutrient. Selenium enters the food chain through incorporation into plant proteins; the concentration present in plant matter is a function of the selenium content of the soil. In the United States, the Eastern Coastal Plain and the Pacific Northwest have the lowest soil selenium concentrations. Selenium has antioxidant activity by virtue of its role in the formation and function of selenium-dependent glutathione peroxidases. It may also have antiinflammatory, immunomodulatory, anticarcinogenic, and detoxification actions in the body. Selenium deficiency appears to be linked to humoral immune suppression. Low immunoglobulin G (IgG) and IgM titers have been reported in association with selenium deficiency; antibody titers have been found to increase with selenium supplementation.[67] Although its role has not been fully elucidated, selenium also appears to be essential for healthy cell-mediated immunity.

In one study, selenium levels were found to be significantly reduced among people with hepatitis C. Patients with CHC who did not have cirrhosis had selenium levels 20% lower than normal, and those patients with cirrhosis had levels 40% lower than normal.[68] Once cirrhosis develops, the degree of serum selenium deficit does not reliably predict disease severity.[69] Patients with chronic hepatitis may benefit from the observed anticarcinogenic effects of selenium supplementation. A large study examining selenium levels in 7342 men with chronic hepatitis B or C and the development of hepatocellular carcinoma found selenium levels were lowest in the men with CHC. Participants with the highest selenium levels were 38% less likely to develop hepatocellular carcinoma than were participants with the lowest selenium levels.[70] Another large-scale study of more than 130,000 people in China found a similar protective effect.[71]

Dosage
The dose is 200 mcg/day in the form of high-selenium yeast or L-selenomethionine.

Precautions
At doses of less than 900 mcg/day, adverse reactions are uncommon. The most frequently reported symptoms associated with acute or chronic selenium toxicity (selenosis) include hair and nail brittleness and loss, rash, fatigue, irritability, nausea, and vomiting. High doses of selenium can decrease gastrointestinal absorption of vitamin C.[72]

S-Adenosylmethionine

S-Adenosylmethionine (SAMe) is a metabolite of the essential amino acid L-methionine. In Europe, SAMe is used medicinally for the treatment of depression, liver disorders, osteoarthritis, and fibromyalgia. It is available over the counter in the United States. SAMe is found in virtually all body tissues. It has a crucial biochemical role, by donating a methyl group in transmethylation reactions. Methylation is one of the key pathways in phase II of the hepatic detoxification system. Transmethylation is also essential in the biosynthesis of DNA, RNA, phospholipids, proteins, epinephrine, melatonin, creatine, and other essential molecules.

The hepatoprotective effects of SAMe are relatively well established. A placebo-controlled, 2-year study of patients with alcoholic cirrhosis found that 1200 mg/day significantly improved survival and delayed the need for liver transplantation.[73] A laboratory model of hepatocellular carcinoma found that SAMe had opposing hepatoprotective effects on normal hepatocytes and proapoptotic effects on hepatoma cells.[74] Clinical trials are under way to determine the possible therapeutic role of SAMe for CHC and for the prevention of hepatocellular carcinoma among patients with cirrhosis. In an open-label pilot study of 29 patients with CHC who had not responded to previous interferon-based combination therapy, coadministration of SAMe and betaine along with peginterferon alfa-2b and ribavirin improved EVR compared with combination therapy alone. SVR, however, was achieved in only 10% of patients receiving the experimental protocol.[75] Studies among patients with chronic viral hepatitis and other chronic liver conditions have found that SAMe helps alleviate symptoms such as itching, jaundice, and fatigue and reduces liver enzymes and bilirubin levels.[76,77]

Depression is a common problem in patients with CHC. SAMe has been used for more than 3 decades in Europe for the treatment of depression. A literature review concluded that the proof of concept is solid, but additional study data are needed before SAMe can be confidently recommended as first-line or adjuvant therapy for depression.[78]

SAMe is expensive and easily oxidized, thus making it an impractical supplement for many patients. In addition, small trials suggested that the oral bioavailability of SAMe may be low. Some clinicians recommend a combination of methionine, trimethylglycine, vitamin B_{12}, and folic acid to support the body's ability to synthesize endogenous SAMe. The high cost of SAMe, its relative chemical instability, and lack of conclusive data to support its use in chronic viral hepatitis preclude recommendation for regular use. In patients with alcohol-related liver disease (alone or in combination with other etiologic factors), however, SAMe supplementation may be advisable.

Dosage
For liver disease, the dose is typically 800 mg twice daily on an empty stomach. Because of its instability with oxidation, SAMe should be individually wrapped in blister packs.

Precautions
Mild gastrointestinal upset, anxiety, hyperactive muscle movement, and insomnia have been reported as side effects of SAMe use. Patients with depression and bipolar disorder should be closely monitored while taking SAMe.

Alpha-Lipoic Acid
Alpha-lipoic acid (ALA) is a fatty acid antioxidant. It is a key metabolite in mitochondrial energy production and acts as a potent free radical scavenger in both aqueous and lipophilic environments. ALA is used as a drug in many European countries, primarily to treat liver disorders and neuropathy. ALA's effect of raising cellular glutathione levels is thought to be important in CHC because patients may suffer from a relative glutathione deficiency.[79,80] ALA also helps recycle and regenerate other antioxidants, including vitamins E and C.[81] Animal models indicate that ALA may impede fibrosis progression associated with chronic hepatitis by reducing the production of reactive oxygen species.[82,83]

ALA is costly and has not been well studied in clinical trials among people with chronic viral hepatitis. Therefore, routine use is not recommended. In patients with unexplained spikes in liver enzymes, however, ALA may be advisable to reduce oxidative stress.

Dosage
ALA 500 to 600 mg/day

Precautions
No side effects have been reported at doses of up to 1000 mg/day.

Glutamine
Glutamine is a conditionally essential amino acid and is the most abundant amino acid in the body. Although the body normally synthesizes adequate amounts of glutamine, endogenous production may be inadequate during periods of metabolic stress. Glutamine is crucial to many metabolic functions, including protein and glutathione synthesis, energy production, acid-base balance, maintenance of optimal antioxidant status, intestinal integrity, immune function, gluconeogenesis, nitrogen transport, and neurotransmitter, nucleotide, and nucleic acid synthesis. Glutamine has been shown to regulate the expression of several genes and to activate several proteins.[84] l-Glutamine is an immunonutrient and is the preferred substrate for energy production in enterocytes and lymphocytes. One study noted that glutamine influences the production of some T-cell–derived cytokines and is thereby important for optimal lymphocyte proliferation.[85] Notably, lymphocytes are unable to produce glutamine. Glutamine deficiency can result in inadequate production of glutathione. If glutamine stores are depleted by ongoing immune system demands, glutathione production will be inadequate. With its many functions, glutamine is an important nutritional supplement when any question exists that metabolic stress may render endogenous synthesis inadequate.

Dosage
Glutamine 2 to 4 g/day during periods of metabolic stress or poor dietary intake. The supplement should be taken between meals.

Precautions
Glutamine supplementation should be approached with caution in patients with hepatic or renal insufficiency.[86]

Zinc
Zinc is an essential nutritional element. It has many important biochemical roles in the body, including acting as an essential cofactor in healthy immunologic function and supporting antioxidant systems. A small, randomized trial of polar zinc supplementation among patients with CHC who were undergoing therapy with peginterferon alfa-2b plus ribavirin found significantly lower ALT levels at 12 weeks among the intervention group.[87] The investigators postulated that the observed effect possibly resulted from enhanced antioxidant activity fueled by the supplemental zinc. Although zinc deficiency is relatively uncommon in developed countries, it may come into play in patients with poor nutritional intake. Routine zinc supplementation is unnecessary for many patients with CHC but should be considered in patients who may be nutritionally deprived because of disease-related symptoms.

Dosage
Zinc 15 mg/day. The recommended UL for zinc is 40 mg/day.

Precautions
Long-term ingestion of high doses of zinc may deplete copper stores, interfere with iron function, and lead to microcytic anemia. Ingestion of large amounts of zinc (more than 30 mg/day) may cause acute toxicity with nausea, vomiting, diarrhea, anorexia, abdominal cramps, a metallic taste, headache, and drowsiness.

Iron
Patients should avoid iron overload. Increased hepatic iron stores (primarily associated with common heterozygous hemochromatosis mutations) are associated with higher grades of inflammation and more severe hepatic fibrosis in patients with CHC, compared with patients without iron overload.[88,89] Patients with reduced iron levels who were treated with interferon had an improved response, as measured by reduction in serum ALT.[90] Iron supplements should be avoided among patients with CHC except in cases of documented deficiency. Iron-binding supplements may be beneficial in patients with increased serum iron.

Botanicals

Milk Thistle (Silybum marianum)
The use of milk thistle for liver disease dates back to the Roman Empire, when this plant was mixed with honey and used for "carrying off bile." Much remains undiscovered

about milk thistle (silymarin), but research has uncovered several mechanisms by which milk thistle may benefit patients with chronic liver disease.

In laboratory models, silymarin has been shown to protect hepatocytes from toxins by stabilizing the cell membrane against free radical attack.[91] A clinical example of this therapeutic use of silymarin is its use in death cap mushroom (*Amanita phalloides*) poisoning. The amatoxins in the mushrooms are taken up by hepatocytes and interfere with messenger RNA and protein synthesis, typically leading to acute fulminant hepatitis. Pooled data from case record studies involving 452 patients with *A. phalloides* poisoning show a highly significant difference in mortality in favor of silybin (the primary isomer contained in silymarin).[92] Investigators believe that silibin binds to the hepatocyte cell membrane and thus prevents toxin penetration. Milk thistle has been found to protect against other toxins, including pesticides, drugs, and halogenated cyclic hydrocarbons.[93]

Silymarin is a potent antioxidant. It was reported to raise liver and intestine glutathione levels by 50% in animal studies[94] and to increase the levels of the antioxidant enzymes superoxide dismutase, glutathione peroxidase, and catalase in a separate animal model.[95] Silymarin also has antifibrotic properties. Among silymarin in the Hepatitis C Antiviral Long-Term Treatment against Cirrhosis (HALT-C) trial, researchers found reduced fibrosis progression but no significant difference in clinical outcome, compared with nonusers.[96] A randomized double-blind 12-month trial of 177 patients with CHC, however, found that although patients taking silymarin supplementation reported improved symptoms and general well-being, no effect was noted on HCV viremia, serum ALT, or serum and ultrasound markers for hepatic fibrosis.[97] Combination treatments with milk thistle as a principal component are being evaluated. In a small study of patients with CHC who were treated with a 3-month course of a concoction of silibin phospholipids and vitamin E, researchers found a significant reduction in aminotransferase levels.[98] Other clinical studies of the effects of silymarin on chronic liver disease have yielded mixed results.[99–101] A 2005 Cochrane Review of 13 randomized trials examining milk thistle concluded that "our results question the beneficial effect of milk thistle for patients with alcoholic and/or hepatitis B or C virus liver diseases and highlight the lack of high-quality evidence to support this intervention."[102]

In summary, research data indicate that many actions of silymarin may theoretically be beneficial to patients with chronic hepatitis. The clinical data to support this supposition, however, are lacking with regard to chronic viral hepatitis. Given that milk thistle has no known serious adverse effects, many clinicians believe that the potential for benefit justifies the recommendation to use this herbal supplement, despite the lack of robust clinical evidence to support this recommendation.

■ Dosage

Milk thistle 300 mg three times a day or 210 mg of silymarin three times daily. The standard dose of milk thistle is based on the silymarin content, which is 70% of the bulk herb (300 mg of milk thistle = 210 mg of silymarin). Silymarin-phosphatidylcholine is absorbed more effectively than regular standardized milk thistle and requires less frequent dosing (240 mg twice daily for active treatment). Alcohol extracts should be avoided in patients with hepatitis.

■ Precautions

Side effects of milk thistle are rare. Reported adverse reactions include stomach pain, nausea, vomiting, diarrhea, headache, rash or other skin reactions, and joint pain. Allergic reactions may occur in patients with hypersensitivity to ragweed or plants in the daisy family.

The potential for interaction between silymarin and peginterferon plus ribavirin has not been thoroughly studied in clinical trials. Some clinicians advise patients to stop taking milk thistle while they are treated with interferon-based therapy to eliminate the possibility of unknown herb-drug interactions.

Licorice Root (Glycyrrhiza glabra)

The licorice plant has been used medicinally since the Scythians introduced it to the ancient Greeks; it has been used in Europe since the Middle Ages. Licorice root preparations have been an accepted treatment for hepatitis in Japan since the 1960s. Glycyrrhizin (an aqueous extract of licorice root) acts primarily as an antiinflammatory and cytoprotective agent; it does not have antiviral properties.[103] Most clinical studies showing benefit have used a form of intravenous glycyrrhizin called Stronger Neo-Minophagen C (SNMC: 0.2% glycyrrhizin, 0.1% cysteine, and 2% glycine). In a multicenter double-blind trial conducted in Japan, investigators found that long-term daily treatment with SNMC among patients with viral hepatitis led to a significantly reduced incidence of cirrhosis and hepatocellular carcinoma.[104] A review article published in 2005 noted that SNMC "improves mortality in patients with subacute liver failure, and improves liver functions in patients with subacute hepatic failure, chronic hepatitis, and cirrhosis with activity. SNMC does not reduce mortality among patients with cirrhosis with activity."[103] A Cochrane Review of medicinal herbs for HCV infection concluded that glycyrrhizin did not demonstrate significant beneficial effects.[105]

The clinician is faced with a decision whether to recommend licorice root for patients with chronic hepatitis. Although promising animal model data and years of experience support its use, clinical data showing efficacy are scant. An open discussion with each patient is advised wherein the clinician presents the information available and helps the patient make an individualized treatment decision.

■ Dosage

Oral forms of licorice root are available over the counter in the United States. The recommended dosage depends on the form taken: 250 to 500 mg three times a day of the solid dry powder; 1 to 2 g three times a day of the powdered root; or 2 to 4 mL three times a day of the fluid extract.

■ Precautions

High doses of glycyrrhizin can lead to an aldosterone effect with potassium loss, water retention, and hypertension. Use can potentiate the effects of diuretics, certain cardiac medications (e.g., digitalis), and corticosteroids. Glycyrrhizin should be used with caution in people with hypertension, ascites, renal insufficiency, or cardiac insufficiency. A diet high in potassium-rich foods is recommended for patients taking a licorice root preparation. Blood pressure and potassium levels should be monitored regularly.

Schisandra (Schisandra chinensis)

Schisandra has been used in China for more than 1000 years to treat liver disorders and other maladies. The medicinal substances are derived from the fruit of the plant and include schisandrine A, B, and C and several gomisins. Schisandra is a potent free radical scavenger, a characteristic that may explain the hepatoprotective effects observed with this botanical. Gomisin A, an active ingredient in schisandra, has been found to promote hepatocyte growth factor, limit lipid peroxidation, and inhibit apoptosis in acute hepatic injury animal models.[106,107] Gomisin A also acts as an anti-inflammatory by preventing the release of arachidonic acid in macrophages in vitro.[108] Laboratory evidence suggests that gomisin A may have anticarcinogenic effects.[109,110] Published clinical trial data examining the use of schisandra in patients with chronic hepatitis are lacking.

■ Dosage

Schisandra extract 100 mg twice daily.

■ Precautions

Schisandra lignans have been reported to induce phase I drug metabolism[111] and competitively inhibit the methylation pathway of phase II detoxification in animal models.[112] Caution should be used if medications metabolized by the cytochrome P-450 system are given with schisandra. Side effects are uncommon and include dyspepsia, anorexia, and urticaria.

Astragalus (Astragalus membranaceus)

Astragalus is an important herb used in Chinese medicine for its effects on the immune system. In vitro studies found that astragalus promotes B-cell proliferation and antibody production and enhances CTL activity.[113] It also acts as a potent antioxidant by increasing superoxide dismutase and decreasing lipid peroxide activity. Astragalus was reported to have protective effects against toxins in animal models.[114] Astragalus injection solution has an inhibitory effect on experimental hepatic fibrogenesis, possibly because of its antioxidant properties.[115] A small trial among patients with chronic hepatitis B found that astragalus supplementation was associated with decreased serum fibrosis markers and liver enzymes.[116] A meta-analysis that included clinical trials from the English and Chinese literature concluded that astragalus and certain other traditional Chinese botanicals may have activity against hepatocellular carcinoma.[117] Whether these agents may have a chemoprotective role for patients with chronic viral hepatitis who are at risk for hepatocellular carcinoma remains a matter of conjecture.

■ Dosage

Astragalus powder 4 to 7 g daily (most commonly used in combination with other herbs)

■ Precautions

Doses greater than 28 g/day may cause immune suppression. Because of its immunostimulatory effects, astragalus should be avoided in patients receiving immunosuppressive therapy and in those with autoimmune disease. Astragalus may contain selenium; ingestion of large amounts over time may lead to selenosis. Astragalus may potentiate the effects of antithrombotic and anticoagulant medications. Side effects of this herb are uncommon.

Herbal Concoctions and Traditional Chinese Medicine

China has a high prevalence of chronic viral hepatitis. Traditional Chinese medicine (TCM) has long described healing remedies for chronic liver maladies. Since the cultural revolution of the 1950s, an integrative form of medicine has been used in China that combines the tenets of both TCM and modern pathophysiology and phytopharmacology.

Chinese medicine relies on individualized constitutional diagnosis and treatment in parallel with biochemical, histologic, and radiologic diagnostic methods. Because constitutional diagnostic methods are used in formulating a treatment plan, individualized herbal concoctions containing several botanicals, each prescribed to address a specific imbalance, are commonly used. Herbal concoctions for chronic hepatitis are likely to include varying doses and combinations of the botanicals discussed earlier in addition to others. Herbal concoction prescriptions are altered according to a patient's changing signs and symptoms. A referral to a qualified TCM practitioner with experience in treating chronic hepatitis may be beneficial for patients who opt to forego interferon-based therapy.

Mind-Body Therapies

Research is beginning to catch up with clinical experience regarding the negative effects of psychosocial stress on health, including liver health. Elucidating the exact mechanisms by which the mind and body interact in the spectrum of health and disease is an arena of active research and an area of healing that has only recently been appreciated from a pathophysiologic perspective.

Two classes of compounds studied in relation to stress and disease are glucocorticoids and catecholamines. Stress activates the hypothalamic-pituitary-adrenal axis and leads to increased glucocorticoid secretion. The sympathetic nervous system is similarly activated by stress, which increases levels of catecholamines.[118] Both groups of substances cause specific cytokine responses that influence the inflammatory response.

A small study in Japan found an association between chronic psychosocial stress related to type 1 personality and increasing hepatitis C severity.[119] Stress has been shown to induce interleukin-6 and tumor necrosis factor-alpha within the liver, thus augmenting the hepatic inflammatory response.[120] Evidence suggests that repetitive stress may aggravate chronic inflammatory diseases to a greater extent than acute stressors.[121] Thus, mind-body therapies that alleviate psychosocial stress may enhance the liver-specific and overall health of people living with chronic hepatitis.

Therapeutic modalities that enhance balance and increase a patient's sense of control, meaning, and purpose may decrease the degree to which psychosocial stress contributes to a patient's disease process. Having a chronic illness is a stressor in and of itself. Whatever we can do to help patients minimize or alleviate this and other stressors in their lives is healing in the broadest and truest sense (see Chapter 93, Relaxation Techniques).

Examples of modalities that may help alleviate stress and enhance peacefulness include meditation, prayer, journaling, counseling, support groups, behavioral therapy, hypnosis, and visualization, as well as art, music, and dance therapy. Relaxation techniques such as deep breathing, biofeedback, and others may also merit discussion. People find respite from the stressors in their lives in many different ways. Practitioners should be mindful of this and tailor recommendations accordingly. Offer suggestions that suit your patient's personality, culture, and belief system. For example, the thought of sitting still for 30 minutes of daily meditation may induce rather than alleviate the anxiety of a goal-oriented type A individual. People with a driving nature may be better suited to more active modalities such as walking or jogging, tai chi, or yoga.

Lifestyle Interventions

Measures to Reduce Toxin Exposure

Exposure to exogenous toxins increases hepatic workload and oxidative stress. When the liver is already in a state of chronic inflammation, this additional burden may exacerbate ongoing injury and accelerate disease progression.

■ Reduce Toxins in the Diet

Oral intake of toxic xenobiotics can be minimized by avoiding prepackaged, ready-to-eat foods, processed meats, and canned foods. Fresh fruit and vegetables are best in terms of nutritional value and minimizing intake of unwanted chemicals. Encourage organically grown foods, but keep in mind that such products may not be affordable for some patients. Washing fresh fruit and vegetables with a brush under running water helps remove pesticides. Filtered water can also reduce the amount of hepatotoxins ingested.

■ Avoid Alcohol

Alcohol abstinence is one of the most important recommendations a clinician can make for patients with chronic hepatitis. Alcohol intake in patients with HCV has been associated with accelerated fibrosis, increased risk of cirrhosis, and reduced response to interferon-based therapy.[122] No "safe" threshold for alcohol intake has been established for people with chronic hepatitis.[6] Patients with an active dependence on alcohol are ineligible for interferon-based therapy; a 6-month period of abstinence is recommended by most clinicians. Clinicians must be prepared to offer patients who have an alcohol problem information about local services available to provide these patients with psychosocial support in becoming alcohol free. Family members may also need to engage in the process. Alcohol in over-the-counter products (e.g., mouthwash, cold preparations, and tinctures) is also to be avoided (see Chapter 81, Alcoholism and Substance Abuse).

■ Avoid Tobacco Products

All tobacco products (chewing tobacco, cigars, pipes, and cigarettes) introduce a wide array of toxins into the body and should be avoided. Smoking reduces glutathione levels through the burden of detoxifying nicotine and neutralizing the free radicals produced by the toxins in tobacco. Smoking increases the risk of hepatocellular carcinoma,[123,124] and it reduces response rates to interferon-based therapy.[125]

■ Avoid Unnecessary Drugs and Supplements

Pharmaceuticals, botanicals, and supplements that are metabolized by the liver can dramatically increase the xenobiotic burden on the liver. Additionally, some of these products

TABLE 19-6. Common Pharmaceuticals and Botanicals With Hepatotoxic Potential

TYPE	SPECIFIC AGENTS
Pharmaceuticals	Acetaminophen Alpha-methyldopa (Aldomet) Amiodarone (Cordarone) Carbamazepine (Tegretol) Diclofenac (Voltaren, Cataflam) Fluconazole or ketoconazole (Diflucan, Nizoral) Hydralazine (Apresoline, Novo-Hylazin) Ibuprofen (Advil, Motrin, Nuprin) Nitrofurantoin (Macrodantin) Phenytoin (Dilantin) Sulfa medications (especially Septra or Bactrim) Amoxicillin (Amoxil) Chlorpromazine (Thorazine) Ciprofloxacin (Cipro) Duloxetine (Cymbalta) Statins/HMG-CoA reductase inhibitors (Caduet, Crestor, Lescol, Lipitor, Mevacor, Pravachol, Simcor, Vytorin, Zocor)
Botanicals	Barberry (Berberis vulgaris) Comfrey (Symphytum officinale): should never be taken internally Golden ragwort (Senecio aureus) Groundsel (Senecio vulgaris) Huang qin (Scutellaria baicalensis) Kava kava (Piper methysticum) Pennyroyal (Mentha piperita officinalis) Sassafras (Sassafras albidum) Senna (Cassia senna) Valerian (Valeriana officinalis) Wall germander (Teucrium chamaedrys) Wood sage (Teucrium scorodonia) Ma-huang (Ephedra equisetina) Jin bu huan (Lycopodium serratum)

have hepatotoxic potential (Table 19-6). All products with hepatotoxic potential should be avoided or prescribed with caution and closely supervised.

Street drugs increase the toxic burden on the liver. Recreational drug use is an important topic to discuss with all patients with chronic hepatitis. Many patients with CHC believe that smoking marijuana is a good way to alleviate symptoms associated with the disease and side effects of interferon-based therapy. In reality, cannabis use dramatically increases the toxin burden on the liver and has been reported to significantly accelerate hepatic fibrosis progression.[126] Additionally, cannabis use may contribute to steatosis, which is independently associated with CHC progression.[127] Patients may be hesitant to mention their marijuana use. Asking about marijuana use in the same manner that you inquire about other lifestyle issues opens the door to a candid discussion.

■ Avoid Environmental and Occupational Exposure to Toxins

Pesticides, herbicides, and other toxic chemicals can damage hepatocytes and elevate liver enzyme levels.[128–130] Protective gear approved by the Occupational Safety and Health Administration is necessary for people whose work exposes them to chemicals, solvents, fumes, pesticides, or herbicides. Home exposure to paint and lacquer, glues, epoxy, and other toxins should be minimized.

Exercise

Exercise enhances portal blood flow, decreases fatigue,[131] and improves overall well-being. Further, exercise may alleviate depression,[132] a common finding in patients with chronic liver disease, especially CHC. Finally, moderate exercise has been shown to improve the immune response.[133,134] Encourage a realistic exercise program that takes into account the patient's current activity level and interests and progresses gradually. Patients who are sedentary and avoidant of "exercise" may respond well to a broadened view: anything that gets one up and moving constitutes exercise.

Nutrition

The adage, "you are what you eat," describes a literal truth. The liver is integral to metabolic homeostasis and is the master processor of all nutritional intake. One's diet can make these jobs easier or more difficult. In general, a diet rich in a wide variety of fresh fruit and vegetables supplies the liver with needed nutrients to support its synthetic and detoxification functions. Adequate high-quality protein intake is needed to support the liver's synthetic functions and the immune system. Low dietary fat helps prevent or counter hepatic steatosis, a condition that accelerates disease progression. Avoiding excessive carbohydrate intake helps stabilize glucose metabolism, which is often disturbed in patients with chronic liver disease secondary to insulin resistance.

■ Encourage Healthy Body Weight

Hepatic steatosis has been reported to increase the rate of hepatic fibrosis in patients with CHC.[135,136] Although patients with genotype 3 disease are more prone to steatosis than are patients with other HCV genotypes, an elevated body mass index is an independent predictor of nonalcoholic steatosis.[137] Further, patients with CHC and significant steatosis have lower response rates to interferon-based therapy, compared with patients without steatosis.[138,139] Overweight and obese patients should be encouraged to engage in a sensible, sustainable weight reduction program that combines moderately reduced caloric intake with increased caloric burn through heightened activity. Fasting and fad diets, especially those that restrict protein or encourage high fat intake, should be discouraged.

> Steatohepatitis is more common with genotype 3 disease and is associated with a lower response rate to interferon-based therapy. Management of metabolic syndrome, high triglycerides, and obesity should be a priority.

■ Encourage Regular Consumption of Cruciferous Vegetables

Cruciferous vegetables are members of the cabbage family of plants and include cabbage, broccoli, cauliflower, Brussels sprouts, kale, mustard greens, collard greens, kohlrabi, rutabaga, turnips, bok choy, arugula, horseradish, radish, wasabi, and watercress. These vegetables are good sources of vitamin C, selenium, folate, carotenoids, lignans, and flavonoids.

Prolonged, high heat can destroy some of the phytochemicals in vegetables. Encourage patients to cook vegetables lightly or eat them raw, when possible and appetizing.

Cruciferous vegetables contain high concentrations of indole-3-carbinol, which can increase the activity of certain phase I and II detoxification enzymes.[140,141] This increase in the activity of biotransformation enzymes is the likely mechanism behind the anticarcinogenic effects associated with consumption of cruciferous vegetables.

■ Encourage Regular Consumption of Fruit

Fruit is a rich source of vitamins C, E, and K, folate, selenium, magnesium, potassium, carotenoids, flavonoids, lignans, terpenoids, and fiber. Eating adequate amounts of a wide variety of fruit helps ensure that the liver has an optimal supply of the substrates needed for detoxification and biosynthesis. Berries, such as cranberries, blueberries, blackberries, and raspberries, contain high concentrations of antioxidants. Peaches, mangoes, and melons are also rich in antioxidants. Citrus fruit (e.g., oranges, tangerines, lemons, and limes) contains high concentrations of the phytochemical D-limonene, a strong inducer of phase I and II of the detoxification system.[142]

■ Avoid Foods That Inhibit the Detoxification System

Foodstuffs that inhibit the detoxification system warrant special mention. Grapefruit contains naringenin, which inhibits the cytochrome P-450 3A4 enzyme of the phase I detoxification system.[143] Capsaicin (the compound responsible for the spiciness of hot peppers), eugenol from clove oil, and quercetin from onions also slow phase I detoxification. Patients with chronic liver disease are best advised to limit their intake of these foodstuffs.

■ Encourage Adequate Protein Intake

Adequate protein intake is essential for healthy immune function and detoxification. Liver disease and chronic inflammation increase the body's need for protein, especially in the presence of cirrhosis. Furthermore, phase II of the detoxification system is especially vulnerable to inadequate protein intake.

Complete proteins contain all the essential amino acids. Healthful sources of complete proteins include eggs, lentils, nuts, lean meats, fish, poultry, and soy. Recommended daily protein intake (in grams) is calculated by multiplying body weight (in pounds) by a factor 0.5 to 0.7.

■ Encourage Healthful Dietary Fat Intake

Fats are easily misunderstood because of confusing terminology. When counseling patients about healthful dietary fat intake, focus on two major points:

1. Limit dietary fat to no more than 30% of caloric intake; 20% is better, and 10% may be best for someone on a weight reduction program.
2. Limit intake of omega-6 polyunsaturated fats and trans fats.

Research has shown that high-fat diets, especially in combination with reduced protein and carbohydrates, increase the risk of steatosis and progression to cirrhosis among patients with chronic hepatitis.[144,145] Hence, patients with chronic hepatitis should be encouraged to limit their overall fat intake.

Advising patients about what fats to eat is somewhat more complicated. Most primary care clinicians are accustomed to promoting the intake of unsaturated fats instead of saturated fats for cardiovascular health. However, patients with chronic liver disease have additional pathophysiologic concerns to be addressed. Unsaturated fats are more volatile (polyunsaturated fats more so than monounsaturated fats) and prone to oxidation than are saturated fats. The oxidative stress in the liver is already high in patients with chronic hepatitis; the additional stress of large quantities of unsaturated fats may exacerbate hepatocyte injury. Particularly important is a reduction in the intake of polyunsaturated omega-6 fatty acids (e.g., safflower oil, sunflower oil, corn oil). Encourage use of predominantly monounsaturated fats such as olive, canola, and peanut oils for cooking. Omega-3 fatty acids should also be encouraged to help reduce inflammation because these oils are known to reduce tumor necrosis factor, a proinflammatory cytokine.[146] Finally, all patients should be advised to avoid trans fats (anything that lists hydrogenated or partially hydrogenated fat on the food label) (see Chapter 86, The Antiinflammatory Diet).

◼ Encourage Dietary Fiber

Dietary fiber helps bind toxins in the gut, thus resulting in excretion through the bowel without hepatic processing. To promote fiber intake, encourage a diet rich in fruit, vegetables, and whole grains. Consider supplementing with a soluble fiber such as methylcellulose or psyllium.

◼ Consume Green Tea

Catechin polyphenols in green tea have antioxidant, antiangiogenesis, and antiproliferative properties that may help reduce inflammation in patients with chronic hepatitis and may potentially slow disease progression and attenuate the risk for hepatocellular carcinoma.[147,148] A study of 124 patients with viral hepatitis who were treated with 3 g of catechins versus placebo resulted in significantly lower AST, ALT, and serum bilirubin levels. Compared with other types of viral hepatitis, people with non-A non-B (presumed HCV) hepatitis showed the greatest response.[149]

◼ Dosage

Prescribe 2 or 3 cups of green tea daily.

◼ Precaution

Many patients think if a little is good, more must be better, but, of course, that is not always the case. Be aware that cases of fulminant hepatitis have been reported after consumption of highly concentrated dry extracts of green tea.[150,151] Caution patients against the use of green tea extracts.

Therapies to Consider

The association of hepatitis B virus (HBV) and HCV with hepatocellular carcinoma has been firmly established. In January 2005, HBV and HCV were added to the list of known human carcinogens in the U.S. Department of Health and Human Services *Report on Carcinogens,* 11th edition.[152] Although the link is clear, the carcinogenic transformation process is poorly understood. Nucleic acid damage by reactive nitrogen and oxygen species is believed to contribute to inflammation-related carcinogenesis in patients with chronic hepatitis.[153] Hepatocyte regeneration in the milieu of chronic inflammation may predispose to such nucleic acid damage. Evidence indicates that virus-specific mechanisms also contribute to hepatocyte carcinogenic transformation.[154,155] Based on the knowledge that the risk of developing hepatocellular carcinoma increases in parallel with the degree of hepatic fibrosis, agents with antifibrotic properties may be useful in delaying progression to cirrhosis and its concomitant risk for hepatocellular carcinoma.

Colchicine

Colchicine, an alkaloid isolated from the autumn crocus, was reported to resolve cirrhotic nodules and extracellular fibers in an animal model.[156] A small study of patients with cirrhosis and ascites reported that survival was three times greater in those taking colchicine versus placebo over 11 years.[157] However, a large, multicenter clinical trial comparing low-dose peginterferon with colchicine as maintenance therapy for patients with CHC and advanced fibrosis or cirrhosis found no significant difference between the treatment groups.[158] Study participants were virologic nonresponders to previous therapy with interferon plus ribavirin. Notably, 49% of the enrolled patients did not complete the 4-year trial. Because colchicine is not standard therapy, clinicians should consult with a gastroenterologist before this treatment is initiated.

◼ Dosage

Colchicine 0.6 mg twice daily

PREVENTION PRESCRIPTION

Hepatitis B Primary Prevention
- ◼ Administer the hepatitis B vaccine.
- ◼ Use universal body fluid precautions.

Hepatitis C Primary Prevention
- ◼ Injection drug users: do not share needles or other drug paraphernalia.
- ◼ Do not share personal care items that may be contaminated with blood, including toothbrushes, razors, and manicure and pedicure equipment.
- ◼ Do not get a tattoo with an unsterilized stylus; be certain that new ink and new or sterilized ink pots are used.
- ◼ If you have multiple sexual partners, avoid contact with blood during sexual activity, and use latex condoms correctly and consistently at every sexual encounter.
- ◼ Use universal body fluid precautions.

Hepatitis C Secondary Prevention
- ◼ Abstain from alcohol.
- ◼ Abstain from tobacco products, street drugs, and unnecessary medications and supplements.
- ◼ Avoid environmental toxins, including pesticides, herbicides, and other toxic chemicals.
- ◼ Achieve and maintain a healthy body weight.
- ◼ Exercise regularly.
- ◼ Establish and maintain ongoing health care to include monitoring for disease progression and screening for the development of hepatocellular carcinoma.

THERAPEUTIC REVIEW

Screening

Because people with chronic hepatitis C (CHC) are likely to be asymptomatic and may not have consistently elevated liver enzymes, all patients should be routinely screened for hepatitis C risk factors.[10] The following list of questions can help elucidate a patient's relative risk for hepatitis C:

- Did you receive any blood or blood products (e.g., packed cells, whole blood, plasma, platelets, clotting factors, gammaglobulin) before 1992?

- Have you ever undergone kidney dialysis?

- Have you had an organ transplant (especially before 1992)?

- Have you ever, even once, injected street drugs?

- Have you ever, even once, shared drug paraphernalia (e.g., needles, cookers, straws)?

- Have you ever been accidentally stuck with a used medical needle?

- Do you have human immunodeficiency virus (HIV)?

- Have you ever held a job (e.g., police officer, fire fighter, emergency medical technician, paramedic, medical or dental worker) or participated in a sport (e.g., hockey, rugby, boxing, football, and other contact sports) that exposed you to blood?

- Did your mother have hepatitis C when you were born?

- Have you ever been incarcerated?

- Have you been in military combat?

- Are you living with or have you ever lived with someone known to have hepatitis C?

- Have you ever shared personal care items that may have been contaminated with blood (e.g., razors, toothbrushes, manicure or pedicure equipment) with others?

- Have you ever had a piercing or tattoo in a noncommercial facility?

- Have you ever had unprotected sex with someone known to have hepatitis C?

- Have you ever had unprotected sex with someone who is or was an injection drug user?

Sexual transmission of hepatitis C is uncommon, especially among people in a long-term, monogamous relationship.[117] However, patients with a history of sexually transmitted infections and multiple, short-term sexual relationships are at increased risk.[159] Sexual behavior that involves contact with blood is the source of potential hepatitis C virus (HCV) exposure (e.g., anal intercourse, fisting, and other practices that can cause bleeding).

Laboratory Testing

Patients with one or more risk factors and those patients who specifically request testing should be screened for hepatitis C by using an enzyme immunoassay for HCV antibodies.[10] A positive serologic test result indicates exposure to the virus but not necessarily active infection. Approximately 25% to 35% of adults infected with HCV spontaneously clear the virus. The remaining 65% to 75% become chronically infected. Patients with a positive antibody screen should be tested for HCV RNA to determine whether they are currently infected. HCV genotype testing is recommended for any patient considering interferon-based therapy because genotype affects the planned duration of treatment and the probability of successful viral clearance.[161]

Although liver biopsy was once considered a standard component of the initial evaluation of patients with CHC, the American Association for the Study of Liver Diseases now recommends that physicians consider obtaining a liver biopsy only if the patient or provider believes that the information will contribute to therapeutic decision making or will provide desired prognostic information.[10] For patients who prefer not to undergo a liver biopsy or who have a contraindication to the procedure, panels of serum markers for fibrosis (e.g., Fibrotest, Fibrosure) may help evaluate the fibrotic state of the liver. These tests are reasonably accurate at differentiating the extremes of the fibrotic spectrum (i.e., little to no fibrosis versus cirrhosis). However, current accuracy of these tests to determine the degree of fibrosis between the extremes of the spectrum is limited.

The following therapeutic review addresses management after a diagnosis of CHC has been made and liver histologic features have been evaluated, directly or indirectly.

Patients With Newly Diagnosed CHC Who Have No Physical, Laboratory, or Histologic Evidence of Advanced Fibrosis or Cirrhosis and Who Are Not Undergoing Interferon-Based Therapy

- Laboratory

  - Obtain baseline markers of liver status (aspartate aminotransferase [AST], alanine aminotransferase [ALT], albumin, bilirubin, and platelet count) and alfa-fetoprotein level.

  - Consider HCV genotype testing to aid in management decisions.

  - Monitor the AST/ALT ratio at least biannually.

- Radiology

  - Obtain a baseline ultrasound study of the liver.

- Lifestyle

  - Reduce toxin exposure (e.g., tobacco, environmental toxins).

  - Urge abstention from alcohol and illicit drug use.

Continued

- Reduce dietary toxins; encourage organic foodstuffs if feasible.
- Encourage achieving and maintaining a healthy body weight.
- Promote regular exercise.
- Counsel patients about how to reduce the risk of spread of chronic viral hepatitis to others.
- Refer for alcohol or drug dependence counseling and treatment as needed.
- Nutrition
  - Fruits and vegetables
    - Increase intake of fruits and vegetables (especially cruciferous vegetables) to six or seven servings daily.
    - Limit grapefruit and other inhibitors of the detoxification system.
  - Dietary fats
    - Limit fat intake (no more than 30%; aim for 10% to 20%).
    - Eliminate trans fats (hydrogenated and partially hydrogenated oils).
    - Use olive, canola, or peanut oil in cooking.
    - Increase intake of omega-3 fatty acids (cold-water fish, nuts, flaxseed).
    - Decrease intake of omega-6 fatty acids (vegetable oils).
  - Dietary fiber
    - Increase fiber intake.
    - Consider supplementation with methylcellulose or psyllium if dietary fiber intake is inadequate.
  - Dietary protein
    - Ensure adequate protein intake (recommended grams of intake = pounds of body weight × 0.5 to 0.7)
- Pharmaceuticals
  - Vaccinate patients without immunity to hepatitis A and B.
- Mind-Body Therapy
  - Encourage lifestyle choices that reduce psychosocial stress.
  - Explore relaxation and meditative techniques tailored to the patient's personality, belief system, and culture to help reduce stress.
- Supplements
  - Selenium: 200 mcg daily
  - Iron-free multivitamin with minerals: daily

- B-complex vitamin: daily
- Vitamin C: 200 to 250 mg twice daily
- Vitamin E (d-alpha tocopherol): 400 units daily
- Precautions: Avoid iron supplementation and excess vitamin A.
- Botanicals to Consider
  - Silymarin phosphatidylcholine: 240 mg twice daily
  - Licorice root: 200 to 500 mg dry powder three times daily or 1 to 2 g powdered root three times daily or 2 to 4 mL of fluid extract three times daily
  - Schisandra: 100 mg of extract twice daily
  - Astragalus: 4 to 7 g of powder daily
- Monitoring
  - See the patient at least twice yearly to monitor for signs of progression or extrahepatic manifestations of disease.
  - Monitor the AST/ALT ratio; a ratio greater than 1 indicates probable disease progression to advanced fibrosis or cirrhosis.[120] Refer for a gastroenterology or hepatology consultation.
  - Consider repeat liver biopsy every 4 to 5 years.
- Consultations
  - An infectious disease consultation and comanagement are highly recommended for patients coinfected with HCV and HIV.
  - A gastroenterology or hepatology consultation is recommended for patients coinfected with HCV and HBV and for patients with HCV and other comorbid hepatic conditions.

■ Patients With Newly Diagnosed CHC Who Have Physical, Laboratory, or Histologic Evidence of Advanced Fibrosis or Cirrhosis

Recommendations are the same as previously described, with the following additions:

- Laboratory
  - Order HCV genotype testing to aid in treatment planning.
  - Order baseline HCV viral load to aid in treatment planning.
- Lifestyle
  - Same as previously described
- Nutrition
  - A nutrition consultation is recommended for patients with cirrhosis.
- Mind-Body Therapy
  - Same as previously described

TABLE 19-7. Contraindications to Pegylated Interferon plus Ribavirin Therapy

TYPE OF ABNORMALITY	SPECIFIC CRITERIA
Hematologic abnormalities	Anemia (hemoglobin less than 12 g/dL in female patients and less than 13 g/dL in male patients), especially patients with hemoglobinopathies Leukopenia (less than $1500 \times 10^3/\mu L$) Thrombocytopenia (less than $100 \times 10^3/\mu L$)
Neuropsychiatric conditions	Unstable depression or other major psychiatric disorder Active alcohol dependence Illicit drug use that interferes with the patient's ability to commit to regular treatment
Comorbidities	Unstable cardiac arrhythmia or cardiovascular disease Uncontrolled cerebrovascular disease or seizure disorder Uncontrolled diabetes mellitus Diabetic retinopathy Renal failure Active autoimmune disease
Hypersensitivity	Hypersensitivity to interferon or ribavirin
Other	Pregnancy or lactation Decompensated cirrhosis Unwillingness or inability to practice reliable contraception

- Pharmaceuticals
  - Recommend peginterferon alfa plus ribavirin treatment for patients without contraindications to this therapy (Table 19-7).
  - For patients with relative contraindications, prepare and execute a management plan to resolve the contraindications.

Monitoring Patients Receiving Peginterferon plus Ribavirin

- Office visits
  - Monitor patients who are receiving therapy at least every 4 weeks for treatment side effects, including depression.
  - Treat side effects aggressively to improve compliance, minimize discomfort, and avoid dose reductions. Encourage patients to call between visits if problems arise.
- Laboratory testing
  - Monitor hemoglobin levels monthly for evidence of hemolytic anemia secondary to ribavirin.
  - Consider determining the HCV viral load at week 4 of treatment to determine whether the

patient has had a rapid virologic response (RVR). This information may help determine the minimum duration of therapy if the patient has difficulty tolerating the planned course of treatment.

- Obtain an HCV viral load measurement at week 12 of treatment to determine whether an early virologic response (EVR) has occurred. In patients without at least a 100-fold drop in HCV viral load (compared with baseline), discontinue therapy. For genotype 1 disease with EVR, continue therapy for a total of 48 weeks. For genotype 2 or 3 disease with EVR, continue therapy for a total of 24 weeks.
- Check the HCV viral load at the completion of a full course of therapy to determine end-of-treatment response. Patients with detectable HCV RNA at the end of treatment are deemed nonresponders. Those without detectable HCV RNA at the end of treatment are viral responders.
- End-of-treatment responders should have an HCV RNA test every 6 months for the first year and yearly thereafter for 5 years to detect possible relapse.

- Botanicals
  - Because the potential interactions among peginterferon, ribavirin, and botanicals have not been evaluated, consider discontinuing all herbal supplements during interferon-based therapy or monitor the patient closely for new or unexpected symptoms or reactions.

- Consultations
  - A nutrition consultation is recommended for patients with cirrhosis.
  - If botanicals are to be continued during interferon-based therapy, consider consulting with a Chinese medicine specialist experienced in the management of patients with CHC who are receiving interferon-based therapy.
  - An infectious disease consultation and comanagement are highly recommended for patients coinfected with HCV and HIV.
  - A gastroenterology or hepatology consultation is recommended for patients coinfected with HCV and HBV and for patients with HCV and other comorbid hepatic conditions.
  - For patients with compensated cirrhosis, a hepatology consultation is strongly recommended before treatment. Interferon-based therapy can push patients with compensated cirrhosis into decompensation.

Patients With Newly Diagnosed CHC and Moderate Fibrosis to Compensated Cirrhosis Who Have Contraindications to or Decline Interferon-Based Therapy

Management of these patients is generally the same as for patients with minimal fibrosis, with a few exceptions. Monitor carefully with periodic biochemical

Continued

testing (AST, ALT, total protein, albumin, bilirubin, white blood cell count, and platelet count). Monitor for development of hepatocellular carcinoma with alfa-fetoprotein testing every 6 months and hepatic ultrasound at least once yearly. Botanical therapy may be advised in these patients.

Additional supplements (not previously mentioned in the recommendations for patients with minimal fibrosis) should be considered to reduce hepatic inflammation, boost hepatic antioxidant capacity, promote robust immune function, and support the detoxification pathway (i.e., glutamine, alpha-lipoic acid, N-acetylcysteine, and S-adenosylmethionine).

■ Patients With CHC and Decompensated Cirrhosis

Refer for a hepatology consultation and possible liver transplant evaluation.

■ Patients With CHC Who Were Previously Treated Unsuccessfully With Standard Interferon plus Ribavirin (Nonresponse and Relapse)

Patients previously treated with standard interferon plus ribavirin or just with interferon who were nonresponders or who relapsed after completion of therapy can be successfully retreated with peginterferon alfa plus ribavirin. Response rates are generally not as high as in treatment-naive patients, especially among previous treatment nonresponders.

The FDA recently approved the protease inhibitors telaprevir (Incivek) and boceprevir (Victrelis), which can be added to peginterferon and ribavirin as triple therapy for patients with genotype 1 CHC. The addition of one of these protease inhibitors increases the probability of response to peginterferon and ribavirin in this difficult-to-treat population.

KEY WEB RESOURCES

For Clinicians

American Association for the Study of Liver Diseases (AASLD). *Practice Guidelines, Diagnosis, Management, and Treatment of Hepatitis C: An Update.* http://www.aasld.org/practiceguidelines/Documents/Bookmarked%20Practice%20Guidelines/Diagnosis_of_HEP_C_Update.Aug%20_09pdf.pdf.

This 2009 update document reviews the relevant peer-reviewed literature and provides evidence-based practice guidelines, which have been endorsed by AASLD, the Infectious Diseases Society of America, and the American College of Gastroenterology.

Centers for Disease Control and Prevention. *Viral Hepatitis.* http://www.cdc.gov/hepatitis.

The CDC viral hepatitis hub provides extensive information for clinicians about the various forms of viral hepatitis, including downloadable publications for your practice, access to articles in *Morbidity and Mortality Weekly Report,* and online study and training resources.

For Patients

National Institute of Diabetes and Digestive and Kidney Diseases. *What I Need to Know about Hepatitis C.* http://digestive.niddk.nih.gov/ddiseases/pubs/hepc_ez/.

This site provides a user-friendly overview of hepatitis C basics, which may be particularly useful for patients with newly diagnosed disease.

American Liver Foundation. http://www.liverfoundation.org.

This site provides online informational materials and webcasts designed for patients and caregivers living with chronic liver disease.

Hepatitis Foundation International. http://www.hepfi.org.

The Foundation is a North American advocacy group that provides an online library of information about various forms of chronic hepatitis, news, and research updates, largely targeted to patients and caregivers.

References

References are available at expertconsult.com.

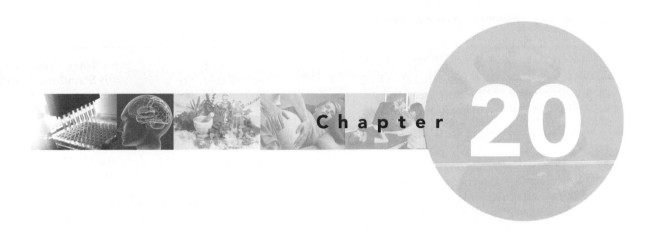

Chapter 20

Urinary Tract Infection

Amy B. Locke, MD

Pathophysiology and Epidemiology

Urinary tract infections (UTIs) are common, with an estimated lifetime incidence of approximately 53% in women and 14% in men.[1] The higher prevalence in women is thought to be related to urethral length. For those who have had a prior infection, the risk of another increases dramatically. One study found a recurrence rate of 44% within 1 year for those women with a history of UTI.[2] The most common pathogens include gram-negative organisms, in particular *Escherichia coli (E. coli)*, which accounts for 80% of infections.[3] Many recurrent infections may actually represent reinfection with the same organism.[4] Despite clearing the bacteria from the urine, the colon may act as a reservoir for pathogenic bacteria.

Simple UTI, or cystitis, involves bacterial colonization of the bladder. Complicated UTIs usually involve structural or anatomic factors, underlying disease states such as diabetes that hinder treatment, or drug-resistant bacterial strains. Ascending infections into the kidneys are not uncommon, particularly with complicated UTIs; pyelonephritis requires urgent medical attention to avoid damage to renal structures and sepsis. Factors that increase the likelihood of disease progression may include delay of treatment, unrecognized infection, asymptomatic bacteriuria in pregnancy, anatomic factors, and systemic diseases that lower immune function, such as diabetes and others. Asymptomatic bacteriuria does not require treatment outside of pregnancy, although debate exists about the utility of treating this condition in patients with diabetes. Although bacteriuria is more common in diabetic patients,[5] treatment has not been shown to alter outcomes.[6] The U.S. Preventive Services Task Force (USPSTF) recommends screening for bacteriuria in pregnancy (A recommendation) and against screening in others (D recommendation).[7] Rapid treatment of pregnant women with clinically diagnosed UTI or asymptomatic bacteriuria is essential because of the high risk of pyelonephritis.

Clinical Presentation

Most episodes of lower UTI manifest with some combination of dysuria, urinary urgency, and frequency. Gross hematuria, suprapubic discomfort, and cloudy urine are not uncommon. Symptoms of fever, myalgia, or low back or flank pain should prompt consideration of pyelonephritis. A history of dysuria, urinary frequency, and absence of vaginal discharge indicates a 90% probability of UTI.[8] Physical examination findings may consist of suprapubic tenderness; however, a physical examination is not required in the evaluation of UTI.

Laboratory testing frequently is isolated to urinalysis. Urinalysis may reveal positive nitrite, positive leukocyte esterase (LE), or hematuria. The presence of nitrite with either LE or hematuria has a positive predictive value of 92%, but a negative predictive value of only 76% when all three values are negative.[9] Urine culture is not required for diagnosis and treatment of simple UTI but may be helpful for recurrent symptoms, to exclude other causes such as interstitial cystitis or when concern exists for a drug-resistant organism. If culture is performed, the finding of more than 100,000 colony-forming units (CFUs) of one organism supports the diagnosis.

The differential diagnosis of dysuria includes *Chlamydia trachomatis* cervicitis and interstitial cystitis, among other disorders in women. Prostatitis and urethritis should be excluded in the treatment of men with UTI. Treatment by telephone for patients with recurrent infection is generally considered acceptable. Many practices have a nurse triage protocol that allows recommendations, including prescriptions to be provided without an office visit. Frequent complicated UTIs or pyelonephritis in women or UTIs in men may benefit from further evaluation by a urologist or further imaging.

Risk Factors

Several factors that may predispose an individual to recurrent UTIs vary across the age spectrum (Table 20-1). Younger women who are sexually active, have a history

TABLE 20-1. Risk Factors for Urinary Tract Infection

YOUNG WOMEN	OLDER WOMEN	MEN	GENERAL
Higher frequency of intercourse	Diabetes	Lack of circumcision	Foreign bodies
History of UTI as child	History of premenopausal UTI	Penetrative anal	Nephrolithiasis
Condom use	Urge incontinence	intercourse	Catheters
Spermicide use	Sexual activity	Female partner with UTI	Family history of recurrent UTI
Diaphragm use	Incomplete bladder emptying	Prostatic hypertrophy	Decreased fluid intake
Pregnancy	Cystocele		
Delayed urination			
Lack of voiding after intercourse			

UTI, urinary tract infection.

of UTIs as children, use condoms (particularly those with spermicidal lubrication), or use diaphragms are at higher risk.[10,11] Frequency of sexual intercourse is an independent risk factor.[10] UTIs have an inverse relationship to voiding after intercourse.[12] Tight clothing and soap preference have not been shown to be related to UTI recurrence in case control trials, although tampon use and soda consumption may be related.[13] Delayed urination in college-age women seems to be significantly related to infection risk.[14] Physiologic changes of pregnancy are associated with a significant increase in UTI.

Postmenopausal women with recurrent UTIs are more likely to be affected by diabetes, a history of premenopausal UTIs, urge incontinence, sexual activity, incomplete emptying of the bladder, or the presence of a cystocele.[15,16]

Some risk factors cross all age ranges, including a family history of recurrent UTIs and foreign bodies such as renal stones and catheters. A family history of recurrent UTIs may be associated with increased risk resulting from the relationship of specific phenotypes and bacterial adherence to the bladder wall.[17]

Risk factors that predispose men to simple UTIs include penetrative anal intercourse, a female partner with UTI, and lack of circumcision.[18] Obstructive symptoms, such as those related to prostatic hypertrophy, predispose patients to complicated UTI.

Integrative Therapy

Nutrition

In general, a diet high in fruits and vegetables, whole grains, and healthy fats will promote good health and may strengthen the immune system. In addition, some foods and food components are thought to have a direct impact on the frequency of UTI.

Bladder Irritants

Many clinicians believe that certain foods cause irritation of the bladder and therefore increase the risk of UTI in some individuals, although case-control studies evaluating dietary factors have not supported this assertion.[12] Possible irritants include caffeine, simple sugars or starches, tobacco and alcohol, and some food additives. For patients with recurrent UTIs, a trial elimination diet to avoid these substances may result in a reduction in the frequency of infections.

Garlic and Onions

Garlic has been used as an antimicrobial agent throughout history for a wide range of conditions. Studies have evaluated its effect on a broad range of organisms, including viral, bacterial, fungal, and parasitic infections. It appears to be active against common urinary pathogens.[19] The most active ingredient in garlic is thought to be the sulfur-containing compound, allicin.[20] Nearly 100 compounds present in garlic may act synergistically, however. In animal models of urinary pseudomonas, garlic appeared to decrease bacterial counts and prevent renal damage.[21] Human trials of garlic for UTI are lacking. Garlic may be useful for acute or recurrent infections.

Chopping or mashing the garlic clove 10 minutes before eating or cooking it seems to maximize the release of allicin, thus increasing effectiveness. Raw consumption is preferred to cooking, because the highest allicin content may be found in raw garlic. Cooked garlic, however, may also have significant health benefits.

Onions also contain allicin and may be helpful in the treatment of UTIs and the prevention of urinary pathogens, although no trials have been conducted. Onions contain many compounds thought to promote health, including flavonoids such as quercetin.

Fluids

Many practitioners recommend significant fluid intake to flush the urinary system, in hopes of preventing UTIs. This practice, however, has not been consistently proved in the literature. Several studies showed an association with decreased fluid intake and susceptibility to UTI,[22,23] while others did not support this finding.[10,12] One review suggested that the issue may be more the combination of fluid intake, frequent voiding, and complete bladder emptying that makes a difference over simply drinking larger volumes.[24] This recommendation is not harmful, and it may be helpful.

Supplements

Probiotics

Because of the colonic bacterial reservoir of pathogenic strains likely involved in recurrent UTIs,[4] it is a logical extension to maximize intestinal health. Probiotic treatments have been evaluated in several studies, although consistent results are lacking. Theoretically, *Lactobacillus* strains provide a barrier in the vagina and on the perineum to prevent bladder colonization. They out-compete pathogenic strains and affect their adhesion.[25] A systematic review in 2009 found five studies that evaluated *Lactobacillus* strains for prevention of UTI, with no consensus.[26] The most efficacious strains in the literature appear to be *Lactobacillus rhamnosus* GR-1 and *Lactobacillus fermentum* RC-14.[27] Several studies showed *Lactobacillus* GG to be less effective.[27] Optimal dosing is unclear but is likely to be at least in the range of 1 billion CFUs. Probiotics can be given orally or vaginally.

Dosage
One billion CFUs daily of *L. rhamnosus* or *L. fermentum*. These probiotics will likely be mixed with other strains in a particular product. The products with these strains are limited in number but are increasingly available.

Precautions
The risk of probiotics in immunocompetent individuals is exceedingly small.

Vitamin C (Ascorbic Acid)
Vitamin C may have a role in the prevention of recurrent UTI. In a single-blind randomized trial of pregnant women, 100 mg of ascorbic acid cut UTI rates by more than half over 3 months (29.1% versus 12.7%).[28] In a case control study, intake of vitamin C correlated with protection against UTI in college age women, however the amounts taken were not noted.[12]

Dosage
Optimal dosage is unknown. Consider 100 mg daily for prevention.

Precautions
Diarrhea may occur in patients taking high doses of vitamin C.

D-Mannose
D-Mannose is a simple sugar found in fruits. It is not broken down in the bloodstream, and it is concentrated in the bladder, where it prevents bacterial adherence to the bladder wall. The cellular receptors of uroepithelial cells to which bacteria such as *E. coli* bind are made of D-mannose.[29] When taken as a supplement, D-mannose binds to the bacterial receptors blocking the bacteria's ability to adhere to the epithelial cell wall.[29] Animal studies showed efficacy in decreasing bacteriuria within 1 day.[30]

The safety of D-mannose was studied in long-term studies of mice, and no evidence of harm was found.[31] D-Mannose has been used in humans for a rare carbohydrate-deficient glycoprotein syndrome. No trials have been done to evaluate the efficacy of D-mannose in humans when it is taken for UTI either as treatment for acute infection or as prophylaxis. D-Mannose shows promise as a potentially safe supplement for treatment of UTI.

Dosage
D-Mannose powder, ¾ to 1 teaspoon one to two times daily, is taken for prevention; and ¾ to 1 teaspoon three times daily is indicated for active treatment.

Precautions
Loose stools and abdominal bloating may occur. High doses over prolonged periods may be nephrotoxic.

D-Mannose is thought to inhibit urinary tract infection by encouraging binding of bacteria to this sugar instead of the bladder wall and thus enhancing evacuation through the urine.

Botanicals
Cranberry (Vaccinium macrocarpon)
Cranberry juice and powder have successfully been used to prevent UTI. The use of cranberry dates back to Native American tribes who used it for urinary conditions. Historically, cranberry was thought to work by acidifying urine, yet studies have shown effects with minimal change in urine pH.[32] The presumed active compounds, proanthocyanidins (PACs), may inhibit bacterial adhesion to the bladder wall and decrease bacterial virulence.[33] In a small trial, a dose of 72 mg of PAC was effective against *E. coli*. This effect appears to be dose dependent,[33] although the optimal dose is unknown.

In one randomized controlled trial, cranberry juice was compared with powder and placebo in sexually active women.[34] Both cranberry groups reduced recurrent UTI by approximately 30%. The doses used in this study were 250 mL of cranberry juice three times daily and concentrated cranberry juice tablets twice daily. The size of the tablets used was not disclosed. Another trial used only 30 mL of cranberry-lingonberry concentrate daily and reported a 20% risk reduction for UTI recurrence.[35] The small studies that have shown success with tablets have used 400 to 800 mg twice daily.[36,37] The size and design of these studies may limit extrapolation to a larger population. Another trial randomized women to 500 mg of cranberry extract or 100 mg of trimethoprim and found equal efficacy in prevention of UTIs.[38]

A 2008 Cochrane Review looked at 10 randomized trials using cranberry juice or capsules and found some evidence that cranberry juice may decrease the frequency of UTI in susceptible women.[39] This review found a high dropout rate, however, likely related to difficulty adhering to daily juice consumption.[39] The optimal dose could not be determined by these studies. Cranberry is not effective in patients with neurogenic bladder.

Although cranberry products are frequently used to treat acute infection, these qualities have not been researched.[40]

Dosage
For prevention of UTI, the dose is 16 oz (500 mL) of unsweetened cranberry juice daily or cranberry extract, 500 mg daily to 400 to 800 mg twice daily.

Precautions
Moderate interaction with warfarin is possible.

Many cranberry beverage products on the market contain only a small amount of cranberry juice and a significant amount of sweeteners. This may have a minimal impact on the urinary tract and potentially a negative impact on overall health.

Uva Ursi (Arctostaphylos uva ursi)

Uva Ursi, or bearberry, leaf has long been used for urinary symptoms, although few human data have evaluated efficacy. The active compound is thought to be arbutin, which is converted into hydroquinone.[41] Alkaline urine is thought to be necessary for efficacy. In vitro studies have suggested activity against typical pathogens.[42]

One preliminary trial showed effectiveness in preventing recurrent UTI when uva ursi was combined with dandelion root and leaf.[43] In this trial, women took an extract for 1 month and then were followed for 1 year. During that time, 18% of women in the placebo group (27 individuals total) and 0% in the treatment group (30 individuals) had a UTI. Unfortunately, because of potential toxicity when uva ursi is used long term, it cannot be recommended for UTI prophylaxis. This toxicity may be related to the component hydroquinone and the inhibition of melanin,[44] although tannins may also play a role. The most common side effects include nausea and gastrointestinal distress. Rarer and more serious side effects may include hepatotoxicity, retinal disease,[44] seizure, cyanosis, and death. These risks are more pronounced with high doses and prolonged use. Many experts recommend limiting use to acute infections for no more than 1 week and restricting use to five times per year.[45]

■ Dosage

Uva ursi is taken as 3 g of dried herb daily or as an infusion (3 g of dried herb steeped in 150 mL of cold water for 12 to 24 hours), 1 cup 4 times daily; the hydroquinone derivative dose is 400 to 840 mg up to four times daily.

■ Precautions

Uva ursi is not safe in pregnancy, in children, or for long-term use. Uva ursi can turn urine greenish brown, which can interfere with urinalysis. It is potentially hepatotoxic with prolonged use.

Berberine

Berberine is an alkaloid found in certain plants. Common in the traditions of traditional Chinese medicine, Ayurvedic medicine, and Native American healing, plant species that contain berberine include goldenseal (*Hydrastis canadensis*), Oregon grape (*Berberis aquifolium*), bayberry (*Berberis vulgaris*), coptis (*Coptis chinensis*), and tree turmeric (*Berberis aristata*). A few studies have been done on this compound. Some have used specific plants, and others have used isolated berberine. In vitro studies showed that berberine sulfate causes inhibition of *E. coli* adhesion to epithelial cells.[46] Studies using berberine for other indications did not show toxicity or significant side effects.[47]

Goldenseal (Hydrastis canadensis)

Goldenseal is a woodland herbaceous plant native to North America. Few data support its use in UTI, but the root has been used for antimicrobial purposes. One study of goldenseal extract showed in vitro activity against several common urinary pathogens.[48] No studies have been conducted in vivo. Concern exists about overharvesting and dwindling populations of goldenseal in the forests of eastern North America.

■ Dosage

The optimal dose is unknown. A common dose of goldenseal is 0.5 to 1 g three times daily of the dried root.

■ Precautions

Berberine (including goldenseal) is not considered safe in pregnancy or for infants because of the risk of kernicterus.[49] It may also effect the cytochrome P-450 system and subsequently the serum levels of other substances.

Other Herbal Preparations

Other traditional herbal preparations that have been used for UTIs include stinging nettles, marshmallow root, echinacea, burdock, slippery elm, dandelion, and lovage. Some of these, such as *Echinacea angustifolia,* have been studied in other conditions. For example, although echinacea has been identified as an immune stimulator, it has not been studied in UTI. Other herbal preparations have little research on any clinical uses.

Pharmaceuticals

Antibiotics

Simple cystitis in women may be treated with a 3-day regimen of any of several antibiotics, including trimethoprim-sulfamethoxazole and ciprofloxacin. Other acceptable antibiotics include nitrofurantoin and amoxicillin. Optimal therapy often depends on antibiotic resistance rates in the individual's community. Complicated UTIs require a longer course. Pregnant women and those with chronic disease such as diabetes should be treated for 7 days. Men with UTI are also usually treated for 7 days, and prostatitis should be excluded.

Recurrent UTIs may be treated with prophylactic antibiotics daily or postcoitally. Either approach has been shown to decrease the frequency of infection. Prophylactic antibiotics are usually continued for 6 to 12 months before a trial off the drugs. In a Cochrane Review, 6- and 12-month regimens appeared to be equal in efficacy.[50] Postcoital antibiotics appear to be as effective against recurrent UTIs as daily therapy for those individuals with symptoms related to intercourse.[50]

■ Dosage

Trimethoprim-sulfamethoxazole, one tablet double strength (DS) (160/800 mg) twice daily for 3 days; ciprofloxacin, 250 mg twice daily for 3 days; nitrofurantoin extended release (ER), 100 mg twice daily for 7 days.

Prophylactic doses are usually given once daily at the same dose used for treatment. Common choices include ciprofloxacin, nitrofurantoin, and trimethoprim-sulfamethoxazole daily.[51] Postcoital doses are given as one tablet at the time of intercourse.

■ Precautions

Frequent or long-term use of antibiotics may be associated with medication side effects and risk of disruption of normal bacterial flora.

Phenazopyridine

Phenazopyridine (Pyridium) can provide pain relief from dysuria and bladder spasms. It is available over the counter and by prescription.

■ Dosage

The dose is 100 to 200 mg twice daily for 2 days.

■ Precautions

This medication turns urine and tears a dark orange that can interfere with urinalysis and can stain contact lenses.

Estrogen

Systemic estrogen replacement does not appear to have an effect on the frequency of UTIs in postmenopausal women,[52] although topical estrogens may be beneficial for postmenopausal women with recurrent UTIs.[53] In one randomized trial, 0.5 mg of vaginal estriol nightly for 2 weeks followed by twice weekly for 8 months compared with placebo resulted in a significant reduction in UTI frequency (0.5 versus 5.9 episodes per patient year). Vaginal estriol was found to be less effective than daily nitrofurantoin (Macrodantin) in preventing recurrent UTI.[54]

■ Dosage

The dose is 0.5 mg vaginal estriol nightly for 2 weeks, followed by twice weekly.

■ Precautions

Vaginal estrogen may be absorbed systemically at high doses, thus prompting the need for endometrial protection. In general, the safest approach is to use the lowest effective dose for the least amount of time needed.

Other Therapies to Consider

Behavioral Changes

Certain behaviors have been thought to be associated with an increased risk of UTI. Many of these behaviors are associated with irritation of the urethra or reflux of urine back into the bladder from the urethra. These include sexual intercourse, wearing of tight clothing, holding of urine, and use of irritants such as bubble bath, douche, or other products. Many of these have no evidence base, but addressing them has little risk of harm.

Acupuncture

In one randomized trial of acupuncture compared with no treatment, women with a history of recurrent UTIs had a 50% reduction in UTIs compared with the control group (73% versus 52% with no UTIs over 6 months).[55] The treatment group received biweekly acupuncture sessions over 4 weeks and were followed for 6 months. Bladder residuals were reduced in the treatment group to 50% compared with baseline, and no change was noted in the control group. An earlier study by the same research team showed similar results, with partial response after sham acupuncture as compared with a no-treatment control.[56]

Mind-Body Skills

Although no specific mind-body skills have been evaluated in the prevention or treatment of UTI, mental health and spiritual health are important components of overall health, including the immune system. These mind-body components, along with other foundations of health, such as nutritional status, adequate sleep, and physical activity, are essential to optimal health. Attention to techniques to improve them, whether yoga, mindfulness, social connectedness, or other strategies, will likely help limit susceptibility to infectious processes.

Biofeedback

In the subgroup of women who suffer from dysfunctional voiding, pelvic floor therapy appears to decrease recurrent UTIs.[57] Dysfunctional voiding is defined as increased external sphincter activity during voluntary voiding. This occurs in individuals without neurologic deficit.

PREVENTION PRESCRIPTION

- Encourage a plant-based diet high in garlic and onions.
- Urge removal of possible bladder irritants such as caffeine, alcohol, and simple sugars.
- Encourage adequate fluid intake.
- Monitor stress, and focus on foundations of health such as optimal diet, physical activity, sleep, and mental and spiritual health.
- Encourage frequent voiding and avoidance of holding urine.
- Consider changing method of birth control if frequent UTIs occur after use of spermicides, condoms, or diaphragms.
- Recommend urination after intercourse.

THERAPEUTIC REVIEW

This is a summary of therapeutic options for UTI both for acute treatment and for prevention. If a patient presents with severe symptoms or has a history suggestive of a complicated UTI, an initial course of antibiotics would be beneficial. For the patient who has mild to moderate symptoms, a ladder approach may be appropriate. Patients should be counseled to seek further care if their symptoms worsen or do not resolve.

■ Acute Infection

■ Nutrition

- Encourage garlic consumption.

■ Supplements

- D-Mannose: ¾ to 1 teaspoon three times daily

■ Botanicals

- Cranberry 16 oz of unsweetened juice daily or extract 500 mg bid

Continued

- Uva ursi: hydroquinone derivative 400-840 mg up to 4 times daily or 3 grams of dried root daily

Pharmaceuticals

- Trimethoprim-sulfamethoxazole: one double-strength tablet twice daily for 3 days
- Nitrofurantoin extended release: 100 mg twice daily for 7 days
- Ciprofloxacin: 250 mg twice daily for 3 days
- Phenazopyridine: 200 mg twice daily for 2 days

Recurrent Infections

Removal of Exacerbating Factors

- Eliminate use of spermicides, and try a change of birth control method.
- Recommend urinating after intercourse.

Nutrition

- Encourage garlic consumption.
- Encourage adequate fluid intake.

Supplements

- Probiotics: 1 billion CFUs daily of *Lactobacillus rhamnosus* or *L. fermentum*
- Vitamin C: 100 mg daily

Botanicals

- Cranberry: 16 oz of unsweetened juice daily or extract, 500 mg twice daily
- Uva ursi
- Other herbal products that have potential benefit, including berberine-containing plants and echinacea

Pharmaceuticals

- Trimethoprim-sulfamethoxazole: one double-strength tablet daily
- Nitrofurantoin: 100 mg daily
- Ciprofloxacin: 250 mg daily

Other Therapies

- Biofeedback for those with dysfunctional voiding
- Acupuncture

References

References are available at expertconsult.com

Recurrent Yeast Infections

Ravi S. Hirekatur, MD

Pathophysiology and Epidemiology

Approximately 55% to 75% of all women experience vulvovaginal candidiasis (VVC) during their lifetime, and up to 40% to 50% of them will have recurrent episodes.[1] Approximately 8% of women will have recurrent vulvovaginal candidiasis (RVVC), as defined by four or more episodes in a year.[2] By age 25 years, half of all college women will have experienced at least one physician-diagnosed case of VVC.[3] African American women are more frequently affected than are others.[4,5]

VVC is extremely rare in premenstrual years and increases in reproductive age. It also tends to be less frequent in postmenopausal women, although women who are undergoing estrogen therapy generally have higher frequency of VVC.[6]

VVC is a spectrum of conditions with variable number of organisms and a variable degree of symptoms. Most highly symptomatic women have a large number of organisms with florid exudative vaginitis or thrush, most likely resulting from a combination of reduced local protective cellular responses and increased immediate hypersensitivity reaction. Other women have minimal symptoms with large numbers of organisms, most likely secondary to reduced local protective immune responses. Still other women are highly symptomatic with a small number of organisms and without thrush, most likely because of an immediate hypersensitivity response.[7]

Candida albicans, the most common pathogen implicated in RVVC, causes approximately 90% of cases. Other species include *Candida glabrata* (second most common), *Candida parapsilosis, Candida krusei, Candida tropicalis, Candida lusitaniae, Saccharomyces cerevisiae,* and *Trichosporon* species.[8] However, approximately 20% to 25% of asymptomatic women are colonized by *Candida* in their vagina, as shown by culture.[9] *Candida* also seems to be part of the normal vaginal flora and is in equilibrium with other bacterial and vaginal defense mechanisms.[10] *Candida* in blastophore form is consistent with asymptomatic colonization, and germinated yeast with hyphae are more common in symptomatic VVC.[7,11] Symptomatic cases of VVC and RVVC appear to be caused by host factors (aggressive innate response by polymorphonuclear neutrophils) rather than by the virulent properties of the organism.[12] Recurrence appears to result from relapse rather than reinfection, in response to a change in normal protective host defensive mechanisms at the vaginal mucosa.[7]

Typical symptoms of VVC include vulvovaginal pruritus (50%), vulvar swelling (24%), and dysuria (33%).[13] Vaginal discharge can be variable, from thin and watery to thick and resembling cottage cheese. Other common symptoms include vaginal soreness, irritation, vulvar burning, and dyspareunia. Examination may show vulvar and labial erythema, edema, and often fissures and peripheral pustulopapular lesions. The cervix is usually normal, often with vaginal mucosal erythema and an off-white discharge.[11]

The diagnosis is based on normal vaginal pH (4.0 to 4.5), clinical findings and symptoms, and positive microscopic findings with 10% potassium hydroxide (KOH). Cultures should be obtained in patients with symptomatic cases and negative KOH findings.[11,13] In recurrent cases, cultures must be obtained.[14] The sensitivity of microscopy is 50% at best,[15] however, and approximately 49% of culture results can be negative.[16] Polymerase chain reaction (PCR) is more sensitive than culture, but costs may be prohibitive.[17] Often, the diagnosis is based on clinical findings, vaginal pH, positive microscopic findings, and yeast cultures. In resistant cases, cultures are useful for isolating candidal species other than *C. albicans* to target the treatment.[14]

Classification of VVC is based on whether the infection is complicated or uncomplicated (Table 21-1).[8,14] Most cases of uncomplicated VVC respond well to a standard course of oral or topical antifungal therapy. In complicated VVC, the clinical situation may be complicated by the risk factors. To achieve a cure, all those factors must be addressed.

TABLE 21-1. Classification of Vulvovaginal Candidiasis

Uncomplicated

- Sporadic or infrequent VVC
- Mild to moderate VVC
- Most likely *Candida albicans*
- Normal, nonpregnant, nonimmunocompromised women

Complicated

- Recurrent (four or more episodes per year)
- Severe VVC
- Non-*Candida albicans*
- Aberrant host (e.g., uncontrolled diabetes, immunocompromised or pregnant women, debilitation)

VVC, vulvovaginal candidiasis.

Risk Factors

The following are considered to be risk factors for complicated VVC.

Nutritional

- Increased ingestion of sweets[14,18]
- Consumption of foods rich in simple carbohydrates[18]
- Decreased milk consumption[19]
- Increased caloric intake, with daily intake of carbohydrates greater than 223 g, and certain fibers[20]

Contraception

- Oral contraception[3,4] (higher risk with high estrogen content[21,22])
- Diaphragm[16,23]
- Intrauterine device[21,22]
- Sponge[21,22]
- Spermicide[4]

Sexual Behavior

- Receiving orogenital sex more than twice in 2 weeks (the most consistent evidence)[4,18,19,24-28]
- Anal intercourse[25]
- Female masturbation with saliva[18,19]
- Age at first intercourse[18,19,25] and frequency of vaginal intercourse[4,18,21,27,28] (conflicting evidence)
- High number of lifetime sex partners[21]
- Sexual intercourse during menstruation[21]
- Male factors: male masturbating with saliva in the past month and lower age of first intercourse[19] (Uncircumcised male patients have a higher risk than do circumcised men.[29])

Hygiene Products

- Douching[21,26,27]

Host Factors

- Immunosuppression/human immunodeficiency virus infection
- Diabetes
- Impaired glucose tolerance in nondiabetic patients[30]
- High body mass index[30]
- Race: blacks > whites > Asians[4]
- Antibiotic use[21,31] (Colonized women are more at risk.[32])
- Noncompliance with medications during previous infection[33]
- Prior diagnosis of VVC in the previous year[4]
- Pregnancy state, as a result of high concentrations of pregnancy hormones[34]

Psychosocial Factors

- High stress and psychosocial factors[35,36]
- Smoking[35]
- Decreased satisfaction in life[36]
- Poor self-esteem[36]

> Receiving orogenital sex and using any form of contraceptive, having a high body mass index, having impaired glucose tolerance, consuming excessive sweets, and having high stress levels constitute some of the risk factors for recurrent vulvovaginal candidiasis.

In addition, women with persistent pruritus may benefit from the addition of antihistamines to main therapy.[37] Some studies have shown that cutaneous systemic hyposensitization of *Candida* antigen may benefit women with RVVC as an alternative approach to antifungal agents.[38,39] Treating male partners has no benefit in VVC recurrence rates.[40-42]

Integrative Therapy

Because RVVC is difficult to treat, incorporating complementary therapies with conventional treatment may be prudent.

Nutrition and Supplements

Given that increased caloric intake and increased consumption of sweets and simple carbohydrates are risk factors for RVVC, a low-fat, low-calorie diet rich in complex carbohydrates with avoidance of simple carbohydrates and sweets is recommended.

Yogurt (Containing Lactobacillus)

Probiotics are supplements that contain live bacteria. They colonize the gut and promote healthy normal flora. Yogurt containing *Lactobacillus acidophilus*, taken orally or intravaginally, has been found effective against VVC. One study found that daily ingestion of 8 oz of yogurt containing

L. acidophilus decreased both colonization and infection by *Candida*.[43] Another study showed that daily ingestion of 150 mL of yogurt containing *L. acidophilus* could increase vaginal colonization of *L. acidophilus*, but not necessarily decrease the incidence of VVC, as compared with pasteurized yogurt.[44]

■ Dosage
The dose is 8 oz of yogurt orally once or twice daily. It can be applied intravaginally with a tampon.

Probiotics
Lactobacillus is considered to be part of the normal vaginal and intestinal flora and may play a large role in the control of microflora and maintenance of the normal state by producing many metabolites that may deter the growth of pathogens, including *Candida*.[45] Among several known species of *Lactobacillus*, *Lactobacillus* GR-1 and *Lactobacillus fermentum* RC-14 have the ability to inhibit or kill yeast.[46,47] They provide resistance against *Candida* by preventing germination by producing bacteriocins and hydrogen peroxide.[48] Women with VVC are shown to have decreased numbers of *Lactobacillus* that produce hydrogen peroxide (*L. acidophilus, Lactobacillus gasseri,* and *Lactobacillus vaginalis*) and increased numbers of non–hydrogen peroxide–producing *Lactobacillus* (*Lactobacillus iners*) in their vaginal flora.[49] Other subspecies of *Lactobacillus* that produce hydrogen peroxide include *Lactobacillus jensenii* and *Lactobacillus crispatus*.[50] One study showed that approximately eight species of *Lactobacillus* have a protective effect against vaginal candidiasis.[51]

The optimum dosage of *L.* GR-1 and *L. fermentum* RC-14 is considered to be 10^9 organisms.[52]

Several clinical studies showed mixed results regarding effectiveness of various species of *Lactobacillus* in the treatment of RVVC. One pilot study showed resolution of RVVC with twice-daily vaginal suppositories containing 10^9 organisms of *Lactobacillus rhamnosus* GG.[53] Weekly intravaginal application of *L. acidophilus* was also found to be prophylactic against VVC in HIV-infected women.[54] However, a large randomized controlled double-blind study found that preparations containing *L. rhamnosus* and *Bifidobacterium longum* oral capsules and *L. rhamnosus, Lactobacillus delbrueckii, L. acidophilus,* and *Streptococcus thermophilus* vaginal pessary taken orally, vaginally, or both during and after the antibiotic administration (for nongynecologic infection) did not prevent VVC in women.[55] The amount of viable organisms was not mentioned in the study, and the duration of treatment after the course of antibiotics was only 4 days. Further large studies involving multiple species of hydrogen peroxide–producing *Lactobacillus* are needed to evaluate the effect on RVVC because *Lactobacillus* show host specificity and colonization potential.

■ Dosage
The dose is not standardized. Recommend using commercially available capsules containing at least 10^9 organisms of multiple species of *Lactobacillus* that produce hydrogen peroxide, such as *L. acidophilus, Lactobacillus* GR-1, *L. fermentum* RC-14, *L. rhamnosus* GG, *L. gasseri,* and *L. vaginalis*. These capsules can be taken orally or intravaginally on a daily basis for RVVC.

■ Precautions
None of the foregoing studies noted any harm or undesirable side effects of *Lactobacillus* used either topically or orally.

> Yogurt or probiotics that contain multiple species of *Lactobacillus* may inhibit the growth of *Candida* species. Oral or topical use of one or two *Lactobacillus* species may not be helpful in preventing recurrent vulvovaginal candidiasis because these species may not have specific action against the organism causing the infection.

Gentian Violet
Gentian violet is a dye and is an old antifungal remedy that is effective as a cure for RVVC.[56] A 0.25% to 0.5% aqueous solution can be applied at home daily for a week, or a 1% solution can be applied in the clinic weekly up to three times.[57] A 1% solution used daily for a week can successfully treat RVVC caused by *C. glabrata*.[58] Most of the commercial products have been discontinued.

■ Dosage
The best way to use gentian violet is to coat the vaginal wall with a swab or soak a tampon in the solution and insert it intravaginally overnight.[59]

Precautions
Gentian violet causes permanent staining of clothes that is almost impossible to remove, and some patients may develop vulvar irritation after application.[57]

Pharmaceuticals
Fluconazole
For uncomplicated infections, topical treatments are as effective as oral treatments, but most women prefer oral treatments with fluconazole for convenience.[40]

Complicated VVC is very difficult to treat and often requires twice the duration of the usual course of treatment; some patients require treatment for weeks or months.[14] One standard treatment is to use fluconazole, 150 mg once every 72 hours for 9 days, followed by maintenance therapy of 150 mg weekly.[14,60] Some patients may need to be treated for 14 days, followed by maintenance therapy. Occasionally, recurrent infections are caused by multiple species, especially *C. glabrata,* which is often resistant to itraconazole (74%) and to fluconazole (16%).[61] *C. glabrata* often requires an increased dose of fluconazole.[61] For recurrent infections, a maintenance regimen with 150 mg of oral fluconazole can be used on a weekly basis for 6 months, followed by 6 months of observation, with disease-free rates at 6, 9, and 12 months of 91%, 73%, and 43%, respectively.[62] Long-term maintenance treatment can reduce the rate of recurrence, but it is difficult to achieve a long-term cure.

Boric Acid and Combination Therapy
Intravaginal application of 600 mg of boric acid once daily for 14 days is effective for *C. glabrata,* with 70% success rate.[60] However, boric acid is associated with fetal anomalies and should not be used in pregnant women or in women who are trying to become pregnant.[60] It should not be taken

orally, either.[63] If boric acid fails to cure an infection, topical nystatin or flucytosine (17%) once daily for 14 days can be used. If that fails, a combination regimen consisting of topical boric acid, flucytosine, or nystatin, with oral itraconazole, is recommended.[64] In severe cases, low-potency topical corticosteroids may be used for symptom relief.[60]

> Recurrent infections that do not respond to standard therapies may be caused by more than one species of *Candida,* and some of these species may be resistant to imidazoles and triazoles. Some patients may need long-term maintenance therapy, and some may require combination regimens.

Botanicals

Garlic (Allium sativum)
Results of in vitro studies showed that garlic has anticandidal properties.[65-68] Oral preparations of both fresh garlic extract and freeze-dried extracts are equally effective. The active ingredient, allicin, is known to inhibit both germination of spores and growth of hyphae.[69] No human studies have been conducted.

■ Dosage
The dosage for garlic has not been well established for VVC. However, one can take commercially available freeze-dried extracts of garlic up to 500 mg two to three times a day orally. Another treatment is to wrap a clove of garlic in unbleached gauze and crush it before inserting it into the vagina and leaving it there overnight. This treatment is repeated for 6 nights.[70]

■ Precautions
Topical applications of garlic can be uncomfortable because it can irritate the mucosa.

Tea Tree Oil (Melaleuca alternifolia)
Tea tree oil is native to Australia, and its main ingredient is terpin-4-ol. Results of in vitro studies have shown that tea tree oil has antifungal activities,[71-75] comparable to those of ketoconazole, econazole, and miconazole.[72] In vitro studies also found tea tree oil effective against fluconazole-resistant *Candida* species.[76] Human studies of tea tree oil for treatment of VVC are lacking.

■ Dosage
A preparation of 5% to 10% tea tree oil is applied topically daily. Alternatively, one to two drops of tea tree oil (commercially available, nonessential oil) can be placed in a gelatin capsule. The remainder of the capsule is filled with calendula oil or vegetable oil or water. Two capsules can be placed intravaginally overnight for up to 6 nights.[77]

Although most of the commercially available tea tree oils do not mention its concentration, patients can make their own preparations from tea tree essential oil. To make 5% tea tree oil, simply add 5 drops of tea tree essential oil to 5 mL of base oil (vegetable oil, coconut oil, or calendula oil) and mix thoroughly. Similarly, adding 10 drops to 5 mL of base oil will make a 10% mixture.

■ Precautions
Tea tree oil is known to cause allergic dermatitis. A skin patch test is recommended before use.[63] Tea tree essential oil should not be applied directly to the vaginal mucosa. It can cause severe irritation and damage because it is highly concentrated.

Mind-Body Approaches and Stress Management

Relaxation methods, meditation, deep breathing, yoga, guided imagery, and self-hypnosis can be used to manage stress and enhance mental and spiritual well-being, thereby improving immune response in patients who experience high levels of stress.

Risk Factor Reduction
Behavioral approaches can be used to reduce the risk factors listed previously. One may not be able to reduce all the risk factors, but addressing as many risk factors as possible may help prevent RVVC. Some of the behavioral approaches include avoidance of orogenital sex and douching, optimal glycemic control in diabetes, weight loss, exercise, and smoking cessation in individuals who warrant it. Unhurried sexual intercourse and extra lubrication for women who have a history of RVVC may help prevent damage to vaginal epithelium and, in turn, may prevent recurrence.[78] Wearing well-ventilated clothing can be beneficial.[11] In patients with severe recurrent cases, discontinuing contraceptives may be recommended. Strict compliance with an antifungal regimen must be emphasized.

> Reducing risk factors for vulvovaginitis may prevent recurrence.

PREVENTION PRESCRIPTION

- Avoid receiving oral sex for recurrent infections.
- Practice unhurried intercourse with extra lubrication to avoid trauma to the vaginal mucosa.
- Avoid using saliva for masturbation.
- Wear well-ventilated clothing.
- Consider discontinuing oral contraceptives with high doses of estrogen.
- Avoid douching.
- Avoid eating simple carbohydrates and sweets.
- Achieve optimal glycemic control in diabetes.
- Follow a diet and exercise program (useful with high body mass index and impaired glucose tolerance for prevention).
- Stop smoking.
- Treat depression, with effective stress management in recurrent cases.
- Ensure daily ingestion of yogurt containing multiple strains of *Lactobacillus.*
- Ensure a daily intake of garlic.

THERAPEUTIC REVIEW

Recurrent vulvovaginal candidiasis (RVVC) is often difficult to cure and may require an integrative approach along with conventional therapy. Some of the integrative approaches include nutrition and supplements, mind-body work, and risk factor reduction, along with longer-term pharmacotherapy.

Mind-Body Therapy

- Deep breathing, relaxation, yoga, and meditation may be useful in highly stressed individuals to prevent recurrences by enhancing immune function.

Nutrition and Supplements

- Ingestion of 8 oz of yogurt containing multiple active species of *Lactobacillus* on a daily basis (Look for the "Live Active Culture" seal on the label, which requires 10^8 viable lactic acid bacteria per gram.)

- Use of probiotics containing multiple active species of *Lactobacillus* (10^9 organisms) on a daily basis

Botanicals

- Tea tree oil (5% to 10%) may be used topically in patients who are not allergic to it.

- Fresh garlic cloves nightly intravaginally or 500 mg of garlic extract may be used orally two to three times daily.

Pharmaceuticals

- For uncomplicated VVC:
  - Fluconazole: 150 mg orally once
  - Clotrimazole vaginal (Gyne-Lotrimin): 200-mg suppository or 2% cream nightly for 3 days
- For potentially resistant *Candida* strains, consider:
  - Terconazole vaginal (Terazol): 80-mg suppository or 0.8% cream nightly for 3 to 7 days
- For complicated VVC:
  - Oral fluconazole: 150 mg every 72 hours for 9 to 14 days
  - Oral ketoconazole: 200 mg once or twice daily orally for 14 days
  - Boric acid: 600 mg intravaginally daily for 14 days
- For RVVC and resistant VVC:
  - Maintenance therapy with fluconazole: 100 or 150 mg once a week long term
  - Combination therapy with topical boric acid, nystatin or flucytosine (17%), and oral itraconazole: may be needed for some patients with recurrent and resistant cases

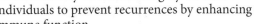

KEY WEB RESOURCES

womenshealth.gov	U.S. Department of Health and Human Services Office on Women's Health
http://www.womenshealth.gov/faq/vaginal-yeast-infections.cfm	Patient education information
http://www.floracopeia.com; http://www.mountainroseherbs.com/aroma/ess.html	For purchasing high-quality tea tree essential oil

References

References are available at expertconsult.com.

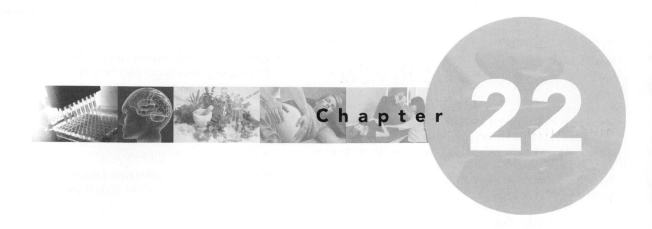

Chapter

22

Lyme Disease

Ather Ali, ND, MPH

Pathophysiology and Epidemiology

Lyme disease is a multisystem infection caused by the spirochetal bacterium *Borrelia burgdorferi*.[1] *B. burgdorferi* sensu stricto is the only species known to cause human infection in the United States, whereas pathogenic species in Europe include *B. burgdorferi* sensu stricto, *Borrelia garinii*, and *Borrelia Afzelii*, among others. Seven pathogenic species have been identified in Asia.[1]

In 1977, Lyme disease was characterized by Steere et al and named for the geographic area (Lyme, Old Lyme, and Haddam, Connecticut) where 39 patients presented with arthritic symptoms of previously unknown cause,[2] although individual cases of Lyme borreliosis were described in Europe in the early twentieth century.[1,3]

Lyme disease is the most common vector-transmitted disease in the United States. Approximately 20,000 cases of Lyme disease are reported to the Centers for Disease Control and Prevention (CDC) each year, although the CDC notes that these rates reflect both overdiagnosis of cases and overall underreporting.[4] Most (95%) reported cases occur in the northeastern and midwestern areas of the United States in 12 states (Connecticut, Delaware, Maine, Maryland, Massachusetts, Minnesota, New Hampshire, New Jersey, New York, Pennsylvania, Rhode Island, and Wisconsin). Figure 22-1 illustrates the distribution of Lyme disease in the United States.

Lyme borreliosis also occurs in some Asian countries and throughout Europe.[1] Connecticut has the highest incidence of Lyme disease in the United States (122 cases per 100,000).[5] The incidence in the other states where Lyme disease is most endemic is 29.2 cases per 100,000.[4]

The principal vectors for transmission of *B. burgdorferi* in the United States are nymphal deer ticks *(Ixodes scapularis)* during the late spring or summer months.[6] Infected ticks need to be attached for at least 24 to 48 hours to be able to transmit the organism.[6] Bites from *Ixodes* ticks are usually painless and are often unrecognized. Figure 22-2 illustrates stages of the life cycle of the deer tick.

Ixodes ticks may also transmit *Anaplasma phagocytophila* (the agent of human granulocytic anaplasmosis [HGA]), *Babesia microti*, other *Borrelia* species, and viruses, either separately or in conjunction with *B. burgdorferi*.[7] The impact of coinfections on the clinical course of Lyme disease is not well defined,[7] although persons with coinfections may present with more symptoms and fever and chills.[8]

Infected persons do not transmit Lyme disease to others. No epidemiologic or clinical data currently confirm sexual or congenital transmission of *B. burgdorferi* between humans.[9]

Clinical Course

Lyme disease is classified into three stages: early localized Lyme disease, early disseminated Lyme disease, and late Lyme disease.[9] Early localized Lyme disease is characterized by a rash (erythema migrans) appearing at the site of the tick bite typically between 7 and 14 days following the bite.[9] Erythema migrans is usually asymptomatic but may become pruritic. Systemic symptoms sometimes may accompany the rash and include fever, myalgia, headache, fatigue, and localized lymphadenopathy.[9]

Early disseminated Lyme disease may manifest as multiple sites of erythema migrans, usually appearing 3 to 5 weeks following the tick bite. Neurologic findings, including meningitis and cranial nerve palsies, may be present along with fatigue, flulike symptoms, and syncopal episodes.[9]

Late Lyme disease is characterized by arthritis, usually affecting the large joints, including the knee, and this arthritis can be monarticular or oligoarticular. Neurologic complications may develop, including polyneuropathy, encephalitis, and encephalopathy.[9,10]

> Persons suffering from chronic persistent symptoms often present with debilitating and severe symptoms. Patients should not be dismissed or disregarded because the pathophysiology of their symptoms is unknown. Effective symptomatic treatments can significantly improve quality of life.

FIGURE 22-1
Epidemiology of Lyme disease. The distribution of Lyme disease corresponds to the distribution of the *Ixodes* ticks that transmit *Borrelia burgdorferi*. (From the Centers for Disease Control and Prevention, Division of Vector-Borne Diseases. *Lyme Disease Transmission*. <http://www.cdc.gov/lyme/transmission/index.html>; 2011 Accessed 27.07.11.)

REPORTED CASES OF LYME DISEASE – UNITED STATES, 2009

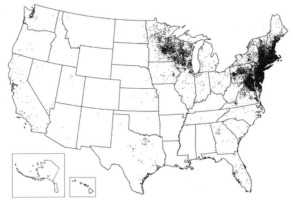

1 dot placed randomly within county of residence
for each confirmed case

FIGURE 22-2
Various stages of the life cycle of the deer tick *Ixodes scapularis*, the vector for Lyme disease in the northern United States. The larval stage is shown on the *left*, followed by the nymphal stage, the adult female, and the adult male on the *right*. Most infections are transmitted from ticks at the nymphal stage. (From Murray TS, Shapiro ED. Lyme disease. *Clin Lab Med*. 2010;30:311.)

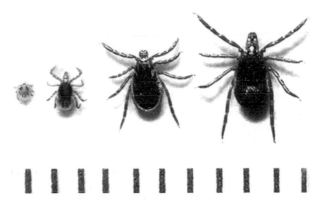

Chronic Persistent Symptoms, Chronic Lyme Disease, and Medically Unexplained Symptoms

Fatigue, arthralgia, and myalgia may persist after initial treatment for Lyme disease. Steere and Glickstein[11] reported that 10% of patients with Lyme arthritis develop persistent synovitis that can last for months or years after initial antibiotic treatment. The impact of persistent symptoms is great. The effect on health-related quality of life is reported to be comparable to or more severe than congestive heart failure and type 2 diabetes.[12]

In a cohort in Westchester County, New York, Asch et al[13] found that 53% of patients reported persistent symptoms following initial treatment for Lyme disease. These

investigators noted that antibiotic treatment within 4 weeks of initial infection was associated with a greater likelihood of full symptom resolution.[13] In a pediatric cohort, 23% of children developed refractory arthritis after initial treatment.[14] These children were subsequently treated with nonsteroidal antiinflammatory drugs, intra-articular steroid injections, or disease-modifying antirheumatic drugs (DMARDs). None developed chronic arthritis or recurrent infections.[14] Polymerase chain reaction (PCR) testing of joint fluid can detect *B. burgdorferi* DNA for several weeks after spirochetes are killed,[15] and thus PCR may not be a good test for effectiveness of treatment. Chandra et al[16] found significantly higher levels of antineural antibody reactivity in persons with persistent Lyme symptoms compared with post-Lyme healthy and normal healthy controls, a finding suggesting that chronic symptoms may be related to a differential immune response.

Chronic Lyme disease is a label used for a constellation of nonspecific symptoms such as fatigue, night sweats, sore throat, lymphadenopathy, arthralgia, myalgia, palpitations, abdominal pain, nausea, diarrhea, sleep disturbance, poor concentration, irritability, depression, back pain, headache, and dizziness, with or without serologic or clinical evidence of previous infection by *B. burgdorferi*.[17-19] The diagnosis of chronic Lyme disease is nebulous; no standard definition exists, although the disorder is understood to be distinct from post-Lyme disease syndrome or late Lyme disease, in which arthralgia and other symptoms persist after documented *B. burgdorferi* infection.[20]

Patients are frequently diagnosed with chronic Lyme disease based on nonstandard interpretations of serology or other testing that has limited validity and reliability or, more often, based on clinical symptoms alone.[20] Chronic Lyme disease is diagnosed throughout the United States, including in areas where Lyme disease is not endemic.[19,21,22] Often, persons self-diagnose using lists of multiple nonspecific symptoms found on the Internet. Treatment usually includes regimens of multiple antibiotics, often administered parenterally, frequently continuing for months or years, in opposition to standard guidelines for treatment of Lyme disease.[20] This approach is far longer in duration and is associated with substantially greater risks than standard treatment for any other spirochetal infection and virtually all infectious agents treated with antibiotics. Chronic Lyme disease regimens often result in considerable out-of-pocket expenses (often amounting to tens of thousands of dollars per year), patient distress, and potential harm,[23] as well as increasing the risk of selecting for antibiotic-resistant bacteria.[19] Some investigators attribute chronic symptoms to drug-resistant reservoirs of *B. burgdorferi*, including atypical intracellular cystic or spherical forms.[24,25] However, no research has correlated the presence of these reservoirs with persistent symptoms, nor has the eradication of these been associated with improvement in symptoms.[26]

One survey found that 2.1% of Connecticut-based primary care physicians diagnose and treat chronic Lyme disease, whereas most were unsure or did not believe in the existence of chronic Lyme disease.[2] The predominant infectious disease, pediatric, and neurology organizations discount chronic Lyme disease as a distinct clinical entity, whereas other academic, professional, and advocacy organizations argue the contrary. The issue has become politicized, with acrimonious debate among academic organizations and advocacy groups.[27]

The symptoms of chronic Lyme disease can resemble other medically unexplained symptoms (also known as functional somatic syndromes) including chronic fatigue syndrome, irritable bowel syndrome, fibromyalgia, sick building syndrome, and chronic unexplained pain,[28,29] as well as neurologic conditions such as amyotrophic lateral sclerosis[30] or multiple sclerosis.[31] The lack of clear pathophysiology in medically unexplained conditions often results in extensive and expensive diagnostic workups and significant iatrogenic complications.[32,33] As in many chronic conditions in which persons are suffering from pain, psychiatric comorbidities are prevalent and are often overlooked.[2,33-35] At least 13% of outpatient visits are attributable to medically unexplained symptoms.[33,36] Suffering is often exacerbated by a self-validated or provider-validated cycle that attributes common somatic complaints to serious conditions.[35] Significant symptomatic and objective overlap occurs in these conditions, as well as high rates of concurrence of different syndromes.[35,37,38] In one sample, nearly half the patients with chronic Lyme disease were diagnosed with fibromyalgia.[39] Many syndromes manifest with similar constellations of nonspecific symptoms such as muscle weakness, arthralgias, and general fatigue.[40] Patients with these conditions regularly seek out complementary and alternative medicine (CAM) therapies and providers.[41-44]

Diagnosis

Lyme disease is diagnosed using historical and physical findings; serologic testing is used to support the diagnosis in persons without erythema migrans. Early Lyme disease is generally diagnosed based on the presence of erythema migrans; persons at this early state are usually seronegative because erythema migrans appears before an adaptive immune response develops.[45] In a case series in Maryland, 87% of patients with early Lyme disease presented with erythema migrans[46]; Of the Lyme disease cases reported to the CDC between 2003 and 2005, 70% manifested with erythema migrans.[4] The Food and Drug Administration (FDA) does not recommend serologic testing in early Lyme disease because of the low sensitivity of tests in early manifestations.[47]

> Be careful to assess the diagnostic workup of any new patient who presents with chronic persistent symptoms attributed to Lyme disease. Patients often diagnose themselves by using unreliable symptom checklists found on the Internet.

The CDC criteria for Lyme disease are (1) erythema migrans alone or (2) at least one late manifestation in addition to laboratory confirmation of infection. Laboratory confirmation, by this definition, includes isolation of *B. burgdorferi* from a clinical specimen or the presence of immunoglobulin M (IgM) or immunoglobulin G (IgG) antibodies to *B. burgdorferi* in serum or cerebrospinal fluid.[48] The CDC recommends a two-tier process when testing blood for evidence of Lyme disease. Initial testing using an enzyme-linked immunosorbent assay (ELISA) or immunofluorescent assay (IFA) is followed by a Western blot for confirmation.[48] It is important to note that the CDC criteria for Lyme disease are not intended for use by clinicians to make a diagnosis of Lyme disease. Rather, they are intended for national surveillance data,[49] though the majority of cases in practice do fulfill this definition.[45]

ELISA testing is associated with many false-positive results,[50] hence the need for confirmation of a positive or equivocal ELISA result by Western blot. A negative ELISA result, conversely, does not warrant further serologic testing.[20,48] Western blot testing is more specific; that is, it will likely be positive when a person is truly infected. IgM antibodies appear first, typically within 1 to 2 weeks of initial infection. IgG antibodies appear later; usually within 2 to 6 weeks after the onset of erythema migrans. At least 90% of persons with late Lyme disease have positive IgG antibodies.[51] These may remain elevated following successful antibiotic treatment and symptom resolution.[45] Steere et al[8] reported that 16% of a large cohort had systemic symptoms of Lyme disease without initially presenting with erythema migrans and later demonstrated positive serologic findings.[8] Persons who fit into this rubric should have objective symptoms such as arthritis or facial palsy, as opposed to arthralgia.

> Enzyme-linked immunosorbent assay (ELISA) testing is associated with many false-positive results,[50] hence the need for confirmation of a positive or equivocal ELISA result by Western blot. A negative ELISA result, conversely, does not warrant further serologic testing.

The sensitivity of two-tier testing is greatest in late Lyme disease; in the acute phase of erythema migrans, sensitivities range from 29% to 40% and increase to 97% in persons with arthritis (with specificity at 99%).[1] Considerable variability exists between the different commercial assays that are cleared by the FDA, especially for the detection of IgM antibodies.[1] Screening persons who do not have evidence of Lyme disease for possible exposure to Lyme disease is not recommended.[45] Seropositivity indicates past exposure and does not prove an active infectious process,[52] and it should not be used to diagnose active Lyme disease. Serologic testing is most useful in persons with a high pretest probability: persons in whom Lyme disease is likely, based on history and clinical presentation. In this population, positive serologic results support the diagnosis of Lyme disease. In late Lyme disease, a positive IgG test result nearly always occurs. In persons with low prior probability of Lyme disease, serologic testing has more false-positive results.

Testing of ticks for *B. burgdorferi* is generally not reliable for determining whether antibiotic therapy should be initiated.[53] Strict use of the standard diagnostic criteria minimizes false-positive test results, but atypical presentations are missed.[54] Less stringent diagnostic criteria incorporating broader clinical symptoms have been proposed and are in use by a minority of clinicians.[55] No literature is available assessing the diagnostic accuracy of these alternative criteria.

Unconventional Testing

Some unconventional (not FDA-cleared) direct-to-practitioner laboratory tests claim to improve on standard Lyme disease assessment and diagnosis methods. To review them all is beyond the scope of this chapter. These are often propriety tests developed and marketed by a single laboratory. These tests are regularly paid for out of pocket by patients, often with extensive markups by practitioners. Besides the marketing materials from the laboratories themselves, few independent data have assessed the validity of these tests. Literature from one representative test included an advertisement for the test that superficially resembled a peer-reviewed journal article. The article promoted incorporating the laboratory's novel testing into existing diagnostic algorithms and claimed that the novel tests have relevance by "...clarifying clinically ambiguous cases, and confirming therapeutic success." No data justifying these claims were presented, although the choices of immunologic markers appeared reasonable.

The alternative tests appear to report positive results at higher rates than do conventional serologic testing. Despite the documented shortcomings of conventional serology that can lead to false-negative results and the appeal of tests that claim more sensitivity, the alternatives cannot be endorsed at this time. It is unknown whether the higher rates of positive results from alternative tests are caused by more true-positive findings or whether the results are (1) affected by selection effects (in which people more likely to be infected are sent to alternative laboratories); (2) less precise or accurate than conventional testing, (3) false positive, (4) affected by confirmation bias, or (5) a combination thereof. Unfortunately, no independent data are available that assess these factors.

Because of the high out-of-pocket cost, and the uncertain benefit of these tests, none of these unvalidated tests[56] can be recommended without documenting adequate human testing, at minimum ensuring the following: (1) high sensitivity and specificity in diagnosing Lyme disease according to established criteria, (2) minimal intrasample variability, assessed independently[5,57,58]; and (3) comparative effectiveness in relation to and in addition to standard ELISA and Western blot testing.

Integrative Therapy for Acute Lyme Disease

Persons with Lyme disease typically seek CAM for three major reasons. Some seek CAM therapies in addition to conventional therapies—a *complementary* or *integrative* approach. Some believe that conventional therapies are ineffective or dangerous and are seeking more "natural" *alternatives* to mainstream therapies. Some patients present after learning about chronic Lyme disease through the Internet or from advocacy groups promoting treatment protocols employing a myriad mixture of long-term antimicrobials (often parentally),[55,59] nutritional supplements, botanicals, and other unconventional therapies such as hyperbaric oxygen[60] or antifungals.[61]

In many conditions, complementary and alternative medicine (CAM) patients and providers are promoting less invasive therapies than the mainstream standard of care. Lyme disease is an unusual case in which CAM patients and providers are often seeking more invasive and elaborate interventions than conventionally provided.

Because the evidence that differentiates chronic Lyme disease from other medically unexplained conditions is unclear, this section focuses on acute Lyme disease, as defined and diagnosed using standard criteria.[20]

Risk Reduction

Reducing the risk of tick bites in endemic areas and proper removal of ticks within 48 hours following a bite are the most effective means to reduce the incidence of Lyme disease (see the Prevention Prescription box).

No major lifestyle interventions such as specific diets or exercise regimens have been shown to reduce risk of contracting Lyme disease.[62] "Immune-boosting" formulas or other natural products have not been shown to affect the incidence of Lyme disease.

Pharmaceuticals

Lyme disease is best treated with antibiotics. Treatment within 4 weeks of symptom onset is strongly associated with complete recovery.[13] Coinfections (HGA/ehrlichiosis, babesiosis) should be addressed as warranted. Persons experiencing symptoms of late Lyme disease with neurologic, rheumatologic, or cardiac manifestations should be treated by an appropriate specialist. No credible alternatives exist to prompt antibiotic treatment; the risks of inadequate treatment are progression to more severe symptoms and greater risk of long-term sequelae.

Antibiotics
Doxycycline is first-line therapy in early Lyme disease. It is effective for the treatment of erythema migrans, as well as for HGA, which may be concurrent with early Lyme disease.

■ Dosage for Adults[20]
Doxycycline: 100 mg twice per day for 14 days (range, 10 to 21 days)
Amoxicillin: 500 mg three times per day for 14 days (range, 14 to 21 days)
Cefuroxime axetil: 500 mg twice per day for 14 days (range, 14 to 21 days)

■ Precautions
Doxycycline should not be used in children younger than 8 years of age or in pregnant or lactating women. Amoxicillin and cefuroxime axetil are also effective for the treatment of early Lyme disease and can be used in children younger than 8 years of age.[20,42]

In persons with early Lyme disease with neurologic manifestations (meningitis or radiculopathy), oral doxycycline[63] or parenteral ceftriaxone is recommended for adults. Cefotaxime and penicillin G are effective alternatives.[20]

■ Dosage and Precautions for Lyme Disease With Neurologic Manifestations
Doxycycline: 200 mg per day for 14 days
Ceftriaxone: 2 g once per day intravenously for 14 days (range, 10 to 28 days)
Cefotaxime: 2 g intravenously every 8 hours
Penicillin G: 18 to 24 million units per day, divided into doses given every 4 hours for patients with normal renal function

Late Lyme arthritis can be treated with somewhat longer regimens than used in early Lyme disease. Some persons may not respond or may require intravenous antibiotics. For recurrent or persistent arthritis, the Infectious Disease Society of America recommends additional 4-week courses of oral antibiotics for persons whose symptoms have improved with initial oral treatment and intravenous therapy for persons not experiencing substantial improvement with oral antibiotics.[20]

Doxycycline can increase photosensitivity. Avoid exposure to sunlight, sunlamps, or tanning beds while using doxycycline. A sunscreen (minimum SPF 15) can also be helpful. Do not take iron supplements, multivitamins, calcium supplements, antacids, or laxatives within 2 hours before or after taking doxycycline.

Supplements

Probiotics

Antibiotic-associated diarrhea occurs in approximately 25% of patients.[64] Probiotic therapy can mitigate this side effect.[65] Because probiotic effects vary by indication and strain, prescriptions need to be strain specific. The strains most likely to be effective in treating antibiotic-associated diarrhea are *Lactobacillus* GG, *Lactobacillus sporogenes*, and *Saccharomyces boulardii*.[65] Some evidence supports the use of *S. boulardii* in treating *Clostridium difficile*–associated colitis.[66]

■ Dosage

The dose is 5 to 40 billion colony-forming units (CFUs)/day,[65] throughout the duration of antibiotic treatment.[67]

■ Precautions

Probiotics are generally safe, but case reports of endocarditis and sepsis in immunocompromised patients exist.[68] In addition, caution should be exercised in patients with a central venous catheter or those who have compromised intestinal mucosa.[64]

Integrative Therapy for Chronic Persistent Symptoms

Assessing whether Lyme disease was adequately treated and whether the patient actually had objective evidence of Lyme borreliosis is important. Persons without an initial diagnosis of Lyme disease that is based on objective criteria should be discouraged from pursuing a diagnosis of chronic Lyme disease. Persistent symptoms may not be caused by continued active borreliosis; rather, such patients can be treated with symptomatic and antiinflammatory measures. Antibiotic-refractory arthritic symptoms may also be autoimmune or attributed to persistent infection.[15]

For persons with unexplained symptoms who have a low prior probability of Lyme disease, the value of alternative testing is minimal because true-positive results are rare. If test results are positive, psychological benefits can be derived from a diagnosis supporting a defined medical process, whether or not the diagnosis is accurate. This potential benefit may be outweighed by the high possibility of negative externalities from identifying with cases of severe, lifelong debilitation (prevalent in the popular media),[69,70] coupled with highly invasive and potentially harmful treatments of unclear benefit. Clearly, benefit exists in a true positive identification of Lyme disease with subsequent treatment resulting in symptomatic relief, reducing the likelihood of long-term sequelae.

Certain unconventional methods are purported to treat acute or, more often, persistent infection. Some of these methods, purporting to detect "vibrations" in the body (e.g., the Rife machine) or electrodiagnostic devices (e.g., the Vega test) have no scientific basis and no validity in treating Lyme disease or any other disorder. Some elaborate alternative protocols exist,[7,72] but they have not been systematically assessed in controlled trials. Other common herbal therapies with some evidence of antimicrobial activity that are safe include *Artemisia annua*, olive leaf, goldenseal (*Hydrastis canadensis*), and grapefruit seed extract, although they have not demonstrated antispirochetal activity. Some other common interventions in Lyme disease protocols include chaparral (*Larrea divaricata*)[73] and colloidal silver,[74] which have significant risks of toxicity and harm; these should be actively discouraged.

The following are a sampling of integrative therapies that can be antiinflammatory or analgesic with a high potential benefit-to-risk ratio. Given the paucity of clinical trials assessing CAM interventions in persons with persistent symptoms following Lyme borreliosis, the therapies chosen here are safe and have demonstrated efficacy in inflammatory conditions or medically unexplained conditions that symptomatically resemble chronic Lyme disease. A more comprehensive list of potential therapies can be found in Chapter 46, Fibromyalgia, and Chapter 47, Effective Treatment of Chronic Fatigue Syndrome, Fatigue Fibromyalgia, and Muscle/Myofascial Pain: A Comprehensive Medicine Approach.

Acknowledging and addressing the real suffering and debilitating symptoms of patients is critical,[69,70] regardless of whether the cause of their symptoms is clear or ambiguous. The benefits of a salutogenic patient-practitioner relationship are described in Chapter 3, The Healing Encounter.

Pharmaceuticals

Antiinflammatory Treatments

Nonsteroidal antiinflammatory drugs (NSAIDs), intra-articular steroid injections, and DMARDs have all been used to treat persistent symptoms associated with Lyme disease.[14]

Antibiotics

Four randomized controlled trials were carried out on patients with post-Lyme disease syndrome who underwent long-term antibiotic regimens.[12,19,75–77] Krupp et al[75] demonstrated improvements in fatigue in persons treated with intravenous ceftriaxone after 28 days compared with placebo, without improvement in cognitive function or a laboratory measure of infection. Six of the 52 patients who began the interventions (11.5%) discontinued the study because of adverse events; of these, 4 patients (3 receiving placebo) required hospitalization for line sepsis.[75] None of the other studies demonstrated significant benefit for long-term antibiotic treatment in patients with ongoing subjective symptoms following standard treatment of initial Lyme disease.[12]

Case reports documenting symptomatic relief using long-term antibiotic therapy are common.[78] Cameron[79] reported significant improvements in quality of life in patients experiencing persistent Lyme disease symptoms when they were treated with amoxicillin for 3 months, although this study was criticized for several methodologic flaws that may render its conclusions moot.[80] Certain antibiotics, including macrolides and tetracyclines, used to treat Lyme disease exhibit antiinflammatory effects,[81] whereas beta-lactams[82] and tetracyclines[83] exhibit neuroprotective effects. Thus, symptomatic relief with antibiotics can be achieved through pharmacologic actions other than antimicrobial effects.

Precautions
The risks of long-term antibiotic therapy are well documented and include anaphylaxis, biliary complications resulting in cholecystectomy,[84] fatal sepsis,[23] and infection of intravenous catheters.[19] Longer courses of antibiotics increase the risk of adverse events.[15] NSAIDs, DMARDs, and intra-articular injections also pose considerable risk and may be undesirable if treatments with a better risk-to-benefit ratio exist.

If the presence of persistent borreliosis cannot be established using objective criteria, nonpharmacologic therapies are initially recommended for symptomatic relief. Pharmaceuticals can be considered if nonpharmacologic means do not provide adequate relief. Antibiotics should be used only if active borreliosis is confirmed.

Gabapentin
In an open pilot study in 10 patients with neuroborreliosis, all 10 patients were treated with gabapentin (starting at 300 mg/day and increasing to a maximum tolerated dose). Weissenbacher et al[85] reported that pain symptoms improved in 90% of patients, and sleep quality and general health improved in 50% of patients.

Dosage
The dose is 300 mg/day, titrating up to a maximum tolerated dose within 4 to 12 weeks. In the study by Weissenbacher et al,[85] the average dose associated with pain reduction was 700 mg, with a maximum doses between 500 and 1200 mg.

Precautions
Gabapentin is associated with various adverse effects, including depression and increased risk of suicide.[86] Abrupt discontinuation of gabapentin can cause withdrawal symptoms.[85]

Botanicals
The herb *Uncaria tomentosa* (cat's claw) is prominent in numerous alternative protocols for Lyme disease.[71] It has antioxidant, antiinflammatory, and immunostimulant activity.[87] No evidence exists for specific antispirochetal activity. In a randomized trial in persons with rheumatoid arthritis, a specific extract of *Uncaria tomentosa* demonstrated efficacy in reducing painful joints.[88]

Dosage
An extract free of tetracyclic oxindole alkaloids is taken at 60 mg daily in three divided doses.[88]

Nutrition
Antiinflammatory Diet
An antiinflammatory diet is characterized by emphasizing omega-3 fatty acids (found primarily in deep-water fish) and minimizing omega-6 fatty acids, with a focus on unprocessed whole grains, beans, and fruits and vegetables. Fish oil, especially eicosapentaenoic acid (EPA), is often added as a supplementary measure. Significant overlap exists between the antiinflammatory diet and the Mediterranean diet that can reduce risk of cardiovascular disease.[89,90]

Antiinflammatory diets have demonstrated clinical benefits in persons with inflammatory diseases such as rheumatoid arthritis.[89,91] More extensive antiinflammatory dietary measures, such as a gluten-free vegan diet, have been shown to reduce inflammatory markers in patients with rheumatoid arthritis,[92] as well as improve symptoms[93] (see Chapter 86, The Antiinflammatory Diet).

Aerobic and Weight-Bearing Exercise
Moderate aerobic exercise was shown to improve physical function, mood, symptom severity, and self-efficacy in patients with fibromyalgia,[94] as well as enhance energy in patients with unexplained fatigue.[95] Other trials confirmed the benefits of aerobic exercise and muscle strengthening for fibromyalgia.[96-98] Pain, the most characteristic symptom of fibromyalgia, was reduced in persons exercising at low-to-moderate intensity two or three times per week, and positive effects on depressed mood, quality of life, and physical fitness were noted.[99] Aerobic exercise, performed twice weekly over 8 months, can alleviate symptoms as well as demonstrate antiinflammatory effects.[100]

A systematic review confirmed that among myriad treatments proposed for fibromyalgia, exercise, specifically aerobic and weight-bearing exercise of mild to moderate intensity, has consistently shown to be effective in alleviating pain, fatigue, and depression and in improving health-related quality of life in persons with fibromyalgia[101] (see Chapter 88, Writing an Exercise Prescription).

Dosage
Mild aerobic exercise with weight training is performed two to three times weekly for at least 4 weeks.[101] Initiate at 15 minutes and increase to 30 minutes as tolerance grows.

Supplements
Probiotics
Preliminary studies suggested efficacy of the probiotic *Lactobacillus casei* strain Shirota (LcS) in treating anxiety associated with chronic fatigue syndrome.[102] Some protocols for chronic Lyme disease include probiotics.[59]

Dosage
The dose is 24 billion CFUs of *Lactobacillus casei* strain Shirota (LcS) per day. This probiotic is available in a fermented milk commercial product (Yakult).

Omega-3 Fatty Acids
Omega-3 fatty acid intake is inversely associated with major depression,[103,104] a strong comorbidity with chronic fatigue syndrome and fibromyalgia.[105] Further, serum levels of EPA

are significantly lower in patients with chronic fatigue syndrome than in healthy controls.[106] Omega-3 fatty acid supplementation has some evidence of efficacy in treating certain nonspecific symptoms associated with persistent Lyme disease including fatigue, arthralgias,[107] depression,[108] and anxiety.[56]

Dosage

The dose is 2500 mg of omega-3 fatty acids (with 50% or more EPA), consistent with a case series[109] documenting clinically significant pain reduction and improved function associated with various conditions, including fibromyalgia.

Intravenous Micronutrient Therapy

A clinical trial of a popular intravenous formula (the Myers cocktail)[110-112] found both a large treatment effect and a large placebo effect in pain, mood, and global function, with effect sizes comparable to those seen with FDA-approved drugs for fibromyalgia.[111]

Dosage

The Myers cocktail is infused intravenously weekly by slow push (10 minutes). Persons responding to the Myers cocktail should experience significant symptomatic relief within 4 weeks. The Myers cocktail contains the following:
5 mL magnesium chloride hexahydrate (20%)
3 mL calcium gluconate (10%)
1 mL hydroxocobalamin (1000 mcg/mL)
1 mL pyridoxine hydrochloride (100 mg/mL)
1 mL dexpanthenol (250 mg/mL)
1 mL B-complex 100, containing: 100 mg thiamine HCl, 2 mg riboflavin, 2 mg pyridoxine HCl, 2 mg panthenol, 100 mg niacinamide, and 2% benzyl alcohol
5 mL vitamin C (500 mg/mL)
20 mL sterile water

Biomechanical Therapies

Acupuncture

Acupuncture[113] and sham acupuncture[114] have been shown to improve pain symptoms associated with fibromyalgia. Although analgesic effects often do not differ from placebo acupuncture,[115] the therapy has minimal risk,[114] reduces anxiety,[115] and may be effective for fatigue[116] in chronic disease.[117]

Dosage

A 20-minute weekly session is typical.

Massage Therapy

Massage therapy demonstrated short-term beneficial effects in treating fibromyalgia symptoms in randomized trials.[118] Despite the lack of a complete understanding of the mechanisms, massage has clearly been shown to improve osteoarthritis pain.[119-123] Massage therapy has been evaluated and found efficacious as an adjunct treatment for pain secondary to cancer,[124-136] low back pain,[137-139] procedural pain,[140,141] rheumatoid arthritis,[142,143] and fibromyalgia.[144,145] It also has been shown to be beneficial for patients with chronic pain following spinal cord injury.[146] In a randomized, open-label clinical trial, a series of classical Swedish massage therapy sessions was found to be as effective as conventional analgesia for chronic rheumatic pain.[142]

Dosage

Swedish massage or another massage approach (30 to 60 minutes) is recommended once or twice weekly.

Mind-Body Therapy

Psychological trauma is associated with persistent Lyme disease symptoms[147] and fibromyalgia,[148] and chronic stress tends to exacerbate symptoms.[149,150] Mind-body therapies are especially attractive when psychological trauma predates the onset of symptoms because both somatic and psychological benefits are often seen[151] (see Chapter 100, Emotional Awareness for Pain, and Chapter 101, Energy Psychology).

Tai Chi

Wang et al[152] demonstrated significant benefits of tai chi, a Chinese mind-body practice involving meditation, deep breathing, and slow, gentle, graceful movements, for fibromyalgia. Tai chi has also shown promise in improving symptoms of rheumatoid arthritis.[61,153]

Dosage

A group course with an experienced teacher is recommended twice weekly for at least 12 weeks.

Mindfulness Meditation

Several trials have assessed the effects of various regimens of mindfulness meditation, with promising results in outcomes ranging from pain severity, physical function, and tender point threshold[154-157] in persons with fibromyalgia.

Mindfulness-based stress reduction (MBSR) is a standardized protocol of mind-body therapies that involves mindfulness meditation, patient education, and group support.[158-160] MBSR was developed by Kabat-Zinn et al at the Stress Reduction Clinic of the University of Massachusetts Medical Center. Several randomized trials demonstrated the benefit of MBSR for various chronic conditions, with improvements in psychological and somatic measures.[161-170]

Dosage

The standard 8-week course of MBSR consists of an instructor delivering group instruction for 2.5 hours weekly (consisting of meditation practice, group discussions, and mindfulness skill-building activities),[160] a single half-day meditation retreat, and daily practice for 30 to 45 minutes 6 days per week.[158]

Therapies to Consider

If chronic persistent symptoms continue without resolution, and if other conditions are definitively ruled out, a consultation with a Chinese medicine practitioner may be helpful. Some traditional Chinese medicine practitioners report treatments for spirochetal infections and related sequelae. No formal studies have assessed the efficacy and safety of such therapies, and caution should be expressed with using Chinese herbal medicines that may be adulterated with contaminants. Only herbal products employing standard quality control measures (e.g., good manufacturing practices) should be used.

PREVENTION PRESCRIPTION

Reduce the risk of tick bites in endemic areas:

- Clear brush and trees, remove leaf litter and woodpiles, and keep grass mowed.
- Wear light-colored clothing that covers the skin to aid in identifying and protecting from tick bites. Tuck pant legs into socks when outdoors in vegetated areas.
- Apply tick and insect repellants containing DEET [*N,N*-diethyl-3-methyltoluamide], although excessive doses have been reported to cause neurologic complications in children.[171]
- Permethrin, a synthetic pyrethroid applied to clothing, is effective in killing ticks. Toxicities have been reported at high doses.[17,172]
- A plant-based insect repellant containing oil of lemon eucalyptus has been shown to protect from mosquitoes, but it has not demonstrated efficacy against ticks.[171]
- The most effective methods shown to reduce the risk of Lyme disease in endemic areas are the use of protective clothing and of tick repellants on the skin and clothing.[173]
- Check skin for ticks after being outdoors in the late spring and summer months in endemic areas.

Figure 22-3 illustrates the life cycle of ticks that can transmit Lyme disease.

- Bathe within 2 hours after spending time in vegetation.[174]
- Pesticides are effective, but recommendations are tempered by environmental concerns and the risk of harming children and wildlife.

Reduce the risk of Lyme disease after a tick bite:

- Remove ticks with fine-tipped tweezers. Using a steady motion, grasp the tick as close as possible to the skin. Pull directly away from the skin. Do not use petroleum jelly, nail polish, or heated instruments to remove a tick.
- Monitor for signs and symptoms of Lyme disease after a tick bite.
- Consider antimicrobial prophylaxis (200 mg doxycycline in a single dose for adults or 4 mg/kg up to a maximum dose of 200 mg for children older than 8 years old, and 250 mg of amoxicillin in children younger than 8 years old) if a tick is attached for more than 48 hours in an endemic area,[20] although risk of *Borrelia burgdorferi* infection is low; 1.2% of untreated children in a large cohort developed Lyme disease after a tick bite in a highly endemic area. Treatment subsequent to symptom onset was associated with a complete recovery.[175]

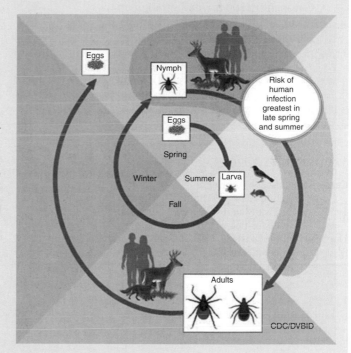

FIGURE 22-3
Life cycle of black-legged ticks that can transmit anaplasmosis, babesiosis, and Lyme disease. (From the Centers for Disease Control and Prevention, Division of Vector-Borne Diseases. *Life Cycle of Hard Ticks That Spread Disease.* <http://www.cdc.gov/ticks/life_cycle_and_hosts.html>; 2011 Accessed 27.07.11.)

THERAPEUTIC REVIEW

▪ Acute Lyme Disease

- Antibiotics for early Lyme disease
  - Doxycycline: 100 mg twice per day for 14 days (range, 10 to 21 days),

  - Amoxicillin: 500 mg three times per day for 14 days (range, 14 to 21 days),
  - Cefuroxime axetil: 500 mg twice per day for 14 days (range, 14 to 21 days),

- Antibiotics for early Lyme disease with neurologic manifestations
  - Doxycycline: 200 mg per day for 14 days

Continued

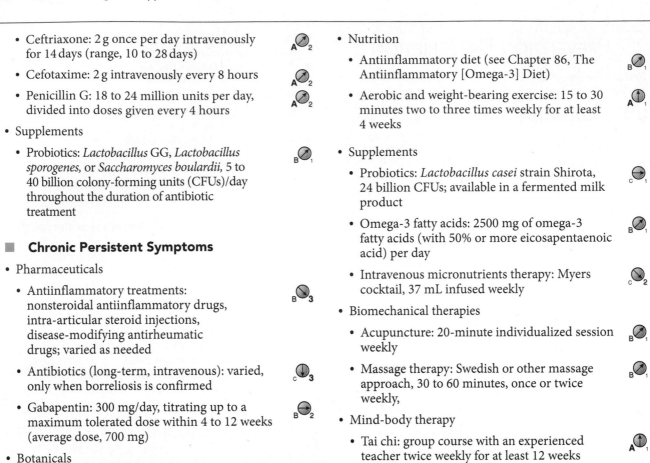

- Ceftriaxone: 2 g once per day intravenously for 14 days (range, 10 to 28 days) A₂
- Cefotaxime: 2 g intravenously every 8 hours A₂
- Penicillin G: 18 to 24 million units per day, divided into doses given every 4 hours A₂
- Supplements
  - Probiotics: *Lactobacillus* GG, *Lactobacillus sporogenes,* or *Saccharomyces boulardii,* 5 to 40 billion colony-forming units (CFUs)/day throughout the duration of antibiotic treatment B₁

▪ Chronic Persistent Symptoms

- Pharmaceuticals
  - Antiinflammatory treatments: nonsteroidal antiinflammatory drugs, intra-articular steroid injections, disease-modifying antirheumatic drugs; varied as needed B₃
  - Antibiotics (long-term, intravenous): varied, only when borreliosis is confirmed C₃
  - Gabapentin: 300 mg/day, titrating up to a maximum tolerated dose within 4 to 12 weeks (average dose, 700 mg) B₂
- Botanicals
  - *Uncaria tomentosa* (cat's claw): 60 mg daily in three divided doses of an extract free of tetracyclic oxindole alkaloids B₂

- Nutrition
  - Antiinflammatory diet (see Chapter 86, The Antiinflammatory [Omega-3] Diet) B₁
  - Aerobic and weight-bearing exercise: 15 to 30 minutes two to three times weekly for at least 4 weeks A₁
- Supplements
  - Probiotics: *Lactobacillus casei* strain Shirota, 24 billion CFUs; available in a fermented milk product C₁
  - Omega-3 fatty acids: 2500 mg of omega-3 fatty acids (with 50% or more eicosapentaenoic acid) per day B₁
  - Intravenous micronutrients therapy: Myers cocktail, 37 mL infused weekly C₂
- Biomechanical therapies
  - Acupuncture: 20-minute individualized session weekly B₁
  - Massage therapy: Swedish or other massage approach, 30 to 60 minutes, once or twice weekly, B₁
- Mind-body therapy
  - Tai chi: group course with an experienced teacher twice weekly for at least 12 weeks A₁
  - Mindfulness meditation or mindfulness-based stress reduction: group course with a weekly meeting and daily practice B₁

KEY WEB RESOURCES

Centers for Disease Control and Prevention, Division of Vector-Borne Infectious Diseases. http://www.cdc.gov/lyme

Lyme Disease Tick Map (iTunes app). http://itunes.apple.com/us/app/lyme-disease-tick-map/id369913510?mt=8

University of Rhode Island Tick Encounter Resource Center. http://www.tickencounter.org/

Acknowledgment

The helpful suggestions from Joshua P. Levitt, ND are appreciated.

References

References are available at expertconsult.com.

Section IV Cardiovascular Disease

Chapter 23

Hypertension

Gregory A. Plotnikoff, MD, MTS, and Jeffery Dusek, PhD

Hypertension is the most important risk factor for cardiovascular morbidity and mortality in industrialized countries. At least 65 million U.S. residents have blood pressures (BPs) that place them at significantly higher risk of coronary artery disease, heart failure, renal failure, thoracic and abdominal aneurysms, myocardial infarction, and stroke. Hypertension is also associated with cognitive dysfunction, erectile dysfunction, and loss of vision. The higher the pressure is, the greater is the risk of complications.[1]

The seventh report of the Joint National Committee on Prevention, Detection, Evaluation, and Treatment of High Blood Pressure (JNC 7) defined a normal BP as less than 120 mm Hg systolic and less than 80 mm Hg diastolic. The report similarly defined stage 1 hypertension as 140 to 159 mm Hg systolic and 90 to 99 mm Hg diastolic. In between normal and stage 1 values is a category the JNC 7 report termed prehypertension. The intent of using this newer term is to heighten awareness of both risk and opportunities for prevention. The JNC 7 report also noted that for persons with diabetes or renal disease and hypertension, the BP treatment goal is less than 130/80 mm Hg[1] (Table 23–1).

> Prehypertension is a condition characterized by systolic blood pressure of 120 to 139 mm Hg and diastolic blood pressure of 80 to 89 mm Hg.

Hypertension has both modifiable and nonmodifiable risk factors. Gender and genetic heritage are certainly nonmodifiable factors. In addition, hypertension is a disease of aging: more than 65% of persons 65 years old or older are hypertensive.[1] Surprisingly, a person who is normotensive at age 55 years still has a 90% lifetime risk of developing hypertension.[2] Although chronologic age is not modifiable, physiologic aging itself may be. Hypertension is certainly also a disease of lifestyle: conventional risk modifications include reducing sodium intake, increasing exercise, moderating alcohol consumption, losing weight, and following the Dietary Approaches to Stop Hypertension (DASH) eating plan. Each of these lifestyle modifications demonstrably reduces BP. Similarly, because smoking, pain, and stress can significantly increase BP, efforts have been made to study the impact of smoking cessation, pain management, and stress management on hypertension.

More than 4 decades of randomized clinical trials have documented that pharmaceutical interventions prevent target organ damage including the number one and number three killers: heart attack and stroke. A reduction of just 5 mm Hg in systolic BP (SBP) is associated with a 7% reduction in all-cause mortality.[3] However, outside of clinical trials, only approximately one third of patients will achieve optimal BP control by using drug therapy.[1] Additionally, lowering of BP itself may not reduce the associated risk of neurocognitive dysfunction.[4] Clearly, an efficacy gap exists between BP reductions achievable in clinical trials and those reductions achievable in clinical practice.

> A reduction of systolic blood pressure of 5 mm Hg is associated with a 7% reduction in all-cause mortality.

This efficacy gap in hypertension treatment represents an ideal opportunity to codevelop with a patient a customized action plan that addresses logical options in diet, exercise, supplementation, smoking cessation, and mind-body skills development. Additional insights may also come from both Ayurvedic and traditional East Asian medicine traditions. This chapter addresses how each of these individual interventions can contribute to improved health and wellbeing. When used in combination, however, these recommendations may be synergistic for other health goals. As an example, for sedentary and overweight or obese persons, the combination of aerobic exercise with the DASH diet and caloric restriction or weight loss not only lowers BP but also improves both insulin sensitivity[5] and neurocognitive function.[6]

TABLE 23-1. Classification and Management of Blood Pressure for Adults*

BP CLASSIFICATION	SBP* (mm Hg)	DBP* (mm Hg)	LIFESTYLE MODIFICATION	Initial Drug Therapy WITHOUT COMPELLING INDICATION	WITH COMPELLING INDICATIONS
Normal	Less than 120	And less than 80	Encourage	No antihypertensive drug indicated	Drug(s) for compelling indications‡
Prehypertension	120–139	or 80–89	Yes		
Stage 1 hypertension	140–159	or 90–99	Yes	Thiazide-type diuretics for most; may consider ACEI, ARB, BB, CCB, or combination	Drugs for the compelling indications‡; Other antihypertensive drugs (diuretic, ACEI, ARB, BB, CCB) as needed
Stage 2 hypertension	160 of higher	or 100 of higher	Yes	Two-drug combination for most† (usually thiazide-type diuretic and ACEI or ARB or BB or CCB)	

From U.S. Department of Health and Human Services, National High Blood Pressure Education Program. *The Seventh Report of the Joint National Committee on Prevention, Detection, Evaluation, and Treatment of High Blood Pressure (JNC VII).* NIH publication no. 03–5233. Rockville, MD: National Heart, Lung and Blood Institute, National Institutes of Health; 2003:3.
ACEI, angiotensin-converting enzyme inhibitor; ARB, angiotensin receptor blocker; BB, beta blocker; BP, blood pressure; CCB, calcium channel blocker; DBP, diastolic blood pressure; SBP, systolic blood pressure.
*Treatment determined by highest BP category.
†Initial combined therapy should be used cautiously in those at risk for orthostatic hypotension.
‡Treat patients with chronic kidney disease or diabetes to BP goal of less than 130/80 mm Hg.

Hypertension frequently is asymptomatic; in the absence of symptoms, elevated numbers may not have any significance for a patient. In many cultures of the world, if no pain is felt, no disease is present. Encouraging any intervention to treat an abstract number, particularly a long-term intervention with no immediate benefit, is inherently problematic. For this reason, exploring the meanings, beliefs, and interpretations the patient brings to the experience of hypertension is crucial. The patient's answers should both guide the clinician's approach and foster a working partnership.

Also key is the patient's awareness of whether a BP issue even exists for him or her. Home BP monitoring with records in a diary is one means of raising awareness. Another method is use a 24-hour home BP monitor with a digital record. These approaches help confirm for the patient and the clinician that what is seen in the clinic is also what is happening at home.

To convey the meaning of the results, SBP values can be entered into the National Cholesterol Education Program Risk Assessment Tool for estimating the 10-year risk of either a myocardial infarction or coronary death (see Key Web Resources, later). Patients and clinicians can follow the risk assessment (based on Framingham Study data) for varying values including age, smoking status, and cholesterol status. These data can make concrete the value of normalizing BP and can show the relative value (and additive value) compared with reducing cholesterol now and as one ages.

Because many persons want to avoid pharmaceutical therapies, they seek integrative clinicians who can counsel from an evidence base on the logical options available to them. What follows are nonpharmaceutical approaches that include and go beyond the basic lifestyle modification recommendations found in the JNC 7 report.

Integrative Therapy

Lifestyle Modification

Smoking Cessation

Smoking cessation, of course, should be part of every comprehensive lifestyle modification plan. Cigarette use causes a 4 mm Hg increase in SBP and a 3 mm Hg increase in diastolic blood pressure (DBP) compared with placebo.[7] Persons with hypertension who smoke, however, have an additional increased risk of cardiovascular events compared with those with hypertension who do not smoke. This risk includes both ischemic stroke and hemorrhagic stroke and correlates directly with the number of cigarettes smoked.[8,9]

Diet

Two very well-studied diets for hypertension prevention and control, the Mediterranean and DASH diets, are quite different from the standard American diet because they are high in vegetables, fruits, and low-fat dairy products and are low in saturated fat and refined grains. This means that they are not high in sodium, but are instead are rich in potassium, magnesium, calcium, and fiber. Unlike the standard American diet, these diets incorporate both healthy fats and more complex, less refined carbohydrates.

▪ Mediterranean Diet

The Mediterranean diet's capacity to prevent or treat hypertension was evaluated in 9408 men and women enrolled in a prospective cohort study from 1999 to 2005.[10] The study documented that, after adjustment for major hypertension risk factors and nutritional covariates, the degree of adherence to the Mediterranean diet over 6 years was associated with modest BP reduction. For study participants with high adherence, mean SBP declined by 3.1 mm Hg (95% confidence interval

[CI], −5.4 to −0.8), and mean DBP declined by 1.9 mm Hg (95% CI, −3.6 to −0.1).[10]

Beyond hypertension, a systematic review of 35 different experimental studies demonstrated that the Mediterranean diet has favorable effects on lipoprotein levels, endothelium vasodilation, insulin resistance, metabolic syndrome, antioxidant capacity, myocardial and cardiovascular mortality, and cancer incidence in obese patients and in those with previous myocardial infarction.[11] Additionally, the study by the National Institutes of Health and AARP (formerly the American Association of Retired Persons) of 214,284 men and 166,012 women demonstrated that, over 10 years, adherence to the Mediterranean diet was associated with approximately a 20% reduction in all-cause mortality in both men and women.[12] In comparing high with low conformity adherence in men, cardiovascular and cancer mortality were 0.78 (95% CI, 0.69 to 0.87) and 0.83 (95% CI, 0.76 to 0.91), respectively. Women similarly demonstrated a reduction of 12% for cancer mortality ($P = .04$).[12] From the HALE (Healthy Aging: Longitudinal Study in Europe) study of persons 70 to 90 years old, adherence to the Mediterranean diet and a healthful lifestyle was associated with a more than 50% lower rate of all-cause and cause-specific mortality[13] (see Chapter 86, The Antiinflammatory [Omega-3] Diet).

■ Olive Oil

One of the main components of the Mediterranean diet is olive oil, which provides both high levels of monounsaturated fatty acids, principally oleic acid, and healthy polyphenols. Oleic acid was shown to have antihypertensive effects in laboratory animals.[14] Phenolic compounds in olive oil prevent lipoperoxidation, induce favorable changes of lipid profile, improve endothelial function, and have antithrombotic properties.[15] In the Prevención con Dieta Mediterránea (PREDIMED) study of 772 asymptomatic persons 55 to 80 years of age who were at high cardiovascular risk, participants allocated to Mediterranean diets supplemented with either nuts or virgin olive oil, compared with participants allocated to a control low-fat diet, demonstrated mean reductions in systolic pressure of 5.9 mm Hg (CI, −8.7 to −3.1 mm Hg) and 7.1 mm Hg (CI, −10.0 to −4.1 mm Hg), respectively.[16]

Olive oil represents a logical substitute for butter and partially hydrogenated vegetable oils. The Food and Drug Administration (FDA) allows manufacturers to state on labels that consuming approximately 2 tablespoons (23 g) of olive oil a day may reduce the risk of heart disease. In general, use virgin olive oil for hot cooking and extra virgin olive oil for cold cooking such as in salad dressing or for dipping.

The consumption of a diet rich in polyphenols, including those found in olive oil and cocoa beans, appears to be important for hypertension prevention and control. Polyphenols can induce nitric oxide–mediated endothelium-dependent relaxation in most arteries including the coronary arteries. They can also induce endothelium-derived hyperpolarizing factor–mediated relaxations in many arteries.[17,18]

■ Cocoa (Theobroma cacao)

In observational studies, regular intake of cocoa-containing foods was linked to lower cardiovascular mortality. In a cohort of 470 Dutch men who were followed up for 15 years, cocoa intake was inversely associated with BP and was positively associated with reduced risk of both cardiovascular and all-cause mortality.[18a]

The first meta-analysis published reviewed five randomized controlled studies of cocoa administration ($N = 173$) with an average intake of 100 g daily (500 mg of polyphenols) for a median duration of 2 weeks.[19] The results demonstrated reductions in the pooled mean SBP and DBP of 4.7 mm Hg (95% CI, −7.6 to −1.8 mm Hg; $P = .002$) and 2.8 mm Hg (95% CI, −4.8 to −0.8 mm Hg; $P = .006$), respectively, compared with controls. Of the five studies cited, only two trials enrolled hypertensive patients.[19]

Following this report, the authors of the meta-analysis enrolled 44 adults with untreated upper-range prehypertension or stage 1 hypertension in a prospective 18-week randomized controlled trial of either 6.3 g (30 kcal) per day of dark chocolate containing 30 mg of polyphenols or matching polyphenol-free white chocolate.[20] Even this low-dose dark chocolate intake reduced the hypertension prevalence from 86% to 68%, with mean SBP decreasing by 2.9 (1.6) mm Hg ($P < .001$) and DBP declining by 1.9 (1.0) mm Hg ($P < .001$). This decrease was accomplished without changes in body weight, plasma levels of lipids, glucose, and 8-isoprostane (a measure of oxidative stress). The BP decrease was also accompanied by a sustained increase of the vasodilative nitric oxide donor S-nitrosoglutathione by 0.23 (0.12) nmol/L ($P < .001$). In comparison, the polyphenol-free white chocolate intake caused no changes in BP or plasma biomarkers.[20]

The benefit of flavanol-containing cocoa appears to extend to persons with diabetes as well. A 30-day, thrice-daily regimen of consumption of flavanol-containing cocoa (321 mg flavanols per dose) versus a matched product with 25 mg of flavanols per dose in 41 persons treated for diabetes increased baseline brachial artery flow-mediated dilation by 30% ($P < .0001$) without evidence of tachyphylaxis or decline in glycemic control.[21]

The most recent pooled meta-analysis included 13 trials (15 treatment arms) and documented the most significant findings for hypertensive or prehypertensive subgroups (SBP: −5.0 ± 3.0 mm Hg; $P = .0009$; DBP: −2.7 ± 2.2 mm Hg; $P = .01$) compared with placebo.[22] BP was not reduced to less than 140 mm Hg systolic or 80 mm Hg diastolic. Daily flavanol dosages ranged from 30 to 1000 mg in the active treatment groups (dark chocolate with 50% to 70% cocoa).[22]

> Consider recommending one fourth of a standard-sized dark chocolate bar consisting of 70% cocoa daily.

■ Red Wine

Although alcohol consumption can cause multiple organ damage and can raise BP, red wine consumption is inversely associated with mortality from cardiovascular diseases.[23] Some studies have shown this effect even at high intakes, as much as 300 mL of wine per day.[24] Risk reduction is greatest for red wine at low to moderate intake.[25] One possible explanation is that red wine is an extremely rich source of bioactive polyphenols. Noteworthy compounds include the flavonoids quercetin, catechin and epicatechin, proanthocyanidins, and anthocyanins and phenolic acids, including gallic, caftaric, and caffeic acid, as well as the trihydroxystilbene termed *resveratrol*. These substances are not found in white wines because the fermentation process for white wines, unlike that for red wines, does not include the polyphenol-rich grape skins, seeds, and stems.[26]

Each polyphenol may play some role in preventing or treating hypertension. For example, quercetin, catechin, and resveratrol promote nitric oxide production by vascular endothelium. Although animal studies documented many potentially beneficial effects with oral administration of quercetin or resveratrol, they did not document a reduction in BP.[27,28]

■ DASH Diet
The DASH diet trial enrolled 459 participants and provided each with all his or her food for 11 weeks.[29] For the first 3 weeks, the participants were provided a control diet that was low in fruits, vegetables, and dairy products, with a fat content typical of the average diet in the United States. Participants were then randomly assigned to receive for 8 weeks the control diet, a diet rich in fruits and vegetables, or a "combination" diet rich in fruits, vegetables, and low-fat dairy products and with reduced saturated and total fat. Sodium intake and body weight were maintained at constant levels. For the 326 participants with prehypertension, the DASH diet resulted in reduced SBP and DBP of 3.5 mm Hg ($P < .001$) and 2.1 mm Hg ($P = .003$), respectively. Among the 133 subjects with stage 1 hypertension, the DASH diet reduced SBP and DBP by 11.4 and 5.5 mm Hg, respectively, more than the control diet ($P < .001$ for each).[29] These results have since been replicated in numerous settings (see Chapter 87, The DASH Diet).

■ Omega-3 Fatty Acids
A diet rich in cold-water fatty fish or grass-fed animals is also rich in omega-3 polyunsaturated fatty acids that may prevent the development of hypertension. Omega-3 fatty acid deficiency contributed to the development of hypertension in animal models.[30] This effect appears to be true for humans as well. A 20-year follow-up of a cohort of 4508 adults 18 to 30 years old who did not have hypertension at baseline documented an inverse association of long-chain omega-3 fatty acid intake with the development of hypertension. For the highest intake quartile compared with the lowest, after adjustment for potential confounders, the hazard ratio was just 0.65 (95% CI, 0.53 to 0.79; P(trend) $< .01$).[31] A double-blind placebo-controlled intervention of 4 g of omega-3 fatty acids for 8 weeks in patients with chronic kidney disease with an initial mean supine BP of 125.0/72.3 mm Hg demonstrated significant reductions in 24-hour SBP (-3.3 ± 0.7 mm Hg) and DBP (-2.9 ± 0.5 mm Hg), along with a 24% reduction in triglycerides.[32]

> Omega-3 fatty acids may be particularly useful in patients with the metabolic syndrome because of the effect of these fatty acids on improving insulin sensitivity and on reducing blood pressure and triglycerides.

■ Fiber
A meta-analysis of 25 randomized controlled trials published up to the year 2004 documented that supplemental intake of dietary fiber significantly reduced both SBP and DBP in hypertensive patients.[33] The degree of reduction was significant: SBP, -9.5 mm Hg (95% CI, -9.50 to -2.40); and DBP, -4.20 mm Hg (95% CI, -6.55 to -1.85). The investigators suggested that a period of at least 8 weeks was necessary to achieve the maximal BP reduction.[33] A 2007 study in hypertensive, overweight patients of psyllium powder, at a dose of 3.5 g 20 minutes before each meal, documented significant SBP and DBP reduction compared with controls.[34]

Exercise
Both JNC 7 and the American College of Sports Medicine recommended aerobic endurance exercise for the primary prevention, treatment, and control of hypertension. BP reductions of approximately 5 to 7 mm Hg systolic can follow an isolated exercise session (acute) or exercise training (chronic). This BP reduction can last up to 22 hours following endurance exercise. The higher the initial BP is, the greater is the response.

The American College of Sports Medicine recommended the following exercise prescription for persons with high BP[35]:
Frequency: on most, preferably all, days of the week
Intensity: moderate (40% to less than 60% oxygen consumption reserve [VO_2R])
Time: 30 minutes or more of continuous or accumulated physical activity per day
Type: primarily endurance physical activity supplemented by resistance exercise[35] (see Chapter 88, Writing an Exercise Prescription)

Weight Loss
A 2008 meta-analysis of all weight loss studies demonstrated that dietary interventions to reduce body weight resulted in better BP reduction than did either of the prescription drugs orlistat or sibutramine.[36] Weight loss of 4 kg (10 lb) by diet reduced SBP by approximately 6 mm Hg. Similar weight loss with orlistat reduced SBP by approximately 2.5 mm Hg. Sibutramine treatment reduced body weight but did not lower BP and may have even elevated it. The investigators noted that no prospective studies demonstrated that mortality or other patient-relevant end points could be lowered by weight reduction.[36]

Supplements

Several limitations exist in the literature on interventional nutrition. First, few studies measure and report serum levels at baseline and conclusion. The failure to document the presence or absence of a serum or intracellular deficiency or functional insufficiency means that dosing is blind. If one size does not fit all, then studies are at high risk for false-negative results because of underdosing. Additionally, treatment of a patient population with sufficient levels presumably means that additional dosing will not bring benefit. Without measurement of serum levels, adherence to the intervention protocol cannot be assessed. Second, few studies intervene with a dose based on achievement of a targeted serum level. Most dosing is extrapolated from in vitro studies or epidemiologic studies of intake in a large population. Individual variability in uptake and metabolism does not enter into dosing considerations. Third, differences in the bioavailability and function of the many forms of a dietary supplement may exist. The result is that much of the interventional nutrition research does not answer the very important clinical question, "Does replenishment of a deficiency to a given serum level result in an improved clinical outcome?" Evidence-based patient-centered care requires significantly better clinical studies.

Coenzyme Q10

Coenzyme Q10 (CoQ10, ubiquinone, or ubiquinol) is a crucial cofactor in the electron transport chain and oxidative phosphorylation for production of adenosine triphosphate (ATP). The highest tissue concentration is found in the heart, and the highest cellular concentration is on the inner membrane of the mitochondrion. CoQ10 can be a potent antioxidant. Reduced levels are associated with aging, hyperthyroidism, cardiovascular disease, total parenteral nutrition, aerobic training, and ultraviolet exposure.[37] Statins and some beta blockers, such as propranolol, can reduce endogenous production of CoQ10 by as much as 40%.[38] Supplementation can reduce two significant drivers of hypertension, oxidative stress and hyperinsulinemia.[39]

> Statin drugs and some beta blockers (propranolol) can reduce the endogenous production of CoQ10 by as much as 40%.

Low serum levels of CoQ10 were first associated with hypertension in 1975.[40] Since then, several studies have documented that supplementation can significantly reduce both systolic and diastolic hypertension. This action happens without affecting plasma renin activity, aldosterone, or sodium and potassium. In 109 symptomatic hypertensive patients, supplementation with CoQ10 (75 to 360 mg/day) to achieve a serum level higher than 2.0 mcg/mL resulted in substantial reduction in mean SBP (from 159 to 147 mm Hg) and DBP (from 94 to 85 mm Hg), with concomitant improvements in New York Heart Association (NYHA) functional class and medication requirements.[41] After an average of 4.4 months, 37% of patients were able to discontinue 1 antihypertensive drug, 11% discontinued 2 drugs, and 4% discontinued 3 drugs. Only 3% required the addition of 1 antihypertensive drug, and none required the addition of more than 1 antihypertensive drug. Twenty-five percent of all patients were able to control their BP with only CoQ10 supplementation.[41]

A 2007 meta-analysis of 12 clinical trials ($N = 352$ patients) concluded that CoQ10 supplementation in hypertensive patients could lower SBP by up to 17 mm Hg and DBP by up to 10 mm Hg without significant side effects.[42] In 3 randomized double-blind controlled trials ($N = 120$), mean SBP in the treatment group decreased by 16.6 mm Hg ($P < .001$) from a mean of 167.7 mg Hg (95% CI, 163.7 to 171.1 mm Hg). The mean DBP decreased by 8.2 mm Hg ($P < .001$) from 103 mm Hg (95% CI, 101 to 105 mm Hg) before treatment. In comparison, the placebo arms of the trials demonstrated minimal and statistically insignificant reductions in SBP and DBP. In the open-label uncontrolled trials included in the analysis, patients were treated at doses of 60 to 120 mg daily for 6 to 12 weeks. Mean SBP declined by 13.5 mm Hg (95% CI, 9.8 to 17.1 mm Hg; $P < .001$), and mean DBP declined by 10.3 mm Hg (95% CI, 8.4 to 12.3 mm Hg; $P < .001$) This meta-analysis noted that in many of the studies included, patients were able to discontinue medication.[42]

■ Dosage

The dose to achieve a serum level greater than 2.0 mcg/mL is 75 to 350 mg a day taken with meals that contain some fat.

■ Precautions

Side effects are infrequent and include abdominal discomfort, nausea, vomiting, diarrhea, anorexia, rash, and headache. CoQ10 has an antiplatelet effect, so theoretically it can increase the risk of bleeding with antiplatelet or anticoagulant agents. Excretion is through the bile, and accumulation can occur in patients with hepatic impairment or biliary obstruction.

Vitamin D

Calcitriol, also known as 1,25-dihydroxyvitamin D, is the activated secosteroid hormone form of vitamin D that has receptors on nearly every tissue, including vascular smooth muscle cells[43] and renin-producing juxtaglomerular cells.[44] Calcitriol regulates hundreds of genes including the renin gene and thus the renin-angiotensin system that controls BP.

Observational data from both the Health Professionals Follow-up Study (613 men) and the Nurses' Health Study (1198 women) associated low vitamin D status with significantly increased risk of incident hypertension over 4 to 8 years. For participants with a serum 25-(OH) vitamin D level lower than 15 ng/mL compared with participants with a level higher than 30 ng/mL, the relative risk for men was 6.13 (95% CI, 1.00 to 37.8) and for women was 2.67 (95% CI, 1.05 to 6.79).[45] In 2010, the Intermountain Heart Collaborative Study Group documented that for 41,504 patients, vitamin D deficiency (less than 30 ng/mL) was associated with highly significant ($P < .0001$) increases in the prevalence of hypertension and the associated cardiac risk factors of diabetes, hyperlipidemia, and peripheral vascular disease. Deficiency also correlated strongly ($P < .0001$) with coronary artery disease, myocardial infarction, heart failure, stroke, and incident-related death.[46]

Despite the potential benefits of vitamin D for cardiovascular health, few prospective trials support the hypothesis that vitamin D replenishment to normal levels reduces BP. For 148 older women with a mean 25-(OH) vitamin D serum level of 10 ng/mL (severe deficiency), 800 units of vitamin D_3 supplementation per day for 8 weeks, compared with placebo, raised serum levels by 12 ng/mL and reduced systolic pressure by 7 mm Hg.[46a] In contrast, for 189 men and women with a mean baseline level of 13 ng/mL, a single dose of 100,000 units of vitamin D_3, compared with placebo, raised serum levels to a mean of 20 ng/mL at 5 weeks but did not change BP.[46a]

The largest prospective trial to date enrolled 438 participants with a mean body mass index of 35, a mean 25-(OH) vitamin D level of 23.2 ± 8.5 ng/mL, SBP of 124 ± 15, and DBP of 75.4 ± 9.7 mm Hg and randomized them into 3 treatment groups: placebo, 20,000 units, or 40,000 units of oral cholecalciferol per week.[47] At the end of 1 year, the low-dose group increased their serum 25-(OH) vitamin D levels to a mean of 40 ng/mL, and the high-dose group increased their levels to a mean of 55 ng/mL with no significant change in BP.[47] Because the main objective of this study was to study the effect of vitamin D supplementation on weight change, the study was not designed and powered for detecting effects on BP. Additional prospective studies are now under way. The most important question at this time is whether a threshold serum level is needed to reduce the risk of incident hypertension or to reduce already elevated BPs. Additionally, the length of time of vitamin D sufficiency required for prevention or reduction must be defined.

◼ Dosage

Until more is known, supplement to keep serum 25-hydroxyvitamin D levels between 40 and 80 ng/mL.

◼ Precautions

Some concern exists regarding increased calcification of blood vessels with aggressive calcium and vitamin D supplementation.

Magnesium

Magnesium is a well-understood and frequently used intervention for the hypertension of preeclampsia. JNC 7 guidelines did not recommend oral supplementation of magnesium. In addition to the potentially high magnesium intake with either a Mediterranean diet or the DASH diet, however, several studies documented that low dietary intake of magnesium correlated strongly with high BP. The Women's Health Study followed 28,349 female U.S. health professionals who were at least 45 years old and were without hypertension for nearly 10 years.[48] Magnesium intake, after adjustment for age and randomized treatment, was inversely associated with the risk of incident hypertension. The highest quintile of intake (median, 434 mg/day) had a relative risk just 0.87 (95% CI, 0.81 to 0.93; P (for trend) < .0001) compared with those in the lowest quintile (median, 256 mg/day). Further adjustment for other risk factors attenuated this inverse association slightly.[48] Natural sources of magnesium include pumpkin seeds, nuts, quinoa, spinach, bran cereal, buckwheat, and beans.

Oral clinical intervention studies have not demonstrated a consistent benefit. As noted earlier, several limitations exist in the literature. For magnesium, few studies have measured serum levels, and even fewer have measured intracellular magnesium levels. Serum magnesium levels do not reflect intracellular magnesium.[49]

Additionally, the many forms of magnesium may have different bioavailability and physiologic activity. The result is a "one size fits all" approach to magnesium studies of varying dosing and varying type of magnesium that prevents any meta-analysis of existing randomized trials. Despite these limitations, magnesium appears to be beneficial and nontoxic.

One clinical trial enrolled 48 patients with mild uncomplicated hypertension and randomized them to 12 weeks of 600 mg/day of oral magnesium pidolate and lifestyle recommendations or a control group of lifestyle recommendations. Mean 24-hour SBP declined 5.6 ± 2.7 mm Hg (P < .001), and DBP declined 2.8 ± 1.8 mm Hg (P = .002) compared with controls.[50] In 82 diabetic hypertensive adults with documented hypomagnesemia who were taking captopril but not diuretics, supplementation of 2.5 g of magnesium chloride over 4 months, compared with placebo, dropped SBP 20.4 ± 15.9 mm Hg versus 4.7 ± 12.7 mm Hg (P = .03). The magnesium intervention reduced diastolic pressure 8.7 ± 16.3 mm Hg versus 1.2 ± 12.6 mm Hg in the placebo group. The adjusted odds ratio between serum magnesium and BP was 2.8 (95% CI, 1.4 to 6.9). A threshold serum level for effect was not reported.[51]

◼ Dosage

The dose is 400 to 800 mg of nonoxide forms of magnesium (e.g., citrate, glycinate, taurate), to achieve a normal intracellular and serum level.

◼ Precautions

Magnesium can cause loose bowel movements. Start at a low dose (120 to 200 mg) and slowly increase as tolerated.

Botanicals

Garlic (Allium sativum)

Garlic has been widely promoted for antihyperlipidemic effects, but both animal and human studies have suggested a BP-lowering effect. Two separate meta-analyses published in 2008 demonstrated significant BP-lowering effects in persons with hypertension.[52,53] The first meta-analysis included 11 of 25 studies from the systematic review. These demonstrated a mean decrease in the hypertensive subgroup of 8.4 ± 2.8 mm Hg for SBP (P < .001), and 7.3 ± 1.5 mm Hg for DBP (P < .001).[52] The second meta-analysis included 10 trials in the analysis, of which 3 had patients with elevated BPs. For hypertensive participants, the garlic interventions reduced SBP by 16.3 mm Hg (95% CI, 6.2 to 26.5) and DBP by 9.3 mm Hg (95% CI, 5.3 to 13.3) compared with placebo.[53]

◼ Dosage

The dose for raw garlic cloves is one half to two per day. Supplements can help prevent garlic breath. Consider a standardized dose of 350 mg twice a day (4000 mcg of allicin).

◼ Precautions

Adverse effects include the following: diaphoresis; dizziness; mouth, esophagus, and stomach irritation; nausea; and vomiting. Allergic reactions are rare. Doses greater than for culinary use may increase the risk of bleeding if they are taken with anticoagulants or antiplatelet agents.

Hawthorn (Crataegus monogyna)

Hawthorn as an herbal extract is a cardiovascular tonic popular in Europe that has been in use since at least the first century AD. Hawthorn is a short deciduous tree whose leaves, berries, and flowers contain high concentrations of flavonoids. Extracts are used for their positive inotropic and vasodilatory properties. Two clinical trials for BP demonstrated very mild changes.[54,55] Hawthorn is most often used for early-stage congestive heart failure (see Chapter 24, Heart Failure).

◼ Dosage

The German Commission E Monographs cites the use of standardized extracts containing 30 to 169 mg of proanthocyanidins (18.75%) calculated as epicatechin or 3.5 to 19.8 mg of flavonoids (2.2%) calculated as hyperoside taken in two to three individual doses for a total of 750 to 1500 mg of hawthorn per day.[56]

◼ Precautions

Transient side effects including dizziness, gastrointestinal complaints, headaches, and heart palpitations have been reported.[57] Results from the HERB-CHF trial of Crataegus extract WS 1442 documented that participants treated with the extract were 3.9 times more likely to experience progression of heart failure at the start of hawthorn therapy compared with placebo. This increased risk decreased over time.[58]

> **Herbs to Avoid in the Treatment of Hypertension**
> Herbs that require close monitoring in the treatment of patients with hypertension include licorice, ephedra, and *Panax ginseng*. These have the capacity to raise blood pressure significantly.

Mind-Body Therapy

Despite numerous historical reports of decreases in BP attributed to mind-body practices,[59-64] a Cochrane Review[65] raised concerns about the impact of these interventions on BP because many studies were conducted in the 1980s and 1990s, and the methodologic quality of these studies was inconsistent. Specifically, not all the studies were randomized controlled trials, the enrollment criteria were not specific to age group, cardiovascular risk factors, or type of hypertension, and the degree of BP reduction varied widely. This important meta-analysis of randomized controlled trials somewhat surprisingly concluded that mind-body practices produced only modest benefits in reducing SBP, even though the investigators reported a roughly 5.5 mm Hg reduction in SBP and a 3.5 mm Hg reduction in DBP.[64] SBP reductions between 2 and 5 mm Hg result in decreased mortality from stroke (14%), coronary heart disease (9%), and total mortality (7%).[66]

Since 1995, additional well-designed randomized controlled trials have demonstrated the efficacy of mind-body interventions, including relaxation response elicitation,[67] biofeedback,[68] transcendental meditation,[69,70] yoga,[71] qi gong,[72,73] and tai chi,[74] on reduction of SBP or DBP. Aggregating these studies, one finds average reductions of roughly 10 mm Hg and 7 mm Hg for SBP and DBP, respectively.

Relaxation Response

One study examined the efficacy of an 8-week relaxation response in hypertensive older adults (mean age, 66.8 years) with elevated SBP and normal DBP who were taking at least 2 antihypertensive medications.[67] Participants were blinded to hypothesis and were randomly assigned to 2 possible interventions to reduce BP: group 1 (relaxation response intervention; $n = 61$) or group 2 (intensive lifestyle modification; $n = 61$). SBP decreased by 9.4 mm Hg and 8.8 mm Hg in the relaxation response and lifestyle modification groups, respectively ($P < .0001$) without group difference. In a second phase of the study, participants who achieved an SBP of less than 140 mm Hg and had at least a 5 mm Hg reduction from baseline entered an antihypertensive medication elimination protocol. Forty-four subjects in the relaxation response group and 36 in the lifestyle modification group qualified for the protocol. Participants in the relaxation response group were more likely to eliminate an antihypertensive medication successfully than were those in the lifestyle modification group (odds ratio, 4.3; 95% CI, 1.2 to 15.9; $P = .03$). The relaxation response intervention not only led to an important decrease in BP comparable to that of intensive lifestyle modification, but also resulted in a significantly greater capacity for participants to eliminate an antihypertensive medication without increasing BP.

Biofeedback

The impact of a biofeedback intervention was tested in unmedicated persons with hypertension (mean age, 50.5 years).[68] Biofeedback ($n = 21$) had a nominal impact on SBP (0.3 mm Hg reduction) and DBP (0.9 mm Hg increase) relative to the control condition ($n = 21$) (0.4 mm Hg reduction in SBP and 3.0 mm Hg reduction in DBP). No differences were shown across groups (see Chapter 94, Enhancing Heart Rate Variability).

Transcendental Meditation

Two studies examined the effect of a 12-week proprietary Transcendental Meditation (TM) intervention on BP in medicated African Americans. In the first study,[69] 111 individuals (mean age, 67 years) were randomized to TM, progressive muscle relaxation (PMR), or health education. Results indicated that TM resulted in a 10.6 mm Hg reduction in SBP and a 6.6 mm Hg reduction in DBP, significantly greater than the 4.0 mm Hg and 2.1 m Hg reduction for PMR and greater than the 1.5 mm Hg reduction in SBP and 0.6 mm Hg increase in DBP for the health education group. In a more recent study enrolling younger subjects (mean age, 48.5 years),[70] the TM intervention ($n = 54$) resulted in a 1.6 mm Hg reduction in SBP and a 4.2 mm Hg reduction in DBP at the end of the 12-week intervention. PMR ($n = 52$) led to a 1.77 mm Hg increase in SBP and a 1.4 mm Hg reduction in DBP, whereas health education ($n = 44$) resulted in a 2.0 mm Hg increase and a 0.5 mm Hg decrease in DBP. In all, the results of these well-controlled trials indicate a significant impact on BP by the TM intervention (see Chapter 98, Recommending Meditation).

Yoga

A study to explore whether a yoga intervention affects BP was conducted in unmedicated persons with hypertension who were 35 to 65 years old.[71] The 33 subjects were equally randomized to yoga intervention, treatment with antihypertensive medications, or a no-treatment control. Yoga resulted in large reductions in SBP (33.3 mm Hg) and DBP (26.3 mm Hg), comparable to the impact of antihypertensive medications on SBP (24.0 mm Hg) and DBP (9.9 mm Hg). Both the active interventions were superior to the smaller reductions exhibited in the no-treatment group (SBP, 4.2; and DBP, 2.0 mm Hg).

Qi Gong

Numerous studies have examined the effect of a qi gong intervention on BP. However, only 2 exist in the English language. In the first study,[72] 58 unmedicated individuals (mean age, 56 years) were randomized to either a 10-week qi gong intervention or a wait list control group. Qi gong led to a significant reduction on SBP and DBP (approximately 10 mm Hg and approximately 3 mm Hg, respectively) compared with increases in SBP and DBP (approximately 3 mm Hg and approximately 1 mm Hg, respectively) in the wait list control group. In the second study,[73] 36 unmedicated participants were equally divided randomly to a 8-week qi gong intervention or a wait list control. Qi gong had a significant reduction on SBP and DBP (approximately 12 mm Hg and approximately 10 mm Hg, respectively) compared with increases in SBP and DBP (approximately 2 mm Hg and approximately 2 mm Hg, respectively) in the wait list control group. Because both studies included a wait list control group, placebo-controlled studies are now needed. Nevertheless, especially if one considers the numerous studies published in Chinese,[74] some support exists for considering a qi gong intervention for hypertension.

Tai Chi

The impact of a tai chi intervention was tested in a group of 76 people with stage 1 hypertension or high-normal BP and no medications (mean age, 51.6 years).[75] The 12-week intervention had a large impact on SBP (15.6 mm Hg reduction) and DBP (8.8 mm Hg decrease) relative to the sedentary control condition ($n = 37$) (6.4 mm Hg increase in SBP and 3.4 mm Hg increase in DBP). Tai chi resulted in significant reductions in BP relative to a sedentary control.

Despite important methodologic concerns raised in meta-analyses from earlier studies, more recent evidence examining the impact of various mind-body approaches on BP supported clinically relevant and persistent reductions. Although it is true that several of the more recent studies also were limited by small sample sizes, the overall consistency of positive results indicates that, as a whole, mind-body interventions do positively affect both SBP and DBP. Many mind-body studies now address the mechanistic and biologic underpinnings of the way in which these approaches reduce BP.[71-73,76] Understanding the mechanisms of how these therapies decrease BP will increase appropriate use of these therapies in clinical contexts.

Therapies to Consider

Ayurveda and traditional Chinese and East Asian medicine are complete paradigms from outside the Western scientific understanding that requires measurement of BP. For this reason, no "traditional" approach exists in either Eastern tradition to the management of the Western diagnosis of hypertension. For Ayurvedic and traditional East Asian medicine practitioners, contemporary approaches to hypertension are extrapolated from ancient texts and modern experience. Their concomitant use may lead patients to a more health-conscious lifestyle.

Ayurveda

Practitioners may use diet, lifestyle adjustments, herbs, breathing exercises, massage, and yoga to balance doshas pertinent to the experience of hypertension such as a state of excess pitta (fire and heat). For many persons with hypertension, a pitta-pacifying diet of cooling foods may be beneficial. Foods that may lead to imbalanced pitta states include coffee, alcohol, and hot, spicy, and oily foods, which can include many nuts, in addition to fermented and pickled foods. These foods may be especially challenging in hot summer months. Patients may also benefit from yoga for hypertension. A study of 57 prehypertensive or stage 1 hypertensive participants randomized to Iyengar yoga or enhanced usual care demonstrated significant reductions after 12 weeks of 6 mm Hg SBP ($P = .05$) and 5 mm Hg DBP ($P < .01$) in the yoga group compared with baseline.[77]

Traditional Chinese and East Asian Medicine

Practitioners may identify persons with the Western diagnosis of hypertension as having one or more Eastern diagnoses such as yin deficiency of liver and kidney, ascendant liver yang, phlegm stagnation, or blood stagnation. Persons with a Western diagnosis of hypertension may be treated for an Asian pattern with acupuncture, moxibustion, or herbs to tonify, expel phlegm and wind, clear heat, resolve blood stasis, or clear dampness. Commonly used herbs in multiple-herb formulas include Gouteng (*Uncaria* species), Niu Xi (*Cyathala* species), Tianma (*Gastrodia* species), Chuanxiong *(Ligusticum sinense),* Fuling (*Poria cocus* Wolf), Zexie (*Alismatis* species) and Juhua (chrysanthemum). The Chinese herb termed Danshen *(Salvia miltiorrhiza),* commonly used for cardiovascular issues, should not be used concurrently with warfarin.[78] Use of any herbal medicines with Western cardiovascular pharmaceuticals warrants close monitoring. Acupuncture may provide positive effects with enhanced regulation of the autonomic nervous system and achievement of a balanced constitutional state. Currently, insufficient evidence exists to support the use of acupuncture,[79,80] moxibustion,[81] or ancient multiple-herb formulas for treating the Western diagnosis of hypertension.

PREVENTION PRESCRIPTION

Michael Pollan advises this: "Eat food. Not too much. Mostly plants." These three guidelines will minimize intake of unhealthy fats including hydrogenated vegetable oils, limit intake of unhealthy sugars including high-fructose corn syrup, and significantly increase soluble fiber intake.

■ Exercise at least 30 minutes a day at least 4 days per week.
■ Limit alcohol consumption.
■ Do not smoke.
■ Breathe: incorporate mind-body practices into your daily routine.

THERAPEUTIC REVIEW

■ **Dietary**

• Follow the DASH diet eating plan with its emphasis on foods rich in potassium, magnesium, and calcium.

• Reduce dietary sodium to less than 2.4 g per day (1 teaspoon).

• Limit alcohol to two drinks or less per day for men and one drink or less per day for women.

• Consider 10 to 30 g per day of 70% cacao dark chocolate (one fourth of a regular-sized chocolate bar).

■ **Exercise**

• Aim for 30 minutes a day of aerobic exercise.

■ **Weight Loss**

• Aim for a weight loss of at least 10 lb (4.5 kg) if overweight.

Continued

■ Supplements

- Maintain serum 25-(OH) vitamin D level greater than 40 ng/mL.

- Ensure 1000 mg a day of eicosapentaenoic acid and docosahexaenoic acid by fish or krill oil.

- Consider coenzyme Q10 to achieve a serum level higher than 2.0 mcg/mL.

- Consider magnesium at 6 mg/kg.

■ Botanicals

- Consider a trial of garlic at 350 mg (4000 mcg allicin) twice daily.

- Consider the tonifying effect of hawthorn at 750 to 1500 mg per day.

■ Mind-Body Therapy

- Attempt to practice any of these approaches for approximately 20 minutes daily.
  - Practices to stimulate the relaxation response
  - Biofeedback
  - Transcendental meditation
  - Yoga
  - Qi gong
  - Tai chi

■ Pharmaceuticals

- Follow the seventh Joint National Committee on Prevention, Detection, Evaluation, and Treatment of High Blood Pressure (JNC 7) guidelines, which emphasize thiazide diuretics as first-line agents.

- Stage 1 hypertension (140 to 159/90 to 99 mm Hg)
  - Start with single-drug treatment (diuretic, angiotensin-converting enzyme inhibitor [ACEI], angiotensin receptor blocker [ARB], or calcium channel blocker)

- Stage 2 hypertension (higher than 160/100 mm Hg)
  - Use two-drug regimen (diuretic, ACE or ARB, beta blocker, calcium channel blocker)

■ Other Therapies

- Consider Ayurvedic assessment for dietary and other means of balancing one's dosha (constitutional state).

- Consider traditional East Asian medicine including acupuncture for balancing one's constitutional state.

  Note: With use of all therapies, including pharmaceuticals, an organized system of regular follow-up and review with self-monitoring and appointment reminders appears to be an effective adjunct for blood pressure control.[82]

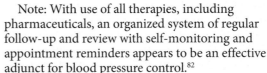

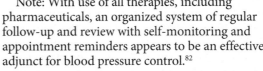

KEY WEB RESOURCES

Risk Assessment Tool for Estimating 10-year Risk of Developing Hard Coronary Heart Disease (Myocardial Infarction and Coronary Death): http://hp2010.nhlbihin.net/atpiii/calculator.asp?usertype=prof.

Systolic blood pressure values can be entered into this National Cholesterol Education Program risk assessment tool.

Your Guide to Lowering High Blood Pressure: Healthy Eating: http://www.nhlbi.nih.gov/hbp/prevent/h_eating/h_eating.htm.

This National Heart, Lung and Blood Institute Web site contains DASH diet instructions.

The DASH Diet Eating Plan. http://dashdiet.org/default.asp.

This Web site is a companion to Marla Heller's The DASH Diet Action Plan. Northbrook, Ill: Amidon Press; 2007.

HeartDecision calculator. https://www.heartdecision.org/index/tool#.

This calculator is used to assess cardiovascular risk and was created by physicians in the Division of Cardiology of the University of Wisconsin School of Medicine and Public Health in Madison, Wisconsin. It also includes helpful patient handouts.

The Eighth Report of the Joint National Committee on Prevention, Detection, Evaluation, and Treatment of High Blood Pressure (JNC 8): http://www.nhlbi.nih.gov/guidelines/hypertension/jnc8/index.htm.

This National Heart, Lung and Blood Institute Web site contains information on the forthcoming eighth report of the Joint National Committee on Prevention, Detection, Evaluation, and Treatment of High Blood Pressure (JNC) (expected availability for public review and comment: 2012; expected release date: 2012).

References

References are available at expertconsult.com.

Chapter 24

Heart Failure

Russell H. Greenfield, MD

Much has changed within a relatively short time span with respect to the management of chronic heart failure. Sadly, much remains largely unchanged. Pharmacologic and technologic advances for the treatment of heart failure helped set the stage for updated treatment guidelines developed jointly by the American Heart Association (AHA) and the American College of Cardiology (ACC) in 2005. The guidelines have undergone gentle refinements since then, and the results of more recent investigations offer great promise for people with chronic heart failure. The reality, however, is that morbidity, mortality, and the escalating financial burden to society associated with heart failure remain unacceptably high. The statistics are sobering. At 40 years of age, the lifetime risk of developing heart failure for both men and women is 20%. Almost 6 million U.S. residents (2.6% of the population) are believed to have had heart failure in 2006, with an incidence approaching 10 per 1000 population after age 65 years. Heart failure is the most frequent Medicare diagnosis-related group,[1] and a conservative estimate of the direct and indirect cost of heart failure in the United States for 2010 is $39.2 billion.[2] The 1-year mortality rate for heart failure is high; 1 in 5 will die, and in 2006, 1 in 8.6 death certificates (282,754 deaths) in the United States mentioned heart failure.[3,4] Most cardiologists and epidemiologists believe that the incidence of left ventricular systolic dysfunction will continue to grow as the population ages and as more people survive heart attacks. These same experts believe that the statistics show that the attention and energy applied by the health care system to the war on heart failure should be equal to those applied to the war on cancer.

Few, if any, medical problems so burden our health care system as heart failure and offer so true a picture of both the need and potential benefit of an integrative approach to care. The single best way to treat heart failure is to prevent its development, because once established, heart failure follows an inexorable progression toward greater infirmity and death within a few years. Prevention, prevention, prevention must be our mantra with respect to heart failure management. Lifestyle and dietary measures that promote heart health should be established early in life, and improved access to preventive medical care across socioeconomic strata should be mandated. Careful surveillance for early signs of hypertension, diabetes, obesity, and coronary artery disease is essential, as well as aggressive treatment of these same maladies, with means both safe and effective drawn from the spectrum of available interventions.

> Integrative treatment of heart failure focuses primarily on prevention.

For people who have already developed symptomatic heart failure, the emphasis rests squarely on conventional medical therapy, with physiologic goals of lowering both preload and afterload, maintaining stable left ventricular function, limiting activation of the renin-angiotensin-aldosterone system, and inhibiting release of neurohormonal factors. Complementary medical therapies with promise of efficacy and evidence of safety can be employed as adjuncts, to the benefit of most patients.

Heart failure exists in various different forms, including acute and chronic, congestive, right and left sided, and systolic and diastolic. This chapter focuses exclusively on chronic systolic heart failure, a disorder marked by impaired left ventricular systolic dysfunction (ejection fraction less than 45%), in which cardiac output is inadequate to meet metabolic demands.

Heart failure most commonly develops as a consequence of long-standing cardiovascular disease, especially hypertension or coronary artery disease, leading to ischemic cardiomyopathy. Once held to be solely a manifestation of the mechanical inability of the heart to pump blood adequately throughout the body, the pathophysiology of heart failure is now recognized to be complex and multifactorial. Initially positive neurohormonal compensatory mechanisms, believed to involve angiotensin II, norepinephrine, aldosterone, natriuretic peptides, vasopressin, and endothelin,[5]

TABLE 24-1. Pathophysiologic Features

- Increased calcium entry into myocytes
- Myocyte hypertrophy and loss with interstitial fibrosis, with resulting ventricular hypertrophy and dilation (structural remodeling)
- Reduced wall motion
- Increased myocardial energy expenditure
- Systemic vasoconstriction
- Sodium retention and circulatory congestion
- Increase in circulating catecholamines
- RAAS activation
- Increased levels of tumor necrosis factor-alpha and atrial and B-type natriuretic peptides

Data from references 6–9.
RAAS, renin-angiotensin-aldosterone system.

TABLE 24-2. New York Heart Association Functional Classification System

NYHA CLASS	DESCRIPTION
I	Physical activity not limited by symptoms such as shortness of breath, fatigue, or palpitations
II	Physical exertion mildly limited, with symptoms of shortness of breath, fatigue, or palpitations developing with typical daily activities
III	Physical activity severely curtailed; symptoms of shortness of breath, fatigue, or palpitations developing with any kind of activity
IV	Symptoms and physical discomfort present even at rest

NYHA, New York Heart Association.

TABLE 24-3. 2005 ACA/AHA Stages of Heart Failure

ACC/AHA STAGE	DESCRIPTION
A	At risk for HF but without structural heart disease or HF symptoms
B	Structural heart disease but without signs or symptoms of HF
C	Structural heart disease with prior or current symptoms of HF
D	Refractory heart failure requiring specialized intervention

Modified from Hunt SA, Abraham WT, Chin MH, et al. ACC/AHA 2005 guideline update for the diagnosis and management of chronic heart failure in the adult—summary article: a report of the American College of Cardiology/American Heart Association Task Force on Practice Guidelines (Writing Committee to Update the 2001 Guidelines for the Evaluation and Management of Heart Failure). *J Am Coll Cardiol.* 2005;46:1116–1143.
ACC, American College of Cardiology; AHA, American Heart Association; HF, heart failure.

The ACC/AHA guidelines do not replace the NYHA system but offer greater utility with regard to cumulative diagnostic and therapeutic intervention (Table 24-3).

Integrative Therapy

The critical message regarding heart failure management cannot be overemphasized—do everything to prevent the disease from ever developing in the first place. Integrative means to help prevent or at least aggressively treat disorders that contribute to development of heart failure (including hypertension, coronary artery disease, diabetes, and dyslipidemia) can be found under appropriate chapter headings in this text. The aims of treatment for established heart failure are straightforward: prevent progressive cardiovascular deterioration, minimize symptoms and enhance the quality of life, and increase survival rates. Figure 24-1 is a flow chart comparing Western, integrative, complementary, and shared approaches to the treatment of heart failure. Figure 24-2 is a treatment algorithm for heart failure by stage of the disease.

Herbs and Supplements

Be sure to advise patients that the agents discussed in the following paragraphs do not act quickly, that 4 to 6 weeks may pass before clinical benefit is evident, and that these agents offer the greatest promise of clinical benefit in people with less severe disease (ACC/AHA stages A to C and NYHA classes I to III). Thus, the use of these agents is not appropriate for acutely worsening heart failure.

Botanicals

Hawthorn (Crataegus oxycantha or Crataegus monogyna)

Long a favored herbal remedy in Europe, hawthorn is a slow-acting cardiac tonic whose active constituents are considered to be flavonoids, such as vitexin and rutin, and oligomeric

among other compounds, ultimately become maladaptive and contribute to clinical deterioration (Table 24-1).[6-9] In the most severe form of heart failure, pulmonary edema, backward pressure is so high within congested capillaries that fluid leaks into lung tissue and compromises gas exchange, thus creating a life-threatening situation. Death most often results from progressive cardiac decompensation and respiratory failure or cardiac dysrhythmia (sudden cardiac death).

Classification systems have been proposed, owing in part to the myriad clinical presentations possible with heart failure. The New York Heart Association (NYHA) system (Table 24-2) defines level of illness according to functional capability and symptoms and is useful, but it does not always help inform therapeutic decision making because symptoms can fluctuate without concomitant change in left ventricular systolic dysfunction. In response to the increasingly complicated nature of caring for people with heart failure, symptomatic and otherwise, the ACC/AHA jointly developed an updated classification system emphasizing the progressive nature of the disease. These guidelines focus on early treatment of risk factors to prevent heart failure, as well as specific interventions recommended at each stage of heart failure development to minimize morbidity and mortality.[10]

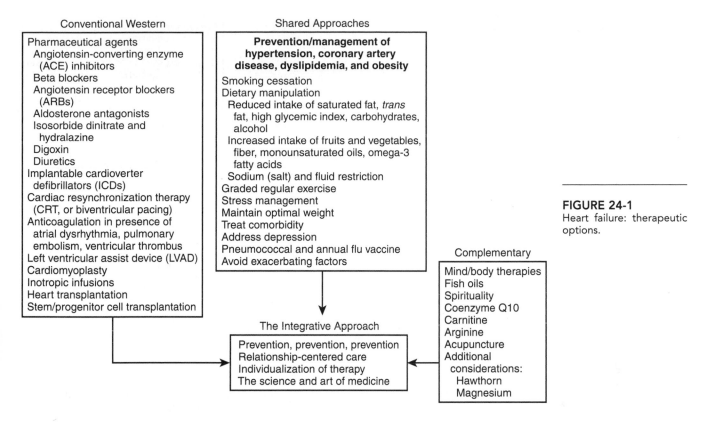

Conventional Western

Pharmaceutical agents
  Angiotensin-converting enzyme
    (ACE) inhibitors
  Beta blockers
  Angiotensin receptor blockers
    (ARBs)
  Aldosterone antagonists
  Isosorbide dinitrate and
    hydralazine
  Digoxin
  Diuretics
Implantable cardioverter
  defibrillators (ICDs)
Cardiac resynchronization therapy
  (CRT, or biventricular pacing)
Anticoagulation in presence of
  atrial dysrhythmia, pulmonary
  embolism, ventricular thrombus
Left ventricular assist device (LVAD)
Cardiomyoplasty
Inotropic infusions
Heart transplantation
Stem/progenitor cell transplantation

Shared Approaches

**Prevention/management of
hypertension, coronary artery
disease, dyslipidemia, and obesity**

Smoking cessation
Dietary manipulation
  Reduced intake of saturated fat, *trans*
    fat, high glycemic index, carbohydrates,
    alcohol
  Increased intake of fruits and vegetables,
    fiber, monounsaturated oils, omega-3
    fatty acids
  Sodium (salt) and fluid restriction
Graded regular exercise
Stress management
Maintain optimal weight
Treat comorbidity
Address depression
Pneumococcal and annual flu vaccine
Avoid exacerbating factors

Complementary

Mind/body therapies
Fish oils
Spirituality
Coenzyme Q10
Carnitine
Arginine
Acupuncture
Additional
  considerations:
    Hawthorn
    Magnesium

The Integrative Approach

Prevention, prevention, prevention
Relationship-centered care
Individualization of therapy
The science and art of medicine

FIGURE 24-1
Heart failure: therapeutic
options.

proanthocyanidins. The German Commission E specifically recommended hawthorn leaf and flower as the plant parts to be used therapeutically.

Numerous beneficial effects have been ascribed to hawthorn based on both animal and human studies,[11-13] including the following:

- Increased coronary artery blood flow

- Enhanced pumping efficiency of the heart (improved contractility)

- Antioxidant activity

- Phosphodiesterase inhibition

- Angiotensin-converting enzyme (ACE) inhibition

- Antidysrhythmic effects (lengthens the effective refractory period, unlike many cardiac drugs)

- Mild reduction in systemic vascular resistance (lowered blood pressure)

Reviews of placebo-controlled trials have reported both subjective and objective improvement in patients with mild forms of heart failure (NYHA classes I and II).[12,14,15] In one study, hawthorn was pitted against the ACE inhibitor captopril in comparable groups of people with heart failure. At trial's end, both groups had improved exercise capacity compared with baseline measurements, with no statistically significant differences between the two treatment arms of the trial. However, the investigators employed a relatively low dosage of captopril.[16] Other studies of hawthorn in people with heart failure revealed improvement in clinical symptoms, pressure-rate product, left ventricular ejection fraction, and patients' subjective sense of well-being.[17-21] A 2008 systematic review suggested significant improvements in symptoms and physiologic outcomes associated with the use of standardized extracts of hawthorn for people with heart failure.[22] Most of the studies with positive results, however, did not include treatment with drugs now accepted as standard medical therapy, such as ACE inhibitors and beta blockers. Later studies employing hawthorn in the setting of chronic heart failure in combination with current standard medical therapy reported less successful outcomes. In one trial, the standardized hawthorn extract WS 1442 was added to conventional medical therapy for heart failure that included ACE inhibition and beta blockade over 6 months. The results for hawthorn showed no significant benefit to patients with respect to a 6-minute walk test, the primary end point, or to secondary end points including indices of quality of life and NYHA classification. A modest improvement in left ventricular ejection fraction was identified.[23] Results of SPICE, a large clinical trial of hawthorn for people with NYHA heart failure classes II and III and left ventricular dysfunction performed over 24 months suggested no statistically significant benefit on the composite end point of cardiac death, nonfatal myocardial infarction, and hospitalization for worsening disease. The trend was toward reduced cardiac mortality in the treatment group, most notably for those with significantly impaired left ventricular function.[24] Perhaps most concerning are the results of a retrospective safety analysis of the use of hawthorn in NYHA class II to III heart failure over 6 months.[25] This analysis revealed that hawthorn use not only failed to impede progression of disease but also appeared in some patients to increase the risk of early heart failure progression. Hospitalization rates were higher, and death rates were slightly higher, compared with those patients who received placebo.[25] In light of a previously good safety record, these findings are both puzzling and concerning.

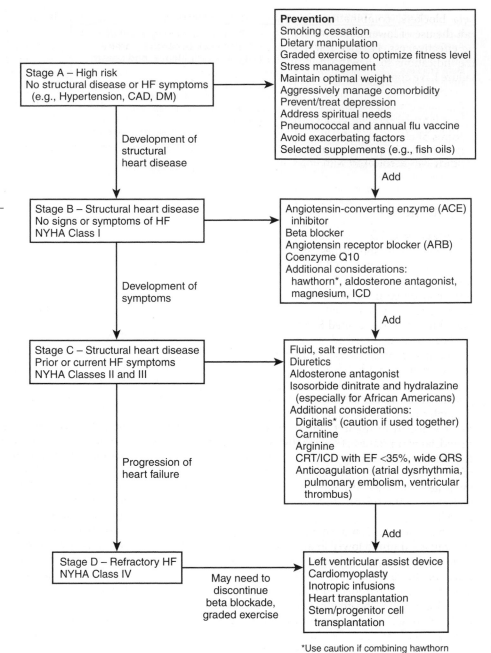

FIGURE 24-2
Clinical pathway: management of heart failure (HF). CAD, coronary artery disease; CRT, cardiac resynchronization therapy; DM, diabetes mellitus; EF, ejection fraction; HF, heart failure; ICD, implantable cardioverter defibrillator; NYHA, New York Heart Association. (Modified from Hunt SA, Abraham WT, Chin MH, et al. ACC/AHA 2005 guideline update for the diagnosis and management of chronic heart failure in the adult—summary article: a report of the American College of Cardiology/American Heart Association Task Force on Practice Guidelines [Writing Committee to Update the 2001 Guidelines for the Evaluation and Management of Heart Failure]. *J Am Coll Cardiol.* 2005;46:1116–1143.)

■ Dosage

Hawthorn is usually standardized to its content of flavonoids (2.2%) or oligomeric proanthocyanidins (18.75%). The recommended daily dose, as reflected in the literature, ranges from 160 to 1800 mg, but most practitioners believe that therapeutic efficacy is greater with higher doses (600 to 1800 mg/day). Again, no noticeable improvement may occur for 6 to 12 weeks.

■ Precautions

With the exception of the one study referenced earlier, few side effects have been associated with the use of hawthorn. Practitioners should remember that hawthorn possesses a mild hypotensive effect. One significant concern regarding a potential herb-drug interaction has largely been allayed.

It was previously suggested that hawthorn could enhance the activity of digitalis glycosides, thus increasing the risk of side effects even though the plant does not contain digitalis-like substances itself. Research suggested no significant interaction between the agents,[26] but the investigators noted that they should still be combined with caution until such a conclusion becomes definitive. Most conventional medical practitioners reflexively state that hawthorn should not be given to people taking digitalis for heart failure. A far more integrative perspective would be one considering the possibility of lowering the therapeutically effective dosage of digitalis and thereby minimizing the side effects associated with its use, by combining it with hawthorn. Similarly, because the purported beneficial actions of hawthorn overlap some of those inherent to medications such as ACE inhibitors and beta blockers, combination therapy possibly would permit the use of lower doses with no diminution of therapeutic effectiveness. Further research is needed. Short of this, the indications for hawthorn in the setting of chronic heart failure have contracted significantly.

> Hawthorn, a long-favored herbal remedy for mild forms of chronic heart failure, possesses actions largely supplanted by conventional medications and in one study was associated with untoward risk.

Supplements

Coenzyme Q10

Coenzyme Q10 (sometimes abbreviated CoQ10) has long been used as a nutritional supplement for cardiovascular disease and at one time was one of the top six pharmaceuticals consumed in Japan under the name ubidecarenone.[27] In more recent years, coenzyme Q10 has become increasingly known in the United States, and significant attention has been paid to published research examining the potential role of this agent in disease management. A naturally occurring substance that behaves like a vitamin, coenzyme Q10 is present in small amounts in most diets. Coenzyme Q10 is also synthesized within the body from tyrosine, partially through a common pathway shared with cholesterol synthesis. It is found in highest concentrations within the mitochondrial membranes of organs that have significant energy requirements, especially the heart, where it acts as a carrier of both electrons and protons, and interacts with enzymes intricately involved with energy production.[28-31] Coenzyme Q10 exerts antioxidant[32] and membrane-stabilizing[33] effects as well.

The concentration of coenzyme Q10 within the plasma and myocardium is lower in subjects experiencing cardiac failure when compared with controls, regardless of the cause of the heart failure.[34-36] The more severe the degree of heart failure as reflected by the NYHA functional classification system, the greater is the deficiency of coenzyme Q10.[37-40] Whether a decreased coenzyme Q10 concentration is causal, as could be the case with idiopathic dilated cardiomyopathy, or secondary, as is likely with ischemic cardiomyopathy, is unclear. Regardless, a demonstrated myocardial deficiency of coenzyme Q10, the knowledge that exogenous administration can correct the deficiency,[36,41] and an appreciation of its necessity for adequate myocardial energy provision together formed the initial rationale for coenzyme Q10 administration in the broad setting of heart failure.

The first clinical application of coenzyme Q10 in cardiovascular disease was reported in 1967.[42] Since that time, numerous studies evaluating coenzyme Q10 use for chronic heart failure have been published. Unfortunately, the studies are of highly variable quality: some were uncontrolled or of short duration (weeks to a few months); they examined only a small number of subjects; they were performed before the widespread use of ACE inhibitors, beta blockers, and aldosterone antagonists; or they measured only functional parameters. Nonetheless, most of the published data suggest a supportive role for coenzyme Q10, with beneficial effects on ejection fraction,[43-45] end-diastolic volume index,[44,46] development of pulmonary edema and hospitalization rate,[47] and symptoms.[45,48,49] Research has shown that withdrawal of coenzyme Q10 supplementation results in worsening cardiac function and symptoms,[50] and two studies suggested a survival benefit when coenzyme Q10 was added to a conventional therapeutic regimen.[51,52] Two more recent studies, however, failed to show clinical efficacy.[53,54] More recently, the authors of a 12-week observational trial combining coenzyme Q10 with a proprietary maritime pine bark extract in a small number of patients with NYHA class II to III heart failure reported improvements in ejection fraction and treadmill walking distances.[55] Large multicenter trials to determine the true efficacy of coenzyme Q10 are needed.

■ Dosage

The optimum dosage of coenzyme Q10 in the setting of heart failure is as yet undetermined. Studies have used doses ranging from 30 to 600 mg/day, but most practitioners initially prescribe 100 to 200 mg daily. Softgel capsules of coenzyme Q10 appear to provide superior bioavailability.[56]

■ Precautions

Coenzyme Q10 has been found to be remarkably free of significant side effects. The most common adverse reaction is gastrointestinal upset (epigastric discomfort, loss of appetite, nausea, and diarrhea), occurring in fewer than 1% of all subjects.[57] Caution is advised for people taking anticoagulation therapy, given that case reports exist of possible procoagulant activity in patients taking warfarin, perhaps because of the compound's structural similarity to menaquinone.[58-60] Patients taking 3-hydroxy-3-methyl-glutaryl-coenzyme A (HMG-CoA) reductase inhibitors (statins) may benefit from supplementation with coenzyme Q10. As alluded to earlier, cholesterol and coenzyme Q10 partially share the mevalonate pathway, the same biosynthetic pathway disrupted by statin drugs. Cholesterol production and the endogenous pathways for coenzyme Q10 production are thus both compromised by HMG-CoA reductase inhibition.[61-65]

Carnitine

Carnitine, another vitamin-like substance, acts as a specific carrier of the fatty acids required for energy production and moves them from the cytoplasm into the mitochondria. Carnitine is synthesized from the amino acid lysine, but it is also available in small amounts in foods such as red meat. Unfortunately, the organs in which carnitine is most highly concentrated (those with high levels of fatty acid metabolism, including the heart and skeletal muscle) are incapable of synthesizing carnitine themselves.[66] Myocardial carnitine is most highly concentrated within the left ventricle.[67,68] Levels of carnitine have been found to be low in patients with heart failure,[69,70] and depletion of myocardial L-carnitine appears to affect cell membrane function adversely, thus translating into impaired myocardial contractility.[71-73]

Only the L-form of carnitine should be used therapeutically. Investigators have suggested that propionyl L-carnitine (PLC; created through the esterification of L-carnitine) is most effective in the setting of heart disease because of its highly lipophilic nature.[74] PLC has been shown to improve muscle metabolism,[75] to stimulate the Krebs cycle,[76] and to improve heart contractility[77,78] in animal models. Studies using L-carnitine in humans with ischemic heart disease or peripheral vascular disease revealed enhanced cardiac performance and increased exercise tolerance.[79-81]

Human trials using PLC in the setting of heart failure provided promising results.[82] Long-term administration of PLC was shown to improve ventricular function, reduce systemic vascular resistance, and increase exercise tolerance.[83,84] Administration acutely lowered pulmonary artery and capillary wedge pressure in one study.[85] Another reported a statistically significant reduced 3-year mortality rate in patients taking PLC.[86] In a well-done study that reported no significant benefit of PLC use in heart failure, the trend was toward beneficial effects for those people with somewhat preserved heart function (ejection fraction between 30% and 40%), and the safety of the agent was confirmed.[87]

◼ Dosage
The dosage of PLC used in most studies is 2 g/day, divided into doses given two to three times daily (range, 1 to 3 g/day).

◼ Precautions
The existing literature strongly suggests that the use of PLC is safe for patients with heart failure. L-Carnitine has been reported to cause an unpleasant body odor in extremely high doses. Most studies that used PLC, however, revealed no side effects, and no major toxicity was reported,[66] although an effect on peripheral thyroid hormone action was posited.[88]

L-Arginine
L-Arginine is an essential amino acid possessing vasodilatory effects that may enhance coronary artery blood flow and lessen the work of the heart by decreasing vascular resistance. Whereas further research is indicated, existing data are promising, albeit inconsistent. Use of L-arginine has been associated with improved hemodynamics and decreased endothelial dysfunction,[89-93] improved exercise tolerance,[89,94,95] improved kidney function,[96] and enhanced quality of life.[97]

◼ Dosage
The typical dose used in heart failure is 2 to 6 g three times daily.

◼ Precautions
L-Arginine increases potassium levels when it is used with other potassium-sparing drugs,[98] and it may increase the incidence of recurrent herpetic lesions. One trial cast doubt on the utility of arginine therapy after myocardial infarction and even raised the suggestion that such an intervention may increase mortality in older patients.[99]

Pharmaceuticals

Angiotensin-Converting Enzyme Inhibitors
Simply put, early institution of maximal therapy with ACE inhibitors saves lives. Numerous studies have shown that treatment with ACE inhibitors slows progression of heart failure and can improve quality of life, as well as long-term prognosis.[100-102] The biggest problem surrounding use of this class of agents is that many patients are not receiving maximal beneficial dosages. Such undertreatment stymies anticipated therapeutic benefits.

◼ Dosage
Initial and target dosages for commonly used agents are as follows[103]:
Captopril: 6.25 to 100 mg three times daily
Enalapril: 2.5 to 20 mg twice daily
Lisinopril: 2.5 to 20 mg daily
Fosinopril: 5.0 to 40 mg daily
Ramipril: 1.25 to 10 mg daily
Quinapril: 5 to 40 mg daily
Trandolapril: 1 to 4 mg daily

◼ Precautions
Many physicians are still wary of potential side effects, such as hypotension, kidney problems (increasing creatinine level), and electrolyte disorders (hyperkalemia). A safe and effective approach is to start with a low dosage, increase that dosage slowly, and periodically check electrolyte levels. Anyone who receives a verified diagnosis of heart failure and can tolerate ACE inhibitors should be taking them, and the dosage should be appropriately maximized. Some people develop a chronic, dry cough with ACE inhibitors that may limit the drug's utility. In this instance, angiotensin receptor blockade and vasodilator therapy are appropriate considerations. However, efforts should first be made to ensure that the cough is not secondary to the development of congestive heart failure.

Angiotensin Receptor Blockers
Angiotensin II subtype I receptor blockers provide more complete blockade of the renin-angiotensin system than do ACE inhibitors, they decrease morbidity and mortality to a degree similar but not superior to that of ACE inhibitors, they have fewer side effects than ACE inhibitors, and they may be of added benefit when combined with ACE inhibitors as part of the standard therapeutic regimen.[104-108] More recent data brought this last point into question, however, by suggesting that the combination of ACE inhibitors with angiotensin receptor blockers (ARBs) should be used with caution; some studies pointed to increased morbidity and mortality, or no significant all-cause mortality benefit, with combined therapy.[107,108] ARBs are a reasonable alternative for patients who cannot tolerate ACE inhibitor therapy.[107,109]

◼ Dosage
Initial and target dosages for commonly used agents are as follows[103]:
Losartan: 12.5 to 100 mg daily
Candesartan: 4 to 32 mg daily
Valsartan: 40 to 160 mg twice daily

◼ Precautions
ARBs are typically well tolerated.

Aldosterone Antagonists
Aldosterone mediates sodium retention, cardiac remodeling, myocardial fibrosis, and baroreceptor dysfunction.[110] Studies addressing the use of spironolactone, a diuretic and nonselective aldosterone antagonist, revealed that the agent reduces

both the need for hospitalization and the risk of sudden death when it was added to standard conventional Western medical therapy.[111-114] Eplerenone is a more selective aldosterone antagonist that has also been shown to reduce morbidity and mortality in heart failure. Although the benefits of aldosterone antagonism in heart failure are well established, this form of therapy remains woefully underused by physicians, perhaps because of the fear of hyperkalemia.[115] Data suggest the possibility of an important role for spironolactone even for people with NYHA class I to II heart failure.[116] All patients with advanced heart failure should be considered for aldosterone antagonist therapy.[117,118]

■ Dosage

Initial and target dosages for commonly used agents are as follows[103]:
Spironolactone: 12.5 to 50 mg daily
Eplerenone: 25 to 50 mg daily

■ Precautions

Spironolactone and eplerenone are known to promote potassium and magnesium retention. Be sure to document adequate kidney function before starting patients on either of these agents, and monitor electrolyte levels frequently.

Beta Blockers

Once contraindicated in the setting of heart failure, beta blockade has clearly been shown to benefit all but the most severe functional classes of heart failure when it is added to a regimen of ACE inhibitors or ARBs, by enhancing left ventricular systolic function, decreasing the rate of hospitalization, and lessening the incidence of sudden cardiac death.[119-125] Beta blockers not only affect the mechanical pump of the heart (improving ventricular function) and provide autonomic balance but also counteract specific neurohormonal processes that contribute to progressively worsening heart function through cardiac remodeling.[126-128] Beta blockade combined with ACE inhibition is now considered a cornerstone of systolic heart failure management.

Three beta blocking agents have been shown most beneficial in the clinical setting, although which agent is most beneficial in specific instances is unclear, as is the existence of a consistent place for beta blocker therapy in stages A or D heart failure. Treatment should be initiated at low doses and gradually titrated upward.[129]

■ Dosage

Initial and target dosages for commonly used agents are as follows[103]:
Carvedilol: 3.125 to 50 mg twice daily
Metoprolol succinate extended release: 12.5 to 200 mg daily
Bisoprolol: 1.25 to 5 mg daily

■ Precautions

Side effects include hypotension and bradycardia.

Angiotensin-converting enzyme (ACE) inhibitors, angiotensin receptor blockers (ARBs), beta blockers, and aldosterone antagonists all have a positive impact on mortality related to heart failure.

Cardiac Glycosides (Digoxin)

Digoxin has been a mainstay of the conventional Western medical armamentarium since the days of William Withering, who first explored the benefit derived from the use of leaves of the common foxglove plant (*Digitalis purpurea*) more than 100 years ago. Digoxin is most commonly employed in the treatment of supraventricular dysrhythmias (atrial fibrillation) and heart failure, especially when the heart failure is associated with hypertension, cardiac valvular disease, or coronary artery disease.

Digoxin has long been known to be a positive inotrope (increase the pumping efficiency of the heart), but more recent work showed it to possess beneficial neurohormonal activity as well. Although the administration of digoxin does not appear to affect overall mortality, when it is added to the standard regimen of ACE inhibitors and diuretics, digoxin has been shown to improve symptoms, enhance exercise capacity, improve patients' quality of life and clinical status, and reduce hospitalization rates.[130-134]

■ Dosage

The initial and target dose is as follows[103]:
Digoxin: 0.125 to 0.25 mg daily in most patients

■ Precautions

Although digoxin is a useful drug, it has a very narrow therapeutic range, and toxicity is not uncommon. Some physicians initiate digoxin therapy early in the course of illness, and others prescribe it only in moderate to severe heart failure. Digoxin can be used both in the setting of acute cardiac decompensation and for chronic maintenance therapy. Do not prescribe digoxin as monotherapy—people with heart failure should almost always be taking an ACE inhibitor and using other interventions, as described previously. A lowered dosage of digoxin is often necessary for patients with significant renal insufficiency.

Isosorbide Dinitrate and Hydralazine

Few therapies underscore the notion that no two people are alike as clearly as the combination of nitrates and hydralazine. The combination of hydralazine and isosorbide dinitrate was the first treatment shown to improve survival in heart failure, but it was subsequently shown to be less effective than ACE inhibition in direct comparisons.[129] African Americans with heart failure, however, do not appear to respond as favorably to ACE inhibitors or beta blockers as do non-African Americans and have a less active nitric oxide system than do non-African Americans. Reevaluation of the Veterans Administration Cooperative Study on Vasodilator Therapy of Heart Failure (V-HeFT trial)[135] showed a significant reduction in mortality for African Americans who were taking nitrates and hydralazine. Subsequently, the African-American Heart Failure Trial (A-HeFT) was performed using the same fixed combination of isosorbide dinitrate and hydralazine in addition to standard therapy.[136] The study was stopped early because the reduction in mortality using the drug combination was so striking—43%. Besides the known vasodilatory effects, isosorbide dinitrate is a nitric oxide donor, whereas hydralazine inhibits breakdown of nitric oxide, and together the drugs act to increase nitric oxide levels. In 2005, the U.S. Food and Drug Administration approved the use of BiDil (a fixed-dose combination of isosorbide dinitrate and hydralazine) for the treatment of heart failure in African Americans. More recent data suggest a possible role for the drug combination as add-on therapy for patients of any race who have advanced heart failure.[137]

Dosage

Initial and target dosages for commonly used agents are as follows[103]:

Hydralazine/isosorbide dinitrate (BiDil): 37.5 mg hydralazine/20 mg isosorbide dinitrate to 75 mg hydralazine/40 mg isosorbide dinitrate three times daily

Precautions

Headaches and dizziness have been reported, as has the potential for hypotension.

Diuretics

Diuretics help lessen cardiac workload by decreasing preload, yet until 2006, few data showed that these agents prolonged survival.[138,139] The most commonly used diuretics in the setting of heart failure are the so-called loop diuretics, such as furosemide, which are especially beneficial once congestion has developed.

Dosage

Initial and maximal dosages for commonly used agents are as follows[103]:
Furosemide: 20 to 600 mg daily
Bumetanide: 0.5 to 10 mg daily
Torsemide: 10 to 200 mg daily
Ethacrynic acid: 25 to 200 mg daily

Precautions

Periodic blood tests are necessary to evaluate electrolyte balance, especially potassium and sodium levels. One challenge is that diuretics may actually increase renin and aldosterone levels and thereby worsen the neurohormonal milieu. Benefits of therapy usually outweigh risks, however, as noted in a review finding that diuretic therapy not only improved symptoms of heart failure but also reduced morbidity and mortality.[138]

Biomechanical Therapy

The risk of sudden cardiac death in patients with heart failure is markedly increased, likely because of the increased incidence of ventricular dysrhythmias. With an eye toward preventing sudden cardiac death, treatment of heart failure is becoming increasingly mechanized. Evidence supporting the use of cardiac resynchronization therapy (CRT, a form of biventricular pacing) to correct dyssynchronous ventricular contraction and associated incomplete ventricular filling, and implantable cardioverter defibrillators (ICDs) either separately or combined, is compelling, with data strongly suggesting improved quality of life and reduced mortality, especially for those patients with stage C disease.[140-150] The use of CRT combined with an ICD in asymptomatic or mildly symptomatic patients with heart disease, reduced ejection fraction, and a wide QRS complex was associated with a 34% reduction in the risk of death or heart failure events as compared with the use of ICD alone.[150] Guidelines recommended

CRT in patients with a left ventricular ejection fraction of less than 35%, NYHA class III to IV symptoms, and a QRS complex duration of more than 0.12 seconds.[1,129] The utility of this approach may be expanding because evidence points to potential health benefits across the spectrum of heart failure presentations, even for patients with mild disease.[151] Drugs remain the mainstay of treatment for people with heart failure and left ventricular dysfunction, but mechanical device therapy is now offering significant benefits to a major subset of patients. Placement of left ventricular assist devices, cardiomyoplasty, revascularization for ischemic heart failure, and heart transplantation represent the most drastic surgical considerations for the treatment of heart failure.

> The most significant recent change in the conventional medical treatment of chronic heart failure is the increased reliance on device therapy (cardiac resynchronization therapy and implantable cardioverter defibrillators).

Bioenergetics

Acupuncture

Investigators have posited that acupuncture may ameliorate conditions that worsen the prognosis for people with heart failure, specifically high sympathetic activity.[152,153] A pilot study of acupuncture offered to 17 subjects with stable NYHA class II to III heart failure and who were receiving appropriate medical therapy reported no benefit with respect to ejection fraction but a marked improvement in 6-minute walk test results for the active group.[154] These results are intriguing, and more research is needed to evaluate the use of acupuncture before it can be recommended for treatment of heart failure.

Mind-Body Therapy

Depression is an independent risk factor for heart failure and is extremely prevalent among patients with established disease.[155,156] Depression-specific activation of inflammatory cytokines occurs in people with heart failure and may lead to worsening morbidity and mortality rates.[157,158] Numerous reports showed that providing adequate means of stress reduction can help relieve depression and anxiety, lessen the risk of developing cardiovascular disease, and improve the health and well-being of people with established heart disease.[159-165] Some of the benefits of mind-body therapies may be related to impacts on the autonomic nervous system.[166] Little research has been performed on the treatment of depression specific to people with heart failure, but this situation has been improving of late.[167] One older study of biofeedback for patients with advanced heart failure reported increased cardiac output and reduced systemic vascular resistance compared with controls.[168] A more recent small trial examining the effects of transcendental meditation compared with health education in African Americans with heart failure found improvements in 6-minute walk scores, depression scores, and measures of quality of life after 6 months, as well as a reduced rate of hospitalization.[169]

Health benefits were also identified in the results of the SEARCH (Study of the Effectiveness of Additional

Reductions in Cholesterol and Homocysteine) trial, which examined the effects of training in mindfulness meditation and coping skills in association with support group discussion for more than 200 adults with reduced ejection fraction or congestive heart failure.[170] Although medical management was not maximized in a small percentage of subjects, measures of anxiety and depression were significantly lower in the active group. The study found no impact on hospitalization or death rates, but symptom improvement persisted at 12 month follow-up. A small study of older patients with heart failure who were receiving maximal medical therapy showed improvements in neurotransmitter levels and quality of life measures after subjects listened to 30-minute meditation tapes twice daily at home for 12 weeks.[166]

Additional studies supporting the benefits of mind-body approaches for patients with heart failure include those focusing on Freeze-Frame stress management,[171] behavior modification,[172] relaxation response training,[173,174] and tai chi.[175,176]

Lifestyle

Community education regarding the adverse effects of smoking, excessive alcohol intake, and obesity must continue and expand. Assistance with tobacco and alcohol cessation, as well as weight management planning, should be made readily available across socioeconomic lines.

Having heart failure is not a contraindication to participating in exercise. Several trials showed that appropriate, graded exercise programming can improve function and quality of life for people with heart failure.[177-180] Lack of improvement after fitness training is associated with a poor prognosis.[181] Results of the HF-Action trial[182] were disappointing, showing at best a modest impact on hospitalization and mortality rate with regular exercise; however, the results reinforced the safety of regular exercise and cardiac rehabilitation for people with heart failure. The combination of physical exertion and a healthy diet can help patients maintain optimal body weight and thereby lessen strain on the heart. Sufficient rest is also important, and asking people to aim for at least 7 to 8 hours of sleep each night is prudent.

Regular participation in spiritual or religious practices may also help fend off heart disease.[183-186] Once heart failure is established, studies reveal that many patients struggle with their spirituality, a struggle that adds to an already stressful situation and perhaps leads to morbidity.[187,188] The burden of symptoms, mood disorders, and spiritual challenges associated with heart failure has been equated with those experienced by people with cancer.[189] Attention to spiritual needs can help people adjust to their new circumstances, address specific regrets with regard to prior lifestyle choices, and search for present meaning and future hope.[190,191]

Nutrition

Adhering to an antiinflammatory diet (see Chapter 86, The Antiinflammatory Diet) may both help prevent development of heart failure and slow progression of established disease. People who have stage C heart failure typically require additional means to keep the illness in check. Fluid and sodium (salt) restriction has been shown to affect cardiac function and symptoms positively in patients with heart failure. In the early stages of heart failure, the degree of restriction need not be severe, and avoiding added salt should be sufficient. With worsening heart function, patients may need to limit sodium intake to 2 g/day and daily ingestion of water to 1.5 to 2 L (see Chapter 87, The DASH Diet).

Supplementation with B vitamins, especially thiamine, should be considered,[192-194] as well as micronutrient supplementation, including magnesium.[195-198] Questions persist about the safety of high-dose vitamin E in patients with established cardiovascular disease.[199]

Future Therapy

Table 24-4 provides a list of future considerations for the therapy of heart failure.[200,201]

TABLE 24-4. Future Considerations

- Calcium sensitizers
- Continuous-flow left ventricular assist devices
- Cytokine inhibitors
- Endothelin receptor blockers
- Erythropoiesis-stimulating proteins
- Fish oils
- Free fatty acid oxidation inhibitors
- Gene expression (miRNA)
- Matrix metalloproteinase inhibitors
- Modified natriuretic peptides
- Nitric oxide–enhancing therapy
- Phosphodiesterase III inhibitors
- Ribose
- Statin therapy
- Stem and progenitor cell transplantation
- Taurine
- Vasopressin antagonists

Data from Jackevicius CA, Page RL 2nd, Chow S, et al. High-impact articles related to the management of heart failure: 2008 update. *Pharmacotherapy.* 2009;29:82-120; and Tang WH, Francis GS. The year in heart failure. *J Am Coll Cardiol.* 2010;55:688–696.

PREVENTION PRESCRIPTION

- Do not smoke. If you do smoke, get help to quit.
- Follow an antiinflammatory or Mediterranean-style diet.
- Participate in regular physical fitness activities.
- Manage stress in healthy ways.
- Maintain a healthy weight for height.
- Work with your doctor to manage medical conditions that may lead to heart failure, especially high blood pressure, coronary artery disease, high cholesterol levels, and diabetes.
- Speak with your doctor about ways to prevent and if necessary, treat depression.
- Attend to your spiritual side.
- Have the pneumococcal vaccination and your annual flu vaccination.
- Avoid overuse of nonsteroidal antiinflammatory medications (NSAIDs).

THERAPEUTIC REVIEW

All patients with heart failure should be started on some combination of angiotensin-converting enzyme (ACE) inhibitor, angiotensin receptor blocker (ARB), or beta blocker, and aggressive management of comorbidity should be undertaken.

Removal of Potential Exacerbating Factors

- Try to discontinue nonsteroidal antiinflammatory drugs and first-generation calcium channel blockers.

Stress Management and Mind-Body Therapy

- Promote proper attention to mood and stress management, and offer instruction in and access to tools such as meditation, relaxation response, and tai chi.

Graded Exercise

- Enroll patients in a certified cardiac rehabilitation program.

Nutrition

- Encourage an antiinflammatory diet or Mediterranean-style diet.
- Urge fluid and salt restriction.

Spirituality

- Inquire about and address needs in an open fashion, and use pastoral care services as appropriate.

Bioenergetics

- Acupuncture

Supplements

- Coenzyme Q10: 100 to 200 mg daily
- Propionyl-L-carnitine: 1 to 3 g daily
- Arginine: 2-6 g three times daily

Botanicals

- Hawthorn: 600 to 1800 mg daily (exercise caution when using with digoxin)

Pharmaceuticals

- ACE inhibitors
- ARBs
- Beta blockers
- Aldosterone antagonists
- Isosorbide dinitrate in combination with hydralazine
- Diuretics
- Digitalis

Surgery

- Cardiac resynchronization therapy or implantable cardioverter defibrillator
- Left ventricular assist device
- Cardiomyoplasty
- Inotropic infusions
- Heart transplantation
- Stem or progenitor cell transplantation

KEY WEB RESOURCES

American Heart Association. http://www.heart.org/HEARTORG/Conditions/HeartFailure/Heart-Failure_UCM_002019_SubHomePage.jsp.	Heart failure management resource
Heart Failure Society of America. http://www.heartfailureguide-line.org/	Guidelines
Agency for Healthcare Research and Quality. http://www.guide-line.gov/content.aspx?id=10587	Heart failure management guidelines
Natural Medicines Comprehensive Database. http://naturaldatabase.therapeuticresearch.com/home.aspx?cs=&s=ND	Evidence-based assessment of vitamins, supplements, and herbs (subscription required)

References

References are available at expertconsult.com.

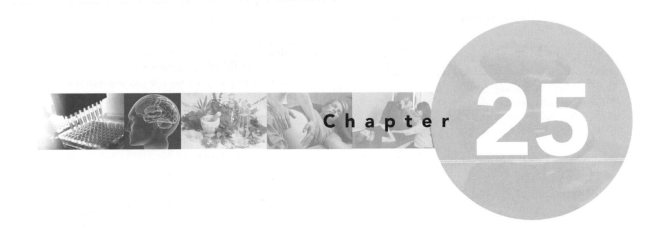

Coronary Artery Disease

Stephen Devries, MD

Despite the many advances, cardiovascular disease is responsible for more than 2000 deaths every day in the United States.[1] Investigators estimate that 1 of 3 U.S. residents is destined to die of cardiovascular cause. Clearly, we have work to do. The causes of cardiovascular disease are diverse but, in large part, are related to lifestyle and environment. Rates of stress, obesity, and diabetes continue to soar. The Centers for Disease Control and Prevention estimates that 1 out of 3 children born in the year 2000 will go on to develop diabetes during his or her lifetime.[2] Consequently, for the first time in history, it is possible that children will have a shorter life expectancy than their parents.[3]

An integrative approach acknowledges the great value and potentially lifesaving benefits of modern pharmacology and procedures while at the same time recognizing the limitations of these approaches when they are used in isolation. An integrative approach is ideally suited for prevention and treatment of coronary disease because it addresses many of the root causes, especially those influenced by lifestyle. The goal of this chapter is to gain perspective into the power of a broader spectrum of therapies beyond those that typically constitute conventional cardiovascular care.

Pathophysiology

What triggers a cardiovascular catastrophe? For many years, investigators believed that a cardiovascular event occurred after many years of progressive narrowing of a coronary artery. This view held that with each passing year, layer on layer of cholesterol-laden deposits accumulated on the surface of a coronary artery. This theory held that, over time, cholesterol deposits accumulated and ultimately stopped blood flow, thus leading to myocardial infarction. In more recent years, this paradigm has been largely upended and replaced by a more complex, and less intuitive, picture.

Angiographic studies have revealed, quite surprisingly, that acute coronary events often arise from "mild"

coronary lesions that are far less than 50% obstructive.[4] The explanation for this paradoxical finding is that vulnerable plaques, those most likely to rupture and evolve into a complete thrombotic occlusion, are those with large lipid cores and thin fibrous caps.[5] Most of the plaques with the largest lipid cores are not severely stenotic (the lipid-laden deposits enlarge the artery and do not always reduce the area of blood flow). Conversely, some of the most severely stenotic plaques are not necessarily the ones with the largest lipid cores and therefore may not be the most "vulnerable."

A useful way of thinking about this concept and of conveying it to patients is that a mild coronary lesion can be considered a "fault line" that, in a quiescent phase, appears quite passive and harmless. However, similar to any fault line, these seemingly harmless plaques may erupt at any moment and cause a potentially lethal cardiac event.

This situation has implications for both detection and treatment of coronary artery disease. With regard to detection, a mildly stenotic coronary lesion is not flow limiting and therefore would not be expected to result in chest pain or provoke abnormal findings on a cardiac stress test. This is the explanation for the anecdote familiar to most clinicians and patients about the individual who sailed through a stress test with "normal" results only to suffer a cardiac catastrophe a short time later.

The finding that a coronary event can rapidly develop from what angiographically appears to be a "mild" coronary lesion emphasizes the need to prevent coronary lesions from developing, rather than to focus on reducing the severity of severe stenoses with interventional procedures.

The triggers of coronary artery disease are both genetic and environmental. Genetic tendencies include inherited metabolic disorders including dyslipidemia and diabetes. Environmental and lifestyle factors include nutritional imbalance, sedentary lifestyle, stress and depression, smoking, and air pollution. These topics are explored in detail in this chapter.

A mild coronary lesion can be considered a "fault line" that, in a quiescent phase, appears quite passive and harmless. However, similar to any fault line, these seemingly harmless plaques may erupt at any moment and cause a potentially lethal cardiac event.

Integrative Therapy

Nutrition

Nutrition is perhaps the most powerful therapy available for prevention and treatment of coronary disease.

Mediterranean Diet

The power of nutritional therapy is highlighted by the striking results of the Lyon Diet Heart study.[6] In this study of individuals who survived myocardial infarction, patients were divided into two groups distinguished only by dietary intervention. The control group was advised to consume a "prudent" diet consisting of reduced cholesterol and total fat. The intervention group, conversely, was advised to eat a Mediterranean-style diet. Patients in this group were counseled to eat more vegetables and fruit and more nuts and fish, to use olive oil and canola-based margarine as their predominant cooking oils, and to reduce their intake of red meat and refined carbohydrates.

The study was intended to last 5 years but was stopped short at 27 months because of a strikingly beneficial effect in the Mediterranean diet group. At that point, a 73% reduction in cardiovascular events, including myocardial infarction and cardiac death, was observed in the Mediterranean-style diet group. A longer-term follow-up study published 5 years later demonstrated a durable benefit of the Mediterranean-style diet with a 72% reduction in cardiovascular events after 5 years.[7]

The substantial benefits of the Mediterranean diet are not surprising, given the proven benefits of its component parts. High consumption of vegetables and fruit is the cornerstone of the Mediterranean-style diet. Daily consumption of vegetables in the Lyon study averaged 427 g (approximately five servings).[8] Increased intake of vegetables, especially dark green leafy vegetables, has been associated with a substantially reduced risk of coronary heart disease. Each daily serving of dark green leafy vegetables, for example, has been linked to a 23% reduction in coronary heart risk.[9] Fruit intake in the Lyon study averaged 271 g (approximately two servings) (see Chapter 86, The Antiinflammatory Diet).

The results of the Lyon Mediterranean diet study underlie my personal recommendation for daily consumption of five servings of vegetables per day and two servings of fruit.

Whole Grains

Other key constituents of the Mediterranean diet are avoidance of refined grains and an emphasis on consumption of whole grains. Refined grains, typically void of fiber, are deleterious in several ways. As compared with their whole grain counterparts, refined grains result in a more exuberant release of glucose into the circulation, thus triggering higher insulin levels and a greater tendency toward atherosclerosis. Higher sugar intake is associated with reduced levels of high-density lipoprotein (HDL) and increased levels of the riskier, more atherogenic small dense low-density lipoprotein (LDL)[10] (see Chapter 85, The Glycemic Index/Load).

The manner in which grains are prepared also has important health implications. Boiled whole grains (e.g., oat, quinoa, barley) are typically a healthier choice than bread made from the flour of whole grains.

Examples of whole grains include barley, buckwheat, quinoa, polenta, and brown rice. A meta-analysis demonstrated a 21% lower risk of cardiovascular events when 2.5 servings per day of whole grains were consumed compared with the absence of whole grain foods in the diet.[11] The manner in which grains are prepared also has important health implications. Consuming pulverized grains, even whole grains, results in a higher blood glucose level than when the intact grain is eaten.[12] Therefore, boiled whole grains are typically a healthier choice than is bread made from the flour of whole grains.

Fish

Fish is another integral component of a heart healthy diet, with benefits in both primary and secondary prevention of heart disease. In the Chicago Western Electric Study, more than 35 g of fish intake/week (approximately three servings) led to a 38% reduced risk of cardiac death.[13] The Diet and Reinfarction Trial (DART) similarly demonstrated a 29% reduction in all-cause mortality in men instructed to eat fish compared with those who did not after only 2 years.[14] Accordingly, substituting chicken or fish for red meat has been shown to reduce the risk of coronary heart disease.[15]

Nuts

Nuts, a part of the Mediterranean-style diet, have potent benefits for reduction of coronary heart disease. Four servings of nuts per week (30 g/serving, or approximately one large handful/serving) have been shown to reduce the risk of coronary heart disease by 37%.[16] Increasing consumption of nuts to two handfuls per day reduces LDL cholesterol (LDL-C) by as much as 10% in those with baseline values of greater than 160 mg/dL.[17]

The success of nutritional interventions is greatly enhanced when the patient perceives that nutrition is a priority of the health care practitioner. At every clinical encounter with a patient, I recommend making a point to inquire about the number of servings of vegetables and fruit consumed every day, the type of grains, the quantity of fish, and the servings of nuts consumed on a weekly basis. Emphasizing the importance of diet during each visit allows obstacles to be identified and progress celebrated.

Exercise

Patients often inquire about "natural" methods for prevention and treatment of heart disease. In concert with dietary changes, no other therapy is more potent than the addition of regular exercise. Surprisingly, intensity of exercise appears to be less important than frequency and consistency. In the Health Professionals Follow-Up Study, walking for 30 minutes per day was associated with an 18% reduction in the occurrence of cardiovascular disease.[18] In the Women's Health Initiative observational study, exercise of as little as 4.2 metabolic equivalent of task (MET)-hour/week resulted in a 27% reduction in heart disease risk. The benefits of exercise were even greater when a higher level of exercise, 32.8 MET-hour/week, were performed.

Although aerobic exercise is generally emphasized for cardiovascular health, resistance training also adds considerable benefit. Resistance training for at least 30 minutes per week resulted in a 23% lower risk of heart disease compared with men who did no resistance training.[18]

Therefore, a reasonable prescription for exercise could start at 30 minutes of brisk walking every day, in addition to two to three sessions per week of light resistance training interspersed with stretching. More vigorous workouts of longer duration are likely to be of even greater benefit. Of course, individual prescriptions must take into account the patient's general health history and cardiovascular status. Stress testing before beginning a program may be appropriate for patients with a history of heart disease or for those with multiple cardiovascular risk factors, especially those who have been previously sedentary.

Pharmaceuticals

In addition to the nutrition and exercise "foundations" of heart health, patients with symptomatic coronary artery disease should receive treatment informed by American Heart Association/American College of Cardiology (AHA/ACC) guidelines. Proven medical therapy for symptomatic coronary disease includes aspirin, nitrates, beta blockers, and calcium channel blockers. Angiotensin-converting enzyme inhibitors are also potent antihypertensives and may provide additional cardiovascular prevention above and beyond antihypertensive properties. Statin therapy should also be considered an essential component of therapy in patients with established vascular disease, as well as in those at high risk for vascular disease both for lipid lowering and for the many "pleotropic" or nonlipid beneficial metabolic effects. A detailed discussion of these therapies is beyond the scope of this chapter but can be found in the AHA/ACC guideline statements (see Key Web Resources, later). Tables 25-1 and 25-2 provide information on interactions of pharmaceuticals and supplements.

Antiplatelet and Anticoagulant Therapies

Aspirin is the most widely prescribed over-the-counter therapy in cardiology and arguably one of the most potent. Aspirin is a mainstay of therapy for patients with established cardiovascular disease and is also frequently recommended for individuals at high risk of disease. Dosing remains a challenge because higher doses have greater antiplatelet

TABLE 25-1. Important Herbal and Supplement Interactions With Antiplatelet Drugs and Warfarin

AGENTS	HERB OR SUPPLEMENT	EFFECTS OF INTERACTION
Antiplatelet drugs (aspirin, ticlopidine, NSAIDs, clopidogrel)	Caffeine	Antiplatelet effect
	Cordyceps fungus	Platelet antagonism
	Curcumin	Antiplatelet effects
	Dong quai	Platelet antagonism
	Feverfew	Inhibition of platelet aggregation
	Fish oil	Platelet antagonism
	Garlic	Inhibition of platelet aggregation
	Ginger	Prolongation of bleeding time
	Ginkgo	Antiplatelet activity, hemorrhage
	Green tea	Antiplatelet effects
	Guggul	Antiplatelet activity
	Horse chestnut	Antiplatelet activity
	Policosanol	Antiplatelet activity
	Resveratrol	Inhibition of platelet aggregation
	Vitamin E	Antiplatelet activity
Warfarin	Coenzyme Q10	Decrease in INR
	Dong quai	Elevation of PT and INR
	Fenugreek	Possible increase in INR
	Fish oil	Elevation of INR
	Garlic	Elevation of INR
	Ginkgo	CNS hemorrhage
	Ginseng	Decrease in INR
	Green tea	Decrease in INR
	L-Carnitine	Potential increase in INR
	St. John's wort	Decrease in INR

From Burleson K. Coronary artery disease. In: Rakel D, ed. *Integrative Medicine*, 2nd ed. Philadelphia: Saunders; 2007:302.
CNS, central nervous system; INR, international normalized ratio; NSAIDs, nonsteroidal antiinflammatory drugs; PT, prothrombin time.

action, as well as a higher risk of gastrointestinal bleeding. Balancing the risks and benefits was addressed in a meta-analysis that recommended 160 mg/day, although individual patient factors must be incorporated in all treatment decisions.[19]

Patients who take warfarin may approach integrative practitioners for recommendations regarding alternative options, including patients with atrial fibrillation who would like to discontinue taking warfarin. Patients frequently inquire about the possibility of replacing warfarin or the antiplatelet agent clopidogrel with over-the-counter products, including nattokinase, fish oil, and vitamin E, among others. Unfortunately, to date, no studies support the use of botanicals or herbs in place of warfarin in clinical situations of high thrombotic risk.[20]

Angioplasty and Stents

Angioplasty and stents are commonly regarded as the most potent interventions available in cardiology. In the past, investigators logically assumed that mechanically opening a severely stenotic coronary artery would reduce the likelihood

TABLE 25-2. Important Herbal and Supplement Interactions With Other Cardiovascular Drugs

CARDIOVASCULAR DRUG	HERB OR SUPPLEMENT	EFFECTS
Digitalis	Hawthorn	Potentially increased serum levels
	Herbal laxatives	Decreased absorption
	Psyllium	Hypokalemia
	St. John's wort	Decreased serum levels
Amiodarone	—	See precautions for digoxin, warfarin, statins, or herbs with hepatic effects
Propranolol	Guggul	Decreased bioavailability
Clonidine	Yohimbine	Both alpha$_2$-antagonists
Calcium channel blockers	Guggul	Decreased bioavailability
Cyclosporine	St. John's wort	Decreased serum levels
Statins	Red rice yeast	Magnified side effects

From Burleson K. Coronary artery disease. In: Rakel D, ed. *Integrative Medicine*, 2nd ed. Philadelphia: Saunders; 2007:303.

of progression to coronary occlusion and myocardial infarction. Surprisingly, however, angioplasties and stents have not been shown to reduce the risk of myocardial infarction and do not prolong life in most patients who receive these therapies—patients who are asymptomatic or those with stable coronary disease. Survival benefit from angioplasties and stents appears confined to patients who are having an acute myocardial infarction or an episode of unstable angina. In the more chronic setting, the benefit is restricted to improvement of chest pain.

This counterintuitive finding was observed in several studies and summarized in a meta-analysis of 11 trials including nearly 3000 patients.[21] More recently, the COURAGE trial confirmed the lack of survival benefit from adding catheter-based coronary intervention to medical therapy alone.[22] The explanation for the lack of expected outcomes benefit from angioplasty and stents in the stable patient is uncertain, but it likely relates to the finding that mechanical interventions are generally directed at one or two of the possibly hundreds of "vulnerable" plaques that exist in an individual's coronary tree.

Despite the evidence, stating that the absence of expected outcomes benefits from catheter-based intervention in stable patients with coronary disease has dramatically altered physicians' practice would be misleading. Numerous reasons exist for this, including patients' (and physicians') emotional discomfort about not intervening on a severe stenosis identified on angiography and fear of medical and legal implications. These concerns are clearly separate from the scientific findings, however.

Lipid Management

Lifestyle changes are the foundation of a solid prevention program, and the role of lipid management is subordinate to optimizing lifestyle measures. Nevertheless, lipid management is an extremely important consideration for both primary and secondary prevention. Among the lipid parameters, the priorities for prevention are as follows, in order of importance: LDL, HDL, and triglycerides. Total cholesterol is not the most useful end point because it is a summated term that may either underestimate or overestimate risk. One third of heart attacks occur in individuals with a total cholesterol value lower than 200 mg/dL[23] (see Chapter 39, Dyslipidemias).

Low-density Lipoprotein

Among all lipid parameters, control of LDL is of primary importance because it is most closely related to cardiovascular risk. Nevertheless, the optimal measurement to describe the risk imparted by LDL is somewhat controversial. LDL is an apolipoprotein that carries the bulk of circulating cholesterol. Traditional measurement of LDL-C, the basis for most treatment decisions, assesses only the cholesterol content of this complex molecule.

Mounting evidence suggests that the cholesterol content of LDL may not be the best reflection of risk, however. Instead, quantification of the number of LDL particles appears to correlate more closely with cardiovascular risk than does the conventional measurement of LDL-C.

To understand more clearly how to relate cholesterol concentration to LDL particle number, consider the following example: imagine filling 2 bathtubs with cholesterol to the same level designated by the LDL-C value. For the purpose of this example, we will designate an LDL-C of 125 mg/dL as corresponding to filling the bathtub halfway with cholesterol balls. In the first tub, 100 large balls are used to fill the tub halfway. In the second, tub, 2000 small marbles are used to fill the tub to the exact same halfway mark. At first glance, both tubs, filled halfway to the same level of 125 mg/dL, would appear to represent equal cardiovascular risk. However, the person with 2000 smaller particles has a much higher risk of cardiovascular disease than the other individual with an identical LDL-C but with many fewer particles. In other words, risk is much more closely linked to the number of LDL particles than to the concentration of cholesterol.[24]

Several tests are available that quantify the number of atherogenic particles (most of which are LDL particles). The most readily available method for estimating the number of atherogenic particles is non–HDL-C, a simple value that is calculated by subtracting HDL-C from the total cholesterol. Calculation of non–HDL-C is especially helpful when triglycerides exceed 200 mg/dL, an environment in which formation of small, dense LDL is more likely. Non-HDL goals are 30 mg/dL higher than LDL-C goals.[25]

A more accurate reflection of the number of atherogenic particles, however, is apolipoprotein B (ApoB). ApoB takes advantage of the fact that each atherogenic particle contains exactly one molecule of ApoB.[26] Therefore, ApoB has been shown to relate more closely than LDL-C to cardiovascular risk. Another option to measure the number of atherogenic particles is LDL particle number, a proprietary test, that was shown in the Framingham Offspring Study to predict cardiovascular risk more closely than LDL-C.[24] Treatment goals for ApoB and LDL particle number have not been well established but are commonly set at percentile rankings in the population (i.e., lower than the fifth percentile for a very high-risk patient).[27]

The most potent agents available for reduction of LDL-C, ApoB, and LDL particle number are prescription 3-hydroxy-3-methyl-glutaryl-coenzyme A (HMG-CoA) reductase inhibitors, or statins. These medications are capable of lowering LDL-C by more than 50% and have been proven to reduce the likelihood of a cardiovascular event by approximately one third in both primary and secondary prevention studies. Some studies with statins have shown overall mortality benefit, but total mortality benefit is not a consistent finding.[28]

■ Statin-Related Myalgias

Despite the proven benefits of statins in high-risk individuals, treatment is not without risk. Myalgias are a particularly frequent adverse reaction that may be more common than described in the package insert for these medications. An observational study of statins in clinical practice reveals that muscle-related adverse reactions occur in as many as 11% of patients.[29] The potential for adverse muscle-related symptoms increases as the dose is raised.

A survey of patients taking statins who reported muscle-related symptoms to their physicians revealed a sobering finding: in only 29% of cases did physicians endorse the possibility of a link between the patients' complaint of muscle pain and the use of statins.[30] In 47% of cases, the physicians dismissed the possibility of such a link. Patients' belief that their symptoms are not acknowledged by their physicians may explain why more than 50% of patients stop taking statins after only 1 year.[31]

> Alternatives to the use of prescription statins can play an important role when prescription statins cannot be tolerated because of adverse reactions and in patients philosophically opposed to the use of prescription statins.

Options for treatment of patients with intolerance to prescription statins include (1) reducing the dose of the prescription statin, (2) changing to a different prescription statin, or (3) using nonprescription lipid-lowering therapy.

Surprisingly, reducing the dose of a statin by half is expected to reduce the LDL-C–lowering impact by only 7%.[32] Nevertheless, adverse reactions, particularly myalgias, are often improved or eliminated by lowering the dose.[29] Therefore, for patients with mild myalgias related to statin use, dosage modification may eliminate the adverse reaction without sacrificing appreciable lipid control.

Another option is to prolong the dosing frequency of the prescription statin. Rosuvastatin, with the longest half-life of any of the available statins, was shown to retain potent LDL-C reductions when it was given as infrequently as once or twice per week.[33,34] In one study, a mean rosuvastatin dose of 10 mg given once a week resulted in a mean 23% reduction in LDL-C.[34]

Another option for the patient intolerant to a prescription statin is to switch to a different statin. Reactions can be idiosyncratic, and one brand may be well tolerated when others are not. Rosuvastatin and pravastatin may be better tolerated in some individuals, possibly related to the hydrophilic nature of these drugs. Fluvastatin can also be considered because it has a metabolic pathway unique among all statins (mostly by 2C9) that may explain the finding that, in a large survey, it had the lowest risk of myalgias among all the statins.[29]

> Water-soluble statins such as rosuvastatin and pravastatin may cause fewer myalgias in some patients. Fluvastatin may also cause fewer muscle symptoms because of its unique metabolism.

High-Density Lipoprotein

HDL is protective against atherosclerotic disease because of its role in removing LDL from plaque (reverse cholesterol transport) and its antioxidant function. Average HDL-C for men is 40 to 45 mg/dL and for women is 50-55 mg/dL. Low HDL levels are associated with significantly increased cardiovascular risk even in individuals with low LDL concentrations.[35]

Lifestyle measures are the primary strategies for raising HDL and include weight loss, exercise, and smoking cessation.[36] Reducing intake of added sugar and food with high glycemic load will also raise HDL.[10]

Alcohol is effective at raising HDL levels, and this effect may explain the lower risk of cardiovascular events associated with moderate alcohol intake (one serving/day).[37] All forms of alcohol, including white and red wine, beer, and hard liquor, are capable of raising HDL. The cardiovascular benefits need to be balanced by the potential for accidents and abuse, as well as the increased risk of breast cancer associated with alcohol intake in women.

The most potent pharmacologic agent available for boosting HDL-C is niacin. The HDL-raising effect of niacin is dose related, with an increase of 20% to 30% observed at the highest doses, generally approximately 2000 mg/day.[38,39] Limited data suggest a very potent, additive, and possibly synergistic benefit when niacin is added to a statin. In the HDL-Atherosclerosis Treatment Study, patients with low baseline HDL who were treated with both a statin and niacin had an unprecedented 90% reduction in cardiovascular events compared with patients treated with placebo.[40] In another study, patients receiving a baseline statin who also received niacin had significantly more regression of carotid intimal/medial thickness compared with patients receiving a statin and ezetimibe.[41] These results were surprising because, with treatment, LDL-C was lower in the ezetimibe group.

Supplements

When none of the dosing options for prescription statins is tolerated (or the patient refuses to consider a prescription statin), nonprescription therapies may be particularly useful.

In order of efficacy, the following nonprescription therapies are useful for control of LDL-C: fiber, stanols or sterols, niacin, and red yeast rice.

In contrast, herbal and botanical preparations often used for cholesterol management that have been shown to have modest benefit or no benefit include policosanol,[42] garlic,[43] and guggulipids.[44]

Fiber

The water-soluble fraction of fiber, soluble fiber, reduces the absorption of cholesterol in the intestinal tract. Therefore, additional fiber, either in food or in supplements, can aid in cholesterol management. Each gram of dietary fiber decreases LDL-C by approximately 2 mg/dL.[45]

■ Dosage

Supplementation with psyllium, totaling 10 g per day, can reduce LDL-C by 7%.[46]

Stanols and Sterols

Plants do not contain cholesterol but are rich in phytosterols and stanols. Sterols and stanols reduce cholesterol by competing with dietary and biliary cholesterol for intestinal absorption. These agents are capable of reducing LDL-C by up to 14% when they are used either as monotherapy or as an adjunct to statin therapy.[47]

■ Dosage

The usual dose of stanols or sterols is 1.8 g/day as a single dose (added in certain margarines or in pill form).

■ Precautions

These agents are generally well tolerated, but they can cause gastrointestinal distress.

Niacin

Niacin, a B vitamin, shifts all lipids in a favorable direction. At higher dosages, niacin can reduce LDL-C by 15% to 20%, shift LDL particle size to the more favorable, larger form, raise HDL, and lower lipoprotein (a). "No flush" or "flush-free" niacin (inositol hexaniacinate) should be avoided because these products do not contain the active form of niacin and consequently have no significant lipid-altering properties for most individuals.[48] Care should also be taken to avoid niacinamide and nicotinamide, products with names resembles niacin but with no lipid-altering properties.

■ Dosage

The usual starting dose is 500 mg per day, titrated upward by 500 mg increments every 6 to 8 weeks as needed, to maximal daily dose of 2000 mg per day. Check liver function tests after each dose adjustment.

■ Precautions

Although niacin has ideal lipid-altering properties, its use is encumbered by frequent adverse reactions, which are typically annoying but harmless. The most common adverse reaction is flushing, which can occur in up to 50% of individuals and is especially likely when initiating therapy or increasing the dosage. The best strategy to reduce the risk of flushing involves taking niacin with food, typically dinner,

and to use aspirin or nonsteroidal antiinflammatory agents just before taking niacin. Additional relief from flushing may be possible by taking niacin with applesauce as an after-dinner snack. The reason that applesauce may be beneficial in reducing flushing is unknown but it may relate to quercetin, an antioxidant found in high concentration in apples and applesauce and shown to reduce niacin-induced flushing in an experimental animal study.[49]

> Strategies to reduce niacin flush:
> Take niacin with dinner, or after dinner with apple sauce.
> Take aspirin or a nonsteroidal antiinflammatory drug with niacin.
> Avoid "no flush" niacin because it is usually ineffective.

Red Yeast Rice

Red yeast rice is the most effective over-the-counter therapy for treatment of elevated LDL-C, with reductions of 20% to 30%.[50,51] The combination of red yeast rice, fish oil, and therapeutic lifestyle changes has been proven to lower LDL-C by 42%, a reduction comparable to simvastatin 40 mg. This supplement, taken in pill form, is the fermentation product resulting from growing the yeast *Monascus purpureus* on rice. Red yeast rice contains a family of cholesterol lowering molecules known as monacolins, the most prevalent of which is monacolin K, better known by the chemical name lovastatin.

The concentration of monacolins varies widely among different preparations of red yeast rice.[52] In addition, some brands have been shown to contain citrinin, a potentially nephrotoxic fermentation byproduct.[52] Therefore, practitioners should become familiar with a particular brand of red yeast rice and advise patients to continue taking the same brand to increase the likelihood of a consistent result.

Red yeast rice may be a useful option for patients who have not been able to tolerate prescription statins, typically because of myalgias. In a study of patients unable to take a prescription statin because of the development of myalgias, 93% of those taking red yeast rice were free of significant muscle symptoms and had an average LDL-C reduction of 21%.[53]

Outcomes data have also been reported with red yeast rice. A Chinese study of 4870 patients who suffered myocardial infarction were followed up for nearly 5 years, and these patients had a proven significant reduction in cardiovascular events, as well as a 33% reduction in total mortality compared with placebo[54] (Table 25-3).

■ Dosage

The usual (and maximal) dose is 1200 mg twice daily. Patients may use a lower starting dose of 600 mg twice daily if they have a history of significant statin intolerance.

■ Precautions

The amount of active ingredient varies by brand. In addition, a few brands have been shown to contain citrinin, a potential nephrotoxin. Obtain baseline liver and renal function tests

TABLE 25-3. Nonprescription Therapies for Reduction of Low-Density Lipoprotein Cholesterol

PRODUCT	PERCENTAGE OF REDUCTION
Psyllium (10 g/day)	7%[46]
Sterol and stanol (1.8 g/day)	14%[47]
Niacin (up to 2 g/day)	15%–20%
Red yeast rice (2400 mg/day)	20%–30%

and repeat laboratory studies 2 months after initiating therapy and twice a year thereafter. Consumerlabs.com has analyzed red yeast rice brands for potency and the presence of citrinin (see Key Web Resources, later).

Fish Oil

High triglyceride values are associated with increased risk in both men and women, but the risk is higher in women.[55] The mechanism of increased risk is not well understood, although it is likely related to the association between high triglycerides and the predominance of the riskier small, dense LDL particles.

Beyond lifestyle changes, the most effective pharmacologic treatment for elevated triglycerides includes fibrates (gemfibrozil and fenofibrates) and fish oil. Fish oil has been shown to reduce triglyceride levels by 50% when baseline levels exceed 500 mg/dL.

■ Dosage

For prevention, a dose of approximately 1000 mg of combined eicosapentaenoic acid (EPA) and docosahexaenoic acid (DHA) is recommended. For treatment of elevated triglycerides, doses of 1000 to 4000 mg combined EPA and DHA are required. This can be achieved with either over-the-counter fish oil or prescription Lovaza. Care should be taken to dose fish oil in terms of combined EPA and DHA content, rather than "total" fish oil labeled on the front of over-the-counter products. For example, if the label lists EPA 300 mg and DHA 200 mg and the serving size is two capsules, then to obtain 1000 mg of EPA and DHA, the dose would be four capsules daily.

■ Precautions

Fish oil can have a mild anticoagulant effect and should be used with caution in patients taking warfarin. It can also cause mild gastrointestinal upset, which may be relieved by storing fish oil in a freezer before use.

> Fish oil dosing:
> Dosage should specify eicosapentaenoic acid (EPA) and docosahexaenoic acid (DHA) content, rather than total fish oil.
> Advise patients to check the nutrition label of products to confirm the EPA and DHA content.
> The typical dosage for prevention is approximately 1000 mg combined EPA and DHA.
> The typical dosage for treatment of hypertriglyceridemia is 1000 to 4000 mg combined EPA and DHA.

Coenzyme Q10

Not controversial: Coenzyme Q10 (CoQ10) is a mitochondrial membrane–bound compound involved in electron transport and energy production. Therapy with statins lowers the level of circulating CoQ10.

Controversial: Supplementing patients who take statins with CoQ10 reduces the risk of statin-related adverse side effects.

Two randomized studies evaluated treatment with CoQ10 to improve statin-related myalgias, and the results were conflicting. One study of 44 patients with a history of statin-related myalgias showed no improvement when CoQ10 at 200 mg/day was added.[56] In contrast, another study of 32 patients demonstrated a significant reduction in myalgias with CoQ10 at 100 mg/day.[57]

Analysis of the possible role of CoQ10 deficiency on statin-related myalgias is difficult. Although blood levels of CoQ10 typically drop with statin therapy, tissue levels are not consistently affected.[58] The majority of circulating CoQ10 is found in LDL, and, therefore, any intervention that lowers LDL also lowers CoQ10.[58] Therefore, despite strongly polarized opinions regarding the need for CoQ10, the role of CoQ10 in patients treated with statins is uncertain. What does appear clear is that no significant adverse reactions have been reported with CoQ10, even when it is used at doses much higher than 200 mg/day.[59]

> Given the high safety margin and evidence of improvement in some patients, many clinicians find it reasonable to attempt a trial of Coenzyme Q10, 100 mg/day, in patients with a history of suspected statin-related muscle symptoms.

■ Dosage

A dose of 100 mg/day may reduce the development of myalgias in patients taking statins. CoQ10 has no intrinsic lipid-altering properties and has not been reported to reduce the likelihood of developing coronary artery disease. Evidence indicates, however, that CoQ10 at doses up to 200 mg/day may improve systolic function for patients in congestive heart failure.[60]

Vitamin D

Receptors for vitamin D have been identified in heart muscle cells, as well as within arterial walls. Activation of these receptors has many beneficial functions that relate to blood pressure regulation and normal arterial function.[61]

Accordingly, deficiency of vitamin D has been associated with increased cardiovascular risk. The Framingham Offspring Study evaluated individuals without known cardiovascular disease and found that a vitamin D level lower than 15 ng/mL was associated with a 62% increase cardiovascular risk. The link between vitamin D deficiency and cardiovascular risk was especially prominent in persons with hypertension.[62]

Vitamin D deficiency also appears to play a role in statin intolerance. The development of myalgias appears to be more prevalent among vitamin D–deficient patients. In one study, the average vitamin D level in patients with statin-related myalgias was 21 ng/mL, as compared with patients without myalgias, who had an average vitamin D level of 30 ng/mL.[63]

This finding was extended by the observation that patients with statin-related myalgias who are vitamin D deficient (mean vitamin D level, 29 ng/mL) may experience resolution of their symptoms with vitamin D replacement.[64]

Dosage

Although much needs to be learned about the relationship between vitamin D and cardiovascular disease, available data suggest that levels higher than 30 ng/mL are desirable. For patients who are vitamin D deficient, replacement can be achieved with daily dosing of over-the-counter vitamin D_3 (doses of 1000 to 5000 units per day, depending on the severity of the baseline deficiency).

Precautions

Excess vitamin D can cause hypercalcemia Thus, levels should be rechecked to assess adequacy of treatment to reduce toxicity.

Folic Acid

Folic acid and other B vitamins have been proposed as useful supplements in patients with coronary artery disease because these substances lower the circulating levels of homocysteine. Elevated homocysteine levels were previously linked to an increased risk of both coronary heart disease and stroke.[65]

Unexpectedly, randomized trials of folic acid, vitamin B_6, and vitamin B_{12} failed to show benefit for secondary prevention despite the achievement of reduced homocysteine levels: the Norwegian Vitamin (NORVIT) trial (3749 individuals following myocardial infarction who were given regimens containing folic acid at 800 mcg per day) and the Heart Outcomes Prevention Evaluation-2 (HOPE-2) trial (5522 patients with vascular disease or diabetes who were taking folic acid at 2500 mcg per day).[66,67] In the NORVIT trial, the trend was toward harm in the group given a combination of folic acid, vitamin B_6, and vitamin B_{12}.

The reason that folic acid has failed to reduce the occurrence of cardiovascular events is unclear. One explanation is that folic acid is simply a marker, as opposed to a target, of increased risk. An alternative explanation is that folic acid causes harm by some unknown mechanism that offsets the benefits of homocysteine reduction.

Although folic acid supplementation has not proven useful, foods rich in folate, particularly dark green leafy vegetables, are strongly associated with cardiovascular benefit. One study demonstrated a 23% reduction in the development of coronary heart disease with each daily serving of green leafy vegetables.[9] Therefore, consumption of foods rich in folate should be encouraged.

> Folic acid supplementation has not proven useful for prevention of cardiovascular events, but foods rich in folate, especially dark green leafy vegetables, are associated with significant benefit.

Vitamin E

Vitamin E was postulated to reduce the risk of coronary disease because of its potent antioxidant properties. An early study, the Cambridge Heart Antioxidant Study (CHAOS), showed benefit in reducing nonfatal myocardial infarction with a median follow-up of approximately 1.5 years.[68] Subsequent studies of longer duration (3.5 to 8 years) and larger sample size (9541 to 14,641 patients) failed to confirm a beneficial effect, with no reduction in cardiovascular events with vitamin E supplementation.[69-71] These trials used 400 to 800 units of alpha-tocopherol per day, mostly from synthetic sources.

Vitamin E exists in eight isomers: four tocopherols and four tocotrienols. One of the concerns of vitamin E studies was the use of the isolated alpha-tocopherol fraction of vitamin E. Some experimental data suggest that gamma- and delta-tocopherol may be more beneficial than the alpha isomer used in clinical trials.[72,73]

> The evidence to date does not support the use of the synthetic alpha-tocopherol isomer of vitamin E for prevention of cardiac disease. Additional research is needed to evaluate the effect of mixed tocopherols and tocotrienols on cardiovascular events.

Mind-Body Therapy

One of the areas in which an integrative approach stands to contribute most to the field of cardiology is in appreciation of the role of the mind-body connection in heart health. Although many people are intuitively aware that thoughts and emotions can influence the body, most conventional medical encounters do not include assessment of the patient's emotional state, let alone offer therapies directed at mind-body interventions.

The emotional states most commonly linked to heart disease are stress, anxiety, and depression. Of equal importance is the known association between happiness and heart health. The link between stress and anxiety with heart disease is strong and far-reaching, so much so that anxiety disorders diagnosed early in life, by age 20 years, independently predict a doubling of heart disease risk more than 30 years later.[74]

The mechanism by which stress affects cardiac function is unclear, but knowledge is increasing rapidly in this area. Stress clearly leads to an increase in catecholamine levels, which are known to increase blood pressure and heart rate, thereby increasing cardiac work.[75] In a fascinating experiment, psychological stress provoked by mental arithmetic produced severely reduced coronary blood flow, identical to that typically observed with strenuous exercise.[75]

A particularly extreme manifestation of stress on heart health is Takotsubo cardiomyopathy. In this fascinating but potentially lethal condition, psychological stress has been shown to lead to a marked increase in circulating catecholamine levels. The jump in catecholamine triggers acute heart failure typically requiring maximal cardiac support. Antecedent psychological stressors documented to trigger "stress cardiomyopathy" include the death of a parent, a surprise birthday party, fear of a medical procedure, and public speaking.[76] Following the acute phase of Takotsubo cardiomyopathy, cardiac function often recovers completely.

Perhaps less well recognized is the influence of stress on lipids. Both acute stress and chronic stress have been linked to unfavorable lipid responses. Within hours of acute psychological stress, total cholesterol has been shown to increase by 7 mg/dL and LDL-C by 5 mg/dL.[77] Furthermore, the acute lipid response to stress was shown to identify those individuals with hypercholesterolemia measured 3 years later, a finding suggesting that stress may be a contributor to chronic dyslipidemia.[77]

Just as emotional factors may contribute to the development of heart disease, they can also be harnessed to promote heart health. Meditation practiced for 5 years in individuals with coronary disease was demonstrated to reduce the combined risk of a cardiovascular event and death by 43%.[78] The mechanism of risk reduction by meditation likely includes a decrease in cardiovascular workload, as demonstrated by the ability of meditation to blunt the expected increase in heart rate associated with infusion of isoproterenol[75] (see Chapter 98, Recommending Meditation). Another study showed that patients assessed as "optimists" had a 55% reduced risk of cardiovascular death, adjusted for traditional risk factors, compared with their less upbeat peers.[79]

> A wide range of therapies is available to assist patients with cardiac disease to manage their stress and anxiety more effectively. In addition to the conventional treatments with psychoactive medication or referral for cognitive-behavioral therapy, the palette available to the integrative practitioner includes meditation, yoga, biofeedback, healing touch, Reiki, massage, and acupuncture.

No one resource is generically superior to another. Instead, referral should be made based on an individualized assessment including the patient's prior knowledge or history with a particular approach, the patient's philosophical inclination, local expertise, and cost. This "matching" process is truly one of the arts of integrative medicine.

Other Therapies

Enhanced External Counterpulsation
Enhanced external counterpulsation is a noninvasive method of improving blood flow to the heart and reducing anginal symptoms. This treatment involves repetitive leg compressions with a pneumatic device that drives blood backward into the aorta and increases coronary blood flow. A study of 1097 patients with coronary disease showed that 73% had improvement in the severity of angina at the completion of treatment, with sustained benefit after 2 years.[80] Another study examined 363 patients with severe angina and depressed left ventricular function.[81] After treatment, 72% patients had a reduction in severity of angina from severe to mild or none, with benefit continued after 2 years.[81]

Protocols generally involve 35 1-hour sessions of treatment spread out over 5 weeks. Patients referred for this treatment historically have been those with refractory angina who have exhausted medical therapy and mechanical revascularization options.

Chelation Therapy
Chelation therapy has been proposed as a treatment for atherosclerotic vascular disease. The hypothesized mechanisms of benefit include the binding of calcium in atherosclerotic plaque, as well as reduction of oxidative stress leading to improved vascular function. Reviews of the limited available data suggest no overall benefit of chelation therapy for the treatment of vascular disease.[82,83] More information will be available when the results of a $30 million National Institutes of Health study, the Trial to Assess Chelation Therapy (TACT), is completed. This study is testing the impact of ethylenediaminetetraacetic acid (EDTA) chelation on approximately 2000 individuals following myocardial infarction.[84]

PREVENTION PRESCRIPTION

- Nutrition (Mediterranean diet)
- Weight management
- Smoking cessation if needed
- Exercise (aerobics and resistance training)
- Tools for management of stress and anxiety
- Lipid management

THERAPEUTIC REVIEW

Nutrition
- Mediterranean-style diet
  - Five servings vegetables/day
  - Two servings fruit/day
  - Whole grains, elimination of refined carbohydrates
  - Two servings fish/week
  - Reduction of red meat consumption
  - Frequent nut consumption

Exercise
- 30 minutes/day walking or more intensive aerobics for a minimum of 30 minutes three times/week
- Resistance training at least 30 minutes/week

Smoking Cessation

Lipid Management
- For low-density lipoprotein cholesterol
  - Fiber supplements (e.g., psyllium, 10 g/day)
  - Stanols and sterols: 1.8 g/day
  - Niacin: 500 to 2000 mg/day
  - Prescription statins: dose varies

Continued

- Red yeast rice: 1200 to 2400 mg/day divided twice daily
- For high-density lipoprotein cholesterol
  - Exercise
  - Weight loss
  - Reduced intake of carbohydrates
  - Niacin: 500 to 2000 mg/day
- For triglycerides:
  - Exercise
  - Weight loss
  - Reduced intake of carbohydrates
  - Fish oil: 1000 to 4000 mg eicosapentaenoic acid and docosahexaenoic acid per day
  - Fibrates: fenofibrate, 45 to 150 mg/day
- To reduce statin-related myalgias
  - Consider coenzyme Q10: 100 mg/day
  - Replete vitamin D deficiency: goal is level greater than 30 ng/mL

■ Stress and Anxiety Reduction

- Breathing exercises
- Biofeedback
- Meditation
- Yoga
- Acupuncture
- Cognitive-behavioral therapy
- Anxiolytics

■ Antianginal Therapy

- Acetylsalicylic acid: 81 to 325 mg daily
- Beta blockers (e.g., metoprolol succinate: usual dose 50 to 200 mg daily)
- Nitrates (e.g., isosorbide mononitrate: usual dose 30 to 120 mg daily)
- Calcium channel blockers (e.g., amlodipine: 2.5 to 10 mg daily)
- Angioplasty and stents (for angina)
- Enhanced external counterpulsation

KEY WEB RESOURCES

American Heart Association practice guidelines. http://my.americanheart.org/professional/StatementsGuidelines/Statements-Guidelines_UCM_316885_SubHomePage.jsp

This Web site from the American Heart Association (AHA) and American Stroke Association (ASA) publishes medical scientific statements on topics related to cardiovascular disease and stroke. Volunteer scientists and health care professionals from AHA and ASA write the statements, which are supported by scientific studies in recognized journals. These statements generally review available data on a topic, evaluate its relationship to the science surrounding cardiovascular disease, and often conclude with an AHA/ASA position on the topic.

Natural Medicines Database. www.naturaldatabase.com.

This site is an excellent resource for detailed information about supplements including the scientific basis (or lack thereof), adverse reactions, and interactions with drugs and supplements.

ConsumerLab. http://www.consumerlab.com.

This site summarizes testing information regarding the content and purity of commonly recommended supplements.

References

References are available at expertconsult.com.

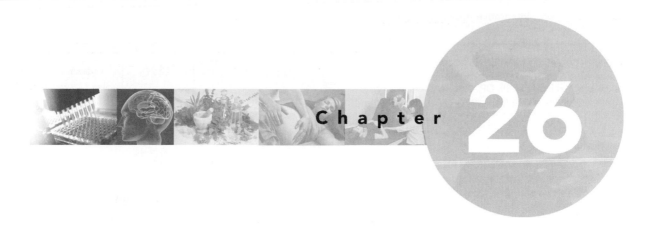

Chapter

26

Peripheral Vascular Disease

Danna Park, MD

Pathophysiology

Peripheral vascular disease (PVD) is a term applicable to several vessel occlusive diseases, whether they stem from the venous system or the arterial system. For the purpose of this chapter, discussion is limited to peripheral atherosclerotic vascular disease, also known as peripheral vascular occlusive disease or peripheral artery disease (PAD), because this entity correlates with coronary artery disease, hypertension, and diabetes. However, PVD can arise from numerous vasculitides and from other venous problems such as chronic venous insufficiency. These conditions would require different assessments and treatment strategies, depending on the underlying cause.

The American Heart Association divides PVD into two categories: functional and organic. Functional PVD is not related to structural problems in blood vessel walls; instead, this type of PVD can stem from vessel spasm or compression. Organic PVD is associated with vessel blockage resulting from fatty infiltrates, inflammation, or tissue damage. PAD is a subset of organic PVD.[1]

Most commonly diagnosed when a patient experiences intermittent claudication, PAD is a peripheral sequela of atherosclerosis in the body, which can affect other systems as well and can result in coronary artery disease, stroke, and renal disease. Other diseases and risk factors that place patients at risk for PAD include diabetes, hypertension, tobacco use, and hyperlipidemia. Estimates indicate that 8 million to 10 million U.S. residents are affected by PAD; concurrent with the diagnosis of PAD is an increased risk of cardiovascular mortality (four to six times greater risk than healthy individuals of the same age).[2] Symptoms of PAD may be variable depending on the vessel involved and range from no symptoms, intermittent claudication (reported in only 11% to 40% of patients), impotence, a feeling of weakness in the hip or thigh, or variable pain in the buttocks, thighs, or feet.[3] Signs on physician examination may also be variable and include the following: ulcerations or nonhealing wounds; loss of hair; skin redness; skin coolness to touch; decreased or absent pulses; impaired capillary refill; and dry, scaly, or shiny skin. The best way to diagnose PAD is noninvasive and can be done in the office setting by using the ankle-brachial index (ABI), a comparison of the systolic blood pressure (SBP) in the dorsalis pedis and posterior tibial arteries in the ankle with the brachial artery of the arm (Fig. 26-1). In comparison with confirmed PAD by angiogram, this simple technique is 95% sensitive and almost 100% specific.[4] A normal measurement is greater than 0.9, whereas any value less than 0.9 indicates the presence of PAD. A patient within the range from 0.9 to 0.7 may be asymptomatic or have very mild intermittent claudication symptoms, whereas patients with an ABI of 0.7 to 0.4 have mild to moderate claudication. Patients with an ABI less than 0.4 have advanced PAD with a high likelihood of rest pain and ulceration complications. In addition to ABI, treadmill testing can be a useful adjunct to determine how fast claudication pain develops, the time to maximal pain, and the effect of exercise on ABI, and it can also be used as a screening tool for atherosclerotic heart disease.[5] Standard of care now emphasizes that all patients with PAD have aggressive treatment and risk reduction therapies regardless of the level of symptom severity, because many patients with PAD are asymptomatic.

Performance measures for PAD were established in 2010 by the American College of Cardiology and the American Heart Association in conjunction with other national associations. The measures include periodic measurement of ABI in at-risk patients, treatment with a statin drug to lower low-density lipoprotein cholesterol (LDL-C) to less than 100 mg/dL (or less than 70 mg/dL in patients with PAD with a very high risk of ischemic events), tobacco cessation treatment, antiplatelet therapy with aspirin or clopidogrel, a supervised claudication exercise program, and serial monitoring of patients with asymptomatic abdominal aortic aneurysms or those who have lower extremity vein bypass grafts.[6]

An ABI less than 0.9 suggests PAD. An SBP value of the posterior tibial artery of 100 mm Hg divided by a systolic brachial artery pressure of 140 mm Hg would give an abnormal ABI of 0.71.

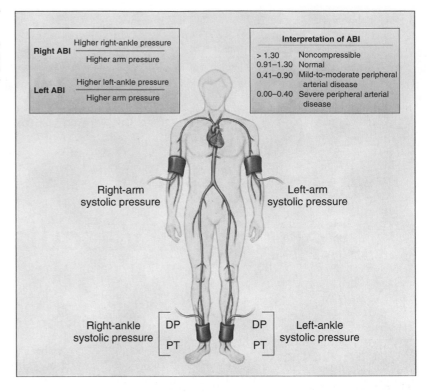

Integrative Therapy

Biomarkers and Genetics

Low-grade inflammation has been implicated as one of the
independent risk factors for PAD, but obtaining a significant
laboratory panel assessment specific and diagnostic for PAD
alone has been elusive. Homocysteine, C-reactive protein
(CRP), fibrinogen, lipid levels, and hypercoagulability markers are all associated with coronary artery disease and atherosclerosis, and they can be elevated in other vascular disorders.
Although ABI is a very low-cost, reasonable tool with high sensitivity and specificity, it has not yet been universally accepted
as a screening tool because it is considered to be technically difficult to perform accurately. Researchers have turned to identification of possible biomarkers specific for PAD that could be
assessed by a simple blood test. Beta$_2$-microglobulin, cystatin
C, high-sensitivity CRP and glucose were shown to be associated with PAD independent of other "traditional" risk factors.[7]

Genetic variants continue to be investigated, because family studies indicate that PAD is heritable. Assessing the impact
of genetic susceptibility is difficult, however, given the many
nonheritable risk factors, such as tobacco use, diabetes, and
hyperlipidemia. Difficulties include the need to screen thousands of patients for adequate study power, the need to look at
more than one single nucleotide polymorphism (SNP) genotype, and the possibility of genotyping errors. Genome-wide
association studies may be more useful for investigating multiple SNPs and relationships with PAD versus no PAD.[8]

Risk Factor Reduction

Because PAD is an indicator of systemic atherosclerosis even
when the patient is asymptomatic, investigators agree that risk
reduction on various levels must be undertaken, especially in
the areas of diabetes control, hypertension, hyperlipidemia,
exercise, and tobacco cessation.

Diabetes increases risk of PAD by fourfold to fivefold, although the often concomitant problems of tobacco
use, high lipid levels, and hypertension seem to play more
important roles in atherosclerosis than does the level of glucose control. However, advising aggressive glucose control
for risk reduction in overall cardiovascular events seems
prudent; a hemoglobin A1c value of 7.0% or less is recommended.[9] Hypertension is associated with a twofold to threefold increased risk of PAD.[9] In the Framingham Heart Study,
risk profiles for intermittent claudication showed a twofold
increase in risk with stage II or greater hypertension (SBP
more than 160 mm Hg or diastolic blood pressure [DBP]
more than 100 mm Hg), and a 1.5-fold risk increase with
stage I hypertension (SBP more than 140 to less than 160 mm
Hg or DBP more than 90 to less than 100 mm Hg). In addition, hypertension is a major risk factor for nonsymptom-
atic PAD found by noninvasive testing (e.g., ABI) as well
as for symptomatic PAD.[10] Risk reduction in this area is of
particular importance for overall cardiovascular mortality
and morbidity—coronary artery disease is associated with a
nearly triple risk for intermittent claudication.[10] Angiotensin-
converting enzyme (ACE) inhibitors are particularly well
suited for hypertension and PAD because of their positive
effects on endothelial remodeling, function, and slowing of
atherosclerotic lesion progression.[3]

Hyperlipidemia plays a significant role in overall cardiovascular morbidity and mortality, as well as in PAD—
recommended target goals for LDL and triglyceride levels
are less than 100 mg/dL (less than 70 mg/dL if many ischemic risk factors are present) and less than 150 mg/dL,
respectively. The evidence for the benefits of statin drugs in
PAD regardless of the patient's coronary artery disease status is significant, so this therapy should be standard of care

for all patients with PAD. A 2005 Cochrane Review had a small number of eligible studies to examine (seven in all) with regard to lipid lowering for lower extremity PAD; however, results showed a reduction in overall mortality, and one study showed a 28% increase in the ABI (an indication of improvement in vessel disease) and improvement in walking distance overall.[11] Subsequent studies have continued to show that statins increase walking time, improve ABI and claudication symptoms, and decrease all-cause mortality, cardiovascular death, and renal failure.[12] In addition to statin therapy, a low-fat diet should be recommended, and lipid-lowering supplements may be considered in addition to drug therapy (see Chapter 39, Dyslipidemias).

High homocysteine levels have been associated with increased risk of coronary artery disease in addition to being an independent risk factor for PAD. Although checking and treating high homocysteine levels were recommended in the past, some more recent studies and meta-analyses evaluating the effectiveness of treatment with folate (with or without other B vitamins) did not show a decrease in myocardial infarction, stroke, sudden death, or vascular disease despite statistically significant decreases in plasma homocysteine levels. Homocysteine may serve as a marker of coronary and vascular disease, rather than a causal factor. Until more evidence is available, current data are insufficient to support screening or treatment of hyperhomocysteinemia.[13,14]

Lifestyle Interventions

Exercise

Studies indicate that exercise helps relieve intermittent claudication, although it must be prescribed in a graduated fashion as the patient tolerates, by increasing the amount of exercise time as claudication symptoms improve. Potential mechanisms by which exercise is thought to improve claudication symptoms include stimulation of angiogenesis, thus causing formation of collateral vessels and increasing blood flow. Improved endothelial vasodilation with exercise was shown in animal models, whereas an increase in the oxygen extraction capacity of exercised leg muscles was demonstrated in patients with claudication.[15] Given that exercise is also indicated for the medical conditions that are most commonly associated with PAD such as heart disease, diabetes, high cholesterol levels, and hypertension, exercise is one of the primary lifestyle interventions. Because patients with PVD are also at high risk for cardiovascular disease, cardiac testing must be undertaken before establishing and individualizing an exercise program. Overall, exercise has been proven to decrease atherosclerotic risk factors such as hypertension, insulin resistance, obesity, and lipid abnormalities such as high triglycerides and low high-density lipoprotein (HDL).[16] One meta-analysis showed that with exercise rehabilitation, walking distance to onset of claudication pain increased by 179%, whereas distance to maximal claudication pain increased by 122%. Greatest improvement occurred with a walking-based exercise program longer than 6 months of at least 30 minutes of walking three or more times per week with intermittent walking to near-maximal claudication pain as the end point.[17] Lower extremity resistance training was shown to increase functional performance in treadmill walking time, quality of life measures, and stair-climbing ability when compared with a control group, so a combination of aerobic and resistance exercise may be optimal.[18]

An exercise prescription should include the foregoing recommendations and should emphasize periods of walking to the point of high to moderate claudication pain interspersed with rest in the 30-minute period. For those patients who do not have access to a supervised exercise program, a self-motivated walking program is also efficacious. One small observational study showed less annual decline in functional walking distance when walking was incorporated as self-directed exercise three or more times per week.[19] Current evidence continues to support the use of cilostazol in conjunction with exercise as the best way to maximize the greatest change in ABI and walking distance to claudication pain; this combination was better for outcomes than conventional medical management, exercise, or drug therapy alone[5] (see Chapter 88, Writing an Exercise Prescription).

> A graduated walking program over 6 months for at least 30 minutes, three or more times per week, can significantly improve claudication pain and exercise endurance.

Tobacco Cessation

That smoking is an enormous risk factor for PAD is universally accepted. The population-attributable risk ranges from 14% to 53%, indicating a huge potential for prevention of PAD if smoking is eliminated.[10] A dose-response relationship has also been established, with an increased prevalence (2.3 times higher) of symptomatic PAD in smokers.[20] Smokers with intermittent claudication have a higher incidence of rest pain, myocardial infarction, and cardiac death; the 10-year survival rate for smokers and nonsmokers with intermittent claudication of 46% and 82%, respectively.[21] Studies show that smoking cessation can cause a 10-fold decrease in the 5-year risk of amputation in patients with PAD, and this finding provides another reason to pursue smoking cessation treatments aggressively in these patients.[22] Surprisingly, radiologic data of patients who continue to smoke heavily after percutaneous transluminal angioplasty (PTA) or stent placement in lower extremity arteries show a reduced restenosis rate. Elevated levels of carbon monoxide resulting from smoking are thought to play antiinflammatory and antiproliferative roles as vascular smooth muscle cell proliferation is inhibited.[23] Obviously, the benefit is far outweighed by the foregoing costs, and smoking cessation should be highly recommended and supported. Options for smoking cessation include nicotine replacement products, counseling, medications such as bupropion and buspirone, hypnosis, acupuncture, and cognitive-behavioral therapy—all these treatments vary in degree of success rates.

Nutrition

Nutrition and weight management are fundamental components of any cardiovascular treatment plan. Dietary recommendations for PVD are in essence the same as for other atherosclerotic conditions, modified by existing risk factors such as insulin resistance or hyperlipidemia as described earlier.[24] Studies looking at dietary factors important in the prevention and management of PVD have focused on dietary fiber and omega-3 fatty acid intake.

Omega-3 Fatty Acids

Omega-3 fatty acids may benefit patients with PVD through lipid-lowering properties, as well as changes in LDL susceptibility to oxidation.[25] A Cochrane Review assessed the benefits as noted in four placebo-controlled randomized trials that used omega-3 enriched foods (e.g., eggs), omega-3–rich fish oils, and supplements.[26] The reviewers concluded that omega-3 fatty acids do have positive effects in this population, as assessed by reductions in triglyceride levels and DBP. However, the effects on clinically relevant outcomes such as pain-free walking distance or ABIs were inconsistent. A study of 60 men with intermittent claudication observed increases in pain-free walking distance and ABI values in those men taking a fortified dairy product that included omega-3 fatty acids, oleic acid, folic acid, vitamin B$_6$, and vitamin E over a 12-month period.[27] To ascertain the significance of each nutrient is difficult, given the multitude included in the supplement.

■ Dosage

Recommend foods abundant in omega-3 fatty acids, such as cold-water fish (salmon, mackerel and sardines), omega-3–enriched eggs, flaxseed products, and fish oil supplements (500-mg capsules, 2 to 4 g/day total dose). Be aware that human enzymatic conversion of plant sources of omega-3 fatty acids, such as flaxseed (an alpha-linolenic acid [ALA] source) into useable eicosapentaenoic acid (EPA) and docosahexaenoic acid (DHA) is very low: in a study of young men, approximately 8% of dietary ALA was converted to EPA and 0% to 4% was converted to DHA.[28] Therefore, the prudent course is not to use flaxseed or other plant sources as the sole sources of omega-3 supplementation in the diet (see Chapter 86, The Antiinflammatory Diet).

■ Precautions

Fish oil in higher doses may inhibit platelet aggregation and increase bleeding risk.

Fiber

Dietary fiber, which includes all plant food parts that the body is unable to digest or absorb, is often divided into those types that do not dissolve in water (insoluble fiber) and those that do (soluble fiber). Soluble fiber is found in oat bran, psyllium, barley, nuts, seeds, beans, lentils, peas, and some fruits and vegetables. Foods high in insoluble fiber include whole wheat breads, wheat cereals, wheat bran, rye, cabbage, beets, carrots, Brussels sprouts, cauliflower, and apple skin.

Several epidemiologic studies examined the relative merits of soluble and insoluble fiber in patients with PVD. A prospective analysis of the relationship between dietary fiber and PAD risk was conducted using sequential food frequency questionnaires among more than 46,000 men with no baseline cardiovascular disease or diabetes. During 12 years of follow-up, 308 cases of PAD were diagnosed. After adjusting for confounding variables, intake of cereal fiber, but not fruit and vegetable fiber, was inversely correlated with PAD risk.[29,30] Other research on fiber in cardiovascular risk identified differential effects: whole grain (cereal) fiber was linked to lower body mass index, blood pressure, and homocysteine; fruit fiber was associated with lower blood pressure and waist-to-hip ratios; vegetable fiber was associated with lower blood pressure and homocysteine; and fiber from nuts, seeds, and dried fruit was associated with less abdominal obesity, insulin resistance, and lower apolipoprotein B levels.

Given the numerous benefits of all dietary sources, recommending adequate fiber intake from various dietary sources as whole foods rather than as supplements is wise. The recommended goal is a total of 25 to 30 g of fiber per day. Specific instructions to help patients achieve this goal may include the following:

- Eat at least 4½ cups of fruits and vegetables daily.
- Replace white bread with whole grain breads and cereals.
- Add ¼ cup of wheat bran to foods such as cooked cereal, applesauce, or meat loaf.
- Eat cooked beans each week.

Caution patients to add fiber to the diet gradually, to avoid excessive abdominal bloating and discomfort (see Chapter 86, The Antiinflammatory [Omega-3] Diet).

Mind-Body Therapy

Biofeedback

Autogenic training, or biofeedback, may be a useful adjunct for the treatment of PAD. Biofeedback training teaches the patient how to control the sympathetic nervous system and leads to relaxation, stress reduction, and decreased nervous system tone. Thermal biofeedback uses temperature sensors to teach how to increase blood flow to the extremities. As muscles relax, peripheral perfusion improves. Two case studies[31] using thermal biofeedback in patients with diabetic intermittent claudication showed improved distal extremity temperatures, ABIs, and walking distance.[32]

Treatment of Depression

Evaluation and treatment for depression should also be considered for patients with PAD because of the correlation between depression and lower extremity arterial disease. One study showed twice the risk of depressed mood in patients with PAD than in controls, with shorter walking distances significantly correlating with the likelihood of depression.[33] A second study in 2003 reinforced these findings and showed a relationship between depression and the prevalence of leg pain at rest and with exertion, shorter walking distance, and slower walking velocity.[34]

If anger proneness is an issue, counseling should be considered. Anger proneness, depression, and lack of social support systems have been shown to be independent risk factors for coronary artery disease. The Atherosclerosis Risk in Communities Study showed a similar association between anger proneness and incident PAD, with relative risk of PAD of approximately 1.4 in the high-anger group. Moderate and high levels of depressive symptoms also increased the risk of PAD, with relative risks of 1.2 and 1.4, respectively.[35]

Pharmacotherapy

All the antiplatelet agents have potentially serious interactions with most of, if not all, the botanical supplements indicated for peripheral artery disease. Using antiplatelet agents in combination with these supplements is not advised.

Antiplatelet agents have known risk reduction and health benefit in patients with PAD. These agents have shown a preventive benefit of limb loss risk and need for revascularization procedures,[22] as well as overall decreased risk (25% reduction) for cardiovascular events such as vascular death, nonfatal myocardial infarction, and nonfatal stroke.[36] Improvement in the ABI and decreased progression of peripheral disease by angiography have also been demonstrated.[37] Because of these findings, standard medical care for PAD now includes an antiplatelet agent.

Aspirin

Aspirin is probably the most cost-effective therapy and is most commonly used in a dose of 160 to 325 mg/day. Evidence indicates that clopidogrel (Plavix), which blocks platelet activation by adenosine diphosphate, has an advantage over aspirin in decreasing the risk of ischemic stroke, myocardial infarction, and vascular death. The Clopidogrel versus Aspirin in Patients at Risk of Ischemic Events (CAPRIE) study showed a 24% risk reduction of the foregoing events in the subgroup of patients with PAD who received clopidogrel (75 mg daily) versus aspirin (325 mg daily).[38] However, the cost difference is substantial: a month's supply of aspirin costs approximately $1.90, and a month's supply of clopidogrel costs $249.00.[39] The low risk of hematologic adverse effects makes clopidogrel the preferred agent over ticlopidine (Ticlid) for aspirin-intolerant or aspirin-allergic patients, because ticlopidine has been associated with serious adverse effects including thrombocytopenia, thrombotic thrombocytopenic purpura, and neutropenia.[40]

Clinical trials evaluating aspirin for PAD have been statistically underpowered, and noncompliance rates in one study (the Aspirin for Asymptomatic Atherosclerosis trial) approached 40%. Despite these limitations, reductions of vascular events were still evident in some trials. Although more studies are needed, evidence favors the use of antiplatelet therapy.[41]

▧ Dosage
The dose for aspirin is 160 to 325 mg/day.

▧ Precautions
Large doses of aspirin have hypoglycemic effects—use caution in diabetic patients. This agent may cause changes in thyroid function tests. Concurrent administration with other antiplatelet or anticoagulant medications increases the risk of bleeding. Do not use aspirin in patients with bleeding disorders, liver disease, vitamin K deficiency, or gastrointestinal bleeding. Use caution in patients with asthma, nasal polyps, or allergic rhinitis. This drug is pregnancy category D.

▧ Adverse Effects
Adverse effects may include gastrointestinal bleeding, dyspepsia, vomiting, diarrhea, hepatotoxicity, tinnitus, vertigo, hematologic dysfunction, urticaria, angioedema, asthma, rash, confusion, and dizziness.

Clopidogrel (Plavix)
▧ Dosage
The dose is 75 mg daily.

▧ Precautions
Clopidogrel is contraindicated if the patient has any active bleeding. Rare reports have noted thrombotic thrombocytopenic purpura even with short exposure (less than 2 weeks). This drug prolongs bleeding time; do not use it in patients with bleeding disorders, gastrointestinal ulcers, or gastrointestinal bleeding, and use it with caution in patients with liver disease and renal disease. Do not use clopidogrel in conjunction with nonsteroidal antiinflammatory drugs. Use with caution in conjunction with aspirin. Clopidogrel inhibits cytochrome P-450 at high concentrations, so use with caution if the patient is taking other drugs that are metabolized using this system.

Drug therapy for intermittent claudication previously included pentoxifylline (Trental) or cilostazol (Pletal). However, as a result of findings from a comparative 24-week study of cilostazol versus pentoxifylline versus placebo for effects on mean and pain-free walking distance in patients with intermittent claudication, cilostazol is now considered more effective. Cilostazol-treated patients had higher increases in pain-free and mean walking distance, and the drug was more effective than placebo or pentoxifylline.[42] In smaller drug withdrawal studies, patients receiving long-term pentoxifylline courses were able to be weaned off their medication without worsening of claudication symptoms. However, one subset of patients does seem to benefit from the drug (approximately 20%)[22] as compared with an estimated benefit of approximately 50% for patients receiving cilostazol.[42]

Cilostazol (Pletal)
▧ Dosage
Give 100 mg twice daily.

▧ Precautions
This drug is contraindicated in congestive heart failure of any severity as a result of phosphodiesterase III inhibition, in patients with active bleeding, or in patients with bleeding disorders. Use caution in patients with renal disease or liver disease. This drug has not been studied in dialysis recipients; reduce the dose if the patient is taking other drugs that inhibit cytochrome P-450, CYP3A4, or CYP2C19; avoid concomitant use with other antiplatelet or anticoagulant medications.

Botanicals

Ginkgo (Ginkgo biloba)
One of the top-selling herbs in the United States, ginkgo has been used medicinally in various cultures for millennia. Strong evidence exists for its use in PVD, evidence attributed to both its inhibition of platelet activating factor and its vascular relaxation by stimulation of endothelium-derived relaxing factor and prostacyclin release and its inhibition of nitric oxide.[43,44] Numerous double-blind randomized trials suggested that Ginkgo biloba extract causes small improvements in pain-free walking distance, maximum walking distance, and plethysmography recordings compared with placebo.[45–50] These results were confirmed as statistically significant in four published meta-analyses.[51–54] With pooled data, however, the increase in pain-free walking was a modest 34 m. Later randomized double-blind controlled studies

varied from not showing any difference in supervised exercise training with 240 mg/day of standardized ginkgo compared with placebo[55] to showing modest but not statistically significant increase in maximal treadmill walking time with 300 mg standardized ginkgo extract daily.[56] Additional evidence is needed.

Dosage

A dose of 120 to 240 mg of standardized leaf extract is taken daily in two or three divided doses. Products used in published clinical trials (available as tablets or capsules) include EGb 761, standardized to contain 24% ginkgo flavone glycosides and 6% terpenoids, and LI 1370, which contains 25% ginkgo flavone glycosides and 6% terpenoids. These formulas are available under many brand names. Three to 6 mL of 40 mg/mL ginkgo leaf liquid extract may also be taken to achieve the same dose.

Precautions

Although ginkgo leaf extract has been generally well tolerated and safe in clinical trials up to 1 year, caution needs to be taken in patients prone to bleeding or bruising. Several case reports have noted spontaneous hemorrhage such as subdural hematoma, subarachnoid hemorrhage, and anterior ocular chamber hemorrhage.[57] Combination with products known to increase bleeding, including herbs (e.g., garlic, ginseng, ginger) and pharmaceuticals (e.g., nonsteroidal antiinflammatory drugs, heparin, and warfarin) should be done with extreme caution or avoided. Although no cases of bleeding have been reported with ginkgo used in conjunction with low-dose aspirin (75 to 325 mg daily), similar concerns apply. Some experts advise stopping ginkgo ingestion 3 to 7 days before surgery to avoid perioperative complications.[58] At high doses, ginkgo theoretically can interact with antidepressants through its inhibition of serotonin and dopamine uptake; concomitant use should thus be closely monitored. Isolated reports of seizure in patients taking ginkgo are of unclear significance.

> Economic data from 2000 showed that a 120-mg daily dose of ginkgo extract in the United States ranged from $0.41 to $0.84 retail. In contrast, costs of the conventional drug pentoxifylline (1200 mg) ranged from $1.83 to $1.93 and for cilostazol (200 mg) from $2.90 to $4.23.[52]

Policosanol

Policosanol is a mixture of alcohols isolated and purified from the outer wax of sugar cane (Saccharum officinarum). It consists of 66% octacosanol, 12% triacontanol, and 7% hexacosanol and smaller amounts of other alcohols. These substances can also be found in wheat germ oil, alfalfa, and some animal products. Research showed that policosanol may lower serum LDL cholesterol, raise HDL cholesterol levels, and reduce platelet aggregation.[59,60] Policosanol is primarily manufactured in Cuba. A single research group in South America has conducted much of the published clinical data in PVD on a uniform population, a situation that casts some concerns about validity and generalizability. Two randomized, controlled trials found improved walking distance by more than 50% at doses of 10 to 20 mg/day taken for 6-month and 2-year durations.[61,62] In addition, small trials by the same researchers found policosanol more effective than the drug lovastatin for treating intermittent claudication and found that policosanol lowered LDL-C, increased HDL, increased the ankle-arm pressure ratio, and also increased walking distance compared with ticlopidine.[63,64]

Dosage

Typical doses of policosanol for PAD range from 10 to 20 mg daily. Consumerlab.com testing of seven policosanol supplements found that four contained only 23% to 78% of the stated ingredient.

Some "policosanol" products on the market use beeswax as the source. Beeswax contains substances similar to policosanol derived from sugar cane, but in different proportions. The relative efficacy of the beeswax products remains unclear.

Precautions

Policosanol appears to be safe at the recommended dose, with only mild short-term side effects reported in the aforementioned trials. In a study that followed 27,879 participants for up to 4 years, only 0.31% reported adverse effects, primarily weight loss, increased urination, and insomnia.[65] Like ginkgo, however, policosanol inhibits platelet aggregation and should be used cautiously, if at all, with herbs and drugs with anticoagulant effects (see earlier). It should be stopped 7 days before and after any surgery, invasive procedures, or dental procedures.

Padma 28

Padma 28 is a complex Tibetan plant preparation composed of 20 different herbs. Its proposed mechanisms of action include lipid lowering, inhibition of platelet aggregation, and antioxidant effects. A meta-analysis of six randomized, controlled trials examining patients with intermittent claudication taking Padma 28 or placebo found an improvement in maximal walking distance of more than 100 m in pooled data in approximately one out of five patients, with good tolerability of the herbal product.[66] Larger studies are needed to clarify long-term safety and efficacy.

Dosage

The dose is 403 mg, two capsules, twice a day. Padma 28 is produced by Padma AG of Zollikon, Switzerland. A related formula, Padma Basic, is available in the United States.

Precautions

Adverse effects reported in studies include mild gastrointestinal disturbances, fatigue, rash, and progression of symptoms.[67]

Supplements

L-Arginine

Arginine is a semiessential amino acid; with the exception of certain conditions and stresses, the body usually synthesizes adequate amounts. Among its many roles, L-arginine is used as a precursor in the formation of nitric oxide, a substance that relaxes the blood vessels. This property led to the postulate that arginine may benefit patients with cardiovascular diseases, including intermittent claudication.[68] A small number of shorter-term studies had found increases in pain-free walking distance. In the most recent and longest randomized clinical trial, the Nitric Oxide in Peripheral Arterial Insufficiency (NO-PAIN) study, 133 patients with PAD were randomized to placebo versus 3 g L-arginine for 6 months, with the primary end point being the change in absolute claudication distance using the Skinner-Gardner treadmill protocol at 6 months. Although plasma arginine levels increased in the study group, nitric oxide availability measures did not. Absolute claudication distance increased in both groups, with the placebo group improving more (28.3%) than the arginine group (11.5%).[69] Arginine does not appear to be useful in PAD for long-term use, perhaps as a result of arginine tolerance and the body's adaptation to higher doses over time.

Dosage
No firmly established dose recommendation exists for arginine. Studies in coronary artery disease and claudication employed 2 to 3 g orally three times a day, for 3 to 6 months. Dietary sources of arginine include nuts, dairy products, poultry, and fish.

Precautions
At moderate doses, oral arginine appears to be safe, with minimal side effects. High-dose arginine is not recommended because it can stimulate the body's production of gastrin, with the potential for gastric ulcers or interaction with other irritants. Arginine may also affect growth hormone, glucagon, and insulin activity and should be used cautiously in diabetic patients. Arginine has the potential to promote low blood pressure and electrolyte and chemical disturbances (e.g., high potassium, low sodium, and high blood urea nitrogen levels). This is a particular concern for individuals who take drugs that also alter potassium balance (e.g., potassium-sparing diuretics and ACE inhibitors), as well as those with severe kidney or liver disease. Arginine can also increase bleeding risk when it is taken with herbs and drugs with anticoagulant or antiplatelet effects (see the earlier discussion of ginkgo). Arginine should be used with caution in combination with nitrates or sildenafil because of potentiating vasodilation and additive hypotensive effects.

Antioxidants
The role of antioxidants, such as vitamin E (alpha-tocopherol), vitamin C, and beta-carotene, in the prevention or treatment of many conditions is an area of active controversy. Initial studies showing benefit were countered by others that demonstrated harmful effects such as increased all-cause mortality.[70] Oxidative stress plays a key role in the initiation and progression of the atherosclerotic process; in theory, antioxidants could act as a defense.[71]

Epidemiologic data support the importance of antioxidants in the diet: the Rotterdam Study performed a cross-sectional analysis of the association of dietary beta-carotene, vitamin C, and vitamin E with prevalence of PVD. Of 4367 subjects with no baseline cardiovascular disease, PVD (diagnosed by ankle-arm SBP index) was found in 204 men and 370 women. Based on analysis of food frequency questionnaires, vitamin C intake was significantly inversely associated with PAD in women, and vitamin E intake was inversely associated with PAD in men.[72] However, the data regarding antioxidant in supplement form are less convincing.

A Cochrane Review identified five trials of vitamin E in PVD that met the eligibility criteria.[73] Each trial reported positive effects on clinical outcomes, yet all were judged to be flawed and of overall poor quality. A double-blind placebo-controlled trial of 1484 individuals with intermittent claudication compared vitamin E (50 mg daily), beta-carotene (20 mg daily), or a combination of the two versus placebo and found no benefit in any of the treatment groups.[74]

> The data for antioxidant use in peripheral vascular disease are currently insufficient to recommend the use of these agents, especially in light of potential safety issues.

L-Carnitine
L-Carnitine plays an important role in energy production by chaperoning activated fatty acids into the mitochondrial matrix for metabolism and chaperoning toxic metabolites out of the intracellular space.[75] L-Carnitine also works indirectly to stimulate the enzyme pyruvate dehydrogenase and increase pyruvate oxidation. By counteracting high levels of free fatty acids, which occur in ischemia, and by enhancing carbohydrate metabolism, L-carnitine may attenuate injury from ischemia.[76]

Clinically, L-carnitine may be of some benefit in intermittent claudication.[77,78] Hemodynamic studies suggest that L-carnitine may increase walking distance by improving energy use in the muscles, rather than by affecting peripheral blood flow.[79]

Several multicenter double-blind placebo-controlled trials in Europe examined the potential utility of a special form of carnitine called propionyl-L-carnitine.[80-82] In a study involving 495 patients, a 44% improvement in walking distance was noted in patients with moderate to severe PVD (initial maximal walking distance of less than 250 m) as compared with placebo.[80] However, patients with milder degrees of PVD did not benefit from supplementation. Another study of 155 patients with disabling claudication in the United States and Russia found significantly improved walking distance and speed (by the Walking Impairment Questionnaire), enhanced physical functioning, and reduced body pain in the treatment group.[85] Many, although not all, other published studies on both L-carnitine and propionyl-L-carnitine also posted positive results. In 2008, a phase IV multicenter clinical double-blind randomized controlled trial of cilostazol and L-carnitine (levocarnitine tartrate) commenced to evaluate peak walking times for cilostazol versus cilostazol plus levocarnitine tartrate. Claudication onset time and quality of life measures were secondary outcome measures. The study, Evaluation of Cilostazol in Combination with L-Carnitine (ECLECTIC), was completed in December 2010.

Dosage
Acetyl-L-carnitine or propionyl-L-carnitine is taken at 500 to 2000 mg daily in divided doses. Dietary sources rich in carnitine include meat, poultry, fish, and dairy products.

Precautions
At recommended doses, carnitine and its derivatives are well tolerated. Possible mild side effects include transient gastrointestinal symptoms and body odor.

Inositol Hexaniacinate

Inositol hexaniacinate, a form of vitamin B_3, is believed to perform the same functions in the body as niacin. Activities include free fatty acid mobilization, a decrease in very low-density lipoprotein and cholesterol synthesis, an increase in HDL levels by decreasing its catabolism, and fibrinolysis. The benefits noted in patients with intermittent claudication have been attributed to the resulting reduction in fibrinogen, improvement in blood viscosity, and improved oxygen delivery. Double-blind studies found that inositol hexaniacinate, typically given at doses of 2 g twice daily, can improve walking distance in people with intermittent claudication.[84,85]

■ Dosage

Recommended doses range from 1500 mg to 4 g daily, in two to four divided doses.

■ Precautions

Although niacin has been associated with many acute and chronic toxic reactions, no adverse effects have been reported from the use of inositol hexaniacinate with intake of up to 4 g daily.[86] Given the strong association of niacin with hepatotoxicity, however, a prudent approach would be to avoid inositol in patients with known liver disease and monitor liver function tests during the initial 3 to 6 months of treatment in other patients. Given its fibrinolytic effect, inositol should be used with caution with other blood thinners.

Mesoglycan

Mesoglycan is a sulfated polysaccharide compound found in many tissues in the body, including the joints, intestine, and the lining of blood vessels. It was shown to have antithrombotic and fibrinolytic activity in laboratory and animal research. A 20-week double-blind placebo-controlled trial that enrolled 242 patients with intermittent claudication (absolute walking distance between 100 and 300 m) evaluated the effects of mesoglycan (100 mg a day orally, after a 3 week course of injected treatment). Half of the mesoglycan-treated group achieved clinical response (defined as greater than 50% improvement in walking distance) compared with 26% of the participants from the placebo group.[87] A double-blind comparative trial between heparin sulfate and mesoglycan demonstrated a 34% improvement in pain-free walking distance.[88] In contrast, a small study comparing defibrotide with mesoglycan (24 mg twice daily for 6 months) showed no improvement in pain-free walking distance or posterior tibial pressure after exercise testing.[89] Further, higher-quality research is needed to clarify the potential role of mesoglycan before it can be recommended for PVD.

■ Dosage

The dose often used in studies of mesoglycan is 100 mg orally daily. In some regimens, an injected or intravenous dose is given initially.

■ Precautions

Mesoglycan was well tolerated in studies, with isolated complaints of headache and diarrhea. However, mesoglycan does act as an anticoagulant and was found to cause a doubling of activated partial thromboplastin time values in more than 80% of patients.[90] Mesoglycan should not be used in conjunction with any drugs or supplements that affect blood clotting.

Interventional Options

Surgery

Surgical intervention is usually reserved for severe disease, as would be expected. Functional outcome and patient satisfaction seem to be greatest when disease is limited to the primary lesion only, the age of the patient is younger than 70 years, the patient is not diabetic, and the ABI normalizes after the procedure.[91] After revascularization, patients commonly are receiving some type of antithrombotic therapy, although the choice of drug (oral anticoagulant versus antiplatelet agent) depends on the type of procedure performed and whether a prosthetic graft was used. Obviously, this situation will affect the integrative practitioner in that it will limit which other integrative approaches, such as botanicals and supplements, may be used.

Angioplasty and Stenting

Percutaneous interventional procedures such as PTA are more commonly being used to attempt limb salvage before more invasive operative approaches or when a patient is not a candidate for surgery. Indications for PTA include claudication symptoms that are functionally limiting, pain at rest, or tissue loss; however, limitations for angioplasty or stenting include the location of the lesion (e.g., stents are not recommended for femoropopliteal lesions because of the high restenosis rate), the length of the lesion, the presence of multiple areas of stenosis, or calcification of the lesion.[92] Other techniques incorporated into PTA for prevention of restenosis include brachytherapy (endovascular radiation therapy) and photodynamic therapy, in which a photosensitive drug is given, followed by endovascular light activation.

Stem Cell Therapy

Bone marrow–derived stem and progenitor cell therapy for revascularization of ischemic limbs is one of the most important areas of research to date in PAD. These cells are thought to help in the normal process of arteriogenesis and capillary growth in the collateral circulation as blood vessel narrowing becomes progressively severe in PAD progression. Animal model studies of ischemic extremities showed incorporation of injected endothelial progenitor cells into capillaries and arteries, improved blood flow, and a higher percentage of limb salvage compared with controls. One small human study in patients with limb ischemia not amenable to revascularization showed that injections of bone marrow–derived mononuclear cells into the lower extremity of the ischemic limb were superior to placebo and peripheral blood mononuclear cells injections, with increases in ABI, transcutaneous oxygen pressure, rest pain, and pain-free walking distance.[93] Nineteen other small human studies showed benefits similar to the foregoing, and at least four studies are currently in progress. Questions that remain to be definitively answered include the cell type to be used, the best cell separation technique, the appropriate dosage of cells, the use of colony-stimulating factors, and safety issues.

Chelation

Intravenous chelation therapy (usually a combination of ethylenediaminetetraacetic acid [EDTA], trace elements, and vitamins) was hypothesized to improve PAD because of the mineral-binding effect of EDTA. Some of the theories of mechanism of action for chelation in atherosclerotic disease are that EDTA is thought to chelate calcium from plaques directly, to chelate other metals involved in free radical formation and the inflammatory response, or to inhibit platelet aggregation.[94] Although few randomized controlled trials of chelation in PAD have been conducted, two systematic reviews, one in 1997[95] and another in 2005, supported the conclusion that chelation is not superior to placebo in the treatment of PAD. The 2005 review from the Cochrane Peripheral Vascular Diseases Group included four studies in which EDTA was compared with placebo. Three of the four studies showed no difference in a variety of PAD outcomes, the first including digital subtraction angiograms,[96] the second including walking distance/subjective walking distance or ABI,[97] and the third including pain-free plus maximal treadmill walking distance and ABI.[98]

Therapies to Consider

Osteopathic Manipulative Treatment

Osteopathic medicine was founded in 1874 by Andrew Taylor Still. This system of medicine uses a holistic view of body systems that focuses on the musculoskeletal system, with manual techniques to affect muscles, bones, joints, and tendons, in addition to other more familiar conventional medical treatments and therapies. The goal of osteopathic manipulative treatment (OMT) is to effect a balance between the parasympathetic and sympathetic nervous systems and thus improve somatic function. Vascular flow improvements have been shown in various manual medicine therapies, probably mediated in part by nitric oxide release. One small case-control study of OMT in 30 patients with PAD used an intervention of 30 minutes of several OMT interventions at the practitioner's discretion to treat any somatic dysfunction findings. Treatments were given every 2 weeks for 2 months, 1 month with no treatment, and then every 3 weeks for 3 months. Techniques included strain-counterstrain, myofascial release, muscle energy, soft tissue, and other osteopathic manual medicine therapies. Assessments included brachial artery flow-mediated vasodilation, ABI, time to onset of claudication pain, and quality of life measures using the Short Form 36 Health Survey (SF-36). At 6 months, the OMT group had statistically significant increases in ABI, time to claudication pain, and quality of life scores. In addition, blood levels of serum interleukin-6, soluble intercellular adhesion molecule-1, and soluble vascular cell adhesion molecule-1 also decreased significantly.[99] Although the study was small, these improvements suggest that OMT may be a useful adjunct for some patients.

Hydrotherapy

Hydrotherapy, or balneotherapy, is an ancient method used for the treatment of disease and injury by many cultures, including those of ancient Rome, China, and Japan. It is now most often employed by naturopaths and in European therapeutic spas. Naturopaths believe that, beyond the vasodilatory effects, hydrotherapy functions by affecting the quality of the blood through detoxification. The technique often recommended involves alternating immersion in hot and cold containers of water. In some cases, minerals are added to the baths.[100] Limited evidence, primarily from German studies in the 1950s, suggests that hydrotherapy may be a helpful adjuvant therapy.

Carbon Dioxide Therapies

European naturopaths may employ subcutaneous carbon dioxide (CO_2) insufflations, during which CO_2 is infiltrated into the subcutaneous tissue through a small-gauge needle. Proponents claim that it works by a vasodilatory effect on nearby capillaries. A systematic review found mixed results from three randomized controlled trials.[101]

Other research looked at the efficacy of CO_2-containing baths (1000 to 1200 mg CO_2/kg water) and CO_2-enriched air. Studies in patients with arterial insufficiency (Fontaine stages II to IV) demonstrated increases in parasympathetic activity, vasodilation, and oxygen use.[102-104] Whether these physiologic effects translate into clinical benefits remains to be seen; only one small study was found reporting an increase in pain-free walking distance after a course of 20 CO_2 bath treatments.[105] These therapies should thus be considered experimental at present.

Traditional Chinese Medicine

Various modalities from traditional Chinese medicine may be beneficial in the management of PVD. Minimal data are available regarding the use of acupuncture for PVD. One study examined lower extremity perfusion after needle stimulation at point N8 for 20 minutes; the results were positive, but whether the difference was statistically significant is not clear.[106] A review of studies looking at peripheral ulcer healing in response to acupuncture concluded that although beneficial effects were reported, the studies were uncontrolled, retrospective, and often without assessment by validated techniques.[107] Other traditional Chinese medicine practices such as qi gong and tai chi may also be considered in the treatment plan.

PREVENTION PRESCRIPTION

- Promote risk factor reduction in the following areas: diabetes, hypertension, and hyperlipidemia.
- Strongly support tobacco cessation.
- Provide an exercise prescription (see Chapter 88, Writing an Exercise Prescription).
- Provide a comprehensive nutritional plan, incorporating the previously mentioned medical issues as needed.
- Add dietary fiber and omega-3 fatty acids (see Chapter 86, The Antiinflammatory [Omega-3] Diet).
- Recommend a total of 25 to 30 g/day of fiber. Specific instructions to help patients achieve this goal may include the following:

- Eat at least 4½ cups of fruits and vegetables daily; replace white bread with whole grain breads and cereals; add ¼ cup of wheat bran to foods (e.g., cooked cereal, applesauce, or meat loaf); eat cooked beans each week. Caution patients to add fiber to the diet gradually, to avoid excessive abdominal bloating and discomfort.
- Recommend foods abundant in omega-3 fatty acids (e.g., cold-water fish such as salmon, mackerel, and sardines), but limit fish intake to two 6-oz portions per week. Include omega-3–enriched eggs, flaxseed products, or fish oil supplements (500-mg capsules, 2 to 4 g/day total dose).
- Evaluate for depression and anger proneness.
- Consider autogenic or biofeedback training.

THERAPEUTIC REVIEW

Risk Factor Reduction A①₁

- Address diabetes control, hypertension, hyperlipidemia, and tobacco cessation.

Nutrition Recommendations and Weight Loss, If Needed

- Include recommendations for dietary fiber, dietary antioxidants (not supplements), and omega-3 fatty acid intake.

Exercise A①₁

- Prescribe a supervised claudication exercise program of 30 to 45 minutes at least three times a week for a minimum of 12 weeks.

Autogenic/Biofeedback Training B⬈₁

Antiplatelet Agent (Standard of Care) A①₁

- Aspirin: 160 to 325 mg daily
- Alternatives include the following:
  - Clopidogrel (Plavix): 75 mg daily (preferred) A①₁
  - Cilostazol (Pletal): 100 mg twice daily
- Precautions: All antiplatelet agents have potentially serious interactions with most of, if not all, the botanical supplements indicated for peripheral artery disease (PAD). Using antiplatelet agents in combination with these supplements is not advised. Statin therapy is indicated to lower low-density lipoprotein cholesterol to less than 100 mg/dL (or less than 70 mg/dL in patients with PAD with a very high risk of ischemic events). Angiotensin-converting enzyme therapy should be highly considered. A①₁

Botanicals

- Ginkgo (*Ginkgo biloba*): 120 to 240 mg of standardized leaf extract taken daily in two to three divided doses A⬈₂
- Policosanol (sugar cane derived): 10 to 20 mg daily B⬈₂
- Padma 28 (Padma Basic in United States): 403 mg, two capsules, twice daily A①₁
- Acetyl-ʟ-carnitine: 500 to 2000 mg daily in divided doses B⬈₁
- Inositol hexaniacinate: 2 g twice daily (Avoid inositol in patients with known liver disease; monitor liver function tests during the initial 3 to 6 months of treatment in other patients.) B→₂
- Mesoglycan: 100 mg by mouth daily (Mesoglycan has an anticoagulant function; do not use in conjunction with any drugs or supplements that affect blood clotting.) B→₂

Percutaneous Interventional Procedures A→₃

- These procedures are indicated for claudication symptoms that are functionally limiting, pain at rest, or tissue loss, for attempted salvage before a more invasive approach, and for patients who are not surgical candidates.

Surgical Intervention A→₃

May include revascularization, angioplasty, or stenting.

KEY WEB RESOURCES

Natural Medicines Comprehensive Database: www.naturaldatabase.therapeuticresearch.com	This peer-reviewed, nonbiased database is regularly updated with information on integrative approaches to medical conditions, as well as information on herbs and supplements. It includes an easy-to-use format for checking drug-herb-supplement interactions.
American Heart Association: www.americanheart.org	This comprehensive site provides general patient information and conventional treatment options for PVD.
National Heart, Lung and Blood Institute: www.nhlbi.nih.gov	This comprehensive site provides information about current research and trials, as well as patient materials (multilingual available) for PVD and heart disease.

References

References are available at expertconsult.com.

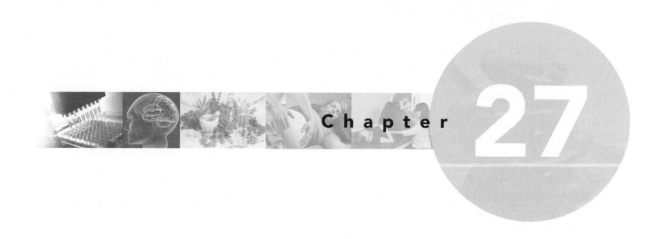

Chapter 27

Arrhythmias

Brian Olshansky, MD

Cardiac arrhythmias are slow (brady), fast (tachy), or irregular heart rhythm disturbances (ectopy, atrial fibrillation, and others). Arrhythmias may be a normal phenomenon related to change in autonomic tone; examples include sinus arrhythmia, sinus bradycardia, and sinus tachycardia. Arrhythmias should be evaluated and treated for interrelated reasons: (1) to eliminate symptoms, (2) to prevent imminent death and hemodynamic collapse, and (3) to offset long-term risk of serious symptoms and death. This chapter focuses on an approach to evaluate and treat arrhythmias by using an integrative approach.

Common arrhythmias encountered in an office-based setting include atrial premature beats, ventricular premature beats, bradycardias, supraventricular tachycardia, nonsustained ventricular tachycardia, atrial fibrillation, and follow-up of already treated sustained ventricular tachycardia or ventricular fibrillation. Potentially symptomatic and dangerous (potentially life-threatening) arrhythmias that require evaluation for possible acute and chronic therapy include (1) sustained ventricular tachycardia in the setting of heart disease, (2) ventricular fibrillation (cardiac arrest), (3) atrial fibrillation, (4) supraventricular tachycardia, (5) sinus bradycardia (and pauses), and (6) atrioventricular (AV) block. Junctional rhythm, AV dissociation, and ectopic beats are common, may cause concern, and may require special attention, further evaluation, and therapy. These latter arrhythmias are generally not serious enough to require long-term aggressive treatment unless they are associated with severe symptoms.

Pathophysiology

Types and Mechanisms

Heart rhythm disturbances have multiple potential mechanisms and causes. The heart rhythm is a mechanical response to electrical activation of specialized fibers and atrial and ventricular myocardium. Electrical activation is generally initiated in the sinus node and then leads to activation through various atrial conductive pathways to the AV node, the His-Purkinje system, and the ventricles. The sinus node may be activated slowly as a result of damage to this structure or because of autonomic effects. Increased vagal tone, for example, slows the sinus node rate. Abnormalities in conduction disturbances throughout the normal pathways can also lead to heart block and bradyarrhythmia.

The autonomic nervous system can influence the sinus node either to slow it or to speed it. The autonomic nervous system can also influence other tissue in the heart to make it more automatic, accelerate faster, and overtake normal sinus node activation. This influence can lead to activation resulting from an ectopic focus.

Tachyarrhythmia

Common rhythm disturbances causing an increase in heart rate are known as tachycardias. Tachycardias include sinus tachycardia. This arrhythmia can be a normal response to stress and exercise, or it can be an inappropriate acceleration for no apparent reason. Supraventricular tachycardias are less common but are tachycardias that require tissue above the His bundle to propagate. Supraventricular tachycardias occur in various forms: atrial flutter, atrial fibrillation, those resulting from abnormal areas in the atria, those secondary to rhythm disturbances in the vicinity of the AV node, and those caused by rhythm disturbances related to extra pathways that connect the atria to the ventricles. These tachycardias are in part related to the underlying mechanisms for arrhythmias that include reentry, triggered automaticity, and normal and abnormal automaticity.

Tachyarrhythmias can result from abnormally fast ventricular activation independent of atrial activation. This arrhythmia is known as ventricular tachycardia. Ventricular tachycardia is often associated with underlying structural heart disease, and the prognosis is often concerning because this arrhythmia can lead to cardiac arrest. This is not always true, however, because in patients with no underlying heart disease (idiopathic cause), ventricular tachycardia can have a benign prognosis. Another serious ventricular arrhythmia is ventricular fibrillation. This rhythm disturbance causes cardiac arrest and, without electrical countershock, is fatal.

Other arrhythmias include ventricular ectopic beats, which can manifest as single ectopic beats, bigeminy (every other beat), trigeminy, quadrigeminy, in a fixed coupled fashion or unrelated to other beats, couplets, triplets, and other forms of nonsustained ventricular tachycardia.

Many potential problems are related to heart rhythm disturbances. Abrupt change in the heart rate, especially with marked slowing or acceleration, can lead to hemodynamic compromise, syncope, and other related symptoms. Rhythm disturbances that are extraordinarily fast or that originate in the ventricles and are associated with structural heart disease can be premonitory signs of cardiac arrest. However, most rhythm disturbances that are seen in clinical practice are benign.

Ectopic Beats

Ectopic beats that trigger palpitations frequently are the result of ventricular ectopic activity (premature ventricular contractions [PVCs]), atrial ectopic activity (premature atrial contractions [PACs]), and atrial arrhythmias such as atrial fibrillation. Ventricular ectopy and atrial ectopy, when not associated with serious underlying structural heart disease, are relatively benign. Although the risk of death may be slightly increased in any patient with PVCs (up to doubling of mortality), the risk remains low in persons with a normal heart. The reason to treat ectopic beats is not to prevent death, but rather to prevent symptoms. Asymptomatic atrial and ventricular ectopy in a patient with no underlying heart disease does not require treatment.

Symptomatic atrial and ventricular ectopy, however, becomes a major problem to treat in clinical practice, for several reasons. First, no good, safe, medical therapies are available.[1-13] Drugs used to suppress ectopy frequently can be proarrhythmic and increase the risk of sudden death or increase the severity of the arrhythmias, and these agents can have numerous other serious complications. Second, the problem can be highly symptomatic and concerning to the patient. It can have a tremendous impact on quality of life. Third, the degree of symptoms from benign arrhythmias varies tremendously, and patients who are highly symptomatic may require several types of therapeutic interventions, which can extend as far as drug therapy and even radiofrequency catheter ablation approaches.

Atrial Fibrillation

Atrial fibrillation is a complex arrhythmia with myriad presentations and therapeutic intervention possibilities. The general approach to atrial fibrillation is threefold: (1) cardiac ventricular rate control, (2) rhythm control, and (3) prevention of thromboembolic events. Although atrial fibrillation is associated with a doubling in mortality, this is not the reason that it is generally treated; yet treatment is directed at prevention of symptoms, and no one has shown that treatment of the arrhythmia alone will decrease mortality (it may even increase mortality). Atrial fibrillation occurs in more than 2.2 million U.S. residents. Ectopic beats are as common, but the extent of their occurrence is not completely known. Not all patients with ectopic beats are symptomatic, and the triggers for ectopic beats can be highly variable. For example, in some patients, caffeinated beverages, chocolate, and even high sugar levels can trigger ectopic activity.[14,15]

> The most important aspect of the history is to inquire about the ingestion of stimulants such as caffeine, simple sugars, chocolate, pseudoephedrine, ephedra, guarana, ginseng, gotu cola, yohimbe, and others.

People with paroxysms of atrial fibrillation, or at least those patients who present to physicians, are highly symptomatic. Perhaps these patients do not represent the great majority of patients with atrial fibrillation, but it is not clear how many patients with paroxysmal fibrillation never frequent a health care provider. In addition, patients with symptomatic atrial fibrillation are not always symptomatic during atrial fibrillation. They often have symptoms when they are in normal sinus rhythm and can be asymptomatic during atrial fibrillation. The presence of persistent paroxysmal or permanent atrial fibrillation frequently inspires long-term treatment and consideration of the threefold treatment approach.

Palpitations

Palpitations are among the most common complaints associated with arrhythmias; the differential diagnosis is extensive. Palpitations can be intermittent or sustained, regular or irregular, and even unrelated to an arrhythmia. Catecholamine excess alone can cause a sensation of palpitations without an arrhythmia even being present.[16]

Some causes of palpitations include the following: anxiety; severe viral syndrome; alcohol; stimulants (cocaine, methamphetamine); stimulant medications including pseudoephedrine; drinks containing caffeine, theobromine, or theophylline; poor sleep (or an irregular sleep cycle); and several supplements (including *Ginkgo biloba,* ephedra, ginseng, guarana, horny goat weed, yohimbe, and others). Hormonal changes and excess thyroid hormone can also lead to palpitations.

Palpitations can represent somatization of a psychiatric disorder. Of 125 outpatients referred for ambulatory electrocardiographic monitoring to evaluate palpitations, 34% had an arrhythmia, whereas 19% had a psychiatric disorder, especially major depression or a panic disorder.[17] Those with psychiatric disorders were younger, more disabled, and more hypochondriacal about their health. Their palpitations were more likely to last longer than 15 minutes, were accompanied by other symptoms, were more intense, and were associated with more emergency room visits. Several reports confirmed the high incidence of psychiatric conditions in association with palpitations.[18,19] Nevertheless, careful evaluation of palpitations must rule out organic disease.

Palpitations only rarely are the result of a life-threatening process, although they can be associated with or represent manifestations of underlying ventricular dysfunction or other structural heart disease. Palpitations in a patient with heart disease, especially coronary artery disease, should raise suspicions that the palpitations are the result of an arrhythmia.[20,21]

Approach to the Patient

Perspective

Arrhythmias may have little meaning if they have no prognostic significance, do not alter hemodynamics or cardiac function, and are not symptomatic. Routine screening of an asymptomatic patient is not recommended. Patients typically seek medical care for palpitations, for an arrhythmia associated with symptoms, for a symptom thought to be caused by an arrhythmia, or for nonspecific symptoms that may result from an arrhythmia.

Initial Evaluation and Diagnosis of the Arrhythmia

The initial evaluation includes a careful, circumspect, and complete history (directed toward the symptoms and any potential relationship with an arrhythmia, as well as an assessment of potential responsible conditions), a physical examination, and a 12-lead electrocardiogram at baseline and, if possible, during the arrhythmia. An unhurried, careful, and complete history is the key to appropriate further evaluation, and the clinician should resist the urge to perform expensive, unnecessary, or potentially risky tests. Several issues should be addressed in the history (Table 27-1).

The electrocardiogram recorded during the arrhythmia or while the patient is symptomatic determines the need for further evaluation and treatment. An ambulatory monitor or an event monitor may be needed, in selected patients, to secure a diagnosis. If the symptoms are sporadic, but occur daily, use of an ambulatory (Holter) monitor is the best approach.[22–25] An event recorder or transtelephonic monitor can help make the diagnosis in a patient with less frequent

---

TABLE 27-1. Historical Features of Importance in the Evaluation of the Patient

- Which arrhythmia is present?
- Does the arrhythmia cause symptoms?
- Does the arrhythmia have prognostic significance?
- Is the problem life-threatening?
- Does the patient require hospital admission or extensive testing?
- Is specialist consultation required, and, if so, how urgently?
- Is treatment required?

---

palpitations. Transtelephonic devices are small, lightweight, and inexpensive. The memory feature allows recording of data without the need for immediate access to telephone transmission. An implantable monitor (Reveal, Medtronic, Minneapolis) is also available.[26] The device can record events triggered by the patient or by preselected criteria automatically. The device can record up to 42 minutes of data. If episodes are associated with exercise or physical or mental stress or when an arrhythmia cannot be documented with ambulatory or transtelephonic monitoring, exercise testing may secure a diagnosis.

Risk Assessment

The clinician should determine whether an arrhythmia has prognostic importance: Is it a premonitory sign of death? Several conditions, ventricular tachycardia and the Wolff-Parkinson-White syndrome (Fig. 27-1), are potentially life-threatening. Not all ventricular tachycardias are life-threatening; a patient without heart disease, for example, who has idiopathic sustained ventricular tachycardia (*not* idiopathic ventricular fibrillation) has little chance of dying. In contrast, even a single episode of nonsustained ventricular tachycardia in a patient with coronary artery disease and poor left ventricular function as a result of prior myocardial infarction may be associated with a poor prognosis.[27]

Rarely, an asymptomatic arrhythmia must be treated urgently. Symptoms and their relationship with the arrhythmia require careful assessment. A correlation of the arrhythmia and symptoms is preferred, although not always possible.

Indications for Inpatient Management

Hospital admission is required if the patient has significant underlying heart disease (e.g., cardiomyopathy with congestive heart failure or coronary heart disease with active ischemia), if the arrhythmia is life-threatening and requires rapid reversion (e.g., rapid tachyarrhythmias, polymorphic ventricular tachycardia, prolonged QT interval in a patient

---

FIGURE 27-1

Six leads of an echocardiograph of a patient with Wolff-Parkinson-White syndrome showing delta waves.

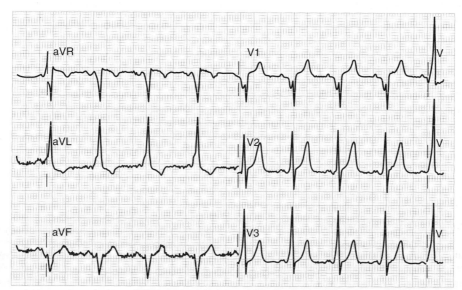

with syncope), or if the arrhythmia is uncontrolled or highly symptomatic. Hospital admission is preferred for older patients, who may have not only underlying heart disease, but also other chronic illnesses such as kidney or liver disease that could affect antiarrhythmic therapy.

Referral to a Specialist

A cardiologist is frequently needed to help manage the complex patient with an arrhythmia; for example, a temporary pacemaker may be needed for a patient with symptomatic bradycardia. Referral to an electrophysiologist may be necessary to institute aggressive acute therapy, such as intravenous amiodarone for life-threatening ventricular tachycardia, antitachycardia pacing for acute reversion of an arrhythmia, or for placement of an implantable cardioverter defibrillator (ICD) or to reprogram a pacemaker or an ICD (Table 27-2).

Integrative Therapy

The decision to start any type of antiarrhythmic therapy depends on the severity and frequency of arrhythmia-related symptoms, the risks of the arrhythmias, and the risks associated with the therapy itself. The need for long-term therapy must be carefully individualized to each patient because the severity and importance of symptoms are highly variable. The symptoms associated with any arrhythmia can have an impact on lifestyle, occupation, driving, and other important daily activities. These issues must be considered for every patient and are evaluated as part of a diagnostic and therapeutic approach.

Diet

Gastric Distention

Dietary interventions in some cases can influence some arrhythmias. A large meal can distend the stomach and stimulate vagal afferents, thus leading to vagal efferent activation causing atrial fibrillation in patients who have vagally mediated atrial fibrillation, hypotension, and bradycardia.

Food as a Trigger

Some foods may even act as triggers, and patients will often report some evidence for this. Alcohol is one of the major triggers for atrial fibrillation and ventricular ectopy.[28,29] Caffeine is frequently another trigger for ectopic beats but not necessarily atrial fibrillation.[14,15] Restriction of alcohol and caffeine may have no effect on arrhythmias. If this is the case, restriction will be of no benefit and may adversely influence the patient's lifestyle. Specific food allergies can trigger a reaction and cause palpitations. Trans fats, particularly of the 18-2 type (found in doughnuts, fried foods, and artificial cheese such as in processed pizza) have been associated with cardiac arrest.[30,31] In contradistinction,[32] omega-3 fatty acids may improve outcomes,[32,33] but data do not indicate an antiarrhythmic effect.[34] Fat balance appears to have an effect on cardiovascular health.[35] Alcohol consumption may enhance the effects of omega-3 fatty acids.[36,37]

The effects of diet on the autonomic nervous system are complex. Several foods increase sympathetic nervous system tone. High levels of sodium also increase the effects of

TABLE 27-2. Reasons for Referral to a Specialist

- Resuscitated ventricular fibrillation
- Sustained ventricular tachycardia
- Atrial fibrillation that is difficult to control or refractory to standard therapies
- Nonsustained ventricular tachycardia
- Symptomatic supraventricular tachycardia that is difficult to control
- Sinus bradycardia (sick sinus syndrome, tachy-brady syndrome)
- Second degree atrioventricular block
- Unexplained ventricular ectopy in the athlete or in a symptomatic patient
- Syncope with a suspected arrhythmic mechanism
- Patients with devices (pacemakers, implantable defibrillators) who are unstable
- Uncontrolled rhythm problems

catecholamines and influence ventricular ectopy.[38-43] It may turn out that caffeine, theophylline, and theobromine present in coffee, tea, and chocolate may be inciting factors, or they may possibly have positive benefit.[44-47] Data that coffee causes atrial fibrillation are questionable.[48,49] Trial and error with these food substances is worthwhile, but no particular reason exists to try to eliminate all these foods if they do not have an effect on the arrhythmia. Patients may complain that a specific food triggers a rhythm disturbance by an unknown mechanism. This is not uncommon and is possibly related to some type of allergic reaction or other related issue.

> Gastric distention from large meals, excessive caffeine, alcohol, high levels of sodium, trans fats, severe fluctuations in blood sugar levels, and possibly food allergies are potential dietary triggers of cardiac arrhythmias.

Botanical Stimulants of Arrhythmia

Specific supplements can trigger arrhythmias. Ma Huang, from the Chinese ephedra plant, contains catecholamines including ephedrine that can initiate ectopic rhythm disturbances and cause life-threatening problems.[50,51] Investigators have even suggested that ambrotose, ginkgo, and other commonly used substances may exacerbate or even cause arrhythmias.

Diet and Anticoagulation

Diet is very important in arrhythmia management, especially in patients who require anticoagulation for atrial fibrillation or other arrhythmias. If the diet changes markedly with significant alterations in vitamin K levels, the prothrombin time will fluctuate tremendously (Table 27-3).

> A balanced diet low in fat and high in roughage that will lead to a moderate level of blood sugar and as little stress as possible on the gastrointestinal tract may improve the arrhythmias.

TABLE 27-3. Assessing the Need for and Risks of Warfarin for Nonvalvular Atrial Fibrillation

Step 1

Is the patient at low or high risk?
Low risk according to the American College of Chest Physicians (ACCP)
None of the following risk factors

☐ Age 75 years or more
☐ Previous stroke or transient ischemic attack (double risk)
☐ Congestive heart failure
☐ Hypertension
☐ Diabetes

If low risk (zero to one of the above): Treat with aspirin.
If moderate risk (two of the above): Consider warfarin in relation to the risk of bleeding in step 2.
If high risk (three or more of the above): Strongly consider warfarin.

Step 2

Is the patient at high bleeding risk?

☐ Age older than 65 years
☐ History of gastrointestinal tract bleeding
☐ History of hemorrhagic stroke
☐ Recent myocardial infarction, hematocrit less than 30, creatinine more than 1.5, or diabetes mellitus

Weigh the potential benefits of warfarin in stroke prevention with the potential risks of bleeding, and make the most appropriate therapeutic decision.

Data from guidelines from the American College of Chest Physicians and Ebell MH. Choosing between warfarin (Coumadin) and aspirin therapy for patients with atrial fibrillation. *Am Fam Physician.* 2005;71:2328–2350.

Exercise

Exercise and physical exertion can trigger various arrhythmias. Maintaining excellent physical health through exercise, however, decreases the effects of the sympathetic nervous system on the heart and the heart rhythm and improves outcomes in almost all circumstances. The sympathetic nervous system often has a major contributory role in the genesis of serious and benign atrial and ventricular arrhythmias. Exercise performed regularly, with enhancement of aerobic capacity, decreases sensitivity to catecholamines, reduces circulating catecholamine levels, decreases sympathetic nervous system tone, and enhances vagal tone. All these effects increase heart rate variability, which decreases the risk of sudden death and the potential for catecholamine-initiated or sympathetically initiated atrial and ventricular arrhythmias (see Chapter 94, Enhancing Heart Rate Variability). Exercise can also modulate other potential rhythm disturbances such as sinus tachycardia. Especially in young women, inappropriate sinus tachycardia and postural orthostatic tachycardia syndrome are potential problems.[52] Inappropriate sinus tachycardia is a condition in which the sinus node appears to be hyperactive; the cause is not completely known. It may be, in part, related to abnormal sympathetic nervous system stimulation, but it could also be an intrinsic problem with the sinus node. Increasing exercise decreases the potential for this problem. Exercise appears to be beneficial in treating many arrhythmias, but it must be used with caution. For

patients with malignant arrhythmias, exercise therapy must be prescribed and supervised by a qualified physician who is knowledgeable about the risks, benefits, and methods of monitoring the patient.

Lifestyle

Lifestyle has a major impact on arrhythmias.[53-55] Cigarette smoking and other forms of nicotine have no potential benefit and may be harmful for any individual.[54,56] Nicotine use can exacerbate the risk of sudden death and malignant and benign arrhythmias of all types. Although alcohol may have a beneficial effect on cardiovascular mortality, myocardial infarction, and cholesterol, it has no benefit for any arrhythmia. The combination of alcohol and nicotine is even more likely to trigger an arrhythmia.

Mind-Body Therapy

Autonomic variations can occur with numerous lifestyle interventions, including meditation and other mind-body therapies.[57,58] The influence can be profound and may occur by several potential mechanisms: (1) change in autonomic function, (2) placebo effect, (3) direct effect on the rhythm, (4) change in perception of the importance of the arrhythmias to the patient, and (5) shifting of the attention from the arrhythmia to some other issue.

Biofeedback can decrease the number, frequency, and severity of palpitations related to arrhythmias. The effects of biofeedback have been known for some time.[59-63] Another issue is the simple process of developing awareness that a patient can learn to identify a rhythm disturbance as not a potentially noxious experience. The interpretation of the severity of the rhythm disturbance amplifies the severity of the effects on symptoms. Having a patient face the problem can actually empower the patient to improve his or her perception of the arrhythmia and its implications. Ultimately, properly used psychosocial therapy can reduce the risk of death.[64] Biofeedback devices can also be used to enhance heart rate variability (see Chapter 94, Enhancing Heart Rate Variability).

Meditation

Meditation has been associated with a decreased risk of sudden death in high-risk patients because of a reduction in ventricular fibrillation.[57,58] Meditation may affect the autonomic nervous system in a beneficial way.[65] It may also change the perception of the arrhythmia for patients who have a benign problem.

Meditation and relaxation techniques may also be useful for individuals who have an ICD for life-threatening rhythm disturbances. If the device is activated frequently, it can cause tremendous grief. Meditation and relaxation techniques can improve outcomes in such patients. These techniques may also allow for better patient acceptance of the shocks (see Chapter 98, Recommending Meditation).

Relaxation appears to have a positive benefit. For years, physicians have used benzodiazepines to treat rhythm disturbances such as atrial fibrillation and supraventricular tachycardia by inducing relaxation. If a patient comes into an emergency room with such an arrhythmia and is allowed to relax, the rhythm will often stop spontaneously (see Chapter 93, Relaxation Techniques).

Acupuncture

Data suggest that acupuncture may be antiarrhythmic for atrial fibrillation.[66] Although acupuncture may affect other arrhythmias beneficially, the data are far from definitive.[67] Acupuncture can also trigger inappropriate shocks in patients with ICDs, and this therapy should be avoided in these patients.[68]

Supplements

Coenzyme Q10

Coenzyme Q10, at a dose of 100 to 300 mg a day, may decrease episodes of atrial fibrillation by an unknown mechanism. Coenzyme Q10 can also have an effect on ventricular and atrial ectopy.[69]

L-Carnitine

L-Carnitine, at a dose of 3 g a day or more, can improve mitochondrial function and left ventricular function and may prevent some atrial and ventricular arrhythmias. Several small randomized controlled trials of carnitine showed a reduction in risk of sudden cardiac death and total death in patients with cardiomyopathy. The mechanism is not clear, but it may be that carnitine improves mitochondrial and myocardial function.[70-72] Carnitine has no known adverse effects. It may reduce ischemia and reperfusion-induced arrhythmias and raise the ventricular fibrillation threshold (of unclear significance).[73]

Calcium and Magnesium

Calcium and magnesium, approximately 1 g a day each of a salt (e.g., magnesium sulfate), have been associated with a decrease in arrhythmias. Magnesium can decrease triggered activity and can slow conduction in the AV node.

Magnesium supplementation given to patients in congestive heart failure in a double-blind placebo-controlled trial showed improvements in arrhythmias. Individuals taking 3.2 g per day of magnesium chloride equivalent to 384 mg per day of elemental magnesium had between 23% and 52% fewer occurrences of specific arrhythmias in a 6-week follow-up period.[43] Although some data suggested that magnesium has a beneficial effect on atrial fibrillation,[74] other data did not support its use.[75] Magnesium may also be associated with reduction in the risk of sudden death in women.[76]

Copper and Zinc

Three cases were reported in which ventricular premature beats disappeared, and PVCs decreased, after copper supplementation at a dose of 4 mg per day.[41] Investigators discovered that zinc made the arrhythmias worse and that extra zinc can lead to copper deficiency. The use of copper has a potential problem, however, in that high copper levels can lead to atherosclerosis.

Selenium

A deficiency in selenium can cause heart problems including arrhythmias. No good data, however, are available to suggest that selenium supplementation in patients with low selenium levels will improve arrhythmia status.[38,77]

Potassium

Potassium supplementation is extraordinarily important, especially if a patient is taking drugs that lower potassium levels. Potassium has been implicated in all types of rhythm disturbances, and potassium deficiencies can lead to torsades de pointes. Anyone with long QT interval syndrome, and specifically those patients who take drugs that lower potassium levels, clearly should take potassium supplements. This can also be done though potassium in the diet, including fruits and vegetables that contain high potassium concentrations (see Chapter 87, The DASH Diet).

Omega-3 Fatty Acids

Omega-3 fatty acids appear to influence several myocardial channels that can affect arrhythmias.[78-82] Specifically, omega-3 fatty acids appear to have an effect on calcium and potassium channels.[83] In men with symptomatic PVCs, omega-3 fatty acids were shown to decrease the risk of PVCs by approximately 70% when supplementation was in the form of fish oil,[84,85] but data are conflicting.[86]

Fish oil was also shown in the second Gruppo Italiano per lo Studio della Sopravvivenza nell'Infarto Miocardico (GISSI2) prevention trial to be associated with a decreased risk of total death and sudden death. This study included 11,324 Italians who had had a myocardial infarction within the preceding 3 months. These patients were randomized to approximately 850 mg of omega-3 polyunsaturated fatty acids (2836), vitamin E (2830), or neither (2828). Patients who were given fish oil had a 45% reduction in sudden death and a 20% decrease in mortality.[83]

The Lyon Diet Heart Study and the Physicians' Health Study both showed a benefit to the use of fish oil. The Diet and Reinfarction Trial (DART) included 2033 men with acute myocardial infarction who were randomized to receive or not to receive advice on diets: decreased fat intake to 30% of total energy, at least two weekly portions (200 to 400 g) of fatty fish (or 1.5 g fish oil capsules if unable to take fish), and cereal fiber to 18 g daily. Patients who were given "fish advice" survived substantially longer and significantly better.[87]

These data inspired the Fatty Acid Antiarrhythmia Trial, which is a randomized placebo-controlled trial of 3 g of fish oil compared with cod-scented olive oil, to look at the incidence of recurrent ventricular arrhythmias in patients who have ICDs and are at risk for sudden death. Many of these patients have malignant ventricular arrhythmias leading to shocks from their device. The aim of this study was to decrease the number of shocks. Fish oil was effective in this study, but data were conflicting.[88]

The data on fish oil in arrhythmias and improving outcomes in patients with heart disease are extensive.[89-91] Although the data in some cases conflict, fish oil is associated with improved autonomic influences,[92-94] reduction in atrial fibrillation[95] (especially after cardiovascular surgery,[96] but not in all studies[97]), reduction in risk of all-cause mortality, reduction in symptomatic ventricular ectopy, and reduction in depression (depression is associated with increased mortality after myocardial infarction).[98] Although some data show benefits for atrial fibrillation,[99] a placebo-controlled study showed no value of fish oil.[100]

In addition, data on patients after myocardial infarction have not shown benefit, likely because present therapy is already so good.[101] The higher-risk patients may be the ones who benefit the most.[102] Concerns also exist about the toxins in some of the supplements, including dioxins, polychlorinated biphenyls, polybrominated diphenyl ethers, and chlorinated pesticides.[103]

Omega-3 fatty acids are available in various forms, not only fish oil.[104] Certain plant oils can be metabolized into omega-3 fatty acids, including flaxseed oil, which also has other potential benefits,[105] including those on mood. Because omega-3 fatty acids can improve mood, they may also have an autonomic affect that can decrease the sensation of arrhythmias or decrease arrhythmias altogether.

> For dosing omega-3 fatty acids, educate the patient to read labels. If you are recommending 1000 mg of omega-3 fatty acids, the user needs to look at the amount of eicosapentaenoic acid (EPA) and docosahexaenoic acid (DHA) per serving size. If the label notes 300 mg of EPA and 200 mg of DHA per two capsules (serving size), the patient would need to take four capsules daily to obtain 1000 mg of omega-3 fatty acids.

Vitamins

A long-standing case of sick sinus syndrome was reported to resolve with supplementation of 800 units per day of vitamin D.[106] However, it is not clear that vitamin D was the cause of this change.

Data indicate that vitamin C given postoperatively to patients at risk for atrial fibrillation and to patients who undergo coronary artery bypass graft surgery may lead to a marked reduction in atrial fibrillation,[107–111] but these data have not been confirmed. By whatever mechanism, vitamin C appears to have antiarrhythmic properties and can prevent atrial fibrillation, at least in some patients. The mechanism may be by clearance of free radicals or by an antiinflammatory effect.

Botanicals

Many of the original antiarrhythmic drugs were derived from herbal therapy: quinidine (a stereoisomer of quinine from cinchona bark), lidocaine, amiodarone (from khellin, derived from the herb *Ammi visnaga*), and digoxin (from foxglove) are a few.[112] Data suggest that several other herbal preparations may have antiarrhythmic effects.

Ciwujia or Siberian ginseng (*Acanthopanax senticosus* Harms), which is used for athletic performance and weight loss, may have antiarrhythmic effects. Ciwujia was studied in isolated rat hearts with transient coronary occlusion.[113] Ciwujia extract reduced reperfusion-induced ventricular fibrillation and ventricular tachycardia. It also reduced the number of cells with abnormal action potential configurations. Ciwujia may reduce the incidence of malignant arrhythmias.[113] Siberian ginseng can cause an apparent increase in digoxin levels.[114] Whether this finding represents a false serum elevation, whether ginseng converts to digoxin in vivo, or whether ginseng alters the metabolism of digoxin is unclear.

Angelica and *Ginkgo biloba* may have a protective influence during myocardial ischemia and reperfusion.[115] In a rat model, the incidence of ventricular premature beats and the total incidence of arrhythmia were greatly reduced.[116]

Licorice root has an antiarrhythmic property.[117] Zhi Gan Cao (prepared licorice) injection can antagonize arrhythmias induced by chloroform, catecholamines, aconitine, strophanthin-K, and barium chloride. Licorice root may slow the heart rate, prolong PR and QT intervals, and antagonize the positive chronotropic response induced by catecholamines. Another component of licorice, sodium 18 beta-glycyrrhetinate, strongly counteracts arrhythmia induced by chloroform, lengthens the appearance time of arrhythmia induced

by $CaCl_2$, slightly retards the heart rate of rats and rabbits, and partly antagonizes the acceleration effect of isoproterenol on rabbit hearts. The clinical significance of these experimental findings is unclear.[118]

Various herbs are now considered potentially useful by some practitioners to treat ventricular and supraventricular arrhythmias. Motherwort contains bufenolide, glycosides (stachydrine), and alkaloids. A dose between 4 and 5 g of motherwort can decrease palpitations, presumably by a mild beta-blocking affect, although the exact mechanism that motherwort exerts on the heart to decrease ectopic beats is unclear. No randomized controlled trial has been performed using motherwort.

Khella (*Ammi visnaga*) has significant antiarrhythmic effects. In the 1950s, a compound known as khella was derived from the *Ammi visnaga* plant. It was used to treat angina resulting from coronary heart disease, with significant improvement in those patients. Khella has also been used over the years by naturopaths to decrease palpitations. Khella is the original substance from which a very potent antiarrhythmic drug, amiodarone, was derived.[119–121]

Hawthorn berry has been used to treat atrial fibrillation, and it may have an effect on other rhythm disturbances as well.[114] Hawthorn contains hyperoside (vitexin, rhamnose), rutin, and oligomeric procyanidins. A dose of 160 to 900 mg of the water ethanol extract is recommended. Exactly how this herb works is unknown, but it may act on the sodium-potassium adenosine triphosphatase pump similar to digoxin. More likely, hawthorn acts as a phosphodiesterase inhibitor. Hawthorn may reduce the risk of sudden death and helps treat patients in heart failure.[122]

Rhodiola may have had some antiarrhythmic effects in a rat model in which arrhythmias were induced by epinephrine and calcium chloride.[123] Rhodiola can increase the ventricular fibrillation threshold,[124] and although this effect may be beneficial, the meaning is uncertain. The antiarrhythmic effect of rhodiola may result from activation of the opioid system and stimulation of kappa-opioid receptors.[125] Rhodiola may affect intracellular calcium handling,[126] and it may even exacerbate palpitations in some instances.

Data suggest that garlic, agrimony, celery, ginger, berberine, corkwort, *Stephania tetandra* root, astragalus, *Fissistigma glaucescens*, Xin Bao, Bu Xin, Yu Zhu, and Mai Dong, among others, are antiarrhythmic under various experimental conditions and for various arrhythmias. At the present time, however, the data are not definitive enough to recommend treatment with any of these herbal therapies for a specific arrhythmia.

Pharmaceuticals

The standard first-line drug therapy approach for benign PVCs, PACs, and episodes of atrial fibrillation is often a beta-adrenergic blocking drug. This drug alters the autonomic nervous system tone on the heart, although the effectiveness of this approach is unclear. Good data suggest that it is not effective whatsoever. Further, side effects are common when using these therapies for ectopic beats.

For atrial fibrillation, various antiarrhythmic drugs are available. Their use depends on the underlying heart disease, link to the episodes, age of the patient, severity of symptoms, and the difficulty in maintaining sinus rhythm. Discussions of antiarrhythmic drug use, anticoagulation, and rate control drugs for atrial fibrillation are beyond the scope of this chapter, but several good references are available.[127]

For ventricular ectopy and PVCs, if beta blockers do not work, various antiarrhythmic drugs can be used, including, for normal hearts without any evidence of ischemic heart disease, class IC antiarrhythmic drugs such as propafenone and flecainide.[5,6] One concern about these antiarrhythmic drugs, like any antiarrhythmic drug, is they can triple the mortality rate if underlying heart disease is present. The use of these drugs is never completely safe, and they can have other, so-called proarrhythmic effects.[1-8]

Numerous other antiarrhythmic drugs can be used, but each one of them has significant side effects. The use of these drugs is discouraged for benign ventricular ectopy unless the patient is severely symptomatic.

Although antiarrhythmic drugs can suppress arrhythmias, the important issues of proarrhythmia and side effects must be considered. All antiarrhythmic drugs have the potential to increase ectopy or induce, or aggravate, monomorphic ventricular tachycardia, torsades de pointes, ventricular fibrillation, conduction disturbances, or bradycardia. This is known as proarrhythmia.[1-8] The use of antiarrhythmic drugs should be reserved for clinicians who are expert in their use.

> The risk of proarrhythmias from medication is greatest in those who need the most protection, specifically those patients with depressed left ventricular function with an ejection fraction less than 30%.

Risk-to-Benefit Ratio

The goal of therapy for any arrhythmia is to eliminate symptoms or prevent a potentially serious outcome, primarily a life-threatening arrhythmia and sudden death. These goals must be balanced against the risks associated with antiarrhythmic therapy, including proarrhythmia and the side effects of individual drugs.

No study has shown that ventricular ectopy suppression in any group of patients with asymptomatic arrhythmia improves survival. The only reason to treat is to suppress symptoms from the arrhythmias as long as treatment does not worsen the arrhythmias and the prognosis.

Antiarrhythmic Drug Therapy and Dose Titration

Therapy with some antiarrhythmic drugs is best initiated in the hospital, primarily to monitor for early proarrhythmia. The decision to hospitalize depends on the presence and severity of structural heart disease, the indication for treatment (e.g., cause of the arrhythmia and type and severity of associated symptoms), and the drug used. If the patient has a life-threatening arrhythmia, drug initiation and dose titration should be performed in the hospital. Follow-up 24 hour ambulatory electrocardiographic monitoring is recommended on a regular basis, for example every 6 months, to assess for continued drug efficacy and safety. An American College of Cardiology/American Heart Association task force published guidelines for the use of ambulatory monitoring in the assessment of antiarrhythmic drug efficacy.[22]

With the advent of newer approaches to the management of serious and sustained arrhythmias, therapy is moving to device-based treatment (implanted defibrillators and pacemakers) and to ablation (to cure the arrhythmias). The use of antiarrhythmic drugs has changed drastically over the years. If a patient has such an arrhythmia, referral to a specialist is in order.

Ablation Therapy

Another potential treatment that is nonpharmacologic is ablation therapy. Occasionally, ablation therapy can be used to remove focal triggers for rhythm disturbances in the atrium or ventricles for eliminating PACs and PVCs.

Occasionally, a patient with ventricular bigeminy does not perfuse with the PVC and therefore has an underlying rapid ventricular rate but without adequate perfusion, especially during the PVC. Such a patient can develop tachycardia-mediated cardiomyopathy, and heart failure will ensue. By treating the PVC, this problem can be eliminated. Ablation therapy is also used to treat various supraventricular tachyarrhythmias. In fact, atrial fibrillation, especially when paroxysmal, can be treated by ablating focal ectopic beats that often originate from the pulmonary veins.

Conclusion

The problem of arrhythmia management is complex and multifaceted. Treatment depends on the arrhythmia, its implications, the symptoms, and the effect on the patient. Patients with serious rhythm disturbances must be referred to a specialist, especially if the arrhythmias are potentially life-threatening. If not, an approach to improve outcomes should involve change in lifestyle and exercise. Following these dietary recommendations may be useful. If this is not enough, mind-body effects can be substantial. Consider meditation. Acupuncture can have a beneficial effects as well. Several herbal preparations may influence the presence of an arrhythmia, but care must be taken because some supplements such as Ma Huang can worsen an arrhythmia or even create a new, life-threatening one.

PREVENTION PRESCRIPTION

- Avoid arrhythmia triggers if identified and definable (e.g., excess caffeine intake).
- Encourage regular aerobic exercise as long as it does not trigger arrhythmias.
- Urge risk factor reduction to prevent the development of structural heart disease (treatment of hypercholesterolemia, hypertension, smoking, excess ethanol intake).
- Moderate balanced caloric intake and maintenance of appropriate weight.
- Prevent stress. Incorporate meditation, yoga, and bioenergy techniques.
- Maintain a regular sleep-wake cycle with at least 7 to 8 hours of sleep nightly.
- Consider supplementing with 1 to 2 g of fish oil and encourage two to three servings of fish each week.
- Avoid the use of drugs or supplements that stimulate or mimic the effect of catecholamines (e.g., over-the-counter decongestants, ephedra [Ma Huang], caffeine).

THERAPEUTIC REVIEW

The treatment of arrhythmias cannot be easily standardized and does not fit into any clearly defined algorithmic pathway. The reason for this is the diverse presentations of arrhythmias, the complexity of management, the great span of problems ranging from completely benign to clearly life-threatening, the lack of randomized controlled clinical data in some instances, the difficulty in diagnosing problems, and the overlap with many other syndromes. Despite these caveats, some rational commonsense recommendations can be set forth to manage patients who have suspected cardiac arrhythmias.

For Patients With Palpitations

- Diagnosis is crucial, and arrhythmias can range from sinus rhythm to various types of ectopy to supraventricular or ventricular tachycardia.

- If no arrhythmia is documented, consider anxiety or panic attacks and treat accordingly.

- Encourage stress reduction techniques such as meditation and yoga.

For Patients With Symptomatic Ectopy or Premature Ventricular Contractions

Lifestyle

- Determine the severity of the symptoms and their relation to the arrhythmia. Assess underlying conditions.

- Determine the risk to the patient.

- For proven benign ectopy, discuss the risks of drug therapy and suggest alternatives first.

Nutrition

- Eliminate dietary or other apparent triggers (caffeine, alcohol, trans-fatty foods, blood glucose fluctuations).

Mind-Body Therapy

- Promote mind-body interventions such as meditation, yoga, Reiki, or qi gong.

- Counsel the patient about the benign nature of the condition. Patients who understand will be able to tolerate the arrhythmia better.

Exercise

- Determine the relation to exercise, and consider a tailored exercise program.

Supplements and Botanicals

- Suggest omega-3 fatty acids: 2 to 3 g/day of eicosapentaenoic acid plus docosahexaenoic acid essential fatty acids

- Magnesium supplementation: 300 to 1000 mg daily

- Consider herbal approaches: motherwort, 4 to 5 g of dried above-ground parts daily

- Consider carnitine: 3 g daily; and then coenzyme Q10: 100 to 300 mg daily with a meal

Pharmaceuticals

- Drug therapy: only if resistant to foregoing measures

- Beta blockade (titrated upward): consider extended-release metoprolol (Toprol XL), 50, 100, or 200 mg daily; or atenolol, 50 to 100 mg daily

- Calcium channel blockers (diltiazem or verapamil): 120 to 360 mg/daily

- Antiarrhythmic drugs: used as last resort (if no structural heart disease, flecainide, propafenone, sotalol are the first choices; then amiodarone, but only in resistant, highly symptomatic cases; risks may outweigh benefits)

Ablation Therapy

- Suggest ablative therapy for motivated patients willing to take the excess risk. (Counsel patients that symptoms are benign.)

For Patients With Paroxysmal Atrial Fibrillation

Lifestyle and Risk Factors

- Correlate symptoms with the arrhythmia. Determine the presence of underlying conditions, including hyperthyroidism.

- Assess the risk to the patient and the need for rate control, anticoagulation, and maintenance of sinus rhythm (see Table 27-3).

Nutrition

- Determine triggers, if possible. If a relationship is determined, eliminate caffeine, alcohol, and any potentially offending drug.

- If arrhythmia occurs at night, consider changes in diet (no large meals causing gastric distention).

Exercise

- If arrhythmia is exercise related, consider an exercise program.

Mind-Body Therapy

- Promote mind-body interventions such as relaxation techniques.

- Counsel patients and educate them about the disease process.

Continued

■ *Acupuncture*

- Suggest acupuncture (not well tested but perhaps effective).

■ *Supplements and Botanicals*

- Omega-3 fatty acids: 1 to 2 g of fish oil daily
- Magnesium supplementation: 300 to 1000 mg daily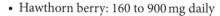
  - Hawthorn berry: 160 to 900 mg daily
  - Motherwort: 4 to 5 g daily
  - Coenzyme Q10: 100 to 300 mg daily with a meal

■ *Pharmaceuticals*

- Beta blockade (to control rhythm and rate): see earlier for dosage
- Calcium channel blockade (to control rate, diltiazem or verapamil): 120 to 360 mg daily
- Digoxin (little effect, but may help in combination with a beta blocker and is safe if used carefully at proper doses)

- Antiarrhythmic drugs depend on the patient and the conditions. The risk-to-benefit ratio is complex and depends on other diagnosed conditions, symptoms, and antiarrhythmic drugs. Amiodarone is the most effective drug but has the greatest risk of side effects. Propafenone and flecainide can triple the risk of death in patients with underlying heart disease and are contraindicated in patients with coronary disease or impaired ventricular function.

■ *Ablation Therapy*

- Ablation of the pulmonary veins or parts of the left atrium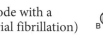
- Ablation of the atrioventricular node with a pacemaker (patient remains in atrial fibrillation) not completely effective
  - Ablation of other inciting arrhythmias

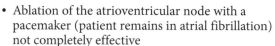
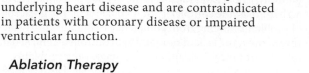

KEY WEB RESOURCES

CHADS2 Score for Atrial Fibrillation Stroke Risk: http://www.mdcalc.com/chads2-score-for-atrial-fibrillation-stroke-risk

This tool calculates the need for warfarin (Coumadin) or aspirin to reduce the risk of stroke in patients with atrial fibrillation.

Surgical Risk Prediction: http://www.surgicalaudit.com/riskcalc.asp

This tool assesses surgical risk of patients seen for preoperative physical examinations.

Risk Assessment Tool for Estimating 10-Year Risk of Developing Hard Coronary Heart Disease: http://hp2010.nhlbihin.net/atpiii/calculator.asp?usertype=prof

This tool from the National Cholesterol Education Program assesses 10-year cardiovascular risk.

emWave by HeartMath: http://www.heartmath.com; and StressEraser: http://stresseraser.com

These biofeedback tools help enhance heart rate variability.

Integrative Medicine Program, University of Wisconsin School of Medicine and Public Health: http://www.fammed.wisc.edu/sites/default/files//webfm-uploads/documents/outreach/im/handout_omega3_fats_patient.pdf

This is a patient handout on omega-3 fatty acids.

References

References are available at expertconsult.com.

Section V Allergy/Intolerance

Chapter 28

Asthma

John D. Mark, MD

Pathophysiology

Asthma, a common chronic respiratory disorder, affects more than 22 million persons in the United States.[1] Asthma is known to be a complex inflammatory process that involves many cell types and cellular elements. Interactions among these cells along with genetic disposition cause asthma symptoms. The symptoms are usually recurrent episodes of wheezing, cough, chest tightness, and breathlessness from widespread but variable airflow obstruction characterized by complete or partial reversibility either spontaneously or with treatment. This chronic inflammation leads to bronchial hyperresponsiveness to various stimuli and results in the clinical manifestations and severity of asthma and the subsequent response to treatment.

Research into the immunologic basis for asthma has shown that, in genetically susceptible individuals, airborne allergens are taken up at the mucosal surface and selective peptides are generated that then influence T cells to develop into type 2 helper T (Th2) cells. The expansion of the proinflammatory Th2-cell population causes a cascade of cytokines to be released, in addition to the up-regulation of adhesion molecules, which trap and activate passing leukocytes, specifically eosinophils, basophils, and monocytes.[2] Finally, these Th2 cells induce the production of allergic antibody immunoglobulin E (IgE), ultimately resulting in the clinical manifestation of allergy and asthma.

Risk Factors and Triggers

Investigators believe that asthma often begins in childhood and may result from an interaction of several factors (Fig. 28-1). Studies of genetic links in families with more than one member with asthma have shown certain regions of chromosomes 5q and 11q to be of interest. However, studies have also shown that in different populations these links are not simple, and susceptibility seems to be determined by several genes that have an effect in different aspects of asthma. Genes have been identified that are linked to the Th2 cytokine signaling pathway, Th2-cell differentiation, airway remodeling, adaptive immune responses, and IgE levels. Thus, the natural course of asthma varies considerably according to asthma phenotype and environmental influences.[3]

Asthma symptoms can be triggered by several factors (Table 28-1). Infections with viruses such as respiratory syncytial virus and rhinovirus have been thought to be triggers not only because of their ability to cause airway swelling and obstruction but also for their influence on the cellular response of the immune system, thus making it more asthma prone. Other key factors associated with poor asthma control include overestimation by patients and physicians of asthma control, improper technique in using inhaled medications, and overall nonadherence to therapies; these factors may lead to increased exacerbations, more hospitalizations, and higher mortality rates.[4] Understanding current asthma guidelines, measuring lung function, and monitoring medication use, in addition to improving adherence and education, would improve asthma control.

Integrative Therapy

Environment

Reducing exposure to environmental triggers such as dust mites and cockroaches, to which many patients with asthma are sensitive, is important. House dust mites, which are microscopic insects that live off dead skin cell flakes, are all around us even though we cannot see them. The mites and their waste products can be allergenic. To limit exposure to dust mites, especially in the bedroom where they are most common, one should (1) enclose pillows and mattresses in airtight polyurethane covers or use

FIGURE 28-1
The condition of a patient's asthma may change with the environment, activities, and other factors. When the patient is well, monitoring and treatment are still needed to maintain control.

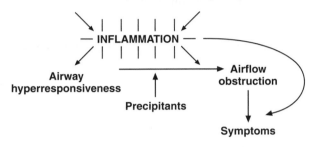

Asthma is a chronic airway inflammation

Environmental risk factors / Genetic predisposition

INFLAMMATION

Airway hyperresponsiveness

Precipitants

Airflow obstruction

Symptoms

TABLE 28-1. Triggers for Symptoms of Asthma

- Allergens such as house dust mites, pets, and pollens
- Colds and viral infections
- Exercise
- Gastroesophageal reflux disease (stomach acid flowing back up the esophagus)
- Medications and foods
- Emotional anxiety
- Air pollutants such as tobacco smoke, wood smoke, chemicals, and ozone
- Occupational exposure to allergens, vapors, dust, gases, and fumes
- Strong odors and sprays such as perfumes, household cleaners, cooking fumes, paints, and varnishes
- Air pollutants such as ozone

fiberfill products instead of down or foam pillows, (2) remove carpeting (hardwood or linoleum floor is better) and curtains, (3) wash sheets and stuffed toys (for pediatric patients) in hot water every week, and (4) clean bedrooms frequently with a vacuum that has a high-efficiency particulate air (HEPA) filter. Cockroaches and their feces represent another trigger for asthma, so cleanliness is important to decrease their presence; in addition, it helps to wash floors and counters frequently, to eliminate cockroach debris. Other important control measures include eliminating exposure to tobacco smoke and removing pets from the home.

Nutrition

Diet therapy or nutritional advice is the most common "alternative" therapy that is given by allopathic physicians for patients with asthma. In theory, diet could modulate intestinal flora, affect immune maturation, and interact with underlying genetic disposition in the development and even the origin of asthma. The literature is difficult to summarize, however, because of the design of many of the studies and the lack of systematic approaches that include the means of diagnosis.[5] Clinicians have long thought that eliminating certain "allergenic" foods and decreasing exposure to foods such as dairy products (believed

to be associated with increased mucus production) will help with chronic asthma symptoms and their severity.[6] The easiest way to conduct an elimination diet is to pick a food to which the patient appears to be sensitive, such as nuts or eggs, and then eliminate it from the diet for 2 weeks. At the end of 2 weeks, gently reintroduce the food into the diet. If a significant change occurs, such as bloating or headaches, the patient may indeed be sensitive to that particular food (see Chapter 84, Food Intolerance and Elimination Diet). Few studies have supported these claims, although one study did suggest a reduction in symptoms in an adult asthmatic patient after adoption of a restricted diet. Some epidemiologic studies suggest that dietary habits influence lung function. The populations with a higher intake of polyunsaturated fatty acids (omega-6 fatty acids) have a higher prevalence of asthma, eczema, and allergic rhinitis.

The following are the nutritional recommendations for patients with asthma:
1. Eliminate potential allergens:
   a. Any food associated with a history of intolerance (gastrointestinal disturbance or eczema)
   b. Sulfites (especially in dried fruits)
   c. Food additives (aspartame, benzoates, and yellow dye no. 5)
   d. Dairy products (for a trial period, as mentioned previously)
2. Increase intake of fruits and vegetables because they are rich in antioxidants, levels of which have been shown to be low in patients with chronic lung problems such as asthma.
3. Increase intake of omega-3 fatty acids by eating cold-water fish (e.g., sardines, herring, and salmon) and reduce intake of omega-6 fatty acids by eliminating vegetable oils and instead using olive oil (see Chapter 86, The Antiinflammatory [Omega-3] Diet).

If intake of dairy products is decreased or eliminated (especially in children), a calcium supplement should be considered.

Exercise

Although exercise in itself can induce symptoms in patients with asthma, numerous studies have shown that asthma can be better controlled in patients who exercise regularly. No study illustrates the superiority of one type of exercise over another. Investigators had long assumed that swimming may be beneficial because the environment is moister, and cold, dry air may actually exacerbate asthma symptoms. Studies did not support this concept, however. Instead, any exercise that the patient will do on a regular basis that does not increase symptoms should be encouraged. In addition, some studies suggest that swimming in highly chlorinated pools or in indoor pools with possible mold exposure may exacerbate asthma symptoms.[7]

The older the patient, the better he or she does with asthma by following an exercise regimen. This effect may, in part, have to do with the better self-image and overall improved health associated with regular exercise in adults.

Breathing Exercises

Breathing exercises and breathing retraining have been used in the management of asthma (Buteyko, yoga, physical therapy). One specific form of breathing therapy, known as the Buteyko breathing technique, has been thought to help asthma by decreasing the respiratory rate and allowing the carbon dioxide concentration in the lungs and blood to rise, thus resulting in bronchodilation. This technique dates back to 1952, when Dr. Buteyko theorized that "hidden" hyperventilation caused asthma symptoms. In vitro studies indicated that having a low alveolar carbon dioxide pressure could result in bronchoconstriction and greater airway resistance. Results of other studies suggested that this breathing technique may be beneficial, but the studies were small. One study did measure end-tidal carbon dioxide ($ETCO_2$) and found no correlation between $ETCO_2$ and breath-holding time; the investigators postulated that this technique may help by improving the biomechanics of breathing.[8] A systematic review concluded that "no reliable conclusions can currently be drawn concerning the use of breathing exercises for asthma in clinical practice."[9] A larger randomized control trial did show that after 6 months of using the Buteyko technique, most subjects in both groups had improved asthma control, and those using Buteyko had an additional benefit of reducing their inhaled corticosteroid use.[10]

Yoga

Yoga embodies many of the previously discussed therapies for improving the health of patients with asthma. Because it is a form of exercise, it has a cardiovascular component. This mind-body method involves using regulated breathing exercises (pranayama), and relaxation and meditation are also included in many yoga practices. One study in adults showed that yoga helped decrease medication use and lower anxiety,[11] and another study showed that yoga reduced airway hyperresponsiveness and improved some aspects of quality of life.[12] A study in 132 adults with mild asthma who were randomized into a yoga group and a control group showed that, after 8 weeks, the yoga group had significantly improved lung function. Both groups continued their regular pharmacologic treatments[13] (see Chapter 89, Breathing Exercises).

Botanicals

Use of botanicals is one of the oldest and most widely used therapeutic approaches in all asthma care worldwide. Historical theories and treatments used in breathing disorders have persisted over thousands of years.[14] Although the amount of knowledge and information regarding herbal or botanical treatment of asthma is large, a significant portion is not based on any well-designed or well-performed clinical studies.[15] In one study, the use of herbal remedies was associated with lower adherence to conventional medications, especially inhaled corticosteroids.[16] Many of the botanicals used are similar to pharmaceuticals in their chemical properties. Many botanicals are used traditionally, and tradition varies by culture.

Boswellia (Boswellia serrata)

Boswellia (also known as salai guggal or Indian frankincense) is a botanical used frequently in Ayurvedic medicine and traditionally used for inflammatory disorders such as asthma and arthritis. Boswellic acid, the major constituent of *Boswellia*, is thought to inhibit 5-lipoxygenase and leukotriene synthesis, and this may be the mechanism for its antiinflammatory properties. *Boswellia* may enhance the effectiveness of conventional leukotriene modifier medications (see later). One small placebo-controlled study in adults did show that subjects taking *Boswellia* had fewer exacerbations and improved lung function.[17]

■ Dosage
A common dosage recommendation is 300 mg three times/day.

■ Precautions
Few precautions have been reported, except for occasional gastrointestinal effects such as epigastric pain, heartburn, nausea, and diarrhea.

Coleus (Coleus forskohlii)

Coleus is a fairly uncommon botanical in the United States, but it has a long history of use for respiratory and asthma problems in India in the Ayurvedic medicine tradition. A member of the mint family, *Coleus forskohlii* grows wild on the mountain slopes of Nepal, India, and Thailand. Traditionally, it was used for numerous purposes, including treatment of rashes, asthma, bronchitis, insomnia, epilepsy, and angina. It is thought to act much like theophylline and has been studied as an effective bronchodilator. Coleus has been shown to increase intracellular cyclic adenosine monophosphate levels and to stabilize cells that release histamine, although its clinical value is still to be determined.[18] One study showed that an inhaled dose of forskolin powder from an inhaler device increased lung function by improving forced expiratory volume in 1 second (FEV_1) in patients with asthma.[18]

■ Dosage
A common dosage recommendation for coleus is 50 mg two or three times/day of an extract standardized to contain 18% forskolin, or a 10-mg dose using an inhaler device.

■ Precautions
No precautions have been reported, but coleus should be used with caution with antihypertensive (beta blocker) and anticoagulant therapy. Pregnant women should not take coleus.

Ma Huang (Ephedra sinica)

Ma Huang, also known as Chinese ephedra and Chinese joint fir, has been commonly used as an asthma remedy in China for thousands of years. The pharmaceutical ephedrine (derived from *Ephedra sinica*) was used in asthma therapy until the advent of more specific beta-agonist medications. Ma Huang may be part of many combinations of other botanicals, including licorice and other antiinflammatory agents. Botanicals and supplements containing ephedra alkaloids have now appeared in many preparations for losing weight and increasing energy.

■ Dosage
Ephedra is not recommended for use in the treatment of asthma because of warnings from the U.S. Food and Drug Administration (FDA) and reports of serious side effects,

especially when it was used in combination with caffeine and other stimulants, such as bitter orange.

■ Precautions

Ma Huang botanicals and its combination products have the most serious potential for side effects. Deaths associated with its use have been reported. Central nervous system problems such as nausea, vomiting, sweating, and nervousness, along with heart palpitations, tachycardia, hypertension, anxiety, and even myocardial infarction, also have been reported.[19]

> Complications, including death, have been reported when Ma Huang is taken in high doses or with caffeine-containing products. Death has even been noted with only one use of this substance.

Licorice (Glycyrrhiza glabra)

Licorice, also known as liquorice, sweet wood, and sweet root, has been used as a cough remedy and asthma treatment. The active ingredient is glycyrrhizin, also called glycyrrhizic acid. Its effect in treating asthma derives from the antiinflammatory nature of licorice and the enhancement of endogenous steroids. Licorice is also thought to be an expectorant, aiding in the expulsion of mucus from the bronchial passages, as well as a demulcent, which can be soothing to irritated airways and bronchioles.

■ Dosage

Licorice is available in several forms such as dried root, which can be used as an infusion or decoction. The dried root dose is usually 1.0 to 5.0 g three times per day. If a licorice tincture is used (1:5 strength is common), the dose is 2 to 5 mL three times a day. Finally, the standardized extract (containing 20% glycyrrhizic acid) dose is 250 to 300 mg three times a day.

■ Precautions

The side effects are minimal if less than 10 mg of the glycyrrhizic acid is taken daily and prolonged use is avoided. Long-term use, however, can cause headache, hypertension, dizziness, edema, and other signs of aldosteronism (through the binding of mineralocorticoids). Licorice may also cause low serum potassium and should be avoided in patients taking cardiac glycosides, blood pressure medications, corticosteroids, diuretics, or monoamine oxidase inhibitors. A deglycyrrhized licorice (DGL) is available, but its effectiveness has not been well studied, and it may not be as effective as other products with glycyrrhizin.

Pycnogenol

Pycnogenol (a proprietary mixture of water-soluble bioflavonoids extracted from French maritime pine) has been used for its antiinflammatory properties in conditions such as asthma. Pycnogenol is a blend of several bioflavonoids—catechin, epicatechin, taxifolin, oligomeric procyanidins, and phenolic fruit acids such as ferulic acid and caffeic acid. This preparation is thought to exert its effect by blocking leukotrienes and other cytokines that increase inflammation and cause asthma symptoms. A study in children with asthma showed that Pycnogenol improved pulmonary function and reduced the need for rescue medications.[20]

■ Dosage

Pycnogenol is supplied in 30-, 50- and 100-mg tablets. The usual dosage is 30 to 100 mg/day for maintenance therapy. The manufacturer recommends 1 mg/kg/day.

■ Precautions

No serious side effects have been reported, but Pycnogenol is recommended to be taken with or after meals because it has an astringent taste. Reports exist of minor side effects, including gastrointestinal discomfort, headache, nausea, and dizziness, which resolve when the botanical is discontinued.

Herbal Mixtures

Japanese combination herbs and remedies (Kampo) such as Saiboku-to blend black cumin, chamomile, cinnamon, cloves, rosemary, sage, spearmint, and thyme into a botanical combination that reduces asthma symptoms. This combination is thought to be effective because of antiinflammatory properties of blocking 5-lipoxygenase and inhibiting platelet-activating factor (PAF).[21] PAF is produced by several inflammatory cells, including eosinophils, thus causing airway hyperreactivity, microvascular leaks, increased airway secretions, and epithelial permeability. Other trials using traditional Chinese medicine herb mixtures also demonstrated a potential for improving asthma control. These mixtures included ASHMI (a traditional herbal mixture) and Ding Chuan Tang, and both showed improvement in asthma control and airway reactivity.[22,23]

■ Dosage

These combination herbal preparations are usually prepared as a tea, taken two to four times/day, depending on the particular mixture and brand used.

■ Precautions

No problems with these combination therapies have been reported.

Supplements

Vitamin and Mineral Overview

In addition to botanical and herbal preparations for the long-term treatment of asthma, vitamins and minerals are used frequently. As with most of the treatments mentioned thus far, few studies support their use, but historically they have been thought to help with asthma and chronic respiratory symptoms.

Vitamin C

Vitamin C has been studied in asthma, and although the results were mixed, one randomized trial did demonstrate reduced asthma symptoms. Vitamin C was also found to be protective against exercise-induced asthma.[24] Another study using vitamin C in 201 patients with asthma for 16 weeks did not show any clinical benefit.[25] Investigators believe that vitamin C inhibits histamine release and promotes vasodilation by increasing production of prostacyclin. A review of 9 studies with 330 participants was analyzed, and the investigators concluded that evidence is insufficient at this time to recommend vitamin C in the treatment of asthma.[26]

■ Dosage

The dose is 250 to 500 mg once or twice a day.

Vitamin D

As with vitamins C and E, numerous studies looked at vitamin D levels and their correlation with asthma. In a survey of 616 children, serum vitamin D levels were associated with airway reactivity, hospitalizations, and the use of antiinflammatory drugs.[27] Lower vitamin D levels were also shown to be inversely associated with recent upper respiratory tract infections, which are a common trigger of acute asthma.[28] Taking supplemental vitamin D to help prevent upper respiratory tract infections could help decrease asthma exacerbations.

■ Dosage

Recommended doses are 400 mg/day for children younger than 4 years of age and 600 mg/day for adults.

■ Precautions

The range for a safe dose of vitamin D is unknown, but an excess of vitamin D may cause abnormally high levels of calcium in the blood that may damage bones, soft tissues, and kidneys.

Vitamin B$_6$

In a double-blind randomized study, vitamin B$_6$ was shown to improve peak flow rates in a group of adults with severe asthma.[29] In patients with low serum pyridoxine (vitamin B$_6$) levels, supplementation helped decrease episodes of wheezing. Lowering of serum vitamin B$_6$ levels may be a side effect of common asthma medications.

■ Dosage

The recommended dose range is 50 to 100 mg/day.

■ Precautions

High doses—usually more than 500 mg/day—and prolonged use of vitamin B$_6$ have been associated with peripheral neuropathy.

Vitamin E

Intake of vitamin E is recommended in the diet or through supplementation because patients who have a high antioxidant intake have fewer pulmonary problems. Poorly controlled asthma has been shown to be associated with low vitamin E levels.[30]

■ Dosage

The recommended dose is 400 units/day of mixed tocopherols.

■ Precautions

The risk of all-cause mortality may be increased with prolonged use of doses greater than 400 units daily.

Magnesium

Magnesium's role in decreasing bronchospasm has been investigated in both the conventional medical and the complementary and alternative medicine communities. Intravenous magnesium is now commonly used for serious asthma symptoms (status asthmaticus). The use of oral magnesium has been studied. In adults, magnesium was shown to decrease symptoms but not to improve pulmonary function in one study and to have no benefit in another.[31] In a more recent study of 55 adults taking 340 mg of magnesium a day for 6 months, objective measurements of lung function, including bronchial reactivity to methacholine and peak flow measurements, improved, as did subjective measures of asthma control and quality of life.[32]

■ Dosage

The dose is 200 to 400 mg/day. Magnesium gluconate and magnesium glycinate are the forms least likely to cause diarrhea.

■ Precautions

One problem with using oral magnesium is the tendency of the preparations to cause diarrhea.

Selenium

Selenium is another potent antioxidant used in many inflammatory conditions, including asthma. One randomized placebo-controlled trial conducted for 14 weeks in 24 patients with asthma found evidence of clinical improvement but no effect on objective markers such as lung function.[33]

Other studies showed inconsistent results. This inconsistency may result from the complex relationship between selenium and asthma because selenium can augment the oxidative stress that accompanies asthma, but it also exerts a significant influence over various immune responses.[34]

■ Dosage

The dose is 100 to 200 mcg/day.

■ Precautions

When selenium is consumed in amounts exceeding 400 mcg/day, symptoms of toxicity may appear, including nausea, vomiting, abdominal pain, fatigue, irritability, and weight loss.

Fish Oil

The use of antiinflammatory medication is now the standard in asthma treatment. If the diet could be altered to decrease the propensity for development of inflammatory precursors, conditions such as asthma would be less problematic. The use of omega-3 essential fatty acids in adequate amounts in the diet may limit leukotriene synthesis by blocking arachidonic acid metabolism. A rich source of omega-3 fatty acid is fish oils. Because eating cold-water oily fish (mackerel, sardines, herring, salmon, and cod) is not common in most Western diets, the use of fish oil capsules has become more standard. Epidemiologic studies in populations that do eat this type of diet have shown it to reduce the risk of asthma significantly and improve pulmonary function. The vegetarian sources of omega-3 fatty acids (flaxseed oil, canola oil, and soy oil) are used even less in most diets, so the study of fish oil in asthma has been investigated.[35]

In one prospective study, dietary supplements of omega-3 fatty acids given to infants who had a high risk for developing asthma showed a small reduction in wheezing episodes in the first 18 months, but by age 5, this association was no longer present.[36,37]

■ Dosage

One 500-mg capsule is taken two to three times/day. Benefit may not be evident for several months.

Pharmaceuticals

Bronchodilators

Bronchodilators have long been used to help alleviate the bronchospasm and difficulty with breathing that are associated with asthma "attacks." Bronchodilators belong to several different classes. Commonly used beta agonists are albuterol and salmeterol or formoterol. A different beta agonist that is similar to albuterol is levalbuterol (Xopenex), which may have fewer cardiovascular side effects. In addition are the methylxanthines (theophylline and aminophylline). The methylxanthines are used as second- or third-line drugs because they have more significant side effects and their use requires serum level monitoring.

■ Dosage

Albuterol: two to four puffs of a metered-dose inhaler (MDI), one to three times/day as needed
Levalbuterol: one inhalation vial (three strengths) per nebulizer three times/day; or by MDI, two puffs one to three times/day as needed
Salmeterol or formoterol (long-acting beta-agonist): one actuation of the dry powder inhaler (DPI) twice a day
Methylxanthines (theophylline): dosage dependent on age and weight

■ Precautions

Beta agonists may cause rapid or irregular heartbeat, insomnia, and nervousness. The anticholinergic medications have few side effects, except for occasional dry mouth or headache. The theophylline-type medications may cause tremor, shakiness, nausea, and vomiting. Overdose of methylxanthines can cause serious problems, such as seizures and cardiac arrhythmias.

Antiinflammatory Medications

Antiinflammatory medications are considered the most important components of the pharmacologic approach to asthma care. Several categories of these medications are available, usually listed as steroidal and nonsteroidal. The steroidal MDIs and DPIs include fluticasone, beclomethasone, mometasone, ciclesonide, and budesonide. Newer proprietary preparations that have been shown to reduce the need for higher doses of the steroidal preparations are combinations of an inhaled steroid (fluticasone, budesonide, or mometasone) with a long-acting bronchodilator (salmeterol or formoterol). Oral preparations, such as prednisone, prednisolone, and methylprednisolone, are also available. The nonsteroidal medications include the leukotriene inhibitors montelukast and zafirlukast. These medications act by blocking certain pathways of airway inflammation once exposure (allergic, irritant, infectious, or emotional or exercise) has occurred. The oral steroids are the most potent agents and have the greatest potential for significant side effects.

■ Dosage

Leukotriene inhibitors differ by the specific type used. The dosage of montelukast, for example, is 10 mg/day for adults and 5 mg/day for children (chewable tablets). For a child younger than 5 years, 4 mg/day is recommended (not to be used in children younger than 12 months).

Dosages for steroidal inhalers are usually two puffs (or one actuation of the DPI) twice/day. Oral steroids are usually taken at 1 to 2 mg/kg or 20 to 40 mg/day (adults) for varying amounts of time. A short "burst" would be 3 to 5 days in total.

■ Precautions

Nonsteroidal medications have few side effects. Leukotriene inhibitors may cause headache, and some cause hepatic dysfunction, so liver function should be monitored. The steroidal medications, especially the oral preparations, may cause problems with decreased height velocity (in children), immune suppression, hypertension, cataracts, and hirsutism (if taken long term). The inhaled forms have rare side effects and have been followed long term in children[38]; they may, however, cause hoarseness, cough, and oral candidiasis unless a spacer is used or thorough mouth rinsing is practiced. Combination medications (corticosteroids plus a long-acting beta agonist such as fluticasone and salmeterol) have a black box warning given by the FDA because of the possibility that some patients may actually do worse when using these types of medications, with more asthma exacerbations and even death.

> The newer antiinflammatory steroidal inhalers, used alone or in combination with a long-acting bronchodilator, constitute the most innovative pharmacologic approach to chronic asthma care.

Biomechanical Approaches

Massage

Massage therapy is an ancient treatment, dating back to the second century in China. It was referred to as the "art of rubbing" and was common until pharmaceuticals began to be heavily used instead, starting in the 1950s. Little material in the literature has investigated the efficacy of massage, and the studies performed before the 1990s had problems with sampling, lack of controls, sample size, and inappropriate use of statistical analysis.[39] Since then, several studies have investigated the use of massage in many areas of medicine that use methods to support the effectiveness of massage. Most of these studies have been conducted by the Touch Research Institute at the University of Miami Miller School of Medicine in Florida. Asthma has been studied in children, and investigators showed that daily massage improved airway caliber and control of asthma.[39] A decrease in anxiety and improved attitude toward the subject's asthma were also noted.

■ Dosage

The time and duration of massage therapy for the average patient with asthma are not known. The study that showed improvement used once-a-day massage for 30 days. The person doing the massage may be another family member or friend who has been taught massage techniques or a massage therapist.

Osteopathy

Osteopathy is another system of medical care that embraces the body as a whole and in which structure and function are closely interrelated. One main premise is that because osteopathy emphasizes that all body systems, including the musculoskeletal system, operate in unison, a disturbance in one system can alter functions of the other systems. Several main categories of osteopathic manipulative treatment (OMT; e.g., craniosacral, strain-counterstrain, and myofascial) involve more than 100 different individual treatments. OMTs in asthma have been used for both chronic and acute symptoms. OMT is used to increase vital capacity and rib cage mobility, improve diaphragmatic function, enhance clearing of airway secretions, and improve autoimmune function. One report proposed that the use of OMTs in the emergency department setting could alleviate acute symptoms.[40] In a randomized controlled trial in 5- to 17-year-old patients with asthma, 90 patients received OMT, and 50 were in the control group. Peak flow improved more in the OMT group than in the control group (measurements were taken before and after OMT).[41] A movement has also been started by the American Osteopathic Association to use OMT in the basic management of asthma.[42]

■ Dosage
The findings of the osteopathic practitioner will determine the form of OMT. Again, the form chosen may affect any part of the body, depending on the physical examination. Often, just helping the patient use various parts of the chest in breathing may help.

Chiropractic
Chiropractic, the third largest regulated health care profession in North America, has been involved in health care for conditions such as asthma since the late 1800s. The theory of chiropractic care is based on the idea that the properly adjusted body is essential for health. Through the use of spinal manipulation therapy for the removal of subluxations, the life force is influenced, and good health is attained.[43]

Some studies involving chiropractic treatments in asthma showed overall improvement in lung capacity. Other findings documented abnormal spinal mechanics associated with asthma. Chiropractic adjustments may produce immediate relaxation of the neck musculature and overall may improve respiratory function. Other chiropractic theories hold that various adjustments may affect respiratory symptoms through the action of treating the subluxations found and subsequent nerve function. Three randomized controlled studies showed benefit in subjective measures, such as quality of life, symptoms, and bronchodilator use; however, the differences between controls and treated groups were not statistically significant.[44]

■ Dosage
The dosage of chiropractic care depends on the practitioner.

■ Precautions
Reported complications of chiropractic manual treatments have been documented, but none were found in the treatment of asthma. Chiropractic care often involves repeated use of radiographs, thus making frequent radiation exposure an issue for some patients.

Manual Therapy
A systematic review of more than 450 citations assessed 3 randomized trials of manual therapies in asthma.[45] The manual therapies included physical therapy, respiratory therapy, chiropractic therapy, and osteopathic therapy. The reviewers concluded that evidence is insufficient to support the use of manual therapies in patients with asthma and suggested the need to conduct adequately sized randomized controlled trials that examine the effects of manual therapies on clinically relevant outcomes. Currently, evidence is insufficient to support or refute the use of manual therapy in patients with asthma.[45]

Mind-Body Therapy

Mind-body therapies have been used in the treatment of asthma in various ways. They are at times referred to as cognitive-behavioral therapies and encompass several approaches. No one therapy has been shown to be superior over another; however, some therapies appear to be more acceptable to individual patients. Discussing several types of therapy with the patient and the family will enhance the success of mind-body interventions. Research in this area started in the early 1960s, and approaches have included relaxation therapy, breathing exercises, biofeedback, and hypnosis and guided imagery.

The theory behind using these therapies is to improve the inflammatory process that can be triggered by the autonomic nervous system through emotions. Numerous studies in both children and adults have shown higher levels of anxiety and even at times panic when asthma symptoms are perceived. In addition to anxiety, stress has been shown to influence the immune response and may promote a higher sympathetic activity, augment IgE production, cause a shift from a Th1 to a Th2 allergic-type response, and promote airway inflammation without overt symptoms.[46] Studies have also shown that using different types of cognitive-behavioral therapies may decrease symptoms and medication use and may reduce the inflammatory response of airway cells.[47,48]

Hypnosis and Guided Imagery
Hypnosis has been used for achieving relaxation, relieving pain, helping with physical discomfort (even chronic pain), and altering moods. It is multidimensional and helps patients develop a heightened concentration of an idea or image. The process may be brief or may involve complex instructions, depending on the subject, the goal, and the therapist. Hypnosis has been shown to be effective in patients whose asthma is mild and those whose symptoms have an emotional component. Studies showed that "motivated" patients had decreases in symptoms and medication use, as well as improvements in pulmonary function.[49]

Guided imagery involves a form of self-hypnosis in which the patient uses an image of her or his own creation after an initial relaxation period to help reduce asthma symptoms. This method is especially effective in children with an active and vibrant imagination. They often can be taught this technique in less than half an hour and do well with their asthma symptoms after a few practice sessions. Guided imagery starts with initial relaxation (using diaphragmatic breathing—"belly breathing") and then progresses to an imagery session. The subject develops an image and then focuses on taking control or command of the perceived airway or lung problem by using this image. An example is moving from a closet to the outdoors, where the child could once again breathe. This emotion-mediated format enables disclosure and subsequent reframing for the child and allows independence from the chronic illness (see Chapter 95, Guided Imagery, and Chapter 92, Self-Hypnosis Techniques).

Dosage
As with relaxation, these therapies are best if used often and especially if used when asthma symptoms are initially mild. This approach prepares the patient for dealing with worse symptoms during an attack.

Disclosure and Journaling
Much like the findings in rheumatoid arthritis, some evidence has indicated that just having the patient with asthma discuss the symptoms may decrease the severity and frequency of the asthma. Journaling, in which one writes about asthma in a journal three to five times a week for 20 to 30 minutes, has been shown to reduce both symptoms and medication use. In one study, patients wrote in their journals about a stressful event that they had not discussed with others or that had been unresolved; the control group just wrote about daily events.[50] The investigators reported a 13% improvement in lung function, as measured by the FEV_1, in patients who wrote about a stressful experience compared with the control group (see Chapter 96, Journaling for Health).

Other Therapies to Consider
Knowing where to put bioenergetic modalities—traditional Chinese medicine (TCM), healing touch and prayer, and homeopathy—in the stepwise approach to asthma care is difficult. These modalities could really fit anywhere in the treatment plan from the most mild to the most severe asthma. These methods should be used in conjunction with the previously discussed therapies if the patient has moderate or severe symptoms, but they are appropriate as first-line treatment in the interested patient with mild or intermittent asthma.

Traditional Chinese Medicine
TCM has been practiced for several thousand years and takes many forms. The basis, however, is the understanding of the connections among body, mind, and spirit in health and disease. The belief in an unseen vital energy that affects the patient's health and in the flow of this energy or qi (chi) through the appropriate channels is the basis of this practice. The practitioner can affect this flow or intensity by manipulating the balance through the use of acupuncture, Chinese herbs, diet, and physical therapy. TCM can successfully treat many medical conditions.

Acupuncture and other forms of TCM are thought to be beneficial in the treatment of asthma. Clinical observations showed that acupuncture and individually mixed Chinese herbs were effective, although clinical trials have not supported these observations. The National Institutes of Health 1997 Consensus Development Conference on Acupuncture recommended acupuncture for many conditions, including asthma.[51] One review showed modest improvement in asthma symptoms by using acupuncture,[52] and another study suggested that acupuncture before exercise protected against exercise-induced asthma symptoms.[53] A systematic review of 11 studies for acupuncture and asthma concluded that evidence is insufficient to make recommendations about the value of acupuncture in asthma treatment. The review went on to recommend further research because of the complexities and different types of acupuncture.[54]

Dosage
The dosage of acupuncture is practitioner dependent, and the effects of TCM usually take several treatments to appear.

Precautions
Adverse side effects of acupuncture are rare but have been reported, including pneumothoraces.

Healing Touch and Prayer
Healing touch and other touch therapies such as therapeutic touch, Reiki, and Johrei are defined as the consciously directed process of energy exchange during which the practitioner uses touch or "nontouch" as a focus to facilitate healing. Prayer, which does not even require touch or the presence of the healer to help with symptoms and medical condition, has been used in nearly every culture for centuries. Few studies have investigated this type of energy healing in the patient with asthma. One small study using "hands-on" healing in adult asthmatic patients did show some reduction in medication use.[55]

Dosage
Dosage depends on the modality (healing touch, therapeutic touch, Reiki, Johrei, prayer); all have different approaches, and practitioners use various assessments.

Homeopathy
Homeopathy is thought to be an energy medicine because it is not based on the usual physical laws found in science, but rather on the premise that the use of "remedies" that would cause the same symptoms (principle of like cure) and are very dilute (the more dilute, the more potent; law of dilution) is the most powerful treatment. Practitioners believe that the dilution in water actually imparts healing energy, and this energy, combined with the patient's vital force or energy, is used in healing.

Several studies have shown efficacy of homeopathic remedies in the treatment of both asthma and allergies.[56] The study in asthma showed a reduction in symptoms but no real difference in pulmonary function. A review of the research in homeopathy for treating asthma (6 trials with a total of 556 subjects were included) concluded that not enough evidence exists to assess the possible role of homeopathy in asthma reliably at this time.[57]

The remedies depend on the particular patient's symptom pattern and should be individually assessed by an experienced homeopath to select the correct constitutional remedy. Some of the commonly used homeopathic remedies are as follows:

Arsenicum album: used for asthma with restlessness and anxiety
Ipecac: used for chest constriction and cough
Pulsatilla: used for chest pressure and air hunger
Sambuscus: used for asthma symptoms that awaken one in the night

Dosage
The dosage depends on the individual and on the guidance of the practitioner (see Chapter 111, Therapeutic Homeopathy).

Precautions
Homeopathy is thought to be safe owing to the extreme dilution, and the treatments are inexpensive.

PREVENTION PRESCRIPTION

- Eliminate potential allergens and triggers in the environment.
- Increase fruit and vegetable intake, along with that of omega-3–rich fats, which are found in cold-water fish, nuts, greens, and ground flaxseed.
- Follow an exercise regimen, and consider other types of activities that incorporate both exercise and meditation, such as yoga and martial arts.
- Take controller medications, such as inhaled steroids and leukotriene-modifier medication, routinely until asthma is no longer persistent and the medications can safely be decreased or discontinued.
- Consider adding a multivitamin with antioxidants (vitamins C, D and E, B-complex, selenium) to the diet.
- Botanicals may be helpful in controlling and decreasing asthma symptoms but are best taken under the guidance of a health care provider with experience in using them.
- Mind-body therapies such as relaxation, visualization, and self-hypnosis may decrease asthma exacerbations and reduce the need for asthma medications.
- Stress reduction in the home, work place, and school may prevent or decrease asthma symptoms and airway inflammation.

THERAPEUTIC REVIEW

The following is a summary of therapeutic options for treating asthma. If a patient is having persistent symptoms (daily wheezing, shortness of breath, difficulty sleeping, or difficulty exercising) or severe symptoms (even if intermittent), it is best to prescribe more aggressive therapy such as the beta-agonist drugs and antiinflammatory medications as controller medications. For the patient who has mild to moderate or intermittent symptoms, this stepwise approach may be considered.

Lifestyle

- As with many chronic illnesses, asthma prevention would be the best treatment. Unfortunately, changing a person's lifestyle, including the environment, is difficult. Because of the cultural and regional differences just in the United States, patient populations differ in how they approach a chronic illness and even in the way they use medical care.

Environmental

- Reducing exposure to asthma triggers can be therapeutic in itself. Such things as house dust mite reduction, frequent cleaning, use of HEPA filters, avoidance of secondhand smoke, and removal of all pets from the home will help decrease the "irritability" of the airways.

Nutrition

- With elimination of allergenic-type foods such as dairy products (at least for a trial period), shellfish, foods with nitrites, sulfites, added food coloring, and artificial sweeteners, asthma symptoms often diminish. Patients should consider increasing intake of organic fruits and vegetables for their antioxidant contribution, as well as foods rich in omega-3 fatty acids while decreasing those containing omega-6 fatty acids (vegetable oils).

Supplements

- Vitamin B$_6$: 100 mg/day
- Magnesium: 200 to 400 mg/day
- Fish oil: 1 g (eicosapentaenoic acid plus docosahexaenoic acid) twice daily
- Vitamin D: 400 units for children younger than 4 years of age and 600 units daily for adults
- Vitamin C: 250 mg twice daily
- Vitamin E: 400 units a day or less of mixed tocopherols

Mind-Body Therapy

- These techniques can be very rewarding in the treatment of asthma, and breathing and relaxation are excellent places to start.

- Guided imagery and hypnosis therapies are readily available in most communities and also help decrease symptoms, medication use, and physician or urgent care visits. Usually, these methods should be used regularly (once or twice daily) until familiar to the patient; they can then be used as needed for asthma symptoms.

- Journaling is also recommended, and patients should spend at least 20 minutes writing about their asthma or other stressors in their lives three times per week.

- Cognitive therapies should not be used in place of medications, especially if symptoms are moderate or severe. If the patient is using a peak flow meter, these therapies can be used if peak flow values are in a safe range.

Exercise

- Not only will routine exercise help with asthma (three to five periods of exercise lasting a minimum of 20 minutes per week), it will also help with self-esteem, weight loss, and cardiovascular health. Exercise should be used with caution in patients with exercise-induced asthma.

Botanicals

- Coleus: 50 mg three times/day

- Kampo (also known as Kanpo) is a mixture of Chinese herbs and found in powder form such as Easy-Breather Tea (Yama's Herbs, New York): 3 rounded teaspoons in warm water two to three times/day

- Pycnogenol: 30 to 100 mg/day or 10 mg/kg/day, taken two to three times/day

Pharmaceuticals

- For patients with mild to moderate symptoms that are persistent, starting with pharmaceuticals with antiinflammatory properties such as fluticasone, two puffs of the 110 metered-dose inhaler (110 mcg/ inhalation) twice daily, or budesonide, one actuation twice daily, will improve symptoms in most patients while the other interventions mentioned previously can be started. For acute symptoms, one should use albuterol, two puffs twice daily, or levalbuterol, two puffs twice daily. These medications should be considered as first-line therapy if a patient has persistent or severe symptoms.

- Other medications, such as leukotriene modifiers (montelukast 10 mg daily), may also be considered.

Biomechanical Approaches

- As adjuncts to other modalities and depending on the patient's preferences, massage, osteopathic manipulative treatment, and chiropractic therapies may be very beneficial. All three have different approaches and regimens, but finding a practitioner who is familiar with treating patients with asthma is the key.

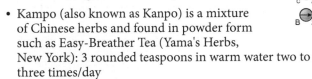

KEY WEB RESOURCES

References

References are available online at expertconsult.com.

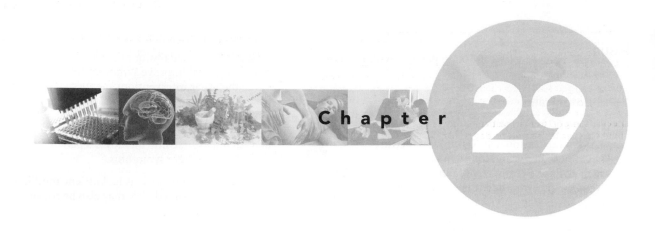

Chapter **29**

The Allergic Patient

Randy J. Horwitz, MD, PhD

More than 20% of U.S. citizens—approximately 50 million people—are estimated to suffer from an allergic condition, and they spend $8 billion annually for prescription drugs to treat allergic symptoms.[1] A nationwide survey found that more than half (54%) of all U.S. citizens test positive to one or more allergens.[2] Although acute and chronic allergic diseases may not rank as a leading cause of mortality in the population, they do constitute a leading cause of work and school absenteeism, and they contribute to significant social and economic costs.

This chapter considers general integrative approaches to the patient with atopy, or environmental allergies, whether seasonal or perennial. Separate chapters in this book deal with some of the more prominent allergic and allergy-related conditions (e.g., asthma, atopic dermatitis, food intolerance, and multiple chemical sensitivities). Some commonalities link these seemingly disparate disorders, however, and knowledge of these common principles may be helpful in devising treatment recommendations for patients with allergies.

Pathophysiology

The wide range of allergic conditions observed in the clinical setting and described in the literature may lead one to believe that an infinite number of discrete mechanisms is responsible for allergic symptoms. Despite the diversity in end-organ effects, however, much of the underlying pathophysiology in allergic diseases is remarkably similar. In addition, such knowledge enables the physician to recognize, and even anticipate, adverse reactions. Knowing that some patients with an anaphylactic reaction or asthma exacerbation may experience a late-phase allergic response, for example, compels the physician to continue intensive therapy until the reaction has completely subsided.

The term allergy, in common usage, connotes a variety of reactions that range from mildly debilitating to life-threatening. In conventional medicine, however, allergy specifically describes a precise cascade of biochemical reactions that, in genetically predisposed (or atopic) individuals,

may result in specific physical symptoms, such as rhinorrhea, sneezing, wheezing, bronchoconstriction, and even life-threatening vasodilation and hypotension (anaphylaxis). Some distinct stages in the development and promulgation of the allergic reaction are well described.

The two-step process by which a genetically susceptible (i.e., atopic) individual initially becomes allergic to a substance begins with *sensitization* (Fig. 29-1). During the initial stage of sensitization, the individual develops significant amounts of immunoglobulin E (IgE) antibodies against an inhaled, ingested, or injected substance. Long-lived memory B cells, which are capable of producing more of this specific IgE antibody immediately when stimulated, appear in the circulation, largely through the action of "allergic" cytokines. The newly formed IgE antibody adheres either to circulating blood basophils or to mast cells located in the mucosal layers of the skin, the gastrointestinal tract, and the respiratory system. Millions of IgE molecules of different specificities (directed against different allergens) are present on the surface of each mast cell and basophil. An individual is considered sensitized only after sufficient levels of IgE antibodies directed against a specific substance have been produced and are bound to the surfaces of these cells. The process of sensitization does not produce any of the symptoms that we equate with allergic disease—in fact, a person is usually unaware of these initial molecular and cellular changes. Not until reexposure to the allergen do allergic symptoms manifest.

> Immunoglobulin E acts as a bridge that crosslinks a specific antigen on the surface of mast cells and basophils to release mediators that foster inflammatory activity.

The second step in the allergic process is the reactivity phase. The allergic reaction requires that a sensitized person be reexposed to the allergen, which now acts as a bridge, cross-linking the IgE molecules on the surface of

FIGURE 29-1

Allergic sensitization and reactivity (degranulation). The process of sensitization and degranulation in mast cells begins with production of antigen-specific immunoglobulin E (IgE) in genetically predisposed individuals. Initial binding of specific IgE to the naive mast cell surface "primes" the cell for activity. Subsequent binding of a specific allergen to the mast cell triggers complex intracellular biochemical events, leading to degranulation and subsequent mediator release.

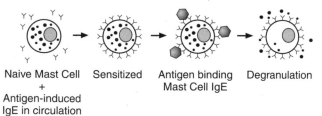

Naive Mast Cell   Sensitized   Antigen binding   Degranulation
       +   Mast Cell IgE
Antigen-induced
IgE in circulation

each basophil and mast cell. This bridging phenomenon induces changes within the cell, typically through the action of multiple complex protein kinase cascades. Ultimately, this cross-linking process leads to degranulation of the mast cell or basophil, a process that releases both preformed mediators (e.g., histamine, serine proteases, and proteoglycans) and newly synthesized compounds (e.g., eicosanoids and cytokines). The activities of these mediators of allergic inflammation are readily observable in a patient experiencing an allergic reaction. Histamine dilates blood vessels and thus causes localized edema in tissues such as the skin and mucosal membranes, as well generalized urticaria. Cytokines lead to the ingress of additional cells to the area of the initial reaction, such as CD4[+] T cells and eosinophils in the lung tissue of an individual experiencing an asthma exacerbation. Overall clinical symptoms vary from negligible rhinorrhea to sudden death (severe anaphylaxis), depending on the degree of exposure and the sensitivity of the person exposed to the allergen. Most cases lie somewhere between these extremes. Although the cellular and molecular events for all immediate hypersensitivity reactions are similar, differences in target organ responses ultimately dictate the clinical patterns of disease activity once a reaction has been induced.

Allergic reactions also produce an inflammatory reaction; indeed, one of the most important research findings from the past few decades is the recognition that most of the pathophysiologic processes of diverse allergic reactions have a common inflammatory pathway. Elucidation of this pathway has resulted in more precise, targeted therapies with which to control allergic inflammation. In the past, treatment with systemic corticosteroids was the only antiinflammatory intervention available. Although remarkably effective, these steroids provide relief at the expense of severe, long-term adverse effects, including bone loss, myopathy, and even psychiatric disturbances. Fortunately, the identification of biochemical intermediates and enzymes in the inflammatory cascade reduced the need for such powerful and nonspecific drugs and led to targeted therapies for interrupting the allergic inflammatory cascade, or at least controlling the allergic symptoms, until the triggered reaction eventually attenuates.

Although analogues for specific pharmacologic activities exist in the conventional and alternative therapeutic realms, the overall approach to treatment more clearly differentiates the two approaches to care. Whereas a conventional physician tends to treat each disease state (and symptom) separately and specifically, an integrative practitioner may additionally consider measures to diminish an atopic predisposition. These additional therapies are described in this chapter and in the chapters on specific allergic diseases.

Integrative Therapy

Nutrition

Specialized Allergen Avoidance Diets

The avoidance of specific foods or food additives that are found to be responsible for gastrointestinal or anaphylactic allergic reactions, such as peanuts in sensitive individuals, is an obvious intervention. Such elimination diets are useful for both true food allergies and food sensitivities (see Chapter 84, Food Intolerance and Elimination Diet). Food avoidance is also useful when one is attempting to control less severe, nongastrointestinal allergies. For example, patients who are troubled by recurrent sinus infections or mild to moderate refractory asthma symptoms often benefit from certain dietary modifications. Usually, these avoidance diets are specific to an individual, but some common classes of foods have been popularly linked to allergic exacerbations, such as dairy products and animal proteins. These foods seem to be associated with a worsening of allergic symptoms in many patients, though published clinical data in this area are scant. A handful of small studies refuted the association between milk and mucus production or allergic symptoms,[3] but biologically plausible hypotheses support such an association.[4] In either case, a brief trial (4 to 6 weeks) of dairy avoidance is helpful to discern such an association in selected individuals.

Omega-3 Fatty Acids

Alterations in the dietary intake of fats are known to affect the fatty acid composition of cell membranes.[5,6] This fact is especially pertinent to inflammatory conditions, because catabolism of cell membrane–derived fats is an initial step in inflammatory mediator production through the arachidonic acid cascade. Omega-3 supplementation decreases the ratio of omega-6 to omega-3 fatty acids in the inflammatory cell lipid membrane and thus creates less substrate for mediator production.[5,6] This process, in turn, decreases the production of many potent bioactive compounds (e.g., leukotrienes) that are intimately involved in allergic inflammation. The level of inhibition of leukotriene production by dietary modification rivals that of pharmacologic agents[7] (see Chapter 86, The Antiinflammatory Diet).

Increased dietary omega-3 intake is a useful clinical intervention, as is a trial of omega-3 supplementation. Published reports used doses of 3.2 g eicosapentaenoic acid (EPA) and 2.2 g docosahexaenoic acid (DHA) daily as a supplement to a standard diet.[5] In one clinical trial, 26 patients with asthma were placed on defined diets of varying omega-3 to omega-6 content.[8] More than 40% of subjects showed marked improvement in airway hyperresponsiveness when they consumed a diet with an elevated omega-3 content. These responders to dietary interventions could be readily identified through analysis of the leukotriene composition of their urine, a measure that predicted which patients were likely to improve with dietary intervention.[8]

Dietary Antioxidants

The association between dietary antioxidant intake and the allergic response has been the subject of much study over many years. Many positive and negative reports exist in the literature, fairly equally divided, thus precluding definitive and global conclusions. Some findings are worthy of mention, however, particularly a few examining vitamin C and selenium intake. A case-control study using a food frequency questionnaire in 1500 people found that apple consumption and dietary selenium intake were negatively associated with asthma prevalence.[9] Further evidence for a role of selenium in modulating allergic diseases is that selenium functions as a cofactor for glutathione peroxidase, which helps prevent peroxidation of cell membranes by consuming free peroxide in the cell. In one report, children with asthma had significantly lower red blood cell glutathione peroxidase activity than a healthy control group.[10] Finally, patients with asthma have higher amounts of oxidized glutathione in their airways, a finding perhaps indicating that patients with asthma are subject to greater oxidative stress.[11]

A study in children found that higher intakes of cooked vegetables, tomatoes, and fruit were protective factors for symptoms of shortness of breath and wheeze during a 12-month observation period.[12] Consumption of citrus fruit, in particular, had a protective role for these symptoms, which may be related to vitamin C intake. In the same study, consumption of bread, butter, and margarine were all associated with an increased risk of shortness of breath and wheezing.[12] These findings are not universally accepted, however, because data in the literature are conflicting.

Finally, no conclusive consensus evidence indicates that antenatal supplementation of any vitamin or mineral during pregnancy will reduce the probability of atopy or asthma later in life for children.[13,14] By definition, these studies are difficult to perform, and the number of confounding variables is extremely high.

Supplements

Quercetin

Quercetin is a bioflavonoid (a plant pigment responsible for the colors found in fruits and vegetables) obtained from diverse sources, including apples, buckwheat, onions, and citrus fruits. Most data supporting its role in attenuating allergic reactivity have been obtained from in vitro studies, as well as from animal models of allergic disease. In vitro, quercetin stabilizes the membranes of mast cells and reduces the release of preformed histamine.[15,16] In animal models, quercetin is able to suppress anaphylactic responses in sensitized rats,[17] and it inhibits asthmatic inflammation in guinea pigs and rats.[18]

Quercetin must be used as a preventative—taken before allergen exposure. Thus, the activity of quercetin is similar to that of cromolyn, a drug that is often prescribed for allergy and asthma prevention (see later). Quercetin also inhibits the production of enzymes responsible for manufacturing

the potent leukotrienes.[19] Practitioners usually recommend that quercetin be used regularly during an individual's entire allergy season, or year-round for those with perennial allergies.

> Quercitin is similar to cromolyn in its mechanism of action. Both are mast cell stabilizers.

■ Dosage

The dose of quercetin is usually 400 to 600 mg of a coated tablet one to three times daily between meals (adjust dose for clinical response). Quercetin is not soluble in water, however, so it is a poorly absorbed nutrient. Bromelain, a protein-digesting enzyme extracted from pineapples, increases the absorption of quercetin, as does vitamin C. Therefore, quercetin is typically sold blended with one or both additives.

■ Precautions

None are reported.

Magnesium

Magnesium is now a standard of care in the emergency treatment of acute asthma exacerbations, and it is usually administered as an intravenous solution. Magnesium has been shown to improve forced expiratory volume in 1 second (FEV_1) in that setting. Inverse associations are also reported between intracellular magnesium levels and asthma severity.[20] Despite this association, little convincing literature supports a role for long-term magnesium replenishment in the care of mild to moderate asthma. Some published reports note an improvement in asthma symptoms for those subjects with higher magnesium intake,[21] while others link dietary magnesium intake with an increased risk of asthma and wheezing in children.[22]

■ Dosage

Magnesium glycinate seems to be less irritating to the gastrointestinal system. The typical dose is 400 mg daily.

■ Precautions

Side effects are primarily gastrointestinal. At standard doses, magnesium exerts laxative effects.

> Some forms of magnesium supplementation have prominent laxative effects. The clinician must be wary of prescribing magnesium citrate, oxide, or hydroxide in a patient for whom diarrhea is a problem.

Botanicals

Butterbur (Petasites hybridus)

Butterbur has traditionally been used to treat migraine headaches but also asthma and bronchitis, because it is thought to reduce mucus production. A study of 132 people with seasonal rhinitis (hay fever) found that an extract of this herb was as effective as cetirizine (Zyrtec), a commonly prescribed, mildly sedating antihistamine, and had fewer side effects (especially less sedating). The study lasted only 2 weeks and required four to five doses of the herb daily.[23] More recently, mechanisms of action were more carefully delineated in a mouse model of asthma.[24] In this study, butterbur was shown to inhibit leukotriene activity and reduce allergic airway inflammation and bronchial hyperreactivity by specifically inhibiting allergic cytokine formation (interleukin-4 [IL-4] and IL-5, and RANTES [regulated on activation, normal T expressed and secreted]).

Dosage
Petasites extracts are typically standardized to contain a minimum of 7.5 mg of petasin and isopetasin. The adult dosage ranges from 50 to 100 mg twice daily for the treatment of migraine headaches. A high-quality, standardized product prepared in Germany is Petadolex. It is prepared using a carbon dioxide extraction, and its content of pyrrolizidine alkaloids is lower than the limits of detection (the German government requires content to be less than 1 mg daily by dosage). In the rhinitis study, participants took one butterbur extract tablet (standardized to 8.0 mg of total petasin per tablet) four times daily. The 50-mg Petadolex tablet is standardized to contain 7.5 mg petasins and may also be used up to four times daily in adults.

Precautions
The main concern in using butterbur is finding a preparation that is free of harmful pyrrolizidine alkaloids. These compounds are capable of causing toxic reactions in humans, primarily venoocclusive liver disease.

Stinging Nettle (Urtica dioica)
Stinging nettle has enjoyed a long history of use as an antiallergy preparation, and it is also used in the therapy of prostatic hypertrophy. The "stinging" hairs and leaves of this plant contain histamine, serotonin, acetylcholine, and 5-hydroxytryptamine, compounds that typically are the cause of allergic symptoms. Some investigators attribute the antihistaminic properties of ingested nettles to an autocoid, or feedback inhibition of histamine and histamine-related compounds. Studies have revealed that nettle extract also inhibits the release of tryptase, a mast cell mediator of allergic inflammation, as well as other proinflammatory mediators, such as cyclooxygenase-1 (COX-1), COX-2, and prostaglandin D_2 synthase (PGDS).[25] More important may be the inhibitory effect of nettle on the transcription of inflammatory genes. Nettle extracts have been shown to inhibit the activity of nuclear factor-kappaB (NF-κB)—a transcription factor, or on-off switch, responsible for the expression of many inflammatory genes (e.g., IL-1, IL-2, IL-6, IL-8, tumor necrosis factor, adhesins, major histocompatibility class I, inducible nitric oxide synthase, and COX-2).[26]

Clinically, few trials have been conducted. In one randomized double-blind study, 57% of patients rated nettles effective in relieving allergic rhinitis symptoms, and 48% said that nettles equaled or surpassed previously used allergy medications in effectiveness.[27]

Dosage
The typical dosage is 300 to 350 mg of a freeze-dried extract used one to three times daily, as needed.

Precautions
Rare allergic reactions and possible gastrointestinal upset have been reported.

Pharmaceuticals
Cromolyn
Cromolyn is a prime example of a drug whose active ingredient was isolated from a botanical source with a historical record of effectiveness. Isolated from an extract of the khella plant (Ammi visnaga), cromolyn demonstrates potent mast cell–stabilizing activity in vitro. When used prophylactically, in advance of allergenic exposure, cromolyn can markedly reduce the rate and degree of mast cell degranulation and thus allergic symptoms. Cromolyn is available by prescription in a nebulized form for inhalation (Intal), as a liquid for oral use in gastrointestinal allergic conditions (Gastrocrom), and without a prescription as a nasal preparation for allergic rhinitis (NasalCrom). Nebulized cromolyn is useful in treating children with asthma and was a mainstay of asthma antiinflammatory medications before the development of inhaled corticosteroids.

Dosage
For the treatment of allergic rhinitis, the dosage is one spray of nasal spray (NasalCrom) into each nostril three to six times/day until the condition is better and then one spray in each nostril every 8 to 12 hours. This preparation can also be used prophylactically approximately 20 to 30 minutes before allergen exposure (e.g., exposure to a cat). For asthma, one ampule (20 mg) is used by nebulizer three to four times daily.

Precautions
Cromolyn is quite safe, and adverse reactions are extremely rare.

Antihistamines
Antihistamines bind to the H_1 histamine receptor and inhibit allergic reactions at the level of the target organs; that is, they do not prevent the initiation of the classic allergic response but can inhibit (or at least reduce) the effects of histamine, a key biochemical mediator of allergy. Many different chemical classes of antihistamines are available, but most clinicians prefer the first- and second-generation pharmaceutical agents.

First-generation antihistamines are safe, over-the-counter preparations that are effective in reducing allergic symptoms, but at the expense of significant central nervous system effects. First-generation compounds tend to be highly lipophilic and readily cross the blood-brain barrier, thus causing sometimes marked sedation. In addition, anticholinergic effects, such as urinary retention, may inhibit the use of these drugs in patients with prostatic hypertrophy or urinary hesitancy from other causes. Because of the longer history of use of first-generation antihistamine products, many practitioners recommend them in certain higher-risk circumstances, such as in pregnancy. Examples of first-generation compounds are diphenhydramine (Benadryl), clemastine (Tavist), and chlorpheniramine (Chlor-Trimeton).

Second-generation antihistamines typically have fewer anticholinergic and antimuscarinic side effects than first-generation agents and are equally effective. The mechanism of action is similar in first- and second-generation drugs, although more research has focused on presumptive antiinflammatory activity of the second-generation compounds. For example, desloratadine down-regulates various inflammatory mediators, including the generation and release of IL-4 and IL-13 by human basophils.[28] Examples of second-generation antihistamines include cetirizine (Zyrtec), loratadine (Claritin), and fexofenadine (Allegra).

Although many advertisements have been devoted to identifying specific and superior uses for differing brands of antihistamines (e.g., better efficacy in treating urticaria or rhinitis), much of this information represents marketing efforts because large head-to-head published comparisons of drugs for specific allergic conditions are lacking.

Finally, topical antihistamines are available as nasal sprays. Although systemic absorption is less than with oral preparations, similar adverse effects can occur. Bitter taste limits use in many patients. Examples of topical antihistamines include azelastine (Astepro) and olopatadine (Patanase).

■ Dosage
The standard dose of antihistamine varies with the particular compound. Follow the label directions.

■ Precautions
Patients should not operate heavy machinery or automobiles while they are taking even mildly sedating antihistamines. A 2000 study compared driving coordination in subjects given standard doses of a first-generation antihistamine (diphenhydramine) with that in subjects given alcohol, fexofenadine, and placebo. Remarkably, diphenhydramine had a greater impact on driving performance than alcohol.[29] In addition, urinary retention, confusion, dizziness, drowsiness, dryness of mouth, or convulsions (seizures) may be more likely to occur in older adults who take the older antihistamines.

Nasal Corticosteroids
Topical (nasal) corticosteroids are relative newcomers to the allergic rhinitis pharmacopeia. They are regarded as first-line therapy for moderate to severe rhinitis symptoms, especially nasal congestion, for which they seem to outperform antihistamines.[30] A brief period (perhaps weeks) often elapses before maximal effects are appreciated. These drugs function as topical antiinflammatory agents and reduce allergic inflammation locally in the nasal mucosa and sinus passages. Many of the newer preparations are regarded as safe because they exhibit first-pass metabolism and thereby lessen the possibility of systemic absorption and long-term adverse effects.

■ Dosage
The dosage varies with each preparation. Typically, one spray in each nostril daily is sufficient for maintenance. Occasionally this dose is doubled for short periods during peak allergy weeks.

■ Precautions
Common side effects include epistaxis (up to 10%). Concern also exists about growth rate declines in prepubescent children, but this observation was noted in very few reports. Higher rates of posterior subcapsular cataracts were also reported. Concerns about systemic absorption

of these steroid compounds and the long-term effects remain, although several studies showed only mild adrenal inhibition.

> I have observed cases of septal perforation as a result of improper spraying of these products in the nares. Advise patients to aim the "nozzle" of the canister or bottle away from the nasal septum (i.e., toward the outside of the nostril).

Immunotherapy

Allergic desensitization is an effective adjunct to drug therapy in selected patients. It is generally reserved for those individuals who show no response to other therapies or for whom life-threatening reactions can occur with unpredictable frequency (e.g., insect sting anaphylaxis). Immunotherapy in the United States usually consists of the subcutaneous administration of gradually increasing amounts of allergic material, given at regular intervals ("allergy shots"). The mechanism by which the injections diminish allergenic sensitivity is not completely clear, but their effectiveness has been demonstrated in cases of allergic rhinitis (and for some types of asthma as well). This therapy is believed by some to be a last resort because the potential for an adverse reaction is always present, and the reaction itself can be life-threatening. From 1985 to 1993 in the United States, 52.3 million administrations of immunotherapy resulted in 35 deaths. These numbers equate to a mortality incidence of less than 1 per million, which is quite low but perhaps unacceptable for patients treated for a non–life-threatening condition such as allergic rhinitis.[31] Moderate to severe systemic reactions are fairly common and warrant close patient supervision immediately after the administration of a desensitization injection.

A newer immunotherapy modality that is rapidly gaining popularity is sublingual immunotherapy. Popularized in Europe when subcutaneous immunotherapy was deemed too dangerous for regular use, sublingual immunotherapy is similar to the subcutaneous route except that the allergen extract is given as drops that the patient self-administers under the tongue (sublingually) on a daily basis. The sublingual route has been shown to be efficacious in numerous studies, and it is very safe, with few mild reactions reported and no deaths.[32] It can be used for aeroallergens as well as for foods.

Mind-Body Therapy

Numerous studies documented the value of mind-body approaches to many allergic conditions. Classic studies from the late 1960s demonstrated that many patients with moderate to severe asthma exhibit severe symptoms when they are exposed to saline mists that they believed were potent allergens. Even more remarkable was their prompt recovery with use of a saline inhaler that they believed to be a beta agonist.[33,34] Even standard skin test reactions that produce classic wheal-and-flare reactions to subcutaneously introduced allergens can be modulated by mind-body techniques. In one study, patients with dust mite sensitivity who were skin tested after viewing a humorous video demonstrated lower wheal-and-flare reactivity to dust mite allergen than did patients viewing a control video (weather documentary).[35] Finally, a randomized controlled study examined the effectiveness of the addition of self-hypnosis to a pharmacologic regimen for allergic rhinitis. Allergic symptoms in 79 patients with "hay fever" showed significant improvement over the course of two pollen seasons compared with those in control groups.[36]

Traditional Chinese Medicine

Until recently, relatively few controlled studies examined the role of acupuncture or Chinese herbs as part of a traditional Chinese medicine approach to allergies. Now, however, owing to several ground-breaking studies, this is perhaps the most exciting area for future innovation. Researchers purified and dissected several ancient Chinese herbal formulations for both asthma and food allergies and uncovered some remarkable results. An herbal preparation, tested in an animal model of asthma, was shown to be as effective an antiinflammatory agent as corticosteroids, but through a novel mechanism and with potentially fewer adverse effects.[37] A similar research initiative by the same workers led to the discovery of a Chinese formula that was completely protective in an animal model of peanut allergy.[38] The therapy also proved to be long lasting. This finding is remarkable because few, if any, therapies exist for this potentially fatal condition.

A human study demonstrated the superiority of a regimen of acupuncture plus Chinese herbs (versus placebo) in the treatment of seasonal allergic rhinitis.[39] The study assessed rhinitis symptoms with several validated scales, which showed significant improvements in quality of life and symptom control in patients who received a standard regimen of acupuncture along with a standardized herbal decoction. The therapy was found to be well tolerated and safe in this study population.

PREVENTION PRESCRIPTION

- Use environmental modification, including reduction of dust mite allergen (mattress and pillow encasements, removal of carpeting as possible, replacement of curtains with shades), removal of allergenic pets from the home (or at least the bedroom), purchase of a high-efficiency particulate air (HEPA) filter, and planning of activities to avoid exposure to early morning peak pollen counts.
- Follow an antiinflammatory diet. Avoid processed foods, partially hydrogenated oils, white sugar, and flour. Replace vegetable oils with olive or canola oil for cooking. Avoid excessive amounts of saturated fat, such as those found in red meat, fried foods, and dairy products.

THERAPEUTIC REVIEW

The following is a summary of general therapeutic options for allergies (e.g., allergic rhinitis). If a patient presents with severe respiratory or anaphylactic symptoms, stabilizing pulmonary function or allergen exposure risk with potent conventional therapies is prudent before introducing supplements or botanical preparations. For the patient with mild to moderate allergy symptoms, however, this stepladder approach is appropriate.

Remove Environmental Triggers From the Home

- With perennial allergens (e.g., dust mites), washing bedclothes weekly in hot water, encasing mattresses and pillows in mite-impermeable covers, and removing carpeting from rooms (especially bedrooms) may be helpful. Regular vacuuming of carpeted areas by someone without allergies is also suggested.

- Pet-sensitive individuals are a special case. The ideal solution, removal of the pet from the household, is typically not an option with pet lovers. In this case, removing pet access to the bedroom is helpful.

- A high-efficiency particulate air (HEPA) filter is useful for light, floating allergens, such as cat allergens; it is less effective with dog allergens.

Avoid Peak Pollen Exposure Outdoors

- Outdoor pollens are ubiquitous; avoidance is nearly impossible. Pollen-sensitive patients can avoid significant exposure by limiting outdoor activities between 5 and 10 AM and on dry, windy days, when airborne pollen levels are highest.

Nutrition

- Decrease dairy (milk protein) and total protein intake. Plant proteins may be preferable.

- Consume omega-3–rich fats found in cold-water fish, nuts, greens, and ground flaxseed. Consider the addition of pharmaceutical-grade (distilled) fish oil capsules or liquid supplements.

- Increase water intake dramatically to maintain adequate hydration.

- Increase intake of natural bioflavonoids and antioxidants by eating more organic fruits (especially berries) and vegetables.

Continued

Mind-Body Therapy

- Clinical hypnosis may markedly attenuate allergic reactivity.

- Consider a trial of homeopathy, which is particularly helpful in individuals with multiple chemical or drug sensitivities. This form of therapy is safe for adults and children.

Traditional Chinese Medicine

- Acupuncture therapy with or without Chinese herbal therapy can be used for allergic rhinitis. Most studies used artificially standardized regimens; individualized therapy may be more efficacious.

- Chinese herbal therapy and acupuncture can be helpful for asthma control.

Supplements

- Quercetin: 400 to 600 mg one to three times daily

- Magnesium glycinate: 400 mg daily

- Vitamin C: 250 mg twice daily

Botanicals

- Freeze-dried stinging nettles: 300 to 500 mg one to three times/day

- Butterbur (Petadolex): 50 to 100 mg twice daily

Pharmaceuticals

- Cromolyn sodium: nasal spray, one spray/nostril three to four times daily; nebulizer, 20 mg (one ampule) two to four times daily

- Second-generation antihistamines (oral)
  - Loratadine: 10 mg daily
  - Fexofenadine (Allegra): 180 mg daily or 60 mg twice daily
  - Cetirizine (Zyrtec): 5 to 10 mg daily

- Nasal antihistamines
  - Azelastine (Astepro), olopatadine (Patanase): one to two sprays/nostril twice daily

- Nasal corticosteroids (may be added if other natural and pharmacologic interventions fail or if nasal congestion or recurrent sinusitis is a prominent problem)

- Fluticasone nasal (Flonase): two sprays/nostril daily

- Budesonide nasal (Rhinocort): one to four sprays/nostril daily

Immunotherapy

- This is typically reserved for those patients with more severe or refractory symptoms, life-threatening allergic reactivity, or coexisting conditions (e.g., asthma, sinusitis).

- Consider sublingual immunotherapy before subcutaneous immunotherapy.

KEY WEB RESOURCES

World Allergy Organization: http://www.worldallergy.org/index.php	This international allergy organization publishes excellent position papers that are highly regarded in the field. The articles are free to all. Look at the sublingual immunotherapy reviews as well.
Allergychoices, Inc.: http://www.allergychoices.com/	This group is the oldest practice in the United States that trains physicians in sublingual immunotherapy. The Web site also contains some good explanations of the theory.
Allergy Control Products: http://www.allergycontrol.com/; and National Allergy: http://www.natlallergy.com/	These two vendors are among the oldest sources for allergy supplies for consumers. They also send health care practitioners order forms and discounts for patient use.
NeilMed Pharmaceuticals, Inc: www.neilmed.com	This company is a great source of nasal irrigation supplies and information for patients and also sends samples to health care practitioners.

References

References are available at expertconsult.com.

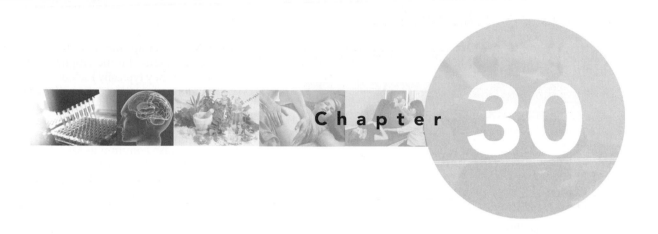

Chapter 30

Multiple Chemical Sensitivity Syndrome

Iris R. Bell, MD, PhD

Pathophysiology

Multiple chemical sensitivity (MCS),[1,2] renamed idiopathic environmental intolerance by its skeptics, is an acquired, chronic, often disabling polysymptomatic condition.[1] The core symptom of MCS consists of flares of illness from exposures to low levels of multiple different chemicals from the environment. MCS involves a two-step process of initiation, followed by elicitation. Typically, patients present with complaints of elicitation, which the clinician may or may not observe directly. Survey data indicate that although the population of patients will report similarly high current reactivity to multiple environmental chemicals and foods at the elicitation phase (the precise eliciting agents and symptom manifestations vary among individuals), the initiation process by history ranges from a single identifiable high-dose chemical exposure to a series of lower-dose exposures to no identifiable chemical initiator at all.[3] Limited data suggest that pesticide-initiated MCS may lead to somewhat more severe clinical pictures than does MCS initiated by indoor remodeling (likely more solvent-related MCS).[4]

Heterogeneous Mechanisms

The pathophysiology of MCS is not well understood. Various investigators have proposed a range of mechanisms, many of which are nonexclusive, and none of which by itself explains the entire clinical presentation. However, the clinician must be aware of the various hypotheses to advise patients on the plausibility of potential treatments they may encounter before rigorous evidence is available on benefit versus risk.

Table 30-1 summarizes the proposed mechanisms of MCS. Leading possibilities, for which some systematic evidence in animals and human subjects exists, include the following: (1) time-dependent or neural sensitization of central dopaminergic pathways[5,6]; (2) neurogenic inflammation involving trigeminal nerve effects mediated by C-fiber irritation, especially in the nasopharyngeal region, leading to sinusitis, or neurogenic vasodilation leading to migraine headache[7–9]; (3) elevated nitric oxide/peroxynitrite as an underlying molecular process contributing to sensitizing and inflammatory events[10,11]; (4) chronic systemic inflammation triggered by exogenous agents[12–14]; and (5) classical conditioning.[15–17] In a simplistic mind-body dualism, proponents and skeptics of MCS have framed the discussion for years as though biogenic and psychogenic mechanisms were mutually exclusive.[18–20]

However, the data support the likelihood that MCS is a mechanistically heterogeneous syndrome with variable degrees of biologic and psychological mechanisms in play.[21,22] To date, the data suggest that various biologic mechanisms contribute to MCS,[14] and psychological mechanisms superimpose their effects[17] and interact with biologic factors in many, but not all, cases.[23,24] For example, controlled animal studies demonstrated that repeated low-level exposures to environmental chemicals such as formaldehyde,[6] toluene,[25] or lindane[26] can sensitize psychomotor activity and, in certain situations, corticosteroid release, as well as increase or delay extinction of classically conditioned fear.[26,27] Thus, the chemical exposures themselves can facilitate classical conditioning processes and can thereby render dualistic models of MCS inaccurate and irrelevant: it is mind and body, rather than mind or body.

Individual difference factors in animals that enhance the ability to become sensitized include parental preference for abusable substances (genetics),[28] female gender (related in part to the progesterone-to-estrogen ratio),[29] hyperreactivity to novel environments,[30,31] and preference for sucrose rather than plain water.[32–35] Human self-report and laboratory studies have repeatedly shown parallel findings in persons with chemical intolerance, including familial substance abuse problems, greater prevalence of women affected, hyperreactivity of acoustic startle blink responses to novel noise stimuli during chemical exposure, and higher scores

TABLE 30-1. Proposed Mechanisms for Multiple Chemical Sensitivity

MECHANISM	STRENGTH OF SUPPORTING EVIDENCE
Time-dependent or neural sensitization	++
Neurogenic inflammation	++
Elevated nitric oxide/peroxynitrite	++
Non-IgE antibodies to food (IgM, IgG)	++
Classical conditioning	++
Misattribution of psychiatric symptoms*	?

IgE, IgG, IgM, immunoglobulins E, G, and M, respectively.
*Psychiatric symptoms are present in a substantial subset of patients with multiple chemical sensitivity, but causality pathways are not well established. Competing hypotheses include the following: (1) mood problems cause environmental chemical reactivity; (2) environmental chemical reactions cause mood problems; (3) some additional factor causes both environmental chemical reactivity and mood problems; (4) patients misattribute their mood-related symptoms to environmental chemical reactions; and (5) mood and chemical reactivity are often concomitant but unrelated.

for carbohydrate and other food cravings on validated questionnaires.[5]

Multisystem Symptoms, Inflammatory Events, and Amplified Reactivity

The key phenomena involve a capacity for nonimmunologically mediated hyperreactivity or amplified responsivity to low-level environmental stimuli from multiple classes of agents (chemicals, drugs, foods, electromagnetic factors). Manifestations include multisystemic inflammatory events and other disturbances of function in target organs, which can include most areas of the body (e.g., central nervous system, heart, airways, gastrointestinal system, and musculoskeletal system). The pattern of symptoms is idiosyncratic to the patient, not to the exogenous agent. In other words, in contrast to conventional toxicants such as heavy metals, the same triggering agent in MCS can cause very different sets of symptoms in different patients; and structurally unrelated agents can cause the same symptoms in a given patient. Thus, although genetic polymorphism data (see later) suggest impaired capacity for metabolic clearance of environmental toxicants in some patients with MCS, classical toxicologic mechanisms also fail to account for the clinical picture in MCS.

Most patients with MCS also report multiple adverse reactions to common foods such as corn, egg, wheat, yeast, milk, beef, tomato, and potato, as well as food additives (colorings, preservatives).[36] Anaphylactoid reactions are less common than are multisystemic symptoms similar to those reported in adverse reactions to environmental chemical triggers. Immunoglobulin E (IgE) antibody mediation is unlikely, based on the evidence, but IgM and IgG antibodies to certain foods in some patients (e.g., those with irritable bowel syndrome) have been demonstrated.[37]

Clinically, MCS overlaps other controversial syndromes such as fibromyalgia and chronic fatigue syndrome.[38] Case definitions vary, but they typically include symptoms of central nervous system dysfunction such as difficulty concentrating, fatigue, migraine headache, irritability, and other mood instability. Arthralgias, irritable bowel syndrome, and rhinitis, as well as sinusitis, ovarian and breast cysts, and menstrual disorders are also common in MCS.[39] Family histories of patients with MCS are notable for an increased prevalence of heart disease and hypertension, diabetes mellitus, sinusitis and rhinitis, and substance abuse, especially alcoholism (e.g., 20% versus 6%).[40,41]

Population-based studies placed the prevalence of MCS in the general population at 2.5% to 4%.[42] Other surveys indicated that 10% to 30% of the general population will self-report some nondisabling problems (e.g., breathing or headache difficulties) during exposures to low levels of environmental chemicals such as scented products.[43,44] Demographically, women report intolerance to environmental chemicals more often than do men, and women comprise 70% to 80% of patients with MCS.[45] The typical age at the time of diagnosis is in the 30s to 40s.[39] Systematic studies suggested that psychiatric comorbidities are common but not universal among patients with MCS, with rates ranging from approximately 25% to 69%, depending on subsets studied.[46] Persons with concomitant MCS, fibromyalgia, and chronic fatigue syndrome have the highest rates of comorbid depression, at 69% (versus 27% in chronic fatigue syndrome alone).[47]

Genetic Polymorphisms

Compared with patients with MCS who can identify an initiating past chemical exposure, the subset of chemically intolerant patients who cannot identify a specific higher level chemical exposure event that initiated their condition presents with higher lifetime rates of psychiatric problems, especially anxiety and depression. The subset of MCS patients ($n = 11$) whose symptoms overlap those of panic disorder exhibits panic-like symptoms during controlled challenges with carbon dioxide, which is a marker of poor indoor air quality, and has cholecystokinin-B receptor alleles, a genetic polymorphism associated with panic diagnoses in persons who do not have MCS.[48] Patients with MCS and normal controls do not differ for a gene coding for the D4 dopamine receptor associated with personality disturbances.

Furthermore, in a larger case-control study of women meeting strict reproducible case definition criteria for MCS ($N = 203$), researchers documented significant differences in genotype distributions for cytochrome P-450 isoenzyme CYP2D6 and N-acetytransferase-2 (NAT2).[49] Odds ratios for being CYP2D6 homozygous active and NAT2 rapid were significantly higher in cases than in controls. Cases also differed from controls for the odds for being heterozygous for paraoxonase 1-55 (PON1-55) and PON1-192. In addition, other studies linked heterozygosity for the PON1 polymorphisms with neurologic symptoms in 1991 Gulf War veterans with chronic illnesses, which partly overlap fibromyalgia and MCS. More recent articles questioned the consistency of the genetic findings in MCS.[14,50] Taken together, however, the genetic polymorphism and biochemical findings suggest that some patients with MCS have inherent susceptibilities to less effective detoxification mechanisms for exogenous substances and increased sensitivity to carbon dioxide triggers (panic-like pictures).

The clinical data raise the possibility of additional individual differences in genetic profiles of patients with MCS in terms of family histories of alcoholism. Although various investigators return to hypothesizing that MCS is "simply" a variant of somatization disorder in psychiatry, such a label does not expand the potential therapeutic armamentarium to help these patients. Mainstream psychiatry has few treatments to offer persons with somatization disorder other than well-structured, predictable contacts with physicians to minimize health service overuse, unnecessary diagnostic tests, and drug side effects. Early twin adoption studies suggested that the daughters of men with alcoholism develop somatoform disorder—but not necessarily alcoholism per se—at higher rates than do controls.[51] In view of the data showing that family histories of patients with MCS include a higher prevalence of alcoholism,[40] the evidence points to potential mechanistic clues that could lead to treatments adapted from the seemingly unlikely area of addiction research. Clinically, patients with MCS report poor tolerance of drugs and alcohol, but addictive-like responses to craved foods, especially those with wheat, yeast, milk, corn, and sugar constituents.[1]

Addiction and Time-Dependent Sensitization

The leading candidate mechanism for MCS from addiction research is time-dependent or neural sensitization.[5,6] This type of nonimmunologic sensitization involves progressive amplification of host behavioral and neurochemical responses to repeated exposures to the same, initially novel or threatening stimulus. Sensitization of the dopaminergic mesolimbic pathway may mediate the development of cravings for drugs of abuse, including alcohol, and sucrose (which cross-sensitizes with stimulant drugs). Both animal studies using formaldehyde, toluene, and pesticides and human research on persons with low-level chemical intolerance demonstrated that low-level environmental chemical exposures initiate mesolimbic sensitization or its psychophysiologic correlates. These correlates include sensitized responding in electroencephalographic alpha or beta frequency activity and progressive increases in blood pressure of human subjects with chemical intolerance versus normal controls.

At the physiologic limits, sensitized systems in animals exhibit a bidirectional or oscillatory capacity.[52] In other words, the response magnitude increases progressively to some biologic ceiling and then reverses direction. Overall, then, patients with MCS may have a biologic susceptibility to sensitize, a process that permits development of addictions to certain foods (in which the craving response remains below the ceiling), as well as intolerance for chemicals (and drugs) (in which the response has reversed into adverse reactions and avoidance or addiction).

Integrative Therapy

Overview

In a useful 2003 study, researchers asked more than 900 persons with self-reported MCS to rate the degree of help versus harm they had experienced in the course of trying each of 101 different treatments to recover from their condition.[53] Thus, although the formal clinical trial evidence for any therapies in MCS per se is very limited, the data from the patients themselves offer revealing information on which to base a treatment plan. Table 30-2 summarizes the top-rated most helpful and bottom-rated most harmful treatments from the patient treatment survey study of interventions tried by these patients with MCS. The reader also is encouraged to review the original article for the comprehensive list of 101 options, with numbers of patients who tried each one.

The evidence indicates that self-management strategies, not supplements or practitioner-administered treatments, are most helpful to the largest proportion of these patients. The most valuable condition-specific options involve reduction of environmental exposures and dietary management (with a rotation diet). Among the nonspecific interventions, spiritual and mind-body approaches, such as prayer and meditation,[23,54] also rank high as much more useful than harmful. Notably lower ranked are supplements and treatments provided by practitioners (acupressure could be either self- or other-administered), although many of these options were rated as more helpful than harmful. Another article proposed use of high-dose vitamin D_3 supplementation for its presumptive antiinflammatory effects,[11] but no studies of this possibility in MCS have been conducted.

Most therapies that would fall into the broad category of complementary and alternative medicine rated at least slightly more helpful than harmful. At the beginning of treatment, however, many patients with MCS do not tolerate botanical agents or nutritional supplements. They also have great difficulty traveling even short distances to appointments with practitioners because of intolerance of vehicle exhaust. As a result, lifestyle and self-management changes are the mainstays of treatment in MCS.

Overall, the coping issues that patients with MCS face include a sense of loss of control, impingement by environmental hazards at every turn, and intolerance of many exogenous substances considered nontoxic as well as toxic by the larger community. As a result, an integrative provider may provide the most help to a patient with MCS by facilitating self-empowering actions, including obtaining advice from other patients, online support groups (for patients who can tolerate being around computers, with necessary modifications such as low-emission screens and well-ventilated boxes to redirect off-gassing of volatile substances from heated plastic components), and other educational resources.[55] For example, support groups were rated as much more helpful than harmful (8.7) by the 520 individuals who had tried them in the 2003 study.[53]

> Self-care lifestyle, mind-body therapy, and constitutional treatments are more helpful and less harmful for environmentally ill patients than are other classes of treatment, such as biochemical therapies. Pharmaceutical drugs, especially antidepressants and anxiolytics, reportedly cause more harm than benefit for a large proportion of individuals.

TABLE 30-2. Patient Ratings of the Most Helpful and Most Harmful Treatments for Multiple Chemical Sensitivity (*N* = 917 Patients)

	NUMBER OF PATIENTS WHO TRIED TREATMENT	RATIO OF HELP-TO-HARM RATINGS*
Most Helpful (Tried by at Least 300 Patients)		
Chemical-free living space	820	155.2
Chemical avoidance	875	118.6
Prayer	609	48.3
Meditation	423	19.2
Acupressure	308	14.9
Air filter	786	13.7
Rotation diet	560	12.7
Lactobacillus acidophilus	661	12.7
Change of residence	513	11.7
Most Harmful (Tried by at Least 100 Patients)		
Sertraline	148	0.1
Fluoxetine	183	0.3
Amitriptyline	149	0.3
Other antidepressants	306	0.5
Diazepam	125	0.5
Alprazolam	134	0.6

*A help-to-harm ratio of more than 1 implies more helpful than harmful effects; a help-to-harm ratio of less than 1 implies more harmful than helpful effects. See the original article for more details on other therapies. (Adapted from Gibson PR, Elms AN, Ruding LA. Perceived treatment efficacy for conventional and alternative therapies reported by persons with multiple chemical sensitivity. *Environ Health Perspect.* 2003;111:1498–1504.)

Much of the research literature has concerned itself with arguing about the reality of the patients' condition and the presence or absence of psychiatric labels. The treatments that patients rated as most harmful were common antidepressant drugs and two benzodiazepines, the conventional treatments most widely used for the depression and anxiety comorbidities that researchers have identified in these patients. Overall, the evidence suggests that these patients need help with emotional disturbances, but they require alternative, nonpharmaceutical approaches to treatment. Psychotherapy to cope with MCS (6.0) rated with a higher helpful-to-harmful ratio than did psychotherapy to cure MCS (1.4).

Apart from the patient-oriented survey study, the controlled data on any of the interventions described here are minimal. In that sense, all the treatments fall into the category of therapies to consider rather than ones with sufficient evidence. Some short-term studies in children with attention deficit disorder, migraine, and epilepsy support comprehensive dietary elimination programs of offending foods,[56–59] but long-term prospective studies in which an intervention leads to clinical improvements are not available in this field. Some retrospective studies and studies documenting changes in proxy variables such as brain neuroimaging

scan patterns support the inference of exposure-dependent, reversible changes in brain function in patients with food or chemical intolerances who have neuropsychiatric symptoms.[60,61] A more recent positron emission tomography scan study found no resting baseline differences between patients with MCS and healthy controls,[62] but no newer controlled study has reported on neuroimaging findings during acute or repeated intermittent chemical exposures. Patients with MCS exhibit significantly greater temporal summation of hyperalgesic responses to intradermal capsaicin compared with controls.[8]

Lifestyle

Chemical Avoidance Programs

The essential feature of chemical avoidance programs is for patients to spend most of their time in chemically less contaminated environments, especially indoors at home and at work.[21] Many affected persons have to work at home or in alternative workspaces. Comprehensive avoidance is key, because continued ambient exposures fluctuate and maintain sensitized states.[63] This approach involves changes in heating and cooking systems (preferring all-electric homes to those with natural gas heat or gas stoves), minimization of volatile organic compounds by using low-outgassing materials such as ceramic tile rather than carpet, glass and metal furniture without glues, untreated cotton-based rather than synthetic fabrics in clothing and home furnishings, glass and stainless steel cookware and dishes rather than plastics; and nonscented products for cleaning and personal hygiene.

Items that have chemical odors are allowed to age outdoors away from living space air, to permit outgassing away from the affected person. Any clothing with residual chemical treatments is washed repeatedly and aired out before use to remove any excess residues. Undyed fabrics are preferable to dyed fabrics for clothing and home furnishings. No pesticide or herbicide use is permitted indoors or outdoors in the vicinity of the affected person. Chemical avoidance reportedly restores a limited amount of ability to tolerate environmental chemicals, but it typically requires at least a year before substantial gains are made.

Patients also often move from homes in more polluted areas to locations in less polluted outdoor air environments, where pesticide and herbicide spraying by neighbors is less common. Many of these patients also report mold sensitivity, and relocating to a home that is mold free is crucial for improvement. Many patients also find air filters helpful to reduce particulate, chemical, dust, and mold levels in indoor environments, but filters alone without significant avoidance programs are rarely effective.

■ Precautions
Social isolation, marital and family disruption, depression, and suicidality are clinical side-effect risks of avoidance programs. Financial losses also develop from overzealous attempts to change home living environments and avoid chemical exposures in a workplace. Interventions to minimize these risks are essential components of any avoidance program.

Nutrition

Rotation Diets
Comprehensive rotation diets involve eating each food no more often than once in 4 to 7 days. Such diets usually start with foods that the patient has eaten less frequently, such as turkey, rice, yams, and nuts (not peanuts). Members of the same botanical food family (e.g., tomato and potato; wheat and rye) are not combined or eaten in close time proximity, to avoid triggering craving reactions or adverse food reactions. Many patients tolerate few foods at first, and meals can consist of a large quantity of a single food by itself, without seasonings or other foods. Rotation diets can reveal "masked" food intolerances, in which the foods that are responsible for chronic symptoms are craved and eaten too often for the cause-and-effect relationship to emerge.

Temporary avoidance of an offending food for 4 to 7 days "unmasks" the process, and challenge tests of the single food typically trigger an enhanced adverse reaction on first reingestion if sensitivity persists. Frequent eating of a food reinstates the masking and chronic symptoms at a lower-grade level. Complete avoidance of an offending food and use of a full rotation diet for months to years clinically restore the ability to tolerate some of the originally offending foods. The ability to tolerate once offending foods can return as early as 3 months after complete avoidance (see Chapter 84, Food Intolerance and Elimination Diet).

If the range of tolerated foods is sufficient to allow selection of antiinflammatory diet foods, these are preferred. Such foods include various less contaminated fishes, organic vegetables, fruits, and nuts on a rotation schedule (see Chapter 86, The Antiinflammatory Diet).

■ Precautions
Undernutrition and malnutrition, including weight loss, are common. Some effort to provide macronutrient and micronutrient supplements (made without common allergens such as wheat, soy, milk, yeast, corn) is appropriate. Some products provide macronutrients in elemental food products (e.g., amino acids rather than proteins with their higher antigenic potential). Many patients do not tolerate any such supplements, however, for long periods after the initial diagnosis.

> Food elimination and rotation diets often foster nutritional deficiencies. However, most environmentally ill patients do not tolerate supplements early in their course. Phase in appropriate multivitamin, multimineral supplementation later in the overall treatment program, as hyperreactivity gradually fades.

Exercise

In view of the evidence that exercise can improve mood as a nonpharmaceutical intervention, aerobic exercise can be a valuable adjunct. For patients with MCS who have comorbid fibromyalgia or chronic fatigue syndrome, data suggest that even walking as exercise is helpful in reducing symptoms.

■ Precautions
Some patients cannot tolerate outdoor environments because of ambient air pollution from vehicle exhaust, pesticides, and herbicides. Provisions for exercising in a chemically less contaminated outdoor or indoor environment will be necessary. Some patients with panic disorder may find their symptoms triggered by stimuli that increase sympathetic discharge or lead to a buildup of carbon dioxide (see Chapter 88, Writing an Exercise Prescription).

Mind-Body Therapy

Prayer, Meditation, Yoga, Self-Hypnosis, Imagery, and Journaling
With or without a spiritual or religious aspect, setting an intention to heal, meditation, and various other mind-body interventions can help patients find a sense of meaning and purpose in their lives, as well as regain a sense of self-efficacy, despite their health problems.

■ Precautions
As with any relaxation program, some patients with anxiety disorders can experience a paradoxical worsening of anxiety during induction of a relaxed or altered state of consciousness.

Energy-Based Therapy

Healing Touch, Reiki, Faith Healing, Polarity Balancing, Craniosacral Work, Acupuncture, and Classical Homeopathy

As an adjunct to avoidance programs alone, constitutionally oriented treatments (e.g., acupuncture and classical homeopathy) have some likelihood of gently, gradually, and persistently reducing the individual's pervasive hyperreactivity to environmental chemicals, foods, and other potentially useful treatments such as supplements. However, patients with MCS are also extremely sensitive and reactive to subtle energy-based therapies. A preclinical study comparing individuals with elevated levels of self-rated chemical sensitivity showed greater variability, exposure to exposure, from repeatedly sniffing a given homeopathic remedy solution, compared with less chemically sensitive controls.[64] Referrals to practitioners with extensive experience in working with highly sensitive patients are highly preferable. Trying one therapy at a time is safer than combining multiple interventions in this class, at least until the effects of a given treatment stabilize.

Forms of these interventions in which the extent of each treatment can be adjusted and titrated are more likely to help than are treatments that are nonindividualized or heroic attempts at treatment. For example, for classical homeopathy, LM potencies whose dosing frequency, amount of dilution, and number of successions can be adjusted daily in the course of treatment are usually preferred over a single high-potency remedy dosing program.

▪ Precautions

Practitioners who are inexperienced in working with this population or who attempt overly aggressive treatments in each encounter are likely to be harmful to patients. Treatment courses are more often long term and gradual, to avoid injuring the individual.

Manual Manipulation

Patients reported that chiropractic with applied kinesiology, followed by massage and traditional chiropractic, were the more helpful versus harmful forms of manual therapies. Patients with more musculoskeletal symptoms may benefit more directly than those with other manifestations of chemical and food intolerances.

▪ Precautions

No specific precautions are necessary, other than awareness that most patients with MCS will not tolerate scented lotions or oils during massage.

Supplements

In addition to *Lactobacillus acidophilus* (12.7), patients rated other supplements as helpful, with a help-to-harm ratio of at least 5.0, as follows: magnesium supplements (8.6); intravenous magnesium (5.8); vitamin C and E supplements (5.5/5.4); mineral supplements other than calcium, magnesium, or chromium (6.4); and milk thistle seed (5.0). The emerging focus on testing multiple antioxidant therapies to reduce oxidative stress and offset chronic inflammation in many different conditions may be a useful consideration in the population with MCS as well.[14]

Practitioners must often delay introducing supplements into the treatment regimen until the patient has experienced some degree of improved tolerance of exogenous substances from constitutional intervention such as acupuncture or LM potencies of classical homeopathy or from prolonged chemical avoidance and elimination or rotation diet programs.

▪ Dosage

Doses vary widely among patients with MCS. The basic rule of thumb for dosing supplements (or drugs) in this population is to treat as though the patient were geriatric regardless of chronologic age (i.e., impaired in liver or renal clearance of, or idiosyncratically highly sensitive to, most exogenous substances). Thus, the guiding principle is start low, go slow in dosing. Doses at one fourth to one half of usual adult doses often make sense for initial trials.

▪ Precautions

Products made without excipients, colorings, flavorings or other additives, or common food allergens (no wheat, dairy, yeast, soy) are generally better tolerated. Patients tolerate supplements with food colorings and other additives less than they do simpler compounds. Use of a compounding pharmacy to individualize tolerated encapsulation materials (e.g., in clear gelatin capsules) may facilitate the patient's ability to tolerate a given substance.

Detoxification

Experts debate the validity of evidence that patients with MCS as a group all have an elevated body burden of environmental chemicals such as volatile organic compounds or heavy metals. Some proponents of detoxification recommend sauna to foster removal of stored toxicants through the skin and other organs.

Heat stress detoxification induces release of fat-stored toxicants. Sauna procedures are not standardized; temperatures, humidity, and duration of administration all vary greatly among different approaches.

One contemporary sauna-based detoxification program (the Hubbard program) involves multiple components: physical exercise; sauna; nutritional supplementation with niacin, as well as vitamins A, D, C, E, B complex, calcium, magnesium, iron, zinc, manganese, copper, potassium, and iodine; water, salt, and potassium repletion; polyunsaturated oil; calcium and magnesium supplements; and a regular balanced meal and sleep schedule (see Chapter 104, Detoxification).

▪ Precautions

Both liver function and kidney function must be monitored. Extreme heat activates sweating and increases circulation at the skin, as well as increases metabolic rate, water and electrolyte losses, and heart rate.

Pharmaceuticals

Despite some case reports of benefit from antidepressant agents and one specific anticonvulsant drug, gabapentin, controlled studies are not available in this area. The only drug with a patient-rated ratio of help-to-harm ratio of 2.0

was nystatin, taken for its presumptive antifungal properties. Fluconazole (Diflucan) rated 1.9, and ketoconazole (Nizoral) rated 1.2. As noted earlier, most psychopharmacologic drugs caused more harm than benefit from the patients' perspective.

For the subset of patients with MCS who have documented elevated levels of heavy metals, oral chelation medications may be indicated, in consultation with a clinical toxicologist knowledgeable in using these drugs.

■ Dosage

Try geriatric doses (one fourth to one half of usual adult doses) of any pharmaceutical agents to start. Doses are titrate by patient tolerance.

■ Precautions

Patients with MCS generally tolerate medications of all types poorly. The help-to-harm ratio ratings are much lower than for many other types of intervention.

PREVENTION PRESCRIPTION

- Choose home and work settings away from highly polluted locations, such as away from major highways.
- Avoid routine use of toxic pesticides and herbicides in and around the home and work environment. Seek safer, less toxic alternatives to deal with pests.
- Ventilate indoor areas undergoing remodeling and do not attempt to spend extended periods of time in the areas until remodeling has been completed and the area has been well ventilated for days to weeks (or even months).
- Avoid any indoor environment that becomes contaminated with molds; find alternate housing or workspace immediately.
- Eat organic and chemically less contaminated foods whenever possible, in a diversified diet plan (in terms of botanical food families).

- Drink environmentally uncontaminated, clean water (tested for consistent purity).
- After acute unavoidable exposure to a toxic chemical that could initiate chemical sensitization, take detoxification steps (discard clothing, wash skin thoroughly, spend extended periods in clean open air; use any facilitating agents as recommended by clinical toxicologist [e.g., vitamin C to acidify urine for some toxicants]) and seek treatment with acupuncture or similar constitutional treatment to rebalance system before the sensitized state takes hold.
- Furnish home and office with glass, metal, less treated woods, and natural fabrics such as cotton rather than synthetics.
- Wear untreated or chemically less treated clothing, especially from natural fabrics such as cotton.
- Avoid or minimize regular use of scented products in home and for personal hygiene.

THERAPEUTIC REVIEW

psychotherapy) on the basis of patient's preferences and personality type (e.g., persons high in trait absorption may prefer meditation over biofeedback).

■ Avoidance or Minimizing of Environmental Chemical Exposures

- Take a comprehensive environmental history and recommend comprehensive avoidance of likely offending substances.

■ Rotation Diet of Less Frequently Eaten Foods

- Eliminate craved foods for at least 3 months; establish a rotation diet for testing and treatment of less frequently eaten foods.

■ Exercise

- Encourage low-impact aerobic exercise, especially for people with overlapping conditions of chronic fatigue syndrome and fibromyalgia.

■ Spiritual and Mind-Body Interventions

- Recommend the specific types (e.g., prayer, meditation, support group, yoga, hypnosis, guided imagery, mindfulness meditation, supportive

■ Constitutional Energy-Based Therapy

- Acupuncture, classical homeopathy, Ayurveda, or a specific energy therapy such as healing touch or qi gong may help gradually and gently lessen susceptibility to environmental substances. Try one type of intervention at a time, and allow adequate time in terms of 6 to 12 months for benefits to emerge unless risks predominate.

■ Manual Manipulation Therapy

- Massage, osteopathy, and chiropractic may be helpful adjuncts, especially in patients with musculoskeletal manifestations of environmental intolerances. Avoid the concomitant use of scented lotions and oils.

■ Supplements

- Patients report good help-to-harm ratios from *Lactobacillus acidophilus,* magnesium, vitamins C and E (presumably mixed tocopherols, but no data exist), and milk thistle seed. Consider adding other antioxidant supplements promoting

Continued

glutathione production such as vitamin C 250 mg and *N*-acetylcysteine 200 mg once or twice a day. Use a geriatric dosing program of one fourth to one half of the usual adult dose, to start.

Detoxification

• Consider referral for oral chelation therapy for patients with a documented heavy metal body burden.

• Consider sauna detoxification referral with appropriate support of electrolytes and nutrients during procedures.

Pharmaceuticals

• Minimize the use of drugs. Patients rate most psychopharmacologic interventions (antidepressants, anxiolytics) as more harmful than helpful, but some find nystatin or fluconazole (Diflucan) for presumptive systemic *Candida*/yeast infection more helpful than harmful. Use a geriatric dosing program of one fourth to one half of the usual adult dose, to start.

KEY WEB RESOURCES

Chemical Injury Information Network: http://www.ciin.org/index.html	This organization offers patient education on potentially toxic chemicals for people with MCS and includes a library of information on chemical health issues.
Chemical Sensitivity Foundation: http://chemicalsensitivityfoundation.org/	This organization focuses on raising public awareness of MCS.
Create Healthy Homes: http://www.createhealthyhomes.com/index.php	This company offers information on testing your home for substances that could trigger sensitivity and tips on creating a healthy home.
MCS Global Recognition Campaign: http://www.mcs-global.org/	This group has helpful resources regarding high-efficiency particulate air (HEPA) filters, masks, food, and building materials for the sensitive individual.

References

References are available at expertconsult.com.

Section VI Metabolic/Endocrine Disorders

Chapter 31

Insulin Resistance and the Metabolic Syndrome

Edward (Lev) Linkner, MD, and Corene Humphreys, ND

The syndrome of insulin resistance (IR) and the metabolic syndrome were coined in the 1980s by Gerald Reaven, MD, an endocrinologist at Stanford Medical School in California. Other names used to describe the condition include syndrome X, prediabetes, dysmetabolic syndrome, and cardiometabolic syndrome.[1]

Metabolic syndrome is associated with a constellation of risk factors for atherosclerosis and type 2 diabetes mellitus (DM), including[2]:

- Elevated fasting glucose
- Elevated triglycerides
- Reduced high-density lipoprotein (HDL) cholesterol
- Hypertension
- Central obesity

When three or more of these risk factors are present, a person qualifies for metabolic syndrome. Following a joint scientific statement by several major organizations, a set of defined cutoff values were determined for all components, with the exception of waist circumference (Table 31-1).[3] According to the National Cholesterol Education Program Adult Treatment Panel III, a waist circumference of more than 40 inches (101 cm) in men and more than 35 inches (89 cm) in women is one of the defining criteria for metabolic syndrome.[4] These values apply to Western cultures only. For information on other ethnic groups, refer to the 2010 article by Lear et al[5] that outlines existing and proposed waist circumference and waist-to-hip ratios. Additional abnormalities include endothelial dysfunction, a procoagulant state, and a proinflammatory state. Table 31-2 provides a list of abnormalities associated with IR.[2,6–8]

IR is the most common clinical finding associated with metabolic syndrome and is thought by many investigators to represent the underlying cause of this condition. IR is defined as a decreased cellular sensitivity to insulin and varies by the cell type, the organ, and the particular metabolic pathway.[1] Research suggests that IR is associated with an inflammatory state and that such activation of inflammatory pathways sustains IR and ultimately leads to the development of metabolic syndrome.[9]

Prevalence

 Information on this topic can be found online at expertconsult.com

Pathophysiology

The etiology of IR and metabolic syndrome is multifactorial and encompasses genetics, nutrient deficiencies, and metabolic defects, as well as lifestyle and environmental factors. The pathophysiology includes a complex cascade of events that occurs intracellularly. Insulin is the major hormone whose action is necessary for proper tissue development, growth, and maintenance of glucose homeostasis.[12] It also affects lipid metabolism by increasing lipid synthesis in the liver and the adipocytes. IR has decreased responsiveness in the tissues to appropriate circulating levels of insulin and is the major factor in the pathogenesis of the metabolic syndrome (Fig. 31-1). Therefore, IR in muscle causes reduced glucose disposal from the bloodstream, and IR in liver causes greater glucose production. Impairment of insulin secretion by the pancreatic beta cells is a critical feature that leads to hyperglycemia when the amount of insulin secreted and the timing of the insulin response to glucose are defective.[13]

TABLE 31-1. Criteria for Clinical Diagnosis of the Metabolic Syndrome

MEASURE	CATEGORICAL CUT POINTS
Elevated waist circumference	Population- and country-specific definitions
Elevated triglycerides (drug treatment for elevated triglycerides is an alternate indicator)	150 mg/dL or higher
Reduced HDL cholesterol (drug treatment for reduced HDL cholesterol is an alternate indicator)	Less than 40 mg/dL for males and less than 50 mg/dL for females
Elevated blood pressure (drug treatment for elevated blood pressure is an alternate indicator)	Systolic 130 mm Hg or higher and/or diastolic 85 mm Hg or higher
Elevated fasting glucose (drug treatment for elevated glucose is an alternate indicator)	100 mg/dL or higher

From Alberti KG, Eckel RH, Grundy SM, et al. Harmonizing the metabolic syndrome: a joint interim statement of the International Diabetes Federation Task Force on Epidemiology and Prevention; National Heart, Lung, and Blood Institute; American Heart Association; World Heart Federation; International Atherosclerosis Society; and International Association for the Study of Obesity. *Circulation.* 2009;120:1640–1645.
HDL, high-density lipoprotein.

TABLE 31-2. Abnormalities Associated With Insulin Resistance[7,8]

Some Degree of Glucose Intolerance
- Impaired fasting glucose
- Impaired glucose tolerance

Abnormal Uric Acid Metabolism
- ↑ Plasma uric acid concentration
- ↓ Renal uric acid clearance

Dyslipidemia
- ↑ Triglycerides
- ↓ High-density lipoprotein cholesterol
- ↓ Low-density lipoprotein particle diameter
- ↑ Postprandial lipemia

Hemodynamic Changes
- ↑ Sympathetic nervous system activity
- ↑ Renal sodium retention
- ↑ Blood pressure (50% of patients with hypertension have insulin resistance)

Hemostatic Changes
- ↑ Plasminogen activator inhibitor-1
- ↑ Fibrinogen

Endothelial Dysfunction
- ↑ Mononuclear cell adhesion
- ↑ Plasma concentration of cellular adhesion molecules
- ↑ Plasma concentration of asymmetric dimethyl arginine
- ↓ Endothelial-dependent vasodilatation

Reproductive Disorders
- Polycystic ovarian syndrome
- Low testosterone in men

Data from Corona G, Monami M, Rastrelli G, et al. Testosterone and metabolic syndrome: a meta-analysis study. *J Sex Med.* 2011;8:272–283; and Reaven G. Metabolic syndrome: pathophysiology and implications for management of cardiovascular disease. *Circulation.* 2002;106:286–288.

FIGURE 31-1
Sites of the three major pathogenic defects that lead to type 2 diabetes mellitus. Insulin resistance in muscle causes reduced glucose disposal from the bloodstream, and insulin resistance in liver causes greater glucose production. Impairment of insulin secretion by the pancreatic beta cells is a critical feature that leads to hyperglycemia when the amount of insulin secreted and the timing of the insulin response to glucose are defective.

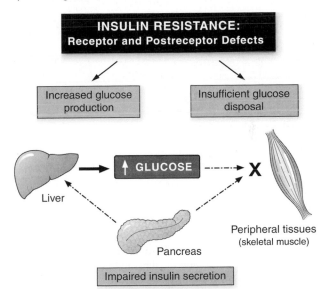

The key targets for insulin actions are predominantly skeletal muscle (75%), cardiac muscle, adipose tissue, and the liver. In the liver, insulin in healthy subjects inhibits the production and release of glucose by blocking gluconeogenesis and glycogenolysis. Defects in glucose transport or in hexokinase II pathways may be the principal impairment of muscle glycogen synthesis. In vivo studies with nuclear magnetic resonance spectroscopy showed that the defect in muscle glycogen synthesis is caused by a defect in muscle glucose itself.[14] The glucose transporter 4 (GLUT4) is the major carrier of glucose into the cell. Stimuli such as insulin and exercise promote GLUT4 activity by embedding it into the cell membrane. Peroxisome proliferator-activator receptors (PPARs) are nuclear hormone receptor transcription factors that cause target genes to be expressed and play an essential role as regulators of insulin action[13] (Fig. 31-2).

Past definitions of IR generally considered it only in terms of the negative effects on glucose metabolism. Such effects include hyperglycemia following a high-carbohydrate meal and overstimulation of the pancreatic beta cells to produce more insulin.

FIGURE 31-2

Insulin signaling pathways. AMP, adenosine monophosphate; ATP, adenosine triphosphate; CLA, conjugated linoleic acid; COX, cyclooxy-genase; GLUT, glutamine transporter; HDL, high-density lipoprotein cholesterol; IL, interleukin; LDL, low-density lipoprotein cholesterol; NFkappab, a B cell–specific transcription factor (nuclear factor kappa B); PPAR, peroxisome proliferator-activator receptor; TNF, tumor necrosis factor.

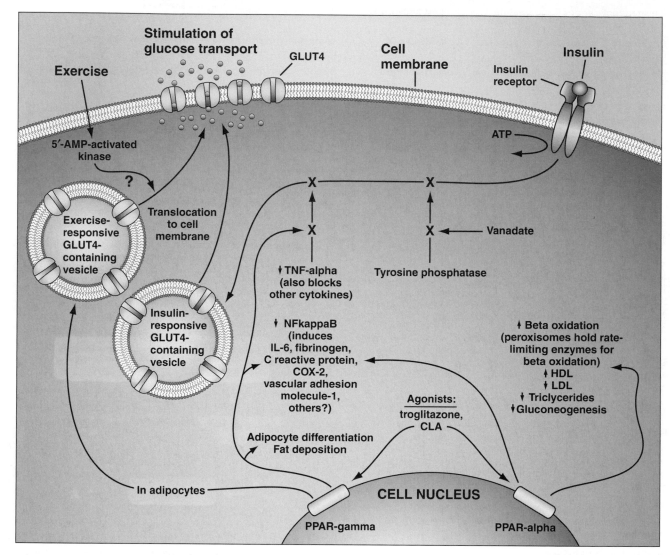

Eventually, these cells are unable to produce enough insulin to maintain normal blood glucose. This inability of the beta cells to produce sufficient insulin generates the transition from IR to type 2 DM.[15] It is crucial to understand that even though the beta cells are dysfunctional, IR still occurs at the cellular level (Fig. 31-3). As further research in the pathophysiology of IR has emerged, the traditional glucocentric view of IR has evolved to include a lipocentric concept as well. Scientists have discovered that abnormalities in fatty acid metabolism cause inappropriate buildup of fat in muscle tissue, the liver, and other organs. Lipotoxicity, with an amplified plasma free fatty acid concentration, is a hallmark of IR. Subsequently, these lipids are associated not only with an abnormal accumulation, but also with increased fat oxidation with further damage to the cell.[16,17]

A likely site of IR may involve the insulin receptor itself. This receptor belongs to the receptor tyrosine kinase family, which also includes molecules such as insulin-like growth factor I receptor (IGF-IR) and the insulin receptor–related receptor (IRR). Therefore, impairment of this

insulin-stimulated glucose uptake may also result from the up-regulation of certain proteins that inhibit these signaling pathways. Furthermore, protein-tyrosine phosphatases (PTPases) may also have a role as negative regulators of this insulin-signaling cascade. A combination of down-regulation of some receptors and up-regulation of others may be a key element in the pathophysiology of IR.[13]

A chronic, low-grade inflammatory condition also has a central pathogenetic role in IR. Research has shown that these proinflammatory cytokines and acute-phase reactants are associated with many of the features of metabolic syndrome. These inflammatory cytokines promote IR through site-specific serine phosphorylation of insulin substrate family.[16]

Therefore, IR, mostly in skeletal muscle, manifests as a reduction in insulin-stimulated glycogen synthesis resulting from decreased glucose transport. Once this occurs, lipid accumulates in many cells, most importantly the liver and pancreas, and causes oxidative damage and destructive cellular metabolism. These multiple defects in insulin signaling

FIGURE 31-3
Natural history of diabetes, depicting the rising blood glucose level with progressive beta cell dysfunction.

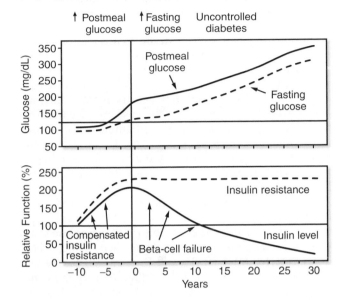

FIGURE 31-4
Summary of insulin resistance and its effects. DM, diabetes mellitus; NA+, sodium.

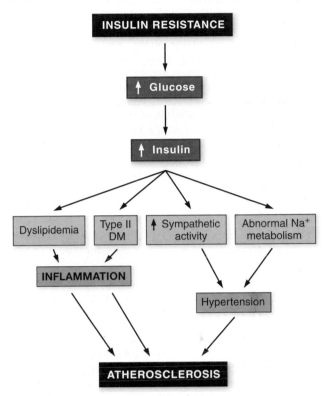

TABLE 31-3. Comorbidities of the Metabolic Syndrome

- Alzheimer disease[19]
- Atrial fibrillation[20]
- Baldness[21]
- Cancer
  - Breast cancer[22]
  - Colorectal cancer (men)[23]
  - Endometrial cancer[24]
  - Pancreatic cancer[25]
  - Thyroid cancer[26]
- Cardiovascular risk[27]
- Chronic fatigue syndrome[28]
- Chronic kidney disease[29]
- Cognitive impairment[30]
- Coronary artery disease[31]
- Depression[32]
- Erectile dysfunction[33]
- Gestational diabetes[34]
- Gout[35]
- Hypothyroid and subclinical hypothyroidism[36]
- Kidney stones[37]
- Nonalcoholic fatty liver disease[38]
- Peripheral artery disease[39]
- Psoriasis[40]
- Sleep apnea[41]

are accountable for the downstream impaired glucose metabolism in most tissues[13,18] (Table 31-3[19–41]). These pathways are summarized in Figure 31-4.

Impact of Environmental Toxins on Metabolic Syndrome and Type 2 Diabetes Mellitus

Newer research points to the role of environmental toxins as etiologic factors in the pathogenesis of IR and type 2 DM. The organic compound bisphenol A (BPA) has been found to have an association between IR and type 2 DM. BPA is used to make polycarbonate and epoxy resins and is found primarily in food and beverage containers. BPA has been used commercially since 1957, and more than 90% of U.S. residents are estimated to have detectable levels in their urine. Findings from the 2003 to 2004 National Health and Nutrition Examination Survey (NHANES) revealed an increased prevalence of liver enzyme abnormalities, DM, and cardiovascular disease with higher urinary concentrations of BPA. After adjustment for confounding variables, the investigators noted a 39% ($P < .001$) increased risk of

type 2 DM with every 1 standard deviation increase in BPA concentrations in the urine.[42]

Persistent organic pollutants (POPSs) may also play a role in the pathogenesis of metabolic syndrome and type 2 DM. Fatty foods, pesticides, and solvents are the main sources of POPs. Because they are lipophilic, these substances are highly resistant to degradation. Some of the most common POPs found in humans include dioxins, polychlorinated biphenyls, dichlorodiphenyldichloroethylene, trans-nonachlor, hexachlorobenzene, and hexachlorocyclohexanes.[43] In the 1999 to 2002 NHANES report, higher concentrations of POPs (mainly pesticides and herbicides) were associated with an increased prevalence of type 2 DM. Subjects in the highest category (more than the 90th percentile) of exposure, as compared with the lowest category (less than the 25th percentile), had a 38-fold ($P < .001$) increased prevalence of type 2 DM. Obesity was not a risk factor for type 2 DM in people with undetectable levels of POPs.[44] A year later, the same research group found a positive correlation between POPs (in particular organochlorine pesticides) and metabolic syndrome.[45] According to a *Lancet* editorial, the findings from Lee et al may imply that "virtually all of the risk of DM conferred by obesity is attributable to persistent organic pollutants, and that obesity is only a vehicle for such chemicals."[43]

Inorganic arsenic is another environmental toxin that appears to be associated with type 2 DM and metabolic syndrome. The primary sources of inorganic arsenic are contaminated drinking water, from naturally occurring arsenic in rocks and soils, and food.[46] Organic arsenic is predominately derived from the ingestion of fish and shellfish and is considered nontoxic, given that it is excreted unchanged in the urine.

Results from the 2003 to 2004 NHANES cross-sectional study revealed a positive association between increasing levels of total urinary arsenic and type 2 DM. Subjects with type 2 DM had 26% higher total arsenic levels than did subjects without DM. In the fully adjusted model comparing subjects in the 80th versus the 20th percentiles of total urine arsenic (16.5 versus 3.0 g/L), the odds ratio for DM was 3.58.[47] No association between organic arsenic and DM was found. Investigators believe that 8% of the public water systems in the United States exceed the U.S. Environmental Protection Agency's standard of 10 mcg/L for drinking water.[47] Wang et al[48] also found an increased prevalence of metabolic syndrome in subjects with elevated hair arsenic levels. After adjustment for confounding variables, subjects with hair arsenic in the 2nd tertile (0.034 mcg/g) had a statistically significant increased risk of metabolic syndrome (odds ratio, 2.54; 95% confidence interval [CI], 1.20 to 5.39; $P < .015$).

> Metabolic syndrome is primarily a phenotypic disorder (92%), as opposed to a genotypic disorder (8%).

Insulin Resistance: A Disease of the Liver or the Pancreas?

Perhaps the liver can be considered the primary factor that produces IR, and the pancreas is an innocent bystander. This hypothesis was supported in a 2007 article by Lim et al,[49] who found a positive association between body mass index and type 2 DM risk only when serum gamma-glutamyltransferase levels were elevated. Liver inflammation and liver IR caused by toxins, xenobiotics, infection, dietary elements (refined carbohydrates, fructose, and fats), and genetic factors end up flooding the body with harmful inflammatory molecules.

Under normal circumstances, insulin stimulates appropriate glucose uptake into cells, inhibits hepatic gluconeogenesis, and decreases adipose tissue lipolysis. Furthermore, insulinsignaling pathways centrally in the brain increase satiety and thus prevent extra glucose production in the liver. In the patient with IR, the liver facilitates the release of free fatty acids directly from adipose tissue, increases hepatic production of very-low-density lipoproteins, and decreases HDL cholesterol. An increase also occurs in the manufacture of free fatty acids, inflammatory cytokines, and adipokines, thus leading to mitochondrial dysfunction and eventually impaired insulin signaling, increased hepatic gluconeogenesis, and poor glucose uptake in skeletal muscle[50] (Fig. 31-5).

Chronic inflammation associated with visceral obesity produces IR in the liver itself, which is characterized by the manufacture of abnormal adipokines and cytokines, including tumor necrosis factor-alpha (TNF-alpha), interleukin-1 (IL-1), and IL-6, as well as free fatty acids, leptin, and resistin. These inflammatory molecules inhibit insulin signaling in the hepatocytes, with subsequent impaired insulin signaling at the insulin receptor and insulin receptor substrate (IRS) levels.[51] Dysfunction of IRS proteins leads to postprandial hyperglycemia, increased hepatic glucose production, and eventually dysregulated lipid synthesis.[52]

At the same time, proinflammatory mediators from adipose tissue migrate through the bloodstream to the increasingly compromised liver, thus triggering a release of adipokines

---

FIGURE 31-5

Causes and consequences of insulin resistance and pathogenesis of the metabolic syndrome. BP, blood pressure; CRP, C-reactive protein; DNL, de novo lipogenesis; FA, fatty acid; HDL, high-density lipoprotein cholesterol; PAI-1, plasminogen activator inhibitor-1; TG, triglyceride; TNF, tumor necrosis factor; VLDL, very-low-density lipoprotein cholesterol. (From Yki-Jarvinen H. Liver fat in the pathogenesis of insulin resistance and type 2 diabetes. *Dig Dis.* 2010;28:203–209.)

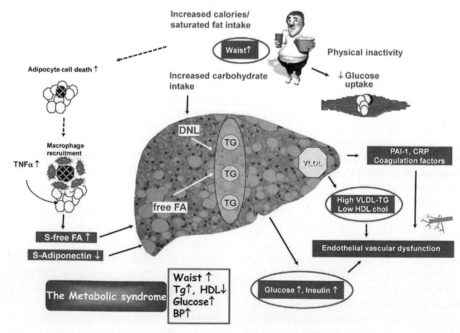

to all organs.[53] The accumulated adipose deposition in the liver causes a vicious cycle that leads to further liver resistance and the flooding of even more inflammatory mediators.[54]

 More information on this topic can be found at expertconsult.com.

Nonalcoholic Fatty Liver Disease

A fatty liver resulting from nonalcoholic causes has become the most common liver disorder seen today. Nonalcoholic fatty liver disease (NAFLD) ranges from steatosis to nonalcoholic steatohepatitis (NASH), which may progress to end-stage cirrhosis.[56]

The fat that goes to the liver is derived from free fatty acids released during lipolysis of visceral adipose tissue. Free fatty acids are the primary sources of hepatic triglycerides that cause NAFLD, whereas hepatic de novo lipogenesis and ingested dietary fat are secondary contributors. Lipid excess, in turn, overwhelms the oxidative capacity of the liver, thus generating reactive oxygen species and increased lipid peroxidation and proinflammatory cytokines.[57] The significant rise in dietary fructose is thought to be one of the major contributors to the obesity epidemic. Fructose is an extremely lipogenic sugar that affects hepatic metabolism by altering gene expression patterns (including liver PPAR-gamma) and increasing portal endotoxin concentrations through Toll-like receptors.[58] Increased fructose intake (e.g., high-fructose corn syrup) is also associated with hepatic IR and fibrosis severity in NASH. High dietary intake of saturated fat is also implicated in NAFLD.[56]

The model that DM can develop as a complication of primary liver disease, called hepatogenous diabetes (HD), makes it apparent that liver dysfunction by itself can promote IR and type 2 DM. Hepatic IR has also been shown to cause defective oxidative and nonoxidative muscle glucose metabolism. NAFLD, alcoholic cirrhosis, chronic viral hepatitis, and hemochromatosis are the most common diseases associated with hepatic IR.[59] A defective insulin response in the liver also adds to the development of clotting disorders resulting from hepatic overexpression of plasminogen activator inhibitor-1 (PAI-1). This up-regulation of PAI-1 expression has been demonstrated in various in vitro and animal liver injury models, as well as in clinical trials.[60,61]

Consolidating all these facts shows that the liver is metaphorically "on fire," spreading inflammation and harmful molecules throughout the body, including the pancreas, which can ultimately lead to beta cell failure. In working with this lipotoxic liver injury hypothesis, a holistic approach must include reducing the burden of fatty transportation to the liver as well as lowering de novo synthesis.[62]

Diagnosis

Metabolic syndrome can be diagnosed with the criteria described in Table 31-1. Outside a research laboratory, the standard of practice is to conduct a 2-hour glucose and insulin tolerance test (GITT), which can easily be ordered through any outpatient laboratory. The protocol is as follows: (1) 2 days of carbohydrate loading, (2) obtaining blood specimens for fasting glucose and insulin measurements, and (3) a 75-g glucose drink. Thereafter, blood specimens for glucose and insulin measurements are obtained (but not always necessarily) at half-hour intervals for the first hour, followed by a final specimen 2 hours later. For most patients, just the fasting and 2-hour measurements are sufficient. Essentially, this is the standard glucose tolerance test (GTT) with concomitant insulin testing. One caveat is that the clinician should make sure that the laboratory used is familiar with diagnostic procedures involving insulin, which is a very unstable hormone in vitro. If only a fasting insulin specimen is obtained, a false-negative diagnosis may be made. Without regular drawing of blood specimens for measurement of insulin, the test is no longer functional. The clinician must learn how the body's insulin serves to manage glucose once it has been ingested. With most laboratories, baseline fasting insulin should normally be less than 15 microunits/mL, and 2 hours following a 75-g glucose load it should be less than 30 microunits/mL.

Even though the most accurate and functional test is the 2-hour GITT, other possibilities for the diagnosis include the following:

- The triglyceride-to-HDL cholesterol ratio: A healthy ratio is less than 2.
- Glycosylated hemoglobin (HbA1c): Values for patients with IR are between 5.7 and 6.4 according to the 2010 American Diabetes Association guidelines.[63]
- Fasting insulin: When this is assessed in isolation, normal values should be less than 15 microunits/mL (140 pmol/L); however, a normal fasting insulin value does not rule out IR. Reference ranges are laboratory specific, so the clinician must check with the clinical laboratory for their specific values. In addition, what is "normal" and what is healthy can be vastly different.

Other markers of importance are elevated high-sensitivity C-reactive protein (hs-CRP), uric acid, small dense low-density lipoprotein cholesterol (sd LDL-C), and inflammatory markers such as IL-6 and IL-8, TNF-alpha, PAF-1, and adiponectin. In working with the hypothesis that IR is a disease of the liver, gamma-glutamyltranspeptidase (GGT) should also be considered because this transaminase enzyme is the most sensitive to detect liver toxicity.

For most clinicians, the 2-hour GITT is the most valuable test for diagnosis and patient education, particularly for normal-weight individuals who may have metabolic syndrome and for women with polycystic ovarian syndrome.

Lifestyle intervention offers the greatest promise for prevention and management of metabolic syndrome.

Integrative Therapy

Lifestyle Factors

Although the cause of IR is multifactorial, lifestyle factors are known to have a profound effect on blood glucose regulation. According to statistics reported in 2009, at least 92% of type 2 DM cases are related to lifestyle choices.[64] Lack of exercise, central adiposity, and a diet high in refined carbohydrates and saturated fats and low in fiber are some of the key lifestyle characteristics associated with IR and type 2 DM. Knowler et al,[65] researchers in the Diabetes Prevention Program, compared lifestyle modification with diet and medication in more than 3000 patients with prediabetes. These investigators assigned patients to three groups who received one of the following: (1) metformin, 850 mg twice daily; (2) a lifestyle modification program with goals of at least 7% weight loss; or (3) placebo. After 3 years of follow-up, the metformin group contained 31% fewer diabetic patients, and the lifestyle modification group contained 58% fewer subjects with DM when compared with the placebo group. Exercise, weight loss, and a healthy diet are the key lifestyle interventions to overcome IR and reducing the risk of type 2 DM.[6]

Exercise

Regular exercise is a vital component of a holistic medical treatment plan and has been shown to reduce the incidence of IR by half.[66] Patients with IR and metabolic syndrome are encouraged to partake in 30 to 60 minutes of moderate-intensity aerobic workouts (e.g., brisk walking) at least five times per week. Resistance training should also be encouraged up to twice weekly.[6] Exercise offers numerous physiologic and mental or emotional benefits. One key benefit is that exercise enhances GLUT4 transporters, which, in turn, helps facilitate glucose entry into the cell while bypassing the need for insulin.[67] This occurs in healthy individuals, as well as those with IR and type 2 DM. Preliminary research also suggests that exercise can improve the inflammatory state associated with IR by reducing proinflammatory chemokines.[68] Other benefits of regular workouts include an increase in lean muscle mass and a reduction in body fat. In addition, this form of therapy promotes a greater sense of well-being and with time becomes an endorphin-inducing experience (see Chapter 88, Writing an Exercise Prescription).

Weight Management

Excessive food consumption, particularly dietary fat and foods with a high glycemic index, is a key pathogenic factor in the pathogenesis of IR and metabolic syndrome.[2] Although most patients with IR are overweight, a small subgroup has a normal body mass index. These people are termed metabolically obese, normal-weight individuals and share the same risks for type 2 DM and cardiovascular disease because they also have increased visceral fat.[69] Increased visceral fat releases an abundance of free fatty acids and sets up a self-perpetuating cycle that increases IR. Affected patients are literally "bathed in cortisol" and can actually look like they have Cushing syndrome. As previously mentioned, this type of fat affects other organs by causing dysfunction and increasing inflammation. Adipose cells are not, as previously believed, just passive depots for energy; rather, they secrete adipokines. Adipose cells also secrete TNF-alpha, adiponectin, resistin, leptin, and other inflammatory substances. These secretions all end up promoting and exacerbating IR. Hu et al[70] found that, irrespective of exercise levels, sedentary behaviors (especially watching television) were associated with significantly elevated risks of visceral adiposity. Studies have shown that even small percentages of weight loss (6% to 10%) can significantly improve IR and reduce the risk of developing type 2 DM by 58%.[65,71]

Nutrition

For the insulin-resistant patient, the dietary focus should be one that is rich in whole grains rather than refined grains, fish and white meat instead of red meat, and plenty of fruits and vegetables along with nuts, legumes, and soy. In 2002, researchers from the Harvard School of Public Health published a set of nutritional guidelines known as the Alternative Healthy Eating Index (AHEI), with an emphasis on the foregoing foods. Results from the Whitehall II Prospective Cohort Study showed that adherence to the AHEI in a middle-aged population was associated with a reversal of metabolic syndrome after 5 years (odds ratio 1.88; 95% CI, 1.04 to 3.41). The effect was more pronounced in subjects with central obesity and elevated serum triglycerides.[72]

> The Mediterranean and low glycemic index/load diets are considered the most effective nutritional regimens for metabolic syndrome and insulin resistance.

Mediterranean Diet

Much has been written about the Mediterranean diet, which is rich in vegetables, legumes, soy products, and essential fatty acids. This type of diet is also low in refined carbohydrates and "junk foods." In a randomized trial, Esposito et al[73] compared a Mediterranean diet with a standard diet in 180 patients with metabolic syndrome. After 2 years, only 40 out of 90 subjects on the Mediterranean diet still had features of metabolic syndrome compared with 78 out of 90 participants in the standard diet group. An article by Salas-Salvadó et al[74] also demonstrated a significant reduction in the incidence of type 2 DM with adherence to a Mediterranean diet. In this trial, nondiabetic subjects 55 to 80 years old were randomly assigned to either a low-fat diet (control group), a Mediterranean diet supplemented with 1 L/week of free virgin olive oil, or a Mediterranean diet supplemented with 30 g/day of nuts. All diets were ad libitum. After 4 years, the incidence of type 2 DM was 18% in the control group, 10% in the Mediterranean plus olive oil group, and 11% in the Mediterranean plus nuts group. When pooling the Mediterranean diet groups, the investigators noted a 52% reduction in the incidence of type 2 DM when compared with the control group. Of particular interest was that the reduced incidence occurred in the absence of any significant alterations in body weight or physical activity (see Chapter 86, The Antiinflammatory [Omega-3] Diet).

Low–Glycemic Index Foods

The glycemic index is a system for classifying carbohydrate-containing foods based on the glycemic response. Carbohydrates range from simple sugars to starches and can all be converted to glucose. The rate at which this occurs is governed by the saccharide chain length, with longer chains constituting complex carbohydrates. The glycemic index value for carbohydrates can vary by more than fivefold; starchy foods have a higher glycemic index than nonstarchy foods such as fruits, vegetables, and legumes. Diets that favor high–glycemic index foods are associated with increased 24-hour glucose and insulin levels, as well as higher levels of C-peptide and glycosylated hemoglobin. These effects occur in both nondiabetic and diabetic individuals.[75]

Research has shown the a combination of exercise and a low–glycemic index diet in obese patients with prediabetes not only improves postprandial hyperinsulinemia, but also reduces pancreatic beta cell stress. Conversely, exercise in combination with a high–glycemic index diet impairs the function of beta cells and intestinal K cells despite a similar reduction in weight loss. These findings emphasize the importance of eating low–glycemic index foods that support beta cell preservation, which is a key factor in the prevention of type 2 DM[76] (see Chapter 85, The Glycemic Index/Load).

Fiber

Dietary fiber, either from whole foods or from dietary supplements, is a vital component of the treatment plan for IR and metabolic syndrome. Fiber helps reduce blood pressure and total and LDL cholesterol, and it modifies inflammatory markers. When taken with meals, soluble fibers such as psyllium have been shown to improve postprandial glycemic index and increase insulin sensitivity. Psyllium appears to work by reducing glucose absorption from the intestine and increasing GLUT4 protein expression in muscles. Regular consumption of dietary fiber also promotes weight reduction by enhancing satiety. Oats and barley are other examples of soluble fiber that have U.S. Food and Drug Administration (FDA)–approved health claims for reducing the risk of heart disease.[4]

Cooking Techniques

 Information on this topic can be found online at expertconsult.com

Therapeutic Foods

Blueberries are rich in phenolic compounds and anthocyanins and have demonstrated certain health benefits, including improved cognition and reduced cardiovascular and cancer risk. Preliminary research suggests that they may also exhibit antidiabetic effects. In a double-blind placebo-controlled randomized trial, consumption of the equivalent of 2 cups of fresh blueberries a day improved IR in nondiabetic and obese insulin-resistant individuals.[78] Consuming this quantity of blueberries has also been shown to reduce

blood pressure, oxidized LDL cholesterol, and lipid peroxidation in patients with metabolic syndrome.[79]

Apple cider vinegar (20 g diluted in 40 g of water) has been shown to reduce postprandial fluxes in glucose and insulin following a carbohydrate-rich meal. The acetic acid in vinegar acts similarly to medications such as acarbose and metformin by suppressing disaccharidase activity and increasing glucose-6-phosphate concentrations in skeletal muscle.[80] Other forms of vinegar such as white vinegar in a vinaigrette sauce can also be used to lower postprandial glucose (20 to 28 g white vinegar mixed with 8 g olive oil).[81,82]

Foods and Substances to Avoid or Consume in Moderation

Table 31-4 outlines a list of foods and substances that should be avoided, given their direct or indirect role in affecting glucose and insulin metabolism.[2,75,83–85]

Research has shown that low to moderate alcohol consumption (one to two standard drinks per day) increases insulin sensitivity and reduces insulin concentrations in nondiabetic postmenopausal women. Regular alcohol consumption in this cohort, however, also increased the steroidogenic hormones dehydroepiandrosterone sulfate (DHEA-S) and estrone sulfate, which are possible risk factors for breast cancer.[86] Alcohol appears to have a U-shaped relationship with metabolic syndrome in which nondrinkers and heavy drinkers have a similar risk profile. This curious finding may in part be explained by an increase in HDL cholesterol observed in heavy drinkers.[87] Given that the potential risks may outweigh the benefits, teetotalers should not be encouraged to start drinking to reduce their risk of developing type 2 DM.

Smoking is a known health hazard and is associated with an increased risk for type 2 DM and should therefore be avoided.[88]

Mind-Body Therapy

Stress Management

Relaxation techniques are valuable in the treatment of IR because they help stabilize adrenal gland function. Stress management lowers both cortisol levels and blood pressure, increases DHEA, improves immunity, and also reduces anxiety and depression. Patients are therefore less likely to abuse their bodies and tend to feel better about themselves.

TABLE 31-4. Foods to Avoid With Insulin Resistance and the Metabolic Syndrome

FOOD/SUBSTANCE	METABOLIC EFFECT
Refined starchy foods	Instant rice, potatoes, white breads, pasta, cereals such as Rice Krispies and corn flakes, corn chips, and canned foods have a high glycemic index and are known to impair glucose metabolism and increase insulin secretion.[75]
"Fast foods"	These foods are calorie rich, given their high sugar and fat content, and contribute to weight gain, insulin resistance, and hyperlipidemia.[2]
Sugar-sweetened beverages	Soft drinks, fruit drinks, iced tea, and energy and vitamin water drinks are often rich in fructose corn syrup and are associated with weight gain and an increased risk of insulin resistance and type 2 DM.[83] Consuming one to two drinks/day is associated with a 26% increased risk of developing type 2 DM.[84]
Artificial sweeteners	Artificial sweeteners such as aspartame, saccharin, and sucralose are associated with obesity and a twofold increased risk of type 2 DM.[85]

DM, diabetes mellitus.

A prescription with an individualized approach involving meditation, relaxation techniques, prayer, visualization, and other stress reducing modalities is indicated.[89]

Stress management and exercise are key therapeutic components.

Depression

A 2009 article by Takeuchi et al[90] suggested that metabolic syndrome may be a predictive factor for the development of depression, but not anxiety. Multivariate analysis indicated that an increase in waist circumference was the main factor influencing the relationship between metabolic syndrome and new-onset depression. Skilton et al[32] also found a positive association between depression (versus anxiety) and metabolic syndrome. In light of their research, these investigators advised screening for depression in patients with this condition.

Supplements

Numerous nutritional supplements have demonstrated a beneficial effect on glucose and insulin metabolism. In general, all adults should take a multivitamin to offset any dietary deficiencies and reduce the risk of developing chronic diseases such as cardiovascular disease. Accordingly, patients with IR and metabolic syndrome should include a multivitamin as a core component of their health regimen. Certain nutrients including antioxidants may be required in therapeutic doses to ensure a physiologic effect in the management of IR and metabolic syndrome.[91–93] Supplementation with the following nutraceuticals should be guided by the patient's overall health, dietary habits, laboratory parameters, and their current IR status.

Vitamin B$_6$

A deficiency in vitamin B$_6$ is associated with a decrease in several important enzymes that contribute to gluconeogenesis (the generation of glucose from nonsugar substrates).[94] In patients taking the drug metformin for polycystic ovarian syndrome, vitamin B$_6$ and folate counteracted the rise in homocysteine levels.[95]

■ **Dosage**
The dose is 50 to 100 mg/day.[96]

■ **Precautions**
None are noted at the recommended dose.

Folic Acid

A combination of IR and elevated plasma homocysteine levels are associated with cardiovascular risk factors. Research has shown that this patient cohort also has disturbed or reduced folate levels, which are thought to lead to the progression of hypertension.[97] Patients heterozygous or homozygous positive for the methylenetetrahydrofolate reductase single nucleotide polymorphism (MTHFR C677T) would benefit from taking L-5-methyltetrahydrofolate rather than folic acid.

■ **Dosage**
The dose is 500 mcg/day.[96]

■ **Precautions**
None are noted. High doses of folic acid administered to patients with a concomitant vitamin B$_{12}$ deficiency may correct megaloblastic anemia but increase the risk of irreversible neurologic damage.[98]

Vitamin B$_{12}$

In patients with metabolic syndrome, taking folate and vitamin B$_{12}$ decreased IR and improved endothelial function. Homocysteine levels also improved with these nutrients, thus affirming their beneficial effect on cardiovascular disease risk factors.[99] Because metformin has been shown to impair vitamin B$_{12}$ status, practitioners should assess and monitor B$_{12}$ levels if patients are taking this medication.[100]

■ **Dosage**
Recommended dose is 500 mcg/day.[101]

■ **Precautions**
None are noted at the dose recommended.

Vitamin C

Individuals with metabolic syndrome have been found to have significantly lower levels of vitamin C.[102] A deficiency of vitamin C is thought to be associated with a greater resistance to fat mass loss.[103] High doses of vitamin C have also been found to reverse the adverse effects of free fatty acids on vascular function.[104,105]

■ **Dosage**
Vitamin C 1000 to 2000 mg/day.[106]

■ **Precautions**
Take with food to reduce the risk of diarrhea.

Vitamin D

Vitamin D is an important fat-soluble vitamin that has been proven to increase the survival rate of patients with cardiovascular disease and type 2 DM. In a study of young adults, an inverse relationship among blood glucose, IR, and serum 25-hydroxy (OH) vitamin D was demonstrated.[107] Other research has confirmed that serum 25(OH) D levels positively correlate with insulin sensitivity.[108,109] Ford et al[110] also found a significant inverse relationship among abdominal obesity, elevated triglycerides, and hyperglycemia.

■ **Dosage**
Dose is 300 to 2000 units/day.[111] Dosing can also be guided by the season of the year and serum 25(OH) D levels (the preferred range is 30 to 60 ng/mL or 75 to 150 nmol/L).[112]

■ **Precautions**
Monitor serum calcium levels in patients taking thiazide diuretics and vitamin D supplements because this combination may cause hypercalcemia.[113]

Biotin

High-dose biotin is considered an important vitamin for preventing and treating IR and obesity.[114] When given in quantities 10 times greater than the physiologic range, it directly activates an enzyme that mimics the action of nitric oxide. One of the ways biotin improves glycemic control is by reducing excessive hepatic glucose output.[115]

▪ Dosage
The dose is 3 mg three times daily.[114]

▪ Precautions
None are known.

Chromium

The trace element chromium is an important nutrient that helps prevent IR and dyslipidemia associated with obesity.[116] Chromium also appears to be important for skeletal muscle IR.[115] This mineral has also been found to improve insulin sensitivity and increase glucose disposal in women with polycystic ovarian syndrome.[117]

▪ Dosage
The dose is 200 to 1000 mcg/day.[117–119]

▪ Precautions
Take half an hour before or 3 to 4 hours after thyroid or levothyroxine medication because chromium may bind to this medication and reduce absorption.[120]

Magnesium

Magnesium within the cell plays a vital role in regulating insulin action, insulin-mediated glucose uptake, and vascular tone.[121] Higher intakes of magnesium are associated with increased insulin sensitivity and a reduced risk of developing metabolic syndrome.[122,123] Conversely, low dietary intake of magnesium is associated with an increased risk of developing IR and type 2 DM.[124,125]

▪ Dosage
A dose of 100 mg/day is recommended to reduce the risk of developing type 2 DM.[126] A dose of 2500 mg/day improves insulin sensitivity.[127] Dosing can also be guided by assessing red blood cell magnesium levels.

▪ Precautions
High-dose magnesium may cause gastric irritation and diarrhea.[128]

Zinc

Although research on zinc has largely focused on type 2 DM, supplementation should be considered in patients with IR and metabolic syndrome, given the role of zinc in insulin production and metabolism. One of the mechanisms by which zinc exerts such valuable effects lies in its antioxidant capacity.[129] Two randomized controlled trials demonstrated a reduction in fasting glucose and insulin, as well as other markers of IR, in obese prepubescent children following zinc supplementation.[130,131]

▪ Dosage
The dose is 20 mg/day.[131]

▪ Precautions
None are noted at the dose recommended.

Alpha-Lipoic Acid

Alpha-lipoic acid (ALA) is a potent antioxidant that is considered important for the treatment of metabolic syndrome. The mechanisms by which ALA exerts its effects include protection against oxidative stress-induced IR, inhibition of hepatic gluconeogenesis, and increased peripheral glucose use.[132] ALA, either alone or in combination with the angiotensin receptor blocker irbesartan, has been shown to improve endothelial function and reduce IL-6 and PAF-1 in subjects with metabolic syndrome.[133]

▪ Dosage
The dose is 100 mg three times daily before each meal.[133]

▪ Precautions
None are reported.

Coenzyme Q10

Coenzyme Q10 (CoQ10) is required for adenosine triphosphate (ATP) synthesis and is therefore important for the conversion of carbohydrates to energy.[134] By enhancing the functioning of the mitochondrial enzyme glycerol-3-phosphate dehydrogenase, CoQ10 helps with glycemic control.[115] A study by Singh et al[135] demonstrated a reduction in systolic and diastolic blood pressure, fasting and 2-hour plasma insulin, and triglycerides. Markers of oxidation such as lipid peroxides, malondialdehyde, and diene conjugates were also lowered, thus indicating a decrease in oxidative stress.[135] Many patients with IR and metabolic syndrome are treated with statin drugs, and these medications have been found to lower plasma and tissue levels of CoQ10.[136]

▪ Dosage
Give 120 mg/day (or 60 mg twice daily).[135]

▪ Precautions
CoQ10 may decrease the anticoagulant effect of warfarin. Monitor clotting time regularly, particularly within the first 2 weeks of taking CoQ10.[137]

Acetyl-L-Carnitine

The amino acid carnitine plays an important role in energy metabolism, largely through its effects on fatty acid oxidation. A deficiency has been associated with various conditions, including obesity and type 2 DM.[138] When fatty acids are unable to enter the cell, triglycerides accumulate in the cytosol, an important factor in the pathogenesis of IR. Administering acetyl-L-carnitine to patients with type 2 DM and to healthy persons improves insulin-mediated glucose disposal.[139]

▪ Dosage
The dose is 1 to 2 g/day away from food.[140]

▪ Precautions
None are documented at the dose recommended.[140]

Omega-3 Fatty Acids

Long-term supplementation with omega-3 fatty acids has been shown to improve postprandial lipoprotein metabolism by decreasing triglycerides and increasing HDL-cholesterol.[2]

Dosage

The dose is 1 g/day of eicosapentaenoic acid and docosahexaenoic acid (EPA and DHA). For patients with elevated triglycerides, it is 2 to 4 g/day of EPA and DHA.[141]

Precautions

None are known at the dose recommended.

Botanicals

Ginseng (Panax ginseng)

The herb *Panax ginseng* has numerous medicinal effects, including antiinflammatory and antioxidant properties, and it has also been used in the treatment of type 2 DM. Ginseng is thought to control and prevent type 2 DM by increasing insulin sensitivity and enhancing insulin secretion.[142] Another proposed mechanism of action lies in the herb's ability to modulate glucose activity by increasing GLUT4 transporter systems.[143]

Dosage

Recommended dose is 100 to 200 mg/day (standardized to contain 4% ginsenosides).[144,145]

Precautions

Ginseng may decrease the effectiveness of warfarin.[146]

Green Tea (Camellia sinensis)

Green tea appears to have a beneficial effect on glucose tolerance and insulin sensitivity.[147] Animal studies suggested that green tea is able to reduce IR by enhancing glucose transport systems, namely GLUT4.[148] Green tea may also support body composition by stimulating thermogenesis and enhancing fat oxidation.[149]

Dosage

Green tea extract (270 mg/day of epigallocatechin gallate)[149]

Precautions

Green tea may decrease the effectiveness of warfarin.[150] Do not combine with ephedrine or other stimulants.[151]

Milk Thistle (Silybum marianum)

Milk thistle is considered an important herb in the treatment of hepatic disorders and also appears to play a beneficial role in glucose and lipid metabolism. Liver dysfunction impairs the efficiency of postprandial hepatic glucose storage and is thought to trigger hyperinsulinemia related to reduced liver clearance of insulin.[152]

Dosage

Give 420 to 600 mg/day (standardized to contain 70% to 80% silymarin).[153,154]

Precautions

Exercise caution in patients taking drugs metabolized by cytochrome P-450 isoenzymes CYP3A4 and CYP2C9 because the silibinin content of milk thistle may inhibit these hepatic isoenzymes.[155]

Pharmaceuticals

Although lifestyle modification is the preferred way of managing IR and metabolic syndrome, at times prescription drugs are necessary. The problem with such medications is that they do not correct the underlying nutrient deficiencies. Medications often merely "treat" the results of the disease; that is, they reduce high serum lipid or glucose levels or high blood pressure, but they do not treat the overall patient. Although no FDA-approved prescription drugs are available for IR, many of the medications used for type 2 DM have been researched for their use with metabolic syndrome. Some of these medications may not specifically address IR or may have unhealthy side effects (e.g., 3-hydroxy-3-methyl-glutaryl-coenzyme A [HMG-CoA] reductase inhibitors [statins] lower serum CoQ10; metformin reduces folic acid and vitamin B_{12} levels and may increase homocysteine levels). In addition, drugs do not correct diet and lifestyle issues. Pharmaceuticals can be an appropriate complementary option, when they are needed.

The most commonly used medications for type 2 DM are insulin sensitizers such as metformin, which reduce glucose output from the liver, and thiazolidinediones, which act as PPAR agonists and support glucose uptake in cells. Alpha-glucosidase inhibitors reduce the intestinal absorption of carbohydrates and thus lower postprandial hyperglycemia. Orlistat, an inhibitor of intestinal lipase that reduces the absorption of dietary fat and is usually used for treatment of obesity, has been shown to improve glucose in obese nondiabetic patients. Newer agents that therapeutically target glucagon-like polypeptide 1 (GLP-1) and gastric inhibitory polypeptide (GIP) are available. Injectable GLP-1 agonists (exenatide and liraglutide) aid glycemic control and often produce weight loss. Dipeptidyl peptidase (DPP-4) inhibitors (sitagliptin and saxagliptin) have not yet been studied in IR.[156]

Colesevelam hydrochloride, a bile acid sequestrant, is used for both hyperlipidemia and type 2 DM. A small study also showed it was helpful for impaired fasting glucose.[157] Commonly prescribed statins may worsen insulin sensitivity and can increase the risk of type 2 DM.[158]

Antihypertensive medications such as angiotensin-converting enzyme inhibitors or angiotensin receptor blockers may mildly reduce IR. The beta blocker nebivolol may actually help decrease IR by its ability to increase nitric oxide production. Most other beta blockers make IR worse. Furthermore, other medications, especially antipsychotic drugs, decrease insulin sensitivity.[156]

A quick-release formulation of bromocriptine mesylate (Cycloset) was approved by the FDA for treatment of type 2 DM. This drug is a dopamine agonist, which acts centrally to reduce resistance to insulin-mediated suppression of hepatic glucose output and tissue glucose disposal. Bromocriptine is also thought to improve glucose tolerance and IR and modulate neurotransmitter actions in the brain by reducing neuropeptide Y and norepinephrine levels.[159]

Some clinicians use one or a combination of prescription medications along with therapeutic lifestyle changes. As the patient improves, these medications can be eliminated.

Surgery

Of course the most dramatic, but at times successful, option is bariatric surgery.[156]

PREVENTION PRESCRIPTION

- Maintain a healthy body weight. People with an increase in visceral (truncal) fat are at higher risk.
- Exercise 30 minutes/day most days of the week for patients with appropriate weight and 60 minutes/ day most days of the week for those needing to lose weight.
- Manage stress and increase the relaxation (parasympathetic) response.
- Follow a low–glycemic load, Mediterranean-type diet.
- Take a high-quality multivitamin that includes minerals and B-group vitamins.

THERAPEUTIC REVIEW

Laboratory Evaluation

- 2-Hour glucose and insulin tolerance test to measure glucose and insulin levels after fasting and 2 hours after a glucose load
- Serum lipid measurements (looking for increased triglyceride level, decrease in high-density lipoprotein cholesterol level, and normal or slightly increased low-density lipoprotein cholesterol level)
- Fasting glucose higher than 100 mg/dL
- High-sensitivity C-reactive protein, a marker for inflammation, and gamma-glutamyltranspeptidase, a marker of liver toxicity

Lifestyle

- Encourage an exercise routine that consists of moderate intensity workouts and resistance training. A_1
- Encourage goals to achieve appropriate weight. A_1
- Encourage the patient to stop using nicotine-containing products. B_1

Nutrition

- Low-carbohydrate, Mediterranean-type diet with a focus on low–glycemic index foods A_1
- High-fiber diet including soluble fiber such as psyllium, oats, and barley B_1
- Decreased consumption of red meat and fried foods B_1

Mind-Body Therapy

- Encourage lifestyle choices to reduce stress and anxiety. Recommend a relaxation technique fitted for the individual. B_1
- *Note:* The preceding recommendations highly outweigh those that follow for the treatment of insulin resistance and metabolic syndrome.

Supplements

- High-quality multivitamin with minerals and B-group vitamins B_1
- Omega-3 fatty acids (eicosapentaenoic acid and docosahexaenoic acid): 1 to 4 g per day to reduce inflammation, blood pressure, and triglyceride levels B_1
- Chromium picolinate: 200 to 1000 mcg/day B_2
- Vitamin C: 1000 to 2000 mg/day B_2
- Vitamin D: 300 to 2000 units/day B_1
- Alpha-lipoic acid: 100 to 300 mg/day B_1
- Coenzyme Q10: 60 to 120 mg/day B_2
- High-risk individuals may need to consider additional supplementation as outlined in the body of the text.

Botanicals

- American ginseng: 100 to 200 mg/day B_2
- Milk thistle: 420 to 600 mg/day B_2

Pharmaceuticals

- Metformin: 500 to 2500 mg each morning or twice daily A_2
- Pioglitazone: 15 to 45 mg/day A_2

National Diabetes Information Clearinghouse (NDIC): http://diabetes.niddk.nih.gov/dm/pubs/insulinresistance	This NDIC link contains information on IR and prediabetes.
myhealthywaist.org: http://www.myhealthywaist.org	This Web site offers education and tools about the importance of reducing large waist lines.
Lipids Online: http://www.lipidsonline.org	This Web site provides educational resources on lipids and health.
Calorie calculator: http://www.mayoclinic.com/health/calorie-calculator/NU00598	This calorie-needs calculator is provided by the Mayo Clinic.
Fitday: http://www.fitday.com	This Web site provides online education, tools, and record keeping to help meet weight loss and exercise goals.

References

References are available at expertconsult.com.

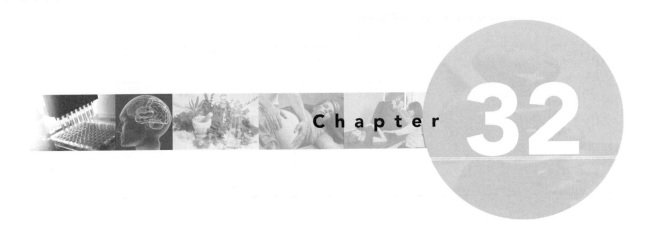

Chapter 32

Type 2 Diabetes

Richard Nahas, MD

Pathophysiology and Epidemiology

We are in the midst of a worldwide diabetes epidemic. World Health Organization estimates of the number of people with type 2 diabetes mellitus (DM) worldwide were 30 million in 1985, 171 million in 2000, and 220 million in 2009.[1] This number represents approximately 5% of the global adult population and is predicted to continue increasing for the foreseeable future. A more rapid increase appears to be occurring in the developing world and is attributed to rising obesity rates, sedentary lifestyles, aging of the population, and improved survival of people with the disease.

The prevalence of diabetes is approximately twice as high in blacks[2] and up to five times higher among indigenous populations in Australia,[3] Canada,[4] and the United States.[5] This prevalence may reflect genetic differences, more rapid changes in nutrition and lifestyle patterns, increased prevalence of vitamin D deficiency (see later), or other unknown factors.

The insulin resistance seen in type 2 DM is just one consequence of a chronic systemic inflammatory response, but type 2 DM is still diagnosed and treated based on derangements in glucose metabolism. This complex process involves multiple transporters, receptors, enzymes, and messenger molecules, which are regulated by hormones, cytokines, and neurotransmitters in multiple tissues. Providing a complete overview of glucose metabolism and the derangements seen in type 2 DM is beyond the scope of this chapter, but some key aspects are relevant to integrative treatment and are reviewed.

The process begins with carbohydrate intake, in the form of simple sugars or starches. This intake is based on feelings of hunger, satiety, cravings, and other signals from the brain, which are influenced by cholecystokinin, leptin, ghrelin, glucagon-like peptide, and other hormones. These brain signals are affected by many factors, including life stress, mood, thirst, circadian rhythms, physical activity, family eating patterns, and even social networks.[6] Overeating and other modern eating habits appear closely linked to the twin epidemics of obesity and type 2 DM, but they can be addressed only with an integrated approach to public health that considers social, economic, and educational policies.

Carbohydrates are long-chain molecules that are cleaved by pancreatic and brush border enzymes in the digestive tract, thus yielding glucose and other sugars. The amount of insulin released by beta cells in pancreatic islets is based on glucose entry into the bloodstream. Rapid sustained rises in serum glucose levels trigger greater insulin release, which has proinflammatory effects throughout the body. Changes in serum glucose and insulin levels after carbohydrate ingestion have been measured for hundreds of different foods, and these changes form the basis of the glycemic index and glycemic load (see Chapter 85, The Glycemic Index/Load).

The primary defect that is most widely associated with type 2 DM is insulin resistance. When insulin binds to the insulin receptor on the cell surface, a cascade of changes occurs to make glucose available for adenosine triphosphate (ATP) generation in mitochondria and shift the balance between glucose and free fatty acids as a fuel source for this process. The best-known action of insulin is to allow glucose entry into cells by triggering translocation of the glucose transporter 4 (GLUT4) from the cytoplasm to the cell membrane. Insulin also decreases protein breakdown and gluconeogenesis in the liver, increases fatty acid uptake and triglyceride synthesis in fat cells, regulates many cytokines and other hormones, activates numerous enzymes, and influences DNA transcription, vascular tone, and brain chemistry.

Extensive research has been undertaken to identify the causes of insulin resistance seen in type 2 DM. Several lines of evidence suggest that a more integrative approach to understanding this process is required (Fig. 32-1). As mentioned earlier, insulin resistance appears to be just one component of a complex systemic derangement in normal physiology that is referred to as chronic inflammation. C-reactive protein has emerged as a key marker of inflammation that is

297

FIGURE 32-1
Pathophysiology of type 2 diabetes mellitus and inflammatory disorders. T2DM, type 2 diabetes mellitus.

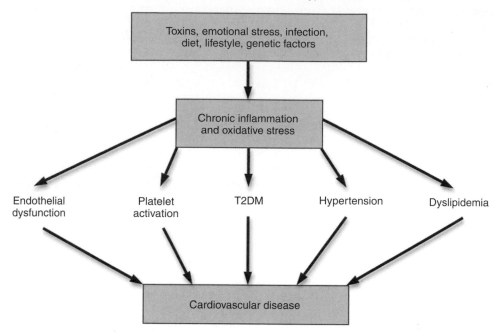

strongly correlated with type 2 DM.[7] Elevated levels of proinflammatory cytokines such as tumor necrosis factor-alpha, interleukin-1 (IL-1), IL-6, IL-8, and interferon-gamma promote a low-grade acute-phase response, including a procoagulant state, platelet activation, vascular adhesion, and other factors that result in endothelial dysfunction. Many of these important mediators are produced by adipocytes and macrophages in adipose tissue, and this may partly explain the link between obesity and type 2 DM.

> Insulin resistance is just one part of the *metabolic syndrome*. Environmental toxins, glycemic load, obesity, emotional factors, certain infections, and other sources of oxidative stress and chronic inflammation likely play a role in the epidemic of type 2 diabetes mellitus.

A key counterregulatory mediator that appears to down-regulate this cascade and protect against diabetes is adiponectin. This collagen-like molecule has pleiotropic effects in multiple tissues. It preserves beta cell function and stimulates insulin secretion in the pancreas, suppresses gluconeogenesis and enhances free fatty acid oxidation in the liver, and increases glucose uptake and fatty acid oxidation in skeletal muscle. Inflammation appears to lead to decreased transcription of this hormone in adipocytes themselves.

Insulin resistance and hyperglycemia appear to be largely responsible for the well-known microvascular complications of retinopathy, neuropathy, and nephropathy seen in type 2 DM. This is why intensive glycemic control slows the progression of microvascular complications. Unfortunately, several large trials demonstrated that intensive glycemic control does not prevent cardiovascular complications or

mortality in type 2 DM.[8] These results call this intensive treatment approach into question. The reason may be that chronic inflammation is a more important therapeutic target than are the resulting insulin resistance and dysglycemia. Most patients with type 2 DM die of these cardiovascular complications,[9] so this is a potentially paradigm-shifting distinction.

An important principle of integrative physiology is that inflammation has many potential causes. One cause is infection. Type 2 DM is well known to be associated with periodontal disease, but this condition has always been assumed to be a vascular complication of the diabetic state. In fact, the relationship is more complex, with clear evidence from the National Health and Nutrition Examination Survey (NHANES) database that periodontal disease is a risk factor for subsequent diabetes.[10] Even more intriguing is evidence that surgical and medical treatment of periodontitis raises serum adiponectin levels[11] and improves long-term glycemic control.[12] The chronic inflammation seen in viral hepatitis also increases the risk of type 2 DM.[13] The fascinating possibility of a bidirectional relationship between inflammation and infection is suggested by the reduced risk of infection seen in users of antiinflammatory statin drugs.[14] Growing evidence suggests that autoimmune diabetes (type 1 DM) may be triggered by various infectious organisms; this evidence is unrelated but worthy of mention.

Environmental pollutants can also trigger inflammation, and their role in type 2 DM is receiving increasing attention. Chronic exposure to inorganic arsenic in drinking water has been associated with type 2 DM in several countries, and in a study of 788 adults from the U.S.-based NHANES study, the prevalence of type 2 DM was 3.58 times higher among those with urine arsenic levels in the 80th percentile than in the 20th percentile.[15] The same study population also had a striking association between type 2 DM and levels of organochlorine pesticides, which was more pronounced in obese individuals.[16] This finding should come as no surprise when one considers that the complex signaling cascade triggered by insulin depends on many conformation-dependent enzymes with the potential to interact with these pollutants. Air pollution is also strongly associated with type 2 DM prevalence in U.S. cities, and the harmful cardiovascular effects of airborne particulate matter are greater in people with type 2 DM.[17] Smoking is another clear toxic source whose impact on type 2 DM risk and progression almost goes without saying. Smokers are at 44% increased risk of type 2 DM, and heavy smokers are at even greater risk.[18]

Emotional stress and inflammation are also closely linked. In the National Comorbidity Survey, childhood neglect was associated with a higher risk of type 2 DM, more so in women.[19] In a Dutch study of 2262 patients, those in the top quintile of self-reported stress were 60% more likely to have undiagnosed type 2 DM.[20] In the Copenhagen City Heart study, men with perceived stress at baseline were also more likely to develop subsequent type 2 DM (odds ratio [OR], 2.36; 95% confidence interval [CI], 1.22 to 4.59).[21] In a review of 13 prospective studies involving 6916 patients, depressed patients were 60% more likely to develop type 2 DM (95% CI, 1.37 to 1.88).[22] Emotional stress can affect insulin, cortisol, glucagon, and other hormones and several proinflammatory cytokines. The role of the renin-angiotensin system in the development and progression of type 2 DM (see the later discussion of angiotensin-converting enzyme [ACE] inhibitors) adds another potential mechanism linking emotional stress to this disease.

Although the increasing prevalence of type 2 DM clearly points to environmental and lifestyle factors, genetic factors may help identify those individuals most at risk. Earlier twin studies overestimated the genetic contribution to type 2 DM because they did not control for shared intrauterine factors. The sheer number of associations reported makes it unlikely that any one association will prove highly relevant to clinical care, but this research will certainly broaden our understanding of the complex set of factors that may contribute to this disease.

Integrative Therapy

Lifestyle Interventions

Most integrative practitioners would agree that type 2 DM treatment plans should include interventions that help patients improve their diet and get regular exercise. In the Action for HEAlth in Diabetes (AHEAD) trial, 5145 overweight adults with type 2 DM were randomized to an intensive lifestyle intervention or a minimal control intervention.[23] The objective was a 7% reduction in body weight, achieved by a diet containing less than 30% of total calories from fat (10% saturated fat), at least 15% of calories from protein, portion control supplemented with liquid meals, and 175 minutes of physical activity per week. Long-term follow-up was twice per month (one visit and one phone call), and regular group sessions were available. After 4 years, the intensive lifestyle group maintained a 6% weight loss and improved their fitness level, glycemic control (glycosylated hemoglobin

[HbA1c] 0.3%), blood pressure, and lipid parameters. Further follow-up will reveal whether this program also improved cardiovascular outcomes.

This kind of comprehensive lifestyle intervention also appears to prevent type 2 DM. The Diabetes Prevention Program assigned 3234 adults with prediabetes (impaired fasting glucose or impaired glucose tolerance) to an intensive lifestyle intervention, metformin, or minimal intervention control.[24] Weight loss was also the goal in this trial; the diet was similar, and the target for physical activity was 150 minutes per week. After 2.8 years of median follow-up, the lifestyle group was 58% less likely than the control group to have type 2 DM. A 10-year follow-up study reported that the lifestyle group was 34% less likely to have type 2 DM; it was 18% less likely in the metformin group.[25]

Exercise

Exercise undoubtedly improves many disease outcomes, and type 2 DM is no exception. The reduction in HbA1c that was reported in a meta-analysis was 0.6%.[26] The question is not whether diabetic patients should exercise, but rather how much—and how to convince people to do it (see Chapter 99, Motivational Interviewing Techniques). One of the main target tissues for insulin is skeletal muscle, so resistance training would be expected to improve glycemic control. Systematic reviews suggest that little difference exists between resistance training and aerobic exercise in terms of HbA1c and glycemic control.[27] Even tai chi helps. This was reported in a 6-month trial involving 99 patients with type 2 DM that included only patients who completed at least 80% of the twice-weekly sessions.[28] Compliance is an issue with any form of exercise, and this may explain why two other tai chi trials reported no benefit.[29,30]

How much exercise is enough? More appears to be better. A dose–response effect has been reported in perhaps the most important outcome measure of all, which is death from any cause.[31] The only real risk that must be considered by diabetic patients just beginning to exercise is hypoglycemia. Close observation is important at the start of any exercise program, and medication doses will likely need to be lowered. Patients should be advised to keep simple sugars within reach during and after exercise (see Chapter 88, Writing an Exercise Prescription).

Behavior Change

Most clinicians have a clear understanding of the importance of diet and lifestyle in the management of type 2 DM and other metabolic signs of chronic inflammation. The difficulty is not in knowing what changes need to be made; making those changes is the hard part. Overall, the evidence on behavior change and lifestyle modification is not encouraging, but this should not deter motivated practitioners or their patients.

One tool I use is to ask patients to record their blood glucose after every single meal for an initial 2- to 3-week period. This powerful educational tool shows them how carbohydrate loads and exercise habits affect glucose levels. Other practitioners have pearls they use to motivate and educate patients. Referring patients to dietitians, personal trainers, psychologists, educators, mindfulness practices, videos, books, Internet-based reminders, and other resources in your community may be appropriate.

Do not make the mistake of assuming that your patients cannot or will not change. Although change is definitely the patients' responsibility, providing thoughtful support and encouragement is ours. A stage-based approach is usually more effective, as described in the Stages of Change model developed by Prochaska et al.[32] An additional tool that is often neglected by busy clinicians is to try and be a role model for patients. Advice about exercise and proper nutrition is much more convincing when it comes from a person who is active and healthy.

Nutrition

Carbohydrates, Glycemic Index, and Glycemic Load

Lifestyle programs may achieve better results in the future as they shift their focus to low-glycemic diets. In a Cochrane Review of 11 trials involving 402 patients with type 2 DM, low–glycemic index diets reduced HbA1c by 0.5%. They also reduced the incidence of hypoglycemic events as compared with the diets mentioned earlier,[33] and they are eventually expected to be incorporated into diabetes education programs worldwide. Systematic reviews suggest that low-glycemic diets also prevent cardiovascular disease[34] and certain cancers.[35]

Low-carbohydrate diets take the principle of glycemic load reduction one step further. They were once considered an unproven fad, but growing evidence suggests that they may be superior to low-fat high-carbohydrate diets in important ways. A systematic review of 19 trials involving 336 patients with type 2 DM found that people who ate low-carbohydrate diets had better glycemic control and lipid profiles than did those who followed a low-fat approach.[36] The Mediterranean diet, which emphasizes whole grains, vegetables, plant protein, and seafood with moderate wine consumption, has also been associated with better health outcomes. This diet may be modified for patients with type 2 DM by moderately decreasing high-glycemic fruits and grains (see Chapter 86, The Antiinflammatory [Omega-3] Diet).

Sugar-sweetened beverages (SSBs) increase the risk of type 2 DM and likely worsen the disease. Whether these drinks are sweetened with sucrose, high-fructose corn syrup, or fruit juice concentrates, they subject drinkers to high glycemic loads that promote beta cell dysfunction and inflammation. In a systematic review of 11 prospective cohort studies involving 310,819 individuals, those in the highest quartile of consumption of sugar-sweetened beverages (one to two drinks per day) had a 26% increased risk of developing type 2 DM.[37] Most researchers do not consider fruit juice to be a sugar-sweetened beverage, but no evidence indicates that it is safer. Fructose may, in fact, be more harmful than glucose because it is metabolized to lipids by the liver. This process increases uric acid levels, which are associated with type 2 DM,[38] and also raises blood pressure.[39]

Specific Foods

Overall nutritional principles can affect the risk and progression of type 2 DM (Fig. 32-2), but so can certain individual foods. Research on functional foods for the treatment of type 2 DM can guide the clinician willing to provide detailed advice to patients who are motivated to make healthy food choices.

Increased protein intake has been associated with an elevated risk of type 2 DM, but this risk appears to be attributed only to animal protein.[40] Vegetable protein does not appear to confer additional risk and may, in fact, improve glycemic control, lipid parameters, and markers of inflammation. This finding has been reported in studies examining intake of chickpeas, beans, lentils and other pulses,[41] soy,[42] and walnuts[43] and other nuts.[44] A growing body of research supports the beneficial effects of vegetarian and vegan diets for patients with type 2 DM.[45] In addition to vegetable protein, whole grains are also rich in minerals and antioxidants. In a large prospective cohort study, fiber from whole grains improved glycemic control in patients with type 2 DM.[46]

Most patients are happy to hear that coffee drinking is a healthy habit. The beans contain chlorogenic acids and other phenolic compounds that reduce oxidative stress and inflammation. Coffee consumption appears to prevent diabetes,[47] and it is associated with improved lipid parameters[48] and a reduced risk of total and cardiovascular mortality in patients with established type 2 DM.[49] Caffeine appears to increase postprandial hyperglycemia,[50] so the prudent course may be to advise patients to drink coffee that is decaffeinated (using steam, not methylene chloride or other chemical processes) or to drink it between meals.

Higher serum carotenoid levels, which reflect dietary intake of carotenoid-rich fruits and vegetables, were associated with markedly lower type 2 DM risk in an Australian study.[51] Although overall fruit and vegetable intake is not a strong predictor of risk,[52] a systematic review suggested that potent benefits are derived from leafy green vegetables.[53]

Moderate alcohol consumption prevents type 2 DM.[54] Guidelines have been cautious about recommending alcohol, for fear of the risk of abuse. This possibility should be kept in mind, but the effects of alcohol on insulin sensitivity and type 2 DM risk are too good to ignore. In a large Dutch cohort of 35,625 adults followed for more than 10 years, moderate drinkers were about half as likely to develop type 2 DM as nondrinkers, even if they were already following other healthy lifestyle habits.[55] The strongest benefit was noted in persons who were not obese, whose risk was reduced by almost two thirds.[55]

People with type 2 DM should probably not eat eggs. A combined analysis of the Physicians' Health Study I and the Women's Health Study found that those who ate more than four eggs per week had a 50% increased risk of developing type 2 DM.[56] Earlier reports noted that people with type 2 DM who ate even a single egg per week had twice the risk of cardiovascular disease as compared with those who did not eat eggs.[57] The consistent trend is for greater risk of egg consumption in men than in women.

Fish intake may increase the risk of type 2 DM. This potentially paradigm-shifting association has been reported in some population studies but not in others,[58] and although omega-3 fatty acids have been implicated, the mercury and polychlorinated biphenyl toxins in modern seafood may also play a role. Providing definite recommendations about fish intake is premature, particularly considering the overall cardiovascular benefits associated with it. The hope is that the issue will be clarified by future research.

Chia (*Salvia hispanica*) is a Mesoamerican and Andean whole grain that was used as a food and medicine by the

FIGURE 32-2
University of Michigan integrative medicine healing foods pyramid. (From Regents of the University of Michigan. Developed by Monica Myklebust, MD, and Jenna Wunder, MPH, RD, 2008.)

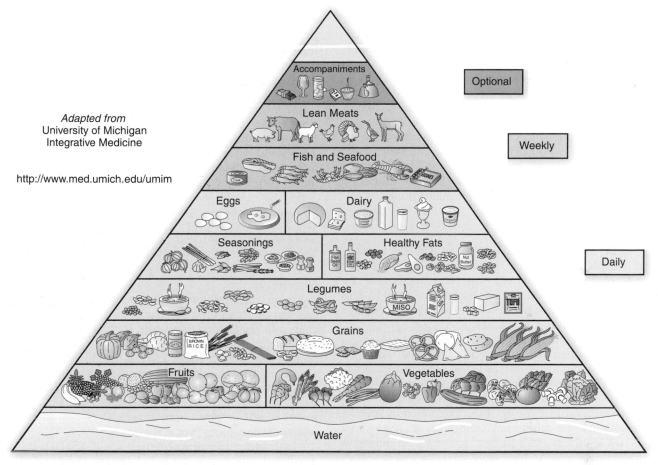

Healing Foods Pyramid

Aztecs for centuries. It has potent antioxidant effects and is the richest source of alpha-linoleic acid in nature. In a 12-week clinical trial, 20 patients with well-controlled type 2 DM who ate 37 g daily enjoyed reduced blood pressure, lower C-reactive protein, and lower HbA1c than did a control group who ate wheat bran.[59]

Onions *(Allium cepa)* and onion extracts demonstrated marked glucose-lowering effects in several animal studies. This finding was confirmed in an unblinded trial in a mixed diabetic population.[60] Although the exact mechanism is unclear, the well-known anticancer properties of onions should make them part of a healthy diabetic diet.

Foods found to be beneficial in type 2 diabetes mellitus include plant protein, whole grains, coffee, carotenoid-rich fruits and vegetables, green leafy vegetables, alcohol in moderation, chia, and onions. Foods found to be associated with increased risk include animal protein, particularly from eggs.

Management, Self-Care, and Education

Several guidelines for prevention and management of type 2 DM provide a good approach to treating these patients and should be consulted by integrative practitioners. These guidelines universally stress the importance of regular visits guided by a diabetic flow chart and the benefit of a diabetic health care team if available. A surveillance schedule should include regular HbA1c measurements, blood pressure and lipid checks, baseline electrocardiograms or exercise stress testing, urine albumin-to-creatinine ratios and serum creatinine levels, monofilament testing for neuropathy, foot inspections, funduscopy by an ophthalmologist, screening for sexual function, depression and anxiety, and immunizations as appropriate.

Self-monitoring of blood glucose is a practice that is widely taught and recommended as an important self-management practice for people with type 2 DM. This expensive habit (approximately $800 per year) is being called into question because good evidence indicates that it has minimal impact on glycemic control, medication changes, or lifestyle habits and is not cost effective by any measure. In a systematic review of 30 randomized controlled trials (RCTs), patients who regularly practice self-monitoring of blood glucose had only slightly better glycemic control (0.21% lower HbA1c), a nonsignificant difference that does not improve clinical outcomes.[61]

Diabetes education is also considered a cornerstone of chronic type 2 DM management, but the evidence of its benefit is also surprisingly scant. A Cochrane Review identified nine RCTs that compared one-on-one education with usual care (six trials) or group classes (three trials). All were low-quality studies, and the only consistent benefit was seen among patients with the worst baseline glycemic control (HbA1c higher than 8%).[62] This result may be partly related to the emphasis placed by most education programs on low-fat diets, which are now known to be inferior to other nutritional approaches. The lack of a systematic approach to knowledge translation of health care research has been an important obstacle for many integrative medicine interventions.

Mind-Body Therapy

Many different mind-body therapies are available to interested patients and clinicians. I find it more appropriate to provide patients with options that seem appropriate for their individual situation and use leading questions to help them make a final choice about which therapy to pursue (see Chapter 93, Relaxation Techniques).

Emotional trauma, current psychological stress, mood disorders, and other factors play critical roles in the development and progression of type 2 DM. The many mechanisms briefly mentioned earlier are the subject of intensive research in the burgeoning field of psychoneuroimmunology. Interventions that reduce stress, promote mindfulness, and strengthen the mind-body connection are even more important to address with patients whose health outcomes are intimately related to their daily choices about how they live their lives. Nonetheless, the evidence to support the use of specific mind-body therapies is relatively limited.

Cognitive-Behavioral Therapy

Cognitive-behavioral therapy helps patients gain insight into the habits and patterns that affect their thoughts and actions and the ways in which these thoughts and actions affect their health and their lives. A sizeable body of research has established the benefits of cognitive-behavioral therapy on glycemic control and self-care. In a systematic review of 25 trials in type 2 DM, 12 trials involving 522 patients used glycemic control as an outcome measure. In those trials, participants who received 6 to 16 group or individual counseling sessions had 0.76% reduction in HbA1c as compared with those receiving various control interventions.[63]

Biofeedback

Biofeedback training can strengthen the mind-body connection by helping patients learn to control specific bodily functions, including muscle tension, skin temperature, sweating, breathing, heart rate, and even regional brain waves. In a published study, researchers randomized 39 patients with well-controlled type 2 DM to receive 10 weekly individual sessions of skin temperature and electromyograph biofeedback or 3 group education sessions. Glycemic control

improved, and HbA1c decreased by 0.8%.[64] This finding may seem surprising, but biofeedback trials have reported changes in plasma cortisol, peripheral vasoconstriction, and other markers of sympathetic nervous system activity.

Sleep

Abnormal sleeping habits increase the risk of type 2 DM. In a systematic review of 13 prospective cohort samples involving 107,756 men and women from around the world, this outcome was seen in people whose average night's sleep was less than 6 hours (relative risk [RR], 1.28) or more than 8 hours (RR, 1.48), as well as in those people who had trouble falling asleep (RR, 1.57) or staying asleep (RR, 1.84).[65] One study found that daytime napping was also associated with an increased risk of type 2 DM.[66] Obstructive sleep apnea is a more serious sleep disorder that increases the risk of many diseases, including type 2 DM.[67] Better sleep is an important independent target for mind-body medicine interventions.

Supplements

Table 32-1 describes the glycemic effects and cardiovascular benefits of different treatments for type 2 DM.

Vitamin D

For more than 1 million years, *Homo sapiens* lived outdoors. Modern lifestyles severely restrict sun exposure, a drastic change in the human environment that has been ignored until recently. Vitamin D synthesis in the skin is triggered by exposure to ultraviolet (UV) light. This stimulus damages DNA, so it should not be surprising to learn that vitamin D activates DNA and cellular repair systems. By binding to nuclear vitamin D receptors, vitamin D actually regulates many aspects of physiology. Investigators now know that vitamin D does more than make bones.

Low serum 25-hydroxyvitamin D (25-OHD) levels are associated with a growing list of serious chronic diseases, including cardiovascular disorders, neurologic diseases, allergic and autoimmune problems, several cancers, and all-cause mortality. Whether this is a cause-and-effect relationship or whether low vitamin D is simply a marker of chronic inflammation, oxidative stress, or some other physiologic disturbance is unclear. Nonetheless, vitamin D trials have reported improvements in chronic pain, blood pressure, pregnancy outcomes, and autoimmune disease risk.

Vitamin D deficiency increases mortality risk in type 2 DM,[68] but the evidence that treating this deficiency improves outcomes in type 2 DM should be considered preliminary.[69] One small study reported that improvements in vitamin D status were associated with reductions in HbA1c in patients with type 1 DM.[70] Large single doses given to patients with type 2 DM significantly reduced blood pressure in a reported trial,[71] and another trial reported improvements in endothelial function.[72] In a study of 24 patients with type 2 DM who were given low doses of vitamin D (400 and 1200 units) for 4 months to treat deficiency, none of their glucose or metabolic parameters improved, but their 25-OHD levels were still low at the end of the study period.[73]

Guidelines for vitamin D supplementation vary widely, and at this time they should be considered in process. I advise patients to supplement in a manner that mimics sunlight exposure. Patients are told to take 10,000 to 15,000 units

TABLE 32-1. Glycemic Effects and Cardiovascular Benefits of Different Treatments for Type 2 Diabetes Mellitus

THERAPY	EFFECTS	CARDIOVASCULAR BENEFITS
Arsenic exposure avoidance	Arsenic exposure increased risk 358% in population studies	—
Emotional stress avoidance	Emotional stress increased risk 60% to 236% in population studies	CV and all-cause mortality
Egg avoidance	Egg consumption increased risk 50% in two population studies	CV disease
Coffee	Reduced risk 40% in meta-analysis	Lipids, CV mortality
Leafy green vegetables	Reduced risk 14% in meta-analysis	BP, lipids, all-cause mortality
Moderate alcohol consumption	Reduced risk 50% in meta-analysis	Lipids, CV and all-cause mortality
Avoidance of sugar-sweetened beverages	Sugar-sweetened beverages increased risk 26% in meta-analysis	—
Treatment of periodontal disease	Periodontal disease increased risk 150% to 225% in population studies	MI and stroke risk
Lifestyle intervention	HbA1c decreased 0.3% in meta-analysis	BP, lipids
Regular exercise	HbA1c decreased 0.6% in meta-analysis	BP, lipids, CV and all-cause mortality
Low-glycemic diet	HbA1c decreased 0.5% in meta-analysis	Lipids, CV disease
Beans and pulses	HbA1c decreased 0.5% in meta-analysis	BP, lipids
Chia	—	BP, C-reactive protein
Cognitive-behavioral therapy	HbA1c decreased 0.78% in meta-analysis	—
Biofeedback	HbA1c decreased 0.8% in one trial	—
Treatment of vitamin D deficiency	May decrease type 2 DM risk	Endothelial function
Chromium	HbA1c decreased 0.6% in meta-analysis	—
Alpha-lipoic acid	Decreased diabetic neuropathy	? Liver, CV disease
Omega-3 fatty acids	—	Lipids, platelets, CV disease
Magnesium	HbA1c decreased 0.3% in meta-analysis Reduces type 2 DM risk 16%	Lipids, endothelial function
L-Carnitine	? Insulin sensitivity	Lipids, lipoprotein(a)
Benfotiamine		Endothelial function
Vitamin K$_2$	? Stimulates beta cells	CV disease
Avoidance of selenium	Selenium may increase risk 55%	—
Avoidance of high-dose vitamin B$_6$, vitamin B$_{12}$, folate	These vitamins may increase nephropathy	Increased CV disease
Berberine	HbA1c decreased 0.9% in one trial	—
Cinnamon	HbA1c decreased 0.5% in one trial	—
Ginseng	Improved glucose parameters	—
Fenugreek	HbA1c decreased 1.4% in one trial	—
Ivy gourd	HbA1c decreased 0.6% in one trial	—
Momordica charantia	Improved glucose parameters in four trials	—
Prickly pear cactus stem	Improved glucose parameters in one trial	—
Pycnogenol	HbA1c decreased 0.8% in one trial	—
Metformin	HbA1c decreased 1.0%	CV and all-cause mortality
Sitagliptin	HbA1c decreased 1.25%	
Sulfonylurea	HbA1c decreased 1.0%	May increase risk
Pioglitazone	HbA1c decreased 1.25%	—
Bariatric surgery	Curative in 78% of patients	? CV and all-cause mortality
Insulin	Dose-dependent	—

BP, blood pressure; CV, cardiovascular; DM, diabetes mellitus; HbA1c, glycosylated hemoglobin; MI, myocardial infarction.

at a time, one to three times per week, until their 25-OHD levels are at the middle of the normal range. Although this range appears to vary from person to person, a reasonable maintenance dose may be 1000 to 4000 units daily. Toxicity is rare unless daily doses of more than 20,000 units are taken for several months. Large, long-term studies will certainly be forthcoming and will help clarify this very important potentially modifiable risk factor.

■ Dosage
The dose is 1000 to 4000 units daily or 10,000 to 15,000 units one to three times a week. Monitor serum 25-OHD levels to keep them between 30 and 80 ng/mL.

■ Precautions
Side effects are rare, but hypercalcemia with subsequent calcification of blood vessels with prolonged use of high doses has been observed.

Chromium
This trace element has several effects on carbohydrate and lipid metabolism. A complex containing trivalent chromium is known as glucose tolerance factor. Evidence suggests that it acts to reduce tissue lipid content and that chromium responders are more likely to be more obese, more insulin-resistant, and have poorer glycemic control regardless of baseline chromium status.[74]

A meta-analysis of 41 trials that evaluated the glycemic effects of various formulations found 14 trials involving patients with type 2DM.[75] The evidence is difficult to interpret because of low study quality and differences in formulation and dose, but the best results were reported in trials that used chromium picolinate or brewer's yeast at doses of at least 200 mcg daily. In these trials, the mean reduction in HbA1c was 0.6% compared with placebo.

■ Dosage
A dose of 200 to 1000 mcg daily is recommended.

■ Precautions
Chromium has no known side effects.

Alpha-Lipoic Acid
Also known as thioctic acid, alpha-lipoic acid (ALA) is a potent lipophilic antioxidant that is found in most eukaryotic cells. It also acts as a cofactor for several mitochondrial and cytosolic enzymes, with the R+ enantiomer being the active form. In addition to its antioxidant activity, it can also regenerate other antioxidants by reducing them; this list includes vitamins C and E, coenzyme Q10, and glutathione. ALA also chelates mercury, arsenic, iron, and other metals that act as free radicals. It is present in trace amounts in organ meats and some vegetables, but these amounts are negligible as compared with usual therapeutic doses.

ALA has been used to treat several diseases in Europe and Japan since the 1950s. A large body of preclinical research supports the potential benefit of ALA in liver disorders, cardiovascular disease, cancer prevention, and neuropsychiatric disorders and for heavy metal and general detoxification.

Good evidence indicates that ALA reduces painful diabetic neuropathy. First used parenterally, ALA in oral form was effective in a multicenter trial involving 181 patients

with type 2 DM who received varying doses for 5 weeks. All doses provided overall 50% symptom reduction, with the lowest dose (600 mg daily) causing the fewest side effects.[76] This finding may be related to reduced lipid peroxidation in neuronal cell membranes or improved endothelial function and microvascular blood flow.[77] ALA also may improve insulin sensitivity through enhanced GLUT4 translocation and glucose uptake in muscle and fat cells.[78] This last effect was seen in intravenous ALA trials and is not yet firmly established with the oral form, but it provides further support for the use of ALA in patients with type 2DM.

Most published trials have used regular ALA (an R-S racemic mixture). R-Lipoic acid is marketed as a superior product because it is the endogenously produced form, but little evidence supports this claim. A sustained-release form is also marketed as superior based on the short half-life of regular ALA, but whether peak levels or total levels are most important is unclear, and evidence of safety and efficacy is similarly lacking. At this time, regular ALA is the recommended form.

■ Dosage
The best dose for neuropathy is 600 mg daily, but a dose of 50 to 100 mg is sufficient for antioxidant purposes. Absorption is best on an empty stomach.

■ Precautions
The most common side effect is nausea, but insomnia, fatigue, diarrhea, and rashes have also been reported.

Omega-3 Fatty Acids
Fish and other marine species are the main sources of eicosapentaenoic acid (EPA) and docosahexanoic acid (DHA) in the human diet. Alpha-linoleic acid is an omega-3 precursor found in walnuts, flax, and other grains. Although they do not affect glycemic control, these fats have antiinflammatory, antithrombotic, and antiarrhythmic effects that appear to prevent and treat cardiovascular disease. For this reason, they offer important benefits to patients with type 2 DM.

A Cochrane Systematic Review of 23 trials involving 1075 patients who used omega-3 fatty acids at an average dose of 3.5 g daily reported improved lipid parameters and platelet function.[79] Small trials have also reported improvements in endothelial function; in one study, impaired flow-mediated dilatation improved significantly after subjects consumed 2 g of omega-3 fatty acids.[80]

■ Dosage
Most cardiovascular benefits of omega-3 fats occur at doses of 1000 mg (EPA and DHA) daily, but higher doses are often used.

■ Precautions
Fishy repeats and mild gastrointestinal upset are the only side effects. Although bleeding in aspirin or warfarin users is often cited as a reason for caution, the literature contains no reports of this effect.

Magnesium
Magnesium affects insulin secretion and action, and it also influences lipid parameters and endothelial function. A systematic review identified 9 trials that evaluated magnesium

supplementation for 4 to 16 weeks in 370 patients with type 2 DM and noted improvements in fasting glucose and high-density lipoprotein cholesterol. In the five trials of sufficient duration to evaluate HbA1c, a nonsignificant reduction of 0.31% (95% CI, −0.81 to 0.19) was reported.[81] A separate review of magnesium for the prevention of type 2 DM found seven cohort studies and reported an overall benefit; an average daily dose of 100 mg decreased risk by approximately 16%.[82] How accurately routine tests reflect total body stores is unclear.

■ Dosage
Usual starting doses are approximately 100 mg daily and can be increased as desired or to bowel tolerance. Magnesium is available as oral liquid or tablets, transdermal lotion, or Epsom salts, as well as in parenteral formulations.

■ Precautions
Gastrointestinal intolerance, mainly diarrhea, is the most common side effect. Chelated magnesium (magnesium glycinate) causes less diarrhea than do other forms of magnesium.

Antioxidants
People who eat diets that are rich in antioxidants have a greatly reduced type 2 DM risk, but commonly used antioxidant supplements do not appear to have the same preventive effect. In 8171 women who were followed for 9.2 years in the Women's Antioxidant Cardiovascular Study, only mild benefit was suggested by a nonsignificant trend with vitamin C, whereas vitamin E increased risk and beta-carotene offered no benefit.[83] The Prevention of Progression of Arterial Disease and Diabetes (POPADAD) trial found no significant benefit in 1276 Scottish adults who took a low-dose mixed antioxidant supplement or placebo for 8 years.[84]

The benefits of antioxidant-rich foods are probably more attributable to the dozens of phytomedicines they contain that we are only beginning to understand. Although antioxidants and multivitamins are commonly prescribed by integrative practitioners as "insurance against deficiency," this practice may not be safe. High doses of vitamins have been shown to interfere with absorption and use of lesser-known but potentially more powerful antioxidants in food; high-profile examples include tocopherols and carotenoids.

Whole food supplements may be a reasonable alternative approach. In one study, an antioxidant supplement derived from pomegranate, green tea, and ascorbic acid improved lipid parameters and markers of oxidative stress in a placebo-controlled trial involving 114 patients with type 2 DM in Turkey.[85]

Vitamin E
Vitamin E is one of the most commonly used specific antioxidants, but no real evidence indicates that it helps patients with type 2 DM. Negative results reported in large cardiovascular and cancer trials have been the subject of media reports, controversy, and debate among integrative medicine practitioners. Alpha-tocopherol supplementation did not decrease the risk of type 2 DM in the large Alpha-Tocopherol Beta-Carotene (ATBC) cancer trial.[86] One small trial actually reported prooxidant effects shortly after ingestion of a single 1200-unit dose.[87]

Although several tocopherols and tocotrienols have vitamin E–like activity, most vitamin E supplements only contain alpha-tocopherol. Some investigators believe that negative results in vitamin E trials can be explained by the decreased absorption of the other, more potent molecules in this family whose absorption is inhibited by alpha-tocopherol supplementation.[88] In fact, one study comparing the effects of alpha- and gamma-tocopherol on markers of oxidative stress and inflammation in patients with type 2 DM found no differences between the two.[89] Single trials reported that gamma-tocopherol increased blood pressure[90] and did not change platelet function.[91]

Greater benefit from alpha-tocopherol has been demonstrated in people who are homozygous for a haptoglobin gene variant that is present in 3% to 4% of the population and increases oxidative stress. In an Israeli double-blind study involving 1434 people with type 2 DM who were homozygous for haptoglobin-2, alpha-tocopherol actually reduced the risk of a combined cardiovascular end point by more than 50%.[92] This is an example of how genetics may improve treatment outcomes in future personalized medicine.

Vitamin E supplements containing mixed tocopherols and trienols are increasingly available, but we cannot provide clear dosing guidelines for their use for type 2 DM. Vitamin E has no known side effects.

L-Carnitine
L-Carnitine shuttles fatty acids into mitochondria. It has been proposed as a potential therapy for type 2 DM based on the known intracellular lipid accumulation that occurs in the disease. A pilot study found no improvements in glycemic control after 4 weeks of L-carnitine use in 12 patients with type 2 DM,[93] but several trials reported that it improved lipid parameters and significantly reduced lipoprotein (a), an important independent inherited cardiac risk factor for which few effective therapies exist.[94]

■ Dosage
The usual dose is 500 to 1000 mg three times daily.

Benfotiamine
Postprandial endothelial dysfunction has been proposed as the link between metabolic syndrome and atherosclerosis. This state is linked to oxidative stress, hyperglycemia, hypertriglyceridemia, and altered nitric oxide function. It is attributed to glucose-protein complexes in food, named advanced glycation end products (AGEs). These complexes are formed at high temperatures and activate AGE-specific receptors, which activate monocytes and endothelial cells and ultimately promote inflammation. Benfotiamine is a synthetic analogue of thiamine that is much more bioavailable. It activates transketolase, an enzyme that helps clear AGEs, thus improving postprandial endothelial function.

In a pilot study, 350 mg of benfotiamine after meals completely eliminated the vascular measures of postprandial endothelial dysfunction in 13 patients with type 2 DM.[95] This important finding has not been replicated since it was reported in 2006, but corroborating evidence seems like a high priority. Several trials suggested that benfotiamine improves diabetic neuropathy,[96,97] a finding that is not surprising considering the neurologic symptoms seen in thiamine deficiency. One trial found no improvement in some markers of diabetic nephropathy,[98] but another reported improvements in microalbuminuria.[99]

Dosage
The 350-mg dose used in the pilot study is higher than that found in most formulations.

Precautions
This early evidence is very promising, but it is probably premature to recommend widespread use of this synthetic thiamine analogue because long-term safety results are not available.

Vitamin K
This fat-soluble vitamin exists as phylloquinone (K_1) in plants and menaquinone (K_2) in animals and in a fermented soybean product named natto. Vitamin K_2 is considered more biologically active and is a cofactor for carboxylation of proteins. It helps make osteocalcin, which strengthens bones by forming a protein scaffold on which it is laid. It also makes matrix Gla protein, which prevents vascular calcification by repairing smooth muscle and endothelium. Vitamin K_2 is receiving growing attention as a target for treatment of diverse disorders in addition to its established role in coagulation factors biosynthesis.

Early studies suggest that vitamin K_2 also stimulates beta cell proliferation and enhances insulin sensitivity. Vitamin K deficiency, as suggested by low levels of carboxylated osteocalcin, is also associated with type 2 DM risk.[100] Recommending vitamin K_2 for glycemic control is premature, but its endothelial and cardiovascular benefits may make it an appealing addition to an integrative type 2 treatment plan.

Dosage
The starting dose of vitamin K_2 is usually 100 mcg daily, but higher doses have been commonly used.

Precautions
Patients taking warfarin will need close monitoring and dose adjustment after starting vitamin K_2, but this ultimately reduces the fluctuations in international normalized ratio results seen in vitamin K_2–deficient patients.[101] Vitamin K has no other known side effects.

Risks of Specific Supplements
Although evidence indicates that selenium has insulin-like actions and may delay microvascular complications, integrative practitioners should know that selenium is associated with increased risk of type 2 DM. In the Nutritional Prevention of Cancer trial, 1202 people with localized melanoma were randomized to receive selenium or placebo for cancer prevention. After 7.7 years of follow-up, selenium users developed type 2 DM more often (hazard risk, 1.55; 95% CI, 1.03 to 2.33), with the greatest risk in people with the highest baseline selenium levels (hazard risk, 2.70; 95% CI, 1.30 to 5.61).[102] Selenium supplementation should be considered only in patients with low baseline selenium levels. The maximum daily dose is 200 mcg. The way in which inorganic and organic forms differ in their effect on type 2 DM risk is unclear.

Practitioners should also exercise caution when using B vitamins in patients with nephropathy. In the Canadian Diabetic Intervention with Vitamins to Improve Nephropathy (DIVINe) trial, 238 patients with type 1 DM and type 2 DM were given a tablet containing folic acid 2.5 mg, vitamin B_6 25 mg, and vitamin B_{12} 1 mg daily or placebo for almost 3 years to treat elevated homocysteine. Although the treatment group had lower plasma homocysteine levels, they had worse kidney function and more cardiovascular events.[103] The investigators postulated that this finding may be explained by cell proliferation induced by folic acid, increased methylation from folic acid and vitamin B_{12}, or nitric oxide–related mechanisms. Earlier reports noted poorer cardiovascular outcomes associated with B vitamins, and one hopes that further study will clarify this issue.

Botanicals

Berberine (Berberis vulgaris)
The barberry plant has been used medicinally for centuries to treat dozens of symptoms, most commonly gastrointestinal and biliary disorders. It contains many physiologically active alkaloids, but the one that has received the most attention is berberine.[104] This compound has antimicrobial, anticonvulsant, and antihypertensive properties. A hypoglycemic effect was first incidentally noted in China in the 1980s, when diabetic patients were given berberine to treat diarrhea, and studies suggest that it may regulate insulin receptor transcription.[105] In a placebo-controlled trial in 116 patients with type 2 DM who were given 1 g of berberine or placebo daily for 3 months, HbA1c decreased from 7.5% to 6.6%.[106] An earlier small trial reported similar impressive benefits.[107] More research on berberine in type 2 DM will undoubtedly be forthcoming.

Dosage
Root or berry extracts at doses of 200 to 500 mg three times daily are commonly used.

Precautions
Berberine can cause uterine contractions, so it should be avoided in pregnancy, but otherwise few side effects have been reported.

Cinnamon
Cinnamon is a culinary spice made from the bark of *Cinnamonum* sp. trees. The aqueous extract appears to improve insulin receptor function by multiple mechanisms, and it also increases glycogen synthase activity.

In a published review, we found three trials evaluating cinnamon in patients with type 2 DM.[108] One was a short-term study that reported changes in fasting glucose,[109] and the two studies that measured HbA1c found no improvement but were of low quality.[110,111] Since then, another trial compared *Cinnamonum aromaticum* (cassia cinnamon) 500 mg twice daily with usual care in 109 patients with type 2 DM for 90 days. The reported average reduction in HbA1c was 0.83% in the cinnamon group and 0.37% in those receiving usual care, a difference that reached statistical significance.[112]

As mentioned earlier, the aqueous extract appears to contain the most active ingredients. Patients may wish to take cinnamon as a hot water infusion. Cinnulin PF is a standardized extract that is widely promoted, but no evidence indicates that it is superior.

Dosage
The optimal dose is unclear, but 1-g doses are commonly prescribed (1 teaspoon of cinnamon = 4.75 g). Most over-the-counter cinnamon is a combination of cassia cinnamon and Ceylon cinnamon.

Precautions
Stomatitis and perioral dermatitis have been reported in some patients.

Ginseng
Several plant species are known as ginseng, including *Panax ginseng, Panax japonicus, Eleutherococcus senticosus,* and *Panax quinquefolius.* They are named after panacea, the Greek goddess of healing, based on their long use as a cure-all for boosting immune function, energy, stamina, and well-being. Ginseng species contain triterpenoid glycosides named ginsenosides that regulate hepatic glucose uptake, glycogen synthesis, and insulin release. Several animal and human trials have demonstrated acute hypoglycemic effects, with no clear difference among tree species. A few small trials have reported improved measures of postprandial insulin and glucose release, but no HbA1c reductions have been reported.[113]

Dosage
Panax ginseng can be used at doses of 1 to 2 g of crude root or powder or 100 to 400 mg of extract standardized to 4% ginsenosides. It can also be used as a hydroalcoholic tincture, hot infusion, or cold decoction.[114]

Precautions
The most common side effect is insomnia, so do not take close to bedtime.

Fenugreek (Trigonella foenum graecum)
Fenugreek is a legume used extensively in India, North Africa, and the Mediterranean. The defatted seeds have been used to treat diabetes for centuries in Ayurvedic and other healing systems. One ingredient, 4-hydroxyisoleucine, increases pancreatic insulin secretion and inhibits glucosidase, and research has demonstrated effects on satiety, gastric emptying, and insulin receptor function. Fenugreek may also have lipid-lowering effects.

In our published review, we identified three small low-quality trials that reported improvements in plasma glucose with fenugreek in patients with type 2 DM.[108] Since then, promising results from a Chinese trial have been reported. Researchers evaluated a fenugreek extract in 69 patients with type 2 DM who had baseline HbA1c of 8.0%. Patients who took 2 g after each meal (equivalent to 32 g crude seeds) for 12 weeks had lower fasting and postchallenge glucose levels and an impressive 1.46% reduction in HbA1c as compared with 0.4% in patients using placebo.[115]

Confirmation of these findings is urgently needed, but this widely used food and medicine certainly deserves attention by integrative practitioners. Optimal dosing, preparation, and use also remain unclear; many different approaches are used in various traditions. One small trial reported improvements when seed powder was added to hot water but not when it was added to yogurt.[116] In addition to the use of fenugreek in food, dry seeds (1 teaspoon) are chewed with meals in many cultures to improve digestion.

Dosage
Until further evidence provides clear guidance, practitioners may use crude powder or extracts at doses equivalent to 20 to 30 g of crude seeds. This dose can be titrated to meal size and individual results.

Precautions
Fenugreek can cause gastrointestinal intolerance with diarrhea, dyspepsia, abdominal distention, and flatulence.

Ivy Gourd (Coccinia indica)
Ivy gourd, a perennial herb in the cucumber family, comes from India but spreads easily and is now distributed worldwide. It is an important Ayurvedic diabetes medicine with additional choleretic, laxative, antiinflammatory, and demulcent properties. The leaves appear to have insulinomimetic effects on lipoprotein lipase, glucose-6-phosphatase, and other glycolytic enzymes.

Results of the first human trial were published in 1980, and the investigators reported glucose-lowering effects.[117] In a more recent trial in 60 patients with well-controlled type 2 DM, 1 g per day of an alcoholic extract for 90 days significantly lowered HbA1c from 6.7% to 6.1%.[118] This dose was equivalent to approximately 15 g of dried leaves and was selected based on traditional practitioners' use of a "handful" of leaves in their patients. Clearly, this is yet another promising botanical medicine worthy of further study.

Dosage
Dried leaves or extracts at doses equivalent to 15 g can be used with meals.

Precautions
Ivy gourd has no known side effects or risks.

Prickly Pear Cactus (Opuntia streptocantha)
The prickly pear cactus was used to treat gastritis and ulcers for centuries by pre-Columbian indigenous peoples in Mexico. The raw stems (cladodes) are liquefied or broiled and consumed with meals to reduce hyperglycemia; in Spanish they are called nopales. In a study of 35 patients with type 2 DM, glucose was measured after three typical breakfasts were eaten with and without nopales. Postprandial rises in glucose were significantly lower after meals with nopales.[119] The glucose-lowering effects of nopales were attributed to its fiber and pectin content, but extracts had the same activity even after filtering out fiber and pectin. Novel compounds are being studied for their possible role.[120] Although no studies have investigated the effects of long-term use on HbA1c, this food medicine is cheap, readily available, and commonly used in the southwestern United States and Mexico.

Dosage
Doses of 85 g or more appear to reduce glucose parameters.

Pycnogenol (Pinus maritima)

Pycnogenol is a standardized extract of French maritime pine bark. It contains procyanidins, catechins, and other compounds with potent antioxidant activity. Cardiovascular benefits have been noted in small trials, but improvements in lipids, blood pressure, and platelet function have been inconsistent. In 48 patients with type 2 DM who used 125 mg of pycnogenol daily or placebo for 12 weeks, those in the treatment group had a 0.8% reduction in HbA1c, along with blood pressure and low-density lipoprotein (LDL) cholesterol reductions.[121] An earlier trial reported similar HbA1c reductions in 77 patients with type 2 DM, but a significant placebo reduction of 0.53% made this finding nonsignificant.[122]

■ Dosage
Optimal benefits have been reported with doses of 100 to 200 mg.

Pharmaceuticals

The standard approach to treating type 2 DM is focused on improving glycemic control, as reflected by serum levels of HbA1c. This approach is based on the assumption that all reductions in HbA1c are of equal benefit, regardless of how they are achieved. Newer evidence contradicts this assumption. More recent systematic reviews clearly indicate that different drugs have very different effects on real-world clinical measures of morbidity and mortality, independent of their ability to lower blood glucose. Growing recognition of this important gap in our understanding of type 2 DM treatment can create confusion for patients and caregivers, but bridging this gap will be crucial to providing more effective integrative treatment in the future.

Metformin

Metformin is a biguanide that is structurally similar to guanidines originally discovered in extracts of *Galega officinalis* (French lilac). Metformin has been in use since the 1950s, thus making it one of the oldest oral hypoglycemic drugs, but it may be the best. Although its exact mechanism of action is unclear, it improves insulin sensitivity and reduces hepatic gluconeogenesis. It is the only drug that has been shown to reduce cardiovascular mortality (OR, 0.74; 95% CI, 0.62 to 0.89) in systematic reviews,[123] and as such it should be considered first-line treatment for diabetes.

■ Dosage
The typical dose range is 500 to 1000 mg twice daily.

■ Precautions
Apart from mild occasional nausea and diarrhea, the only drawback of metformin use is impaired vitamin B_{12} absorption in the terminal ileum, which can lead to vitamin B_{12} deficiency.[124] Metformin can also cause lactic acidosis in patients with renal insufficiency or alcoholism.

> Improving glycemic control does not always improve cardiovascular outcomes. Metformin is the only hypoglycemic drug with proven cardiovascular and mortality benefits.

Sulfonylureas

Sulfonylureas increase insulin secretion by pancreatic beta cells by binding to membrane channels. These drugs have also been used for several decades, but they do not appear to improve cardiovascular outcomes. One problem is that they cause weight gain. They also cause more frequent hypoglycemic episodes, which can lead to arrhythmias and cardiac ischemia.[125] A systematic review found that glyburide was almost twice as likely as other sulfonylureas to cause hypoglycemia, but cardiovascular outcomes were the same for all drugs in the class.[126] Patients using sulfonylureas and metformin in combination are also at greater risk of cardiovascular mortality than are patients using metformin alone.[127]

■ Dosage
The usual dose of glyburide is 2.5 to 10 mg twice daily.

■ Precautions
Hypoglycemia and weight gain.

Thiazolidinediones

Thiazolidinediones increase insulin sensitivity by activating peroxisome proliferator-activated receptor gamma, a nuclear receptor with salutary effects on fatty acid balance, adipocyte differentiation, adiponectin, and other factors involved in glucose and lipid metabolism. The use of rosiglitazone has decreased dramatically since it was found to increase the risk of heart attacks by more than 40% in patients with type 2 DM, possibly because of drug-related LDL rise or congestive heart failure. Pioglitazone (Actos) is the only drug in this class that clinicians can use. Its impact on cardiovascular outcomes is still unclear, but a systematic review did find that it improved glycemic control by 0.58% HbA1c when it was added to metformin.[128]

■ Dosage
The dose of pioglitazone is 15 to 30 mg once daily.

■ Precautions
The average weight gain is 7 lb, and mild edema is commonly noted. Another problem with long-term use is osteoporosis; in a meta-analysis of 10 trials involving 13,715 participants, fracture risk was more than doubled (OR, 2.23; 95% CI, 1.65 to 3.01).[129] Pioglitazone can increase cardiac disease risk.

Incretins: Sitagliptin

Incretins are hormones produced in the small intestine during a meal that enter the vasculature and trigger insulin release by pancreatic beta cells. The two incretins are glucagon-like peptide (GLP-1) and gastric inhibitory peptide (GIP). A newer class of drugs inhibits dipeptidyl peptidase-4 (DPP-4), an enzyme that degrades GLP-1 and GIP, thus leading to increased insulin and decreased glucagon levels. The most widely studied drugs in this class are sitagliptin (Januvia) and, to a lesser extent, vildagliptin.

■ Dosage
The recommended dose of sitagliptin is 100 mg once daily.

Precautions

The only side effects noted in trials have been nasopharyngitis and headache, but because DPP-4 degrades dozens of other enzymes and the drugs have not been evaluated in long-term trials, questions about safety remain. The impact of these drugs on cardiovascular events and mortality also is unclear, but meta-analyses suggest HbA1c reductions of 0.7%.[130]

Exenatide

Exenatide (Byetta) is a GLP-1 analogue that is administered as a weekly injection. In comparison trials with insulin and other oral hypoglycemics, it reduced HbA1c by approximately 1.0% without causing hypoglycemia or weight gain.[131] More research on long-term use and clinical outcomes will likely follow for this promising drug, but this drug is limited by having to be injected.

Dosage

The dose is 5 mcg twice daily for 1 month and is then increased to 10 mcg twice daily as needed.

Precautions

Reported side effects include diarrhea, nausea, and vomiting. Cases of pancreatitis have also been reported. No cardiovascular outcomes are available.

Alpha-Glucosidase Inhibitors

Alpha-glucosidase inhibitors prevent enzymatic cleavage of oligosaccharides into glucose and other simple sugars. They improve glycemic control by reducing glucose absorption when they are taken with meals. Systematic reviews have reported HbA1c reductions of approximately 0.8%,[132] but no clear cardiovascular benefits have been seen.

Dosage

A dose of 25 to 100 mg three times daily can be used, but no additional benefit is seen with doses greater than 50 mg.

Precautions

The most unpopular side effect is flatulence, but these drugs can also elevate liver enzymes.

Insulin

Although insulin administration can be lifesaving, insulin is a proinflammatory hormone. Every effort should be made to optimize glycemic control, but it is probably best to use the lowest possible doses of exogenous insulin to achieve this goal. Insulin-dependent patients with type 2 DM can often greatly reduce their dose requirements by following an integrative treatment protocol, as described in this chapter.

One important mechanism of risk is stimulation of insulin-like growth factor-I (IGF-I) and other growth hormones. IGF-I levels predict cancer risk, and the first suggestion that insulin users may be at increased risk of cancer was published in 1967.[133] For reasons that are unclear, people with type 2 DM have a 20% increased risk of breast cancer[134] and a 30% increased risk of colon cancer.[135] Some studies suggest that glargine, a long-acting insulin analogue, may be more carcinogenic by stimulating IGF-I much more than other types of insulin. The hope is that the International Study of Insulin and Cancer, funded by Sanofi-Aventis (the makers of glargine) will clarify this issue.

Many insulin protocols, regimens, and analogues are available; their use is beyond the scope of this chapter. Practitioners should be aware that although these regimens may allow patients to take their insulin in a more convenient or practical manner, no evidence indicates that any one approach is superior to another. Short-acting insulin analogues are commonly used, but meta-analyses suggest that they do not provide any advantage over regular human insulin.[136] Similarly, no evidence indicates that the long-acting insulin analogues glargine and detemir are superior to regular insulin.[137] Continuous infusion pumps are a newer technology that may be superior, but their benefit has been demonstrated only in type 1 DM.[138]

Other Drugs That Improve Outcomes

Angiotensin-Converting Enzyme Inhibitors

ACE inhibitors prevent and treat diabetes. This startling fact makes it clear that integration between seemingly disparate physiologic systems can have a powerful impact on health and disease. Exactly how the renin-angiotensin system influences glucose metabolism is unclear, but multiple lines of suggestive evidence exist. Angiotensin II is known to mediate vasoconstriction and hypoperfusion of skeletal muscle and pancreatic islets. It also appears to affect insulin signaling and glucose transport in ways that are still unknown. In a systematic review of 13 trials involving 93,451 patients with hypertension, the use of these drugs reduced the risk of incident type 2 DM by an impressive 26%.[139] Many ACE inhibitors are available; the most widely studied is ramipril, at a recommended dose of 2.5 to 10 mg once daily.

Statins

Statins are universally recommended for patients with type 2 DM, but their effect on this disease now seems complicated. As a drug class, 3-hydroxy-3-methyl-glutaryl-coenzyme A (HMG-CoA) reductase inhibitors are known for their ability to improve lipid parameters. The clear cardiovascular benefits of these drugs are actually more strongly associated with antiinflammatory effects, however. The absolute risk reduction seen with these drugs is very compelling in people who have already had a cardiovascular event, but it is unimpressive in those who have not. patients with type 2 DM fall somewhere in between; the higher baseline vascular risk in diabetes makes statin therapy much more appropriate.[140] Red yeast rice is a natural source of several statin compounds, and it may be considered a reasonable alternative for patients who cannot tolerate or do not want to use a statin drug.

Unfortunately, newer evidence suggests that some statins increase type 2 DM risk. In a meta-analysis of 13 trials involving 91,140 adults, the overall increase in type 2 DM risk was 9% (95% CI, 1.02 to 1.17).[141] Subgroup analysis revealed that different statins have very different effects. Simvastatin, atorvastatin, and rosuvastatin increase the risk of type 2 DM, whereas pravastatin reduces the risk.[142] This finding suggests that pravastatin may be a better choice in patients with type 2 DM until this issue becomes clearer. Recommended dose is 20 to 80 mg once daily.

■ Aspirin

Low-dose aspirin has long been advocated for cardiovascular prevention, but it appears to offer little benefit in patients with type 2 DM. This conclusion was noted in a joint position paper published by the American Heart Association, the American College of Cardiology, and the American Diabetes Association and was based on a meta-analysis of nine RCTs. A nonsignificant benefit and the risk of major gastrointestinal bleeding make aspirin recommended only for men older than 50 years and women older than 60 years who have at least one cardiac risk factor.[143]

Mechanical Therapies

Bariatric Surgery

Various surgical procedures induce weight loss by resecting, tightening, shrinking, or bypassing the stomach and upper digestive tract. These forms of so-called bariatric surgery lead to profound weight loss, and they may be the most important advance in the treatment of type 2 DM in decades. Although surgery is not the most philosophically appealing solution to the worldwide epidemic of type 2 DM and other metabolic diseases related to obesity, it is increasingly recognized by governments and insurers worldwide.

In a review of 103 clinical trial treatment arms involving 3188 patients with type 2 DM, 78% had complete resolution of clinical and laboratory manifestations of diabetes after surgery; 87% of patients improved significantly and reported an average weight loss of 38.5 kg.[144] Long-term reductions in all-cause morbidity and mortality are increasingly reported.

Short-term complications include gastric dumping syndrome, hernias, wound infections, and pneumonia. The most important long-term consideration is nutrient malabsorption. Deficiencies of vitamins A, C, D, K, and B_{12} and folate and of iron, selenium, calcium, zinc, and copper should be expected.[145] All patients who have undergone bariatric surgery should take a daily multivitamin and multimineral supplement. Anemia, hyperparathyroidism, and peripheral neuropathy are common. Patients who have undergone bariatric surgery and who report vague symptoms should be evaluated for nutrient deficiency and reminded of the importance of supplementation.

> Metformin, angiotensin-converting enzyme inhibitors, statin drugs, and bariatric surgery appear to offer proven benefits in type 2 diabetes mellitus, but other hypoglycemic drugs do not.

PREVENTION PRESCRIPTION

- Manage psychological stress and treat emotional trauma or mood disorders if present.
- Obtain 6 to 8 hours of restful sleep per night.
- Eat a low-glycemic Mediterranean diet that includes whole grains, vegetable protein, vegetables and some fruit, coffee, and moderate alcohol.
- Avoid sugar-sweetened beverages, animal protein, and eggs.
- Practice daily exercise, aerobic or resistance.
- Manage weight and treat obesity.
- Avoid air pollution by maintaining safe distance from high-traffic roads at work or home.
- Maintain proper oral hygiene and treat periodontitis if present.
- Treat hypertension with ramipril (2.5 to 10 mg daily) or another angiotensin-converting enzyme inhibitor.
- Treat prediabetes with aggressive lifestyle intervention and consider metformin, 500 to 1000 mg twice daily.
- Treat vitamin D deficiency if present.
- Take omega-3 fatty acids at 1 to 2 g daily.
- Take magnesium at 100 to 300 mg daily.
- Avoid selenium supplementation if serum levels are adequate.

THERAPEUTIC REVIEW

■ Lifestyle

- Consider referral to a comprehensive lifestyle program if available.

■ Exercise

- Encourage daily aerobic, resistance, or mindfulness-based (e.g., tai chi) exercise.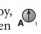
- Provide behavioral support tailored to patients' stage of readiness to change.

- Strive to inspire patients with your own lifestyle choices.

■ Diet

- Low-glycemic diet and moderate carbohydrate reduction
- Avoidance of sugar-sweetened beverages and juices, animal protein, and eggs
- Consumption of more lentils, beans, pulses and soy, chia and other whole grains, onions and leafy green vegetables, and walnuts and other nuts
- Moderate coffee and wine consumption

Mind-Body Therapy

- Ask about and treat disordered sleep, stress, anxiety, and depression. B₁

- Discuss stress reduction options and facilitate the chosen modality. B₁

- Refer patients to a psychologist you are comfortable with as needed. A₁

Supplements

- Vitamin D: 1000 to 4000 units daily unless deficient B₁
- Alpha-lipoic acid: 50 to 100 mg daily B₁
- Chromium: 200 to 1000 mcg daily A₁
- Benfotiamine: 350 mg with meals B₂
- Omega-3 fatty acids: 1 to 4 g daily B₁
- L-Carnitine: 500 to 1000 mg three times daily C₁
- Magnesium: 200 to 500 mg daily A₂
- Vitamin K: 100 mcg daily (caution with warfarin) B₂

Botanicals

- Berberine *(Berberis vulgaris):* 200 to 500 mg three times daily B₁
- Ivy gourd *(Coccinia indica):* 15 g powdered dried leaves or equivalent extract) B₂

- Fenugreek *(Trigonella foenum-graecum):* 30 g seed powder or equivalent extract with meals B₂
- Cinnamon: 1 to 5 g ground bark with meals or equivalent extract B₁
- *Panax ginseng:* 1 to 2 g ground root or 100 to 400 mg extract B₂
- Prickly pear cactus *(Opuntia streptocantha):* 85 g broiled or liquefied stems with a meal B₁
- Pycnogenol *(Pinus maritima):* 100 to 200 mg daily B₁

Pharmaceuticals

- Metformin: 500 to 1000 mg twice daily A₂
- Ramipril: 5 to 10 mg daily (or another angiotensin-converting enzyme inhibitor) A₂
- Pravastatin: 20 to 80 mg daily (or other statin or red yeast rice) A₂
- Other drug classes as needed to achieve a glycosylated hemoglobin level lower than 7.0%, including thiazolidinediones, sulfonylureas, incretins, and insulin

Surgery

- Bariatric surgery for morbidly obese patients A₃

KEY WEB RESOURCES

Glycemic Index Foundation (an international glycemic index database): http://www.glycemicindex.com.

California Academy of Family Physicians list of diabetes flow sheets: http://www.familydocs.org/new-directions-diabetes-care/tools-and-resources/flow-sheets-forms-signs-and-charts.php.

National Center for Alternative and Complementary Medicine, National Institutes of Health diabetes Web site: http://nccam.nih.gov/health/diabetes.

References

References are available online at expertconsult.com.

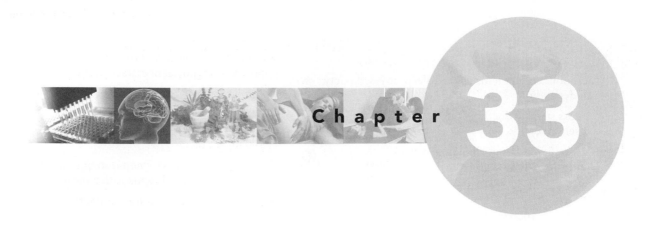

33

Hypothyroidism

Leslie Mendoza Temple, MD

Pathophysiology

Hypothyroidism is the insufficient synthesis of thyroid hormone, necessary for metabolic processes throughout the body. Worldwide, iodine deficiency is the most common cause of *primary hypothyroidism,* the most common type of hypothyroidism. In iodine-sufficient countries, autoimmune destruction of the gland (Hashimoto disease) is the leading cause of primary hypothyroidism. The second leading cause of primary hypothyroidism is iatrogenic, including surgery, radioactive iodide, medications (i.e., lithium, amiodarone), overconsumption of goitrogens, and external-beam radiation. Primary hypothyroidism accounts for approximately 95% of cases compared with less than 5% from secondary and tertiary types.

Secondary hypothyroidism results from decreased thyroid-stimulating hormone (TSH) secretion from pituitary tumors (adenomas most commonly), pituitary surgery, or other pituitary disease, such as Sheehan syndrome. *Hypothalamic or tertiary hypothyroidism* results in decreased thyrotropin-releasing hormone secretion related to infiltrative processes such as sarcoidosis, infection, or congenital defect. *Transient hypothyroidism* may occur after abrupt withdrawal of long-term thyroid hormone therapy or from silent or subacute thyroiditis.

Clinical Presentation

Common symptoms of hypothyroidism include fatigue, dry skin, cold intolerance, hair loss, concentration problems, constipation, weight gain, carpal tunnel symptoms, dyspnea, hoarseness, and menorrhagia. Physical signs include dry and coarse skin, brittle nails, cool extremities, thinning of the lateral eyebrows and hair, myxedema, delayed tendon reflexes, and diminished hearing.[1] In addition to these physical findings, basal metabolic rate may be estimated using axillary temperature measurements and assessment of Achilles tendon reflexes. A series of morning basal body temperatures less than 97.4 °F and delayed Achilles tendon reflexes may add to the clinical diagnosis.[2]

Laboratory Studies

The laboratory evaluation of hypothyroidism remains a controversial topic in the medical community. The minimal evaluation should include TSH, free triiodothyronine (T_3), free thyroxine (T_4), and thyroid peroxidase antibodies (TPO Abs). Additional testing may include measuring nutritional cofactors and related hormone pathways such as urinary iodine levels and adrenal gland function, although these tests are not commonly performed in conventional endocrinology (with respect to hypothyroidism). Some clinicians also check reverse T_3, which is a much less active form of T_3 hormone.

TSH secretion varies in a circadian pattern, with highest levels between 10 PM and 4 AM and the lowest levels between 10 AM and 6 PM.[3] Hence testing at a consistent time of day is best for serial comparisons, preferably during the morning before caffeine consumption.

The normal TSH reference range is wide, from 0.45 to 4.5 milliunits/L. Some investigators suggested lowering the upper limit of serum TSH concentration to 2.5 milliunits/L.[4-6] Every individual has an endogenously set TSH value that determines that person's optimum level with respect to thyroid function. Significant variation of TSH measurements in a symptomatic but euthyroid patient deserves further investigation of cofactors and treatment, depending on symptoms.

Primary Hypothyroidism

In primary hypothyroidism, serum TSH is elevated with decreased serum free T_4. The thyroid secretes mostly T_4 and 10% to 20% T_3. Approximately 80% to 90% of circulating T_3, the most active thyroid hormone, is derived from peripheral deiodination of T_4. Serum free T_3 levels are normal in approximately 25% of hypothyroid patients. This reflects the body's adaptive responses to hypothyroidism through increased peripheral conversion of T_4 to the active T_3. Thus, serum free T_3 measurements should not be used in isolation to confirm or exclude the diagnosis of hypothyroidism. Serum T_3 levels are frequently lower in euthyroid patients with nonthyroidal disease and during food restriction. These lower free serum T_3 levels occur because of a decreased peripheral conversion of T_4 to T_3.[7,8] Measuring serum free T_3 levels, however, may help with titrating thyroid hormone dosages, particularly in patients taking combination T_4 and T_3 medication. One must evaluate and treat for other causes of hypothyroid-like symptoms, including adrenal insufficiency, hypogonadism, anemia, and depression, which may be comorbid conditions in a single patient.

> Serum triiodothyronine (T_3) is generally not used to confirm the diagnosis of hypothyroidism. It may be useful for guiding thyroid hormone dose titration in patients taking a combination of thyroxine (T_4) and T_3 medication.

Secondary and Tertiary Hypothyroidism

Patients may present with symptoms consistent with primary hypothyroidism but with evidence of pituitary hormone imbalance. TSH levels may vary from low, normal, or even slightly elevated values, whereas the free T_4 level is low. Generally, serum TSH concentrations are low in patients with pituitary disease and normal or high in patients with hypothalamic disease. Clinical correlation and magnetic resonance imaging of the hypothalamus and pituitary are necessary for proper diagnosis.

Subclinical Hypothyroidism

In subclinical hypothyroidism, TSH is elevated but free T_4 is in the normal range. The thyroid gland is stimulated to work harder while still keeping up with the body's metabolic needs. The prevalence of subclinical hypothyroidism is variable, with 8% of women and 3% of men affected, increasing to 15% to 18% in women older than 60 years of age.[9] Annually, 2% to 5% of patients with subclinical hypothyroidism will progress to overt hypothyroidism.[4]

In subclinical hypothyroidism, the clinical decision to prescribe thyroid hormone is based mainly on the presence of symptoms and laboratory results. If a patient is symptomatic, checking TPO Ab may help identify an autoimmune cause (Hashimoto disease) and the risk of progression to overt hypothyroidism. If the TPO Ab test result is positive and the patient is symptomatic, then treatment with low-dose thyroid hormone may be indicated. If the patient has significant symptoms with a borderline TSH level but negative TPO Ab, a low dose of thyroid hormone may still be warranted for several months' trial.

Possible consequences of untreated subclinical hypothyroidism are coronary atherosclerosis, elevated low-density lipoproteins (LDLs), and progression to overt hypothyroidism.[10] Statin-induced myopathy may be associated with mild thyroid insufficiency, so thyroid hormone may be useful for high-risk cardiovascular patients starting statin medication, particularly if their TSH concentration is elevated.[11,12]

The risks of cardiac arrhythmias (atrial fibrillation) and osteoporosis must be weighed against the benefits of receiving thyroid hormone therapy.[4]

Other abnormal laboratory findings in hypothyroidism may include increased creatine phosphokinase, elevated cholesterol and triglycerides, and normocytic or macrocytic anemia.

Integrative Therapy

Tenets of an integrative, functional medicine approach to improving thyroid health include the following[13]:

- Reduce chronic stress from physical, emotional, nutritional, and environmental sources that can promote an overactive immune system, particularly in patients with positive antithyroid antibodies.
- Provide nutrients that are needed for adequate thyroxine (T_4) manufacture, proper T_4 to triiodothyronine (T_3) conversion, and optimal T_3 binding activity to intracellular receptors.
- Exercise and follow a heart-healthy nutrition program to increase energy and maintain weight (or at least stop gaining weight).
- Use appropriate testing, monitoring, and medications as needed to treat hypothyroidism.

Exercise

Along with a heart-healthy, antiinflammatory nutrition plan, exercise is absolutely critical for hypothyroid patients to maintain healthy weight (or stop gaining weight), elevate mood, modify cardiac risk, and increase bone density, especially when they have a decreased metabolic rate (see Chapter 88, Writing an Exercise Prescription).

Nutrition

Foods to Avoid or Limit
Brassica Vegetables

Patients should avoid eating very large amounts of *Brassica* vegetables (e.g., cabbage, turnips, Brussels sprouts, rutabagas, broccoli, cauliflower, bok choy). Millet, peaches, peanuts, pine nuts, strawberries, spinach, and cassava root have small levels of goitrogens as well. These foods are rich in dietary sulfhydryl and thiocyanate compounds that can adversely affect the iodination of thyroglobulin if they are consumed in high amounts.[13,14] An observational study of 37 healthy subjects looked at a high daily soybean intake of 30 g or more over 1 to 3 months. The subjects had within normal range increases in TSH levels and more hypothyroid-like symptoms that normalized 1 month after soybean cessation.[15] When eating a reasonable amount of soy and *Brassica* vegetables (less than 30 g per day), steaming or cooking these foods briefly may help reduce their goitrogenic effect while preserving their nutrient content.[16,17]

Steaming or cooking *Brassica* vegetables and soy briefly may help reduce their goitrogenic effect while preserving their nutrient content.

Soy

Isoflavones are iodinated by TPO, which may be the mechanism for their competitive interference with thyroid hormone production.[14] Genistein, the major soy isoflavone, can be goitrogenic as seen in iodine-deficient neonates exclusively fed soy formula. Soy isoflavones can also aggravate hypothyroidism in iodine-deficient adults.[18] Adequate supplementation of at least 150 mcg of iodine and 200 mcg of selenium may counteract this risk. For adults receiving thyroid hormone replacement therapy who eat soy or take soy supplements, the thyroid hormone may require more frequent dosage surveillance and higher dosing. Ideally, soy foods (in limited amount) and thyroid medication should be taken several hours apart.[19]

A small double-blind randomized placebo-controlled study of iodine-replete healthy postmenopausal women showed that soy supplementation did not significantly affect TSH or serum T_4 or T_3 levels compared with placebo. The supplement used was Novasoy by Archer Daniels Midland (ADM) that contained 40% isoflavones (50 mg isoflavones per capsule), at three capsules a day for 6 months.[20] More research is necessary to determine the effect of soy and goiter development in healthy iodine-sufficient individuals.

Supplements

Several minerals and trace elements are essential for proper thyroid function and metabolism.

Iodine: Too much or too little can cause hypothyroidism; too much can also cause hyperthyroidism.

Iodine Deficiency

Underconsumption of iodine deprives the thyroid gland of manufacturing active thyroid hormones through the organification of iodine. Repleting with iodine is the treatment of choice for iodine deficiency, and it is achieved with varying success in areas of the world by the iodination of refined salt. Iodine lost from salt is estimated to be 20% from production site to table, with another 20% lost during cooking.[21] Thus, iodine should also come from sources such as fresh ocean fish, seaweed, and unrefined sea salt. (Tables 33-1, 33-1e, and 33-2). Short-term iodine repletion with supplements is discussed later for appropriate patients. A minimum of 150 mcg of iodine should be consumed on a daily basis for adults (200 mcg for pregnant women and 290 mcg for lactating women).[22]

 Table 33-1e, which compares seaweed iodine by genus, location, and study, can be found online at expertconsult .com.

Iodine Testing

If a patient is suspected to have iodine deficiency caused by dietary restrictions (e.g., seafood avoidance, low salt consumption), iron deficiency, medication use, or heavy metal toxicity, iodine testing may be useful. Because public health programs to iodize salt have occurred worldwide,

TABLE 33-1. Iodine Content of Selected Foods

FOOD	CONTENT (mcg)
Salt, iodized, 1 teaspoon	400
Bread made with iodate dough conditioner and continuous mix process, one slice	142
Bread, made with regular process, one slice (most widely available)	35
Haddock, 3 oz	104–145
Shrimp, 3 oz	21–37
Egg, one	18–26
Cottage cheese 2%, ½ cup	26–71
Cheddar cheese, 1 oz	5–23
Ground beef, 3 oz	8

Adapted from U.S. Department of Agriculture. *Composition of Foods.* USDA handbook no. 8 series. Washington, DC: Agricultural Research Service; 1976–1986.

TABLE 33-2. Commonly Used Seaweed Preparations*

TYPE OF SEAWEED	COMMON USE	AMOUNT TO MEET MINIMUM IODINE DOSE OF 150 mcg/day	AMOUNT TO MEET MAXIMUM IODINE DOSE OF 1100 mcg/day
Nori	Sushi wrapper, rice balls	9 g/day	69 g/day
Wakame	Miso soup	2 g/day	17 g/day
Dulse	Seaweed chips, soups, sauces	2 g/day	15 g/day
Kelp/kombu	Hot pot dishes, soups	9 mg/day	710 mg/day

Adapted from Teas J, Pine S, Critchley A, et al. Variability of iodine content in common commercially available seaweeds. *Thyroid.* 2004;14:839.
*Minimum and maximum daily iodine amounts are based on U.S/Japanese source values.

one may assume that most individuals are iodine replete in targeted countries. However, cases of iodine deficiency have been identified in the United States, a country that has largely eradicated iodine deficiency. The *24-hour urine iodine test* (unprovoked) is the standard test for checking iodine status.[23]

Some clinicians use the *iodine loading test*, a provoked measure of body iodine stores. The test consists of consuming 50 mg of an iodine/iodide combination followed by a 24-hour urine collection. An iodine loading test result is normal if 90% or more iodine was excreted in the urine. If the test resulted in a 75% excretion rate, this would imply that the body needs more iodine.[24,25] If an iodine deficiency is noted from this test, some clinicians have used kelp tablets or iodine/iodide replacement (Lugol's solution or Iodoral). However, the risk of iodine toxicity, transient hyperthyroidism, and hypothyroidism increases with this approach. Iodine supplementation should be recommended for short term only, with iodine sources coming from food thereafter.

The *iodine skin patch test* is unreliable and should not be used in isolation for determining iodine status. The test consists of painting a 3×3 inch square of iodine tincture on the inner forearm or abdomen at bedtime. A normal body iodine level is supposedly diagnosed if the orange color of the patch takes longer than 24 hours to disappear. If the patch disappears in 10 hours or less, it implies a significant iodine deficiency. However, the iodine skin patch test fails to take into account the differences in an individual's skin moisture, ambient temperature, and atmospheric pressure, all of which may affect iodine evaporation rate and patch color intensity.

> The 24-hour unprovoked urine iodine test is the standard test for checking iodine status.

Iodine Excess

The tolerable upper intake level (UL) for adults is 1100 mcg/day (1.1 mg/day).[26] The UL is the highest level of a daily intake that is likely to pose no risk of adverse health effects to almost all individuals in the general population. Chronic overexposure to iodine reduces organic binding of iodine by the thyroid gland. A daily iodine intake of 10 times (more than 1500 mcg/day) the minimum daily adult requirement may cause iodine goiter in some people, especially in individuals with underlying thyroid abnormalities such as Hashimoto disease.[27-29] Difficulty arises in determining the cumulative daily dose of iodine one is exposed to in food (i.e., kelp, seaweed, food preservatives) and in iodine-containing substances (i.e., medications, contaminated drinking water, topical antiseptics).

Some practitioners believe in using iodine doses much higher than the UL to overcome measured deficiencies for hypothyroidism and even other conditions such as breast cancer.[25] The evidence base on this practice needs larger randomized controlled studies than the current literature offers.

The recommended iodine replacement dose far exceeds the UL, but the UL is not meant to apply to individuals who are treated with the nutrient under medical supervision or to individuals with predisposing conditions that modify their sensitivity to the nutrient.[26] Hence patients with a documented iodine deficiency who are closely monitored should receive dietary or medical iodine replacement. The best dosage and duration of oral iodine replacement vary with the individual patient. A dosing regimen is suggested in the following section. Multiple factors such as a low-salt/low-seafood diet, high goitrogen consumption, and exposure to chlorine, bromine, fluoride, perchlorate, and certain medications, as well as heavy metal toxicity, can negatively influence the iodination steps necessary for thyroid hormone production.[13]

The clinician must use caution in repleting high doses of iodine in a person with a low-iodine state because this can temporarily trigger iodine-induced hyperthyroidism (Jod-Basedow phenomenon) or iodine-induced hypothyroidism (Wolff-Chaikoff effect).

Patients who are taking iodine supplements or kelp tablets should be counseled to report side effects that are consistent with either a worsened hypothyroid state or, conversely, a hyperthyroid state.

■ Dosage: Dietary Iodine for the General Population

Adult men: 150 mcg up to 1100 mcg
Adult women: 150 mcg up to 1100 mcg
Pregnant women: 220 mcg up to 1100 mcg
Lactating women: 290 mcg up to 1100 mcg[22,26]
The iodized salt equivalent is up to 2.75 teaspoons per day (based on 400 mcg of iodine per 1 teaspoon).

■ Caution

Do not recommend iodized salt for individuals with congestive heart failure, hypertension, or salt sensitivity. Recommend fish or seaweed for natural iodine supply in these patients.

■ Dosage: Iodine Tablets or Drops for Documented Iodine Deficiency

For adults with iodine deficiency documented by a 24-hour urinary iodine test, monitor closely for iodine toxicity if oral iodine/iodide is prescribed, and use the supplement for the short term only. Iodine should then be replaced by food sources, and substances that deplete iodine stores should be avoided when possible. See Table 33-1 for selected foods high in iodine.

Lugol solution: two drops contain 5 mg iodine and 7.5 mg iodide as potassium iodide. The dose is two drops orally daily for 1 to 3 months, and then retest.

Iodoral tablet: Each 12.5-mg tablet contains a combination of 5 mg iodine and 7.5 mg iodide as potassium iodide.[30] The dose is one half to one tablet orally daily for 1 to 3 months, and then retest.

■ Precautions

Monitor for signs of iodine toxicity: brassy taste in the mouth, increased salivation, gastrointestinal upset, and acne. Chlorophyll tablets may ease the metallic taste side effect.[25]

Selenium

Selenium is an essential trace element required for the deiodination of T_4 to active T_3 hormone.[31,32] At least 55 mcg per day of selenium is recommended for adults. A handful of Brazil nuts (six to eight raw nuts) contains approximately 543 mcg of selenium, the highest natural food source of this mineral. See Table 33-3 for foods containing high levels of selenium.[33]

■ Dosage

Adult men: 55 mcg up to 400 mcg
Adult women: 55 mcg up to 400 mcg
Pregnant women: 60 mcg up to 400 mcg
Lactating women: 70 mcg up to 400 mcg[22,26]

■ Precautions

The UL for adults is 400 mcg per day, based on the risk of selenosis.[34,35] Excessive intake of selenium (selenosis) can cause discoloration of the skin, deformation and loss of nails, reversible baldness, excessive tooth decay and discoloration, garlic breath odor, weakness, lack of mental alertness, and listlessness.[36]

Vitamin A

Vitamin A is a fat-soluble vitamin obtained directly from animal sources (preformed vitamin A known as retinol) or synthesized from beta-carotene from plant sources. Beta-carotene is a provitamin A precursor that is converted to retinol in the gut.

In persons with vitamin A and iodine deficiency from malnutrition, hypothyroidism risk can be reduced with vitamin A supplementation.[31,37] Vitamin A is involved in T_4 manufacture and in intracellular receptor formation for T_3.[38] In the United States, vitamin A deficiency is most often associated with excess alcohol intake and strict dietary restrictions. Vegetarians who avoid dairy and eggs should be able to meet their vitamin A requirements through beta-carotene by eating at least five servings of fruits and vegetables daily. At least 3 to 6 mg of beta-carotene daily (equivalent to 833 to 1667 units of vitamin A) may

maintain blood levels in the range associated with a lower risk of chronic diseases. The highest yielding sources of carotenoids are carrots, cantaloupes, sweet potatoes, and spinach. Most U.S. residents consume enough retinol in milk, margarine, eggs, meat, liver, and fortified ready-to-eat cereals.[39]

■ Dosage: Vitamin A (Preformed)

One microgram retinol is equivalent to 3.33 units vitamin A (on a label) and equivalent to 12 mg beta-carotene (from food).

Adult men: 900 mcg (approximately 3000 units) up to 3000 mcg (approximately 10,000 units) preformed vitamin A

Adult women: 700 mcg (approximately 2300 units) up to 3000 mcg (approximately 10,000 units) preformed vitamin A

Pregnant women: 770 mcg (approximately 2500 units) up to 3000 mcg (approximately 10,000 units) preformed vitamin A

Lactating women: 1300 mcg (approximately 4300 units) up to 3000 mcg (approximately 10,000 units) preformed vitamin A[22,26]

■ Precautions

Too much preformed vitamin A can lead to toxic symptoms, namely birth defects, liver abnormalities, reduced bone mineral density, and central nervous system disorders. No published UL is available for carotenoids.[26]

Zinc

Abnormal zinc metabolism has been linked to hypothyroidism.[31,40,41] Zinc participates in more than 300 enzymatic reactions, along with multiple functions in transport, immunity, metabolism, and cell structure. Zinc is involved in conversion of T_4 to T_3 through the deiodinase enzyme. Zinc is also necessary to synthesize retinol-binding protein, which transports vitamin A to body tissues, an important factor in T_3 binding to intracellular receptors in the body. Severe zinc deficiency often accompanies vitamin A deficiency in malnutrition or severe dietary restriction. For most of the U.S. population, most zinc in the diet comes from meat, fish, poultry, fortified breakfast cereals, dairy, oysters, liver, dried beans, ginger, soy, and nuts. Good protein intake correlates with zinc intake.[42] The UL for zinc is 40 mg/day for adults.[26]

■ Dosage

Adult men: 11 mg up to 40 mg
Adult women: 8 mg up to 40 mg
Pregnant women: 11 mg up to 40 mg
Lactating women: 12 mg up to 40 mg[22,26]

■ Precautions

Doses greater than 40 mg/day can lead to copper deficiency and gastrointestinal irritation.

Iron

Iron deficiency impairs thyroid hormone synthesis by reducing the activity of TPO. In a deficient state, iron supplementation improves the efficacy of iodine

TABLE 33-3. Selenium Content of Selected Foods

FOOD	CONTENT (mcg)
Brazil nuts, unblanched, dried, 1 oz (six to eight nuts)	543
Halibut, Atlantic or Pacific, half fillet (159 g weight)	88
Pearled barley, raw, 1 cup	75
Wheat flour, whole grain, 1 cup	74
Lobster, 3 oz	62
Sardines, Atlantic 3 oz	45
Couscous, 1 cup	43

Adapted from U.S. Department of Agriculture (USDA), Agricultural Research Service. USDA National Nutrient Database for Standard Reference. Release 23. Nutrient Data Laboratory. <http://www.ars.usda.gov/ba/bhnrc/ndl>; Accessed 12.08.11.

supplementation.[31] Animal sources provide the most potent iron content, with liver, seafood, organ meats, and poultry in descending order of potency. Vegetarian sources of iron are most potent in dried beans, iron-fortified cereal and bread, blackstrap molasses, spinach, peas, and dried apricots. Concomitant intake of vitamin C–rich food or vitamin C as a supplement enhances the gastrointestinal absorption of iron. Laboratory evaluation should include serum ferritin, which reflects the body's iron storage pool. Ferritin is the carrier protein for iron.[42] The UL for iron is 45 mg/day for adults.[26]

■ Dosage

Adult men and postmenopausal women: 8 mg up to 45 mg/day
Adult premenopausal women: 18 mg up to 45 mg/day
Pregnant women: 27 mg up to 45 mg/day
Lactating women: 9 mg up to 45 mg/day[22,26]

■ Precautions

Long-term overdose of iron can create abnormal iron accumulation in the liver. Hemochromatosis may result, causing tissue damage. Iron overload can also favor oxidation of LDL cholesterol and the generation of free radicals that may also damage body tissues.[42]

> Soy, calcium, and iron supplements should be consumed at least 2 to 3 hours separately from thyroid medication because they may interfere with their bioavailability. Thyroid medication is typically most effective when taken on an empty stomach in the morning, at least 30 minutes before eating breakfast for maximum absorption.

Botanicals

Seaweed

Seaweed is a rich source of naturally occurring iodine and is a good source for meeting daily iodine requirements. Seaweed may aggravate thyroid conditions if too much is ingested, however, as is seen in Asian populations that regularly consume seaweed.

Seaweed iodine content varies by many factors, and this poses a challenge in terms of determining safe consumption levels. The part of seaweed used, cooking method, genus, geographic location, climate, and stage of growth all play a role in seaweed's iodine content. Iodine content is lowest in certain types of seaweed, such as nori and dulse. Iodine is also lowest in seaweed harvested dried on the beach or free-floating in bunches. Iodine level can be reduced by boiling seaweed for 15 minutes and discarding the water. Iodine content is highest if the seaweed is harvested from young plants, stored in watertight and airtight containers, and eaten roasted rather than boiled.[43]

Exercise caution in patients taking blood thinners who consume bladderwrack, an edible brown kelp, which may have some anticoagulant activity.[44] Depending on local pollution levels, edible seaweeds may contain heavy metals such as arsenic and cadmium. Hence selection of high-quality kelp and seaweed from reputable harvesters is ideal to reduce the risk of toxic ingestion.[45] Table 33-1e [online at expertconsult.com] compares differences in seaweed iodine content based on genus and location, and Table 33-2 outlines commonly used seaweed preparations and iodine content based on U.S and Japanese source values.[43]

Guggulu (Commiphora mukul)

Some animal studies showed that the Ayurvedic herb guggulu, a gum resin of the *Commiphora mukul* tree, may stimulate thyroid function. It seems to increase T_3 synthesis by increasing conversion of T_4 to T_3.[46-48] Asian studies showed that guggulu may also improve the hyperlipidemia that often accompanies hypothyroidism.[49]

A double-blind randomized controlled trial in the United States, however, showed that hyperlipidemic patients ingesting a standard Western diet who took a standardized dose of guggulu experienced a rise in LDL cholesterol levels compared with placebo. TSH levels were not significantly different after treatment with guggulu.[50] The differences in medical traditions of Ayurvedic and Western medicine and diet must be considered with respect to these differing results. More research is necessary to study the effects of guggulu in the context of an Ayurvedic treatment plan as opposed to its incorporation as a single ingredient in a conventional Western medicine regimen. Take great care in recommending Asian-source Ayurvedic herbs because some brands commonly found in the United States were found to have significant levels of lead, mercury, and arsenic.[51]

Pharmaceuticals

Synthetic Hormone Replacement: T_4 Alone Versus Combination T_4 Plus T_3

The use of combination T_4 (levothyroxine) plus T_3 (liothyronine) therapy versus T_4 alone has been controversial.[52-56] The conventional medicine treatment of choice for hormone replacement in hypothyroidism remains T_4 alone.[57]

Proponents of combination therapy have advised the use of sustained-release T_3 plus T_4, or the use of porcine thyroid (e.g., Armour, Nature-Throid, Westhroid), which contains natural T_3 and T_4 plus other iodinated compounds. Another good option is to use compounded T_3 and T_4 from a reliable compounding pharmacy. The best candidates for this kind of combination therapy typically have had unsatisfactory results from T_4 therapy alone despite proper dosage titration and TSH monitoring.[2,55,56]

Desiccated Porcine Thyroid Replacement

Porcine thyroid hormone (e.g., Armour, Nature-Throid, Westhroid) is an older medication used in hypothyroidism considered by some in the medical community to be obsolete and by others as equally efficacious or superior to synthetic hormones. Desiccated porcine thyroid contains approximately 20% T_3 and 80% T_4, as well as other iodinated compounds, diiodotyrosine (T_2) and monoiodotyrosine (T_1), which may play a role in providing additional relief of symptoms. As with its synthetic T_4

TABLE 33-4. Adult Thyroid Hormone Dosage Recommendations

THYROID HORMONE	GENERIC (TRADE NAME)	STARTING ORAL DOSE	AVERAGE DAILY DOSE AND TITRATION
Synthetic T_4 alone	T4 levothyroxine (Synthroid, Unithroid, Levoxyl) Note: Stick with one formulation (generic or name brand) throughout the course of treatment because of dose variability	100 mcg daily[a] or 25–50 mcg daily in older or sensitive patients	200–300 mcg daily[a] Titrate every 6 weeks until symptoms improved and TFTs normalize Follow TFTs every 6 months or sooner if symptoms arise[a]
Synthetic T_4 + T_3 separate tablets or compounded together by a reliable compounding pharmacy	T_4 levothyroxine + T_3 liothyronine (Cytomel)	100 mcg T_4 + 25 mcg T_3 daily[a] or 25–50 mcg T_4 + 12.5 mcg T_3 daily in older or sensitive patients	Titrate T_4 as above Titrate T_3 by 12.5–25 mcg/day every 1–2 weeks to a maximum of 100 mcg/day;[a] sustained-release T_3 may be more effective[b]
Synthetic T_4 + T_3 combination tablet (Liotrix)	Liotrix (Thyrolar) Liotrix is a uniform mixture of synthetic T_4 and T_3 in 4:1 ratio by weight	1 tablet = 50/12.5 mcg of T_4 and T_3 Various proportions available Start with 1–2 tablets daily[a]	Use if simplification of dosing is necessary; no therapeutic advantage over using T_4 + T_3 as separate doses[a]
T_4 and T_3 desiccated porcine thyroid gland	Armour, Nature-Throid, or Westhroid 1 grain = 60 mg = 38 mcg T_4 + 9 mcg T_3	Start with ¼–½ grain = 15–30 mg daily[c]	60–120 mg (1–2 grains) daily Titrate by 15 mg (¼ grain) orally every 2–3 weeks[c]

T_3, triiodothyronine; T_4, levothyroxine; TFTs, thyroid function tests (thyroid-stimulating hormone, free T_4, free T_3).
[a]Data from Lexi-Comp Online.[58]
[b]Data from Blanchard[55] and Henneman et al.[56]
[c]Data from Gaby[2] and Armour Thyroid Web site.[59] For converting synthetic T_4 and T_3 to desiccated porcine thyroid, see http://www.armourthyroid.com.

and T_3 counterparts, close monitoring of symptoms and a regimen of thyroid function tests are important when taking care of a patient prescribed porcine thyroid replacement. Recommended thyroid hormone dosages are shown in Table 33-4.[2,55,56,58,59]

> 1 grain (60 mg) desiccated porcine thyroid = 100 mcg thyroxine (T_4) and 25 mcg triiodothyronine (T_3).

Other Endocrine Factors to Consider When Treating Hypothyroidism

The thyroid gland does not work in isolation and requires inputs from a complex web of chemical messages, notably from the brain, gut, gonads, and adrenal glands. Balancing the interplay of hormones (and reducing the stressors that diminish their function) is important in the holistic treatment of thyroid disease. Chapter 47 (Effective Treatment of Chronic Fatigue Syndrome, Fatigue, Fibromyalgia, and Muscle/Myofascial Pain: A Comprehensive Medicine Approach) specifically addresses the evaluation and treatment for adrenal gland insufficiency, which plays an important role in thyroid dysfunction.

Therapies to Consider

Traditional Chinese Medicine

In the traditional Chinese medicine (TCM) system, the diagnosis and treatment of individuals with a conventional medicine diagnosis of hypothyroidism depend on the history, tongue, and pulse diagnosis. Hypothyroidism is generally considered to be a deficiency of spleen or kidney "yang"

energy, especially if the disorder is characterized by cold sensation, lack of appetite, fatigue, and weight gain. Weight gain is evidence of "dampness," which is a complication of spleen or kidney yang deficiency. The spleen and kidney are considered too weak to transform excess dampness, thus causing accumulation of fat and swelling. The clinician should appreciate that these findings are classic and may not adequately describe an individual's complete TCM diagnosis.[60]

Herbal treatment in hypothyroidism aims to strengthen qi and yang deficiency. Qi and yang tonics may include codonopsis, astragalus, epimedium, curculigo, cinnamon bark, and cuscata, to name a few.[61]

TCM therapies include acupuncture, herbs, moxibustion, nutrition, massage, and movement. The therapeutic effect of these therapies on hypothyroidism may result from promotion of T_4 deiodination with production of more active T_3.[62-65] Research in this area is necessary to understand the mechanisms of action of TCM in the treatment of thyroid disease more fully.

Yoga

Hatha Yoga is a component of the philosophical doctrine of Yoga. Hatha Yoga is the physical training that prepares the body for a spiritual path through poses (asanas), breathing exercises, and asceticism (self-denial and active self-restraint). The body is prepared with this physical practice so that the mind can meditate without obstacles. Asanas are special positions of the body that may strengthen, purify, and balance the endocrine, nervous, and circulatory systems. Although asanas are rarely prescribed to treat specific illnesses, they may have healing properties.

The shoulder-stand asana (Sarvāngāsana) may help stimulate the thyroid and parathyroid glands because these glands receive increased blood flow from the firm chin lock of the pose.[66] In this pose, the body is positioned more or less perpendicular to the floor, with the head and neck tucked under, the chest brought forward to touch the chin, and the hands strongly supporting the back (Figs. 33-1 and 33-2). Frequent practice with a skilled instructor and strengthening of the neck, back, and core muscles allow the body gradually to straighten and become more perpendicular to the floor. Contraindications to this pose include spinal osteoarthritis, cervical disk disease, neck injury, hypertension, glaucoma, stroke, and vertebrobasilar syndrome. Inversion poses such as the shoulder stand should be avoided in women who are menstruating and after the first trimester of pregnancy.[67,68]

FIGURE 33-2
Sarvāngāsana. (Courtesy of Ms. Polly Liontis, RYT.)

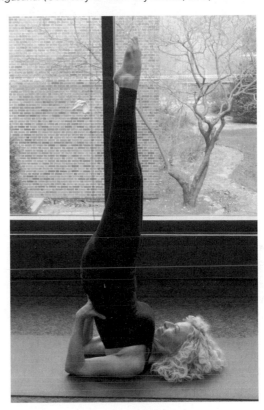

FIGURE 33-1
Modified Sarvāngāsana. (Courtesy of Ms. Polly Liontis, RYT.)

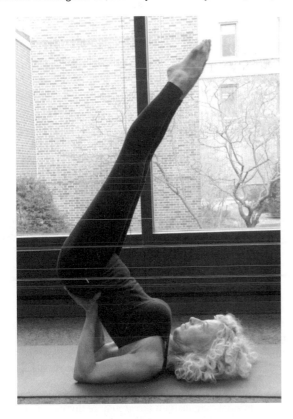

PREVENTION PRESCRIPTION

- Consume a diet with adequate amounts of iodine, selenium, iron, vitamin A, and zinc.
- Do not consume excessive amounts of iodine for long periods of time.
- Avoid substances that block thyroid hormone synthesis, such as chlorine, bromine, perchlorate, and certain medications, as well as radiation to the head and neck area when possible.

THERAPEUTIC REVIEW

Exercise

- Maintain a regular aerobic and weight-bearing exercise routine.

Nutrition

- Eat a heart-healthy, antiinflammatory diet to maintain proper body weight and reduce cardiovascular risk.

- Limit goitrogenic foods and avoid substances that interfere with thyroid activity.

- Limit vegetables from the *Brassica* family (cabbage, turnips, Brussels sprouts, rutabagas, broccoli, cauliflower, bok choy), millet, peaches, peanuts, pine nuts, strawberries, spinach, and cassava root. Cook vegetables briefly to reduce goitrogenic substances and consume at least 2 to 3 hours separately from thyroid medication.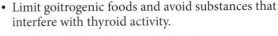

- Avoid the following medications and toxins, if possible: lithium, thionamides, amiodarone, interferon-alpha, interleukin-2, cholestyramine, perchlorate, expectorants, aluminum hydroxide, raloxifene, heavy metals, chlorine, fluoride, and bromine.

Continued

- Avoid topical antiseptics (Betadine) and radiocontrast dyes when possible.

Supplements

- Vitamins and minerals (preferably consumed in food)
  - Iodine*: 150 to 1100 mcg/day
  - Iron: 8 to 45 mg/day
  - Selenium: 55 to 400 mcg/day
  - Vitamin A†: 2300 to 10,000 units/day
  - Zinc: 8 to 40 mg/day

Botanicals

- Seaweed: Total iodine content should not exceed 1100 mcg/day for the general population unless on targeted megadose therapy. See Table 33-2 for assistance in determining allowable grams per day, depending on the variety of seaweed.

- Guggulu: Consider using it in the context of an Ayurvedic treatment regimen and not as an isolated treatment for hypothyroidism or hyperlipidemia. Take care to avoid heavy metal toxicity in certain Asian formulations.

Pharmaceuticals

- Levothyroxine alone (T_4): gold standard of therapy

- Synthetic combination T_3 plus T_4: considered if T_4 alone fails to control symptoms adequately; may use compounded formulations

- Desiccated porcine thyroid: considered if synthetic T_3 plus T_4 fails to control symptoms adequately or based on patient preference or physician experience

Traditional Chinese Medicine

- Qi and yang tonics include codonopsis, astragalus, epimedium, curculigo, cinnamon bark, and cuscata. A traditional Chinese medicine practitioner with a strong background and certification in Chinese herbalism should prescribe these combinations.

Mind-Body Therapy

- Advise yoga therapy with an emphasis on thyroid-enhancing poses such as the shoulder stand (Sarvāngāsana) if the patient has no contraindications.

- Yoga practice may be helpful even without challenging poses such as the shoulder stand, for the purposes of stress reduction, meditation, enhanced flexibility, and strength.

---

* Consider testing for iodine deficiency. Use Lugol solution or Iodoral tablet for documented deficiency for a limited time when the patient is unable to increase iodine through diet or is unable to reduce exposure to iodine-depleting medications or substances.
†Most people in the United States receive an adequate supply of preformed vitamin A (retinol) in milk, liver, margarine, and fortified cereals. Beta-carotene from plants is an excellent source of vitamin A.

KEY WEB RESOURCES

MedlinePlus information on thyroid diseases. http://www.nlm.nih.gov/medlineplus/thyroiddiseases.html.

This Web site from the U.S. National Library of Medicine of the National Institutes of Health provides patient information for the conventional diagnosis and treatment of thyroid disease.

American Thyroid Association. http://www.thyroid.org.

This Web site provides patients and physicians with guidelines for the conventional diagnosis and treatment of thyroid disease.

About.com information on thyroid disease. http://www.thyroid.about.com.

This patient advocate Web site provides a forum for patients to discuss integrative therapies for managing thyroid disease through novel testing, nutrition, supplements, and alternative thyroid medication use.

References

References are available online at expertconsult.com.

Hormone Replacement in Men

Alicia Stanton, MD

Pathophysiology

Testosterone Production

Conversion of cholesterol and steroid hormones occurs in only three organs: the adrenal cortex, the testis in men, and the ovary in women. Whereas most endocrine texts discuss adrenal, ovarian, testicular, placental, and other steroidogenic processes in a gland-specific fashion, steroidogenesis is better understood as a single process that is repeated in each gland with cell type–specific variations on a single theme.[1] The relative activity of the steroidogenic enzymes in each of the three organs determines the major secreted product. This is not absolute, however, and other organs are capable of secreting small amounts. In pathologic situations such as a defect in steroidogenesis or a steroid-secreting tumor, a very abnormal pattern of steroid secretion may be observed.[2]

Testosterone is made primarily by the testes. Testosterone production depends on intact hypothalamus, pituitary gland, and testicular Leydig cells.[3] These Leydig cells make up less than 10% of the testicular volume and produce 95% of circulating testosterone.[4] A small amount of testosterone is also produced in the adrenal glands and other tissues such as the fat cells by conversion from adrenal androgens such as dehydroepiandrosterone (DHEA) and androstenedione into testosterone.[5]

Testosterone is produced from the conversion of cholesterol, a 27-carbon molecule, by using enzymes that are cytochrome P-450 proteins requiring oxygen and reduced nicotinamide-adenine dinucleotide phosphate (NADPH). The biosynthetic pathway is largely made up of cleavage of carbon-carbon bonds and hydroxylation reactions.[1] The first and rate-limiting step in steroidogenesis is the conversion of cholesterol to pregnenolone, a 21-carbon molecule, by a single enzyme, P450scc (CYP11A1), but this enzymatically complex step is subject to multiple regulatory mechanisms.[6] Chronic quantitative regulation is principally at the level of transcription of the CYP11A1 gene encoding P450scc, which is the enzymatically rate-limiting step. Acute regulation is mediated by the steroidogenic acute regulatory protein (StAR), which facilitates the rapid influx of cholesterol into mitochondria, where P450scc resides.[1] Cholesterol is converted to pregnenolone, which produces other possible precursors such as progesterone, 17-alpha hydroxy-progesterone, androstenedione, 17-alpha hydroxy-pregnenolone, DHEA, and androstenediol. These reactions can be seen in Figure 34-1.

The anterior hypothalamus secretes gonadotropin-releasing hormone in a pulsatile fashion. This hormone then stimulates the pituitary to secrete luteinizing hormone (LH) in a pulsatile fashion as well. Investigators have established that steroidogenesis in Leydig cells is mainly regulated by LH, through the interaction with its receptors coupled to the adenylate cyclase–cyclic adenosine monophosphate signaling pathway.[6] The LH stimulates the Leydig cells in the testes to produce testosterone, a 19-carbon corticosteroid. Testosterone can then be aromatized in adipose tissue to estradiol, an 18-carbon corticosteroid. Testosterone can also be converted, by 5-alpha-reductase, to dihydrotestosterone (DHT).

Dihydrotestosterone

DHT, one of the two important androgens in boys and men, is synthesized in the prostate, testes, hair follicles, and adrenal glands. In men, approximately 5% of testosterone undergoes 5-alpha reduction to form the more potent androgen DHT. DHT has three times greater affinity for androgen receptors than does testosterone.[7] During embryogenesis, DHT has an essential role in the formation of the male external genitalia, and in the adult, DHT acts as the primary androgen in the prostate and hair follicles.

DHT is generated by reduction of testosterone by the enzyme 5-alpha-reductase (Fig. 34-2). Two isoenzymes of 5-alpha-reductase have been discovered. Type 1 is present in most tissues of the body where 5-alpha-reductase is expressed and is dominant in sebaceous glands. Type 2 5-alpha-reductase is dominant in genital tissues, including

FIGURE 34-1

The steroidogenic pathways. DHEA, dehydroepiandrosterone; DHT, dihydrotestosterone.

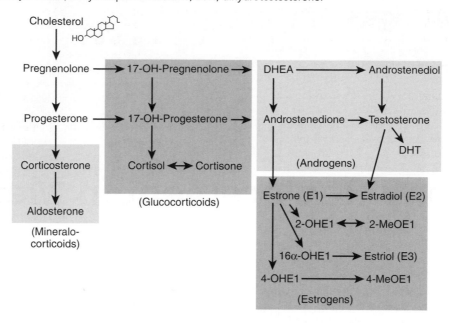

FIGURE 34-2

Androgens. DHEA, dehydroepiandrosterone; DHT, dihydrotestosterone.

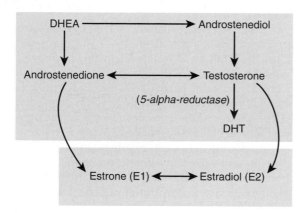

BOX 34-1. 5-Alpha-Reductase Inhibitors

Finasteride
Dutasteride
Zinc
Progesterone
Saw palmetto
L-Lysine
Epigallocatechin gallate (ECGC)
Linolenic acid

the prostate.[8] Because DHT is the primary prostatic androgen, it may have a significant role in prostate disease pathogenesis.[9] In reality, the prostate has only one function, which is to secrete seminal fluid to support the sperm, assisting in reproduction. This process requires an extremely high concentration of androgens in the tissues. This allows DHT, with its greater affinity for testosterone receptors, to enhance the tissue response to androgens in the prostate.

Benign prostatic hypertrophy (BPH) seems to be related to long-term exposure of the prostate to DHT and possibly to estrogens.[10] Serum DHT levels are not elevated in humans with BPH; they remain at a normal level with aging despite a decrease in plasma testosterone.[8] Investigators hypothesized that DHT may provide an amplification mechanism for testosterone that could be a beneficial effect in men with low

circulating testosterone. Since then, the essential role of DHT in the development of BPH has been recognized; treatment has focused on blocking the 5-alpha-reductase enzymes (Box 34-1).[11,12]

The normal level of DHT in the blood is approximately one tenth that of testosterone, but the affinity of DHT for androgen receptors is three times greater. Amory et al[13] looked at the effects of reduction of serum DHT on bone mineral density, serum lipoproteins, hemoglobin, prostate-specific antigen (PSA), and sexual function in healthy young men. By blocking 5-alpha-reductase using dutasteride and finasteride, these investigators significantly suppressed circulating DHT levels. They found that this therapy did not affect bone mineral density, markers of the metabolism, serum lipoproteins, or hemoglobin. Serum PSA and self-assessed sexual function decreased during treatment with both 5-alpha-reductase inhibitors but returned to baseline during follow-up.[13] Therefore, sexual function has some relationship with the circulating serum level of DHT, and aggressively lowering that level, even without lowering testosterone, may potentially affect libido and sexual arousal.

Dehydroepiandrosterone

DHEA is not a hormone. It is a very important prohormone secreted in large amounts by the adrenals in humans and other primates, but not in lower species. DHEA is secreted in larger quantities than cortisol and is second in blood concentration only to cholesterol.[14] Humans are unique in that their adrenal glands can secrete large amounts of DHEA and its sulfate (DHEA-S), which are converted to androstenedione and then into androgens and estrogens and peripheral tissues. This gives the tissues autonomous intracrine control, so they can adjust the formation and metabolism of active sex steroids according to local requirements. Investigators have estimated that 30% to 50% of total androgens in men are synthesized in peripheral intracrine tissues from an adrenal precursors.[15]

> Intracrinology, a term coined in 1988, describes local formation, action, and inactivation of the sex steroids from the inactive sex steroid precursor dehydroepiandrosterone.[16]

When human development is completed and adulthood is reached, DHEA and DHEA-S levels start to decline from age 25 years. By 70 to 80 years of age, peak DHEA-S concentrations are only 10% to 20% of those in young adults.[14,17] The marked reduction in the production of DHEA-S by the adrenals during aging results in the dramatic fall in the availability of active sex steroids in peripheral target tissues. This change is thought to be associated with age-related illnesses such as insulin resistance, obesity, osteoporosis, cardiovascular disease, loss of muscle mass, cancer, and other diseases.[15] Genazzani et al[17] discussed the findings that DHEA appears to be beneficial in hypoandrogenic men, as well as in postmenopausal and aging women.

DHEA administration has been shown to reduce accumulation of abdominal visceral fat and protect against insulin resistance. Villareal et al[18] showed that DHEA therapy, when compared with placebo in a randomized double-blind placebo-controlled trial, resulted in a significant decrease in visceral and subcutaneous fat, as well as in a significant increase in insulin sensitivity. A possible explanation for the findings is that DHEA is an activator of peroxisome proliferator-activated receptor-alpha (PPAR-alpha). Activation of PPAR-alpha induces transcriptional up-regulation of fatty acid transport proteins that facilitate fatty acid entry into cells and the enzymes involved in the beta oxidation of fatty acids. This process favors increased fat oxidation and reduced fat deposition.[18] Hernández-Morante et al[19] took this one step further and focused on gender-specific fat distribution. They found that serum DHEA-S was inversely and specifically associated with visceral fat area, as assessed by computed tomography in men and with waist-to-hip ratio (WHR) in women. Therefore, DHEA-S promotes lipolysis preferably in subcutaneous fat in women and in visceral fat in men.[19]

The activation of PPAR-alpha also gives DHEA-S a role in inhibition of vascular inflammation in human aortic endothelial cells. Altman et al[20] found that DHEA-S can reduce inflammation in vascular endothelial cells by a mechanism involving the PPAR-alpha receptor that inhibits transcription factors involved in endothelial cell inflammation. In addition, treatment of endothelial cells with DHEA-S dramatically inhibited the tumor necrosis factor-alpha–induced activation of necrosis factor (NF)-kappa beta-alpha, an inflammatory transcription factor. These results signified the ability of DHEA-S to inhibit the inflammatory process and showed potential direct effects on vascular inflammation.[20] DHEA was also shown to increase endothelial cell proliferation and enhance large and small vessel endothelial cell function.[21,22]

Because visceral fat, inflammation, and endothelial cell function are all related to cardiovascular disease, correlation of DHEA levels with the risk of cardiovascular disease makes sense. In fact, this association was seen in several studies. In 2003, Thijs et al[23] looked at a total of 12 studies and calculated the pool relative risk associated with levels of DHEA-S. These investigators found a 13% increase in fatal coronary heart disease with a 2 micromol/L decrease in DHEA-S.[23] Barrett-Connor et al[24] studied the relationship of baseline circulating DHEA-S levels with subsequent 12-year mortality from any cause, from cardiovascular disease, and from ischemic heart disease in a cohort of men aged 50 to 79 years at the start of the study. The mean DHEA-S levels decreased with age and were significantly lower in men with a history of heart disease. In addition, these investigators found that an increase in DHEA-S was associated with a reduction in overall mortality from any cause and an even greater reduction in mortality from cardiovascular disease. These investigators concluded that DHEA-S concentration is independently and inversely related to death from any cause and death from cardiovascular disease in men older than 50 years.[24] These results were confirmed in 2010 by Ohlsson et al[25] after studying a cohort of 2644 men, age 69 to 81 years, with a mean follow-up of 4.5 years. These investigators concluded that low serum levels of DHEA-S predict death from all causes, from cardiovascular disease, and from ischemic heart disease in older men.[25] What we do not know at this time, however, is whether supplementing with DHEA reduces risk or is safe with regard to other risks, such as prostate cancer.

Estrogen

Testosterone can be converted into estradiol by an aromatase enzyme. Androstenedione can also be converted into estrone, which can then be converted into estradiol through a reversible reaction. Androgen-to-estrogen conversion, however, is irreversible. Because aromatase enzymes are seen in fat cells, obesity is associated with increased conversion of testosterone to estradiol. Aromatase levels are known to rise with age.[26] This increase often causes a relative imbalance of estrogen and testosterone in men as they grow older. In addition to having a decreased output of testosterone with age, the age-related increase of aromatase causes older men to convert what testosterone they do produce into estrogen.

Other possible mechanisms for increasing aromatization to estradiol include liver dysfunction, zinc deficiency, and excessive alcohol consumption.[27] Excess estrogen or an elevated estrogen-to-testosterone ratio can cause gynecomastia, breast tenderness, BPH (from estrogenic stimulation of the prostate stromal tissue), and impotence (from blockage of DHT receptors by estradiol).[28]

However, estrogen plays several very important roles in men. These roles were elucidated when a few men who lacked aromatase or estrogen receptors were studied. Investigators found that these men had problems including osteopenia, abnormal lipid profiles, hyperinsulinemia, and glucose intolerance.[29,30] When appropriately balanced with testosterone, estrogen also appears to have a role in libido and sexual desire in men. In a study by Carani et al,[31] a man who lacked aromatase enzyme was followed during the course of testosterone therapy, estradiol therapy, and combination therapy with estradiol and testosterone. His libido significantly improved only with combination therapy.[31]

> To help maintain an optimal balance of estradiol and testosterone naturally, the patient should appropriately manage his weight, with a focus on limiting central adiposity. In addition, he should limit alcohol, caffeinated beverages, and tightly fitting undergarments because these stimulate conversion of testosterone to estradiol. If lifestyle changes are not enough, the use of aromatase inhibitors may be necessary (Box 34-2).

Testosterone Decline

The daily average production of testosterone in healthy young men is 7 mg. Testosterone levels peak for men in their 20s. After the age of 40 years, a 0.2% to 2% annual decline is observed in morning total testosterone.[32] Half the healthy men between the ages of 50 and 70 years have a bioavailable testosterone level lower than the lowest level seen in healthy men who are 20 to 40 years of age.[33] At the age of 75 years, the mean total testosterone level in the morning is approximately 66% of the mean level at age 20 to 30 years. However, the mean free testosterone and bioactive testosterone (free testosterone plus albumin-bound testosterone) levels are only 40% of the mean levels in younger men.[34] Testosterone levels decline because of decreased production secondary to reduced Leydig cell activity and decreasing LH, as well as increased binding of available testosterone by sex hormone–binding globulin.[35]

Testosterone has a circadian rhythm. Testosterone levels are approximately 20% higher in the morning than in the evening. Investigators noted that the circadian rhythm in serum testosterone levels found in normal young men is markedly attenuated or absent in healthy older men. The early morning rising testosterone levels characteristic of young men is not present in the older men.[36] Research suggests that the decline in nocturnal testosterone secretion appears to involve a combination of testicular and pituitary hypogonadism.[32]

In 2006, Travison et al[37] observed that recent years had seen a substantial and yet unrecognized age-independent population level decrease of testosterone in men in the United States. These investigators reported that a population level decline was greater in magnitude than the cross-sectional decline in testosterone typically associated with age. They hypothesized that the observed age-matched decline resulted from an undocumented historical or contemporary or environmental influence that had not yet been identified.[37] Obesity, stress, medication use, metabolic syndrome, and environmental toxins such as bisphenol A (BPA) and phthalates are known to contribute to low testosterone.[38-43] Therefore, patients should be monitored for signs and

BOX 34-2. Aromatase Inhibitors

Anastrozole (Arimidex)
Letrozole (Femara)
Quercetin
Chrysin*
Resveratrol/grape seed extract
Zinc
Progesterone

*Many studies show limited usefulness.

symptoms of low testosterone. Helping them understand that things they can do in everyday life may to help maintain optimal testosterone levels is even more important. Besides aging alone, lifestyle and different comorbidities are associated with the decline in total testosterone level. This finding suggests that the age-related decline in total testosterone may be at least partly prevented through the management of potentially modifiable risk factors and health-related behavior.[11]

> Obesity, stress, metabolic syndrome, and environmental toxins (bisphenol A, phthalates) can lead to low testosterone levels. Exercise, avoiding weight gain, and not smoking can reduce the rate of decline of testosterone.

Mortality

Several studies have linked androgen deficiency to increased mortality in men.[44] In 2007, Maggio et al[45] looked at the mortality rate of men over the course of 6 years in the InCHIANTI study compared with their levels of testosterone, DHEA-S, and insulin-like growth factor-I (as an indicator of growth hormone level). These investigators stated: "Multisystem disorders that are widely prevalent in aging, such as the metabolic syndrome, frailty syndrome, and chronic heart failure, are more significantly associated with multiple hormonal dysregulation rather than a single hormonal derangement. Studies have found that the risk of death increases progressively with the number of dysregulated hormones and becomes 2.5 times higher when 3 hormones are dysregulated compared with no dysregulation."[45] Laughlin et al,[46] in the Rancho Bernardo study, followed 794 men for up to 20 years (average, 11.8 years) and found that men with total testosterone and bioavailable testosterone levels in the lowest quartile were 40% more likely to die of all causes than were men with testosterone levels in the highest quartile.

Symptoms Associated With Low Testosterone

Approximately 30% of men 60 years old and older are estimated to have low testosterone,[47] which is often accompanied by undesirable signs and symptoms such as low bone and muscle mass, increased fat mass (especially central adiposity), low energy, low libido, and impaired physical, sexual, and cognitive function. That these complaints have clinical consequences is supported by prospective cohort studies showing that men with low testosterone are at increased risk of falls[48]; hip fracture, if estradiol is also low[49]; anemia[50]; type 2 diabetes[51]; depressive illness[52]; and, in some studies, Alzheimer disease.[53,54] Table 34-1 is a review of evidence regarding testosterone and specific conditions.[26,44,47,51,54-73]

TABLE 34-1. Evidence of Androgen-Deficient Effects on Specific Conditions

CONDITION	EVIDENCE
Obesity	BMI is inversely associated with free testosterone. This may be related to the increased conversion of testosterone to estrogen by aromatase that occurs in visceral fat.[26]
Metabolic syndrome	Low TT may predict the onset of diabetes and has been associated with increased risk.[55–57] High TT is associated with less risk.[51] Low TT is associated with insulin resistance and risk of metabolic syndrome.[44,58] A meta-analysis of 20 studies found that testosterone therapy resulted in a reduction in FBS, TG, and waist circumference and a rise in HDL.[58]
Heart disease	TT is lower in men with CVD.[44] Low TT is associated with visceral obesity, insulin resistance, low HDL, and high TG and LDL.[59] Low TT is associated with an increased risk of aortic atherosclerosis independent of BMI, lipids, smoking, and ETOH intake.[54,60] Low TT is associated with hyperlipidemia including TC, LDL, and TG.[61,62] Low TT is associated with higher mortality in men with CAD.[63]
Alzheimer disease	Androgens and estrogens have a neuroprotective effect and have been associated with less beta amyloid plaque and enhanced neuron survival in AD.[64] AD patients treated with testosterone improved over the course of a year.[65] High TT levels have been associated with better performance in memory, executive function, and spatial ability.[66,67]
Depression	Some studies suggest low TT in depressed men.[68,69] Men with low TT often present with depressive symptoms.[70] In men with refractory depression, those treated with testosterone gel versus placebo had greater improvement in Hamilton depression scores, a finding suggesting potential benefit in augmenting therapy in this population.[71] This gel appears less beneficial as monotherapy.[72]
Osteoporosis	Low TT is found in 20% of men with symptomatic vertebral fractures and in 50% of older men with hip fractures.[73] Testosterone therapy along with calcium, vitamin D, weight-bearing exercises, smoking cessation, falls prevention, and limited ETOH intake, should be considered in men with osteoporosis.[47]

AD, Alzheimer disease; BMI, body mass index; CAD, coronary artery disease; CVD, cardiovascular disease; ETOH, ethyl alcohol; FBS, fasting blood sugar; HDL, high-density lipoprotein; LDL, low-density lipoprotein; TC, total cholesterol; TG, triglycerides; TT, total testosterone.

BOX 34-3. Physical Signs of Testosterone Deficiency

Dry eyes
Reduced muscle tone
Depressed attitude
Poor concentration and memory
Decreased axillary and pubic hair
Pale skin
Anemia
Increased fat deposits in breast, abdomen, and hips
Nervousness and irritability

BOX 34-4. Signs and Symptoms of Low Testosterone

Decreased muscle mass and strength
Decreased sex drive
Reduced frequency and firmness of erections; reduced ejaculate volume
Hot flushes
Excessive emotions and sensitivity to difficulty
Unnecessary worry, anxiety, and fear
Depression
Loss of self-confidence
Joint pains
Persistent fatigue that increases with activity

From Hertoghe T. *The Hormone Handbook*. Walton-on-Thames, UK: International Medical Publications; 2006:219.

Diagnosis of Testosterone Deficiency

The diagnosis of testosterone deficiency rests on physical signs, symptoms, and laboratory values demonstrating symptomatic, inadequate testosterone levels. Men with acquired hypogonadism, as seen after trauma or orchiectomy, note certain well-documented changes in body composition, mood, strength, libido, and erectile function. Because testosterone levels naturally decrease with aging, it can be difficult to define which older men are actually androgen deficient and should have testosterone therapy. Therefore, each individual patient should be treated based on specific signs and symptoms (Boxes 34-3 and 34-4) combined with laboratory assessment showing low testosterone levels.

■ Laboratory Testing for Testosterone Deficiency

Testosterone can be evaluated by several testing modalities. These include tests of serum, urine, saliva, and capillary blood spot. However, most published studies on testosterone use serum levels. That being said, follow-up testing should be done with consideration for the therapeutic modality being used. For example, serum levels are excellent ways to measure testosterone therapy that uses injections, pellets, transdermal gels, and oral micronized testosterone. However, transdermal creams do not readily equilibrate in the serum for several weeks and thus may be more difficult to evaluate. Saliva and urine tests are better for evaluating transdermal creams.

> Serum testing is best for measuring testosterone therapy given by injection, pellets, transdermal gels, and oral micronized oral formulations. Saliva and urine tests are better modalities for evaluating transdermal creams.

Testing should be done at the same time of the day each time, preferably first thing in the morning. For optimal results, the patient should avoid sexual intercourse, vigorous exercise, or intense emotional stress for 24 to 72 hours before testing. In addition to testing testosterone levels, evaluation of other hormones should be done as well, especially before starting testosterone therapy. Because metabolic syndrome and cardiovascular disease are so closely tied to testosterone deficiency, evaluations of insulin sensitivity and cardiovascular risk factors are important. The function of the hypothalamic-pituitary-adrenal (HPA) axis is also closely tied to testosterone level and to the success of therapy. Therefore, I recommend a four-point cortisol level to evaluate diurnal cortisol rhythms in the health of the HPA axis (Box 34-5).

Integrative Therapy

Supplements

Zinc
Zinc is an important cofactor in many metabolic reactions within the body. In addition, zinc has been implicated in testicular development, sperm maturation, and testosterone synthesis. Therefore, zinc deficiency may affect testosterone production and male fertility.[74] Hartoma et al[75,76] were able to demonstrate a significant positive correlation between serum zinc and serum testosterone in men 36 to 60 years old.

In rats, cadmium toxicity was used to induce testicular disease that resulted in significant decreases in plasma testosterone level, sperm count, and motility. The addition of zinc and selenium to the cadmium caused reductions in the serum and testicular cadmium concentrations and offered more efficient protection against testicular damage.[77] Another article by He et al[78] showed that supplementation with zinc and selenium are "favorably related to androgen deficiency and sperm production." Netter et al[79] looked at men with idiopathic infertility of more than 5 years' duration. These investigators found that when serum testosterone was low, administration of oral zinc increased testosterone, DHT, and sperm count. In the group whose testosterone level was within normal limits, administration of oral zinc did not increase testosterone or sperm count. However, DHT increased significantly.[79]

BOX 34-5. Recommended Baseline Laboratory Testing for Testosterone Deficiency (Serum)

Total and free testosterone
Sex hormone–binding globulin (SHBG)
Dihydrotestosterone
Dehydroepiandrosterone (DHEA)
Ultrasensitive estradiol
Luteinizing hormone and follicle-stimulating hormone (LH and FSH)
Prolactin (prolactinoma can suppress testosterone levels)
Prostate-specific antigen (PSA)
Complete blood cell count (CBC)
Chemistry panel with liver functions tests (LFTs)
Lipid panel
Fasting insulin
Fasting glucose
Hemoglobin A1c
Cardiovascular C-reactive protein
Homocysteine
Vitamin D
Zinc level
Salivary diurnal cortisol

The relationships among chronic renal disease, zinc deficiency, low libido, and testosterone levels have been studied for decades. In 1977, Antoniou et al[80] looked at impotent men who were undergoing hemodialysis and who had low plasma zinc levels, low libido, and low plasma testosterone. These investigators compared administration of zinc with that of placebo and found that, "dialytic administration of zinc strikingly improved potency in all patients and raised the plasma testosterone to normal in those with low testosterone. Zinc deficiency is a reversible cause of gonadal dysfunction."[80] In 2010, Vecchio et al[81] also studied sexual dysfunction in patients with chronic kidney disease. These investigators found that "oral zinc improved the end of treatment testosterone levels."[81]

■ Dosage
Usual dose is 15 to 30 mg daily.

■ Precautions
Zinc should not be given with other minerals because of inhibition of absorption (particularly copper).

Botanicals

Saw Palmetto
Saw palmetto (Serenoa repens) is a weak inhibitor of 5-alpha-reductase. Therefore, it could reduce the conversion of testosterone to DHT. It may also have a role in reducing the number of estrogen and DHT receptors. Sinescu et al[82] showed that long-term treatment with 320 mg Serenoa repens proved to be efficient in reducing urinary obstruction and improving symptoms and quality of life in patients with BPH.

Wilt et al[83] stated that the evidence suggests that Serenoa repens improves urologic symptoms and flow measures.

Compared with finasteride, *Serenoa repens* produced similar improvements in urinary tract symptoms and urinary flow and was associated with fewer adverse treatment events. Further research is needed using standardized preparations of *Serenoa repens* to determine its long-term effectiveness and ability to prevent complications of BPH despite recent research showing limited benefit.[83]

Bonvissuto et al[84] studied the antiinflammatory effects of *Serenoa repens,* lycopene, and selenium on prostate inflammation in rats. These investigators showed that, in comparison with single agents, the combination of *Serenoa repens,* lycopene, and selenium in vivo reduced prostate inflammation induced in rats by bladder outlet obstruction.[84]

■ Dosage
The dose is 160 mg twice daily or 320 mg daily.

■ Precautions
Side effects are mainly gastrointestinal, including nausea, vomiting, constipation, and diarrhea. Saw palmetto can also cause dizziness.

Chrysin
Chrysin is a naturally occurring flavone that can be chemically extracted from the blue passion flower *(Passiflora caerulea).* It is also reported in *Oroxylum indicum* or Indian trumpet flower. Flavones, or flavonoids, have been used as drugs and food supplements and are reported to have antioxidant, antibacterial, antiinflammatory, and antiviral properties.[85,86] Chrysin (5,7-dihydroxyflavone) was once believed to be an effective aromatase inhibitor, inhibiting the conversion of testosterone to estradiol and decreasing the levels of estrogen in the body. Several in vitro studies supported the aromatase inhibitory activity of chrysin. In the 1980s, Kellis et al[87,88] found that chrysin had significant aromatase-inhibitory activity when it was tested with placental microsomes. Afterward, several other studies drew similar conclusions.[89-94]

However, the growing consensus is that chrysin has limited effect on estrogen levels in either animals or humans. Unfortunately, follow-up studies have determined that cell membranes effectively block chrysin from entering the cells and having any effect at all on estrogen levels in biologic organisms.[90,95,96] In vivo studies involving biologic organisms lend support to the observation that chrysin has no effect on estrogen levels, but it may have other detrimental effects on the body, particularly on thyroid function.[97]

Lifestyle Overview

Lifestyle plays a critical role in the balance of male hormones. The hypogonadal axis is very closely tied to diet, amount and quality of sleep, level of stress, and toxin exposure. Therefore, whether or not hormone therapy is to be instituted, lifestyle factors need to be evaluated and corrected.

Toxin Exposure

Increasing numbers of reports suggest that chemical and physical agents in the environment affect testosterone levels and male fertility. The different potential toxin exposures include pesticides, food additives and preservatives, organophosphates, polychlorinated biphenyls (PCBs), electromagnetic radiation, heavy metal toxicity, phthalates, and BPA. The additives in our food and processed foods, such as refined sugar and high-fructose corn syrup, create a strain in the detoxification system as we try to handle foods our body was never intended to use. In addition, many of these additives, such as hydrogenated fats, high-fructose corn syrup, artificial sweeteners, flavor enhancers, and preservatives, do not contain beneficial nutrients. Therefore, we are eating foods that may add calories without providing nutrition, thus creating hormone imbalance.

Phthalates
Phthalates are esters of phthalic acid and are mainly used as plasticizers. Billions of pounds of phthalates had been produced worldwide. Phthalates were introduced in the 1920s and are currently used for enteric coatings, viscosity control agents, lubricants, and binders.[98] We come in contact with phthalates every day in our shampoos, colognes, detergents, cleaning materials, paints, food packaging, and many other places. In 2008, the United States Research Council[41] recommended investigating the cumulative effect of phthalates and other antiandrogens. The Council stressed that the effect of phthalates should be examined together with other antiandrogens, which otherwise may have been excluded, because their structures were different. Various effects on the development of the reproductive system can be observed in boys and men at much lower doses than previously observed after exposure to various phthalates. Phthalate syndrome has been described and includes infertility, decreased sperm count, cryptorchidism, hypospadias, and other reproductive tract malformations.[41]

Bisphenol A
BPA has been used in commerce since the 1960s and is primarily used to make plastics. It is currently used in polycarbonate bottles (clear, flexible plastic) such as water bottles. It is also found in baby bottles, dental sealants, sports equipment, eyeglasses, CDs and DVDs, and in the lining of aluminum cans.[99] BPA is a known endocrine disrupter and can mimic estrogens.[100] Early development appears to be the time of greatest sensitivity to its effects. In 2007, a consensus statement by 38 experts on BPA concluded that the average levels in people are higher than those that cause harm to animals in laboratory experiments.[101] BPA and phthalates appear to be related to obesity. In 2008, Elobeid et al[102] concluded that obesity may be increased as a function of BPA exposure. In 2009, Rubin et al[103] stated that in a review of available studies, perinatal BPA exposure acts to exert persistent effects on body weight and adiposity. The relationship is strong enough that another review in 2009 concluded that eliminating exposures to BPA and improving nutrition during development offered the potential for reducing obesity and associated diseases.[104]

BPA is also linked to prostate disease. A 2006 study in rats showed that neonatal BPA exposure at 10 mcg/kg levels increased prostate gland susceptibility to adult-onset precancerous lesions and hormonal carcinogenesis.[105] In 2007, Richter et al[106] did an in vitro study showing that BPA exposure is associated with permanently increased prostate size. The correlation was confirmed again in 2009, when

Prins et al[107] found that newborn rats exposed to a low dose of BPA (10 mcg/ kg) had increased prostate cancer susceptibility as adults.

Organophosphates and Polychlorinated Biphenyls

Organophosphates and PCBs are also creating problems. Several studies suggested that human semen quality has declined over the past decades, and some investigators associated this decline with occupational exposure to pesticides. In 2008, Recio-Vega et al[108] evaluated the effect on semen quality of organophosphate pesticides at three occupational exposure levels. The worst semen quality was found among subjects with the highest organophosphate exposure and the highest urinary organophosphate levels.[108] PCBs are a class of persistent organic pollutants that were widely used in the midtwentieth century. Although their production and use was banned in most countries several decades ago, the general population continues to be exposed because of the persistence and accumulation of PCBs. Regardless of study design or measurement method, the adverse association between PCB level and sperm motility may suggest a lack of exposure threshold for PCB-related effect on sperm motility. In addition, some studies also reported an adverse association between PCBs and circulating testosterone levels in men.[109,110]

Reducing Toxin Exposure

Although many of our foods come in packaging that contains BPA, we can still reduce our exposure. Plastic should not be heated, given that heating can trigger release of chemicals. This is true even for microwave-safe containers because, although they do not disintegrate, they may still leach toxins into the food. Plastic storage containers are also labeled depending on the type of resin used to make the container. The bottom of plastic containers usually has a triangle with a number that identifies the type of resin used. Containers marked with a number 2 (high-density polyethylene), number 4 (low-density polyethylene), or number 5 (polypropylene) are designed to be reused and do not leach chemicals. Bottles marked number 1 (polyethylene terephthalate) are for one-time use and should not be reused; however, they are safe for the one-time use. Containers marked number 3 (polyvinyl chloride), number 6 (polystyrene), and number 7 (polycarbonate) leach chemicals into the food and should be avoided. Polycarbonate plastics (number 7) leach the most BPA. Some plastics made from corn husks and other plants are a more environmentally safe, sustainable option. These are labeled number 7 PLA (polylactide biodegradable corn), and they should be used when available. Plastic wrap, freezer bags, and sandwich bags may or may not leach chemicals. It depends on the brand. The National Geographic Society produces the Green Guide (www.TheGreenGuide.com), which provides an updated list of specific safe brands of freezer bags and sandwich bags.

> Plastics marked with a number 2, 4, 5, and 7 PLA are the safest to use. Those marked with a number 1 should be used only once, and those marked with a 3, 6, or 7 should not be used at all. Those marked as 7 PLA (made from corn husks) appear to be safe.

Mind-Body Therapy: Stress Reduction

The HPA axis, the mediator of cortisol, plays an essential role in hormone balance and general homeostasis. That acute distress activates the sympathetic nervous system and HPA axis is well documented. In addition, chronic stress, with its prolonged high cortisol levels and subsequent increases in visceral adipose tissue, can create a vicious circle. Visceral fat leads to increased inflammation and cytokine production, which creates increased demand for cortisol and increased visceral adipose tissue. Studies have shown that patients with central obesity have increased cortisol secretion. A high WHR is associated with low production of sex steroids, such as testosterone in men.[111] In addition, studies of the HPA axis and the hypothalamic-pituitary-testicular (HPT) axis have revealed a reciprocal relationship between these two endocrine pathways. Stress can have varying effects on testosterone secretion, and increased levels of glucocorticoids can abolish normal HPT rhythmicity.[112] Rivier[113] hypothesized that cytokine release by inflamed tissues, an event that may precede any symptoms, is responsible for activation of the HPA axis and, independently, for decreased activity of the HPT axis.

Long-term overactivation of the HPA axis results in low diurnal cortisol variation and blunted dexamethasone suppression, findings that indicate abnormal regulation of the HPA axis. This HPA axis abnormality has been reported to be a characteristic consequence of frequently repeated or chronic environmental stress challenges. Rosmond et al[114] studied men with normal cortisol variability as compared with those with low variability (abnormal HPA regulation). These investigators showed that in men with low diurnal cortisol variability, stress-related cortisol secretion showed a strong negative relationship with testosterone, insulin-like growth factor-I, high-density lipoprotein, and obesity factors (body mass index, WHR) and blood pressure.[114] The close association of HPA axis dysfunction may explain the previously reported powerful risk of abdominal obesity on low testosterone, cardiovascular disease, type 2 diabetes, and stroke.[115]

Sleep

A very strong relationship exists between sleep efficacy and testosterone production. In addition, increased concentrations in HPA axis hormones have been noted in sleep-deprived individuals. Changes in nocturnal testosterone are sleep related, with levels rising during sleep and falling on waking. Peak testosterone levels coincide with rapid eye movement (REM) sleep onset. The decreasing sleep efficacy in numbers of REM sleep episodes with altered REM sleep latency is associated with lower concentrations of circulating testosterone. This situation is normally seen in older men. In addition, sleep curtailment has been shown to lead to reduced levels of circulating androgens in healthy young men as well.[116] Penev[117] objectively measured differences in amount of nighttime sleep and showed that the amount of nighttime sleep was an independent predictor of the morning total testosterone levels of his subjects. Reduced sleep duration is also associated with an increased incidence of type 2 diabetes. Short sleep times of 5.5 hours per night were associated with weight gain, reduced oral glucose tolerance, and reduced insulin sensitivity[118] (see Chapter 8, Insomnia).

A poor sleep-wake cycle is associated not only with low testosterone but also with abnormalities in progesterone, prolactin, cortisol, dopamine, norepinephrine, and adrenocorticotropic hormone. Improving the sleep-wake cycle is vital in improving hormone balance.

Nutrition

Following a diet focused on limiting insulin resistance is important. As previously described, low testosterone is closely associated with insulin resistance, metabolic syndrome, and type 2 diabetes. I recommend that my patients eat smaller meals every 2 to 3 hours to maintain a steady blood glucose level. The meals and snacks should consist of lean proteins (e.g., poultry, fish, beef, nuts, eggs, and beans), vegetables and high-fiber fruits, and monosaturated and polyunsaturated fats. To avoid pesticide, antibiotic, and xenohormone exposure, consumption of organic foods is important.

In addition, patients should avoid refined carbohydrates and sugar as found in sweets, soft drinks, cookies, breads, and pastas (see Chapter 85, The Glycemic Index/Load). Ethanol is known to increase cortisol, reduce LH, and reduce testosterone production. It was originally thought to do so by directly affecting the hypothalamic-pituitary axis.[119,120] However, a study by Emanuele et al[121] demonstrated that the suppression of the reproductive axis is independent of the hypothalamic-pituitary axis. Therefore, limitation of alcohol also optimizes testosterone therapy and treatment.

Exercise

Exercise, especially resistance training, is an important adjunct to testosterone therapy and prevention of osteoporosis. Testosterone is one of the most potent androgenic-anabolic hormones, and its biologic effects include promotion of muscle growth. In general, testosterone concentration is elevated directly following heavy resistance exercise in men.[122] Resistance exercise has been shown to elicit a significant acute hormonal response. Anabolic hormones such as testosterone and growth hormone have been shown to be elevated 15 to 30 minutes after exercise as long as adequate stimulus has been given. Protocols high in volume, moderate to high in intensity, with easy short rest intervals and stress in a large muscle mass, tend to produce the greatest acute hormone elevations.[123] Specifically, training involves frequent repetitions of moderate weight, and the dynamic components tend to produce its beneficial results.[124]

One of the most efficient ways to increase endogenous testosterone is through regular resistance exercise.

Kraemer et al[125] were able to show that trained individuals could exhibit early-phase endocrine adaptations during a resistance training program. Their protocol consisted of 1 week of preconditioning orientation followed by 8 weeks of heavy resistance training. Serum total testosterone concentrations were significantly higher for men at all points measured, and exercise-induced increases in growth hormone over the preexercise values were observed at all phases of training.[125] Another study looked at the effect of circadian rhythm in the interactions of cortisol and testosterone with resistance training.[126] Elevated postexercise testosterone concentrations can be modulated by dietary nutrients such as adequate fat and an appropriate protein-to-carbohydrate ratio.[127,128]

Pharmaceuticals: Hormonal Therapy

Testosterone Therapy Overview

Testosterone therapy has been shown to alleviate certain symptoms associated with low testosterone. Before prescribing testosterone therapy, the clinician should document the diagnosis of hypogonadism, make a list of signs and symptoms to support a diagnosis, and evaluate the patient for possible causes and complications of hypogonadism. A complete hormone profile and general health panel should also be reviewed, and attention should be paid to balancing all hormones, especially cortisol and insulin. Pay close attention to the prolactin level because a prolactinoma can cause low testosterone. In addition, as previously described, the patient must optimize lifestyle factors to support testosterone therapy further.

Box 34-6 lists considerations before initiating testosterone therapy. The clinician should discuss with the patient the possible therapeutic modalities including creams, gels, patches, injections, and so on, to determine which modality he wishes to use. If the patient wishes to maintain his fertility, hCG must be used to stimulate his natural production of testosterone. Testosterone replacement will reduce sperm count and inhibit fertility. For hCG to work, testicular function must be intact. Therefore, the LH level should be in the normal range. Contraindications to therapy are listed later in this chapter. Obviously, it is prudent not to start testosterone therapy in a patient with a contraindication.

Testosterone Cypionate, Propionate, and Enathenate Esters

The most commonly used forms of androgen replacement therapy include 17β-hydroxyl esters of testosterone administered with slow-release, oil-based vehicles. Commonly used intramuscular injectable testosterone esters are testosterone enanthate, propionate, and cypionate.[129-131] The different esters absorb at various rates and have different half-lives.

BOX 34-6. Considerations for Initiating Testosterone Therapy

What form will the patient use (gel, injection, pellet, patch)?
Does the patient wish to maintain his fertility?
What is the testicular function?
What lifestyle changes does the patient need to make?
Does the patient have a contraindication to therapy? (see Box 34-8)

Dosage

Testosterone cypionate is one of the most widely used intramuscular testosterone esters. At a dose of 200 to 250 mg, the optimal injection interval is 2 to 3 weeks, but peak and trough values are clearly higher and lower than the normal range.[129] More often, it is dosed more frequently at 50 to 100 mg once or twice a week, to avoid the high peaks and troughs. In addition, it can be dosed subcutaneously at 30 to 50 mg twice a week. Many of my patients tolerate subcutaneous administration well. It is easy for them to self-administer and does not cause significant peak or trough symptoms.

Topical Testosterone Creams and Gels

Commercially available testosterone products on the market include testosterone gels, AndroGel and Testim, and the Androderm testosterone patch. Transdermal administration delivers testosterone at a controlled rate into the systemic circulation by avoiding hepatic first pass and reproducing the diurnal rhythm of testosterone secretion, without the peak and trough levels observed in long-acting testosterone injections.[132] These patches have a reservoir containing testosterone with a permeation-enhancing vehicle and gelling agents. Clinical efficacy is as good as with conventional testosterone ester injections.

Dosage

Testosterone gels and creams can be made by compounding pharmacies in any dosage requested. I find that my compounded dosages are much lower than those currently available on the market. Transdermal creams are well absorbed in most men and are easy to apply. These creams should be applied to the upper torso in areas with a reduced amount of hair. Because hair follicles and the skin of the scrotum contain 5-alpha-reductase, keeping cream or gel application away from those areas will limit testosterone conversion to DHT. I usually compound testosterone creams and gels in dosages from 10 to 30 mg per day. However, dosages reported in the literature range from 10 to 300 mg per day.[133]

Patients should be counseled to rub cream or gel in carefully for maximal skin absorption. In addition, they should avoid putting creams, lotions, or bath oils over the area where the testosterone has been applied, so these substances do not interfere with absorption. Special consideration should be given to men who have small children or animals in the house because the testosterone creams and gels can be transferred to others. He should avoid applying the testosterone to the skin areas with a large potential for contact with others. It is best to apply it to the upper chest and arms, immediately put a shirt on to cover the area, wash hands with soap, and use a separate hand towel.

Precautions

The most common adverse effect is local skin reactions. Fifty percent of men participating in a clinical trial reported transient, mild to moderate erythema at some time during therapy.[134]

Testosterone Pellets

Subdermal pellet implantation was among the earliest effective treatment modalities for clinical use of testosterone and became an established form of androgen replacement by 1940. Testosterone pellets, or subdermal implants, offer the longest duration of action with prolonged, zero order, steady-state characteristics. Implantation requires a minor office procedure, and, once implanted, the pellets last 4 to 7 months, depending on activity and stress level.

Dosage

The standard dosage is 800 to 1000 mg subdermally every 4 to 7 months.

Precautions

Potential drawbacks of the pellet include the need for the physician to be trained in its insertion, the risk of infection from the procedure, the inconvenience of pellet extrusion, and the inability to remove the pellet if a contraindication to testosterone therapy develops.[135]

Human Chorionic Gonadotropin

Human chorionic gonadotropin (hCG) is a polypeptide hormone produced by the placenta, containing an alpha and a beta subunit. The alpha subunit is essentially identical to the alpha subunits of LH and FSH, so it has the ability to stimulate the testes to produce more testosterone. In addition, because exogenous testosterone is not being given, it can avoid the testosterone replacement side effects of lower sperm count and loss of testicular volume. hCG alone, with no exogenous testosterone, is the preferred therapy for hypogonadal men younger than 40 years old who have adequate testicular function. Tsujimura et al[136] discussed a testosterone replacement method using 3000 units subcutaneously every 2 weeks. These investigators noted that total, free, and bioavailable testosterone increased by 25%, and symptoms improved.[136] Saez et al[137] showed that after the administration of hCG, plasma testosterone increased sharply within 4 hours and then decreased slightly and remained at a plateau for least 24 hours. A delayed peak of testosterone was seen between 70 and 96 hours. Thereafter, testosterone declined to the initial levels at 144 hours.[137]

Dosage

The most common dosages used are between 2000 and 5000 units subcutaneously per week. I usually use approximately 1000 units subcutaneously once to twice per week.

Precautions

Although hCG can increase testosterone and avoids the side effects of testicular atrophy and low sperm count, the long-term risks of giving men a female pregnancy hormone is unknown, and precaution should be taken.

Progesterone

Progesterone has not been as thoroughly studied in men as it has in women. Progesterone is the third hormone in the cascade starting from cholesterol and is the precursor to cortisol, testosterone, and estrogen. In healthy men, progesterone production is approximately 1.5 to 3 mg per day, and the hormone is produced almost entirely by the adrenal glands. As men age, progesterone production decreases.[138] However, it does not decline as rapidly as DHEA or pregnenolone. Progesterone helps reduce the level of estradiol in the blood by increasing the conversion of estradiol and estrone, which is 10 to 12 times less active than estradiol.[139] Thus, progesterone deficiency can be seen in diseases that are associated with estrogen excess such as gynecomastia, ischemic heart disease, BPH, and, possibly, prostate cancer.[140]

Progesterone is also known to reduce the level of DHT in the blood and the prostate by competing for the 5-alpha-reductase enzymes where it is converted into 5-alpha-dihydroprogesterone. This, in turn, limits the ability of 5-alpha-reductase to turn testosterone into DHT.[141] Progesterone also has a calming effect on the body. When it is given orally, its metabolites, pregnenolone and allo-pregnenolone, increase relaxation by stimulating the gamma-aminobutyric acid receptors. Progesterone has been used in men to help reduce insomnia.[142]

Possible Side Effects of Testosterone Therapy

The clinician must follow up the patient for the potential risks of testosterone therapy. Gynecomastia may occur if conversion of testosterone to estradiol is high. Therefore, clinicians should monitor estradiol levels, and as gynecomastia occurs, consider reducing testosterone dose, inhibiting aromatase (weight loss, quercitin, zinc, resveratrol, progesterone), and evaluating for other possible reasons of elevated estrogen such as alcohol use. Polycythemia is more likely to occur with injections. Hemoglobin and hematocrit should also be monitored, especially earlier in therapy. If the patient has a hematocrit greater than 55, testosterone therapy should be stopped, or therapeutic phlebotomy should be recommended (donate 1 unit of blood). This situation is more often seen in men with chronic obstructive pulmonary disease or sleep apnea and in smokers. Rhoden and Morgentaler[143] noted that "it is reassuring that as far as we can determine, no testosterone associated thromboembolic event has been reported to date." Reduced testicular volume may be a cosmetic issue to some men but is reversible with cessation of therapy (Boxes 34-7 and 34-8).

Prostate-Specific Antigen

PSA is a 34-kDa glycoprotein manufactured almost exclusively by the prostate gland. PSA is produced for the ejaculate, in which it is thought to help with the liquefaction of the semen in the seminal coagulum, which allows sperm to swim freely.[144] PSA is also believed to be useful in dissolving the cervical mucus cap, thus allowing the entry of sperm. It is present in small quantities in the serum of men with healthy prostates, but it is often elevated in prostate cancer and in other prostate disorders. PSA levels can increase with prostatitis, irritation, BPH, and recent ejaculation, thereby producing a falsely elevated result.[145]

BOX 34-7. Potential Adverse Effects of Testosterone Therapy

Polycythemia
Gynecomastia
Fluid retention
Reduced testicular volume
Decreased sperm count
Elevated prostate-specific antigen
Stimulated prolactinoma growth

BOX 34-8. Contraindications to Testosterone Therapy

Active prostate carcinoma
Breast cancer
Prostatic nodules or indurations
Unexplained prostate-specific antigen (PSA) elevation
Erythrocytosis (hematocrit greater than 50)
Unstable congestive heart failure
Severe, untreated sleep apnea

From Bassil N, Alkaade S, Morley JE. The benefits and risks of testosterone replacement therapy: a review. *Ther Clin Risk Manag.* 2009;5:427–448.

PSA should not rise significantly as a result of testosterone therapy. With the start of therapy, patients may have a small increase of approximately 0.2 ng/mL. The first 3 to 6 months after initiating testosterone therapy is the most critical time for moderate effects on the prostate. Therefore, PSA levels should be monitored every 3 months for the first year of treatment. The clinician must also be mindful when comparing PSA levels from different laboratories or different techniques of measure.

Benign Prostatic Hypertrophy, Prostate Cancer, and Testosterone Therapy

BPH, a common disease in older men, is believed to be related to the androgens DHT and estrogens. The incidence tends to increase when serum testosterone levels fall and estrogens increase. Testosterone replacement therapy appears to have little effect on prostate tissue androgen levels and cellular function and causes no significant adverse effects on the prostate. At the present time no conclusive evidence indicates that testosterone therapy increases the risk of prostate cancer or BPH.[67,143]

Today, as documented in many reviews, nothing has been found to support the evidence that restoring testosterone levels within normal range increases the incidence of prostate cancer. In fact, the incidence of prostate cancer in men with primary or secondary hypogonadism who are treated with testosterone is lower than the incidence observed in the untreated eugonadal population.[146] Mounting evidence demonstrates a lack of association between testosterone therapy and prostate cancer progression.[147,148] Gould and Kirby[149] looked at the risk of testosterone therapy inducing prostate cancer as they reviewed 16 studies, some of which were placebo controlled. These investigators found no increased risk of prostate cancer over the background prevalence with up to 15 years of follow-up.[149] Rhoden and Morgentaler[143] concluded that there is "no compelling evidence at present to suggest men with higher testosterone levels are at greater risk of prostate cancer or that treating men who have hypogonadism with exogenous androgens increases the risk. In fact, it should be recognized that prostate cancer becomes more prevalent exactly at the time in a man's life when testosterone levels decline."

Monitoring Therapy

Before starting testosterone therapy, clinicians must adequately diagnose and document male hypogonadism, with documentation of symptoms and physical examination with a digital rectal examination. In addition, clinicians should obtain necessary laboratory tests (see Box 34-5), and discuss lifestyle factors. Once therapy has started, I have follow-up in 1 month to discuss symptom improvement, potential side effects, lifestyle issues, and any other concerns. Patients then come in for a follow-up visit every 3 to 6 months until they are stable. After that time, they follow up every 6 months. During their follow-up visits, we review laboratory test results for total and free testosterone, complete blood cell count, PSA, estradiol, DHT, and any other laboratory abnormalities that are specific for the patient. I titrate testosterone and estradiol to stay within the physiologic range. I recommend that the patients undergo digital rectal examination every 6 months to monitor prostate health (Box 34-9).

Low free testosterone with a high estradiol level (greater than 30 pg/mL) suggests excess aromatase activity with conversion of testosterone to estradiol. Because most aromatase is found in fat cells, weight loss in the overweight patient is a key therapeutic tool (see also Box 34-2 for a list of aromatase inhibitors).

BOX 34-9. Recommend Urologic Consultation

Verified serum prostate-specific antigen (PSA) greater than 4.0 ng/mL

Increase in serum PSA concentration more than 1.4 ng/mL within any 12-month period of testosterone therapy

PSA velocity greater than 0.4 mg/mL/year using PSA after the first 6 months of testosterone therapy

Detection of prostate abnormality on digital rectal examination

American Urological Association prostate symptom score higher than 19

From Bassil N, Alkaade S, Morley JE. The benefits and risks of testosterone replacement therapy: a review. *Ther Clin Risk Manag.* 2009;5:427–448.

PREVENTION PRESCRIPTION

- Manage stress levels (see Chapter 93, Relaxation Techniques).
- Avoid sugars and refined carbohydrates to maintain insulin sensitivity.
- Eliminate food additives such as trans fats and high-fructose corn syrup.
- Eat whole foods every 3 hours by consuming lean proteins, vegetables, high-fiber fruits, and healthy fats.
- Get adequate sleep every night.
- Maintain ideal weight.
- Engage in interval and strength training exercises.
- Limit consumption of alcohol, which can increase the conversion of testosterone to estradiol.
- Avoid pesticides and environmental toxins: bisphenol A.
  - Do not microwave in plastic containers.
  - Use only containers marked with number 2, 4, or 5.
  - Do not use containers marked with number 3, 6, or 7 (PC).
  - Use number 7 (PLA) bottles when available.
  - Drink filtered water from BPA-free bottles or from ceramic or stainless steel bottles.
  - Limit canned soups, juices, and sauces; buy them in glass containers.
  - Do not drink or eat out of Styrofoam containers.
- Avoid pesticides and environmental toxins: phthalates.
  - The best way to avoid phthalates is to locate less toxic products and begin to use them.
  - A number of Web sites (e.g., www.LessToxicGuide.ca) provide information on phthalate-free products including cosmetics, shampoos, soaps, and household cleaning ingredients.

THERAPEUTIC REVIEW

■ Lifestyle

- Avoidance of toxin exposure
  - Encourage organic food consumption to reduce exposure to pesticides and persistent organic pollutants.
  - Encourage reduction in exposure to bisphenol A and phthalates.

- Stress reduction
  - Encourage the patient to practice the stress reduction techniques in Chapter 93, Relaxation Techniques.

- Maintenance of ideal weight
  - Specifically avoid buildup of abdominal and visceral fat that increases conversion of testosterone to estradiol.

- Adequate sleep

- Encourage the patient to get at least 7 hours of sleep at night.
- Diet
  - Encourage the patient to eliminate refined carbohydrates and sugars.
  - Encourage the patient to eat smaller meals and snacks every 2 to 3 hours consisting of lean proteins, vegetables, high-fiber fruits, and healthy fats to maintain stable blood glucose levels.
- Exercise
  - Encourage regular resistance training.

Note: If the patient is successful with the foregoing recommendations, replacement therapy is often not necessary.

Supplements

- Zinc: 25 to 50 mg per day (balance with 2 mg copper per day)
- Saw palmetto: 160 mg once or twice per day
- Chrysin: 1000 to 2000 mg per day orally; 100 to 200 mg per day transdermally

Hormonal Therapy

- Testosterone
  - Testosterone cypionate injections: 50 to 100 mg once or twice per week intramuscularly; 30 to 50 mg once or twice per week subcutaneously
  - Testosterone creams and gels: 10 to 30 mg per day (literature ranges from 10 to 300 mg per day)
  - Testosterone patch (commercial products more expensive than compounded products): Androderm, 2.5- to 5-mg patch each evening, starting with the 2.5-mg patch to the back, abdomen, thigh, or arm; AndroGel, 25 to 50 mg (25 mg/2.5 g, 50 mg/5 g) each morning; Testim, 50 mg/5 g applied each morning
  - Testosterone pellets: 800 to 1000 mg every 4 to 7 months (depending on symptoms and levels of testosterone)
- Human chorionic gonadotropin: 1000 units 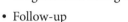 once or twice per week (as a single therapy); 250 units once or twice per week (when used as an adjunct to testosterone therapy)
- Progesterone: 25 mg at night orally
- Follow-up
  - Follow-up visits are scheduled every 3 months until levels are stable and then every 6 months.
  - Laboratory tests include total and free testosterone (bring up to physiologic levels), estradiol (bring down to physiologic levels), complete blood cell count (watch for polycythemia, hematocrit greater than 50), prostate-specific antigen (watch for elevation greater than 1.4 ng/mL in 12 months while on testosterone therapy), DHT (if elevated, reduce testosterone dose or increase 5-alpha-reductase inhibition [see Box 34-1]).
  - Titrate testosterone to stay within the physiologic range.
  - If estradiol is high, encourage therapies that inhibit aromatase (weight loss, progesterone, zinc, grape seed extract) or reduce the testosterone dose if levels are elevated.
  - Patients should undergo digital rectal examination every 6 months to monitor prostate health.
- Contraindications to testosterone therapy
  - Active prostate carcinoma
  - Breast cancer
  - Prostatic nodules or indurations
  - Unexplained prostate-specific antigen elevation
  - Erythrocytosis (hematocrit greater than 50)
  - Unstable congestive heart failure
  - Severe, untreated sleep apnea

KEY WEB RESOURCES

WorldHealth.net information on testosterone: www.WorldHealth.net/list/news/testosterone

Endocrine Society: www.endo-society.org

The American Academy of Anti-Aging Medicine is dedicated to the advancement of technology to detect, prevent, and treat aging-related disease and to promote research into methods to retard and optimize the human aging process. The section of this Web site on testosterone offers some articles and insights from leaders in the field.

Founded in 1916, this group is the world's oldest, largest, and most active organization devoted to research on hormones and the clinical practice of endocrinology. Members of the Endocrine Society represent the full range of disciplines associated with endocrinologists: clinicians, researchers, educators, fellows and students, industry professionals, and health professionals who are involved in the field of endocrinology.

American Urological Society: www.auanet.org.

This organization, founded in 1902, is the premier professional association for the advancement of urologic patient care. It works to ensure that its more than 17,000 members are current on the latest research and practices in urology. If you search "testosterone" on the Web site, you gain access to articles and other information.

Harvard Newsletter on Male Hormone Replacement: http://www.health.harvard.edu/newsweek/Hormone-replacement-the-male-version.htm.

Harvard Health Publications is the publishing division of the Harvard Medical School of Harvard University. The goal is to bring people around the world the most current health information that is authoritative, trustworthy, and accessible, by drawing on the expertise of the 9000 faculty physicians at Harvard Medical School in Boston.

Environmental Working Group: www.EWG.org.

This organization's mission is to use the power of public information to protect public health and the environment. The group specializes in providing useful resources to consumers while simultaneously pushing for national policy change.

References

References are available online at expertconsult.com.

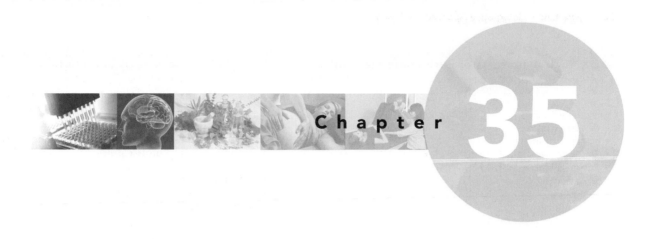

Chapter **35**

Hormone Replacement in Women

Pamela W. Smith, MD, MPH

A woman's hormonal response is as unique to her as her own fingerprints. Hormonal replacement at any age should not be considered without a thorough understanding of all the hormones in a body. The hormones are part of a symphony, and everything needs to be playing in tune. If one hormone is not in concert, then the patient will have a difficult time achieving optimal health. This chapter discusses the functions, symptoms of hormone deficiency, and symptoms of hormone excess with regard to estrogen, progesterone, and testosterone. Hormone replacement of estrogen, progesterone, and testosterone is also examined. Other hormones such as dehydroepiandrosterone (DHEA), cortisol, insulin, pregnenolone, prolactin, and thyroid are also part of the hormonal web but because of space constraints are not discussed in this chapter. Hormonal dysfunction can occur at any age. This chapter focuses on hormone replacement therapy (HRT) for women in the perimenopausal and menopausal years.

Perimenopause and Menopause

Menopause is defined as no menstrual cycle for 12 months. If a woman's hormones are out of balance, symptoms may begin many years before menopause. The symptoms of both perimenopause and menopause are similar (Box 35-1).

The normal age for a woman to go through menopause ranges from 35 to 55 years. Therefore, a woman may easily live one half of her life without a menstrual cycle. Some women have premature ovarian failure, which occurs when their ovaries stop producing an adequate amount of sex hormones before the age of 35 years (Box 35-1e).[1]

 Box 35-1e, which lists causes of premature ovarian failure, can be found online at expertconsult.com.

Estrogen

Estrogen has 400 crucial functions in the body (Box 35-2).[2-54] The body has receptor sites for estrogen in many locations: brain, muscles, bone, bladder, gut, uterus, ovaries, vagina, breast, eyes, heart, lungs, and blood vessels (Box 35-2e).

 Box 35-2e, which identifies symptoms of low estrogen, can be found online at expertconsult.com.

The patient can have excess estrogen levels in the body in relation to progesterone. This condition is called estrogen dominance. Estrogen dominance can result from the overproduction of estrogen or from an imbalance of progesterone to estrogen ratio. The symptoms of estrogen excess may also be the result of estrogen transformation, rather than the absolute amount of estrogen in the system (see the section on estrogen metabolism) (Box 35-3).[55]

Integrative Therapy (Hormones)

Synthetic Estrogens

Synthetic estrogens do not have the same chemical structure as hormones produced by the body and consequently do not fit into the estrogen receptors exactly as do natural estrogens.[56] Estradiol (E_2) that is produced naturally in a woman's body is eliminated within a few hours. Conversely, some synthetic estrogens (conjugated equine estrogen [Premarin]) have been shown to stay in the body for up to 13 weeks because the enzymes designed to metabolize the body's own estrogen do not break down synthetic estrogens as effectively.[57] Furthermore, the potency of synthetic estrogen is approximately 200 times that of natural E_2.[58]

BOX 35-1. Symptoms of Perimenopause and Menopause

- Hot flashes
- Night sweats
- Vaginal dryness
- Vaginal odor
- Mood swings
- Irritability
- Insomnia
- Depression
- Loss of sexual interest
- Hair growth on face
- Painful intercourse
- Panic attacks
- Excessive dreaming
- Urinary tract infections
- Vaginal itching
- Lower back pain
- Bloating
- Flatulence
- Indigestion
- Osteoporosis or osteopenia
- Aching ankles, knees, wrists, shoulders, or heels
- Hair loss
- Frequent urination
- Snoring
- Sore breasts
- Palpitations
- Varicose veins
- Urinary leakage
- Dizzy spells
- Panic attacks
- Skin feeling crawly
- Migraine headaches
- Weight gain
- Memory lapses or lack of focus and concentration

BOX 35-2. Functions of Estrogen

- Stimulates the production of choline acetyltransferase[7-11]
- Increases metabolic rate[12]
- Improves insulin sensitivity[13-16]
- Regulates body temperature
- Helps prevent muscle damage[17]
- Helps maintain muscle[18,19]
- Helps one sleep deeply[20]
- Reduces the risk of cataracts[21]
- Helps maintain the elasticity of arteries[22]
- Dilates small arteries[22,23]
- Increases blood flow[22-25]
- Inhibits platelet stickiness[22]
- Decreases the accumulation of plaque on the arteries[22]
- Enhances magnesium uptake and use[26]
- Maintains the amount of collagen in the skin
- Reduces vascular proliferation and inflammatory responses and thereby decreases heart disease risk[27]
- Lowers blood pressure[28]
- Decreases low-density lipoprotein and prevents its oxidation[29,30]
- Helps maintain memory[31-36]
- Increases reasoning and new ideas[24,37]
- Helps with fine motor skills[24,37]
- Increases the water content of the skin and is responsible for its thickness and softness[38]
- Enhances the production of nerve growth factor[39]
- Increases high-density lipoprotein by 10% to 15%[40]
- Reduces the overall risk of heart disease by 40% to 50%[40]
- Decreases lipoprotein (a)[40]
- Acts as a natural calcium channel blocker to keep the arteries open[41]
- Enhances energy[42]
- Improves mood[43-47]
- Increases concentration[43]
- Maintains bone density[43,49]
- Increases sexual interest[43]
- Reduces homocysteine[49,50]
- Decreases wrinkles[51]
- Protects against macular degeneration[51]
- Decreases the risk of colon cancer[51]
- Helps prevent tooth loss[51]
- Aids in the formation of neurotransmitters in the brain such as serotonin[43,52]

Obesity and alcohol increase estrone-to-estradiol ratio and may thus increase the risk of breast and uterine cancer.

Natural Estrogens

The body makes many kinds of estrogens. The three main estrogens are as follows:

- E_1, called estrone
- E_2, called estradiol
- E_3, called estriol

Estrone (E_1)

E_1 is the main estrogen the body makes postmenopausally. It is derived from E_2. High levels stimulate breast and uterine tissue, and many researchers believe it may be related to an increased risk of breast and uterine cancer.[42,59]

Before menopause, E_1 is made by the ovaries, adrenal glands, liver, and fat cells. Premenopausally, E_1 is converted to E_2 in the ovaries. Postmenopausally, little E_1 becomes E_2 because the ovaries stop working. In later years, E_1 is then made in the fat cells and, to a lesser degree, in the liver and adrenal glands.[42] Therefore, the more body fat one has the more E_1 will be manufactured. Consequently, obese women have an increased E_1:E_2 ratio.[60] In addition, routine alcohol consumption shifts the estrogen production to E_1.[61,62]

Estradiol (E_2)

E_2 is the strongest estrogen. It is 12 times stronger than E_1 and 80 times stronger than E_3. It is the main estrogen the body produces before menopause. Most E_2 is made in the ovaries. High levels of E_2 are associated with an increased risk of breast and uterine cancer. E_2 is the main estrogen the patient loses at menopause. However, two thirds of postmenopausal women up to the age of 80 years continue to make some E_2.[54] E_2 levels are lower in women who have had a surgical procedure that affected their ovaries. Even with one or both ovaries remaining, these patients may still have a decrease in hormonal function and may have menopausal symptoms[63] (Box 35-3e).[64-66].

 Box 35-3e, which lists the functions of estradiol in the body, can be found online at expertconsult.com.

Estriol (E_3)

E_3 has a much less stimulating effect on the breast and uterine lining than does E_1 or E_2. E_3 has been shown not to promote breast cancer, and considerable evidence indicates that it protects against the disease.[67] In Western Europe, E_3 estrogen has been used for decades.[68-73]

E_3 is an adaptogen, meaning that it adapts in the body to the ambient environment. E_3 given by itself has few estrogenic effects.[74-77] When given in a tenfold amount in relation to E_2 (biest; see later), E_3 antagonizes the effect of E_2.[78] Studies of E_3 since the 1970s revealed that E_3 given experimentally to women with breast cancer decreased disease recurrence. This group includes one study in the 1970s in which women with metastatic breast cancer were given E_3. Thirty-seven percent of the women had remission of the metastatic lesions or their cancer spread no further.[70] More research is needed in this area before E_3 can be recommended for women with a history of hormonally related breast cancer (Box 35-4).[72,79-83] Asian and vegetarian women have high levels of E_3 and much lower rates of breast cancer.[84]

Although E_3 does not have the major bone, heart, or brain protection of E_2,[42,85] it does have some minor positive effects on bone[72] and heart health by lowering cholesterol.[86,87]

Estrogen prescribed for HRT should be applied transdermally and not orally. In part because of the first-pass effect through the liver, estrogen given by mouth can have the following effects[88,89]:

- Elevate blood pressure
- Increase prothrombic effects[90]
- Increase triglycerides
- Increase E_1
- Cause gallstones
- Elevate liver enzymes

- Decrease growth hormone
- Interrupt tryptophan metabolism and consequently serotonin metabolism[91]
- Increase C-reactive protein[44]
- Increase sex hormone–binding globulin (which can decrease testosterone)
- Increase carbohydrate craving[92]
- Increase weight gain[92]

Estrogen replacement therapy should be administered by the transdermal route. Oral dosing can increase the risk of heart disease, a finding that may help explain the elevated risk in the Women's Health Initiative study.

Consequently, as HRT, estrogens should be applied transdermally. Many studies have been conducted on transdermal application of E_2. Transdermally given E_2 has been shown to have the following effects[90]:

- Does not have the same impact on liver synthesis of proteins as estrogen given by mouth[93-95]
- Does not have negative effects on the health of the heart
- Does not negatively affect blood clotting[96-98]
- Lowers triglycerides and thus decreases the risk of heart disease in women[99]

Estrogen Receptor Sites

Estrogen has two main receptor sites to which it binds in the body: estrogen receptor alpha, which can increase cell growth; and estrogen receptor beta, which decreases cell growth and helps prevent breast cancer development. E_2 equally activates estrogen receptors alpha and beta. E_1 selectively activates estrogen receptor alpha sites in a ratio of 5:1, which can increase cell proliferation. E_3 binds preferentially to estrogen receptor beta in a 3:1 ratio, which may be one of the reasons that E_3 may help prevent breast cancer development.

Estrone (E_1) selectively activates estrogen receptor sites that increase cell proliferation and has the greatest risk of stimulating breast cancer.

Estrogen Metabolism

A growing body of research shows that it is not simply the amount of total estrogen circulating in the body that is critical to women's health. How estrogen is metabolized in the body may also play an important role in causing various estrogen-dependent conditions, including osteoporosis, autoimmune disorders, and cancer.

After menopause, the metabolism of estrogen can change. Consequently, a woman may respond differently to exogenous estrogen.[100]

Estrogen is metabolized in the body in the following ways (Fig. 35-1):

- Two major competing pathways
  - 2-Hydroxyestrone
  - 16-Hydroxyestrone
- One minor pathway
  - 4-Hydroxyestrone

2-Hydroxyestrone is sometimes called the good estrogen.[101] It does not stimulate the cells to divide, which can cause damage to DNA and cause tumor growth.[101] Furthermore, by latching onto available estrogen cell receptors, 2-hydroxyestrone may exhibit a blocking action that

FIGURE 35-1
Steroid hormone metabolism. (Courtesy of Sahar Swidan, PharD, BCPS.)

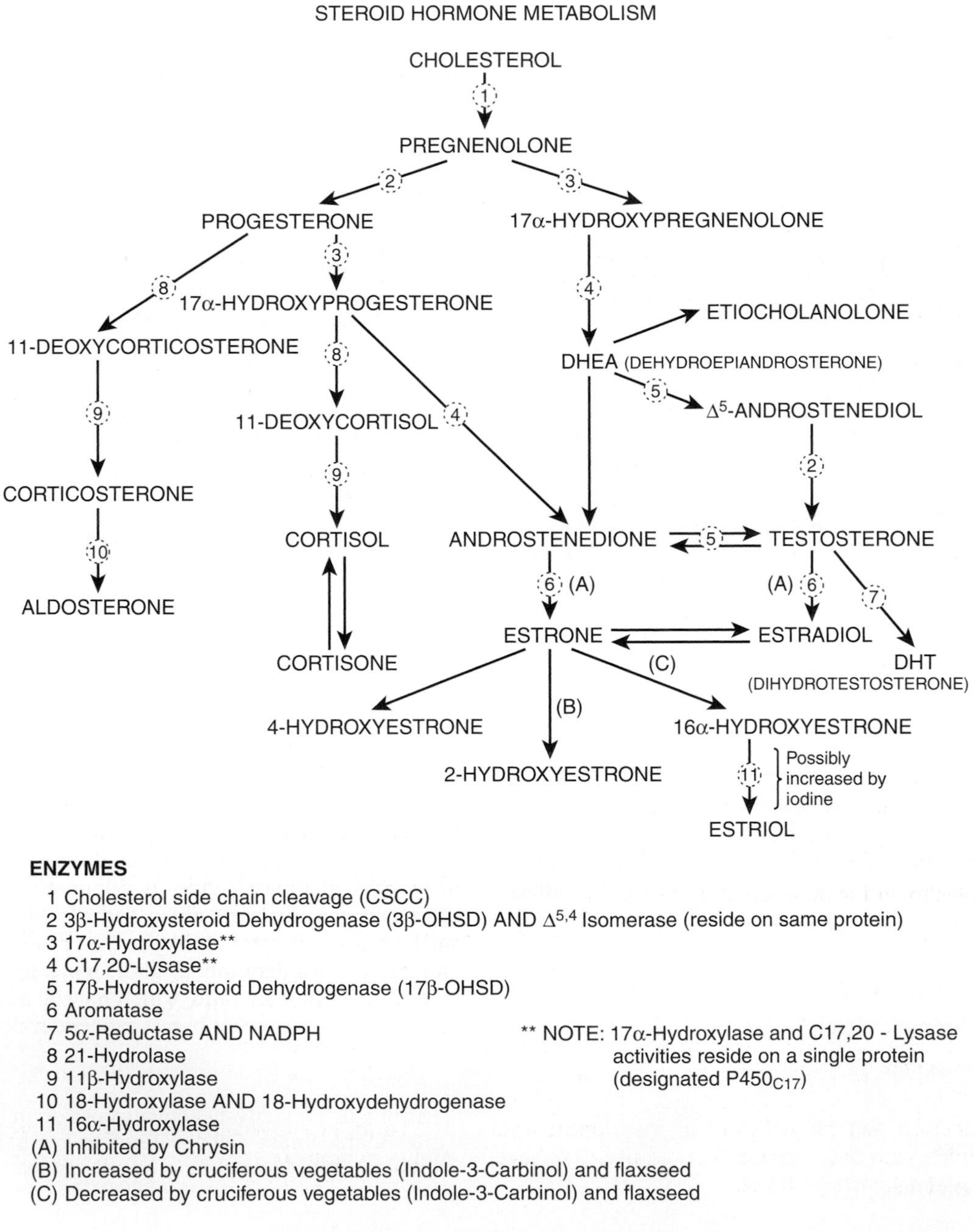
STEROID HORMONE METABOLISM
CHOLESTEROL
1
PREGNENOLONE
2
3
PROGESTERONE
17α-HYDROXYPREGNENOLONE
3
8
4
17α-HYDROXYPROGESTERONE
ETIOCHOLANOLONE
11-DEOXYCORTICOSTERONE
8
DHEA (DEHYDROEPIANDROSTERONE)
5
9
11-DEOXYCORTISOL
4
Δ5-ANDROSTENEDIOL
2
9
CORTICOSTERONE
CORTISOL
ANDROSTENEDIONE
5
TESTOSTERONE
10
6 (A)
(A) 6
7
ALDOSTERONE
ESTRONE
ESTRADIOL
CORTISONE
(C)
DHT
(DIHYDROTESTOSTERONE)
(B)
4-HYDROXYESTRONE
16α-HYDROXYESTRONE
2-HYDROXYESTRONE
11
Possibly increased by iodine
ESTRIOL
ENZYMES
1 Cholesterol side chain cleavage (CSCC)
2 3β-Hydroxysteroid Dehydrogenase (3β-OHSD) AND Δ5,4 Isomerase (reside on same protein)
3 17α-Hydroxylase**
4 C17,20-Lysase**
5 17β-Hydroxysteroid Dehydrogenase (17β-OHSD)
6 Aromatase
7 5α-Reductase AND NADPH
8 21-Hydrolase
9 11β-Hydroxylase
10 18-Hydroxylase AND 18-Hydroxydehydrogenase
11 16α-Hydroxylase
(A) Inhibited by Chrysin
(B) Increased by cruciferous vegetables (Indole-3-Carbinol) and flaxseed
(C) Decreased by cruciferous vegetables (Indole-3-Carbinol) and flaxseed
** NOTE: 17α-Hydroxylase and C17,20 - Lysase activities reside on a single protein (designated P450C17)

prevents stronger estrogen products from gaining a foothold into the cells. Therefore, 2-hydroxyestrone is suggested to be anticancerous.[102]

The other major pathway of estrogen metabolism is 16-hydroxyestrone. This metabolite is much more active and has a strong stimulatory effect. 16-Hydroxyestrone binds to special receptors inside the cells that can increase the rate of DNA synthesis and cell multiplication.[103] Consequently, 16-hydroxyestrone is proposed to have significant estrogenic activity and to be associated with an increased risk of breast cancer. [104–113] Furthermore, 16-hydroxyestrone permanently binds to the estrogen receptor. Other estrogens attach briefly and then are released.[114] Other reasons may also exist for the association of 16-hydroxyestrone with a higher rate of cancer. High levels of 16-hydroxyestrone are associated with obesity, hypothyroidism, pesticide toxicity (organochlorines), omega-6 fatty acid excess, and inflammatory cytokine production. For the body to make a small amount of 16-hydroxyestrogen is advantageous, however, because 16-hydroxyestrone decreases the risk of osteoporosis. Therefore, a small amount of 16-hydroxyestrone production is desirable. Extensive endogenous and exogenous estrogen production through the 16-hydroxy pathway may put the patient at higher risk for breast cancer than when the 2-hydroxy pathway breaks down more estrogen.[115]

Studies have shown that low 2:16 hydroxyestrogen ratios are associated with elevated breast cancer risk. One study of postmenopausal women who went on to develop breast cancer had a 15% lower 2:16 hydroxyestrogen ratio than did women in control groups.[111] Similarly, in women who already have breast cancer, the survival rate is greater in women with higher ratios.[116,117] 2-Hydroxyestrone is protective against cancer only when this substance is methylated by catechol-O-methyltransferase (COMT) into 2-methoxyestrone. The ratio of 2-methoxyestone to 2-hydroxyestrone can be measured in the urine and is a good gauge of the body's ability to methylate. Another way of evaluating the body's ability to methylate is by measuring the serum homocysteine level. If it is elevated, this suggests poor methylation. Low ratios of 2:16 hydroxyestrogen are also associated with an increased rate of developing lupus.

Factors that support methylation are numerous:

- *S*-Adenosyl-L-methionine (SAMe)
- Methionine
- Vitamins B_2, B_6, and B_{12}
- Folic acid (also as folinic acid, 5-formyl THF, or 5-methyltetrahydrofolate)
- Trimethylglycine (TMG)
- Reducing catecholamine production by decreasing stress

A minor pathway of estrogen metabolism is 4-hydroxyestrone. It may also enhance cancer development. 4-Hydroxyestrone may directly damage DNA by causing breaks in the molecular strands of DNA.[118] Furthermore, the 4-hydroxyestrogens have the ability to convert to metabolites that react with DNA and cause mutations that can be carcinogenic.[119] In addition, 4-hydroxyestrone is present in greater quantities in patients deficient in methionine and folic acid. Women who have uterine fibroids also may have increased levels of 4-hydroxyestrone.

Equine estrogens increase metabolism to 4-hydroxyestrones.[120,121] Studies have shown that 4-hydroxyestrone from equine estrogen causes mutagenic damage five times more rapidly than do other forms of 4-hydroxyestrogens.[122]

Therefore, the metabolism of estrogen through the 2-hydroxy pathway is of critical importance in lowering the risk of cellular damage and possible development of cancer. It is consequently very important to measure the patient's levels of 2-hydroxyestrone and 16-hydroxyestrone, as well as the ratio between these two metabolites. Equally important is to measure 4-hydroxyestrone levels. The goal is to normalize estrogen metabolism. Follow-up testing is also suggested to assess the clinical impact of dietary and lifestyle changes, as well as HRT.[123] Even patients not receiving HRT should have an estrogen metabolism test, particularly if they have a family history of breast cancer.

What can elevate 2-hydroxyestrone levels?

- Moderate exercise[124,125]
- Cruciferous vegetables[105,126–135]
- Flax[136,137]
- Soy[138]
- Kudzu (source of isoflavones)
- Rosemary, turmeric
- Exercise
- Weight loss
- Broccoli derivatives[130,139–146]
  - Indole-3-carbinol
  - Diindolylmethane (DIM), a breakdown product of indole-3-carbinol
  - Sulforaphane glucosinolate
- High-protein diet[147]
- Omega-3 fatty acids[101,108,148]
- Vitamins B_6 and B_{12} and folate[149,150]

All the foregoing have been shown to increase the 2:16 ratio significantly and decrease 4-hydroxyestrone production, thus reducing the risk of estrogen-dependent health problems by shifting estrogen metabolism toward the less active 2-hydroxyestrone pathway.

Other factors affect how the body metabolizes estrogen. The first is obesity, which increases the action of estrogens in three ways[151]:

- Estrogen production and storage occur in fat cells.[152,153]
- Concentrations of sex hormone–binding globulin are decreased in obese patients. This change increases the amount of unbound estrogen available for use by the body.[154]
- Obesity decreases 2-hydroxyestrone and increases 16-hydroxyestrone production.[139,155]

The second factor is the presence of xenoestrogens. Researchers have identified 50 chemicals that imitate estrogen.[101,156–159]

Third, excessive alcohol intake interferes with the body's ability to detoxify estrogen and increases E_2 levels and, consequently, the risk of breast cancer.[160]

Finally, even antibiotics found in the food may be associated with an elevated risk of breast cancer development by changing the gut flora involved in the enterohepatic circulation of estrogens.[161]

> Measuring estrogen metabolism (the 2-hydroxyestrone-to-16 alpha-hydroxyestrone ratio, 4-hydroxyesterone) is a key component to therapy.

Estrogen Receptor Modulators

Selective estrogen receptor modulators (SERMs) are also a type of HRT. SERMs decrease total cholesterol by 5% and low-density lipoprotein (LDL) by 10%. They are not as effective in lowering triglycerides, however, and they do not increase high-density lipoprotein (HDL) as effectively as does standard HRT.[162] Furthermore, because estrogen receptor modulators are not neuroprotective, they do not have the same positive effect on memory and mood as does natural estrogen.[163]

Progesterone

Progesterone is made in the ovaries before menopause. After menopause, some progesterone is made in the adrenal glands (Box 35-5 and Box 35-4e).[164–169]

 Box 35-4e, which identifies the causes of low progesterone levels, can be found online at expertconsult.com.

Natural progesterone is biologically identical to what the patient's own body produces. Synthetic progesterone, called progestin, is very different from natural progesterone because it does not have the same chemical structure. Consequently, progestins do not reproduce the actions of natural progesterone.[170] Further information on progesterone is available in the literature.[171–189]

One study showed that the use of synthetic progesterone increased the risk of breast cancer by 800% as compared with the use of estrogen alone.[190–193] Furthermore, an article published in *JAMA* (the official journal of the American Medical Association) discussed a risk of breast cancer that was predicted to rise by nearly 80% after 10 years of use of estrogen-progestin HRT and 160% after 20 years.[192] Similarly, Dr. Stephen Sinatra, a well-known cardiologist, found that synthetic progestins can lead to serious cardiac side effects in patients, including shortness of breath, fatigue, chest pain, and high blood pressure.[177] Progesterone (bio-identical) does not share the same risk seen with progestins (Box 35-6).[67,164,187,188,194–217]

BOX 35-5. Symptoms of Decreased Progesterone Levels

- Anxiety
- Depression
- Irritability
- Mood swings
- Insomnia
- Pain and inflammation
- Osteoporosis
- Decreased high-density lipoprotein
- Excessive menstruation
- Hypersensitivity
- Nervousness
- Migraine headaches before cycles
- Weight gain
- Decreased libido

Data from Smith P. *What You Must Know About Women's Hormones.* Garden City Park, NY: Square One Publishers; 2010:20.

BOX 35-6. Effects of Bio-Identical Progesterone

- Helps balance estrogen
- Leaves the body quickly
- Improves sleep hygiene
- Stimulates the production of new bone
- Has a natural calming effect[205]
- Lowers high blood pressure
- Helps the body use and eliminate fats
- Lowers cholesterol
- May protect against breast cancer by inhibiting breast tissue overgrowth
- Increases scalp hair
- Normalizes libido
- Helps balance fluids in the cells
- Increases the beneficial effects of estrogens on blood vessel dilation in atherosclerotic plaques[206–208]
- Has an anti-proliferative effect on all progesterone receptors, not just receptors in the uterus[187,188]
- Does not change the good effect of estrogen on blood flow[177]
- Increases metabolic rate[209]
- Is a natural diuretic
- Enhances the action of thyroid hormones
- Prevents migraine headaches that are cycle related
- Is a natural antidepressant
- Improves libido
- Helps restore proper cell oxygen levels
- Induces conversion of estrone (E_1) to the inactive E_{1S} form
- Promotes helper T-cell (Th2) immunity
- Is neuroprotective by promoting myelination
- Is antiinflammatory
- Relaxes smooth muscle
- Promotes bone formation or turnover[210]

The hormonal symphony is very important. If the body has too much synthetic or natural progesterone, then some of the following effects can occur[206,211,212]:

- Increases fat storage
- Decreases glucose tolerance and increases insulin levels, which may lead to insulin resistance
- Increases cortisol
- Increases appetite
- Increases carbohydrate cravings
- Relaxes the smooth muscles of the gut and thus can cause bloating, fullness, and constipation; can also contribute to gallstone formation[213]
- Suppresses the immune system[214]
- Causes incontinence[215]
- Causes ligaments to relax and can cause backaches, leg aches, and achy hips[216]
- Decreases growth hormone levels[217]

This discussion clearly shows that natural (bio-identical) progesterone offers a safer approach than synthetic progesterone (progestin).[187] Moreover, the level of progesterone must be measured before the patient begins HRT and then again on a regular basis to confirm that the patient is receiving an optimal dose in balance with other hormones.

Progesterone can be prescribed as a pill or a topical cream. If the patient has insomnia, then oral progesterone is the preferred route of administration because it crosses the blood-brain barrier and affects the gamma-aminobutyric acid receptors in the brain to produce a calming effect that helps the patient sleep.[205,214] Prometrium is a natural progesterone preparation available from a pharmaceutical company. This preparation is made from peanut oil. More commonly, natural progesterone is prescribed by a health care practitioner and is then made by a compounding pharmacy, to facilitate customizing the patient's dosage. This form of natural progesterone is made from an extract of yams. The compounded formulation of progesterone has an enzyme added to convert the diosgenin in the yam into progesterone. Over-the-counter progesterone frequently does not contain this enzyme unless it appears on the label.[218] The absorption rate of oral progesterone increases as one ages; consequently, patients may need less medication as they grow older.[219] Some women have side effects of oral progesterone such as nausea, breast swelling, dizziness, drowsiness, and depression resulting from first-pass effects on the liver and gastrointestinal tract.[220,221] Lowering the dose or optimizing gastrointestinal tract health usually resolves these symptoms. Progesterone may be given transdermally, although no studies have shown that transdermal administration of progesterone aids in the prevention of endometrial hyperplasia.

Finally, epinephrine also interacts with progesterone as part of the hormonal symphony. Epinephrine surges, which occur with stress, can block progesterone receptors and can prevent progesterone from being used effectively in the body.[222]

Estrogen-to-Progesterone Ratio

As discussed, the risk of breast cancer is increased when estrogen metabolism favors the 16-hydroxyestrone or 4-hydroxyestrone pathway. Patients with a low progesterone-to-estrogen ratio, otherwise known as estrogen dominance, also have a higher risk of breast cancer.[223]

Important facts about the estrogen-to-progesterone ratio are as follows:

- Progesterone and E_2 (estrogen) work together in the body. E_2 lowers body fat by decreasing lipoprotein lipase. Progesterone increases body fat storage by increasing lipoprotein lipase.[224]

- Estrogen and progesterone work together to control the body's release of insulin. Women with diabetes must be prescribed the smallest amount of progesterone that will balance E_2.[225] E_2 increases insulin sensitivity and improves glucose tolerance, whereas excess progesterone decreases insulin sensitivity.

- A progesterone-to-estrogen ratio that is too high in progesterone breaks down protein and muscle tissue.[226] This process may worsen symptoms of diseases such as fibromyalgia.

Prolonged use of progesterone without adequate estrogen can have the following effects[226]:

- Increased weight gain
- Increased total cholesterol
- Decreased HDL
- Increased LDL
- Increased triglycerides
- Increased risk of developing insulin resistance
- Depression
- Fatigue
- Decreased libido

Progesterone must balance with estrogen in the body.

Testosterone

Testosterone is made in the adrenal glands and ovaries. As women age, their ovaries produce less testosterone. Of testosterone women produce, 1% is unbound, and the remainder is bound to sex hormone–binding globulin. Women with increased androgens have more free testosterone available for the body to use. Therefore, measuring hormone levels is important (Box 35-7).[227-233]

Research is showing that for testosterone to work well, E_2 must also be optimized. Without enough estrogen, testosterone cannot attach to brain receptors.[232] Testosterone given

BOX 35-7. Functions of Testosterone in Women

- Increases sexual interest (86% of women state they have a decrease in sexual interest with menopause.)[227]
- Increases sense of emotional well-being, self-confidence, and motivation[228]
- Increases muscle mass and strength
- Helps maintain memory[229]
- Stimulates the growth of pubic hair and underarm hair at puberty
- Increases muscle tone so the skin does not sag[230]
- Decreases excess body fat
- Decreases bone deterioration and helps maintain bone strength[231]
- Elevates norepinephrine in the brain[232]
- Has cardiovascular benefits[233]
  Low testosterone levels can occur at any age and can be caused by the following:
- Menopause
- Childbirth
- Chemotherapy
- Surgical menopause[234]
- Adrenal stress or burnout
- Endometriosis
- Depression
- Psychological trauma
- Birth control pills (increases sex hormone–binding globulin)
- Cholesterol-lowering medications[235]

with E_2 lowers cardiac risk.[232,236] If given alone (and a women's own estrogen level is low), testosterone increases plaque formation in the coronary vessels and thereby increases the patient's risk of myocardial infarction. If testosterone is given with estrogen, it has a beneficial effect on the arterial walls.[237]

> Testosterone increases plaque formation in the coronary vessels unless it is balanced with estrogen.

Prescription natural testosterone is the preferred method of testosterone replacement. Methyltestosterone (synthetic) use may increase the risk of liver cancer in women.[238–240] Testosterone should be applied transdermally to decrease negative effects on the liver. The patient should be instructed to rotate application sites. If the patient applies testosterone to the same location daily, she will have an increase in hair growth at the site of application.

A woman can have excess testosterone levels. Excess androgen production may come from the ovaries or the adrenals. Almost 10% of women have had some kind of androgen imbalance in their lifetime (Box 35-5e).[67,241,242]

 Box 35-5e, which lists the symptoms of increased testosterone production, can be found online at expertconsult.com.

For the patient to have optimal health, her level of testosterone should be in balance with all the other hormones. Levels that are too high or too low are not desirable (Table 35-1).

PREVENTION PRESCRIPTION

The body is designed not to need HRT postmenopausally. The adrenal glands produce enough dehydroepiandrosterone (DHEA) to make sufficient estrogen and testosterone to maintain function. Similarly, pregnenolone makes adequate progesterone, estrogen, testosterone, DHEA, and cortisol to maintain function in most patients. This function can be maintained best by the following recommendations:

- Encourage regular exercise.
- Maintain optimal weight.
- Maintain an adequate sleep-wake cycle with 7 to 8 hours of uninterrupted sleep each night.
- Decrease exposure to xenobiotics that can have hormonal influences by eating organic foods, drinking filtered water, avoiding petroleum-based cosmetics, storing food in glass (not plastic), avoiding eating animal fat, and avoiding diesel exhaust.
- Make changes to avoid chronic emotional stress (see Chapter 93, Relaxation Techniques).
- Eat a diet rich in protein, ground flaxseed, green tea, omega-3 fatty acids, and cruciferous vegetables. Obtain protein from plant sources (beans, nuts) more than from animal sources (see Chapter 86, The Antiinflammatory Diet).

TABLE 35-1. Twenty-four–Hour Production Rates of Sex Steroids in Women at Different Stages of the Menstrual Cycle

SEX STEROIDS	EARLY FOLLICULAR	PREOVULATORY	MIDLUTEAL
Progesterone (mg)	1.0	4.0	25.0
17-Hydroxyprogesterone (mg)	0.5	4.0	4.0
Dehydroepiandrosterone (mg)	7.0	7.0	7.0
Androstenedione (mg)	2.6	4.7	3.4
Testosterone (mcg)	144.0	171.0	126.0
Estrone (mcg)	50.0	350.0	250.0
Estradiol (mcg)	36.0	380.0	250.0

THERAPEUTIC REVIEW

Hormone replacement therapy (HRT) is all about balance and individualized treatment dosages. Needs change over time, and ongoing reevaluation is beneficial through relationship-centered care.

■ Laboratory

- The levels of all three estrogens (along with progesterone, testosterone, dehydroepiandrosterone [DHEA], cortisol, and thyroid hormones) must be measured before the patient is prescribed HRT, and regularly thereafter, to help maintain the patient on the optimal amount of each hormone.

▦ Lifestyle

- Many positive lifestyle behaviors can be protective by increasing 2-hydroxyestrone levels.

  - Regular moderate exercise.

  - Weight loss is encouraged if the patient is overweight. This is one of the most important goals in balancing hormones in overweight women.

▦ Nutrition

- Cold water fish twice weekly

- Cruciferous vegetables including broccoli, cabbage, Brussels sprouts, kale, and cauliflower

▦ Botanicals

- Kudzu (rich in isoflavones): 100 mg daily

- Turmeric extract: 500 to 1000 mg two to three times a day

▦ Supplements

- If homocysteine is elevated, suspect poor methylation. Supplement with the following: vitamin B$_6$, 50 mg daily; vitamin B$_{12}$, 1000 mcg weekly; and folic acid, 800 mcg daily to increase 2-hydroxyestrone levels.

- Fish oil with eicosapentaenoic acid and docosahexaenoic acid: 1000 mg daily

- Zinc if deficient: 15 to 30 mg daily (needed for testosterone metabolism)

- Indole-3-carbinol 300 mg daily or diindolylmethane (DIM) 225 mg daily

▦ Mind-Body Therapy

- Chronic stress and anxiety are foundational elements in hormone imbalance because the perception of stress has a direct effect on the hypothalamic-pituitary axis (see Chapter 93, Relaxation Techniques).

▦ Pharmaceuticals (Hormones)

A practitioner usually begins by prescribing 20% estradiol (E$_2$) and 80% estriol (E$_3$). Then the percentages of E$_2$ and E$_3$ are adjusted according to repeated laboratory testing. The combination of E$_2$ and E$_3$ together is called biest and is a prescription that a compounding pharmacist can formulate. Any percentage of these two estrogens can be used because the dosage is individualized. Start low and go slow.

▦ Progesterone

- For premenstrual syndrome

  - Consider progesterone alone cyclically.

- Oral administration of sustained-release capsules (compounded) or micronized progesterone (Prometrium; comes in 100- and 200-mg formulations), at 25 to 400 mg (most common, 50 to 200 mg) given cyclically from days 12 to 24 of the menstrual cycle

- Topical administration, at 5 to 50 mg applied daily on days 14 to 25 of the cycle

- For perimenopause

  - Oral administration and topical application with doses same as for premenstrual syndrome. The patient should use this cyclically alone or combined with estrogen.

  - Use the lowest possible dose of progesterone in patients with obesity or metabolic syndrome.

- For postmenopausal or surgical menopause status

  - Oral sustained-release capsules (dose at bedtime because of sedation) 50 to 200 mg or topical compounded cream, at 20 to 50 mg daily. Patients may also use 100 mg of Prometrium at bedtime if this dose is needed (lowest dose available is 100 mg).

  - Treatment may be continuous or stopped for 5 days a month.

▦ Estrogen

- For perimenopause

  - Bi-estrogen (80% E$_3$, 20% E$_2$). Compound 2 mg E$_3$ with 0.5 mg E$_2$ per gram and start at 0.25 mg cream topically daily or twice daily, if progesterone alone does not control symptoms.

- For postmenopausal status and surgical menopause

  - Bi-estrogen (50% E$_3$, 50% E$_2$). Compound 1 mg E$_3$ with 1 mg E$_2$ per gram and start 0.25 mg cream topically daily or twice daily. Patients may use it continuously or stop 5 days a month.

▦ Testosterone

- For postmenopause

  - Topical compounded cream, at 0.25 to 2.0 mg once daily

- For surgical menopause

  - Topical compounded cream, at 0.25 to 2.0 mg daily

▦ Converting Administration Routes

- Approximate ratio for transdermal to sublingual to oral

  - For progesterone, estrogen, and DHEA: transdermal 1 to sublingual 2 to oral 4 to 5

  - For testosterone: transdermal 1 to sublingual 2 to oral 5 to 6

Continued

■ **Other Considerations**

- After hormones are prescribed, the patient should have hormone levels checked again in 90 days and then every 6 to 12 months.

- The evidence/harm rating for hormones is a 2. If the recommendation were equine estrogen with progestin, as used in the Women's Health Initiative study, the rating would be a 3 because of the increased risk of myocardial infarction, stroke, deep vein thrombosis, and breast cancer.

- As with any therapy, hormones should be matched to the unique needs of the patient to provide the most benefit with the least amount of harm.

KEY WEB RESOURCES

International Academy of Compounding Pharmacists: http://www.iacprx.org.	This Web site includes a directory of compounding pharmacists in the United States.
Professional Compounding Centers of America: http://www.pccarx.com.	This site also includes a directory of compounding pharmacists in the United States.
Laboratories (see Appendix in This Text for a Complete List) Genova Diagnostic Laboratory: www.genovadiagnostics.com.	This laboratory performs salivary and 24-hour urine hormone testing, as well as estrogen metabolism testing.
Metametrix Clinical Laboratory: www.metametrix.com.	This laboratory conducts estrogen metabolism testing.
NeuroScience, Inc.: www.neurorelief.com.	This laboratory performs salivary testing of hormones.
ZRT Laboratory: www.zrtlab.com.	This laboratory also performs salivary testing of hormones.

References

References are available online at expertconsult.com.

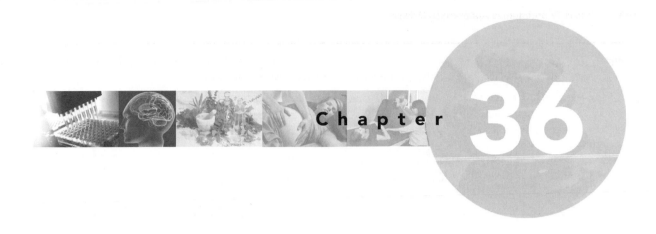

Chapter 36

Polycystic Ovarian Syndrome

Melinda Ring, MD

Polycystic ovarian syndrome (PCOS) is the most common female endocrine disorder, affecting 10% of women of reproductive age, yet it is frequently overlooked.[1,2] PCOS affects young women with oligo-ovulation (which leads to oligomenorrhea in more than 75% of affected patients), infertility, acne, and hirsutism. It also has notable metabolic sequelae, including an elevated risk of diabetes and cardiovascular disease, and attention to these factors is important.[3] The heterogeneous nature of the condition and the diversity of presentations led to a symptom-based approach to treatment, because PCOS manifests differently, depending on many interacting factors including environmental exposures, genetics, and lifestyle (Fig. 36-1). This chapter discusses the pathophysiology and integrative approach to treatment of women with PCOS.

Pathophysiology

When PCOS was first described (as Stein-Leventhal syndrome) in the 1930s, the presence of cysts in the ovaries was believed to be a defining factor in the origin of the syndrome.[4] Since then, research has shown that, in fact, the cysts are only one potential expression of what begins as a disorder in the endocrine system. On pelvic ultrasound, 90% of women with biochemical features of PCOS will have characteristic changes; however, 20% to 30% of women without the hormonal issues of PCOS will have similar ultrasound features.[5] Our current understanding, albeit incomplete, is that PCOS phenotypic expression results from primary hormone imbalances. The three prevalent theories for the pathogenesis of PCOS are as follows:

1. Hypothalamic-pituitary dysfunction results in gonadotropin-releasing hormone and luteinizing hormone dysfunction, which then has downstream effects on ovarian hormone production.
2. A primary ovarian defect (with or without an adrenal defect) in steroidogenesis results in hyperandrogenism.
3. A metabolic disorder characterized by peripheral insulin resistance exerts adverse effects on the hypothalamus, pituitary, ovaries, and, possibly, adrenal gland.

Variables including genetic factors and lifestyle choices contribute to the wide range of manifested symptoms and make the diagnosis challenging unless the clinician is attuned to the potential problem.

Criteria for PCOS have been debated among leading organizations since 1990. The differences reflect the controversy over the origin of the syndrome, as well as its heterogeneous manifestations (Table 36-1).[6-8] The diagnostic criteria have unifying trends, however. All require the presence of at least one of the stigmata of ovarian disease: a history of anovulation or the finding of classic polycystic ovaries on ultrasound. All three schemata are consistent in the inclusion of hyperandrogenism, through either clinical expression (hirsutism or acne) or laboratory confirmation. Finally, all guidelines also require exclusion of hormonal disorders that may mimic PCOS. Although insulin resistance has been noted consistently among women with PCOS, it is not included in any of the diagnostic criteria.

Based on current data, evaluation for PCOS should include a search for both primary markers and secondary dysfunctions. History and physical examination focus on symptoms and signs such as oligomenorrhea, acne, hirsutism, and central obesity, as well as searching for manifestations of other confounding diseases. Laboratory tests should include androgen levels (dehydroepiandrosterone [DHEA] sulfate and total and free testosterone measured by equilibrium dialysis) and tests to rule out alternative diagnoses as warranted (e.g., congenital adrenal hyperplasia, androgen-secreting tumors, Cushing syndrome, 21-hydroxylase–deficient nonclassic adrenal hyperplasia, androgenic or anabolic drug use or abuse, syndromes of severe insulin resistance, thyroid dysfunction, or hyperprolactinemia). Laboratory testing for antimüllerian hormone is a newer diagnostic tool, not yet widely available, that holds promise as a confirmatory test. A search for evidence of metabolic syndrome and cardiovascular risk should also be performed (e.g., insulin resistance measurement by oral glucose tolerance test including glucose and insulin levels and measurement of lipids and inflammatory

FIGURE 36-1
Proposed relationships leading to phenotypic expression of polycystic ovarian syndrome.

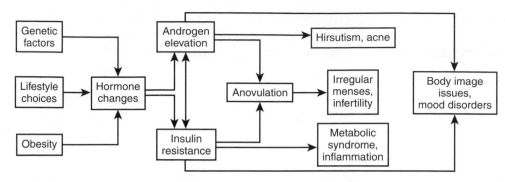

TABLE 36-1. Differing Criteria for Polycystic Ovarian Syndrome Among Organizations

ORGANIZATION	CRITERIA	OVARIAN DYSFUNCTION	OVARIAN MORPHOLOGY	HYPERANDROGENISM
National Institutes of Health (1990)[6]	Both of the following and exclusion of related disorders	Oligo-ovulation (less than 6 menses per year)		Clinical or biochemical (not specified)
Rotterdam Group (2003)[7]	Any two of three of the following and exclusion of related disorders	Oligo-anovulation (nonspecified)	Polycystic ovaries (> 12 follicles 2 to 9 mm, or ovarian volume > 10 mL)	Clinical or biochemical (free testosterone or free testosterone index)
Androgen Excess Society (2006)[8]	Hyperandrogenism as critical, with addition of at least one ovarian marker and exclusion of related disorders	Oligo-anovulation and/or polycystic ovaries	Oligo-anovulation and/or polycystic ovaries	Clinical or biochemical (free testosterone)

markers such as C-reactive protein and fibrinogen). Pelvic ultrasound can also support the diagnosis.

> A thorough clinical assessment is critical both to confirm the diagnosis and to identify risk factors for long-term health maintenance. This information helps the clinician prioritize integrative approaches when creating a management plan by elucidating the primary metabolic targets. The plan should take into equal consideration each woman's unique concerns such as weight management, acne, hair loss, or infertility.

Integrative Therapy

A holistic approach to PCOS addresses not just the patient's immediate symptoms and risk management, but also the impact of the syndrome on her mental state and sense of self.

Lifestyle

Weight Management
Weight management plays a central role in the expression of symptoms and long-term consequences in women with PCOS. Fifty percent to 70% of women with PCOS are obese

and should be informed that even 5% to 10% weight loss of body mass is associated with significant improvement in clinical metabolic and hormonal markers.[9–11] Guiding women in this arena can be challenging because insulin resistance may inherently make weight loss more difficult, and women are often frustrated by repeated failed attempts to lose weight. Current evidence suggests that the approaches described in the next sections may be most successful.

Physical Activity
Exercise is an important lifestyle approach in PCOS, with diverse benefits such as improved insulin sensitivity and preservation of lean body mass. A 2010 systematic review of exercise therapy in PCOS identified eight studies (five randomized controlled and three cohort) involving moderate intensity physical activity (aerobic and/or resistance) for 12 to 24 weeks.[12] The most consistent improvements included improved ovulation, reduced insulin resistance (9% to 30%), and weight loss (4.5% to 10%). The optimal exercise regimen for PCOS has yet to be defined, so current theories regarding interval training and full-body exercise should be used (see Chapter 88: Writing an Exercise Prescription).

A study published in *Human Reproduction* compared the effects of exercise versus a low-calorie diet in 40 women with PCOS.[13] The exercise group had higher ovulation rates, better insulin sensitivity, and greater reduction in waist measurements despite less absolute weight loss.

Nutrition

Macronutrients

Although caloric restriction is clearly needed for weight loss, to date only a few small studies have examined the impact of macronutrient composition in PCOS. Several studies ranging from 1 to 6 months that compared a high-protein and low-carbohydrate diet with a high-carbohydrate and low-protein diet showed no significant difference in terms of weight loss, improvements in circulating androgens, glucose metabolism, and leptin.[14,15] Conversely, two pilot studies showed that low-carbohydrate diets were associated with improved depression scores and self-esteem ratings, as well as lower fasting insulin levels and lower rates of acute insulin response to glucose.[16,17] None of these studies took into account the glycemic index of the carbohydrates or the source of protein (animal versus plant based), which may be important factors in insulin resistance and hormone regulation. In 2010, the first study examining impact of glycemic index in overweight and obese premenopausal women with PCOS ($N = 96$) randomized these women to either an ad libitum low–glycemic index diet or a macronutrient-matched healthy diet and followed the women for 12 months or until they achieved a 7% weight loss. The attrition rate was high in both groups (49%). Among the women who completed the study, those on the low–glycemic index diet showed greater improvements in insulin resistance ($P = .03$), menstrual cyclicity (95% compared with 63%; $P = .03$), and serum fibrinogen concentrations ($P < .05$). At this point, no firm recommendations can be given about macronutrient content, although trends suggest that women may do best on a low-carbohydrate diet with inclusion of low–glycemic index, high-fiber carbohydrates (see Chapter 85: The Glycemic Index/Load).

Soy

Soy intake in PCOS is a controversial topic. Soy is a plant food that is also a complete protein, meaning that it has all the required amino acids. It is also low in fat and contains essential fatty acids, numerous vitamins, minerals, and fiber. Soy foods include soy milk and cheese, tofu, tempeh, miso, soy sauce, and edamame. Soy contains phytoestrogens, which led to the debate of its benefits versus risks in PCOS.

Currently, very few studies have actually looked at PCOS and soy intake. One study showed favorable results for PCOS in improving cholesterol.[18] Twelve obese women with PCOS who had high insulin and high cholesterol levels consumed 36 g of soy each day for 6 months. The results showed favorable improvement in reducing low-density lipoprotein cholesterol. The investigators noted no effect on weight loss, hormones, or menstrual cycle in this study. Conversely, many animal studies showed that soy intake can negatively affect fertility. A review of seven soy intervention studies done on women using 32 to 200 mg/day of isoflavones showed increased menstrual cycle length.[19] Current evidence does not imply that soy prevents ovulation, but soy may delay it.

More studies need to be conducted on soy consumption in polycystic ovarian syndrome (PCOS). Women with PCOS who struggle with infertility, consume few calories, or eat a poor diet may want to avoid or limit soy products. Otherwise, a moderate to low intake of soy (once a day or several times a week) can be part of a healthy diet for women with PCOS.

Omega-3 Fatty Acids

Inflammation has been identified in patients with PCOS, whether as a consequence or a contributing factor remains unclear.[20,21] In comparison with control subjects, patients with PCOS have decreased fibrinolytic activity, higher levels of plasminogen activator inhibitor-1, and increased C-reactive protein levels (in both obese and nonobese women), all of which are markers for inflammation.[20,21] Attention to reduction of cardiovascular risk should probably be more aggressive in those women with PCOS who have increased C-reactive protein levels. Including omega-3 fatty acids will help combat the inflammatory component of PCOS, as well as support cardiovascular health (see Chapter 86, The Antiinflammatory Diet). The lignans in flaxseeds may provide additional benefit through support of estrogen elimination.

Supplements

Inositol Family

Investigations into the cause of insulin resistance in PCOS led some researchers to investigate whether derangements in insulin signal transduction could be overcome by oral administration of D-*chiro*-inositol (DCI), a mediator of insulin action that forms naturally in the human body from the metabolism of pinitol and myoinositol (commonly known as inositol) in the diet. In several early studies, evidence favored a benefit of this supplement in improved insulin sensitivity, triglyceride and testosterone levels, as well as improved blood pressure, ovulation, and weight loss.[5,22,23] Forty-four obese women with PCOS were randomly assigned to receive placebo or DCI (1200 mg once a day) for 8 weeks. Supplementation with DCI resulted in an improvement in insulin resistance ($P = .07$), a 55% reduction in the mean serum free testosterone concentration ($P = .006$), and an increase from 27% to 86% in ovulation compared with placebo ($P < .001$). The more readily commercially available D-pinitol (D-*chiro* (+)-O-methyl inositol) was shown to raise DCI serum levels; however, results of clinical end points such as impact on insulin sensitivity were mixed.[24,25] In an important study of this nutrient in diabetic patients, 600 mg of pinitol twice per day for 3 months lowered blood glucose levels by 19.3%, lowered average glucose levels by 12.4%, and significantly improved insulin resistance.[24] In another study, 25 women received inositol for 6 months. Twenty-two of the 25 (88%) patients had a single spontaneous menstrual cycle during treatment, of whom 18 (72%) maintained normal ovulatory activity. Ten pregnancies (40% of patients) occurred.

■ Dosage

DCI: 600 mg daily if less than 60 kg (130 lb) or 1200 mg daily if heavier; pinitol: 600 mg twice daily

Precautions

No interactions with herbs and supplements are known. There is concern that high consumption of inositol might exacerbate bipolar disorder.

Chromium

Chromium is an essential trace mineral that enhances the action of insulin. Although supplementing with chromium has been shown in studies to improve the blood glucose control in type 2 diabetes mellitus, little research has focused specifically on the PCOS population.[26] A pilot study of six women with PCOS concluded that 1000 mcg per day of chromium for as little as 2 months improved insulin sensitivity by an average of 38% (significant) and decreased baseline insulin by 22% (not statistically significant).[27]

Dosage

Chromium picolinate: 600 to 1000 mcg in divided doses daily. Picolinate, a byproduct of the amino acid tryptophan, is combined to support absorption of chromium. Dietary sources include Brewer's yeast, liver, mushrooms, wheat germ, oysters, and some fresh fruits.

Precautions

The daily adequate intake for women ranges from 20 to 45 mcg, depending on age. Laboratory animals have tolerated 350 times this dose without adverse effects, although a question of possible mutagenicity exists with prolonged use. In humans, short-term use of chromium at 1000 mcg daily is safe; these doses are not recommended in pregnancy or renal insufficiency. Prolonged use should be avoided due to concerns about adverse effects.

Vitamin D

Vitamin D plays a role in insulin resistance and egg follicle maturation and development. In a small trial of 13 women with PCOS and vitamin D deficiency, normal menstrual cycles resumed within 2 months in 7 of the 9 women who had irregular menstrual cycles after vitamin D repletion with calcium therapy.[28] Two women even established pregnancies. The authors of the study suggested that abnormalities in calcium balance may be responsible, in part, for the arrested follicular development in women with PCOS and may contribute to the pathogenesis. Vitamin D also plays a key role in glucose regulation, notably in decreasing insulin resistance.[29,30] Low levels of vitamin D have been negatively correlated with the incidence of type 1 and type 2 diabetes.

Dosage

Vitamin D_3: 2000 units daily. Higher doses may be prescribed based on serum 25-OH vitamin D levels. Overweight individuals have a greater risk of vitamin D deficiency because, as a fat-soluble vitamin, vitamin D may not be as bioavailable in high amounts of fat tissue.

Precautions

Vitamin D is well tolerated. Gastrointestinal side effects are most common.

N-Acetylcysteine

Many studies of N-acetylcysteine (NAC) have shown benefit in diabetes and several showing benefit in PCOS. NAC has multiple actions, including increasing the antioxidant glutathione, lowering inflammatory markers such as tumor necrosis factor-alpha, and improving insulin sensitivity.[31,32] A study in clomiphene-resistant patients showed improved ovulatory rates (49.3% versus 1.3%) and pregnancy rates (21% versus 0%).[33]

Dosage

Give 1200 to 1800 mg/day in divided doses.

Precautions

NAC is well tolerated, with occasional reports of nausea.

Botanicals

Cinnamomum Cassia

Cinnamomum cassia (not *Cinnamomum zeyanicum* or *Cinnamomum verum*) has been studied in vitro and in humans for lowering glucose levels in diabetes.[34-36] A pilot study published in the July 2007 issue of *Fertility and Sterility* showed that ¼ to ½ teaspoon of cinnamon powder reduced insulin resistance in 15 women with PCOS.

Dosage

The dose is 1 to 6 g powdered cinnamon (¼ to 1 teaspoon) or 200 to 300 mg cassia extract.

Precautions

Cinnamon is well tolerated. Gastrointestinal side effects are most common.

Licorice

Licorice root and glycyrrhetinic acid have antiandrogen effects that may support goals in PCOS. Licorice root as part of a traditional Chinese medicine formula has also been associated with reduced serum testosterone and ovulation induction in women with PCOS.[37,38] Licorice additionally is synergistic with spironolactone; its impacts on potassium loss, hypertension, and fluid retention counteract the opposing actions of spironolactone. Thirty-two hirsute women with PCOS were given 100 mg of spironolactone per day; half also received 3.5 g/day of a licorice root extract standardized to 7.6% glycyrrhetinic acid for 2 months.[39] Licorice use was associated with amelioration of orthostatic symptoms, polyuria, and systolic blood pressure drops, especially during the first 2 weeks of treatment.

Dosage

Glycyrrhiza glabra: 500 mg standardized to 6% to 15% glycyrrhizin (approximately 3.0 to 8.0 g of crude plant material).

Precautions

At lower doses or normal consumption levels, few adverse reactions are evident. A no-observed effects level has been proposed as purified glycyrrhizin, 2 mg/kg/day, and the acceptable daily intake for glycyrrhizin is suggested at 0.2 mg/kg/day. Toxicity from excessive licorice ingestion is well established, with hypokalemia, hypertension, and fluid retention. Licorice is contraindicated in pregnancy.

Chaste Tree Berry (Vitex Agnus-castus)

Vitex is one of the most popular botanicals for PCOS, although data from well-done studies are not available. *Vitex* is believed to shift the estrogen-progesterone balance in favor of progesterone through increased luteinizing hormone and mild inhibition of follicle-stimulating hormone secretion. *Vitex* also reduces prolactin secretion, which when elevated may inhibit fertility. A small study involving women with fertility disorders examined pregnancy rates from a chaste berry–containing herbal blend versus placebo twice daily for 3 months.[40] Women with secondary amenorrhea or luteal insufficiency in the active treatment group achieved pregnancy twice as often as in the group receiving placebo. However, the total number of patients conceiving was small (15 women).

Two other publications explored the benefits of a *Vitex*-containing blend on progesterone level, basal body temperature, menstrual cycle length, pregnancy rate, and side effect profile.[41,42] The designs were double-blind placebo-controlled trials of a proprietary nutritional supplement containing chaste berry, green tea, L-arginine, and vitamins and minerals. The treatment group ($n = 53$) demonstrated increased mean midluteal progesterone, especially among women with very low pretreatment levels. Cycle length and luteal basal body temperatures improved significantly. After 3 months, 14 women in the treatment group were pregnant (26%) compared with 4 of the 40 women in the placebo group (10%; $P = .01$). These studies are difficult to extrapolate given the proprietary nature of the supplements, although the trends toward improvement with no side effects warrant further consideration. Several small studies in the German literature also reported a benefit of *Vitex* for acne, with self-reports of improvement of up to 70%.[43]

■ Dosage
Vitex products are available in many different dosage forms, including fresh and dried berries, capsules containing powdered chaste berries, and liquid preparations such as extracts and tinctures. The German Commission E recommends a daily intake of 30 to 40 mg of dried herb. *Vitex* should be standardized to 0.5% agnuside and 0.6% aucubin per dose.

■ Precautions
Animal and human studies suggest that *Vitex* may interfere with oral contraceptives and hormone therapy. Based on in vitro data, *Vitex* may also interact with dopamine agonists (e.g., bromocriptine, levodopa). Use during pregnancy is not recommended.

Other Herbs: Saw Palmetto and Green Tea
Herbalists recommend several other herbs for PCOS based on biochemical activity. Minimal research has been done to verify benefits or identify appropriate doses, however.

■ Saw Palmetto
Elevated 5-alpha-reductase activity has been demonstrated in women with PCOS.[44] Saw palmetto inhibits 5-alpha-reductase and thereby reduces the conversion of testosterone to dihydrotestosterone, the more potent form. Although saw palmetto has the potential for benefit in reducing acne, excess facial and body hair, and androgenic hair loss, no research has been done in women, and saw palmetto has potential interactions with drugs such as oral contraceptive pills (OCPs). Saw palmetto should not be recommended at present.

■ Green Tea (*Camellia sinensis*)
Green tea extracts have been proposed as a natural remedy for PCOS based on several pathways. Polyphenols may reduce inflammation and insulin resistance, stimulate thermogenesis, and increase production of sex hormone–binding globulin, thus leading to reduced free testosterone. However, a study from Asia of high-concentration polyphenol extracts for 3 months did not find improvements in laboratory or clinical measures.[45] At this point, green tea extract should not be recommended, although drinking 3 cups of organic green tea daily is a healthy option.

Complementary Healing Approaches

Acupuncture
Acupuncture has the potential to influence PCOS through its effects on the sympathetic nervous system, the endocrine system, and the neuroendocrine system.[46,47] In a 2009 study, one group of women with PCOS was treated for 4 months with electroacupuncture, another group of women was given heart rate monitors and told to exercise three times a week, and a third, control group was educated about the importance of exercise and a healthy diet but received no instructions. The investigators found that the women who received acupuncture or who exercised had decreased sympathetic activity. The women who received electroacupuncture treatments also had more regular menstrual cycles, reduced testosterone levels, and reduced waist circumference. Experimental observations in animal and clinical data suggest that acupuncture exerts beneficial effects on insulin resistance and ovulation. Although research studies are limited, acupuncture as an adjunctive therapy may be considered in many women for the direct impact not only on PCOS parameters, but also on associated mood disorders and stress.

Mind-Body Therapy
Women with PCOS have a significantly increased prevalence of depression and anxiety.[48–50] Mood disorders may be directly related to biochemical imbalances (androgens, insulin resistance), and they may also be exacerbated by stress related to body image issues and infertility. Addressing concerns through mind-body approaches, self-care, and cognitive-behavioral therapy should be encouraged for all women.

Pharmaceuticals
Medication decisions should be based on a woman's predominant symptoms and goals. Major classes include insulin sensitizers, weight loss medications, and hormone modulators.

Insulin Sensitizers
Metformin improves insulin resistance and hyperandrogenism.[51] It is also associated with regulation of menstruation and ovulation and may benefit up to 79% of women attempting to conceive. Metformin is considered weight neutral, as opposed to many other medications used for glucose regulation.

■ Dosage
Start with 500 mg daily for 1 week; titrate to 500 mg twice daily in week 2 and as needed thereafter. The maximum daily dose is 2.5 g in two or three divided doses.

■ **Precautions**

Side effects are gastrointestinal and include nausea and diarrhea. Metformin should be avoided if creatinine clearance is less than 30 mL/minute. *Thiazolidinediones* are less thoroughly studied in PCOS compared with metformin. This class of medications is associated with weight gain, thus making it an unattractive choice for many women struggling with PCOS. Studies of troglitazone (now off the market because of hepatotoxicity), pioglitazone, and rosiglitazone demonstrated improvements in insulin sensitivity, hyperandrogenemia, and ovulatory rates. Given the potential for adverse effects, this class of medications is best reserved for patients with established diabetes mellitus.

Weight Loss Medications

Orlistat, given with an energy-restricted diet, was shown to improve insulin resistance, as well as lower free testosterone markers, in obese women in some but not all studies.[52-54] The trials were short term (3 to 6 months), and orlistat needs further investigation to determine its utility in patients with PCOS.

■ **Dosage**

A dose of 120 mg, three times daily before meals, was used for 3 to 6 months in the studies.

■ **Precautions**

Orlistat may cause fat-soluble vitamin deficiency and greasy stools.

Hormone Modulators
■ **Oral Contraceptives**

Oral contraceptive pills (OCPs) are first-line options for androgen excess issues such as hirsutism and acne, in accord with the 2008 Endocrine Society Clinical Practice Guidelines. OCPs reduce luteinizing hormone secretion and thus ovarian androgen secretion; additional reductions in free androgen concentration occur through increased levels of sex hormone–binding globulin.[55] OCPs provide additional benefit by protecting against endometrial hyperplasia in amenorrheic women with excess estrogen exposure.

■ **Dosage**

Appropriate choices include OCP preparations containing 30 to 35 mcg of ethinyl estradiol combined with a progestin with minimal androgenicity, such as norethindrone, norgestimate, desogestrel, or drospirenone.

■ **Precautions**

Risks and side effects of OCPs are similar to those for women without PCOS. The concern also exists that OCPs may increase some cardiovascular risk factors such as inflammatory markers and insulin resistance. Absence of pregnancy should be documented before OCPs are begun. If the woman has had no menstrual period for 6 or more weeks, withdrawal bleeding should be induced by administration of 5 to 10 mg of medroxyprogesterone acetate daily for 10 days before initiation of OCP treatment (to minimize breakthrough bleeding when starting the pill).

Although oral contraceptive (OCP) use helps many women overcome the troublesome symptoms of polycystic ovarian syndrome (PCOS), these drugs have been associated with higher risk of cardiovascular disease in the general population.[56,57] The risk of cardiovascular disease is associated with increased age, smoking, and hypertension. Additional concerns include a negative impact on inflammatory markers and diabetes risk. Studies are needed in the PCOS population to assess the long-term benefit-to-risk ratio of using OCPs. For now, increased awareness and attention to regular follow-up of metabolic and cardiovascular markers are critical in any woman taking OCPs.

■ **Progestins**

Progestins are appropriate for women who need endometrial protection but who are not interested in or appropriate for OCPs. Cyclic progestins promote withdrawal bleeding and prevent endometrial hyperplasia.

■ **Dosage**

Synthetic progestin: medroxyprogesterone acetate: 10 mg orally daily for 7 to 10 days every 1 to 2 months. Bio-identical progestin: micronized progesterone: 400 mg orally daily for 10 days every 1 to 2 months. Bio-identical progesterone cream has not been used in research studies, and whether the creams can provide consistent levels sufficient for uterine protection is unclear.

■ **Precautions**

Sedation or confusion may occur.

■ **Antiandrogens**

Antiandrogens, which block androgen binding to receptor, are often used off label for hirsutism.[58] Most commonly prescribed is spironolactone. Flutamide is another option, although it is associated with more side effects.

■ **Dosage**

Spironolactone: 50 to 200 mg/day; flutamide: 250 mg two to three times a day

■ **Precautions**

Contraception is essential, because if pregnancy occurs, an antiandrogen such as spironolactone could be teratogenic; discontinuation 3 months before conception is recommended. If spironolactone alone is used, endometrial protection may be needed.

■ **Clomiphene Citrate**

Clomiphene citrate is an antiestrogen and an effective option to stimulate ovulation induction for women with PCOS. Approximately 80% of women with PCOS ovulate in response to clomiphene citrate, and approximately 50% conceive.

■ **Dosage**

The strategy is to use the lowest dose of clomiphene possible to initiate ovulation, starting with 50 mg/day, for 5 days (usually days 5 to 9). If no follicle development occurs with this dose, the dose or duration of treatment can be increased.

Statins

Statins are an area of debate in the literature regarding their cardiovascular and endocrine benefit in women with PCOS. An initial study was very promising: 40 patients with PCOS were randomly assigned to atorvastatin at 20 mg daily or placebo.[59] After 12 weeks, the researchers reported an absolute reduction in free androgen index (−32.7%) and total testosterone (−24.6%) and increased sex hormone–binding globulin (+13.7%) in the atorvastatin group, but none in the placebo group. Patients in the atorvastatin group had lower serum insulin levels and homeostasis model of insulin resistance (HOMA-IR) compared with increases in the placebo group. Conversely, a study published in 2010, in which 20 patients with PCOS who had low-density lipoprotein levels higher than 100 mg/dL took atorvastatin at 40 mg/day or placebo for 6 weeks of treatment, showed reduced androgen levels, biomarkers of inflammation, and blood pressure.[60] However, atorvastatin worsened hyperinsulinemia and failed to improve endothelial function in women with PCOS. Until the full picture is defined, reserving statin use for women only for treatment of hyperlipidemia and not as an attempt to treat hyperandrogenemia or insulin resistance seems prudent.

■ Dosage

Doses are prescribed per usual recommendations for hyperlipidemia.

■ Precautions

Statins are considered possibly teratogenic in pregnancy. The usual concerns regarding liver and muscle issues apply.

Surgery

When severe symptoms are not controlled with the therapies described earlier and a patient has morbid obesity, bariatric surgery may be considered. Results of two small studies on the effects of bariatric surgery have been published.[61] A retrospective study evaluated 30 women with PCOS who underwent laparoscopic Roux-en-Y gastric bypass. Postoperative benefits included resolution of menstrual irregularity (100%), improvement in hirsutism (75%), resolution of type 2 diabetes, and ability to cease medications for hypertension (78%) and hyperlipidemia (92%). These results were confirmed in a prospective study evaluating 17 women with PCOS.

Surgery may also be performed for ovulation induction in the management of clomiphene citrate–resistant anovulatory women with PCOS. Various types of ovarian surgery are employed (e.g., wedge resection, electrocautery, laser vaporization, multiple ovarian biopsies), and all procedures result in an altered endocrine profile after the procedure. One plausible mechanism postoperatively is that the rapidly reduced secretion of all ovarian hormones restores feedback to the hypothalamus and pituitary and results in appropriate gonadotrophin secretion. These surgical procedures provide an option, albeit one used less often now, when natural and pharmaceutical approaches are not successful in anovulatory patients with PCOS.

PREVENTION PRESCRIPTION

- Maintain appropriate weight and a regular aerobic exercise routine.
- Avoid excessive amounts of saturated fat such as those found in red meat, fried foods, and dairy.
- Replace vegetable oils with olive or canola oil for cooking.
- Consume omega-3–rich fats found in cold-water fish, nuts, greens, and ground flaxseed.
- Encourage soy-based foods such as soy milk, edamame, tempeh, miso, soy nuts, and nongenetically modified tofu. Try to eat 1 to 2 oz a day.
- Avoid dietary supplements or environmental exposures that may increase circulating hormone levels such as pesticides, herbicides, and bovine growth hormone–rich dairy products.
- Avoid supplements or drugs that include dehydroepiandrosterone, androstenedione, testosterone, and human growth hormone.

 # THERAPEUTIC REVIEW

Lifestyle approaches are first-line recommendations for PCOS, both in conventional and integrative medicine approaches. Many women with PCOS do well with attention to diet, exercise, supplements, and acupuncture. Some women need medications to achieve needed improvements when metabolic derangements are greater.

■ Lifestyle

- Remove exacerbating factors. Minimize exposure to hormone-disrupting chemicals.

■ Nutrition

- Promote weight loss to achieve an ideal body weight. Start with achievable goals and provide adequate support.
- Eat 1 to 2 servings of soy-rich foods daily. Each 1-oz serving (approximately the size of the palm of the hand) provides approximately 25 mg.
- Encourage a low-carbohydrate diet that takes into account the glycemic index of foods.
- Encourage foods rich in omega-3 fatty acids (e.g., salmon, nuts, or ground flaxseeds).

Continued

▪ Physical Activity

- Recommend moderate exertion 30 to 60 minutes daily.

▪ Supplements

- Vitamin D₃: 2000 units daily (dose based on serum 25-OH vitamin D level)
- Chromium picolinate:1000 mcg daily
- D-*chiro*-inositol/pinitol: 600 mg once or twice per day

▪ Botanicals

- *Cinnamomum cassia*: ¼ to 1 teaspoon
- Licorice root in conjunction with spironolactone for amelioration of side effects and complementary action
- Chaste tree berry (*Vitex*): 60 drops of tincture or 175 mg of extract, standardized to 0.6% agnusides

▪ Complementary Therapies

- Acupuncture may reduce sympathetic nervous system tone and improve menstruation. It has additional benefits for stress reduction and mood.

- Mind-body therapies can help women cope with stress, depression, and anxiety related to PCOS.

▪ Pharmaceuticals

- Insulin sensitizers include metformin, at 500 to 1000 mg twice daily.
- If the patient is unable to achieve satisfactory weight loss, consider support with orlistat.
- Medications such as clomiphene may be prescribed in consultation with a reproductive endocrinologist for ovulation induction.
- Antiestrogens for hirsutism include spironolactone, at 50 to 200 mg/day, or flutamide, at 250 mg two to three times a day.
- Oral contraceptive pills are prescribed for amenorrhea, hyperandrogenism, and uterine protection.

▪ Surgical Therapy

- If the patient has morbid obesity with significant comorbidities despite the foregoing measures, consider referral for bariatric surgery.
- Ovarian surgery may be indicated for infertility.

KEY WEB RESOURCES

American Association of Clinical Endocrinologists: www.aace.com.	This Web site contains a position statement on metabolic and cardiovascular consequences of PCOS, as well as practice management forms for new and follow-up visits for patients with PCOS.
Womenshealth.gov: www.womenshealth.gov/faq/polycystic-ovary-syndrome.cfm.	This Web site, from the U.S. Department of Health and Human Services Office on Women's Health, provides patient education materials on PCOS.
American Society for Reproductive Medicine: www.asrm.org.	This Web site describes medical and surgical options for PCOS.

References

References are available online at expertconsult.com.

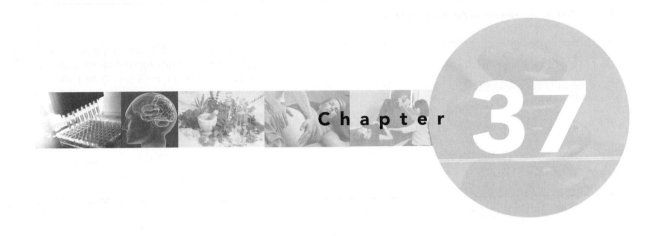

Chapter **37**

Osteoporosis

Louise Gagné, MD, and Victoria Maizes, MD

Osteoporosis is defined as a generalized skeletal disorder characterized by compromised bone strength, which predisposes individuals to an increased risk of fracture. It is a significant cause of pain, disability, and death throughout the world. That treatment strategies are limited and imperfect heightens the importance of preventive strategies. Integrative medicine emphasizes the use of lifelong exercise habits and an antiinflammatory diet to prevent the development of osteoporosis.

Pathophysiology and Epidemiology

The incidence of osteoporotic fractures varies widely across populations. The Chinese have relatively low rates, whereas in Iceland rates are high.[1] More than 10 million people in the United States have osteoporosis, and more than 2 million osteoporotic fractures occur each year.[2] Women are at higher risk than men and account for approximately 75% of all cases. However, men are at greater risk of dying of a hip fracture should they sustain one (20.7% versus 7.5%.).[3]

To assess bone health, the World Health Organization (WHO) uses only the dual x-ray absorptiometry (DEXA) scan, which measures bone density but not quality. By this criterion, approximately 7% of postmenopausal women 50 years old or older have osteoporosis, and 40% have osteopenia. The costs to the U.S. health care system are significant, totaling more than $16 billion annually. As the population ages, the costs related to osteoporosis prevention and treatment are expected to continue to climb.[4]

Osteoporosis is a multifactorial disease arising from genetic, hormonal, metabolic, mechanical, and immunologic factors (Fig. 37-1). Our bones provide the support structure for our bodies, protect vital organs, and play a central role in mineral and acid-base balance. The two main types of bone cells are osteoblasts (which synthesize the organic bone matrix and its calcification) and osteoclasts (which resorb bone to allow for metabolic requirements and for repair and remodeling).

Bone mass reaches its peak at approximately 30 years of age and begins to decline after age 40 years. Repair and renewal of bone continue throughout adult life, however, with approximately 15% of bone mass turning over each year. Bone is dynamic, constantly responding to a range of hormonal, metabolic, neurologic, and mechanical signals. Bone mineral density (BMD) is a function of bone gained during growth and lost during aging.

Bone loss begins in both men and women in the fourth decade. Women lose an average of 35% of their cortical bone and 50% of their trabecular bone. Because men reach higher peak bone mass, have a larger cortical thickness, and have better preservation of bone microstructure, they are half as likely as women to experience a fracture. Women typically lose 0.5 to 0.9% of bone density per year during the perimenopause, 1% to 3 % during the menopausal years, and 1% per year into old age.[3]

Screening and Diagnosis

Assessing Bone Strength

Bone strength is determined by bone quality as well as by bone mass. Bone quality is influenced by bone microarchitecture and the composition of the bone matrix and mineral.[5] No established way exists to assess bone quality in a clinical practice setting. Bone mass or BMD is most commonly assessed using a DEXA scan.

Osteoporosis is defined as a BMD more than 2.5 standard deviations (SD) below the mean for young adults. Osteopenia is defined as a BMD 1 to 2.5 SD below the young adult mean.

The usefulness of screening for fracture risk with DEXA has been questioned. Some studies did not show BMD measurement to be helpful in predicting nonvertebral fracture risk.[6] Other studies showed a strong correlation between low femoral neck BMD and risk of hip fracture.[7] In addition, evidence indicates a significant inverse relationship between BMD and vertebral fracture risk.[8] Nonetheless, a wide overlap exists between the bone densities of women who will eventually suffer a fracture and those who will not.[9]

353

FIGURE 37-1
Pathophysiology of osteoporosis. 1,25-(OH)$_2$D, 1,25-dihydroxyvitamin D (vitamin D component that aids calcium absorption); PTH, parathyroid hormone.

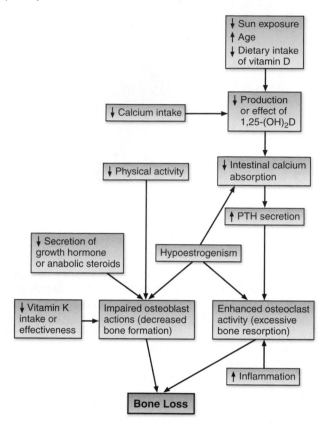

Measuring biochemical markers of bone turnover combined with BMD may provide a more accurate prediction of future fracture risk.[10] Other known risk factors for osteoporotic fracture should be assessed as well.

The North American Menopause Society (NAMS) recommends that BMD be measured in all women 65 years old or older, in younger postmenopausal women with one or more risk factors, and in all women with medical conditions associated with an increased risk of osteoporosis.[11]

Risk Factors for Osteoporotic Fracture

The focus of osteoporosis screening programs is to reduce the risk of fracture. In addition to bone density, many other factors influence fracture risk. The Women's Health Initiative (WHI) investigated whether an algorithm could be created that would predict the 5-year risk of hip fracture among the 93,676 postmenopausal women who participated in the observational component. Eleven factors were found to be predictive: age (number of years older than 50), self-reported health, weight, height, race or ethnicity, self-reported physical activity, fracture at 55 years old or older, parental hip fracture, smoking status, corticosteroid use, and treated diabetes.[12]

Other factors that increase the risk of a fracture include nutritional deficiencies, high alcohol intake, excessive caffeine consumption, premature menopause, malabsorption disorders, autoimmune disease, small body frame, white

/Caucasian or Asian descent, impaired vision, dizziness or balance problems, fainting or loss of consciousness, physical frailty, vitamin D deficiency, and use of medications, including corticosteroids, aromatase inhibitors, anticonvulsants, sedatives, anticholinergics, antihypertensives, heparin, cyclosporine, and medroxyprogesterone acetate.

Role of Inflammation

Chronic inflammation is implicated in the process of aging,[13,14] and it plays a role in the development of a wide range of chronic diseases, including cardiovascular disease, Alzheimer disease, diabetes, and cancer.[15,16] Growing evidence indicates that osteoporosis is also, in part, a result of chronic low-grade inflammation.[17-21] Women with chronic inflammatory diseases such as rheumatoid arthritis and inflammatory bowel disease are known to be at increased risk of developing osteoporosis.[22] However, elevated levels of high-sensitivity C-reactive protein (hsCRP) are associated with lower BMD in healthy women, as well as in women with inflammatory conditions.[19]

Proinflammatory cytokines such as interleukin-6 (IL-6), IL-1, and tumor necrosis factor-alpha (TNF-alpha) promote accelerated bone loss by activation of osteoclasts, inhibition of collagen production in osteoblasts, and enhanced breakdown of the extracellular matrix.[16] Furthermore, suppression of proinflammatory cytokines appears to support the growth of new bone. For instance, TNF-alpha inhibitors such as Etanercept have been found to improve BMD in patients with spondyloarthropathy.[23]

Additionally, diets rich in fruits, vegetables[24] and omega-3 fatty acids[25] have been found to decrease the risk of developing osteoporosis. Fruit and vegetable consumption is associated with both increased peak bone mass and improved bone health in older populations.[26-29] The bone-building effects of fruits and vegetables may result from several factors: antiinflammatory and antioxidant properties; alkalinizing effects; the nutrients, such as potassium, vitamin K, and vitamin C, that they provide; and the presence of other unknown compounds and synergistic effects. For all these reasons, an antiinflammatory diet is recommended as the foundation of an integrative bone health plan.

Integrative Therapy

Nutrition for Bone Health

Calcium

Calcium is an essential nutrient for building and maintaining healthy bones; 99% of calcium in the body is in bone, and 38% of bone matrix consists of calcium. Surprisingly, however, high calcium intakes do not ensure strong bones, and low calcium intakes do not necessarily lead to weaker bones.[2,30] Calcium is absorbed in the small intestine by a transcellular transport mechanism that requires adequate vitamin D. Calcium may also be absorbed by passive diffusion when calcium intakes are high. Calcium excretion increases as dietary protein[31] and sodium intakes rise.[32] Vegetarians excrete less calcium in their urine than do omnivores.[33]

Calcium absorption can be improved and excess excretion can be decreased by the following: maintaining a 25(OH)D concentration higher than 34 ng/mL (85 nmol/L),[34] avoiding

TABLE 37-1. Dietary Reference Intakes for Calcium and Vitamin D

	CALCIUM			VITAMIN D		
Life Stage Group	Estimated Average Requirement (mg/day)	Recommended Dietary Allowance (mg/day)	Upper Level Intake (mg/day)	Estimated Average Requirement (mg/day)	Recommended Dietary Allowance (Units/Day)	Upper Level Intake (Units/Day)
Infants 0–6 mo	*	*	1,000	†	†	1,000
Infants 6–12 mo	*	*	1,500	†	†	1,500
1–3 yr	500	700	2,500	400	600	2,500
4–8 yr	800	1,000	25,000	400	600	3,000
9–13 yr	1,100	1,300	3,000	400	600	4,000
14–18 yr	1,100	1,300	3,000	400	600	4,000
19–30 yr	800	1,000	2,500	400	600	4,000
31–50 yr	800	1,000	2,500	400	600	4,000
51–70 yr (M)	800	1,000	2,000	400	600	4,000
51–70 yr (F)	1,000	1,200	2,000	400	600	4,000
Older than 70 yr	1,000	1,200	2,000	400	800	4,000
14–18 yr, pregnant or lactating	1,100	1,300	3,000	400	600	4,000
19–50 yr, pregnant or lactating	800	1,000	2,500	400	600	4,000

From Committee to Review Dietary Reference Intakes for Vitamin D and Calcium. In: Ross AC, Taylor CL, Yaktine AL, Del Valle HB, eds. *Dietary Reference Intakes for Calcium and Vitamin D.* Washington, DC: National Academies Press, 2011.
*For infants, adequate intake is 200mg/day for 0 to 6 monthsof age and 260mg/day for 6 to 12 monthsof age.
†For infants, adequate intake is 400mg/day for 0 to 6 monthsof age and 400mg/day for 6 to 12 monthsof age.

excess animal protein, increasing consumption of fruits and vegetables, limiting dietary sodium to less than 2400 mg/day,[35] avoiding excess caffeine,[36] eating fewer highly refined carbohydrates,[37] and having an adequate intake of essential fatty acids.[38]

In the United States, the Institute of Medicine (IOM) issued a 2010 update of the dietary reference intakes (DRIs) for calcium and vitamin D (Table 37-1).

A *Lancet* meta-analysis published in 2007 reviewed 29 randomized trials with more than 63,000 patients and found good evidence that the use of calcium, alone or in combination with vitamin D, prevented osteoporosis in women and men 50 years old and older.[39] The meta-analysis also showed a 12% reduction in the risk of fractures, with treatment more effective at higher doses of calcium (higher than 1200 mg) and vitamin D (higher than 800 units). Calcium sources in the diet extend significantly beyond dairy products (Tables 37-2 and 37-3). An estimate of calcium intake from all dietary sources should be made before supplements are added.

In postmenopausal women with low calcium intakes, the addition of 500 mg per day of calcium citrate has been found to significantly reduce bone loss in the femur, radius,

TABLE 37-2. Dairy Calcium Sources

FOOD	AMOUNT (oz)	CALCIUM (mg)
Milk	8	300
Yogurt	8	275–325
Hard cheeses high in calcium (cheddar, Swiss, Edam, Monterey Jack, Provolone, Parmesan, Romano, part-skim mozzarella)	1	200–300
Soft cheeses low in calcium (Brie, Neufchatel)	1	20–50

and spine.[40] Milk consumption[41] and higher calcium intakes alone may not favorably affect fracture risk, however.[42] Accordingly, calcium supplementation should be part of a broader strategy that includes adequate vitamin D and other bone-building foods and nutrients.

TABLE 37-3. Nondairy Calcium Sources

FOOD	AMOUNT	CALCIUM (mg)
White beans	1 oz cooked	161
Spinach	½ cup	122
Turnip greens	½ cup	99
Soybeans	½ cup cooked	90
Broccoli	1 cup cooked or fresh	90
Bok choy	½ cup cooked or fresh	80
Almonds	1 oz dry-roasted	80
Salmon	3 oz, canned with bones	180
Dried figs	10	269

A 2010 meta-analysis in *BMJ* (the *British Medical Journal*) suggested increased cardiovascular events in women taking calcium. The studies, conducted in patients with osteopenia, were not controlled for risk factors for heart disease, however. In addition, when calcium was administered with vitamin D (as is recommended), it did not lead to any increased risk.[43]

Large tablets may be difficult to swallow and may not fully disintegrate in the stomach. Some people tolerate calcium supplements better in the form of powders, capsules, and liquids. Calcium supplementation should not exceed 500 mg at any one time, to maximize absorption. Avoid taking calcium supplements along with psyllium or with foods high in oxalic acid (e.g., spinach) or phytic acid (e.g., wheat bran). Chewable calcium supplements are well tolerated by children.

Calcium carbonate is best taken with meals and is less expensive than calcium citrate. Calcium carbonate provides 40% elemental calcium. Calcium citrate is well absorbed with or without meals,[44] and it is the best form for older adults with reduced stomach acid. Calcium citrate provides 21% elemental calcium. Calcium from dolomite, oyster shell, or coral is not recommended.

Acid-Base Issues

The skeleton plays a key role in acid-base homeostasis.[45] Eating animal protein generates acids that are excreted in the urine. High intakes of animal protein can lead to significant calcium resorption from bones to buffer the acids.[4,46] Urinary losses of calcium rise in proportion to net renal acid secretion. In contrast, fruits and vegetables generate bicarbonate, which can buffer the acidifying effects of animal protein, alkalinize the urine, and significantly lower urinary calcium excretion.[4] A study by Buclin et al[46] revealed that acid-forming diets increased calcium excretion by 74% when compared with base-forming diets.

In bone, minute downward shifts in the local pH can stimulate osteoclast activity and impair the activity of osteoblasts.[47] The typical Western diet tends to produce chronic low-grade metabolic acidosis that is harmful to bone health.[48–50] Diets with less animal protein and increased amounts of fruits and vegetables are therefore recommended.

Muhlbauer described 25 plant foods as bone resorption inhibitory food items (BRIFI). These include garlic, rosemary, Italian parsley, sage, thyme, parsley, dill, onion, arugula, prune, fennel, orange, leek, yellow boletus, wild garlic, field agaric, red cabbage, celeriac, red wine, and lettuce.[51] In addition to effects on acid-base balance, the benefits of plant foods also appear to be related to the pharmacologically active compounds they contain. Certain specific monoterpenes,[52] flavonoids, and phenols[53] may be responsible for the observed beneficial effects on bone.

Vitamin D

Vitamin D is essential for calcium absorption and for bone health. The hormonally active form of vitamin D, 1,25(OH)D, induces active transport of calcium across the intestinal mucosa. Vitamin D also stimulates the absorption of phosphate and magnesium ions and acts synergistically with vitamin K to stimulate bone mineralization directly.

Vitamin D deficiency and insufficiency are widespread throughout North America.[54–56] Breast-fed infants, women, older adults, obese persons, and people with darker skin tones are at higher risk of deficiency. An international epidemiologic study found that 64% of postmenopausal women seeking medical care for osteoporosis had inadequate vitamin D concentrations (less than 30 ng/mL).[57] Supplementation with vitamin D at doses of 700 to 800 units/day has been shown to reduce fracture risk in older adults.[58,59] Vitamin D also reduces the risk of falls[60–62] and improves lower extremity function[63] in older adults.

Current recommended intakes of vitamin D are considered too low by many researchers.[64,65] All patients should be screened at least once for vitamin D deficiency with a measurement of their serum 25(OH)D concentration. Although in 2010 the IOM revised the vitamin D deficiency level to 20 ng/mL, data support higher levels for bone health. For example, a 2005 meta-analysis found that optimum fracture prevention was reached at a level of 40 ng/mL (100 nmol/L).[59] Each incremental increase in 25(OH)D is associated with an increase in BMD.[66–68]

Vitamin D can be obtained through sunlight exposure, from a limited number of foods, or from supplements. Sunlight exposures of 10 to 15 minutes, without sun block, at the appropriate latitude and season, can be a good source of endogenously produced vitamin D. A few foods are naturally rich in vitamin D: fatty ocean fish such as salmon, sardines, and black cod, as well as sun-exposed mushrooms. Fortified foods include some brands of orange juice, fortified milk, and some yogurts. Vitamin D supplementation is an inexpensive and reliable way to ensure an optimum serum concentration of 40 ng/mL (100 nmol/L). For most adults older than age 65, a supplement of at least 700 units/day is needed to achieve this serum concentration.[69,70] Vitamin D_3 (cholecalciferol) is the preferred form to use,[71] and it should be taken with meals.

Essential Fatty Acids

Both omega-6 and omega-3 polyunsaturated fatty acids are essential nutrients. They are incorporated into cell membranes, where they influence membrane characteristics and become precursors for eicosanoids such as prostaglandins, leukotrienes, and thromboxanes. An ideal ratio between omega-6 and omega-3 fatty acids is thought to be 1:1 to 2:1.[72] However, Western diets tend to be relatively high in omega-6 fats and low in omega-3 fatty acids, and typical ratios are approximately 10:1 (omega-6 to omega-3).[73] These fats perform opposing roles in the body, and the balance between them plays a significant role in regulating the inflammatory response.

Omega-3 fatty acids are known to have antiinflammatory effects and act to suppress production of IL-1-beta, TNF-alpha, and IL-6.[74,75] Certain omega-6 fatty acids, such as gamma-linolenic acid (GLA) are also known to possess antiinflammatory effects. In contrast, the omega-6 fatty acid linoleic acid (LA) tends to have proinflammatory effects and leads to increased production of IL-1, TNF, and IL-6 cytokines.

The intake and ratio of essential fatty acids in the diet appear to play important roles in bone health. In animal studies, fish oils rich in omega-3 fatty acids have been found to attenuate bone loss associated with estrogen withdrawal.[76] Animal studies have also shown that the omega-3 fatty acid eicosapentaenoic acid (EPA) enhances calcium absorption, reduces calcium excretion, and increases calcium deposition in bone.[77]

Limited human studies of omega-3 supplementation for osteoporosis prevention or treatment have been conducted. One small study found that supplementation with calcium, EPA, and GLA resulted in a decrease in bone turnover and an increase in lumbar and femoral bone density in older women.[77] In the Rancho Bernardo study, higher ratios of omega-6 to omega-3 fatty acids were associated with lower BMD in the hip for all women studied and with lower BMD in the spine for women not taking hormone replacement therapy (HRT).[78] Overall, omega-3 fatty acids appear to enhance calcium absorption, reduce calcium excretion, and improve mineralization of bone matrix and bone strength.[38]

Protein

Protein is required for bone formation, and adequate protein intake, particularly in the premenopausal years, is essential.[79] However, high levels of animal protein in the diet are associated with increased fracture rates and accelerated bone mineral loss.[80-82] In the Nurses' Health Study, protein intakes higher than 95 g/day were associated with significantly higher forearm fracture rates than were protein intakes lower than 68 g/day.[81] In another study, lowering protein intakes to current recommended dietary allowance (RDA) guidelines (0.8 g/kg) resulted in significant reductions in urinary calcium excretion and in markers of bone resorption.[83] Several studies also showed that an increased ratio of vegetable to animal protein was protective against fractures.[84-86] To support bone health, an adequate but not excessive intake of protein is recommended. Some protein-rich vegetarian foods such as tofu and edamame should be included.

Vitamin K

The two naturally occurring classes of vitamin K are phylloquinone (K_1), which is synthesized by plants, and menaquinone (K_2), which is synthesized by bacteria. Both forms are useful in the prevention and therapy of osteoporosis. Vitamin K plays a key role in carboxylating osteocalcin and other bone proteins.[87] As mentioned, vitamins K and D act synergistically to stimulate bone mineralization.[88,89]

Epidemiologic studies consistently show a link between higher vitamin K status and reduction of fracture risk. Booth et al[90] reviewed data from the Framingham Heart Study and found that elderly men and women in the highest quartile of dietary vitamin K had a relative risk for hip fracture of 0.35. Women in the Nurse's Health Study who consumed one or more servings of lettuce per day (a source of vitamin K_1) had a relative risk of 0.55 for hip fracture.[91] Patients with osteoporotic fractures of the spine and femoral neck were found to be markedly deficient in vitamin K_1 and in the MK-7 and MK-8 forms of vitamin K_2.[92] Other studies have shown similar findings.[93] Most vitamin K intervention studies also showed a reduction in BMD loss and improved bone biomarkers.[94]

The Vitamin K Supplementation in Postmenopausal Women with Osteopenia (ECKO) trial was a 2-year randomized controlled trial of 440 postmenopausal women with osteopenia. The women were treated with 5 mg of vitamin K_1 daily. No significant difference in changes in BMD was noted between the two groups. Although fewer women in the vitamin K group had clinical fractures (9 versus 20, $P = .04$), the study was not sufficiently powered to measure fractures.[95]

Subclinical vitamin K deficiency is common, and typical dietary intakes are lower than the levels associated with decreased fracture risk.[96] The current DRI for adult women is 90 mcg, but amounts of 450 mcg/day or higher may be needed for optimum bone health.[87] The best food sources of vitamin K_1 are green leafy vegetables such as lettuce, collards, spinach, and kale, as well as other vegetables rich in chlorophyll, such as broccoli. Other plant sources include vegetable oils, nuts, and fruits. Animal foods such as chicken, soft cheeses, and butter contain relatively small amounts of vitamin K_2. Natto, a fermented soybean food, is a very rich source of vitamin K_2. Vitamin K is fat soluble, and foods rich in vitamin K should be eaten with some healthy fat, such as olive oil. Patients taking anticoagulants should aim for a consistent intake of vitamin K–rich foods.

Vitamin K supplementation does not have an overcoagulation effect, and it has an excellent safety profile. In 2001, the IOM showed no evidence of toxicity with vitamin K supplementation, and in Japan, vitamin K_2 is prescribed at doses of 45 to 90 mg (1000 times the RDA) without side effects. Vitamin K supplements should not be used by patients taking anticoagulants.

Magnesium

Epidemiologic studies have linked higher magnesium intakes with increased BMD.[11,12] Some intervention trials of magnesium supplementation have also shown an increase in BMD, as well as reduced fracture rates.[97,98] In the WHI trial, however, participants in the highest quintile of magnesium intake had the highest rate of wrist and lower arm fractures.[99]

Therefore, the data on the relationship between magnesium intake and bone remain inconclusive. The average magnesium intake for U.S. women is 228 mg/day, whereas the DRI for magnesium is 320 mg/day, so insufficient intakes are common. Magnesium deficiency may impair osteoblast function and induce bone resorption by osteoclasts.[100] Magnesium is also required for the conversion of vitamin D to 1,25-dihydroxycholecalciferol (calcitriol).[101] Good sources of magnesium include nuts and seeds, soybeans, dark green leafy vegetables, and dairy products.

Trace Minerals

Several trace minerals including zinc, copper, boron, and manganese act as cofactors in specific enzymes related to bone metabolism. Serum concentrations of zinc and copper have been found to be lower in osteoporotic women than in controls.[102] A varied, whole food diet in addition to a good-quality multivitamin/mineral supplement should ensure an adequate supply of these nutrients.

Vitamin C

Vitamin C (ascorbic acid) is a required nutrient for collagen formation. Although vitamin C deficiency is often unrecognized, it is relatively common in the United States; 18% of adults consume less than 30 mg/day.[103] Vitamin C, along with calcium intakes of 500 mg/day or more, appears to support an increase in BMD.[104]

Soy

Studies of soy's effects on bone have shown mixed results.[105] Unfortunately, as outlined in a 2006 meta-analysis, these studies have many flaws. Of the 11 randomized controlled trials, no two studies used identical products; they studied isoflavones rather than soy as a whole food; some studies used very low doses of isoflavones, whereas others did not specify the amounts; and most trials lasted for only 6 to 12 months, too short to detect effect on BMD.[106]

An exception to these poorly designed trials is the Shanghai Women's Health Study. This study, which examined food frequency questionnaires of 75,000 Chinese women 40 to 70 years old, found a relative risk of fracture of 0.63 in the highest quintile of soy protein intake (13 g/day or more).[107] In fact, a significant reduction in fracture risk was seen beginning in the second quintile, at soy protein intakes of 5 g/day (21 mg/day of isoflavones). This study examined the intake of traditionally eaten whole soy foods, such as tofu and fresh soybeans, rather than isolated isoflavones. This is also one of the few studies of soy to look at the key end point of fracture risk, as opposed to BMD or markers of bone turnover.

Soy appears to have certain beneficial effects on bone: stimulating production of osteoprotegerin by osteoblasts, suppressing activation of osteoclasts, and increasing production of insulin-like growth factor-I.[108,109] On the whole, the evidence from in vitro, animal, and human studies supports a beneficial effect of soy on bone health.[110,111] Based on the available evidence, one to two servings/day of whole soy foods can be recommended.

Substances That May Be Harmful to Bone Health

Sodium

Average sodium intakes in the United States (3500 mg/day) exceed the recommended intake of less than 2400 mg/day, and high-salt diets are known to increase urinary calcium excretion.[12] The Dietary Approaches to Stop Hypertension and Sodium Reduction (DASH II) diet, which included 9.5 servings of fruits and vegetables per day, low-fat dairy products, whole grains, and reduced meat and sodium intake, resulted in decreased calcium losses and reduced bone turnover.[112] However, the bone benefits of DASH II diet appear to be related to its overall effects rather than specifically to the reduction in sodium. Increasing calcium and potassium intakes can substantially offset the urinary losses of calcium caused by high sodium intakes.[32] Because there are cardiovascular benefits to moderating sodium intake and because many diets do not contain sufficient calcium, patients should be advised to stay within the recommended sodium intake of less than 2400 mg/day.

Caffeine

Excessive caffeine intake is associated with a modest increase in the risk of osteoporotic fracture.[36] The increased risk appears to occur in women who consume more than 300 mg of caffeine/day or approximately 4 cups of coffee, and who also have low calcium intake. Excessive caffeine intake should be avoided.

Phosphorus

Phosphorus is required to form hydroxyapatite, a key component of bone. The RDA is 700 mg; however, typical North American diets contain amounts ranging from 1000 to 1600 mg per day. Furthermore, additives in processed foods such as hot dogs and processed cheese can add as much as 1000 mg/day of additional phosphorus to the diet. Total phosphorus intake may be underestimated because phosphorus from food additives is often not included in food composition tables.[113] Excessive intake of phosphorus may be harmful to bone health; it has been shown to depress serum calcium levels, increase secretion of parathyroid hormone, decrease markers of bone formation, and increase markers of bone absorption.[114] The Brazilian Osteoporosis Study found that a higher intake of phosphorus was associated with an increased risk of fragility fractures in women older than 40 years.[115] Although human studies are few, preventing excessive phosphorus intake by reducing intake of processed foods and by avoiding excess animal protein in the diet seems to be a prudent approach.

Vitamin A

Vitamin A (retinol) intakes of more than 3000 mcg/day are associated with a significantly increased risk of hip fracture.[116] This increased risk exists for retinol intake from foods and from supplements.[117] Although not all studies support these findings, consumers should choose supplements that contain less than 2000 mcg of retinol, or preferably, products that contain only beta-carotene or mixed carotenoids.

Smoking

Cigarette smoking is a known risk factor for osteoporosis, but the underlying mechanisms for this association are not fully understood. The effect of smoking on fracture risk is not closely linked to BMD, and it may be related to lower body mass, earlier age of menopause, estrogen-lowering effects, impaired calcium absorption, or increased production of free radicals.[118] In the Nurses' Health Study, smokers had a relative risk of 1.2 for hip fracture, and this figure rose to 1.4 for those who smoked 25 or more cigarettes/day.[119] A meta-analysis involving more than 59,000 men and women found that smokers had a relative risk of 1.13 for any fracture and a relative risk of 1.6 for hip fractures.[120] Clearly, for many reasons, people should be encouraged not to begin smoking. Current smokers who quit will obtain benefits to their bone health after a period of 10 years.[119]

Alcohol

Animal studies showed that chronic heavy alcohol consumption, especially during adolescence and young adulthood, can significantly damage bone health.[121] In contrast, low or moderate consumption of alcohol in adulthood appears to have protective effects on bone.[122] Moderate alcohol consumption has recognized cardiovascular benefits,[123] but it can also increase the risk of breast cancer in women,[124] and it has other potentially detrimental effects on health.[125] Men may benefit from a daily alcoholic beverage; women should be advised to have fewer than seven alcoholic drinks per week.

Botanicals

Numerous in vitro and animal studies and a smaller number of human trials have examined the potential of herbal medicines to enhance bone health.[53] A study of Shen Gu (Mixture for Nourishing Kidney and Strengthening Bone) in 96 osteoporotic patients found significant beneficial effects on bone as compared with controls.[126] The Ayurvedic herbal-mineral preparation Reosto, which contains a mixture of botanicals and organic calcium, was studied in a randomized double-blind placebo-controlled trial. BMD increased significantly in the treatment group versus controls over the study period of 12 months.[127] A 12-week study involving 62 postmenopausal women found that black cohosh (Actaea racemosa) increased concentrations of bone-specific alkaline phosphatase (a metabolic marker for bone formation) and stimulated osteoblast activity.[128] Dioscorea spongiosa,[129,130] Astragalus membranaceus,[131] walnut extract (Juglans regia L.),[132] and curcumin, a compound found in turmeric root (Curcuma longa),[133] have also shown osteoprotective effects in laboratory and animal studies. Further research is needed to assess the role of botanical medicines in supporting bone health.

Tea (Camellia sinensis)

Tea has antiinflammatory effects, cardiovascular benefits, and cancer protective properties.[134,135] Several studies have linked tea consumption to modest increases in BMD.[135,136]

Mind-Body Connection

Chronic stress, through activation of the sympathetic nervous system, tends to exert catabolic effects on the body that result in the breakdown of energy stores and body tissues. In animal studies, both chronic stressors and the administration of glucocorticoids were shown to stimulate bone resorption.[137,138] Major depression[139,140] and anorexia nervosa[141] are both associated with elevation of serum cortisol levels and with increased bone loss. Increased sympathetic nervous system activity stimulates resorption of bone by osteoclasts and inhibits bone formation by osteoblasts.[142]

Bone remodeling appears to be influenced by input from the central nervous system, as well as by previously recognized local factors and hormonal signals.[143] Stress reduction, using mind-body practices such as meditation, self-hypnosis, guided imagery, breath work, or biofeedback, is highly recommended as part of an integrative plan to support bone health and overall well-being.

Exercise

In addition to high-quality nutrition, exercise is the other major factor needed to build and maintain strong bones. Bone is dynamic tissue that responds to the physiologic and biomechanical signals it receives. Both general physical activity and mechanical loading contribute to building peak bone mass, beginning in the prepubertal years.[144,145]

Bone density at all skeletal sites is strongly correlated with muscle mass, and muscle mass is strongly linked to physical activity.[146] Muscle mass generally increases until approximately the age of 30 years and begins to decline after 50 years of age. Muscle strength losses tend to be most striking after the age of 70 years. Investigators have proved, however, that regular exercise at any age, even in very old persons, can result in increased muscle strength, balance, and functional capacity.[147,148]

Exercise training programs in premenopausal and postmenopausal women have been shown to prevent or reverse bone loss consistently in both the lumbar spine and the femoral neck.[149] The Bone Estrogen Strength Training (BEST) Study found that postmenopausal women who received 800 mg/day of calcium citrate, along with a structured exercise program, increased their muscle mass by 11% to 21% and increased their BMD by approximately 2%.[150] Even women with established osteoporosis can improve their bone mass with a low-impact exercise program.[151] Fracture risk can also be decreased with exercise programs. Walking for at least 4 hours per week has been found to decrease hip fracture risk by 41%.[152] Another study of postmenopausal women found a reduced risk of vertebral fractures after a 2-year program of back-strengthening exercises.[153]

In the Senior Fitness and Prevention (SEFIP) study, 246 women who were older than 65 years old were randomized to an 18-month exercise program or a wellness program. Participants in the exercise program showed an increase in BMD at the spine of 1.77% (controls increased 0.033%) and at the femoral neck of 1.01% (controls decreased 1.05%). Fewer falls occurred in the exercise group (1.0 per person compared with 1.66 in the control group). In addition, health care costs were lowered in the exercise group (€2225 versus €2780 in controls).[154]

Recommended physical activities include walking, gentle and vigorous aerobic exercise, jumping, running, weight training, and racquet sports. Ideally, people should aim for 30 to 45 minutes of exercise, five or more times per week. Weight training is best done on alternate days. Tai chi is highly recommended to reduce the number of falls in older adults.[155–157]

Considerations in Younger Women

Ideally, every young woman should reach her own highest possible peak bone mass by age 30 to 35 years. Peak bone mass is influenced by genetic factors, as well as by diet and physical activity during childhood, adolescence, and young adulthood. Young women should be counseled about the importance of a healthy diet, adequate calcium and vitamin D, and regular weight-bearing exercise. Maintaining an ideal body weight and engaging in regular physical activity may be the most important modifiable factors in the development of optimum bone mass.[158]

Young women who use depot medroxyprogesterone acetate (DMPA) for contraception are at risk for bone loss. Women 18 to 21 years old who use DMPA have been found to lose bone at a rate of 1.5% per year during a time when control groups gained bone at an average rate of 2% per year.[159] BMD tends to recover after discontinuation of DMPA.[160] Smoking, heavy alcohol consumption, anorexia nervosa,[141] late-onset menarche, amenorrhea,[161] primary ovarian failure, and autoimmune diseases[162] are other risk factors that may prevent young women from achieving their optimum peak bone mass.

Some bone loss normally accompanies pregnancy and lactation and is then usually recovered after infants are weaned.[163] Epidemiologic studies show that multiple pregnancies and periods of lactation are not associated with lower bone mass or increased fracture risk.[164]

Pharmaceuticals

Osteoporosis is best approached with a lifelong, comprehensive prevention program. Women of all ages should be aware of the diet and lifestyle choices that support bone health. Ongoing strategies should include optimum diet, appropriate supplementation, regular physical activity, and fall prevention. Secondary causes of osteoporosis should be corrected when possible.

In addition, pharmacologic therapy for prevention or treatment of osteoporosis may be recommended. Guidelines for initiating therapy vary among different organizations. The NAMS guidelines recommend treatment in all postmenopausal women with prior vertebral or hip fracture or with hip or spine T-scores lower than −2.5 and in postmenopausal women with T-scores between −2.0 and −2.5 and with one or more additional risk factors.[165] Some women may wish to begin an extensive bone-building program and continue to monitor their bone density before making a decision to begin medication.

The number needed to treat (NNT) and, when available, the number needed to harm (NNH) are useful communication tools for discussing the benefit of any medication used for prevention. These numbers are especially useful in osteoporosis in which the NNT tends to be quite high, thus making the decision much less clear and more closely related to a patient's values. (Some patients like to do everything possible to prevent a possible problem, whereas others prefer to take as few medications as possible.)

Role of Estrogen

As estrogen levels fall in the years following menopause, bone loss accelerates. The primary action of estrogen on bone is to inhibit the osteoclast by increasing the amount of osteoprotegerin produced by osteoblasts.[166] Estrogen also has antiinflammatory effects and suppresses the production of bone-resorbing cytokines.[167-169] Consequently, at the time of menopause, the concentration of inflammatory cytokines that can induce osteoclastogenesis rises.[170,171]

Postmenopausal HRT has beneficial effects on bone, reduces the risk of colon cancer, and can alleviate hot flashes and vaginal dryness. Conversely, women who use HRT have an increased risk of cardiovascular disease, stroke, thromboembolic events, and breast cancer.[172] In the WHI trial, women receiving hormone therapy with conjugated equine estrogen, alone or with medroxyprogesterone acetate, had increased BMD and lower fracture rates. However, the study investigators concluded: "When considering the effects of hormone therapy on other important disease outcomes in a global model, there was no net benefit, even in women considered to be at high risk of fracture."[173] Some leading health organizations recommend against the use of HRT for the prevention of chronic disease.[174] Thus, treatment with HRT

should be individualized, based on a careful exploration of the risks and benefits for each woman.

Bisphosphonates

Antiresorptive therapies reduce fracture risk by inhibiting the activity of osteoclasts and reducing bone turnover, thus increasing bone mass. High bone turnover is particularly relevant in the pathogenesis of vertebral fractures.[39] Bisphosphonates are indicated for both prevention and treatment of postmenopausal osteoporosis. The most common side effects are dyspepsia, nausea, and abdominal pain. Osteonecrosis of the jaw is a serious, rare event associated with bisphosphonate use (most often when bisphosphonates are prescribed intravenously as a component of cancer treatment). Some concern also exists that bisphosphonates may impair microdamage repair and thus increase the brittleness of bone.[175,176]

Alendronate has been shown to increase BMD and to reduce the incidence of fractures of the spine and hip in women with osteoporosis.[177] Esophagitis may occur with alendronate. The usual dose range is 35 to 70 mg once weekly. Risedronate also increases BMD and reduces vertebral and some nonvertebral fracture rates.[178] The usual dose is 35 mg once weekly. Ibandronate has indications and side effects similar to those of the two other bisphosphonates discussed. Ibandronate may be given as a once-per-month dose of 150 mg.[179] Of the three oral forms, alendronate has the lowest 3-year NNT to prevent vertebral fractures (NNT = 15) (Tables 37-4 and 37-5).[165,180]

TABLE 37-4. Vertebral Fracture Prevention Studies

MEDICATION	DOSE	3-YEAR NNT TO PREVENT VERTEBRAL FRACTURE	TRIAL
Alendronate (Fosamax)	5 mg/day for 2 yr then 10 mg/day	15/34	FIT
Ibandronate (Boniva)	2.5 mg/day or 20 mg eod for 12 doses every 3 months	21	BONE
Risedronate (Actonel)	2.5 or 5 mg/day	20	VERTA-NA
Zoledronic acid (Reclast)	5 mg IV every yr	14	HORIZON
Raloxifene (Evista)	60 or 120 mg/day	29	MORE
Strontium ranelate	2 g/day	9	SOTI
Teriparatide (Forteo)	20 mcg sq/day	12	—

BONE, oral iBandronate Osteoporosis vertebral fracture trial in North America and Europe; eod, every other day; FIT, Fracture Intervention Trial; HORIZON, Health Outcomes and Reduced Incidence with Zoledronic Acid Once Yearly; IV, intravenously; MORE, Multiple Outcomes of Raloxifene Evaluation; NNT, number needed to treat; SOTI, Spinal Osteoporosis Therapeutic Intervention; VERTA-NA, Vertebral Efficacy with Risedronate Therapy—North America.

TABLE 37-5. Hip Fracture Prevention Studies

MEDICATION	DOSE	NNT TO PREVENT A HIP FRACTURE	TRIAL
Alendronate	5 mg/day for 2 yr then 10 mg/day	91	FIT
Risedronate	2.5 or 5 mg/day	91	HIP
Zoledronic acid	5 mg IV/yr	91	HORIZON
Strontium ranelate	2 g/day	48	TROPOS

FIT, Fracture Intervention Trial; HIP, Hip Intervention Program; HORIZON, Health Outcomes and Reduced Incidence with Zoledronic Acid Once Yearly; IV, intravenously; NNT, number needed to treat; TROPOS, Treatment of Peripheral Osteoporosis.

Selective Estrogen Receptor Modulators

Selective estrogen receptor modulators act as estrogen agonists on bone and lipid metabolism while also having antagonist actions on breast and endometrial tissue. Raloxifene has been shown to be effective at reducing postmenopausal bone loss and at decreasing the risk of vertebral fractures.[181] The 3-year NNT to prevent vertebral fractures is 29. Raloxifene also significantly reduces the risk of breast cancer and improves lipid profiles.[182] The usual dose is 60 mg/day. Side effects include deep vein thrombosis and pulmonary embolism.

Calcitonin

Calcitonin is produced by thyroid C cells and acts to inhibit bone resorption by inhibiting osteoclast activity. Calcitonin from salmon may be used to treat osteoporosis in women who have been postmenopausal for at least 5 years. Calcitonin is effective in reducing the pain associated with acute compression fractures of the vertebrae,[183] and it may reduce the incidence of vertebral fractures. It is normally given as a daily intranasal spray of 200 units. Side effects are usually minor and include flushing, nausea, and diarrhea.

Teriparatide

Teriparatide (PTH 1-34) is a medication that includes a sequence of 34 amino acids contained in parathyroid hormone. Teriparatide has anabolic effects on bone and stimulates osteoblast cell proliferation. This agent is useful in reducing the incidence of new vertebral and nonvertebral fractures in postmenopausal women.[179,184,185] The 3-year NNT to prevent vertebral fractures is 12. Teriparatide is given as a once-daily subcutaneous injection (20 mcg) for a period of up to 2 years. This therapy may be followed by an antiresorptive agent. Side effects include nausea and headaches.

Strontium

Strontium ranelate is a promising medication that is currently used in Europe for the treatment of postmenopausal osteoporosis. Several studies found it to be an effective agent in reducing vertebral and nonvertebral fracture risk in both younger postmenopausal women and very old

adults.[186,187] The 3-year NNT to prevent vertebral fractures is 9, the lowest of all currently available therapies. Strontium ranelate acts both to stimulate bone formation and to reduce bone resorption. Adverse effects include nausea and diarrhea.[188]

Pharmaceuticals to Avoid

Many pharmaceuticals can negatively affect bone density. In May 2010, the U.S. Food and Drug Administration added a warning label to proton pump inhibitors and stated that these drugs were associated with possible increased risk of fractures of the hip, wrist, and spine.

Conclusion

Osteoporosis is a costly and potentially disabling condition affecting millions of people. An integrative approach encompassing diet, exercise, supplements, and mind-body therapies, as well as pharmaceutical medications when indicated, is recommended to prevent and treat this disorder. The good news is that essentially the same strategies that help people build healthy bones will also protect them against heart disease, diabetes, depression, and a host of other chronic conditions.

PREVENTION PRESCRIPTION

Recommendations to build and maintain healthy bones:

- An antiinflammatory diet that includes an abundance of deeply colored fruits and vegetables, healthy fats, whole grains, and antiinflammatory herbs, teas, and spices
- Elemental calcium intake from diet in addition to supplements adding up to at least 800 mg per day
- A serum 25-OH vitamin D concentration in the range of 40 ng/mL (100 nmol/L)
- A balanced ratio of omega-6 to omega-3 fatty acids
- Adequate but not excessive protein (0.8 g/kg), including some vegetarian protein sources
- One to two servings per day of whole soy foods
- A good-quality multivitamin and mineral supplement
- Physical activity for 30 to 45 minutes most days of the week that includes weight-bearing, aerobic, and weight-lifting exercise
- A daily mind-body practice
- Avoidance of smoking, excess alcohol intake, excess caffeine consumption, and vitamin A (retinol) in amounts greater than 2000 mcg/day
- Reduction of the risk of falls and, if possible, avoidance of prescribing medications that harm bone or increase the risk of falls
- Pharmaceutical therapies that are individualized, with risk and benefits explored with each patient

THERAPEUTIC REVIEW

Osteoporosis is a costly and potentially disabling condition affecting millions of people. An integrative approach encompassing diet, exercise, supplements, and mind-body therapies, as well as pharmaceutical medications when indicated, is recommended to prevent and treat this disorder. The good news is that essentially the same strategies that help people build healthy bones will also protect them against heart disease, diabetes, depression, and a host of other chronic conditions.

Laboratory Evaluation

- 25-Hydroxy vitamin D level with a goal near 40 ng/mL

- Dual x-ray absorptiometry bone scan

- Consider highly sensitive C-reactive protein, thyroid-stimulating hormone, calcium, and alkaline phosphatase.

- To assess metabolic markers of bone turnover, consider urine levels of N-telopeptides or deoxypyridinium.

Lifestyle

- Avoid first-hand and second-hand smoke exposure.

Exercise

- 30 to 45 minutes/day of aerobic, weight-bearing, and weight-lifting exercise (Patients with osteoporosis should consult with a health professional to plan an appropriate, safe exercise program.)

Nutrition

- Limit
  - Sodium
  - Caffeine
  - Phosphorus (including phosphoric acid in soda)

- Encourage
  - Antiinflammatory diet
  - Calcium-rich diet (see Table 37-2)
  - Adequate protein intake from plant sources more than from animal sources; one to two servings a day of whole soy foods

- Vitamin K_1–rich foods. These include any green plant with chlorophyll such as green leafy vegetables such as lettuce, collards, spinach, kale, and broccoli. Other plant sources include vegetable oils, nuts, and fruits. Animal foods that include vitamin K_2 include chicken, soft cheeses, and butter. Natto, a fermented soybean food, is a very rich source of vitamin K_2.

- Tea (*Camellia sinensis*), 2 cups a day

Supplements

- Vitamin D: 1000 to 2000 units/day

- Calcium citrate or carbonate as required so that total daily intake from diet, in addition to supplements, is at least 800 mg/day

- Multivitamin and multimineral: Minerals should include zinc, copper, magnesium, boron, and manganese.

Mind-Body Therapy

- Meditation, self-hypnosis, guided imagery, biofeedback, and breath work

Pharmaceuticals

- Consider a bisphosphonate in patients with a previous osteoporotic fracture, or a T-score between 2.0 and −2.5 and one or more additional risk factors.

- Consider a selective estrogen receptor blocker such as raloxifene, at 60 mg daily, in patients also at risk for breast cancer.

- Consider calcitonin in postmenopausal women. This can also reduce pain associated with vertebral compression fracture. The dose is one spray (200 units) in alternate nostrils daily.

KEY WEB RESOURCES

Bayer HealthCare BEST strength training videos: http://cals.arizona.edu/cpan/	This is the Web site for University of Arizona Center for Physical Activity and Nutrition. Detailed information is available on the Bone Estrogen Strength Training study, and a training guide book and continuing education course is available.
Foundation of Osteoporosis Research and Education 10-Year Fracture Risk Calculator (FORE Fracture Risk Calculator): http://riskcalculator.fore.org	This easy-to-use fracture risk calculator requires that you enter a BMD score, age, height, and weight, in addition to some other basic lifestyle information.
National Osteoporosis Foundation: http://www.nof.org	This Web site provides detailed information for health care professionals and patients about osteoporosis prevention and treatment.

References

References are available online at expertconsult.com.

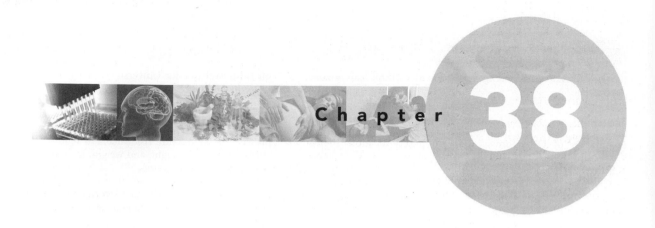

Chapter 38

An Integrative Approach to Obesity

James P. Nicolai, MD; Junelle H. Lupiani, RD;
and Andrew J. Wolf, MEd

Overview: The Danger and the Crisis

 Information on this topic can be found online at expertconsult.com.

Pathophysiology

Definition of Overweight and Obesity

In 2004, obesity was reclassified by Medicare as a chronic disease. Obesity is characterized by an excess of body fat and is most often defined by the body mass index (BMI), a mathematical formula that correlates well with excess weight at the population level. The BMI is measured by taking weight in kilograms, divided by height in meters squared (kg/m^2). Worldwide, adults with a BMI of 25 to 30 are categorized as overweight, whereas obesity is classified according to stages or grades (Table 38-1). Grade III obesity was formerly known as morbid obesity, but the term was appropriately changed for several reasons: morbidity may not occur at a BMI higher than 40 but certainly can be found at BMIs lower than that. BMI can sometimes be inaccurate because it does not distinguish between fat and muscle, nor does it predict body fat distribution. On a population level, however, BMI does seem to track trends in adiposity as opposed to muscularity, and those individuals with large muscle mass with resulting high BMIs are easily distinguishable from those with large amounts of adipose tissue.

In a clinical setting, the most valuable measurement strategy for classifying weight other than the BMI is waist circumference. The presence of extreme abdominal fat has been shown to be an independent risk factor for diabetes, high blood pressure, and cardiovascular disease. [6] Waist circumference is obtained by placing a measuring tape in a horizontal plane around the waist at the level of the umbilicus and the superior iliac crests.

> Risk of obesity and associated diseases is increased if waist circumference is greater than 40 inches in male patients and more than 35 inches in female patients.

In children, the term obesity is generally not used because of the potential prejudicial issues that may ensue when a child is labeled with such a title. As a result, overweight in children is defined conservatively as being at or higher than the 95th percentile of age- and sex-adjusted weight. At risk for overweight falls under the classification of those children who are at the 85th to 94.9th percentile. Increasing concern about the potentially high numbers of overweight children not classified correctly has prompted an ongoing initiative to revise the definition.

Obesity-Related Health Risk and Morbidity

The disease risk profile based on BMI and waist circumference is described in Table 38-2. Evidence shows that obesity is a proinflammatory state that increases the risk of several chronic diseases, including hypertension, dyslipidemia, diabetes, cardiovascular disease, asthma, sleep apnea, osteoarthritis, and several cancers. [7] Excess weight may also promote gallstone formation, fatty liver, gastroesophageal reflux, menstrual abnormalities, infertility, stress incontinence, gout, carpal tunnel syndrome, and low back pain. [8–12] Obese adults have more annual admissions to hospitals, more outpatient visits, higher prescription drug costs, and worse health-related quality of life than do adults of normal weight. [13]

More information on this topic can be found online at expertconsult.com.

Pathogenesis

The challenge with understanding the etiology of obesity is that obesity is the result of a relatively straightforward series of outcomes achieved by a set of complex and dynamic interactions. Obesity is a direct result of long-term mismatches in energy balance, with daily intake of energy greater than daily output. This condition puts people in a state of positive energy balance, and the longer they are there, the more weight they will gain. The complexity lies in how that energy balance is maintained.

Calories encompass the value of energy that determines this state of balance. We eat food, and various metabolic processes in our bodies break it down into energy. The relationship between energy and matter is under the control of the laws of physics, specifically the first law of thermodynamics, proved by Sir Isaac Newton, which states that all energy in the universe is conserved. In relation to food, when more energy is taken in by the body relative to the energy consumed, the surplus is ultimately converted into matter. This works well in a vacuum, but it may not be easily translated into the real world. Although energy intake is relatively determined by food and drink, with each having a particular caloric value, the nature of that matter can vary. Thus, calories may not be equal and can translate into differing amounts of energy burned by the body over a fixed period of time. Although a pound of lead and a pound of feathers may drop in a vacuum at the same speed, when a similar experiment is conducted outside, air resistance causes the lead to drop like a stone and the feathers to float to the earth at a leisurely pace. Calories operate in a similar fashion. The calories you eat are absorbed at different rates and have different amounts of fiber, carbohydrates, protein, and fat, along with other chemicals and nutrients that may translate into different metabolic signals that affect the energy equation.[23] Consequently, if it is true that calories are not equal, calorie type may influence energy balance as much as amount. A study from the Harvard School of Public Health confirmed this to be true; overweight patients fed 300 more calories per day actually lost more weight than did their counterparts who were eating food of different composition.[24]

Whereas we are beginning to discover the inherent complexity on the left side of the energy equation (calories in), measuring energy output has always been a much more intricate calculation because of the number of variables that determine the consumption of calories. Energy output is expressed as the sum of various processes, including resting energy expenditure, basal metabolic rate, physical activity, rates of growth, and thermogenesis. Studies have confirmed that macronutrient distribution, endocrine factors, and diverse genetic predispositions may contribute important mitigating influences at any given level of calorie consumption.[2]

Although the pathogenesis of obesity involves a set of complex multifactorial details to explain a relatively simple

TABLE 38-1. Adult Classification of Overweight

CLASSIFICATION	BODY MASS INDEX (kg/m²)
Underweight	18.5
Normal weight	18.5–24.9
Overweight/preobese	25.0–29.9

Obese
  Class I
  Class II
  Class III
	
	30.0–34.9
	35.0–39.9
	40.0 or higher

Adapted from the National Heart, Lung and Blood Institute, National Institutes of Health. *The Practical Guide: Identification, Evaluation, and Treatment of Overweight and Obesity in Adults.* NIH publication no. 00–4084. Bethesda, MD: U.S. Department of Health and Human Services, 2000.

TABLE 38-2. Classification of Overweight and Obesity and Associated Disease Risk

CLASSIFICATION*	BMI (kg/m²)	OBESITY STAGE	Disease Risk (Relative to Normal Weight and Waist Circumference)† WAIST CIRCUMFERENCE Men: up to 40 in. (up to 102 cm); women: up to 35 in. (up to 88 cm)	WAIST CIRCUMFERENCE Men: more than 40 in.; women: more than 35 in.
Underweight	Lower than 18.5	—	—	—
Normal	18.5 to 24.9	—	—	—
Overweight	25.0 to 29.9	—	Increased	High
Obese	30.0 to 34.9	I	High	Very high
	35.0 to 39.9	II	Very high	Very high
Extremely obese	40.0 or higher	III	Extremely high	Extremely high

Adapted from World Health Organization. *Preventing and Managing the Global Epidemic of Obesity.* Report of the World Health Organization Consultation of Obesity. Geneva: World Health Organization; 1997.
BMI, body mass index.
*For persons 20 years old and older.
†Disease risk for type 2 diabetes mellitus, hypertension, and cardiovascular disease. Increased waist circumference can be a marker for increased disease risk, even in persons of normal weight.

condition, what should not be forgotten is that human physiology is much the same as it has always been. The increase in obesity prevalence in the past few decades cannot be explained by changes in the human gene pool, but rather by environmental changes that have not been seen previously in our collective history. An environment that promotes excess food intake of poor quality and discourages physical activity will most surely produce obesity in a species that has adapted itself to survive by responding to caloric scarcity within the confines of a world that demands a significant level of energy expenditure.[13]

Integrative Assessment

People living in the United States average 2.7 office visits to a physician per person per year, and 60% of these visits occur within a primary care setting. Patients regard physicians as a primary resource for preventive health information and recommendations. Moreover, when physicians counsel patients to make a change in their lifestyle, they are more likely to make an attempt.[25] Ideally, assessment and treatment of obesity should be done within the setting of a multidisciplinary team designed to manage medical, nutritional, emotional, and exertional components of the desired lifestyle intervention—in this case, weight loss. This ideal setting is often unavailable or unrealistic, however, and in a primary care setting, an obesity management strategy can still be implemented successfully with simple interventions by a single practitioner. Initial goals should focus on modest weight loss of 5% to 10% of total body weight over a 12- to 16-week period of time. Such weight loss has been shown in studies to improve blood glucose control in obese patients with type 2 diabetes.[26] Modest weight loss has also been found to prevent the progression of diabetes and cardiovascular disease in those obese individuals with impaired glucose tolerance and insulin resistance.[27] Improvements can be seen in most obesity-related conditions, from lipid disorders and hypertension to joint pain, muscle weakness, and lung function, after such a modest 5% to 10% reduction in total weight.

An integrative assessment of obesity should include a thorough medical history and physical examination with anthropomorphic measurements, weight history, nutritional and dietary history, assessment of current and past physical activity, diagnostic laboratory evaluation, electrocardiogram (if considering weight loss medications), and screening for current levels of motivation, emotional status, availability of support systems, and potential barriers to treatment.

A medical history should inquire about the presence of obesity-related conditions in the individual or family: asthma and sleep apnea, coronary artery disease with or without dyslipidemias, diabetes, hypertension, thrombophlebitis and cellulitis, chronic pain, muscle and joint disorders, impingement syndromes, menstrual abnormalities, infertility, and stress incontinence, along with obesity-related cancers of the esophagus, colon, rectum, and pancreas and hormonally related cancers such as breast, ovarian, endometrial, and prostate. Metabolic syndrome should be identified because it is often a marker for insulin resistance, which ultimately leads to type 2 diabetes (Table 38-3). Current medical history, physical examination, and laboratory information allow an accurate diagnosis of metabolic syndrome. Abdominal obesity and hypertriglyceridemia may be particularly early markers of the syndrome and represent a readily detectable indicator of diabetes risk.[28]

TABLE 38-3. Clinical Identification of Metabolic Syndrome

RISK FACTOR	DEFINING LEVEL
Abdominal adiposity	Waist circumference
Men	102 cm (40 inches)
Women	88 cm (35 inches)
Triglycerides	150 mg/dL
HDL cholesterol	
Men	40 mg/dL
Women	50 mg/dL
Blood pressure	130/85 mm Hg or higher
Fasting blood glucose level	110 mg/dL or higher

Adapted from National Heart, Lung and Blood Institute, National Institutes of Health.
Third Report of the Expert Panel on Detection, Evaluation, and Treatment of High Blood Cholesterol in Adults (Adult Treatment Panel III): *National Cholesterol Education Program*. Bethesda, MD: National Institutes of Health; 2004.
HDL, high-density lipoprotein.

Current medications should be assessed for their potential promotion of weight gain. Psychiatric medications are notorious for contributing to weight gain and include antipsychotics, some antidepressants, and antiseizure medications. Other commonly used drugs that promote weight gain include long-acting steroid medications, some oral contraceptives, certain diabetic medications, and drugs for the treatment of blood pressure. Weight-neutral alternatives are available and should be attempted if weight loss is a priority (Table 38-4).

Weight history should assess the progression of weight gain over time to illustrate the use of any previous weight loss strategies such as special diets, exercise programs, meal replacements, nutritional supplements, medications, or surgical procedures. The practitioner should understand how much weight was lost and over what period of time, what was the period of weight maintenance, and what promoting factors caused weight regain, if any. "Yo-yo" dieting, consisting of repetitive patterns of weight loss followed by weight regain, may provide information about previous successful strategies, as well as recurrent negative behavioral patterns.

Laboratory testing is an important adjunct to information obtained from a patient's history, and patients should be screened for obesity-related conditions such as hypothyroidism, liver disease, metabolic syndrome, dyslipidemia, glucose intolerance, insulin resistance, diabetes, and, if suspected, polycystic ovarian syndrome (PCOS) and Cushing syndrome. Because obesity is a proinflammatory condition, the prudent approach may be to assess inflammatory markers such as high-sensitive C-reactive protein. Serum 25-(OH) vitamin D levels should be obtained in light of research demonstrating the trend toward significant vitamin D deficiency and decreased bioavailability of vitamin D in the obese population.[29] Vitamin D deficiency is associated with muscle weakness, fatigue, and pain in bones, joints, and muscles, among other things. Normalizing vitamin D status in the obese population should be a priority.

TABLE 38-4. Medications Associated With Weight Gain

DRUG CLASS	MEDICATIONS THAT MAY PROMOTE WEIGHT GAIN	ALTERNATIVE DRUGS THAT MAY BE WEIGHT NEUTRAL OR PROMOTE WEIGHT LOSS
Psychiatric/Neurologic		
Antipsychotics	Olanzapine, clozapine, risperidone	Ziprasidone, quetiapine
Antidepressants	SSRIs, tricyclics, lithium	Bupropion, nefazodone
Antiepileptics	Valproate, gabapentin, carbamazepine	Topiramate, lamotrigine, zonisamide
Diabetes Agents	Insulin Sulfonylureas Thiazolidinediones	Metformin, exenatide* Acarbose, miglitol
Steroid Hormones	Hormonal contraceptives Corticosteroids Progestational steroids	Barrier methods NSAIDs
Miscellaneous Agents	Antihistamines	Decongestants, inhalers
	Alpha-antagonists, beta blockers	ACE inhibitors, calcium channel blockers

Adapted from the North American Association for the Study of Obesity, Obesity Research, Stanford University Libraries, Stanford, CA.
ACE, angiotensin-converting enzyme; NSAIDs, nonsteroidal antiinflammatory drugs; SSRIs, selective serotonin reuptake inhibitors.
*Incretin mimetic.

> Laboratory tests to consider in the evaluation of obesity include fasting blood sugar (100 to 125 indicates prediabetes); triglycerides (high in metabolic syndrome), high-density lipoprotein (low in vitamin D deficiency); 25-hydroxyvitamin D; thyroid-stimulating hormone (hypothyroidism); cortisol, 8 AM spot or 24-hour urine (Cushing disease); high-sensitive C-reactive protein (inflammation); and aspartate aminotransferase, alanine aminotransferase, and gamma-glutamyltransferase (steatohepatitis).

Nutritional assessments and evaluations of physical activity can be done concurrently by other members of the weight loss team (dietitians and exercise specialists) or with simple diagnostic tools and lines of questioning. Dietary recall over the course of 1 to 2 days can provide an idea of food intake, eating patterns, and quality of choices. This approach is limited by the tendency of most people to underreport intake of food, as well as uncertainty about identifying a representative day or so in an individual's typical routine. Various software programs and online tools are available for performing nutrient analyses of dietary records and for calculating calories, macronutrient and micronutrient profiles, fiber, essential fats, and sources of each. This information can be useful to provide to clients who are undergoing nutritional counseling.

Further inquiry is often necessary to obtain more details from food records that are often vague and nonspecific. Even when reports of food intake are underreported or somewhat inaccurate, however, viewing the amount of calories one consumes over a 24-hour period can often be surprising and revelatory to the individual who is unaware of portion sizes and the nutritional content of food. Providing patients with a visual illustration of this can be valuable.

Ultimately, for an intervention to be successful, it must closely match the individual's readiness to change. Commitment to such behavioral change is maximized when goals are self-selected and fit with personal lifestyle and values. Gaining clarity on these values is obtained through interactions that allow the practitioner to understand and appreciate the world of the client. Such techniques as motivational interviewing and the Pressure System model (PSM) can provide primary providers with the kinds of counseling tools they need to improve the likelihood that their patients will implement the suggested strategies[30] (see Chapter 99, Motivational Interviewing).

 More information on this topic can be found online at expertconsult.com.

> Interventions must match readiness to change. Commitment to behavioral change is maximized when goals are self-selected and fit with personal lifestyle and values. Patient ambivalence is universal and should be recognized and acknowledged. Doing so will encourage the patient to argue for instead of against change.

Integrative Therapy

In general, the primary clinical intervention for weight management involves lifestyle modification. This includes attention to levels of activity, nutrition, stress management, sleep, sexual activity, relationships, and motivation. Lifestyle modification should be part of any program addressing excess weight, regardless of BMI. More aggressive approaches that include weight loss medications, low-calorie diets with or without liquid meal replacements, and various methods of fasting require a BMI of 30 or higher without comorbidities or of 27 or higher with the presence of one or more comorbid conditions (see Table 38-4). These strategies require frequent monitoring and, if implemented for longer than 3 months, should be administered by a medical professional trained in supervised weight loss strategies (i.e., a physician certified by the American Board of Bariatric Medicine). For patients who have given serious attempts to their weight loss without appropriate long-term results, surgical interventions should be evaluated as a viable option.

Therapeutic Counseling

Once the assessment has been made and initial treatment goals have been established, a regular visit schedule should be proposed and agreed on by the management team and patient. The more contact patients have with practitioners, the longer they will remain in a program, and the greater potential they have to achieve and maintain their weight loss goals. Frequent visits with physicians and ancillary staff (dietitians, exercise physiologists or trainers, counselors) are recommended and promote greater compliance, as do group support programs.[31-34] Behavioral and nutritional counseling can be done by physicians or dietitians and coded for using Current Procedural Terminology (CPT) codes for individuals (97802) or groups (97804). A minimum of one visit per month is encouraged, and weekly or twice-monthly visits are recommended. Programs offering combination visits with a physician followed by ancillary practitioners can allow for efficient delivery of information in a multidisciplinary fashion without having to extend doctor visits. Obese individuals with eating disorders or who have comorbid psychological conditions such as depression or anxiety should be provided with the opportunity for psychotherapy and other counseling by licensed mental health professionals.

Nutrition

Diet and its role in weight loss have been studied abundantly over the decades, with evidence to support restriction of calorie-containing macronutrients (carbohydrates, fats, and proteins) as an effective means of achieving weight loss.[35] However, further research suggests that macronutrient-restricted diets may be no better than overall calorie-restricted diets for achieving long-term results.[36-38] Moreover, dietary adherence, rather than type of diet, predicts the greatest success regarding weight lost over time.[39] These three points suggest that personal preference is an important consideration when tailoring individualized dietary interventions for successful weight loss. Assessment tools such as 24-hour dietary recall and food frequency questionnaires are important methods for identifying personal preference as a means of recommending dietary approaches to reduce calorie intake.

Popular Diets and Common Weight Loss Programs

Many people seek out recommendations from popular diets and common weight loss programs, most of which have minimal evidence or formal studies to show their effectiveness. However, evidence studying the efficacy of four popular diets (Atkins, Zone, Weight Watchers, and Ornish) for weight loss showed modest reduction in body weight. The study showed that increased adherence was associated with greater weight loss and cardiac risk factor reduction for each diet group.[40] This finding further supports individualized dietary interventions based on personal preference as an important factor in recommending therapy.

Although questions remain about long-term effects and mechanisms, data suggest that a low-carbohydrate, high-protein, high-fat diet may be considered a feasible alternative recommendation for weight loss.[41] Three popular examples are the Atkins diet, the South Beach diet, and the Zone diet. The Atkins diet focuses on eliminating the majority of carbohydrate sources with no modification of fat or protein calories. The South Beach diet offers a 2-week elimination of all carbohydrates followed by the addition of low-glycemic sources in moderate amounts. The Zone diet encourages physical activity, exercise, and hydration and limits carbohydrates. Another popular diet that achieves weight loss by what is most likely calorie restriction is the Ornish diet, mainly a very low-fat vegetarian plan that combines dietary approaches with group support, stress reduction, and moderate exercise. Research from Stanford University in California studied the Atkins, Zone, LEARN (Lifestyle, Exercise, Attitudes, Relationships, Nutrition), and Ornish diets, by specifically looking at macronutrient quality, and concluded that weight loss diets focusing on macronutrient composition should attend to the overall quality of the diet, including the adequacy of micronutrient intakes. Concerning calorie-restricted diets, those providing moderately low carbohydrate amounts and containing nutrient-dense foods may have a micronutrient advantage.[41]

Each year, millions of U.S. residents enroll in commercial and self-help weight loss programs. Health care providers and their patients know little about the clinical utility of these programs because of the absence of systematic reviews. The University of Pennsylvania in Philadelphia performed an evaluation of major commercial weight loss programs in the United States (eDiets.com, Health Management Resources, Take Off Pounds Sensibly, Optifast, and Weight Watchers). The outcome of the systematic review showed that use of the major commercial and self-help weight loss programs involved in the trial, with the exception of Weight Watchers, is suboptimal.[42] The study noted limitations related to lack of control for high attrition rates. The investigators also reported that many of the programs were associated with high costs and a high probability that participants will regain 50% or more of lost weight in 1 to 2 years. This study further supports the need for controlled trials to assess the efficacy and cost effectiveness of commercial weight loss interventions. Additional commercial programs that lack research but continue to gain popularity are Jenny Craig and LA Weight Loss. These programs, like Weight Watchers, provide weight loss services including prepackaged food, planned menus, and psychological support. Limitations are cost, sales promotions that encourage on-the-spot commitment to prepaid contracts, and the cost of food and additional vitamins.

In February 2011, the Department of Geriatrics and Metabolic Diseases in Naples, Italy, evaluated the effect of Mediterranean diets on body weight in randomized controlled trials using a meta-analysis. This research found that the Mediterranean diet could be a useful tool to reduce body weight, especially when it is calorie restricted, associated with physical activity, and followed for more than 6 months. The Mediterranean diet was not found to promote weight gain, a finding that removes the objection to its relatively high fat content.[43] This research further supports evidence suggesting that macronutrient-restricted diets may be no better than overall calorie-restricted diets in achieving long-term weight loss. Key components of the Mediterranean diet emphasize exercise, primarily plant-based foods (fruits, vegetables, whole grains, legumes, and nuts), olive oil and canola oil, two or more servings of fish and seafood weekly, and limitations

FIGURE 38-1
Mediterranean diet pyramid. (From Oldways Preservation and Exchange Trust. <www.oldwayspt.org;> 2009 Accessed 04.08.11.)

MEDITERRANEAN DIET PYRAMID

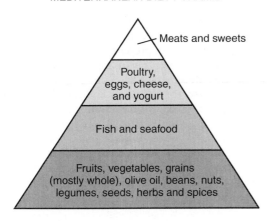

Food groups	Guidance
Meats and sweets	Less often
Poultry, eggs, cheese and yogurt	Moderate portions, daily to weekly
Fish and seafood	Often, at least two times a week
Fruits, vegetables, grains (mostly whole), olive oil, beans, nuts, legumes, seeds, herbs and spices	Base every meal on these foods

on red meat (Fig. 38-1). The diet also recognizes the importance of enjoying meals with family and friends.

The antiinflammatory diet designed by Andrew Weil, MD, based on principles found in the Mediterranean diet, is not intended as a weight loss program, although people have found they have lost weight while adhering to it. General dietary recommendations include eating as much whole, fresh, and unprocessed food as possible (fruits, vegetables, whole and cracked grains, beans and legumes, nuts, avocados, and seeds), with an emphasis on variety of these foods. The diet also limits consumption of processed foods, "fast foods," and foods high in saturated fat sources. The elimination or significant limitation of these foods is most likely an important factor contributing to weight reduction. The diet is based on a 2000 calorie per day plan that provides adequate vitamins, minerals, essential fatty acids, dietary fiber, and protective phytonutrients. At this point, no research has been conducted to study the effects on weight loss associated with the Weil antiinflammatory diet (see Chapter 86, The Antiinflammatory Diet).

Ultimately, dietary restriction as a management strategy for weight reduction can often be used as a sole intervention. Evidence suggests, however, that its use in combination with other strategies such as exercise, behavioral therapy, surgery, and pharmacologic treatments may increase overall success.

The best nutritional plan for weight loss is the one to which the patient will adhere.

Exercise

When consulting with someone who is interested in using exercise as a weight management tool, assessment is essential to setting attainable goals and creating an action plan. For sedentary individuals who are starting an exercise program, the initial goal is simply to start moving. Creating a habit of exercise or movement that emphasizes enjoyment and adherence is an important first step. During this phase, the intensity of exercise is not of paramount importance, but adherence to a modest volume of movement is. Even with modest amounts of movement, one can experience favorable functional changes in strength and endurance that can be a positive and encouraging first step. After a pattern of regular movement has been established and exercise tolerance has improved, the notion of increasing the frequency, duration, and intensity of activity becomes more realistic. Improvements to the thermoregulatory, muscular, and cardiovascular systems of the body operate synergistically to make higher intensities and longer durations more easily tolerated. Ratings of perceived exertion, pedometers, and heart rate monitors are all tools that can be used when making the transition to this next phase of exercise. Although this more detailed phase of exercise prescription is not absolutely needed for managing obesity, it can be very helpful. Exercise has only mild effects on resting metabolic rate, but exercise of sufficient intensity can alter aerobic capacity and improve an individual's capacity to burn calories. Given that most exercise bouts are limited to the 20- to 60-minute window, the productivity of an exercise session can be key to success.

Aerobic capacity or Vo_2max refers to the number of liters of oxygen that can be consumed per minute at maximal aerobic workloads. This workload has been traditionally expressed in terms of metabolic equivalents (METs) or in terms of milliliters of oxygen consumed per minute per kilogram (mL O_2/min/kg). The more oxygen someone can consume per minute or the more METs they can produce per minute, the more calories they can burn. For example, two people seem identical on the surface. Both women are 55 years old, are 5 foot 4 inches tall (165 cm), and weigh 165 pounds (75 kg). Subject number 1 can produce 12.8 METs (45 mL O_2/min/kg) during a treadmill test, whereas subject number 2 can produce 8 METs (28 mL O_2/min/kg) during her treadmill test. Both women achieve maximal heart rates of 165 beats per minute at the end of the tests. Translated into exercise (30 minutes on a treadmill) at a comfortable heart rate for both women (127 beats per minute), the differences are substantial. Subject 1 will burn approximately 13.0 calories per minute for 30 minutes and 390 calories during the 30-minute exercise bout. Subject 2 will burn approximately 8 calories per minute and 240 calories for the 30 minutes. Having a very clear picture of what your clients' abilities are—even determining their aerobic capacity—before creating an exercise prescription is a powerful tool for anyone facilitating weight loss.

During a period of weight loss, clients will inevitably have some losses in lean mass, as well as losses in fat mass. Given the protein-sparing effects induced by resistance training, the addition of resistive muscular work makes sense. Full body exercise routines that engage as many muscles as possible not only save time but also can have beneficial effects on the hormonal response to resistance training.[44] A twice-weekly regimen is sufficient to produce these results.

Supplements

Omega-3 Fatty Acids

Omega-3 fatty acids have been shown in various studies to have significant positive effects on cardiovascular health.[45] They are an integral part of an antiinflammatory diet, as well as having an indication for the treatment of elevated triglycerides.[46] Omega-3 fatty acids should be considered in the obese patient with cardiovascular comorbidities because clinical studies show that disease risk decreases as the ratio of omega-3 to omega-6 in the diet increases.[47] Supplements are available in prescription form as omega-3-acid ethyl esters under the trade name Lovaza.

■ Dosage

For improvement of cardiac disease risk, the recommended dose is 1 to 3g daily, and the ratio of eicosapentaenoic acid (EPA) to docosahexaenoic acid (DHA) should be greater than 1. For the treatment of high triglyceride levels, the recommended dose is higher, at 2 to 4g of combined EPA and DHA.

■ Precautions

Individuals with allergies to fish or shellfish should use caution when taking fish oil. Omega-3 fatty acids have antiplatelet and antithrombin effects, which may cause bruising or may interact with additional blood thinning agents. However, bleeding effects of fish oils taken alone have not been shown to be clinically significant even in large doses.[46] Side effects include a fishy aftertaste and mild gastrointestinal upset.

Vitamin D

Overweight individuals tend to have lower blood levels of vitamin D because excess adipose tissue absorbs and stores this fat-soluble vitamin. In addition, unlike normal-weight individuals who turn over fat tissue, those with relatively immovable fat stores cannot liberate the vitamin D they have. As a general rule, obese individuals are less active outdoors and are exposed to less ultraviolet radiation, a situation that compounds their vitamin D deficiency. Studies have validated that obese individuals tend to have significantly low levels of vitamin D, with symptoms of muscle weakness, muscle aches, bone pains, and fatigue, all of which are potential manifestations of vitamin D deficiency.[48] Additional research has validated the lower comparative bioavailability of vitamin D in obese individuals; they need more of it compared with nonobese subjects.[29] Higher levels of calcium in the presence of adequate serum vitamin D levels has been shown to inhibit fatty acid synthase, an enzyme that converts calories into fat, whereas diets low in calcium increase the enzyme by as much as fivefold.[49]

■ Dosage

First, the clinician should determine the patient's serum 25-hydroxyvitamin D level in the blood. Recommended adequate blood levels of vitamin D are between 40 and 60ng/mL.[50] Supplementation should be adequate to correct deficiencies if present. Obese individuals may need two to three times more vitamin D daily than those of normal weight, somewhere between 3000 and 6000 units daily, without posing any risk of toxicity.[49]

■ Precautions

Gastrointestinal effects of larger doses of vitamin D have been reported. Some suggestion exists that this effect may result from the gelatin capsule of prescription formulations and not the preparation itself. These symptoms may be remedied by opening the capsule and ingesting the liquid form. Vitamin D toxicity is often difficult to diagnose. This condition depends on blood levels of calcium (usually above 10.4mg/dL) and occurs when 25-hydroxyvitamin D levels are usually higher than 200ng/mL. Hyperphosphatemia and hypercalcemia that occur in vitamin D toxicity can cause constipation, confusion, depression, increased thirst, urination, and electrocardiographic changes, with ultimate calcification of organs and tissues leading to damage and organ failure.[49]

Conjugated Linoleic Acid

Conjugated linoleic acid (CLA) is a polyunsaturated fatty acid in the omega-6 category found naturally in beef and whole-fat dairy products. CLA supplements have been widely promoted as being beneficial for weight loss in some individuals. CLA has been shown to be an effective supplement for reducing fat mass in animal models, but results in humans have been inconsistent. One meta-analysis found that CLA produces a modest loss in body fat in humans.[51]

■ Dosage

Modest weight loss (between 1.1 and 2.6kg) in human studies was achieved at a dose of 3.2g daily.

■ Precautions

Although no serious adverse effects have been related to the use of CLA, this substance has been linked to slight increases in inflammatory markers, including C-reactive protein and white blood cell counts. This finding contradicts research in animal models, which suggested that CLA is more of an antiinflammatory substance. CLA was also reported to be linked to an increased risk of insulin resistance in certain individuals, as well as greater gastrointestinal upset.[51]

Green Tea and Green Tea Extract

Animal studies suggested a fat-burning, weight loss, and cholesterol-lowering effect of green tea extracts. This effect seems to be synergistically improved with the addition of exercise. A small Asian study validated significant reductions in body weight, BMI, waist circumference, body fat mass, and subcutaneous fat area after 12 weeks of consuming one bottle of tea with 690mg catechin antioxidants per day.[52] Another Japanese study found that green tea contains ingredients besides caffeine that stimulate thermogenesis and burn fat.[53]

■ Dosage

Studies found that fat-burning results occurred with tea containing 690mg of catechins daily. Depending on the brand, the recommended dose consists of 2 to 3 cups of green tea per day (for a total of 240 to 320mg polyphenols) or 100 to 750mg per day of standardized green tea extract. Caffeine-free products are available.

Precautions

One cup of green tea typically contains approximately 50 mg of caffeine as compared with 90 to 150 mg of caffeine for a percolated cup of coffee. People with heart problems, kidney disorders, stomach ulcers, anxiety, and sleep disorders should not take green tea. When considering green tea, pregnant and breast-feeding women should consult their obstetricians.

People who drink excessive amounts of caffeine for prolonged periods may experience irritability, insomnia, heart palpitations, and dizziness. Caffeine overdose can cause nausea, vomiting, diarrhea, headaches, and loss of appetite.

Mind-Body Therapy

Mind-body therapies such as mindfulness and mindful eating programs, meditation, hypnosis, and biofeedback are popular strategies used to facilitate weight loss plans with a specific target on emotional eating patterns. Stress reduction and improved emotional regulation can potentially allow individuals to make better food choices, feel fuller faster, and recognize abnormal eating habits. By accessing the parasympathetic nervous system more often, the balance of stress hormones, including epinephrine and cortisol, can be shifted in a positive direction. Studies have confirmed that stress-induced cortisol secretion is linked to abdominal obesity, endocrine abnormalities such as increased insulin, metabolic derangements in blood lipids, and hemodynamic changes in blood vessels.[54] Decreasing cortisol levels can aid in a positive strategy to address weight gain proactively.

Unfortunately, the available literature on these therapies in the obese population is relatively scarce. Preliminary studies showed mindfulness meditation to reduce episodes of binge eating and nighttime eating disorder.[55] Some studies looking at the role of biofeedback techniques and hypnosis in weight loss showed a mildly positive effect.[56] At present, recommending these strategies to the right individuals who are open to them seems prudent as an adjunct to an ongoing lifestyle management program.

Pharmaceuticals

Pharmacologic treatment may be considered an adjunct to lifestyle modification in those patients who have not lost at least 1.1 lb (0.5 kg) per week after 3 to 6 months of implementing their lifestyle program.[57] These medications are appropriate for patients with a BMI 30 or higher or 27 or higher in the presence of comorbid conditions. At present, two classes of drugs are used for weight control: (1) drugs that suppress appetite and augment thermogenesis (phentermine) and (2) drugs that prevent the absorption of fat through the gastrointestinal tract (orlistat). The withdrawal of sibutramine by Abbott Laboratories from both the U.S. and European markets because of an increased risk of stroke and heart attacks raised concern about the long-term effects of stimulant medications and prompted petitioning for higher standards of review for weight loss medications.[58] When considering drug therapy, the clinician should conduct a careful review of medical history, drug interactions, and potential side effects before prescribing weight loss medications. Evaluation of a recent electrocardiogram is recommended to assess a patient's cardiac health before administering medications with known stimulant effects, and aggressive regular monitoring (1- to 2-week visits) should be done during initial treatment to assess vital signs and tolerance to therapy. Longer-term therapy should also prompt regular medical supervision with at least monthly visits.

Phentermine

Phentermine (Adipex-P) is a norepinephrine reuptake inhibitor with schedule IV identification (debated in some medical circles) that has been approved by the U.S. Food and Drug Administration (FDA) for short-term use (12 weeks) since 1959. Phentermine is the most commonly prescribed weight loss medication to date, probably because of its low cost, its long history of use, and, contrary to popular belief, its low addictive potential. To illustrate this point, the *Drug Abuse Warning Report (DAWN)*, published in 2006 by the Substance Abuse and Mental Health Services Administration of the U.S. Department of Health and Human Services, showed that anorectics such as phentermine had among the lowest drug misuse or abuse rates per 100,000 emergency room visits, even lower than ibuprofen.[59] Unfortunately, many of the current guidelines for prescribing phentermine reflect recommendations that are more than 50 years old, rather than current evidence of efficacy and safety.[60] Because it has a molecular structure similar to that of amphetamine, phentermine was originally labeled a schedule IV drug; however, over many decades of clinical use, phentermine has proved to have little to no addictive value, and no abuse or withdrawal syndromes are associated with its use.[59] Continuous use beyond 12 weeks is a common off-label use pattern in bariatric medicine and has validation in the international literature.[61] Putting time limits on medication use for the treatment of a chronic illness such as obesity seems inappropriate when (and only when) the risk of taking the medication is less than the risk of leaving the illness untreated. Weight loss during drug therapy should perhaps not be considered an indication to stop treatment any more than a positive outcome would be for the treatment of other chronic diseases. For this to happen, however, the long-term safety of agents must be assessed and documented in the literature.[62] The literature suggests the effectiveness of phentermine in helping patients lose weight and maintain that loss for at least a year, if not longer.[63]

Dosage

Phentermine is often prescribed in doses of 15 to 37.5 mg once daily, typically in midmorning. It is sometimes prescribed in half doses given early in the morning then at midmorning, to extend its effects toward evening, when individuals tend to have higher calorie intake.

Precautions

Side effects include insomnia, dry mouth, palpitations, hypertension, and constipation.

> Contrary to popular belief, phentermine has a low addiction potential.

Orlistat

Orlistat (Xenical) works by inhibiting lipases in the gastrointestinal tract such that fat absorption is partially blocked. It is FDA approved for up to 2 years of continuous use, and it has been shown to be effective for significant and sustainable weight loss, as well as for improving lipid levels, enhancing glucose metabolism, and lowering blood pressure.[64] The discontinuation rate is relatively high because of gastrointestinal side effects related to fat malabsorption and roughly equates to 33% in various studies.[65] In one study, lifestyle intervention and orlistat treatment for 4 years delayed the development of type 2 diabetes in obese subjects by 37%, a finding perhaps suggested to result in part from the weight loss achieved.[66] Orlistat is now available in half strength (60 mg per dose) over the counter under the brand name Alli.

■ Dosage

Orlistat is prescribed in doses of 120 mg taken three times daily with meals, and the dose can be omitted when patients ingest a low-fat meal. Starting orlistat once daily with the fattiest meal (usually dinner) and then advancing the dose to three times daily as needed can help lessen the intensity and frequency of side effects.

■ Precautions

Common adverse effects include bloating, flatulence, and fatty or oily stools. Oily spotting, increased fecal urgency or incontinence, and abdominal pain can also be experienced, especially when patients are noncompliant with a low-fat diet. Use of fiber supplements, especially psyllium, can be helpful in reducing side effects. Patients should also take a daily multivitamin, independently of orlistat, to compensate for the potential decreased absorption of fat-soluble vitamins (A, D, E, and K).

Off-Label Use of Medications for Weight Loss

Physicians commonly prescribe a wide variety of drugs for other indications. An estimate suggests that 21% of all prescriptions are issued for off-label use.[67] Physicians certified in the treatment of obesity often use phentermine on a long-term basis, as has been validated by studies demonstrating safety in patients after more than 10 years of continuous phentermine use.[62]

Additionally, three drugs with other indications besides weight loss are being investigated: bupropion, topiramate, and metformin. Bupropion (Wellbutrin) is a norepinephrine and dopamine reuptake inhibitor that is approved for the treatment of depression and was shown to have a dose-dependent weight loss effect in a double-blind placebo-controlled study. In this study, 83% of patients achieved weight loss of more than 5% of initial body weight when they took 400 mg/day of sustained-release bupropion as compared with 59% of subjects taking 300 mg/day and 46% treated with placebo.[68] Topiramate (Topamax) is an antiepileptic drug that has shown positive weight loss effects during clinical trials in smaller doses than achieved for seizure control.[69] Metformin (Glucophage) is indicated for the treatment of type 2 diabetes, but it has also been used off-label for the treatment of insulin resistance syndromes, especially PCOS. Studies have suggested a mild weight loss effect in abdominally obese women with PCOS.[70] Metformin has also been shown to promote weight loss in morbidly obese children and in men with normoglycemic hyperinsulinemia.[71]

Surgery

Bariatric surgery is well established as the most effective treatment for obesity; however, it is indicated only for the management of severe obesity with or without comorbidities, when other therapies have been tried without long-term success.[72] Surgical interventions are currently indicated for patients with a BMI of 40 or higher or 35 or higher with comorbid conditions and reduced quality of life (i.e., hypertension, sleep apnea, diabetes). Typically, reimbursement for surgical procedures will be granted only after at least a 6-month trial of medically supervised weight loss.

Bariatric surgery rapidly evolved with the advent of laparoscopic approaches in the mid-1990s. Currently, most bariatric surgery is initially attempted in laparoscopic fashion. Surgical weight loss falls into the category of restrictive procedures, malabsorptive procedures, or a combination of the two. Strictly malabsorptive procedures such as jejunoileal bypass and duodenal switch are seldom performed. Purely restrictive procedures include the vertical banded gastroplasty (rarely done these days), adjustable gastric banding, and vertical sleeve gastrectomy (an emerging procedure). The Roux-en-Y gastric bypass, involving restriction of stomach size along with bypassing a large part of the stomach and duodenum, is an example of a combined restrictive and malabsorptive procedure. It is still the most popular procedure; however, restrictive techniques are beginning to emerge as competitive procedures that are less invasive and have fewer side effects.

A Cochrane Review compared different surgical procedures, all of which were found to be more effective in promoting weight loss than were nonsurgical methods.[73] Roux-en-Y gastric bypass was more effective than laparoscopic adjustable gastric banding and just as effective as vertical sleeve gastrectomy. Weight loss of up to 33% has been maintained after gastric bypass surgery for up to 10 years, and loss of 50% or more of excess weight is achieved with either of the procedures, again an outcome superior to that of nonsurgical approaches.[73] In addition, resolution of comorbidities is often common. Meta-analyses demonstrated complete resolution of type 2 diabetes in 31% to 77% of patients who underwent laparoscopic banding and in 72% to 100% of patients who had Roux-en-Y bypass.[74] Similar resolution of blood pressure abnormalities has been verified. A Swedish study demonstrated a substantially reduced 10-year mortality rate with bariatric surgery as compared with nonsurgical treatment of obesity.[75]

Bariatric surgery is typically safe, with surgical mortality approaching as low as 0.1% to 0.3%, whereas postoperative complications occur in 4% to 10%.[76,77] Emerging evidence indicates that bariatric surgery may be beneficial for patients with BMIs lower than 35 and comorbidities; however, it is still too early to recommend surgery to those individuals.[78]

Individuals considering bariatric surgery require thorough preparation for the effects of such a procedure on their long-term lifestyle. This preparation should be facilitated by a multidisciplinary team of surgical and nonsurgical practitioners. Coordination of treatment has been cited as one of the most important advances in the care of patients undergoing these surgical procedures.[79] Postoperative challenges include malabsorptive nutritional deficiencies, dumping syndrome that involves profuse diarrhea and stomach pain after overeating refined carbohydrates in patients who underwent bypass procedures, changing dietary patterns to accommodate effects of the procedure, and the physical and emotional changes that occur when experiencing large amounts of weight loss. Regular close monitoring by nutritionists is necessary to provide assistance with safe and efficacious dietary advancement along with guidance of supplement needs for those individuals exhibiting vitamin and mineral deficiencies, a potential problem for all patients after bypass procedures. Preoperatively, all patients need psychological evaluation to assess whether they are appropriately motivated, likely to be compliant in their long-term program, and prepared to accept the changes that often occur with dramatic reductions in weight. Regular access to behavioral experts is essential for patients as they lose weight. Often, maladaptive patterns of eating are a defense mechanism used by patients to deal with elevated levels of emotional stress. When those options are eliminated by a surgical process, the potential for other patterns of behavior to emerge is evident. Having a management strategy to support patients through these psychological adaptations and providing them with proactive alternatives to stress response other than with food can create life-changing opportunities. Support groups are often used as adjuncts to individual behavioral therapies and can be helpful in long-term weight management after surgery.

Therapies to Consider

The clinical literature contains few substantiated claims to document the effectiveness and safety of over-the-counter weight loss aids.[80,81] Even so, use of supplements for weight loss is a popular practice. As of 2004, more than 50 individual dietary supplements and more than 125 commercial combination products were available for weight loss.[81] In 2002, retail sales of weight loss supplements were estimated to be more than $1.3 billion.[82] The literature also points out that some individuals use over-the-counter aids while continuing to take their prescription weight loss drugs.[83] This situation emphasizes the need for practical navigation by medical practitioners as they monitor and counsel their patients about the use of anorectic supplements. The well-publicized toxicity of ephedra highlights the potential dangers of relying on such supplements and botanicals as a sole weight loss strategy [84] Given the widespread use of these agents, clinicians who treat obesity should be familiar with the risk-to-benefit profile of common products, to counsel patients about their use or avoidance more accurately. Table 38-5 summarizes the evidence for efficacy and safety of common weight loss supplements.

TABLE 38-5. Evidence Summary and Clinical Advice for Common Individual Weight Loss Supplements

| SUPPLEMENT | Evidence Summary | | CLINICAL ADVICE |
	PRODUCT EFFICACY	PRODUCT SAFETY	
Apple cider vinegar	U[a]	U	Counsel and caution
Cascara	U[a]	U	Counsel and caution[b]
Chitosan	A	P	Discourage
Chromium	U[c]	U	Counsel and caution
Conjugated linoleic acid	U[c]	U	Counsel and caution
Dandelion	U[a]	U	Discourage[b]
Ephedra alkaloid-caffeine combinations[d]	P	A	Discourage
Ginseng	U[a]	U	Counsel and caution
Glucomannan	U[e]	P	Counsel and caution
Green tea	U[a]	P[f]	Counsel and caution
Guar gum	A	P	Discourage[g]
Guggul	U[a]	U	Counsel and caution
Hydroxycitric acid	U[h]	U	Counsel and caution
Laminaria	U	U	Counsel and caution
L-Carnitine	U[a]	P	Counsel and caution
Licorice	U[a]	U	Counsel and caution
Psyllium	U[a]	P	Counsel and caution

Continued

TABLE 38-5. Evidence Summary and Clinical Advice for Common Individual Weight Loss Supplements—cont'd

| | Evidence Summary | | |
SUPPLEMENT	PRODUCT EFFICACY	PRODUCT SAFETY	CLINICAL ADVICE
Pyruvate	U[e]	U	Counsel and caution
St. John's wort	U[a]	U	Counsel and caution
Vitamin B$_5$	U[a]	P	Counsel and caution

Adapted from Saper R, Phillips R, Eisenberg D. Common dietary supplements for weight loss. *Am Fam Physician.* 2004;70:1731–1738.
A, absent; P, present; U, uncertain.
Note: If strong evidence indicates the presence of efficacy and safety, then the suggested clinical advice to provide the patient is to recommend the supplement actively. None of the weight loss supplements meet these criteria. If strong evidence indicates the absence of efficacy or safety, then the suggested clinical advice is to discourage use of the supplement actively. If the evidence does not meet the criteria to recommend or discourage (i.e., evidence for efficacy or safety is uncertain with no strong evidence against efficacy or safety), then the suggested clinical advice is to counsel and caution the patient on the available scientific information.
[a]No or few human weight loss trials.
[b]Given the inadvisability of using conventional diuretics or laxatives for the purpose of weight loss, it is reasonable to discourage these agents if they are used by the patient only for losing weight. If overweight patients are using these supplements for other indications (e.g., hypertension, constipation), to counsel and caution may be reasonable.
[c]Most or all trials do not show weight loss, but the small number of trials and subjects precludes definitive efficacy conclusions.
[d]Also includes country mallow, bitter orange, guarana, and mate.
[e]Most or all trials demonstrate weight loss, but the small number of trials and subjects precludes definitive conclusions.
[f]If taken in appropriate doses (the equivalent of less than 5 cups of green tea daily).
[g]"Discourage" refers to the use of guar gum as an antiobesity agent only. Guar gum and other fiber agents may have a role, however, in obese patients for the treatment of comorbidities such as diabetes, glucose intolerance, or hyperlipidemia.
[h]Efficacy data are contradictory.

PREVENTION PRESCRIPTION

■ The basis for prevention of weight gain is learning how to follow an antiinflammatory diet that emphasizes vegetables and fruits from all parts of the color spectrum, whole grains, fish and other sources of omega-3 fatty acids, vegetable protein more than animal sources, monounsaturated fats, and low-fat dairy. To make this a long-term lifestyle change, fruits, vegetables, and high-fiber grains must be used to displace high-calorie processed foods of poor nutritional content (see Chapter 86, The Antiinflammatory Diet).

■ Fostering a healthy relationship with food and becoming aware of reactive, habitual patterns of eating are vital to preventing weight gain. Learning techniques of mindful eating can facilitate this process.

■ Physical activity may play a role in the prevention of weight gain[85]; 30 minutes/day, 5 to 7 days/week of any physical activity should be encouraged (see Chapter 88, Writing an Exercise Prescription).

THERAPEUTIC REVIEW

All patients should undergo the following assessments. Appropriate therapy can then be determined.

■ Medical History

• Assess for comorbid diseases and concomitant medications that induce weight gain.

■ Nutrition History

• Determine previous weight loss attempts and use 24-hour recall and food frequency questionnaires.

• Rule out clinically significant eating disorders (anorexia and bulimia nervosa, binge-eating disorder, nighttime eating syndrome).

■ Anthropometric Measurements

• Weight, height, BMI, waist circumference, body composition, blood pressure, heart rate

■ Laboratory Tests

• Complete blood count, metabolic profile, fasting lipids, thyroid-stimulating hormone, liver function tests, fasting serum glucose and insulin, hemoglobin A1c (if diabetic), high-sensitive C-reactive protein, 25-(OH) vitamin D

• Electrocardiogram, unless recent one (within 6 to 12 months) is available for review

■ General Evaluation

• Assess for motivation, importance, and confidence for weight loss, barriers to change, and realistic weight loss goals.

• Assess exercise history, sleep patterns, relevant stressors, and social support.

■ Therapeutic Options

- BMI 25 or higher

  - Promote a balanced hypocaloric diet and physical activity, and provide behavioral modification counseling.

  - Reduce caloric intake from baseline by 500 to 1000 cal/day to yield a 1- to 2-lb weight loss per week.

  - Encourage purposeful activity for at least 60 minutes daily 6 to 7 days of the week. Total time may be broken into short bouts of 10 to 15 minutes each during the initial adoption of an exercise program only.

  - Stress management techniques include mind-body therapies such as meditation, biofeedback, or hypnosis.

  - Ensure adequate sleep and treatment of any concomitant sleep disorders.

  - Suggest interactive individual or group support sessions for nutrition education and behavioral modification.

  - Refer to a dietitian, mental health professional, or exercise specialist as needed.

- BMI 30 or higher or 27 or higher with comorbid conditions

  - Full liquid fast, protein-sparing modified fast, and pharmacotherapy with dietary intervention are suitable for this BMI level.

  - Orlistat, 120 mg orally three times daily, is the first option. This medication is localized to the gut and can be used in combination with phentermine.

  - Phentermine can be taken alone (15 to 37.5 mg daily) or in combination with orlistat (approved for 3-month use by the Food and Drug Administration).

  - Suggest omega-3 fatty acids, at 2 to 4 g/daily.

  - Treat vitamin D deficiency appropriately to achieve serum 25-(OH) vitamin D levels between 40 and 60 ng/mL.

  - Other dietary supplements should be used, if at all, on an individualized basis determined by risk-to-benefit ratio and by evaluating the efficacy and safety of each product or combination.

- BMI 40 or higher or 35 of higher with comorbid conditions

  - Weight loss surgery, if other treatment modalities are ineffective, is suitable for this BMI level.

KEY WEB RESOURCES

Procedures for Collecting 24-Hour Food Recalls: http://www.csrees.usda.gov/nea/food/efnep/ers/documentation/24hour-recall.pdf.

This useful handbook from the U.S. Department of Agriculture describes the procedures for conducting a 24-hour diet recall, which is an in-depth interview that collects detailed information on all foods and beverages consumed by a participant during the previous 24 hours. These recalls are best administered "unannounced" (not scheduled on a specific day) so that participants cannot change their eating habits based on anticipation of the interview.

NutritionQuest assessment and analysis services: http://www.nutritionquest.com/assessment.

This company is a leader in the field of diet and physical activity assessment, and their Web site is the official source of the Block Food Frequency Questionnaire and other dietary and physical activity questionnaires developed under the guidance of Dr. Gladys Block. Block Assessment Tools are designed and tested for usability and have a long history of validation in various demographic subpopulations. These tools are available in both paper and electronic format.

Basal metabolic rate calculator: http://www.calculator.org/calculate-online/health-fitness/basal-metabolic-rate.aspx.

This tool calculates how many calories your body requires each day.

Mayo Clinic calorie calculator: http://www.mayoclinic.com/health/calorie-calculator/NU00598.

This calculator includes individual activity in the calculation.

FitDay.com: http://www.fitday.com/.

This Web site allows you to track your nutrition and fitness goals online.

The Center for Mindful Eating: http://www.tcme.org/.

This organization helps people learn how to use eating as a mindful process that brings awareness to what we are eating, thus leading to healthier food choices and reduced calorie consumption.

References

References are available online at expertconsult.com.

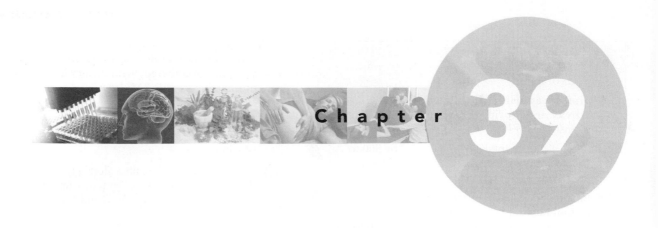

39

Dyslipidemias

Gail Underbakke, RD, MS, and Patrick E. McBride, MD, MPH

Pathophysiology

Dyslipidemias, including lipoprotein overproduction or deficiencies, are a common clinical problem. Approximately 25% to 30% of adults in the United States have total cholesterol levels of 240 mg/dL or higher, and more than half of all U.S. residents have a total cholesterol level that exceeds 200 mg/dL.[1] The number of patients with dyslipidemias and cardiovascular disease (CVD) is expected to increase because of an aging U.S. population and an increasing incidence of diabetes and obesity. The National Cholesterol Education Program (NCEP) Adult Treatment Panel (ATP) III guidelines recommend that all adults 20 years old and older have a baseline fasting lipoprotein profile followed by appropriate management if lipid levels are abnormal, or repeat testing approximately every 5 years if lipid values are normal. The current recommendation is that high-risk children be screened starting at the age of 10 years, although universal screening is being considered by the National Institutes of Health. All adults and high-risk children (those with diabetes, obesity, or a family history of premature CVD or dyslipidemia) should have a complete lipid evaluation. Although routine screening of all children remains controversial, children or adolescents who have parents, grandparents, or siblings with premature atherosclerosis or dyslipidemias can be considered for lipid screening.[2,3]

Many clinical prevention trials have demonstrated that cholesterol treatment leads to prevention of atherosclerosis, stabilization of atherosclerotic plaque, improved function of arteries, regression of existing plaques, and reduction of cardiovascular events and total mortality.[4,5] High-risk patients benefit most from cholesterol treatment. High-risk patients include those with the following:

- CVD or noncoronary atherosclerosis

- Genetic dyslipidemias

- Diabetes mellitus

- Multiple risk factors, including lipoprotein abnormalities[1]

The NCEP ATP III guidelines recommend evaluation for underlying atherosclerosis and comprehensive risk assessment for all patients before determining lipoprotein goals, by using history, physical examination, and overall risk assessment. Consideration is given to other methods of screening (stress tests or imaging of blood vessels) if the patient has symptoms or is considered high-risk (greater than a 20% 10-year risk of coronary heart disease [CHD]). Low-density lipoprotein cholesterol (LDL-C) treatment goals are risk stratified using 10-year risk estimates from NCEP ATP III guidelines. Clinicians can estimate CHD risk with risk calculators for desktop or handheld computers available at the NCEP Web site (see Key Web Resources).

Table 39-1 outlines the ATP III classification of LDL-C, total cholesterol, high-density lipoprotein cholesterol (HDL-C), and triglycerides (TGs). HDL-C and LDL-C continue to be important risk factors in adults older than 65 years of age.[1] Clinicians should consider each older adult for dyslipidemia treatment individually, based on the patient's motivation, prognosis, comorbidities, and potential improvement in quality of life. Table 39-2 outlines classifications of lipids for children and adolescents.

Measuring Cholesterol and Lipoprotein Levels

Note that total cholesterol and HDL-C levels are not influenced by fasting and can be measured at any time of day. Lipoprotein profiles must be done after a 12- to 14-hour fast because TG measurements are variable in the nonfasting state. When total cholesterol, TG, and HDL-C are measured, and serum TG levels are less than 400 mg/dL, LDL-C can be estimated using this formula:

$$LDL\text{-}C = \text{Total cholesterol} - (HDL\text{-}C + TG/5)$$

Dividing the clinical TG levels by 5 provides an estimate of very-low-density lipoprotein cholesterol (VLDL-C). However, the LDL-C calculations are not accurate if the TG level exceeds 400 mg/dL.[1]

TABLE 39-1. Adult Treatment Panel III Classification of Total, Low-Density Lipoprotein, and High-Density Lipoprotein Cholesterol and Triglycerides

CHOLESTEROL AND TRIGLYCERIDES (mg/dL)	DESCRIPTOR
Total cholesterol	
Less than 200	Desirable
200–239	Borderline high
Greater than 240	High
LDL-C*	
Less than 100	Optimal
100–129	Near optimal/higher than optimal
130–159	Borderline high
160–189	High
Greater than 190	Very high
HDL-C	
Less than 40	Low
Greater than 60	High
Triglycerides	
Less than 150	Normal
150–199	Borderline high
200–500	High
Greater than 500	Very high

Data from National Cholesterol Education Program Expert Panel on Detection, Evaluation, and Treatment of High Blood Cholesterol in Adults (Adult Treatment Panel III). Third Report of the National Cholesterol Education Program (NCEP) Expert Panel on Detection, Evaluation, and Treatment of High Blood Cholesterol in Adults (Adult Treatment Panel III) final report. *Circulation.* 2002; 106:3143–3421.
HDL-C, high-density lipoprotein cholesterol; LDL-C, low-density lipoprotein cholesterol.
*Primary target of therapy.

A lipoprotein profile is usually sufficient to develop a clinical classification and treatment approach for dyslipidemias. When the TG level is more than 400 mg/dL, however, lipoprotein phenotyping to determine the specific biochemical abnormality may be useful to direct treatment. In addition, newer technology and research have found that the LDL particle number is a better predictor of CVD risk than the LDL-C level (or the total amount of cholesterol available in LDL particles).[6,7] Research shows that small LDL (type B) particles are easily oxidized, thus leading to greater penetration of the arterial wall and resulting in the development of atherosclerosis. Small LDL particles are common when TG levels exceed 80 to 100 mg/dL.[6] Special testing is needed to determine whether a patient has small LDL or the less atherogenic large LDL particles. This determination is most accurate with nuclear magnetic resonance testing, which is emerging as a more sensitive and predictive test for cholesterol risk. More research is under way regarding the best use of this test and the assessment of LDL particles.[6]

Factors That Can Affect Cholesterol Measurements

Certain patient-related factors, including the following, can influence cholesterol measures and should be considered when interpreting test results[1]:

- Acute or chronic illness (e.g., heart attack, viral illness, bacterial infection)
- Recent general surgery
- Pregnancy or lactation
- Poor nutritional status or ongoing significant weight loss
- Nonfasting state (affects TG levels, not HDL-C or total cholesterol)
- Improper fingerstick technique ("milking the finger")
- Day-to-day or seasonal variation

TABLE 39-2. Classifications of Lipid and Lipoprotein Concentrations for Children and Adolescents*

	ACCEPTABLE (mg/dL)	BORDERLINE (mg/dL)	HIGH RISK (mg/dL)
Total cholesterol	Less than 170	170–199	200 or greater
LDL-C	Less than 110	110–129	130 or greater
TG			
0–9 yr	Less than 75	75–99	100 or greater
10–19 yr	Less than 90	90–129	130 or greater
HDL-C	Greater than 45	40–45	Less than 40

(LDL-C), high-density lipoprotein cholesterol (HDL-C), and non–HDL-C by 38.6; for triglyceride (TG), divide by 88.6. Data from National Institutes of Health. *Integrated Guidelines for Cardiovascular Health and Risk Reduction in Children and Adolescents.* http://www.nhlbi.nih.gov/guidelines/cvd_ped/index.htm. Accessed 18.1.12.
*To convert mg/dL to SI units, divide the results for total cholesterol, low-density lipoprotein cholesterol

Secondary Causes of Dyslipidemias

Before conducting extensive testing or making treatment decisions, clinicians must evaluate patients to rule out the following potential secondary causes of dyslipidemias:

- Poorly controlled diabetes mellitus
- Obesity and metabolic syndrome
- Medications (steroids, including estrogen, progesterone, prednisone, anabolic steroids, beta blockers, or *cis*-retinoic acid)
- Obstructive liver disease
- Nephrotic syndrome
- Multiple myeloma
- Hypothyroidism
- Excess dietary alcohol, saturated fat, carbohydrate, or caloric intake

A directed medical history, nutrition history, thyroid-stimulating hormone assay, and fasting blood chemistry survey (including glucose, liver enzymes, and creatinine) can rule out most of the common secondary causes. Treating the secondary cause usually markedly improves or normalizes abnormal cholesterol levels.

Dyslipidemia Classifications

Table 39-3 presents a practical system for classifying dyslipidemias based on clinical, genetic, and biochemical parameters. This approach uses results from the lipoprotein profile and is compatible with the more complex Fredrickson-Levy system.

High Low-Density Lipoprotein Cholesterol Levels

Elevated LDL, with normal TG, is considered either primary or familial hypercholesterolemia, a relatively common disorder caused by defects in the LDL receptor gene. Familial hypercholesterolemia is expressed during childhood and is autosomal dominant, with selective elevation of LDL, usually higher than 180 mg/dL in adults or higher than 170 to 200 mg/dL in children. Most adult patients with isolated LDL-C elevations greater than 180 mg/dL have familial hypercholesterolemia and are considered to have primary hypercholesterolemia, which is probably attributable to multiple causes, including nutrition, obesity, and behavioral and genetic factors.

High Triglyceride Levels

High TG levels (higher than 500 mg/dL) result from elevations of chylomicrons, intermediate-density lipoproteins, or VLDLs. Fasting TG levels higher than 1000 mg/dL can result from either genetics or a combination of genetics and a secondary cause, such as alcohol abuse, poorly controlled diabetes, estrogens, obesity, renal disease, or steroid use. Because patients with a TG level higher than 1000 mg/dL have a high risk of developing pancreatitis, this is the priority of treatment.

Low High-Density Lipoprotein Cholesterol Levels

HDL-C is an independent risk factor and is the most powerful predictor of premature CHD.[1] Low HDL-C (less than 40 mg/dL, TG less than 150 mg/dL) is associated with genetic factors, male sex, smoking, obesity, and a sedentary lifestyle. Familial hypoalphalipoproteinemia (low HDL-C), a syndrome found in 7% to 10% of patients with CHD who are younger than

TABLE 39-3. Dyslipidemia Classifications

Lipoprotein Levels (mg/dL)				
LDL-C	HDL-C	TG	CLASSIFICATION	GENETIC DISORDER
Greater than 130	Greater than 40	Less than 150	High LDL-C	Familial hypercholesterolemia (LDL-C greater than 200 mg/dL)
				Primary hypercholesterolemia (LDL-C 130–199 mg/dL)
NA	NA	Greater than 500*	High triglycerides	Lipoprotein lipase deficiency
				Apoprotein C III deficiency
				Familial hypertriglyceridemia
Less than 130	Less than 40	Less than 150	Low HDL-C	Hypoalphalipoproteinemia
				Tangier disease
				Fish-eye disease
Greater than 130	Less than 40	Greater than 150	Combined dyslipidemia	Familial combined hyperlipidemia
				Familial dysbetalipoproteinemia

NA, not applicable.
*Low-density lipoprotein cholesterol (LDL-C), high-density lipoprotein cholesterol (HDL-C), and total cholesterol measurements are not accurate when triglyceride (TG) is higher than 400 mg/dL. Ideally, weight loss is accomplished through a modest, consistent reduction in calorie intake (approximately 500 cal/day) and an increase in physical activity (at least 150 minutes/week of moderate physical activity).

60 years of age, is characterized by an HDL-C level lower than 40 mg/dL, normal TG, and autosomal dominant inheritance. Other genetic forms of low HDL-C exist, but they are far less common. Medications, including beta blockers (nonsympathomimetic), retinoids, progestins, and anabolic steroids, can significantly lower HDL-C. Weight loss, lowering TG, exercise (if HDL-C exceeds 30 mg/dL), smoking cessation, and some medications (niacin, fibrates) can raise HDL-C levels.

Combined Dyslipidemia

Combined dyslipidemia is common and important; it is frequently found in patients who survive myocardial infarction or who undergo coronary revascularization. Combined dyslipidemias include abnormalities of several lipoproteins, usually elevated LDL-C and TG, with low HDL-C. Moderately elevated TG (TG 150 to 499 mg/dL) is usually associated with small atherogenic LDL particles, low HDL-C, and altered HDL effectiveness.[1,6]

Metabolic syndrome is a common, high-risk syndrome that resembles combined dyslipidemia and includes multiple risk factors related to abnormal metabolism caused by the central deposition of body fat and secondary insulin resistance resulting in hyperinsulinemia. This situation causes glucose intolerance or type 2 diabetes and hypertension, in addition to combined dyslipidemia, all of which are considered important CVD risk factors (see Chapter 31, Insulin Resistance and the Metabolic Syndrome).

In addition to the metabolic syndrome, other causes of combined dyslipidemias include the following:

- Lack of physical activity
- Hypothyroidism
- Diabetes mellitus
- Alcohol abuse
- Nephrotic syndrome
- Use of glucocorticoids

Integrative Therapy

Lifestyle: Weight Management

Overweight and obesity increase the risk of CVD in part because of negative effects on lipid levels, by increasing LDL-C and TG and decreasing HDL-C. Although separating the effects of weight loss from the effects of the diet changes made to achieve the weight loss is difficult, a modest 10% weight loss leads to reductions of approximately 15% for total cholesterol and 20% for TG. HDL-C levels may be reduced during active weight loss but are often increased after weight has stabilized at a lower level.[8] Weight loss also reduces risk by increasing LDL particle size.[8]

Exercise training trials have demonstrated 3% to 10% increases in HDL-C and modest reductions in LDL-C (1% to 5%) and TG (4% to 15%) levels, with greater improvements in lipid levels if weight loss occurs.[9,10] In addition to lipid and overall cardiovascular benefits, regular exercise is important for effective long-term weight management because it increases calorie expenditure, maintains or increases muscle mass, and helps maintain metabolic rate.

Although many popular diet books suggest that specific diet patterns or food choices are more effective for weight loss, body weight depends primarily on energy balance. If calories consumed are greater than calories expended, weight gain will occur; conversely, if calories consumed are less than those expended, weight loss will occur. Higher-protein diets may lead to better control of appetite and lower calorie intake, but they are often lower in cardioprotective foods such as whole grains, fruits, and some vegetables.[11] An evaluation of several popular diets revealed that the degree of adherence to the diet plan, rather than the plan itself, predicted weight loss.[12]

Generally, an intake of 1800 to 2000 calories/day for men and 1500 to 1800 calories/day for women represents the recommended 500 calories/day energy deficit, although these numbers vary with body size and activity level. Calorie reduction can be accomplished by counting calories (i.e., keeping a list of food intake and tallying calories to stay within the prescribed limit), but an emphasis on portion control and adjustments in meal composition also lead to weight loss. Reducing portions of calorie-dense foods (meats, starchy foods, salad dressings, spreads, sweet drinks, desserts, and snack foods) by approximately one fourth to one third while increasing quantities of foods of lower calorie density (vegetables, fruits) can be effective. The plate method helps control calories by emphasizing meal composition and encouraging patients to visualize their meal on a plate. One quarter of the plate should be dedicated to a protein food and another quarter to a starchy food (grains, potato, corn, peas), whereas the remaining half of the plate is dedicated to nonstarchy vegetables (anything other than potatoes, corn, or peas).[13]

Nutrition

Recommendations for lifestyle changes to improve serum lipids are based on a vast body of epidemiologic investigations, metabolic studies, and clinical trial evidence. Diet trials have demonstrated significant reduction in heart disease risk and improvement in lipid values with a variety of dietary approaches.[14,15] Diet guidelines published by the American Heart Association (AHA) and the NCEP are based on a review of currently available evidence and are generally regarded as the standard of treatment.[1,16] Ongoing and future research will add to our understanding of the complex effects of lifestyle on serum lipids and heart disease risk.

The NCEP ATP III defines lifestyle modification as the critical first step in the management of dyslipidemia.[1] Table 39-4 lists levels of LDL-C at which lifestyle change should be initiated based on a patient's risk. In most situations, a trial of nutrition and exercise changes should be recommended for at least 3 to 4 months before supplements, botanicals, or pharmaceuticals are considered. Effective lifestyle modifications vary depending on the type of dyslipidemia and may include weight management, exercise, smoking cessation, changes in specific dietary components (saturated fat, carbohydrate, fiber, alcohol, and soy), and the addition of supplements or botanicals (Table 39-5).

Macronutrient Distribution

Extensive research has demonstrated that the proportion of fat, carbohydrate, and protein in the diet affects serum lipids. Very-low-fat diets (10% to 20% of calories) often lead to a reduction in LDL-C, primarily because of the smaller

TABLE 39-4. Low-Density Lipoprotein Cholesterol Goals and Cut Points for Initiating Lifestyle Changes or Medical Therapy: National Cholesterol Education Program Adult Treatment Panel III Guidelines

PATIENT RISK GROUP	LDL-C GOAL (mg/dL)	LDL-C LEVEL (mg/dL) AT WHICH TO START LIFESTYLE CHANGES	LDL-C LEVEL (mg/dL) AT WHICH TO CONSIDER STARTING MEDICAL THERAPY
CHD or CHD risk equivalent (10-yr risk less than 20%)*	Less than 100 (less than 70 optional)	Greater than 100	Greater than 100
2 or more risk factors (10-yr risk 10%–20%)	Less than 130	Greater than 130	Greater than 130 (10-yr risk 10%–20%) Greater than 160 (10-yr risk < 10%)
0–1 risk factor†	Less than 160	Greater than 160	Greater than 160 (160–189: medical therapy optional)

Data from Grundy SM, Cleeman JI, Merz CN, et al. Implications of recent clinical trials for the National Cholesterol Education Program Adult Treatment Panel III guidelines. *Circulation.* 2004;110:227–239.
*A coronary heart disease (CHD) risk equivalent is a condition that carries an absolute risk for developing new CHD equal to the risk for having recurrent CHD events in persons with established CHD. Evidence now supports the use of low-density lipoprotein cholesterol (LDL-C)–lowering medications in this category even if LDL-C levels are less than 100 mg/dL; statin clinical trials demonstrated risk reduction at any LDL-C level for patients with CHD. Medications that primarily modify triglycerides and high-density lipoprotein (e.g., nicotinic acid or fibrate or fish oil) are indicated when those values are abnormal.
†Almost all people with zero to one risk factor have a 10-year risk lower than 10%; thus, 10-year risk assessment in people with zero to one risk factor is not necessary.

TABLE 39-5. Nutrition Priorities for Different Lipid Abnormalities

LIPID ABNORMALITY	NUTRITION PRIORITY
LDL-C elevation	Limit saturated fat to 7% of calories and cholesterol to 200 mg/day
	Avoid trans fats
	Increase dietary fiber, especially soluble fiber
	Weight management
	Consider psyllium and plant sterol or stanol supplements
TG elevation 150–500 mg/dL	Weight management and exercise
	Limit sugars, sweet drinks, and alcohol
	Moderate total carbohydrate intake (up to 60% of calories)
	Moderate unsaturated fat intake
TG elevation >500 mg/dL	Limit total fat intake to 10%–15% of calories
	Avoid alcohol
	Weight management and exercise
Low HDL-C	Weight management and exercise
	Moderate unsaturated fat, moderate carbohydrate (avoid very low-fat diets)

HDL-C, high-density lipoprotein cholesterol; LDL-C, low-density lipoprotein cholesterol; TG, triglyceride.

amounts of saturated fat in the diet. However, the higher carbohydrate content (65% to 75% of calories) found in these diets may increase TG, as well as reduce HDL-C and LDL particle size, thus making a very-low-fat diet inappropriate for patients with elevated TG or low HDL. Moderate-fat diets (30% to 40%) result in a lower carbohydrate intake (40% to 55%), which can help reduce TG and maintain or increase HDL-C.[17] Diets higher in fat do not increase LDL-C as long as saturated fat is controlled, but because fat is calorie dense, these diets can make weight loss more of a challenge. The Therapeutic Lifestyle Change (TLC) diet from the NCEP ATP III recommends a moderate-fat, moderate-carbohydrate diet with 25% to 35% of the calories as fat, 15% to 20% as protein, and 45% to 60% as carbohydrate.[1]

Type of Fat

Based on the number of double bonds in the fatty acid chain, fats in food can be classified as saturated or unsaturated. Trans fat, a term describing the fatty acid structure resulting from partial hydrogenation, is technically a monounsaturated fat (MUF), but it has negative effects on CVD risk. Saturated fats raise LDL-C and HDL-C levels, whereas trans fats raise LDL-C, reduce HDL-C, and may reduce LDL particle size.[8,18] Unsaturated fats can be divided into two categories: MUF, with one double bond; and polyunsaturated fat (PUF), with more than one double bond. Within the PUF category, fats can be further divided into omega-3 and omega-6 fats, based on the distance of the first double bond from the omega end of the carbon chain. Unsaturated fats of all types reduce LDL-C when they are substituted for saturated fat.[19] Fats of all types raise HDL-C when they are substituted for carbohydrate, but unsaturated fats substituted for saturated fats either reduce or maintain HDL-C.[17,20] Omega-3 fats reduce TGs and have positive nonlipid effects on inflammation, oxidation, and thrombosis (see Chapter 86, The Antiinflammatory Diet).[19] When TG levels are higher than 1000 mg/dL, dietary fat of any form will raise TG levels because of the lack of lipoprotein lipase activity. Limiting total fat intake to 10% to 15% of calories is necessary to reduce TG levels and decrease the risk of pancreatitis in these situations.

The U.S. Department of Agriculture National Nutrient Database is an excellent free resource to determine the fat and other nutrient content of individual foods. Go to http://www.nal.usda.gov/fnic/foodcomp/search/

Saturated Fat

Considering all available evidence, the TLC diet and the 2006 AHA diet goals recommended a saturated fat limit of 7% of calories for management of lipid disorders and intensive reduction of CVD risk.[1] Dairy fat (butter, cream, cheese, ice cream, whole milk), which is approximately 60% saturated, and meat fat (fatty beef or pork, chicken skin, sausage, hot dogs, bologna), which is approximately 30% saturated, are the major sources of saturated fat in the U.S. diet. In addition, the fats found in coconut oil, palm oil, palm kernel oil, and chocolate contain a significant amount of saturated fat. Research has shown that not all saturated fatty acids have the same influence on lipids. Of the four main saturated fats in our food supply (lauric, myristic, palmitic, and stearic), the myristic and palmitic acid found in meats, dairy, and palm oil appear to have the greatest negative lipid effects. Lauric acid, found in coconut and palm kernel oil, raises both LDL-C and HDL-C, whereas stearic acid, found mainly in beef and chocolate, reduces LDL-C.[21] Because foods contain a mixture of saturated fatty acids and because research is currently limited, recommending specific intakes of each fatty acid is not possible.[22-24] Current recommendations to reduce saturated fat from high-fat dairy products, fatty meats, and tropical oils (palm, palm kernel, coconut) are appropriate.

Trans Fat

Trans fats are found in liquid vegetable oils that have been partially hydrogenated to produce a solid or semisolid fat. These fats are popular in the food industry because of their long shelf life, solid consistency, and stability for deep frying. Trans fat should be avoided as much as possible. Food labels have included trans fat content as of January 2006, thus making it easier for the consumer to make choices based on trans fat content. As a result of consumer demand for trans fat–free products, many food producers have nearly eliminated trans fat from their products. Unfortunately, to maintain the desired texture and stability of processed foods, saturated fats are often substituted for trans fat.[25] Reading labels for trans and saturated fat content and limiting the use of processed foods in general are recommended for management of dyslipidemia and reduction of CVD risk.

Unsaturated Fats

The benefits of MUF versus PUF have been debated for many years. Both types of fats appear to reduce LDL-C to approximately the same degree when they are substituted for saturated fat, and although MUFs seem to maintain HDL-C more effectively than PUFs, PUFs are associated with a greater overall reduction in cardiovascular risk.[19] MUFs are found primarily in olive oil, canola oil, avocado, nuts, and olives. PUFs are found in corn, soybean, safflower, sunflower, and flaxseed oil, as well as fish and some nuts and seeds. Because unsaturated fats come primarily from plant foods, some of the cardiovascular benefits noted with higher unsaturated fat intake may possibly relate to other plant constituents.

PUFs can take the form of omega-3 or omega-6 fats and are essential for good health because they cannot be manufactured by the body. The omega-3 fats influence the inflammatory pathways that affect cardiovascular risk and are discussed further in Chapter 86 (The Antiinflammatory Diet). Eicosapentaenoic acid (EPA) and docosahexaenoic acid (DHA) are the primary omega-3 fats obtained from marine sources including fish and fish oil, whereas the omega-3 alpha-linolenic acid can be obtained from plant sources, including flax, canola, walnuts, soy, mustard oil, and hemp. From 2 to 4 g of EPA and DHA per day can lower TG levels by 20% to 40%, usually accompanied by a slight increase in LDL-C and HDL-C.[26-28] The AHA recommends two fish meals per week, with an emphasis on fatty fish.[16] Because many types of fish may be contaminated with polychlorinated biphenyls and heavy metals, recommendations to increase fish intake should be carefully considered, especially for children and for women of childbearing age.[29] Many fish oil capsules are guaranteed for purity and can be safely used to increase EPA and DHA intake. Investigators have estimated that only 10% to 15% of the omega-3 fats from plant sources (alpha-linolenic acid) are converted to EPA or DHA, and whereas alpha-linolenic acid may offer some protection against CVD, the TG-lowering effect of plant omega-3 fats is not as significant as the effect of marine omega-3 fats.[17,30,31]

Dietary Cholesterol

Individual serum lipid response to dietary cholesterol intake varies widely and is difficult to separate from the effects of dietary saturated fat. Dietary cholesterol is found only in foods from animal sources, and the most significant source is egg yolks. Cohort studies have reported no significant relationship between egg intake and heart disease risk, but metabolic studies have shown a 10-mg/dL increase in serum cholesterol with a 200-mg increase in dietary cholesterol.[25] The ATP III TLC diet recommends a daily limit of 200-mg dietary cholesterol, which equates to approximately two egg yolks per week.[1]

Carbohydrate

Carbohydrates provide a ready source of energy and are found in grains, fruits, vegetables, and legumes, foods that also contain various cardioprotective nutrients. The TLC diet guidelines recommend that carbohydrates provide approximately 50% of the calories to achieve optimal lipid levels.[1] As carbohydrate intake increases, TG levels increase and LDL size and HDL-C levels decrease, so diets containing more than 60% of the calories as carbohydrate are not recommended for persons who have elevated TG levels, low HDL levels, or a predominance of small dense LDL particles.[32] The TG-raising effects of carbohydrates are reduced by fiber and are increased by sugar in the diet.

Based on 2000 calories/day, a diet containing 50% carbohydrate would include 250 g of carbohydrate per day:

$$2000 \times 0.5 \div 4 \text{ calories per gram of carbohydrate}$$

Aiming for an even distribution of the carbohydrate intake, meals would contain 60 to 75 g of total carbohydrate, and snacks would contain 15 to 25 g.

Sugar

A diet that contains more than 20% of the calories as sucrose (approximately 8 tablespoons of table sugar per day in a 2000-calorie diet) will raise TG and probably reduce HDL levels.[33] Large amounts of sugar are absorbed so rapidly that the normal pathways for carbohydrate metabolism are overwhelmed, thus leading to greater synthesis of fatty acids.[32] High-fructose corn syrup is a widely available, inexpensive sweetener used in many processed foods.[34] Fructose may have a greater effect on lipids because the metabolism of fructose encourages the production of VLDLs more than other sugars. Sugar alcohols such as mannitol and sorbitol are commonly used in "low-sugar" foods, but because they are converted to fructose, they can also contribute to the overproduction of TG.[33]

For patients with elevated TG levels, aim for the total carbohydrate goals described earlier, with specific limits on sugar-containing beverages (no more than 8 to 12 oz of regular soda, fruit juice, or fruit drinks per day). Modest amounts of desserts and other sweet foods can be incorporated if they fit within the total carbohydrate goals.

Glycemic Index

The glycemic index ranks carbohydrate-containing foods based on their effect on blood glucose when a prescribed dose of a food is eaten in isolation.[35] The glycemic index of a food is influenced by the type of starch it contains, the amount of fiber present, and the other foods eaten at the same time.[36] Studies suggest the risk of CHD is higher for people who consume high–glycemic index foods, especially if those people have underlying insulin resistance or metabolic syndrome[37,38] (see Chapter 85, The Glycemic Index/Load).

Fiber

Dietary fiber can be classified as insoluble (primarily cellulose found in wheat) or soluble (viscous) fibers including beta-glucan, pectin, and gums. Food contains a mixture of fibers, with an average U.S. diet containing approximately two-thirds insoluble and one-third soluble fiber. Although insoluble fibers have significant benefit for digestion and satiety, the beneficial effects of fiber on cholesterol levels are primarily attributed to soluble fibers. The mechanisms are not clearly understood, but they probably include binding of bile acids in the viscous intestinal contents and fermentation of soluble fiber by colonic bacteria, thus leading to inhibition of hepatic cholesterol synthesis.[39] The TLC diet recommends 10 to 25 g of soluble fiber per day, which has been shown to reduce LDL-C by 3% to 10%.[1,40] The most significant dietary sources of soluble fiber are legumes, oats and oat bran, barley, flax, and fruits. One fourth of the fiber in flaxseed is soluble fiber, and consumption of 1 to 2 oz of ground flaxseed per day can reduce total cholesterol and LDL-C by 2% to 3%, with no effect on TG and HDL-C. Flax oil void of lignan fiber does not have the same lipid-lowering effects as ground flaxseed.[41] Studies show that a higher intake of whole grains is associated with a lower risk of CVD, a finding suggesting that components other than soluble fiber (vitamins, minerals, phytoestrogens) are also important.[42]

Adding 1 to 2 teaspoons of a soluble fiber (psyllium, guar gum, ground flaxseed, bran) before meals has multiple benefits. This practice lowers cholesterol, reduces the glycemic index of the carbohydrates eaten (lowers triglycerides), and stimulates satiety by soaking up water in the stomach, with resulting mild weight loss from reduced calorie intake.

Soluble fiber found in legumes, oats, oat bran, barley, and pectin (apples and oranges) has a greater benefit on cholesterol than does insoluble fiber such as cellulose found in wheat.

Protein

For many years, most dietary guidelines assumed that the amount of protein in the diet had no impact on serum lipid levels. Research suggests, however, that if protein low in saturated fat is substituted for carbohydrate, the risk of CHD is reduced, possibly through improved lipid levels.[43]

Soy Foods

Soy protein substituted for animal protein can reduce total cholesterol, with little effect on TG or HDL-C. Cholesterol-lowering effects of soy are greatest in people with the highest initial cholesterol levels.[41] In general, 25 g of soy protein per day reduces LDL-C levels by approximately 5% and may produce a modest reduction in TG.[44] The mechanisms for the LDL-C reduction are not well understood but may include increased excretion and synthesis of bile acids, reduction of cholesterol absorption, and increased LDL receptor activity.[41] Studies to determine whether the soy protein or the isoflavones found in soy (primarily genistein and daidzein) are responsible for hypolipidemic effects have produced mixed results. A meta-analysis found that soy protein containing isoflavones had a greater lipid-lowering effect than soy protein without isoflavones, but soy isoflavones without soy protein showed no significant lipid-reducing effects.[45] For maximum benefit, minimally processed soy foods (soy nuts, tofu, soy burgers, soy milk, tempeh) are recommended as the primary source of soy protein, rather than isolated soy protein or isoflavone supplements.

Alcohol

Consumption of one or two alcoholic drinks per day is associated with a 30% to 50% reduction in CHD risk.[46] About half of the beneficial effect of alcohol is likely the result of an average 12% increase in HDL-C with one or two drinks per day.[47] In susceptible people, however, one or two drinks per day can raise TG levels, increase blood pressure, and provide extra calories that will make weight loss more difficult. Certain alcoholic drinks (red wine, dark beer) contain phytochemicals that have benefits for cardiovascular health but do not alter lipid levels.[47]

Other Bioactive Food Components
Phytosterols

Phytosterols are naturally occurring sterols present in plants that may enhance the cholesterol-lowering effects of vegetable oils.[48] Typical consumption of plant sterols in the United

States is 200 to 400 mg/day, primarily from vegetable oils, legumes, and nuts and seeds.[49] Studies show that approximately 2 g/day of plant sterols can reduce serum cholesterol levels by approximately 10%.[49] Because this dose is impractical to obtain from food on a daily basis, plant sterols are concentrated and added to foods, including some margarines, orange juice, and soy milk. These products are discussed later under Supplements.

Nuts

Nuts are a rich source of unsaturated fatty acids, plant protein, fiber, vitamins and minerals, plant sterols, and flavonoids, all of which may have health benefits. Numerous studies have shown an inverse relationship between nut consumption and CHD risk, with CHD risk reduced by up to 50% by consumption of 1 oz of nuts or more per day.[50] Studies of walnuts, almonds, pecans, peanuts, macadamias, and pistachios showed modest changes in serum lipids when compared with diets with similar fatty acid profiles but showed significant improvement when nuts were substituted for saturated fat or carbohydrate.[51-55] Similar to other foods rich in unsaturated fat, nuts help maintain HDL levels. To control calorie intake, moderate quantities of nuts should be substituted for other foods, because 1 oz of nuts (approximately ¼ cup) contains 170 to 190 calories. Recommend a handful (not a canful) daily.

Garlic

Garlic is valued for the flavor it adds to food and has been assessed for its lipid-lowering effects, but results are difficult to interpret because of the instability of the active ingredients and variations in preparations used in research studies. Garlic cloves (one half to one per day) and garlic oil may reduce LDL-C by up to 10%, probably related to a reduction in cholesterol synthesis and absorption, whereas the effects of garlic powder are more variable.[50,56] In addition to lipid-lowering effects, garlic seems to have a positive impact on platelet aggregation, which may reduce CVD risk.[20,37]

Eating Patterns

Research on specific nutrients is critically important, but the translation of this research into food and eating patterns will ultimately influence CVD risk. The 2006 AHA guidelines focused on a balanced diet emphasizing vegetables, grains, and fruits while simultaneously limiting saturated fat and cholesterol intake.[17] Emphasis on eating patterns acknowledges that people eat food, not nutrients, and encourages recognition of the potential additive and synergistic effects of various dietary components.[57]

Mediterranean Diet

A Mediterranean diet is described as a diet rich in plant foods (vegetables, fruits, legumes, nuts) and including fish, some poultry, limited red meat, and primarily unsaturated vegetable oils. Interest in this diet plan grew when epidemiologic studies noted that populations with this dietary pattern had lower risks of CVD. The macronutrient composition of the Mediterranean diet is variable but is generally 45% to 55% of calories as carbohydrate, 25% to 35% as fat, and 15% to 20% as protein, with a high content of fiber and omega-3 fatty acids, similar to the TLC diet recommendations of the ATP III.[1] The Lyon Diet Heart Study studied diet plans consistent with a Mediterranean diet and found significant reduction in CVD risk, only partially accounted for by lipid improvements.[15] More recently, a study comparing the effects of a plant-based diet having Mediterranean characteristics with a diet higher in refined convenience foods but low in saturated fat and cholesterol found that the plant-based diet offered additional lipid benefits, likely because of constituents of whole plant foods.[57]

Portfolio Diet

The Portfolio diet study used a Mediterranean-type diet enhanced with foods and nutritional supplements to achieve optimal LDL-C reduction. The diet was vegetarian, with less than 7% of calories as saturated fat, and included foods high in soluble fiber (oats, barley, eggplant, okra), 1 oz of almonds per day, and generous amounts of soy protein (approximately 50 g/day). In addition, participants took supplements of plant sterols and psyllium fiber. All foods were provided for the participants in the 1-month study, which produced LDL-C reductions almost equal to those achieved with 20 mg of lovastatin (28.6% versus 30.9%), a response greater than in any previous dietary study.[58] A year-long follow-up study was conducted, with participants preparing their own foods. Adherence to diet varied significantly, and the mean LDL reduction was 12% to 15%; closer adherence led to LDL-C reductions of greater than 20%.[59] Although these results are encouraging, routine adherence to the Portfolio diet requires a committed patient and a wider availability of dietary products similar to those used in the study.

> The Portfolio eating plan is a vegetarian/Mediterranean-type diet with less than 7% of calories from saturated fat. It consists of 2000 calories/day and includes the following key ingredients:
>
> - 30 g of almonds (approximately 23 almonds)
> - 20 g of viscous fiber from foods such as oats, barley, psyllium, and certain fruits and vegetables
> - 50 g of soy protein from foods such as tofu, soy meat alternatives, and soy milk
> - 2 g of plant stanols or sterols from supplements, avocado, soybeans, olive oil, and green leafy vegetables
>
> The results of this regimen are equal to the reduction in low-density lipoprotein cholesterol obtained with 20 mg of lovastatin (approximately 30%).[53,54]

Supplements

Plant Stanols and Sterols

The plant sterol mixtures typically used in supplements to reduce cholesterol levels are usually extracted from pine tree wood pulp or soybean oil. Plant sterols are often hydrogenated, forming stanols, and both sterols and stanols can be esterified to make them soluble in fats, forming stanol and sterol esters. Plant stanols and sterols decrease cholesterol absorption by displacing cholesterol from the intestinal micelles and increasing fecal elimination of both dietary and biliary cholesterol.[41] Stanol or sterol esters in doses of 2 to 3 g/day reduce LDL-C by 8% to 14%, with the greatest reductions occurring when they are added to a high-fat diet.[50,60]

Doses higher than 3.4 g/day provide no additional benefit.[61] Supplements of stanol and sterol esters can be obtained in capsules or "chews," as well as in fortified food products, including margarines, juice, and rice or soy milk. The stanol or sterol content of each supplement or fortified food should be checked because some items contain only small amounts and will not provide the desired lipid reductions.

Safety concerns relate to decreased plasma levels of carotenes, tocopherol, and lycopene when stanol or sterol ester supplements are used.[60] At present, the significance of these changes is not known. In addition, concerns exist about the absorption of plant sterols and the resulting elevations in serum sterol levels, which may increase the risk of heart disease. This occurs in people affected by the rare condition (fewer than 100 cases worldwide) sitosterolemia, characterized by an inability to clear dietary sterols, but studies suggest that this situation may also occur to a lesser degree in the general population. The clinical significance of elevations in serum sterol levels is not clear. Plant stanols do not seem to aggravate sitosterolemia or increase serum sterol levels and may be the safer choice.[62,63]

■ Dosage

The dose of beta-sitosterol is 800 mg to 1 g, taken 30 minutes before meals three times daily. Benecol chews, four chews per day, are spread over the day. Take Control or Benecol margarine is consumed at 2 tablespoons per day (1 g plant sterol or stanol per tablespoon).

■ Precautions

Stanol and sterol supplements are generally well tolerated. In some patients, they can cause nausea, indigestion, gas, diarrhea, or constipation. Long-term use may negatively affect plasma levels of sterols, carotenes, tocopherols, and lycopene.

Psyllium

The LDL-C–reducing effect of soluble (viscous) fiber found in food can be enhanced by using supplements high in viscous fiber. Psyllium husk is a well-tolerated, readily available source of soluble fiber that has been extensively studied. LDL-C levels were reduced approximately 7% when 10.2 g of psyllium was added to a diet low in saturated fat.[64] Study subjects taking 10 mg of simvastatin achieved an additional 6% LDL-C lowering when they added 15 g of psyllium per day.[65] Psyllium has a minimal effect on HDL-C or TG levels. Because psyllium supplementation can lead to gastrointestinal symptoms, gradual introduction is recommended, starting with 1 teaspoon/day for a week and increasing the dose by 1 teaspoon/day each week until reaching a maximum dose of 4 to 6 teaspoons/day. Each teaspoon of plain (no sugar added) psyllium powder contains approximately 3.4 g of psyllium husk. Adequate fluid intake is important to prevent choking and improve tolerance. Flavored psyllium supplements may contain undesired sugar and calories, but artificially sweetened or unflavored supplements are available. Other soluble fibers, including guar gum and pectin, have been shown to reduce LDL-C but are less readily available to consumers.[50]

■ Dosage

Numerous sources of psyllium are available: powder, capsules, wafers); 1 teaspoon of unsweetened powder equals 3.4 g of psyllium husk. Slowly titrate up to 15 to 20 g/day (approximately 4 to 6 teaspoons or 1.5 to 2 tablespoons in divided doses daily).

■ Precautions

Taking soluble fiber with inadequate fluid intake can lead to constipation and possible fecal impaction.

Fish Oil

Omega-3 fatty acids have multiple cardioprotective mechanisms, but their major lipid effects are reduction of TG and increase in HDL-C. The minimal effective dose of EPA and DHA for TG reduction is slightly more than 1 g/day; a dose of 2 to 4 g/day reduces TG by 25% to 50%.[17,66,67] Patients should begin with a dose of 1 to 2 g/day and titrate to the level that provides adequate TG control. Fish oils reduce production of VLDLs, result in smaller VLDL particles by reducing TG transport, and increase VLDL clearance. Fish oil reduces the absorption and synthesis of cholesterol but may produce a slight increase in LDL-C related to down-regulation of LDL receptors.[66]

Consumption of two to three fatty fish meals per week (as recommended by the AHA) provides approximately 250 to 400 mg of EPA and DHA per day, which is less than the dose required for significant TG reduction. Higher dietary intake of fish is a potential source of heavy metals and other contaminants.[17] Fish oil capsules checked for purity can safely be used to achieve higher doses of omega-3 fatty acids. The omega-3 fatty acid content varies with different fish oil preparations but is often 120 mg of DHA and 180 mg of EPA per 1-g capsule. Thus, 7 to 13 capsules per day would be required to achieve a dose of 2 to 4 g of EPA and DHA per day. This sometimes results in gastrointestinal upset, burping, and a fishy taste. Patients can minimize these symptoms by using fish oil capsules with a higher concentration of DHA and EPA, by taking fish oil with meals, by freezing capsules, or by using enteric-coated fish oil capsules. Some fish oil preparations are more concentrated in EPA and DHA, thus making fewer capsules necessary and possibly minimizing side effects. Cod liver oil is a popular fish oil supplement, but it is high in vitamin A and has a lower concentration of EPA and DHA (190 mg/g) than do oils from fish flesh. Consuming the large amount of cod liver oil necessary to meet omega-3 fatty acid goals on a regular basis could lead to dangerously high vitamin A intakes.

■ Dosage

A dose of 1 to 4 g of EPA and DHA daily is recommended. Higher doses (3 to 4 g) are needed to treat hypertriglyceridemia.

■ Precautions

Avoid acquiring omega-3 fatty acid from cod liver oil because of the risk of high vitamin A intake with high doses.

Red Yeast Rice

Red yeast rice is the fermented product of rice on which red yeast (Monascus purpureus) has grown. Red yeast rice has been used as a preservative, colorant, and spice in China for centuries. Studies in China and the United States have shown that red yeast rice may reduce cholesterol levels by up to 30% and TG levels by approximately 12% to 19%, because of the presence of monaclins.[68] Red yeast rice has the same potential side effects as 3-hydroxy-3-methylglutaryl–coenzyme A (HMG CoA) reductase inhibitors, including a risk of myopathy. In 1998, the

U.S. Food and Drug Administration (FDA) sought to regulate supplements containing red yeast rice because of the presence of lovastatin, which is identified by the FDA as a drug. Red yeast rice supplements are still available to consumers, but the monaclin and lovastatin contents are highly variable and often unknown, thus making dosing difficult and raising safety concerns. In addition, these products contain other inhibitors of the cytochrome P-450 isoenzyme CYP3A4, which can inhibit the metabolism of the statins and other medications.

▣ Dosage
A standard dose is 1200 mg twice daily, with doses ranging from 600 to 3600 mg daily. A dose of 2400 mg of RYR contains approximately 9.6 mg total statins, of which 7.2 mg is lovastatin. Special care should be taken to ensure a product low in citrinin.

▣ Precautions
Because standardized dosing and reliable preparations of red yeast rice and monaclins are not available, red yeast rice should be used with caution for lipid reduction.[31,69] Inappropriate fermentation practices can result in a chemical contaminant, citrinin, that can be nephrotoxic. Although associated with less myopathy, this supplement should be treated like a statin drug and liver enzymes should be monitored with long-term use.

Guggulipid
Guggul gum is an extract from the resin of the mukul myrrh tree that has been widely used in Asia for centuries. The active ingredients are not clearly defined but may be the plant sterols, guggulsterones, or sesamin, a lignan component, suggesting a mechanism involving reduction in cholesterol absorption or bile acid reabsorption.[70] Most of the research on guggulipid has been conducted in India, with few randomized, controlled studies. One controlled study showed reduction in LDL-C, total cholesterol, and TG,

whereas a study in the United States showed no improvements in lipid values.[71]

▣ Dosage
The suggested dosage is 75 to 100 mg daily divided into three doses. This supplement likely works similarly to viscous fiber.

▣ Precautions
Guggulipid may cause gastrointestinal upset, headache, and rash.[21]

Pharmaceuticals

Pharmaceuticals for dyslipidemias should be used for patients at moderate risk after an adequate trial of lifestyle changes and supplements, usually 3 to 6 months. High-risk patients, such as those with genetic cholesterol disorders, very high TGs, or atherosclerosis, may require pharmaceutical treatment at the onset of the diagnosis. Treatment should be individualized for patients, depending on personal characteristics such as the following:

- Overall risk
- Type of dyslipidemia
- Associated medical conditions
- Prognosis
- Patient motivation
- Cost of treatments

The cholesterol-lowering medications have specific lipoprotein actions. Currently, four classes of medications are used to treat dyslipidemias: (1) statins (HMG CoA reductase inhibitors), (2) fibrates, (3) niacin, and (4) cholesterol absorption inhibitors (ezetimibe and bile acid resins. Table 39-6 lists the available medications and provides

TABLE 39-6. Cholesterol Medications

MEDICATION	DOSE RANGE	LDL-C REDUCTION (%)	COST	SIDE EFFECTS AND SPECIAL CONSIDERATIONS
Statins[a]				For all statins: most LDL-C reduction with statins occurs with initial dose Increased hepatic, transaminases and other minor GI effects (2%–3%) May continue if liver function tests are elevated but less than two to three times normal—remonitor Myalgias or arthralgias (2%–3%)
Atorvastatin (Lipitor)	10 mg daily min 80 mg daily max	35–38 50–60	$$$–$$$$	
Fluvastatin (Lescol)	20 mg nightly min 40 mg twice daily or 80 mg XL max	20–25 35–38	$$ or more	[b,c] [b,c]

Continued

TABLE 39-6. Cholesterol Medications—cont'd

MEDICATION	DOSE RANGE	LDL-C REDUCTION (%)	COST	SIDE EFFECTS AND SPECIAL CONSIDERATIONS
Lovastatin (Mevacor, Altocor, generic)	10 mg nightly min 80 mg nightly or 40 mg twice daily max	25–30 34–40	$–$$	[b,c]Lovastatin now available as a generic medication
Pravastatin (Pravachol)	10 mg nightly min 80 mg nightly max	25–32 30–35	$$$	[b]Only statin without CYP450 metabolism; less interaction with other medications; now available as a generic medication
Rosuvastatin (Crestor)	5 mg daily min 40 mg daily max	54–61 35–40		
Simvastatin (Zocor)	10 mg nightly min 80 mg nightly max	45–50	$–$$	[b,c]Simvastatin now available as a generic medication
Bile Acid Sequestrants[d]				
Colestipol (Colestid)	4–8 g two to three times daily	10–25	$$$–$$$$	May increase TG; bloating, constipation
Cholestyramine (Questran)	5–10 g two to three times daily (start at low dose)	TG may increase moderately	$$–$$$	Interference with some medications and fat-soluble vitamin absorption
Colesevelam (WelChol)	6–7 capsules daily (3 capsules twice daily or 6 daily with meal)		$$$$	Less GI toxicity and possibly less interference with absorption of other medications
Niacin				
Niacin plain (crystalline)	500–1,500 mg two to three times daily (starting dose: 100 mg)	20–25 (at high dose); also 50% TG reduction	$	Flushing, dry skin, rash, glucose intolerance, hepatitis, elevated uric acid
Extended-release niacin (Niaspan, only SR formulation recommended)	Starting dose 500, max dose 2,000 mg nightly	Also 50% TG decrease and 25% HDL-C increase	$$–$$$	Dyspepsia or ulcer; caution use in diabetes, gout, history of gastritis or peptic ulcers
Fibrates				
Gemfibrozil (generic, Lopid) Fenofibrate (TriCor, Lofibra, Antara, Lipofen, Triglide)	600 mg twice daily 50–201 mg daily	10% increase to 20% decrease; also 50% TG decrease and 5%–20% HDL-C increase	$–$$$ $$–$$$	Nausea, rare hepatitis, myositis (2%–6%) with statins and cyclosporine; caution use in renal failure
Other				
Ezetimibe (Zetia)	10 mg daily	15–20	$$$	Angioedema, pancreatitis, hepatitis, diarrhea, abdominal pain
Red yeast rice	1200 mg twice daily	25–35	$$ (OTC)	Similar to statins; avoid products with the nephrotoxin citrinin
Guggulipid	50–75 mg twice daily	10–12	$ (OTC)	Headache, nausea, loose stools, bloating, hiccups

$ to $$$$, least expensive to most expensive; GI, gastrointestinal; HDL-C, high-density lipoprotein cholesterol; LDL-C, low-density lipoprotein cholesterol; max, maximum; min, minimum; OTC, over the counter; PO, orally; TG, triglyceride.
[a]All statins have moderate TG-lowering (15% to more than 40%) and HDL-raising (5% to 12%) effects.
[b]Increased myositis occurs with gemfibrozil, fenofibrate, and niacin.
[c]Cytochrome P-450 (CYP450) metabolism leads to interactions with other medications that are metabolized there. The results may be higher statin levels and possible myositis or rhabdomyolysis.
[d]This second-line treatment for LDL-C disorders is a potent combination with statins.

information on their use. To treat dyslipidemias effectively, health professionals should become familiar with all the medication classes. Medications within each class have similar intraclass effects and side effects. However, because pharmacokinetics will vary, if side effects occur, medications may be cautiously substituted within a class.

Choosing the Right Medication for Specific Dyslipidemias

The pattern of dyslipidemia dictates the choice of medication for each patient. Figure 39-1, a dyslipidemia treatment summary, can help the clinician choose an appropriate therapy.

■ Treating Elevated Low-Density Lipoprotein Cholesterol

- Statins are the most effective treatment for LDL-C elevations, and they also moderately reduce TGs and moderately raise HDL-C.

- Ezetimibe (Zetia) is effective as monotherapy (18% LDL-C reduction) but is more effective in combination with statins (25% LDL-C reduction and 14% TG decrease) and is used only in the 10-mg dose.

- The bile acid resins primarily lower LDL-C but may exacerbate TG elevations.

- Niacin is a potent and inexpensive LDL-C agent, especially in low-dose combination with bile acid resins, but high doses are usually required to lower LDL-C significantly (niacin 2000 mg daily total reduces LDL-C 20% to 25%). The use of niacin is somewhat limited by side effects.

- "No flush" preparations of niacin, such as nicotinamide, have no effects on lipids and should not be substituted for niacin.

■ Treating High Triglyceride Levels

After secondary causes are evaluated and treated, niacin, gemfibrozil, fenofibrate, and fish oils are the most effective and cost-effective treatments for patients with hypertriglyceridemia (TG higher than 400 mg/dL).

FIGURE 39-1
Dyslipidemia treatment summary. *Exception*: Immediate medication (gemfibrozil or niacin) for patients with triglyceride (TG) higher than 1000 mg/dL because of the high risk of pancreatitis, or low-density lipoprotein cholesterol (LDL-C) higher than 220 mg/dL because of genetic disorders and resistance to nonpharmacologic treatment after ruling out secondary causes. [†]*Notes*: (1) goal LDL-C lower than 100 mg/dL (70 mg/dL optional) with coronary heart disease (CHD)/noncoronary atherosclerosis, diabetes mellitus, or 10-year CHD risk greater than 20%; (2) goal LDL-C lower than 130 mg/dL if no known CHD or noncoronary atherosclerosis but high risk; (3) goal LDL-C higher than 160 mg/dL with two or more risk factors or LDL-C higher than 190 mg/dL in isolation. [‡]*See text*: Statins and fibrates or niacin may be used in combination with close monitoring for hepatitis or myositis (risk of interaction, 2% to 6%). HDL, high-density lipoprotein. (Modified from McBride PE, Underbakke G, Stein DH. Dyslipidemias. In: Taylor RB, ed. *Family Medicine: Principles and Practice*. 6th ed. New York: Springer; 2003:1019–1029.)

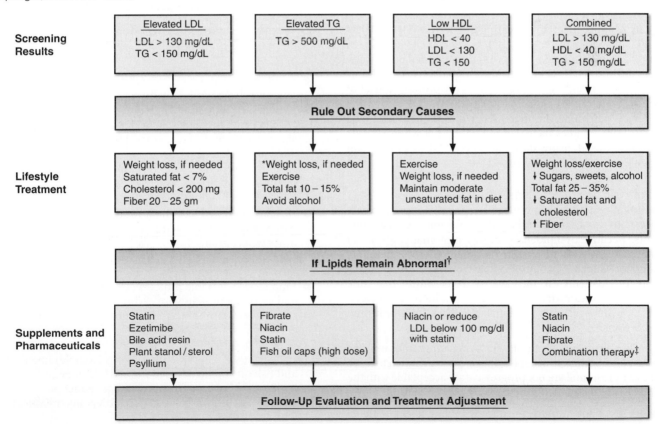

Specific guidelines for treating hypertriglyceridemia include the following:

- The fibrates, including gemfibrozil and fenofibrate, primarily reduce TGs and subsequently raise HDL-C. However, they may also elevate LDL-C.

- Fenofibrate is effective for TG, HDL, and LDL if the baseline TG is lower than 200 mg/dL.

- Estrogens, progestins, and other steroids are contraindicated for patients with hypertriglyceridemia because they elevate the TG level and may cause pancreatitis.

- Fibrates are the treatment of choice for hypertriglyceridemia associated with diabetes, gout, gastritis, or ulcer disease because niacin may worsen these conditions.

- Patients with well-controlled diabetes may tolerate niacin without significant worsening of hyperglycemia, but caution and careful monitoring are advised.

■ Treating Combined Dyslipidemia

The treatments of choice for combined dyslipidemia are statins, niacin, gemfibrozil, and fenofibrate.

- To reduce LDL-C effectively, use a statin, ezetimibe, or bile acid resin.

- Statins may not be effective if the TG level is higher than 300 to 400 mg/dL. In that case, treat with a TG-lowering medication such as niacin (Niaspan), fibrates, or fish oil capsules.

■ Treating Low High-Density Lipoprotein Cholesterol

Niacin is highly effective in treating isolated low HDL-C (less than 40 mg/dL). Isolated low HDL-C deficiencies are slow to respond to treatment. Patients with documented atherosclerosis and low HDL-C should have a goal LDL-C of lower than 70 mg/dL and may be candidates for prolonged trial of low- to moderate-dose niacin (500 to 1000 mg) to determine whether HDL-C can be increased without significant side effects. Some studies have demonstrated that when HDL-C cannot be raised, using statins to lower LDL-C to less than target levels can reduce CVD.[1,4]

Monitoring Medications

Treatments should be monitored regularly, approximately every 4 to 6 weeks, to adjust the dose and evaluate side effects. Because dyslipidemias are asymptomatic, an initial visit 4 to 6 weeks after therapy is initiated provides an opportunity for valuable patient feedback on medication effectiveness. If patients do not have feedback within that time frame, a significant drop in medication adherence occurs.[1] The following are some additional guidelines for monitoring medications:

- Levels of liver function tests, such as alanine transaminase or aspartate aminotransferase, that are less than two to three times normal and are not progressive are acceptable with the use of cholesterol medications, especially the statins.

- More frequent monitoring is recommended for patients with severe underlying clinical disease, liver enzyme elevations, or underlying liver disease and for patients taking combination therapy.

- Statin drugs lower coenzyme Q10 serum levels, but research has not found that supplementation reduces the incidence of myalgias.

- Because physical activity often causes benign elevations of creatine kinase, measuring creatine kinase levels is recommended only if patients complain of generalized myalgias.

- When lipoprotein levels reach treatment goals, monitoring every 4 to 6 months (to assess the side effects, check laboratory studies, and verify diet and medication adherence) is appropriate.

If a statin is causing myositis, fatigue, or difficulty with memory, consider switching to a water-soluble statin such as pravastatin or rosuvastatin. Also consider adding coenzyme Q10, 100 to 200 mg daily.

PREVENTION PRESCRIPTION

- Choose a whole foods, plant-based diet that includes generous amounts of vegetables, whole grains, fruits, and legumes, as well as some fatty fish, nuts and seeds, vegetable oils, and possibly poultry or lean meat.
- Maintain appropriate weight by reducing portions of higher-calorie foods and increasing physical activity.
- Limit foods that are high in saturated fats, trans fats, and cholesterol: fatty meats, butter, cheese, ice cream, other whole milk dairy products, egg yolks, coconut and palm oil, hardened vegetable shortenings, commercially fried foods, snack foods, and bakery items.
- Include food sources of unsaturated fats in moderate quantities: fatty fish, flaxseed, nuts and seeds, and liquid vegetable oils.
- Increase intake of high-fiber foods, especially oats, barley, and legumes, as well as fruits, vegetables, and other whole grains.
- Limit use of high-sugar foods such as sweetened drinks and fruit juices.
- Emphasize vegetable proteins (soy and legumes), and combine protein with carbohydrate at meals and snacks to minimize blood glucose changes and control appetite.
- Use alcohol in moderation, if at all.
- Add plant stanols or sterols, viscous (soluble) fiber, and fish oil supplements as needed to achieve additional cholesterol or triglyceride reduction.
- Add pharmaceutical agents if the foregoing measures do not result in adequate control.

THERAPEUTIC REVIEW

The approach to the therapy of dyslipidemia varies, depending on the patient's cardiovascular disease risk assessment and the severity of the dyslipidemia.

Check for Secondary Causes

- Blood tests for thyroid status, blood glucose, and renal or liver disease
- Review of medications

Lifestyle

- Weight management (initial goal, 5% to 10% weight loss) is a priority for all lipid disorders. $A^{①}_1$
- Regular exercise is prescribed, with a goal of 150 minutes of moderate intensity exercise per week. $A^{①}_1$

Nutrition

- Emphasize limits on saturated fat (less than 7% of total calories), trans fat, and cholesterol (less than 200 mg/dL), with increases in fiber and soy for low-density lipoprotein (LDL) elevations. $A^{①}_1$
- Recommend limits on sugar intake, moderation of total carbohydrate intake, and low–glycemic index foods for triglyceride (TG) elevations. $A^{①}_1$
- Encourage substitution of monounsaturated fats for high-carbohydrate foods to maintain or increase high-density lipoprotein (HDL) levels. $A^{①}_1$

Supplements

- Add fish oil supplements to reduce TG levels. Start with 1 g of eicosapentaenoic acid and docosahexaenoic acid per day and increase as needed and tolerated. $A^{①}_1$
- Use 2 to 3 g/day plant stanols or sterols for LDL-C elevations (1 g before meals). $B^{⊖}_2$
- Add psyllium supplements to increase viscous fiber, including recommended amounts of fluid. Start with 1 teaspoon/day and increase gradually to 4 to 6 teaspoons/day, as tolerated. $B^{⊖}_2$

Pharmaceuticals

- For LDL elevations, consider
  - Statins $A^{⊘}_2$
  - Ezetimibe: 10 mg/day $A^{⊘}_2$
  - And bile acid sequestrants $A^{⊘}_2$
- For TG elevations, consider
  - Niacin: titrated slowly up to 1000 mg $A^{⊘}_2$
  - Fibrates (see Table 39-5) $A^{⊘}_2$
  - Or fish oil: 1 to 4 g/day $A^{⊘}_2$
- For low HDL cholesterol therapy to improve the LDL-to-HDL ratio, consider
  - Niacin $A^{⊘}_2$
  - And/or an additional statin $A^{⊘}_2$
- When TG is higher than 400 mg/dL, TGs must be controlled before total cholesterol and LDL cholesterol can be successfully lowered.

KEY WEB RESOURCES

HeartDecision: www.heartdecision.org

This University of Wisconsin Web site provides a CVD risk calculator, management guidelines, and patient education materials.

National Cholesterol Education Program10-year cardiac risk calculator: http://hp2010.nhlbihin.net/atpiii/calculator.asp?usertype=prof.
Third Report of the Expert Panel on Detection, Evaluation, and Treatment of High Blood Cholesterol in Adults (Adult Treatment Panel III): www.nhlbi.nih.gov/guidelines/cholesterol/index.htmwww.nhlbi.nih.gov/guidelines/cholesterol/index.htm

This National Institutes of Health site includes guidelines, risk calculator, and patient education materials.

My.AmericanHeart for professionals: my.americanheart.org/professional/guidelines.jsp

HeartHub for patients cholesterol information: www.hearthub.org/hc-cholesterol.htm

This American Heart Association Web site includes a learning library, consensus statements, and guidelines.

This American Heart Association Web site has handouts, videos, and newsletters.

National Lipid Association: http://www.lipid.org

This Web site includes references, tools, protocols, and guidelines.

FamilyDoctor cholesterol information: www.familydoctor.org/online/famdocen/home/common/heartdisease/risk/029.html

This American Academy of Family Physicians Web site has patient education materials.

University of Wisconsin Integrative Medicine program module on nonpharmaceutical methods to lower cholesterol: http://www.fammed.wisc.edu/integrative/modules/cholesterol

This site also includes patient handouts.

References

References are available online at expertconsult.com.

Section VII Gastrointestinal Disorders

Irritable Bowel Syndrome

Patrick J. Hanaway, MD

Pathophysiology and Epidemiology

Irritable bowel syndrome (IBS), one of the most common symptom complexes seen by the primary care physician, affects 30 to 50 million people in the United States.[1] Based on the Rome Foundation's Rome III criteria (Table 40-1),[2] the prevalence of IBS has been estimated to range from 10% to 18% in Western countries.[3] IBS has a major impact on modern industrialized societies in terms of economic costs from lost days of employment and health care expenditures, as well as impaired quality of life because of symptoms and impaired psychosocial functioning.[4] In the United States, $10.5 billion is spent each year on direct medical costs and an additional $20 billion on indirect medical costs associated with IBS and related conditions,[5] with an additional $20 billion in indirect costs and absenteeism. Several studies have highlighted that patients with IBS cost insurers 50% more annually than do patients without IBS.[6] Patients with IBS visit their physicians three times more often for symptoms not related to the gastrointestinal (GI) tract than do patients without IBS.[7] Symptoms are reported by 12% to 15% of the U.S. population and are the reason for 30% to 50% of referrals to gastroenterology clinics.[8] IBS is often not seen as a serious medical condition, but patients with the disorder experience a poorer quality of life than described by U.S. norms and than experienced by patients with asthma, diabetes, or migraine headaches.[9]

Functional changes in bowel patterns are the hallmark of IBS, described by Hippocrates as the triad of abdominal discomfort, irregular bowel movements, and various degrees of bloating and rectal urgency. IBS is generally considered a diagnosis of exclusion, defined by the presence of symptoms (abdominal pain or discomfort, bloating, and diarrhea or constipation) and the lack of a known disorder. The Rome III diagnostic criteria are used to define this functional bowel disorder in research, but these criteria are not useful in determining treatment options. As a result, treatment options focus on symptom suppression, rather than on an integrated approach to the person with GI dysfunction that is based on a current understanding of pathophysiologic changes.

The pathogenesis of IBS is multifactorial, with contributions from diet,[10] visceral hypersensitivity,[11] neuroendocrine dysfunction,[12] psychosocial factors,[13] stress,[14] enteric infection,[15] altered GI flora,[16,17] food sensitivities or allergies,[18] and other factors.[19] Research on the treatment of IBS has emphasized diet and nutrition, psychoneuroendocrinologic factors, gut microflora, and the immune system.[20] Research has focused primarily on the gut-brain interactions that highlight visceral perception and autonomic response. However, newer studies of postinfectious IBS, low-grade inflammation, small intestinal bowel overgrowth, and altered gut microflora have yielded more effective clinical improvements.

Gut Microflora and Inflammation

Studies increasingly indicate that a substantial subset (25% to 30%) of patients will develop IBS after an enteric infection.[21] This form of postinfectious IBS is noted to have greater mucosal inflammation extending into the myenteric plexus.[22] The presence of inflammation (even low-grade inflammation) within the GI tract potentiates activation of visceral perception, motility, and hypersensitivity, even after the original infection has cleared.[23]

The role of GI flora in relation to immune activation is currently being explored across the continuum of GI dysfunction, from IBS to inflammatory bowel disease.[24] In IBS, culture and molecular studies have demonstrated decreased diversity of the gut microflora, particularly in aerobic species.[25] Probiotic and dietary prebiotic therapies have been used to correct these deficiencies, with mixed results. Each species and strain of probiotic is unique, with different biochemical effects and specific interactions with the mucosal immune and enteric nervous systems (see Chapter 102, Prescribing Probiotics).

An interesting counterpoint to concerns about gut microflora in IBS is seen in the work of Pimentel et al,[26] who reported that the eradication of bacterial overgrowth of the small intestine eliminated IBS symptoms in 41% of patients. This type of overgrowth could provide a better understanding of the bloating and distention common in IBS.

TABLE 40-1. Rome III Criteria for the Diagnosis of Irritable Bowel Syndrome (IBS)

Symptoms present for at least 3 days per month in the past 3 months (with symptom onset at least 6 months previously) with at least two of the following features:

- Pain improved with defecation
- Onset of pain associated with a change in stool frequency
- Onset of pain associated with a change in stool form

From Longstreth GF, Thompson WG, Chey WD, et al. Functional bowel disorders. *Gastroenterology.* 2006;130:1480–1491.

Additionally, stress produces an inflammatory phenotype in patients with IBS. In response to chronic stress, patients with IBS have helper T cell (Th1 and Th2) suppression and increased interleukin-6. As stress and inflammation increase, so do symptoms. Treatment strategies must consider each of these phenotypic subsets.

Stress

Since the eighteenth century, IBS (formerly known as irritable or spastic colon) was believed to be a nervous disorder that developed in response to external stress and internal neuroses such as depression and anxiety.[27] Early epidemiologic studies demonstrated a 2:1 female-to-male predominance, as well as a higher prevalence of emotional, physical, or sexual abuse in patients with IBS.[28] These vulnerability factors are part of the enhanced stress responsiveness observed in IBS that manifests as an inability to turn off the stress response.[29] Higher cortisol levels in morning urine and saliva have been reported in subjects with IBS than in controls, a finding indicating a state of chronic stress.[30] Stress increases intestinal permeability and susceptibility to colonic inflammation.[14]

The evolution of mind-body medicine and research into psychoneuroimmunoendocrinology helps us better understand the intrinsic relationships among external stressors, emotions, and physiologic changes. Integrative treatment of IBS requires an array of therapeutic approaches that treat the patient on mental, emotional, and physical levels. The studies described here tend to evaluate a single parameter in the treatment of IBS. Intuitively, comprehensive treatment approaches will be of greater benefit.

Enteric Nervous System

Clinicians clearly understand that stress and emotions affect GI function and worsen symptoms in patients with IBS.[31] In addition to elevations in cortisol, patients with IBS have significantly higher postprandial serotonin levels,[32] which are associated with altered gastric emptying, increased small bowel contractions, faster small bowel transit time, and altered pain perception.

Dr. Michael Gershon first described the enteric nervous system as the "second brain"[33] that detects nutrients, monitors the progress of digestion, and modulates the pressure and motility of the GI tract. Alterations in the gut-brain axis observed with positron emission tomography[34] and functional magnetic resonance imaging[35] highlight the role of emotions and mood on the perception of pain in patients with IBS. Studies have recognized the importance of gut

microflora, as well as diet, in bidirectional communication with the brain. In other words, brain signaling changes the gut environment, whereas changes in gut microflora can affect both emotions and pain perception by central nervous system signaling through vagal afferent nerves.[36] A synergistic effect on signaling occurs when inflammatory mediators are also present, thus leading to a further increase in visceral hypersensitivity.[37] In addition, 95% of the serotonin (i.e., 5-hydroxytryptamine) in the body is in the GI tract, not in the brain.

Putting it all together: gut signaling arises from gut microflora, serotonin-producing enterochromaffin cells, and localized inflammation. Pharmacologic approaches have focused on the use of agents to bind enteric serotonin receptors, but untoward side effects of these agents create a high risk-to-benefit ratio. Integrative medicine takes the root cause of individual imbalance into account and leads to therapies that focus on the aforementioned areas of diet, inflammation, gut microflora, infection, stress, and mood.

> Ninety-five percent of the body's serotonin is in the gut and not the brain.

Diagnosis

Conventionally, the symptom-based determination of IBS is based on the Rome III criteria, as well as a complete history and physical examination. No diagnostic testing is necessary to confirm the diagnosis. Careful attention should be paid to potential alarm signs that should initiate further investigation for cancer or inflammatory bowel disease (Table 40-2). Given the multifactorial nature of IBS, however, this descriptive definition of disease does little to target treatment recommendations. The updated Rome III criteria place greater emphasis on subtypes (IBS-C, constipation; IBS-D, diarrhea; and IBS-M, mixed), which further suggests the importance of symptom-based treatment. More recent studies, however, indicate that IBS subtypes are not stable over time.[38] Similar to the Rome III criteria, this subtype stratification does not facilitate integrative treatment based on the underlying physiologic changes. IBS is diagnosed according to the exclusion of other disease, so it remains necessary to rule out specific illnesses that could mimic IBS. GI imbalances to consider include celiac disease, lactose intolerance, fructose intolerance, food sensitivities, food allergies, small

TABLE 40-2. Alarm Signs in the History of a Patient With Irritable Bowel Syndrome

- Weight loss
- Fever
- Overt or occult blood in stool
- Frequent nocturnal bowel movements
- Abnormal laboratory test results
- Family history of inflammatory bowel disease
- Family history of early colon cancer
- Onset of symptoms after age 50 years

From Thompson WG, Longstreth GF, Drossman DA, et al. Functional bowel disorders and functional abdominal pain. *Gut.* 2000;45(suppl 2): S243-S247.

intestinal bacterial overgrowth, dysbiosis, pancreatic insufficiency, acute infection (bacterial, viral), parasitic infection (acute or chronic),[39] *Clostridium difficile* infection, inflammatory bowel disease, and colorectal cancer.

Diagnostic considerations include, first and foremost, an extensive health history with an understanding of dietary inputs, food intolerances and allergies, and use of antibiotics, laxatives, fiber, and herbs. In addition, the clinician must elicit the current pattern of bowel movements including frequency, history, abdominal pain, gas, bloating, relation to meals, and duration. It is amazing how many patients consider their altered bowel movements to be normal. Western medicine does not have a defined norm of bowel movement frequency, whereas other forms of healing such as Ayurveda and traditional Chinese medicine view the regular functioning of the GI tract to be a critical barometer of health and well-being, with one well-formed bowel movement per day as the norm.[40]

> Etiologic factors—infection, parasites, pancreatic insufficiency, celiac disease, food sensitivities, and *Clostridium difficile* infection—should be considered in the differential diagnosis of irritable bowel syndrome before treatment is begun.

Integrative Therapy

We must look beyond symptom-based diagnosis and suppression-based treatment to understand the underlying causes of imbalance and illness. IBS represents an imbalance within the digestive system. The essential components of that system—nutrition, gut flora, immune system, constitution, thoughts, and environment—work optimally when they are in balance and harmony. This integrative approach highlights the unique needs of the individual patient.

Nutrition

Diet

Dietary factors can cause all the symptoms of IBS—pain, bloating, discomfort, and alterations in bowel pattern. More than 70% of patients with IBS describe a worsening of symptoms after meals.[41] Cordain et al[42] described the dietary patterns most common today and compared them with the characteristics of ancestral diets. These investigators noted significant alterations in glycemic load, fiber content, essential fatty acid composition, pH balance, and macronutrient and micronutrient composition. All these factors have tremendous effects on the balance of the commensal flora and the nutrient delivery within the GI tract. This observation is an important reference point, as are the unique and simple food rules that author Michael Pollan has offered: "Eat food. Mostly plants. Not too much."[43] Many patients with IBS experiment with their diet, particularly by removing wheat, corn, dairy, eggs, coffee, tea, and citrus, before they seek medical attention.[44]

Dietary approaches provide the most effective means of returning balance to dysfunction within the GI system, and clinicians have many opportunities to bring these tools to patients. However, the profound dietary changes that humans have adopted over the past 10,000 years, changes that have accelerated over the past 100 years, have created discord with the nutritional input that our genetic structure has evolved to maximize.[42] This discordance creates a much more complex set of clinical opportunities required to regain balance and optimal function.

Food Allergies and Sensitivities

Conventional research has noted that food allergies (mediated by immunoglobulin E [IgE]) and food sensitivities (IgG-mediated) account for approximately 8% of patients with GI symptoms,[45] although many integrative practitioners would remark that the rate of food sensitivity is higher, based on clinical experience. IgE-mediated food allergies can be measured but are present only 2% to 4% of the time. Typically, this diagnosis is made with an elimination diet, during which the symptoms resolve when the patient has removed the offending food and symptoms recur when the offending food is returned to the diet. Atkinson et al[46] used enzyme-linked immunosorbent assay to evaluate food sensitivity in patients with IBS. These investigators used a therapeutic diet in one cohort (based on the IgG assay results identifying foods to which subjects had raised IgG levels) and a sham diet (i.e., the foods eliminated were not those identified as those to which subjects had sensitivities, according to the IgG assay results) in the control population. A 26% decrease in IBS symptoms occurred when test subjects consumed the therapeutic diet, and symptoms returned when they resumed an unrestricted diet.

In a patient with IBS, a diet history should be taken, and a therapeutic diet should be formulated on the basis of results of a targeted elimination-challenge diet (see Chapter 84, Food Intolerance and Elimination Diet).

Gluten Sensitivity and Celiac Disease

Gluten sensitivity is a term used to describe a condition in which gluten leads to a clinical or serologic reaction that improves with gluten elimination. This condition is not exclusive to those who are genetically predisposed through human leukocyte antigen (HLA) DQ2/DQ8.[47] Approximately 4% to 5% of patients with IBS have celiac disease, more than fourfold higher than people without IBS.[48] Investigators have also demonstrated that people without celiac disease who have IgG antigliadin antibody (ABA) feel significantly better when gluten is removed from their diet.[49] Antibody testing for celiac disease is quickly becoming a standard of care in patients with IBS.

Lactose and Fructose Intolerance

The most common form of food intolerance is lactose intolerance, which affects approximately 25% of adults in the United States and 35% to 40% of patients with IBS. Of the patients with IBS who restrict lactose in their diets, more than half will have symptom improvement.[50] Fructose and sorbitol intolerances have also been noted, with similar rates of carbohydrate malabsorption in patients with IBS and controls. However, one study found that patients with IBS had significantly more symptoms because of their carbohydrate malabsorption; these symptoms resolved in 40% of the study subjects after intake of the offending sugar was restricted.[51] The clinician should perform a 14-day trial of a fructose-free, lactose-free, sorbitol-free diet to determine whether the patient's symptoms resolve. Foods with these constituents should be added back with a dietary challenge one at a time every 3 days.

> Sorbitol-containing chewing gum can be a common trigger of irritable bowel syndrome, and the clinician should screen for its use when taking the patient's history.

Fermentable Carbohydrates

An extension of the idea to avoid simple sugars is the concept of a diet restricting fermentable oligosaccharides, disaccharides, monosaccharides, and polyols (FODMaPs). These fermentable substrates (apples, pears, dried fruit, sugar alcohols, mushrooms, avocado, milk, cheese, wheat, rye, onions, artichokes, and inulin) act as prebiotics and stimulate bacterial growth and gas production.[4] This diet is similar to the specific carbohydrate diet that has been anecdotally effective for IBS and inflammatory bowel disease.[52]

Dietary fiber intake in the United States averages less than 15 g/day, well short of the recommended intake of 25 to 35 g/day, or the 115 g/day found in the Paleolithic diet. Although fiber seems to ease constipation symptoms in some patients, the ability of dietary fiber to help with abdominal pain and diarrhea has been limited. Multiple randomized controlled trials (RCTs) have failed to show benefit of soluble and insoluble fiber supplementation together for the multiple symptoms of IBS.[53] Many studies have been complicated by the use of significant amounts of wheat bran as a source of fiber; wheat has been noted to be a common source of food sensitivity, thus potentially altering symptom measures in these studies. Partially hydrolyzed guar gum, a soluble fiber derived from ispaghula, has also been shown to reduce IBS symptoms.[54] Soluble fiber and insoluble fiber have been found to have different effects on IBS symptoms. In one study, soluble fiber (psyllium, ispaghula, calcium polycarbophil) led to significant improvement, whereas insoluble fiber (corn, wheat bran), in some cases, worsened the clinical outcome.[55] The clinician should recommend soluble fiber (e.g., 1 tablespoon psyllium seed with 8 oz of water daily) for patients with constipation. This dosage can be titrated to 30 g/day of soluble fiber in food (or as a supplement). The patient should be told to avoid eating insoluble fiber alone or on an empty stomach, but instead to eat it with a larger quantity of soluble fiber.

> Soluble fiber (psyllium, ispaghula, calcium polycarbophil) improves symptoms, whereas insoluble fiber (corn, wheat bran) can worsen symptoms in some cases.

Exercise

Regular physical exercise has been demonstrated to improve stress coping, enhance well-being, and decrease feelings of depression and anxiety. Light to moderate exercise is recommended and encouraged for all patients with IBS.

Sleep

Poor sleep quality, which has been reported and quantitated in patients with IBS, further compromises their quality of life. Good sleep hygiene is an important consideration and often requires supporting the entire family unit to adopt this approach.

Supplements

Probiotics

Awareness is growing that the human gut microflora plays a critical role in maintaining host health both within the GI tract and systemically through the absorption of metabolites. An optimal gut microflora establishes an efficient barrier to the invasion and colonization of the gut by pathogenic bacteria, produces a range of metabolic substrates that are used by the host (e.g., vitamins and short-chain fatty acids), and stimulates the immune system in a noninflammatory manner.

The fecal microflora has been shown to be abnormal in IBS. Patients have high numbers of facultative anaerobic organisms and lower amounts of *Lactobacillus* and *Bifidobacterium*. Changes in the colonic flora may lead to altered fermentation and immune dysregulation of the intestinal mucosa.

Trials have focused on altering gut microflora with the therapeutic use of probiotics, which are live microbial organisms that are administered in foods or supplements. Probiotics are nonpathogenic, of human origin, resistant to gastric acid and bile, adhere to intestinal epithelium, and they can colonize the GI tract.[56] Probiotic action appears to decrease fermentation, improve competition against imbalanced and potentially pathogenic flora, and stimulate proper immune functioning. Probiotics have been shown to improve the symptoms of IBS[57] and to balance inflammatory cytokines in patients with IBS.[58] A systematic review in the journal *Gut* evaluated 19 RCTs. Results showed clear benefit, although only one strain (*Bifidobacterium infantis* 35624) demonstrated statistical significance in reductions of pain, bloating, and inflammatory cytokines.[59] Information and studies on clinical utility cannot be transferred across different strains and different bacteria. Initial studies focused on several strains of probiotic, with positive effects reported for *Lactobacillus plantarum*, *L. plantarum* in combination with *Bifidobacterium breve*, *Streptococcus faecium*, and VSL#3.[53]

■ Dosage

Recommend a mixture of 50/50 *L. plantarum* with *B. breve* at 25 billion colony-forming units (CFUs) twice daily for 6 to 8 weeks; then decrease to 10 billion CFUs/day. Other probiotic combinations may be considered on the basis of fecal flora (see Chapter 102, Prescribing Probiotics).

■ Precautions

Avoid probiotics in the severely immunocompromised host.

> Altered gastrointestinal flora (also known as dysbiosis) is considered a critical factor in immune dysregulation and altered function. Correction of dysbiosis is necessary in the treatment of irritable bowel syndrome.

Prebiotics

Prebiotics are simple carbohydrate molecules that selectively stimulate normal GI flora to proliferate and thus compete with abnormal flora and pathogens for space, food, and adherence. Synbiotics are the combination products of prebiotics and probiotics. Fructo-oligosaccharides and inulin are the most commonly used prebiotics at this time; they increase bifidobacteria in the stool. Animal studies have demonstrated beneficial effects on microflora balance,[60] and human studies have shown in vivo activation of bifidobacteria,[61] but no improvement in IBS.[62]

■ Dosage

See the earlier discussion of the FODMaP diet. Do not recommend prebiotics unless or until rebalancing of the gut flora occurs. Common food sources include apples, pears, dried fruit, mushrooms, avocado, milk, cheese, wheat, rye, onions, artichokes, and inulin.

Pancreatic Enzymes

One of the conditions to be considered diagnostically with IBS is pancreatic insufficiency. This disorder can be a primary process, with depletion of exocrine pancreatic function, or it can be secondary to villous atrophy and insufficient cholecystokinin stimulation of the exocrine pancreas. Both conditions lead to a decrease in the production of pancreatic elastase and chymotrypsin in the stool, identification of which will help determine the need for supplemental pancreatic enzymes. Laboratory data reveal that approximately 20% of patients with IBS have mild pancreatic insufficiency, whereas 8% have moderate to severe pancreatic insufficiency. Studies of pancreatic enzyme supplementation in patients with IBS symptoms are now under way.

> Testing the stool for pancreatic elastase is a relatively inexpensive way to check for pancreatic insufficiency.

Botanicals

Peppermint Oil

Peppermint (Mentha piperita) has been used for GI disturbances for millennia. Menthol and methyl salicylate, the main active ingredients, have antispasmodic actions, with calming effects on the stomach and GI tract. Peppermint also has analgesic properties, mediated through activation of kappa-opioid receptors to help block transmission of pain signals. Peppermint oil has been evaluated in several randomized trials, and a meta-analysis performed by Pittler and Ernst[63] demonstrated a beneficial effect after 2 weeks of therapy. A 2006 Cochrane Review confirmed these initial reports; 79% of patients with IBS noted alleviation of abdominal pain.[64]

■ Dosage

The recommended dosage is one to two 0.2-mL (200 to 400 mg) enteric-coated capsules three times/day between meals; smaller doses (100 to 200 mg) are effective in children.[65]

■ Precautions

Non–enteric-coated capsules and peppermint oil can decrease the tone of the lower esophageal sphincter and can lead to heartburn. Skin rash has also been reported approximately 2% of the time.

Fennel

Fennel (Foeniculum vulgare) has antispasmodic properties and is particularly helpful in the treatment and prevention of bloating and gas, as a result of the volatile anethole oil.

■ Dosage

Fennel is best used with food (1 teaspoon), but it can also be taken as a tea, oil capsule, or alcohol extract. Caraway seeds are noted to have similar properties.

Ginger

Ginger (Zingiber officinale) can be used nutritionally, in cooking, or as an herbal remedy and has been evaluated in the treatment of postoperative nausea and vomiting. No studies have been conducted with ginger in IBS, although the active gingerols act as an antispasmodic and improve the tone of intestinal muscles. Ginger is available in many forms, and ginger root tea is particularly helpful after overeating.

■ Dosage

The dose of powdered root is 250 to 500 mg three to four times/day. Prepare ginger tea by chopping a piece of ginger the size of the patient's fifth digit; place in 150 mL of boiling water for 5 to 10 minutes and strain. Drink 1 cup before meals.

Aloe

Aloe (Aloe spicata and Aloe vera) is commonly considered safe for internal ingestion and is used commonly in patients with IBS. Aloe vera is classified by the U.S. Food and Drug Administration (FDA) as a class 1 harsh stimulant laxative because the anthraquinones in aloe significantly increase colonic peristalsis. Aloe should be regarded as being in the same class as other anthranoid laxatives, such as cascara (Cascara sagrada) and senna (Cassia senna). Although these agents may be used for short-term relief of constipation, they are not suitable for use in IBS because of their powerful action and tendency for dependency.[66]

Combination Herbal Therapies

Traditional Chinese Medicine

One of the most often cited studies of integrative medicine in IBS was published by Bensoussan et al in JAMA.[67] These researchers demonstrated a beneficial effect of a combination Chinese patent medicine (Tong Xie Yao Fang [TXYF], a generic prescription for presumed spleen qi deficiency and liver-spleen disharmony) used for 16 weeks. Symptoms improved significantly during treatment but returned after the medicine was stopped. Individualized herbal therapies demonstrated sustained improvement, however, even 14 weeks after the individualized herbal medicines were stopped. Thus, individualized traditional Chinese medicine treatment is recommended. An additional study of TXYF in 120 patients with IBS showed decreased mast cell activation, but the trial was not placebo controlled.[68]

Padma Lax

Padma Lax is a complex Tibetan herbal formula for constipation; it contains aloe extract, calumba root, cascara bark, frangula bark, rhubarb root (all known laxatives), and other herbs and minerals with antispasmodic and antidiarrheal effects. Several studies have demonstrated the effectiveness of this treatment in constipation-predominant IBS.[69]

Dosage

For IBS with constipation, the dose of Padma Lax is two capsules/day for 3 months; then decrease dosage to one capsule daily if loose stool is noted.

STW 5

STW 5 is a mixture of aqueous ethanolic plant extracts from *Iberis amara* (Clown's mustard), chamomile flower, caraway fruit, peppermint leaves, greater celandine, licorice root, lemon balm leaves, angelica root, and milk thistle fruit. In a 2001 randomized multicenter study of 208 patients with IBS, STW 5 reduced total abdominal symptoms by approximately 54%, compared with 27% for placebo, at 4 weeks.[70]

Dosage

A common brand name of this product is Iberogast. It can be mixed with water in the following dosage:

Adults and children older than 12 years of age: 20 drops, three times/day

Mind-Body Therapy

Mind-body therapy, in the form of relaxation therapy, biofeedback, hypnosis, counseling, or stress management training, has been shown to reduce symptom frequency and severity and to enhance the results of standard medical treatment of IBS. Most of these therapies focus on correcting maladaptive coping skills that engender emotional stress, which then manifests as GI symptoms.

Stress Management

Lifestyle changes that incorporate stress reduction and stress management strategies, along with progressive muscle relaxation, have proved to be more effective than medical therapy[71] (see Chapter 93, Relaxation Techniques).

Hypnosis

Trials conducted in the United Kingdom found that weekly hypnosis sessions, in combination with self-hypnosis techniques for 12 weeks, improved the symptoms of abdominal pain, bloating, and disturbed defecation, as well as anxiety scores, but did not alter rectal tone or pain threshold.[72] Specific gut-directed hypnotherapy programs are now available (see Chapter 92, Self-Hypnosis Techniques).

Psychotherapy and Cognitive-Behavioral Therapy

Cognitive-behavioral therapy (CBT) combines cognitive therapy and behavioral therapy. Behavioral therapy helps a person weaken the connections between troublesome situations and habitual reactions to them. Cognitive therapy teaches how certain thinking patterns are causing symptoms. When combined into CBT, these therapies provide powerful tools for eliminating symptoms. CBT has been shown to improve symptoms significantly in patients who had moderate to severe IBS in comparison with education alone.[73] A Cochrane Review confirmed the positive data noted earlier but indicated that more research is needed to draw a conclusion about the effectiveness of hypnotherapy for IBS.[74] Additionally, the review of psychological treatments for IBS

stated that most of the studies have been suboptimal, so physicians should choose individualized therapies.[75]

> Persons with irritable bowel syndrome symptoms often have a combination of mental and emotional stressors and alterations in the psychoneuroimmunologic axis. Ensuring a proper gut milieu, along with stress management strategies, is necessary for optimal gut function.

Acupuncture

In 2006, the Cochrane Review analyzed six RCTs using acupuncture in IBS. No evidence supported the use of acupuncture in treating IBS.[76] A more recent study was performed by Lembo et al[77] that demonstrated a benefit of both real and sham acupuncture. The nonspecific placebo effects of acupuncture seemed to be therapeutically effective.[77]

Placebo Effects

The high placebo response rates noted in RCT research in the treatment of IBS have been well documented. Kaptchuk et al[78] developed a unique study to evaluate the benefit of openly offering a placebo treatment, which was found to be efficacious.

Pharmaceuticals

Oral Cromolyn

Several studies compared oral cromolyn with placebo in randomized double-blind crossover trials; in one study, an 8-week treatment resulted in significant symptom reduction and a long carryover effect in the group initially treated with cromolyn.[79] Two large unblinded studies compared oral cromolyn with elimination diet. The largest trial involved 409 patients with well-defined IBS who were monitored for 4 months.[80] Symptom improvement was noted in 60% of patients treated with elimination diet and in 67% of those receiving cromolyn.

Dosage

The recommended dose is 200 to 400 mg (one to two gel caps) four times/day, before meals and 30 minutes before bedtime.

Antibiotics

The "shotgun" use of antibiotic treatments leads to significant alterations in the GI microflora that can be deleterious in the long term.[81] Rifaximin (a nonabsorbable antibiotic) has been demonstrated to improve IBS symptoms significantly.[82] Rifaximin has also been shown to be useful in treatment of small intestinal bacterial overgrowth, a source of bacterial fermentation, gas, and bloating. Small intestinal bacterial overgrowth can be diagnosed with a lactulose or glucose breath test.

Dosage

The recommended dose of rifaximin is 550 mg three times/day for 14 days in patients with small intestinal bacterial overgrowth.

Precautions

Rifaximin is not absorbed systemically, so most of the side effects are related to GI function, including flatulence, abdominal pain, and stool urgency.

Antidepressants

A meta-analysis reported that tricyclic antidepressants significantly lessened abdominal pain and diarrhea in patients who had diarrhea-predominant IBS.[83] Patients who can tolerate these medications are likely to have symptomatic benefit, but many patients experience unacceptable side effects. Although the neuroendocrine role of serotonin in the GI tract is understood, no support exists for selective serotonin reuptake inhibitor treatment of IBS at this time.[84] A Cochrane Review from 2005 found no evidence to suggest that antidepressants are effective for the treatment of IBS.[85]

Therapies to Consider

Betaine Hydrochloride

A basic evaluation of digestion and absorption is often excluded from the initial evaluation of GI function in patients with IBS. Factors that affect digestion of food include mastication, hypochlorhydria, and pancreatic insufficiency. Mastication is a simple clinical point to make with patients and is often overlooked. Pancreatic insufficiency and the benefit of digestive enzyme supplementation have already been discussed. Data indicate that stomach acid declines with age, even as proton pump inhibitor prescriptions are increasing. Decreased pH limits the activation of peptidases and other critical enzymes necessary for digestion and absorption. Betaine hydrochloride can be used as a supplement to support the reactivation of proper digestion.

Dosage

The dose is 325 to 650 mg before a protein-containing meal.

Homeopathy

In classic homeopathy, an extensive historical interview is performed that seeks to identify the totality of the patient on physical, emotional, and mental levels. To this picture the practitioner matches a remedy that best suits the individual patient. This remedy is administered in small and infrequent doses, and follow-up is performed to determine whether the chosen remedy should be repeated, changed, or allowed to continue its work.

Osteopathic Medicine

A common view is that osteopathy and other related manual therapies are used only for musculoskeletal problems. However, recognition of a somatovisceral pathway amenable to manipulation has led to use of these approaches for relief of symptoms in people with IBS. The somatic areas commonly affected include the following: external oblique muscles (especially the lower portion), internal oblique muscles, and rectus abdominis muscle; lower segments of the thoracic spine (T10 to T12); iliocostalis thoracis and lumborum and longissimus thoracis and lumborum muscles; and quadratus lumborum muscles. Persons with this somatovisceral connection are often not aware of these tender points until they are discovered by careful palpation. This indirect technique seeks to release the strained somatic segments through initiation of a reciprocal counterstrain of the antagonist muscles (see Chapter 106, Strain/Counterstrain).

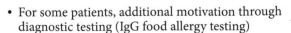

THERAPEUTIC REVIEW

An initial diagnostic evaluation is necessary to target effective therapies for irritable bowel syndrome (IBS). For the patient with mild to moderate symptoms of no clear cause, this ladder approach is appropriate.

■ Mind-Body Therapy

- Cognitive-behavioral therapy
- Hypnotherapy

■ Nutrition

- Elimination/challenge diet (see Chapter 84, Food Intolerance and Elimination Diet)

- For some patients, additional motivation through diagnostic testing (IgG food allergy testing)

■ Probiotic Supplements

- 50 billion CFUs/day as 25 billion CFUs/day of *Bifidobacterium* and 25 billion CFUs/day of *Lactobacillus*; or *Bifidobacterium infantis* 36524 at 5 billion CFUs/day

- Soluble fiber (psyllium, guar gum): 15 g/day with meals

Botanicals

- Peppermint oil: one to two enteric-coated capsules 3 times/day between meals
- Traditional Chinese medicine herbs: Tong Xie Yao Fang
- Tibetan herbs/Padma Lax for IBS with constipation: two capsules/day for 3 months

- STW 5: 20 drops three times/day for 4 weeks

Pharmaceuticals

- Oral cromolyn: 200 mg (two capsules) four times/day before meals and before bedtime
- Antibiotic: rifaximin, 550 mg three times/day for 14 days, if evidence of small intestine bacterial overgrowth[86]
- Tricyclic antidepressants: lower doses to start, such as amitriptyline at 10 to 25 mg/day

KEY WEB RESOURCES

International Foundation for Functional Gastrointestinal Disorders: www.iffgd.org.	The aim of this nonprofit education and research organization is to inform, assist, and support people with functional GI disorders. The Web site offers patient information, as well as recent publications and current research on IBS.
Institute for Functional Medicine: www.fxmed.com.	This Web site offers educational opportunities to help health care practitioners develop personalized approaches to understand and find the root cause (i.e., the core clinical imbalances) for various chronic diseases, including IBS.
American Board of Integrative Holistic Medicine: www.holistic-board.org.	This Web site offers digital education tools, online learning modules and educational conferences on integrative (the what) holistic (the how) medicine. In addition, the organization has defined the new standard of care through its Board Certification in Integrative Holistic Medicine process.

References

References are available online at expertconsult.com.

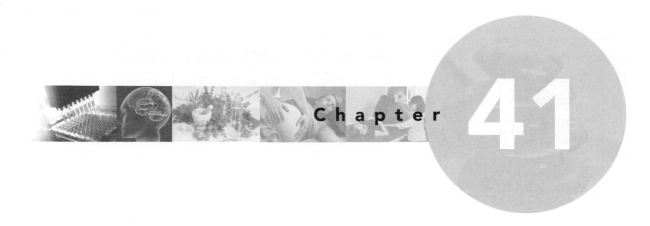

41

Gastroesophageal Reflux Disease

David Kiefer, MD

Gastroesophageal reflux disease (GERD) occurs when there is abnormal passage of acidic stomach contents, or refluxate, into the esophagus, causing symptoms or complications. It is one of the primary causes of the informal name and symptom "heartburn," and GERD is a common phenomenon. Estimates are that 15% to 20% of people in the United States have heartburn or regurgitation at least once a week, and 7% of people suffer from those symptoms daily.[1-3]

Symptoms of GERD may include any or all of the following: retrosternal burning, acid regurgitation, nausea, vomiting, chest pain, laryngitis, cough, and dysphagia.[3] The injury to the esophagus can include esophagitis, stricture, the development of columnar metaplasia (Barrett esophagus), and adenocarcinoma.[2] A poor correlation exists between the severity of symptoms and the pathophysiologic findings in the esophagus.[2] For example, GERD is not the only phenomenon in the differential diagnosis of heartburn. Many people with GERD do not have endoscopic evidence of esophagitis, and up to 40% of people with Barrett esophagus in one study did not report heartburn.[2] The confusing nature of this condition makes it a challenge to develop concrete screening recommendations for advanced disease.

People may turn to complementary and alternative medicine to help with their gastrointestinal symptoms. The 2002 National Health Interview Survey, based on 31,044 interviews in the United States, documented that 3.7% of people used complementary and alternative medicine for stomach or intestinal illnesses.[4]

Pathophysiology

Symptoms of GERD result from the interplay of many factors, including the amount of time the esophagus is exposed to refluxate, the degree of refluxate causticity, and the susceptibility of the esophagus to damage.[5] Three main mechanisms or factors prevent refluxate from entering the esophagus: the lower esophageal sphincter (LES), the crural diaphragm (which acts as an external esophageal sphincter), and the location of the gastroesophageal junction below the diaphragmatic hiatus.[1] Dysfunction or malalignment in any or all of these structures could lead to symptoms of GERD, although the major pathologic mechanism is some abnormality in tone of the LES.

The LES normally exists in a contracted state, but it relaxes during the swallow mechanism to let material into the stomach (Fig. 41-1). The LES also relaxes to vent swallowed air and allow retrograde expulsion of material from the stomach.[5] For approximately an hour after meals, people may normally have up to five transient episodes of reflux, but if these episodes continue, symptoms of GERD may develop.[5]

Decreased tone of the LES occurs with many substances, medications, and other factors (Table 41-1).[1] Certain beverages may exacerbate symptoms of GERD, some by affecting LES tone. For example, coffee, including instant coffee, decaffeinated, and ground coffee, decreases LES initially and, in some people with sustained decreased tone, for up to 90 minutes after ingestion. Caffeinated coffee seems to cause more gastric acid production,[6] and it decreases LES tone more at lower pH.[7] Another study found an association between pH and titratable acidity and the frequency with which some beverages, such as juices, sodas, coffee, and tea, caused heartburn symptoms in 394 people with GERD.[8] Caffeine itself has some ability to decrease LES tone.[9]

Symptoms of GERD may result from other factors. For example, increased intra-abdominal and gastric pressure, such as from obesity, ascites, pregnancy, or even tight clothes, may lead to GERD.[1,10] In addition, GERD may occur when the gastric contents are located near the gastroesophageal junction, such as in the recumbent position, while bending

FIGURE 41-1

Normal swallow mechanism. A continuous tracing of esophageal motility showing two swallows, as indicated by the pharyngeal contraction associated with relaxation of the upper esophageal sphincter (UES) and followed by peristalsis in the body of the esophagus. The lower esophageal sphincter (LES) also displays transient relaxation (*arrow*) unassociated with a swallow. An episode of gastroesophageal reflux (*asterisk*) is recorded by a pH probe at the time of the transient LES relaxation. (From Behrman RE, Kliegman RM, Jenson HB, eds. *Nelson Textbook of Pediatrics.* 17th ed. Philadelphia: Saunders; 2004.)

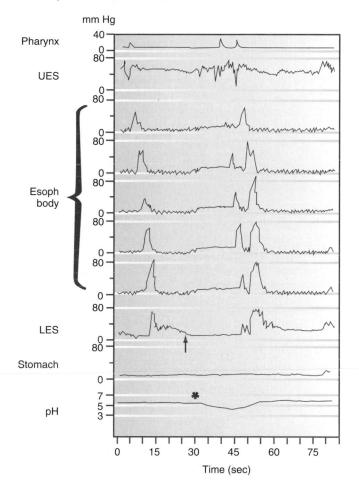

TABLE 41-1. Factors Associated With Decreased Tone of the Lower Esophageal Sphincter

FACTOR	EXAMPLES
Dietary supplements	Arginine may cause lower esophageal sphincter relaxations through the nitric oxide system Carminative herbs such as peppermint (*Mentha piperita*), spearmint (*Mentha spicata*), and other mint family (Lamiaceae) plants Essential oils (high doses)
Foods and beverages	Alcohol Chocolate (probably through the methylxanthines) Coffee (caffeinated more than decaffeinated) Cow's milk Fat Orange juice Spicy foods Tea Tomato juice
Lifestyle	Smoking
Medications	Aminophylline Anticholinergics Beta-adrenergic agents Calcium channel blockers Nitrates Phosphodiesterase inhibitors, including sildenafil
Physiologic, by stomach dilatation	Acid hypersecretion After meals Gastric stasis Pyloric obstruction
Trauma, irritation, and miscellaneous factors	Esophagitis Scleroderma-like diseases Surgical damage

Data from references 1, 16, 17, and 27.

over, or in patients with a hiatal hernia.[1] Furthermore, any conditions that decrease the production of saliva may predispose to GERD because of the neutralizing effect of saliva on acid.[1]

People report that stress exacerbates GERD, a finding that has borne out in clinical trials. For example, stress was shown to increase GERD symptom reports, without necessarily being correlated with objective physiologic changes such as increased esophageal acid exposure or duration of acid exposure.[11,12] This phenomenon occurs especially in people with high levels of anxiety.[12]

Diagnostic testing can be used to determine the cause of a patient's symptoms and any pathophysiologic correlates. For example, barium swallow, upper endoscopy, ambulatory pH, and a trial of proton pump inhibitor (PPI) medications are the most commonly used diagnostic tests.[13] Ambulatory pH testing, estimated to have a sensitivity of 79% to 96% and a specificity of 85% to 100% for GERD, may also be used with impedance testing to explore the correlation of symptoms with refluxate volume regardless of acidity (weakly acidic or nonacid reflux).[2,13] One approach is to consider diagnostic testing (upper endoscopy, ambulatory pH, or impedance testing) if a patient is unresponsive to PPI therapy.[13]

Special Considerations for Pediatrics

In children, GERD is the most common esophageal disease.[5] In infants, symptoms often peak at 4 months of age and resolve by 12 to 24 months, whereas in children, the clinical course may wax and wane, resolving in about half the cases.[5] Infants may present with postprandial regurgitation, irritability, arching, choking, gagging, feeding aversion, failure to thrive, obstructive apnea, or stridor; signs and symptoms in older children are abdominal pain, chest pain, asthma, laryngitis, and sinusitis.[5] Studies in infants with suspected GERD have found both a high incidence of allergy to cow's milk protein[14] and symptomatic improvement when infants with intractable symptoms were changed to a diet free of cow's milk protein.[15]

Cow's milk protein is a common cause of gastroesophageal reflux disease in infants, and a trial of elimination should be considered.

Integrative Therapy

Lifestyle

In mild cases of GERD, lifestyle modifications are the first line of therapy and can lead to improvement or elimination of symptoms. For example, GERD symptoms may improve if smokers quit and if obese patients lose weight.[1,16] Patients should avoid the foods and supplements and, if possible, the medications mentioned in Table 41-1 because of their relaxing effect on the LES. In addition, patients should avoid eating large meals or consuming large quantities of fluids with meals.[1]

If nighttime symptoms are present, patients should elevate the head of the bed 4 to 6 inches, by using blocks under the bed posts rather than extra pillows. Use of extra pillows could compress the abdomen and increase intra-abdominal pressure, thereby exacerbating symptoms.[1,2,16]

Demulcent Botanicals

Several types of botanical treatments are useful for GERD (Table 41-2). Demulcent, or mucilaginous, botanical medicines can be used as mucoprotection of the esophageal mucosa, both to soothe irritated tissues and promote healing.[16,17]

Licorice (Glycyrrhiza glabra)

Licorice is a well-known demulcent botanical used for GERD, gastritis, and duodenal and peptic ulcers. For long-term use, it should be prescribed as deglycyrrhizinated licorice, to prevent the side effects of one of its phytochemicals, glycyrrhizin (see later).

■ Dosage

Two to four 380-mg tablets of deglycyrrhizinated licorice should be taken before meals.[18]

The prolonged use of decoctions or infusions of dried, unprocessed licorice root can cause hypertension, hypokalemia, and edema because of the mineralocorticoid action of a saponin glycyrrhizin, also called glycyrrhizic acid.[19]

Slippery Elm (Ulmus fulva) Root Bark Powder

Slippery elm root bark powder is one demulcent botanical that can be used for symptomatic relief and promotion of healing of irritated esophageal or gastric mucosa. Most health food stores, integrative pharmacies, and herbal dispensaries with botanical products for sale in bulk will have slippery elm.

■ Dosage

One to two tablespoons of the powder should be mixed with a glass of water and taken after meals and before bed. The proportions should be carefully titrated because the preparation can be very thick and difficult for some people to tolerate. To increase palatability, this supplement can be sweetened slightly with honey or sugar.

■ Precautions

This botanical is described by most sources as very safe, although the hydrocolloid fibers may bind simultaneously administered medications and decrease their absorption.[19]

TABLE 41-2. Botanical Medicines Useful in Gastroesophageal Reflux Disease

COMMON NAME	SCIENTIFIC NAME (FAMILY)	MECHANISM OF ACTION	DOSE	ADVERSE EFFECTS
Chamomile	*Matricaria recutita* (Asteraceae)	Antiinflammatory, antispasmodic	1–3 g of an infusion of the flowers three to four times daily	Occasional allergic reactions in people allergic to plants in the daisy family (Asteraceae)
Licorice	*Glycyrrhiza glabra* (Fabaceae)	Mucoprotective	Two to four 380-mg DGL tablets before meals	Mineralocorticoid side effects avoided when DGL form is used
Marshmallow	*Althea officinalis* (Malvaceae)	Mucoprotective	5–6 g of tea daily, in divided doses	Decreased drug absorption
Skullcap	*Scutellaria lateriflora* (Lamiaceae)	Antianxiety	1–2 g of the herb as infusion three times daily, 1–2 mL tincture three times daily	Confusion, stupor, and twitching with high doses
Slippery elm	*Ulmus fulva, Ulmus rubra* (Ulmaceae)	Mucoprotective	1–2 tablespoons per glass of water, three to four times daily	Decreased drug absorption
Valerian	*Valeriana officinalis* (Valerianaceae)	Antianxiety	1–2 g root infusion two to three times daily, or 150-mg capsule two to three times daily	Possibly increased effects of alcohol, barbiturates, benzodiazepines

DGL, deglycyrrhizinated licorice.

Marshmallow (Althea officinalis)

Marshmallow is another mucilaginous herb for GERD symptomatic relief. Its demulcent properties also make it useful for pharyngitis, wound healing, cough, and bronchitis.

■ Dosage

It is usually taken at 5 to 6 g daily, in divided doses, as an infusion of the leaves or root.[18]

■ Precautions

As with slippery elm, a decrease in absorption of orally administered drugs taken simultaneously with marshmallow may occur.[19]

Antiinflammatory Botanicals

Antiinflammatory herbs are often used for GERD symptom relief and to improve healing of the irritated esophageal mucosa.[17] Examples are meadowsweet *(Filipendula ulmaria)*, which also reduces acidity, chickweed *(Stellaria media)*, and chamomile *(Matricaria recutita)*.

Chamomile (Matricaria recutita)

Chamomile is well known for its mild sedative actions and for its antispasmodic effects on the gastrointestinal tract. In GERD, it is used as a nondemulcent antiinflammatory agent.[16,17]

■ Dosage

Chamomile is most commonly prepared as a hot water infusion (tea) of 1 to 3 g of the flowers, steeped in a cup covered with a saucer, taken three to four times daily.[18]

■ Precautions

Chamomile is generally well tolerated, although individuals allergic to other plants in the daisy family (Asteraceae) may experience an exacerbation of their allergic symptoms with consumption of chamomile.

Antianxiety Botanicals

Many herbal experts recommend botanicals as part of an overall approach to anxiety management, given the connection between anxiety and GERD. Examples are valerian *(Valeriana officinalis)* and skullcap *(Scutellaria lateriflora)*[17] (see Chapter 5, Anxiety).

Pharmaceuticals

Both histamine-2 (H_2) receptor antagonists or blockers (H2Bs) and PPIs are commonly used for the symptoms of GERD. A meta-analysis showed that both H2Bs and PPIs are effective in GERD symptomatic improvement, but PPIs are significantly more effective than H2Bs.[20] PPIs are also used in a 1-week therapeutic trial to test and diagnose GERD empirically.[1] The optimal dosing time for PPIs is 30 minutes before a meal, although adherence to the ideal dosing regimen may or may not lead to better symptom control.[21] Some clinicians use H2Bs or PPIs indefinitely as necessary to control symptoms.[2]

> Aggressive, long-term acid suppression can decrease the absorption of vitamin B_{12}.[1] Consider regular intramuscular injections of vitamin B_{12} for those individuals requiring long-term treatment with histamine-2 receptor blockers or proton pump inhibitors. Use of these drugs can also lead to iron malabsorption, increased risk of hip fracture, and community-acquired pneumonia.

In one study, between 10% and 40% of people who took PPIs for GERD failed to respond symptomatically, partially or completely, whereas another study found that 85% of people taking PPIs had persistent GERD symptoms even though 73% of those patients were still satisfied with the treatment.[21] Some debate exists about the reasons that certain patients may not respond to PPIs. Investigators have theorized that these patients may actually have functional or nonerosive reflux disease, or they may have weakly acidic or alkaline refluxate.[21]

Some nuances with the prescribing of the two primary classes of pharmaceuticals for GERD, PPIs and H2Bs, are noted in Table 41-3. Box 41-1 describes the protocol for tapering PPIs.

Biomechanical Therapy

Some naturopathic physicians recommend hernial reduction adjustments, an abdominal manipulation technique, when GERD symptoms are complicated by the presence of a hiatal hernia.[16] Although no clinical trials have examined this treatment, referral to an experienced practitioner could be considered for patients with a documented hiatal hernia and symptoms of GERD. Aside from surgery, no documented allopathic interventions exist for the treatment of hiatal hernia.

Mind-Body Therapy

Relaxation training can improve symptoms of GERD, by addressing the issue that stress exacerbates GERD symptoms, especially in people suffering from chronic anxiety.[21]

Other Therapies to Consider

Homeopathy

Homeopathy can be a therapeutic consideration. Many of the symptoms associated with GERD, such as indigestion and heartburn, or even associated disorders such as hiatal hernia, are mentioned in homeopathy sources and treated with a wide variety of short-term remedies, such as phosphorus, nux vomica, pulsatilla, carbo vegetabilis, arsenicum, bryonia,

TABLE 41-3. Proton Pump Inhibitors versus Histamine-2 Receptor Blockers for Gastroesophageal Reflux Disease

PPIs	H2Bs
Greater rate of healing from esophagitis than H2Bs	Greater rate of healing from esophagitis than placebo
Slight benefit in healing esophagitis with twice the standard dose	
Unclear whether PPIs heal heartburn, as a symptom, more than H2Bs	Both PPIs and H2Bs heal heartburn more than placebo
Complete resolution of heartburn in approximately 40% of people (compared with 15% for placebo)	

Data from Kahrilas PJ. Gastroesophageal reflux disease. *N Engl J Med.* 2008;359:1700–1707.
H2Bs, histamine-2 receptor blockers; PPIs, proton pump inhibitors.

BOX 41-1. Helping Taper off a Proton Pump Inhibitor

For those patients who have made positive lifestyle changes and may not need continued chronic acid suppression, it can often be difficult to discontinue proton pump inhibitors (PPIs) because they often cause rebound hyperacidity even if the underlying condition has resolved.[1]

Plan:

1. Slowly taper off the PPI over 2 to 4 weeks (the higher the dose, the longer the taper).
2. While the taper is being completed, use the following for bridge therapy to reduce the symptoms of rebound hyperacidity:

   Encourage regular aerobic exercise.

   Encourage a relaxation technique such as self-hypnosis for gastrointestinal disorders (see Chapter 92, Self-hypnosis Techniques) or meditation (see Chapter 98, Recommending Meditation).

   Suggest acupuncture one to two times per week.[2]

   Add one or more of the following:

   Deglycyrrhizinated licorice, two to four 380-mg tablets before meals or Sucralfate (Carafate) 1 g before meals.

   Slippery elm, 1 to 2 tablespoons of powdered root in water three to four times per day

   A combination botanical product, Iberogast (Clown's mustard, German chamomile, angelica root, caraway, milk thistle, lemon balm, calendine, licorice root and peppermint leaf), 1 mL three times per day[3]

3. If the taper is successful, slowly taper the foregoing supplements (except for positive nutritional changes, exercise, and stress management). If symptoms return, start with one of the foregoing or a histamine-2 receptor blocker. If symptoms are still difficult to control, consider adding back the PPI.
4. Ideally, it is beneficial to avoid long-term acid suppression if possible because this can be associated with malabsorption of vitamin B$_{12}$ and iron,[4] increased risk of community-acquired pneumonia,[5] hip[8,9] and spine[10,11] fracture, and *Clostridium difficile* diarrhea.[12]

---

china, anacardium, argentum, sepia, lycopodium, graphites, and kali bichromium[22] (see Chapter 111, Therapeutic Homeopathy).

Traditional Chinese Medicine

Traditional Chinese medicine, which provides a complete assessment based on a unique cultural, diagnostic, and therapeutic approach, may offer relief for people suffering from GERD. In a study comparing acupuncture with doubling the dose of a PPI for GERD, acupuncture was found to be more effective in reducing symptoms.[23] With treatment suggestions incorporating diet, lifestyle, botanical medicines, and acupuncture or acupressure,[24] traditional Chinese medicine should be considered a therapeutic option, based either solely on a patient's personal preference or on the need for adjuncts to incomplete or ineffective allopathic therapeutics.

Surgery

Surgical treatment is considered by many experts to be an option for people in whom lifestyle modification or adequate medical therapy fails or who are unwilling to take long-term medication.[1,3,25] The most common surgical procedure is the Nissen fundoplication, either open or laparoscopic, whereby the fundus of the stomach is wrapped wholly (total fundoplication) or partially (partial fundoplication) around the lower esophagus to create an area of high pressure meant to prevent refluxate from entering the esophagus and causing symptoms. Laparoscopic fundoplication provides long-term disease control similar to that seen with the open approach but with fewer incisional hernias.[25] One review examined health-related quality of life and GERD symptoms after 1 year in 4 studies involving 1232 people who underwent medical management versus laparoscopic surgical management.[3] Overall, the surgical approach seemed to improve symptoms of GERD more effectively than did medical management, although in some cases dysphagia (8% to 12% postoperatively),[25] costs after 1 year, and adverse effects were more pronounced in the surgical group. One review and meta-analysis found that the partial laparoscopic fundoplication was associated with less postoperative dysphagia than was total fundoplication.[25]

Special Considerations in Pediatrics

The treatment of GERD in infants usually involves dietary interventions such as the normalization of feeding techniques, volumes, and frequency, if these are abnormal.[5] Formula can be thickened with a tablespoon of rice cereal per ounce, to decrease the number of regurgitation events, increase calorie density, and reduce the number of crying times.[5] One meta-analysis supported the concept that thickened feedings improves GERD symptoms in infants.[26] A short trial of a hypoallergenic diet, in particular to exclude milk and soy, can be helpful in children suspected of having allergies to those foods. Older children with GERD are advised to avoid tomatoes, chocolate, mint, and classically offending beverages (juices, sodas, caffeinated beverages) and to lose weight, if applicable.

With respect to positioning during meals, infant GERD is worse when infants are seated, supine, or on their side and better when they are prone or carried upright. Because of the risk of sudden infant death syndrome, a prone position cannot be recommended for sleep.[5] Older children may have some relief from GERD when they lie on their left side or with the head of the bed elevated. As with adults, children experience some symptomatic improvement with H2Bs and PPIs; the dose of PPIs is higher per kilogram than for adults (0.7 to 1.5 mg/kg/day).[5]

PREVENTION PRESCRIPTION

- Avoid foods and supplements, and, when possible, medications known to decrease lower esophageal sphincter tone (see Table 41-1).
- Maintain ideal body weight.
- Reduce stress as much as possible, through lifestyle change and stress management and mind-body techniques.
- Avoid large meals and consuming large quantities of liquids with meals.

THERAPEUTIC REVIEW

This summary of possible therapies is for patients with mild to moderate, short-term GERD. Patients with long-standing, more severe GERD should undergo an appropriate diagnostic workup, which may include a referral to a gastroenterologic specialist and upper endoscopy to rule out esophagitis, ulcers, Barrett esophagus, or adenocarcinoma.

▨ Removal of Exacerbating Factors

- Avoid foods, supplements, and, when possible, medications known to decrease lower esophageal sphincter tone (see Table 41-1).
- If applicable, quit smoking.
- If applicable, lose weight.

▨ Lifestyle

- For nocturnal symptoms, elevate the head of the bed 4 to 6 inches.
- Avoid large meals and consuming large quantities of liquids with meals.

▨ Mind-Body Medicine

- Practice stress management and relaxation techniques.

▨ Botanical Medicines

- Deglycyrrhizinated licorice: two to four 380-mg tablets before meals
- Slippery elm: 1 to 2 tablespoons of powdered root in a glass of water, three to four times daily
- Other botanical medicines that have potential benefit include chamomile, marshmallow, skullcap, and valerian (see Table 41-2).

▨ Pharmaceuticals

- Start with a proton pump inhibitor, both for symptomatic relief and for diagnostic purposes.
- Histamine-2 receptor antagonists
- Over-the-counter antacids, such as calcium carbonate, aluminum hydroxide, and magnesium hydroxide, can be helpful.

▨ Surgery

- For people with intractable symptoms, fundoplication should be considered.

KEY WEB RESOURCES

American College of Gastroenterology clinical updates: www.acg.gi.org/physicians/clinicalupdates.asp.

This collection of allopathic, evidence-based reviews covers numerous topics relevant to GERD, including diagnosis, management, reflux testing, and surveillance of Barrett esophagus.

References

References are available online at expertconsult.com.

Chapter 42

Peptic Ulcer Disease

Joseph Eichenseher, MD, MAT

Pathophysiology

Peptic ulcer disease (PUD) is caused by disturbances of the gastrointestinal (GI) mucosa secondary to loss of protective elements or to damaging insults, resulting in mucosal erosions, most commonly located in the duodenum or stomach. People with PUD most often complain of epigastric pain (especially a few hours after meals), bloating, nausea, early satiety, altered bowel habits, and heartburn. Pain is often improved with food or antacids. PUD can also occur without symptoms, especially in older adults. Peptic ulcers can cause GI bleeding, which is potentially a life-threatening emergency necessitating urgent endoscopy and intensive care unit consideration. Rarely, ulcers can also perforate, leading to intense pain and acute peritonitis, which is a surgical emergency. Patients with significant weight loss and PUD symptoms also deserve endoscopy to investigate for potential malignant diseases.

Loss of mucosal integrity is usually multifactorial, with diminished protective elements (mainly decreased acid buffering, reduced immune system functioning, and slowed wound healing) and increased insults (primarily *Helicobacter pylori* infection, nonsteroidal antiinflammatory drugs [NSAIDs], increased acidity, and inflammation). Treatment efforts are focused on restoring these protective factors and reducing harmful affronts.

> Nonsteroidal antiinflammatory drugs should be avoided in patients with a history of peptic ulcer disease (PUD) and also minimized in people with PUD symptoms who lack a formal ulcer diagnosis.

Approximately half a million people in the United States are newly diagnosed with PUD each year.[1] Peptic ulcers can occur at any time in life, although the incidence gradually increases with age.[2] In the early twentieth century, PUD was diagnosed in men at twice the rate as in women, yet it is now nearly equally distributed by gender; gastric ulcers tend to be more common in women, and duodenal ulcers occur more often in men.[3]

Historically, investigators knew that smoking, stress, NSAIDs, and family history (risk increases three times with an afflicted first-degree relative)[4] contributed to peptic ulcer formation. Before the late 1970s, however, allopathic medicine had limited success in addressing PUD until the arrival of two revolutionary developments: the invention of pharmaceuticals that reduced the amount of acid the stomach produced and the discovery of *H. pylori* (Figure 42-1).

The development of gastric acid–suppressing medications, with the advent of histamine-2 receptor antagonists (H₂ blockers) in the late 1970s and proton pump inhibitors (PPIs) in the late 1980s, heralded a new chapter in Western medicine's management of PUD. Previous efforts had focused on reducing risk factors, giving acid buffers (e.g., calcium carbonate) for symptom relief, and surgery (with significant morbidity and mortality). With the invention and administration of acid-reducing medications, most cases of PUD were quickly attenuated. This drastically reduced the need for surgery and dramatically increased the role of pharmaceuticals in PUD therapy.

H. pylori was identified in 1982 (a discovery for which Drs. J. Robin Warren and Barry J. Marshall won the Nobel Prize for medicine in 2005), and the more the medical world learned about this unique bacterium, the more it revolutionized how we thought about PUD. Having an *H. pylori* infection has been shown to increase the rate of PUD by at least four times.[5] Living in the harsh acidic environment of the human stomach, *H. pylori* seems to increase the risk of PUD by directly damaging the protective mucus lining of the GI tract and allowing for more acidic damage. *H. pylori* also triggers an immune response that causes damaging inflammation. Rates of *H. pylori* infection are stratified worldwide by age and economic status. Younger, more affluent people have rates as low as 20%, whereas up to 60% of all people in the developing world and 50% of people who are older than 60 years in the United States are colonized by the bacterium.[6] With an estimated 4 billion people infected worldwide, the goal of complete global eradication is likely logistically impractical, if not impossible, even though *H. pylori* only

FIGURE 42-1
Helicobacter pylori, the discovery of which revolutionized medical understanding and management of peptic ulcer disease. (Courtesy of Yutaka Tsutsumi, MD.)

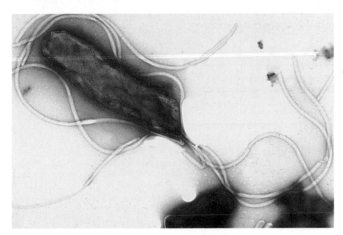

resides in humans. The drastic impact of *H. pylori* on PUD has triggered management strategies focused on eradication with antibiotics. However, only 10% to 20% of *H. pylori*–infected people ever develop PUD.[5]

Altogether, *H. pylori* and NSAIDs account for most peptic ulcers.[1] The remainder is attributed to other risk factors and a few "zebras," such as Zollinger-Ellison tumors, carcinoid syndrome, other drugs, radiation, cytomegalovirus, and systemic mastocytosis.

These two developments, pharmaceutical acid suppression and the discovery and subsequent antibiotic treatment of *H. pylori*, had PUD morbidity and mortality riding off into the sunset near the end of the twentieth century. Yet more recent discoveries (increasing resistance of *H. pylori* to antibiotics and further knowledge of the harms of long-term pharmaceutical acid suppression, mixed with more evidence of botanical anti-*H. pylori* approaches and growing patient preference for more alternative therapeutic options) promise an increasing need for more integrative PUD approaches in the years and decades ahead.

Diagnosis

The overlapping constellation of PUD symptoms with such diseases as gastritis, irritable bowel syndrome, gastroesophageal reflux disease, Crohn disease, pancreatitis, gallstones, and malignancies makes a first-time diagnosis of PUD challenging, especially because the best current standard diagnostic test is endoscopy (an invasive, costly procedure) and the next best tool for diagnosis is a barium GI series (with resulting radiation, cost, and potential inaccuracy). One study even showed that a physical examination finding of epigastric tenderness to palpation lessens the likelihood of PUD.[7] Thus, it is not surprising that many practitioners, as well as patients without signs of serious disease (bleeding or weight loss), hesitate to pursue these invasive diagnostic measures. The likely result is that most cases of PUD are never diagnosed with certainty. More frequent *H. pylori* testing increases the number of people diagnosed with *H. pylori* infection, but a positive test result indicates only bacterial

infection (and 80% to 90% of *H. pylori*–infected people will not develop ulcers).[5] Once a diagnosis of PUD is established, recurrence is reported in up to 74% of patients.[8] Much PUD management therefore focuses on prevention and symptomatic treatment, a good fit for an integrative approach (Fig. 42-2).

Integrative Therapy

Nutrition

Diet was linked to PUD long before the discovery of *H. pylori,* and with research demonstrating the anti–*H. pylori* properties of certain foods, nutrition is even more of a key component of ulcer prevention and symptom management.

Meal timing has a reported relation to PUD. Skipping breakfast is an established risk factor,[9] and consuming large meals shortly before bedtime can also increase the chance of PUD.[10]

Fruit and vegetable intake reduces the risk of developing ulcers, and epidemiologic studies demonstrated that a diet high in plant-based fiber and vitamin A (e.g., carrots, spinach, mango, sweet potatoes, apricots) helps protect against PUD.[11] Flavonoids, which are compounds found throughout the plant world, show anti–*H. pylori* properties and are present in concentrated amounts in citrus, berries, onions, parsley, green tea, red wine, and dark chocolate.[12] Sulforaphanes, which are phytochemicals found in vegetables such as Brussels sprouts, cabbage, cauliflower, bok choy, turnips, radishes, and in especially high concentrations in broccoli sprouts, also have anti–*H. pylori* properties.[13]

Foods containing capsaicin (chili) are shown to be protective against ulcers,[14] and chilies (fruit of the plant genus *capsicum*) are reviewed in the botanical section of this chapter for acute symptom relief. Other foods demonstrating anti–*H. pylori* properties include honey and garlic.[15]

> Foods found to be associated with a reduced risk of *Helicobacter pylori* infection include fruits and vegetables rich in carotenoids (yellow, orange), flavonoids (purple, blue, red wine, green tea), sulforaphanes (cruciferous veggies, including cabbage and broccoli), capsaicin (chili), and fermented foods rich in probiotics (yogurt, miso, aged cheese, and sauerkraut),

Milk increases PUD risk, likely because of increased stimulation of acid production.[16] Nonetheless, fermented dairy products and other food with probiotics, such as yogurt, aged cheeses, and sauerkraut, are shown to be protective against *H. pylori.*[17,18]

Coffee and caffeine, long thought to be risk factors for PUD, have so far eluded convincing data to that effect but are known risk factors for reflux disease.

Physical Activity

Multiple studies have demonstrated that regular physical activity, when compared with a more sedentary lifestyle, is protective against PUD.[19,20] One study specifically

FIGURE 42-2
Integrative management flow chart for peptic ulcer disease (PUD). Neg, negative; NSAIDs, nonsteroidal antiinflammatory drugs; Pos, positive; PPI, proton pump inhibitor.

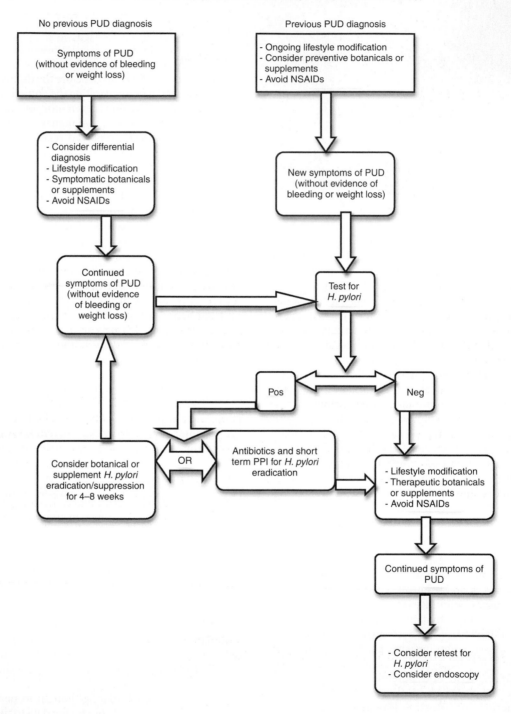

Integrative PUD management
(If evidence of bleeding or significant weight loss occurs at any time, pursue endoscopy)

Stress Reduction

demonstrated that the risk for duodenal ulcers was 62% less in men who cumulatively walked or ran more than 10 miles per week.[20] Routine exercise should be recommended for almost all patients, especially those with a previous history of PUD.

The relationship between stress and PUD is a classic example of why clinicians must keep in mind the social determinants of health (Fig. 42-3), over which our patients have varying degrees of control. Stress is largely a product of this social and environmental milieu, and convincing evidence

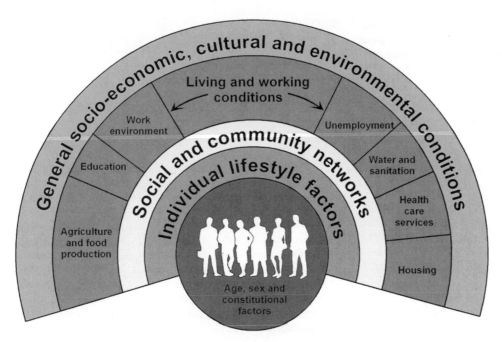

indicates that stress plays a role in PUD. This connection is established early in life. Childhood stress, in the form of traumatic events such as an illness of a family member, financial strain, or family conflict, causes nearly 50% higher rates of PUD in adulthood.[21] Studies have also shown that GI ulceration increases with both chronic stress and in times of acute stress, such as during an earthquake or war (e.g., during the bombing of London in World War II).[22,23] A multipronged approach to stress reduction, in comparison with any single method, appears to provide more protection against PUD.[24] As a clinician, recommending individually tailored stress reduction programs, including yoga, tai chi, and other coordinated movements, as well as meditation, focused breathing, and any other culturally applicable relaxation methods, will likely be beneficial (see Chapter 93, Relaxation Techniques, and Chapter 98, Recommending Meditation).

Sleep

Inadequate sleep is a risk factor for PUD.[9] This is probably the result of increased stress levels, which cause immune dysfunction and impaired lifestyle decisions. Maintaining good sleep hygiene is an important key to ulcer avoidance (see Chapter 8, Insomnia).

Tobacco Cessation

Smoking increases rates of PUD up to four times when compared with nonsmokers.[19] This added risk is likely because of decreased wound healing in smokers. Accordingly, smoking cessation is essential in addressing PUD.

Alcohol Avoidance or Moderation

Alcohol, in large amounts, has been shown to be a risk factor for ulcers, likely because of mucosal damage. One epidemiologic study showed that people who had more than 42 drinks per week had more than 4 times the rate of bleeding ulcers compared with people who had 1 drink per week or less.[25] However, red wine has anti–*H. pylori* properties in animal models, possibly because of bioactive compounds such as flavonoids.[26] Avoiding large quantities of ethanol, especially higher-percentage drinks, is prudent in patients with a history or symptoms of PUD, whereas moderate red wine consumption should not necessarily be discouraged.

Nonsteroidal Antiinflammatory Drugs

Evidence shows that NSAID use increases baseline risk of PUD by up to five times, and it also increases the risk of bleeding ulcers in patients with established PUD by five times.[27] NSAIDs inhibit prostaglandin production and thus decrease mucoprotective elements in the GI tract. Although evidence indicates that administration of medications such as sucralfate or misoprostol with NSAIDs can help ease ulcer symptoms and prevent ulcer recurrance,[28,29] NSAIDs should be avoided as much as possible in patients with PUD symptoms and an existing history of PUD disease. More than 80% of people taking NSAIDs never develop PUD,[30] and thus these drugs should not necessarily be avoided in patients who do not have PUD.

Supplements

Probiotics

These helpful microorganisms have proven versatile in the realm of PUD. They have been shown to reduce ulcer recurrence,[31] and people with higher intakes of probiotics have correspondingly lower rates of *H. pylori* infection.[17] Although no clinical trials currently exist with convincing evidence that probiotics eradicate *H. pylori* by themselves, probiotics can reduce the severity of infection.[32] Probiotics are likely effective in combating *H. pylori* as a result of increased GI mucus production, competition for mucosal binding sites, and production of anti–*H. pylori* compounds, and they were also shown in animal models to decrease the inflammatory response from *H. pylori*.[32] Most studies were conducted with *Lactobacillus* strains commonly found in yogurt, yet evidence indicates that other strains of probiotics are also helpful.[33] Thus, incorporating yogurt and other probiotic-containing foods, such as aged cheeses and sauerkraut, into a diet on a regular basis can be beneficial for PUD prevention and avoidance of ulcer recurrence. Probiotics, including both *Lactobacillus* and *Saccharomyces boulardii*, have also demonstrated synergy with antibiotic for *H. pylori* eradication and can decrease antibiotic side effects such as diarrhea[29,34,35] (see chapter 102, Prescribing Probiotics).

■ Dosage
During *H. pylori* eradication antibiotic therapy, the regimen is as follows: either *Lactobacillus (acidophilus* or GG) capsules, containing at least 1 billion organisms, twice daily, or *Saccharomyces boulardii*, 500 mg, twice daily.

■ Prevention
Probiotic-containing foods are recommended on a regular basis for people with a previous history of PUD, a family history of ulcer disease, or other risk factors for PUD.

■ Precautions
Patients sensitive or intolerant to lactose may have GI discomfort with dairy products containing probiotics.

Vitamin C
Ascorbic acid (vitamin C) has been shown to have potential for *H. pylori* eradication; one study demonstrated a 10% eradication rate with 2 weeks of 1000 mg daily.[36] Vitamin C also has additive effects on antibiotic regimens for *H. pylori* eradication.[37] This anti–*H. pylori* capability has been supported by in vitro studies.[38] A 5-year Japanese study demonstrated lower PUD rates in persons taking vitamin C supplementation.[39] A steady dietary intake of vitamin C is recommended for anyone with current symptoms, a previous history or a family history of PUD, or other risk factors for ulcer disease.

■ Dosage
For *H. pylori* eradication or suppression (in addition to daily dietary intake), the dose is 500 mg twice daily.

■ Prevention
Eat foods containing vitamin C on a regular basis, including citrus, kiwi, broccoli, strawberry, and cauliflower.

■ Precautions
Dose-related potential adverse effects include kidney stones, diarrhea, nausea, and gastritis. Use with caution in patients with kidney disease.

Zinc
A clinical trial showed zinc to accelerate the healing of gastric ulcers up to three times faster than seen with placebo.[40] This finding was also supported by more extensive animal studies.[41] Enhanced healing is likely the result of the fundamental role of zinc in repair of damaged tissue. A compound not available in the United States, zinc acexamate, has been used in East Asia and Europe for PUD and has been found effective in numerous studies.[42]

■ Dosage
For gastric ulcer treatment, the dose is 40 mg daily for 4 weeks.

■ Precautions
Potential effects include nausea, vomiting, diarrhea, and altered taste. Zinc inhibits the absorption of other minerals, particularly copper.

Polyunsaturated Fatty Acids
Multiple polyunsaturated fatty acids (PUFAs) have been shown to have anti–*H. pylori* effects in vitro (including alpha-linolenic acid, eicosapentaenoic acid [EPA], gamma-linolenic acid [GLA], and linoleic acid).[43] A clinical study administering 2 g a day of a 1:1 mixture of fish oil (EPA and docosahexaenoic acid) and black currant seed oil (GLA), for 8 weeks, cleared *H. pylori* in more than 50% of patients.[44] Although elimination rates are significantly lower for PUFAs when compared with antibiotics, PUFAs are reasonable to recommend for patients desiring *H. pylori* eradication without antibiotics.

■ Dosage
For *H. pylori* suppression or elimination, 1 g of fish oil and 1 g of GLA-containing oil (evening primrose, black currant seed, borage, or hemp seed oils) are taken daily for 8 weeks.

■ Precautions
PUFAs may cause GI upset. Higher doses of omega-3 fatty acids (more than 3 g/day) may increase the risk of bleeding from anticoagulant effects.

Glutamine
In clinical trials, glutamine has been shown to prevent and cure PUD. A study of patients with burn injury demonstrated that glutamine can help prevent stress ulcers.[45] Another trial showed more rapid healing of peptic ulcers in patients given 400 mg of glutamine four times a day.[46] This limited clinical research has also been supported by animal studies.[47,48] Glutamine supplementation is likely successful because it is a necessary amino acid for the repair and new growth of cells lining the GI tract. Dietary sources of glutamine include beef, chicken, fish, eggs, wheat, cabbage, beets, beans, spinach, and parsley.

■ Dosage
For PUD treatment, the dose is 400 mg of glutamine powder in water four times daily.

■ Precautions
No significant adverse effects have been reported.

Botanicals

Turmeric (Curcuma longa)
Turmeric has been used for centuries in Chinese and Ayurvedic medicine for treatment of dyspepsia and epigastric pain. One clinical trial administered 600 mg of turmeric root five times daily to people with PUD and demonstrated 48% ulcer resolution at 4 weeks and 76% at 12 weeks.[49] The same study also showed that turmeric markedly improved symptoms of dyspepsia in 1 to 2 weeks.[44] Turmeric and

curcumin, a commercially available turmeric derivative, are known to have anti–*H. pylori* properties in vitro.[50,51] One clinical trial failed to show turmeric's ability to eradicate *H. pylori* completely, yet it demonstrated relief of dyspeptic symptoms.[52] Turmeric has been found to have H_2 blocking properties, which likely also explains much of its healing potential.[53]

Dosage

For PUD treatment and for symptoms of PUD, the dose of whole turmeric root or powder (capsules) is 600 mg five times daily for 12 weeks.

Precautions

Turmeric potentially can cause nausea, diarrhea, heartburn, or kidney stones. Some evidence exists that it may increase the risk of bleeding secondary to antiplatelet activity.

Mastic (Pistacia lentiscus)

Mastic is a member of the pistachio tree family found throughout the Mediterranean, and its resin has been harvested for more than 2000 years as a spice, for chewing gum, and for medicinal purposes. A double-blind placebo-controlled trial of 350-mg capsules, taken three times a day for 3 weeks, demonstrated clinically significant improvement of dyspepsia.[54] Mastic is known to have anti–*H. pylori* properties in vivo and in vitro.[55] A separate double-blind trial showed that mastic significantly improved duodenal ulcer healing when compared with placebo.[56]

Dosage

For dyspepsia, the dose is 350-mg capsules three times a day for 3 weeks. For duodenal ulcer healing, the dose is 500-mg capsules twice daily for 2 weeks.

Precautions

Avoid in people with pistachio allergies. Use with caution in patients taking angiotensin-converting enzyme inhibitors because it may cause hypotension.

Cabbage (Brassica oleracea)

Clinical studies in the 1950s demonstrated the effectiveness of cabbage juice for gastric and duodenal ulcer healing. Participants drank 1 L of fresh cabbage juice over the course of a day for 10 days.[57,58] Because this research was completed more than 50 years ago, and in light of subsequently improved diagnostic studies and further understanding of PUD, new studies in the years ahead are warranted. Because of its safety profile and accessibility, however, cabbage still deserves recommendation for PUD treatment. Cabbage has been shown to be a rich source of glutamine and sulforaphanes, likely accounting for much of its healing power.

Dosage

For PUD, the dose is 1 L of fresh juice (pasteurized juice was found ineffective) divided over the course of a day for 10 days.

Precautions

Because of its vitamin K content, cabbage can potentially decrease the anticoagulant efficacy of warfarin.

Deglycyrrhizinated Licorice (Glycyrrhiza glabra)

Licorice has been used for medicinal purposes, including epigastric pain and dyspepsia, since ancient Egyptian times and for at least 4000 years in China.[59] Deglycyrrhizinated licorice (DGL) does not include the adrenocorticoid effect of glycyrrhiza (sodium retention leading to hypertension) and is less hepatotoxic than the native plant. A small clinical trial demonstrated DGL to be as effective as H_2 blockers for duodenal ulcer resolution at 12 weeks, with fewer episodes of relapse.[60] Licorice derivatives also have anti–*H. pylori* properties in vitro.[61] This effect is possibly explained by the bioactive flavonoids found in licorice. Many good-quality studies have compared licorice, in combination preparations with other botanicals, with placebo in the treatment of PUD. Determining the efficacy of a single ingredient or estimating their synergistic properties is impossible, however, because all these combination products have three or more ingredients. More placebo-controlled individual studies are warranted.

Dosage

For PUD, the dose is 380 mg three times per day for 12 weeks.

Precautions

Use with caution in patients with liver disease, renal insufficiency, and hypokalemia. Avoid in pregnancy because of a theoretical risk of preterm labor.

Chili (Capsaicin)

Capsaicin is the active component of chili peppers (the fruits of plants of the genus *Capsicum*). Historically, chilies were thought to exacerbate PUD, but more recent research is proving the opposite. Epidemiologic studies have shown that people with higher dietary intakes of capsaicin have correspondingly lower rates of PUD.[14,62] A double-blind trial, in which patients took 2.5 mg of chili pepper in capsules daily for 5 weeks, demonstrated that chili was effective for epigastric pain and other symptoms of functional dyspepsia.[63] Animal models also showed capsaicin, by decreasing gastric acidity, to be protective against ulcer formation.[64]

Dosage

For epigastric pain and functional dyspepsia, the dose is 2.5 mg daily of chili pepper capsules (can divide doses) for 5 weeks. For PUD prevention, patients should follow a diet rich in capsaicin, as tolerated.

Precautions

Avoid in people with pepper allergies. Use with caution in patients with diabetes (may cause hypoglycemia) and heart disease (may increase blood pressure). Chilies may cause GI upset. Skin contact may cause irritation.

Cranberry (Vaccinium oxycoccos)

A double-blind clinical trial in *H. pylori*–positive patients demonstrated the ability of cranberry to suppress and eradicate *H. pylori* in patients who drank 500 mL of cranberry juice for 90 days. Although the study demonstrated only a 14% eradication rate, that rate was many times higher than results seen with placebo.[65] In vitro studies of human gastric cells showed cranberry's ability to impair *H. pylori* adhesion to gastric cell walls, similar to its ability to prevent *Escherichia coli* from binding to the bladder wall in the prevention of urinary tract infections.[66]

■ Dosage
For *H. pylori* suppression or eradication, the dose is 500 mL of cranberry juice daily for 90 days.

■ Precautions
Patients with diabetes should consider sugar-free juice. High doses may cause stomach distress. Cranberry may affect warfarin efficacy.

Neem (Azadirachta indica)
In Ayurvedic medicine, the neem tree has been used for thousands of years for multiple purposes, including for epistaxis, parasites, asthma, diabetes, fever, and epigastric pain. This versatility has earned neem the nickname "the village pharmacy."[67] Clinical studies demonstrated that 30 mg of neem bark extract, taken for 10 days, reduced gastric acid secretion by 77% while additionally causing significant duodenal ulcer healing when taken for 10 weeks.[68] Animal studies also demonstrated the antiulcer properties of neem,[69] and they elucidated that neem inhibits the proton pump, similar to pharmacologic PPIs.[70]

■ Dosage
For duodenal ulcers, the dose is 30 mg bark extract twice daily for 10 weeks.

■ Precautions
Use cautiously in patients with liver disease. Avoid use in pregnant women (because of abortifacient properties). Avoid in infants and children because of potential toxicities.

Additional Botanicals
Some other botanicals demonstrate in vitro anti–*H. pylori* properties. The list keeps growing, and more clinical trials are needed. These botanicals include the following: broccoli sprouts (*Brassica oleracea*),[13] peppermint (*Mentha piperita*),[71] silver wormwood (*Artemisia ludoviciana*),[71] garlic (*Allium sativum*),[72] yarrow (*Achillea millefolium*),[73] chamomile (*Matricaria recutita*),[73] ginkgo (*Ginkgo biloba*),[73] nutmeg (*Myristica fragrans*),[73] ginger (*Zingiber officinale*),[73] hops (*Humulus lupulus*),[74] goldenseal (*Hydrastis canadensis*),[75] sage (*Salvia officinalis*),[75] green tea (*Camellia sinensis*),[76] and red ginseng (*Panax ginseng*).[76]

Additional mucoprotective therapies, which are traditionally used and have animal model evidence but lack sufficient clinical trials, include the following: pectin,[77] aloe (*Aloe vera*),[12] fenugreek (*Trigonella foenum-graecum*),[78] banana powder (*Musa paradisiaca*),[79] and mugwort (*Artemisia douglasiana*)[80].

Pharmaceuticals

Antibiotics
Overwhelming evidence indicates that *H. pylori* eradication with antibiotics, in patients with PUD, dramatically improves symptom resolution and reduces ulcer recurrence.[81] Recommended eradication regimens usually include two to three antibiotics and a PPI and historically demonstrated up to an 80% to 90% eradication rate.[82] Years after antibiotic treatment of *H. pylori* began, however, the bacterium has proven tenacious and has developed more and more resistance to standard regimens. With traditional three-drug therapies, most studies now show less than 80%

eradication rate, with some less than 50%.[82] Specifically, metronidazole and clarithromycin have demonstrated marked resistance, thus necessitating newer and potentially more toxic antibiotics.[83] Because of the significant geographic differences in resistance patterns, prescribers should be aware of local susceptibilities before patients are administered one of the numerous anti–*H. pylori* antibiotic regimens.[84] In light of this trend of increasing resistance, it is becoming more practical to look to other methods of *H. pylori* eradication or suppression, such as the integrative therapies discussed in this chapter.

■ Dosage
A typical *H. pylori* eradication regimen is as follows: amoxicillin, 1 g; clarithromycin, 500 mg; and omeprazole, 20 mg; this combination is taken twice per day for 14 days. (Probiotics are also recommended as adjuvant therapy.) Check regional susceptibilities when choosing antibiotics.

■ Precautions
Common side effects of antibiotics used include diarrhea, altered taste, headache, and allergic reactions.

Acid-Suppressing Drugs
Since their introduction in the late 1970s, gastric acid suppression medications, in the form of H_2 blockers and later PPIs, have dramatically assisted in the relief of PUD symptoms and ulcer healing. PPIs have been shown to be more effective than H_2 blockers and are used more frequently today.[85] Accumulating evidence, however, shows that chronic acid suppression (longer than 2 to 3 months) has potential adverse effects, including increased rates of pneumonia, *Clostridium difficile* infections, and bone fractures; these drugs also decrease absorption of certain minerals and nutrients, specifically calcium, vitamin B_{12}, iron, and magnesium.[86-88] Animal models also demonstrated an increased gastric cancer rate with extended periods of gastric acid suppression.[87]

■ Dosage
For PUD and PUD symptoms, the regimen is as follows: PPI (e.g., omeprazole, 20 mg) or H_2 blocker (e.g., ranitidine, 150 mg) once or twice daily, per individual drug, for up to 8 weeks.

■ Precautions
Potential adverse effects of H_2-blockers include nausea, headache, dry mouth, rash, and confusion. PPIs can cause headache and nausea. Extended use may cause the adverse effects discussed earlier.

> Long-term pharmaceutical acid suppression (especially with proton pump inhibitors) is increasingly associated with adverse effects, such as infections and decreased nutrient absorption, and should be limited to 8 weeks or less.

Antacids
Likely millions of years ago, our ancestors figured out that eating chalk or other natural acid buffers relieved epigastric pain and symptoms of PUD. Antacids are still potentially useful today in helping with symptom relief, and they are found in various nonprescription forms, including calcium

carbonate, aluminum hydroxide, magnesium hydroxide, and sodium bicarbonate. Theoretically, antacids cause increased gastric acid production as a result of rebound, and although some studies support this hypothesis, the research demonstrates antacids to be safe in recommended doses.[89]

Dosage
For PUD symptoms, patients may take over-the-counter antacids according to individual product instructions.

Precautions
High doses of calcium-containing antacids may cause kidney stones, constipation, renal failure, alkalosis, or hypercalcemia. Carbonate-containing antacids may cause alkalosis. Aluminum antacids, in high doses, may cause hypophosphatemia, osteomalacia, constipation, and renal insufficiency. Magnesium antacids should be used in caution in people with renal disease, and they may cause hypermagnesemia.

Sucralfate
An older synthetic compound, sucralfate, has been shown effective in promoting ulcer healing and has been used since the late 1960s as a PUD treatment. It has an impressively complex chemical formula of $C_{12}H_{54}Al_{16}O_{75}S_8$, yet most of its beneficial effects are attributed to two properties: its ability to act as an acid buffer and its ability to bind to ulcer sites, thus protecting them from further insult. In clinical trials, sucralfate has been shown to be as effective as H_2 blockers for treatment of duodenal ulcers.[90]

Dosage
For duodenal ulcers, the dose is 1 g four times daily, 1 hour before meals and bedtime, for up to 8 weeks.

Precautions
Sucralfate can cause bezoar formation and constipation.

Acupuncture

Controlled trials have shown that acupuncture is an effective treatment for epigastric pain.[91] Case studies and animal models have also shown acupuncture to be specifically useful for PUD and prevention of ulcer recurrences, yet more clinical trials are needed.[92]

Therapies to Consider
Traditional Chinese Medical Massage
In a limited study, 74.5% of patients with PUD who received 20 sessions (every other day) of traditional Chinese medical massage demonstrated complete ulcer resolution.[93] This trial was not randomized, however, and more rigorous investigations are warranted.

Osteopathy
Although adequate clinical trials are lacking, osteopathy has potential in PUD for symptom relief and prevention. Manual medicine, in theory, can help the GI system to maintain sympathetic and parasympathetic balance, thus reducing excess acid production and restoring homeostasis. Osteopathy can also lead to relief of symptoms by manipulating somatovisceral pathways, and it is worth considering in patients with access to clinicians experienced in these techniques.

PREVENTION PRESCRIPTION

- Eat a diet rich in fruits and vegetables (especially those containing vitamins A and C).
- Eat foods containing capsaicin (chili), as well as those with flavonoids and sulforaphanes.
- Eat probiotics: yogurt, sauerkraut, active yeasts, and aged cheeses.
- Avoid nonprobiotic dairy products such as milk.
- Eat breakfast every day, and avoid eating large meals shortly before sleeping.
- Minimize use of nonsteroidal antiinflammatory drugs.
- Avoid smoking cigarettes.
- Avoid excessive alcohol consumption.
- Maintain a moderate exercise routine.
- Obtain adequate sleep.
- Develop and incorporate stress reduction activities.

THERAPEUTIC REVIEW

The following integrative therapeutic options are useful for different niches on the peptic ulcer disease (PUD) spectrum, from prevention, symptom relief, and *H. pylori* elimination to active ulcer healing. Being mindful of the individual end goals of therapy will guide clinical choices. Evidence of a bleeding ulcer or significant weight loss is a reason to refer patients for endoscopy and can constitute a medical emergency.

Lifestyle
- Tobacco cessation
- Adequate sleep
- Routine exercise
- Stress reduction interventions
- Abstention from heavy ethanol intake

Nutrition
- Eat breakfast daily.
- Avoid eating shortly before sleeping.
- Avoid milk.
- Eat probiotic-containing foods, such as yogurt, aged cheeses, miso, and sauerkraut.
- Eat foods containing chili (capsaicin).
- Eat fruits and vegetables, especially those with vitamins A and C.

Continued

■ Supplements

- Probiotics during *H. pylori* antibiotic therapy: either *Lactobacillus (acidophilus* or GG) capsules, containing at least 1 billion organisms, twice daily, or *Saccharomyces boulardii,* 500 mg, twice daily A↑₁

- Vitamin C for *H. pylori* suppression: 500 mg twice daily B→₂

- Zinc for gastric ulcers: 40 mg daily for 4 weeks B→₂

- Polyunsaturated fatty acids for *H. pylori* eradication: 1 g of fish oil and 1 gram of gamma-linolenic acid–containing oil (evening primrose, black currant seed, borage, or hemp seed oils) taken daily for 8 weeks B↗₁

- Glutamine for peptic ulcers: 400 mg four times daily B↗₁

■ Botanicals

- Turmeric for peptic ulcers and PUD symptoms: whole root or root powder (capsules), 600 mg five times daily for 12 weeks B→₂

- Mastic for dyspepsia: 350-mg capsules three times a day for 3 weeks B↗₁

- Mastic for duodenal ulcers: 500-mg capsules twice daily for 2 weeks B↗₁

- Cabbage for duodenal or gastric ulcers: 1 L of fresh juice divided over the course of a day for 10 days B↗₁

- Deglycyrrhizinated licorice for duodenal ulcers: 380 mg three times per day for 12 weeks B→₂

- Chili (*Capsicum* fruit) for epigastric pain and dyspepsia: 2.5 mg daily of chili pepper capsules for 5 weeks B→₂

- Cranberry for *H. pylori* eradication: 500 mL of cranberry juice daily for 90 days B↗₁

- Neem for duodenal ulcers: 30 mg bark extract twice daily for 10 weeks B→₂

■ Pharmaceuticals

- Eliminate nonsteroidal antiinflammatory drugs for patients with PUD A↑₁

- Antibiotics and proton pump inhibitors (PPIs) for *H. pylori* eradication: amoxicillin, 1 g; clarithromycin, 500 mg; and omeprazole, 20 mg; combination to be taken twice daily for 14 days (check regional bacterial susceptibilities) A↗₂

- Acid suppression therapy for PUD and PUD symptoms: PPI (e.g., omeprazole) or histamine-2 (H₂) receptor blocker (e.g., ranitidine) once or twice daily, per individual drug, for up to 8 weeks A↗₂

- Antacids for PUD symptoms: over-the-counter antacids, per individual product instructions B→₂

- Sucralfate for duodenal ulcers: 1 g four times daily for up to 8 weeks A↗₂

■ Acupuncture

- Acupuncture for epigastric pain B↗₁

■ Therapies to Consider

- Traditional Chinese medical massage for peptic ulcers C→₁

- Osteopathy for PUD C→₁

KEY WEB RESOURCES

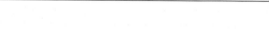

http://digestive.niddk.nih.gov/ddiseases/pubs/hpylori/index.aspx	National Digestive Diseases Information Clearinghouse updated allopathic information on PUD
www.umm.edu/altmed/articles/peptic-ulcer-000125.htm	University of Maryland Medical Center integrative info on PUD for patients
http://www.nobelprize.org/nobel_prizes/medicine/laureates/2005/ warren-slides.pdf	2005 Nobel Prize for Medicine winner, Dr. J. Robin Warren's, slideshow on the discovery of H. pylori

References

References are available online at expertconsult.com.

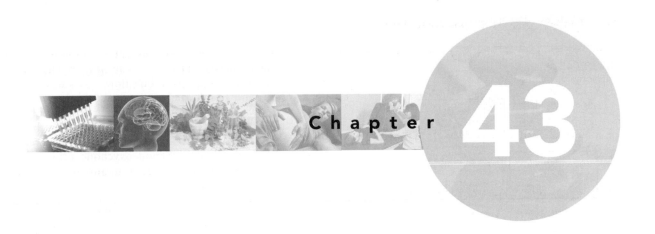

Chapter 43

Cholelithiasis

Ann C. Figurski, DO

Pathophysiology

According to the third National Health and Nutrition Examination Survey, more than 20 million people in the United States have gallbladder disease.[1] The occurrence of gallstones varies greatly, ranging from 2% to 70% among different populations. The highest incidence is among Pima Indian women older than 30 years of age.[2]

Bile aids in the digestion and absorption of lipids from the intestines. Made by the liver, bile is composed of bile acids, cholesterol, and phospholipids, and it is stored in the gallbladder until stimulation by cholecystokinin causes its release. Conditions that lead to gallstone formation include supersaturation of bile with cholesterol, decreased bile acids that dissolve cholesterol, excess mucus production, and gallbladder dysmotility and stasis (Fig. 43-1). Gallstones are classified as either cholesterol or pigment. In industrialized countries, cholesterol stones account for up to 85%. Most people with gallstones remain asymptomatic. Approximately 20% will develop true biliary symptoms, such as severe pain in the right upper quadrant that can radiate to the back or shoulder, and 1% to 2% will develop a complication that requires surgery.[2]

Epidemiologic research has revealed many risk factors for gallstones. Some of these conditions are not modifiable: sex, age, and ethnicity. Many conditions can be changed, however, such as obesity, physical inactivity, medications, nutrition, and stress.[2,3] Table 43-1 provides a list of conditions that increase risk.

Integrative Therapy

Lifestyle

Gallstones can be added to a long list of diseases heavily influenced by lifestyle. The profound rise in chronic conditions, such as diabetes, hypertension, and heart disease, has caused Western medicine to reevaluate its treatments and enhance prevention methods. The causes of these conditions are multifactorial, but a lifestyle of inadequate physical activity and the standard U.S. diet are major culprits. These chronic conditions are not isolated; they have similar causes, related to a proinflammatory state of imbalance. Gallstones can be grouped with these other diseases such as diabetes and heart disease, because evidence shows that lifestyle factors such as diet (macronutrient and micronutrient intake) and exercise are also linked to gallbladder disease.

Maintenance of a Healthy Weight

Obesity, especially abdominal, is a well-known risk factor for gallstones. It is associated with increased cholesterol secretion into bile.[2] Gradual weight loss is important for obese individuals because rapid weight loss may also promote gallstone formation secondary to increased biliary cholesterol and bile stasis from gallbladder hypomobility. Weight loss should not exceed 1.5 kg (3.3 lb) per week to avoid this risk.[4]

Exercise

Physical activity is a necessary component of a healthy lifestyle and has a significant impact on many diseases. Studies have also shown that exercise can increase gallbladder motility.[5] In postmenopausal women, physical activity is inversely related to the development of gallstone disease.[6] In one report, women who sat for more than 60 hours a week were 2.32 times more likely to have a cholecystecomy.[7] Fortunately, even modest amounts of physical activity have a positive effect; an observational study of more than 2000 people found that just 2 hours of activity a week reduced the risk by 40%.[8]

Stress Reduction

Even without having randomized placebo-controlled trials to prove it, stress is likely a factor in most diseases. Evidence indicates that stress causes gallbladder dysfunction and bile stasis in animal studies.[3] The general benefits of stress reduction on both mind and body may extend to the gallbladder, too; after all, it is all connected. Consider recommending counseling, meditation, or other stress reduction techniques as appropriate.

FIGURE 43-1
Pathophysiology of gallstones.

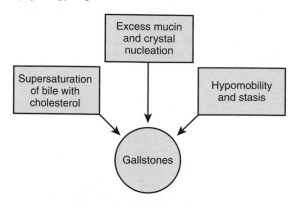

TABLE 43-1. Conditions That May Increase the Risk of Gallbladder Disease	
Increased cholesterol saturation	Estrogen (endogenous: pregnancy; or supplemented: hormone replacement therapy, oral contraceptives) Obesity High-cholesterol diet
Decreased bile salts (or increased ratio of secondary bile acids)	Low-fiber diet Ileal inflammation (Crohn disease) Cirrhosis Cystic fibrosis Fibrates Age
Stasis of bile flow	Parenteral nutrition Low-fat, weight loss diets Hypertriglyceridemia (impaired motility) Physical inactivity Ceftriaxone (biliary sludge)[2] Octreotide[2] Stress[3] Iron deficiency anemia[51]

Nutrition

Several areas of nutrition overlap in gallbladder disease. For example, vegetarians have a lower rate of cholelithiasis.[9] The reason could be related to higher consumption of fruits and vegetables, which are good sources of vitamins, minerals, fiber, and antioxidants, all of which have been linked to inhibition of gallstone formation. In a study looking at diet differences, patients with gallstones consumed less fish, fruit, fiber, folate, magnesium, calcium, and vitamin C; they also ate more cereal, sugar, calories, and saturated fat.[10] Specific components of diet are separated for research, but of course the sum is likely greater than the individual parts. Encouraging healthy, well-balanced nutrition (e.g., the Mediterranean diet) full of colorful vegetables and including healthy fats may be a good place to start.

Fats

The type of fats consumed is important in gallbladder disease. The diet should be low in saturated fats, but it should have sufficient sources of polyunsaturated fats and omega-3 fatty acids. Animal studies showed that monounsaturated and polyunsaturated fats act as inhibitors of cholesterol cholelithiasis.[11] Fish oil can decrease biliary cholesterol saturation and enhance bile flow.[12] A study comparing fish oil with fibrate therapy in men with hypertriglyceridemia showed that both approaches lowered triglyceride levels, but only the fish oil increased bile acid synthesis. The same research also demonstrated that fish oil increased the ratio of cholic acid to chenodeoxycholic acid, which improves cholesterol solubility.[13] Proinflammatory, arachidonic acid–rich saturated fats can increase cholesterol saturation and disrupt the gallbladder epithelium.[14] Another study revealed that men with the highest consumption of long-chain saturated fatty acids (which includes arachidonic acid) had a 40% increased risk of cholecystectomy.[15] The goal is to replace this fat with the antiinflammatory effects of healthy fats, such as omega-3 fatty acids (see Chapter 86, The Antiinflammatory Diet).

Fiber

A higher intake of fiber is associated with a lower prevalence of gallstones. Fiber reduces the absorption of deoxycholic acid by decreasing its formation by intestinal bacteria. Deoxycholic acid is a secondary bile acid, and it increases the lithogenicity of bile.[16] Water-soluble fiber found in fruits, vegetables, pectin, oat bran, and guar gum can bind this acid and may be helpful in preventing and treating gallstones.[14] A prospective study of 77,000 women demonstrated that those consuming the most fruits and vegetables reduced their risk of gallstones by 21%.[17]

A good source of fiber is to mix 1 teaspoon of ground flaxseed (lignan) into 8 oz of apple juice or applesauce (pectin) and consume daily. This recipe has the added benefit of being a good source of omega-3 fatty acids.[14]

Legumes are a good source of fiber, yet their role in gallbladder disease is uncertain. They have been shown to increase biliary cholesterol saturation and decrease phospholipids, which can lead to gallbladder disease.[16] However, a case-control study found a negative association with legume intake and gallbladder disease, but the population studied had a relatively small legume intake.[18] The risk that legumes may cause gallstone disease should be weighed against their other known health advantages when considering recommendations.

Nuts

In the Nurses' Health Study, a large prospective study, women who consumed nuts frequently had a more than 20% reduced risk of cholecystectomy. This relationship persisted after controlling for multiple confounding variables, including fat intake.[19] Other research showed similar results in men. Men who frequently ate nuts had a reduced risk of gallstone disease. This inverse relationship existed independently of consumption of peanuts, other nuts, or a combination of both.[20]

Simple Sugars

Refined sugars increase the cholesterol saturation of bile and reduce the ratio of beneficial cholic acid to deoxycholic acid.[21] Although consumption of refined sugars is also a factor in obesity, evidence indicates that simple sugars (monosaccharides and disaccharides) promote gallstone formation independent of obesity.[15] A relationship also appears to exist between glucose intolerance and gallstones.

Hyperinsulinemia may cause supersaturation of cholesterol in bile and gallbladder dysmotility. The prevalence of cholesterol gallstones is higher in diabetic patients; even in women without diabetes, fasting serum insulin levels are positively associated with gallstones.[22] Sugar intake is positively related to triglycerides and inversely related to high-density lipoproteins, and this effect on lipoprotein metabolism may contribute to gallstone formation.[23] Additionally, diets with high glycemic load have been linked to increased rates of cholecystectomy in women[24] (see Chapter 31, Insulin Resistance and the Metabolic Syndrome, and Chapter 85, The Glycemic Index/Load).

> Foods associated with a reduced risk of gallstones include fiber-rich fruits and vegetables, whole grains, nuts, coffee, and moderate alcohol.

Coffee

Often, people with gastrointestinal symptoms are told to avoid coffee. Interesting research has demonstrated that coffee can play a role in preventing gallstones, however, and numerous epidemiologic studies support this finding.[2] Coffee and its components have been shown to stimulate cholecystokinin release, enhance gallbladder contractility, and decrease cholesterol crystallization in bile.[25] A large prospective study demonstrated a 40% lower risk of cholecystectomy in men who drank 2 to 3 cups of coffee a day over a 10-year period.[26] Other prospective research found that intake of caffeinated coffee was associated with a significantly reduced risk of cholecystectomy in women. This is not the case for other caffeinated beverages; in fact, a positive association was noted with caffeinated soft drinks.[22] Some studies have not demonstrated this link,[27,28] but many have, and so it is reasonable to continue coffee according to a patient's preference.

Food Allergy

Interest is growing in food allergies and the effects they may have on health and wellness. A small amount of research from as early as the 1940s noted that food allergy is a cause of gallbladder disease.[16] In an uncontrolled study of 69 patients with gallstones or postcholecystectomy syndrome, 100% of these patients reported symptom resolution after 1 week of starting an elimination diet. The foods that most commonly evoked symptoms were eggs, pork, onions, fowl, milk, coffee, citrus, corn, beans, and nuts.[29] Thus, the clinician should keep in mind, when giving dietary advice to patients with gallstones, that it may not be as simple as saying "avoid fatty foods." An elimination diet may be a good option for those patients with biliary colic who want to avoid surgery (see Chapter 84, Food Intolerance and Elimination Diet).

Water

Drinking 6 to 8 cups of clean water a day will ensure the water content of the bile and help prevent crystal agglomeration.[14]

Alcohol

Epidemiologic evidence shows that gallstones are among a handful of diseases that are less common in people who consume a moderate amount of alcohol.[1,30] A large prospective study found that moderate alcohol intake was associated with a decreased risk of cholecystectomy in women.[31] Health benefits are associated with regular consumption of small amounts of alcohol, rather than heavy sporadic drinking. The many hazards and potential health consequences of alcohol consumption must also be considered. Any recommendation for moderate alcohol intake must be evaluated carefully for each person.

Supplements

Vitamin C

Ascorbic acid is involved in the conversion of cholesterol to bile acids, and vitamin C deficiency has been associated with gallstones in numerous studies.[32,33] Vitamin C supplementation, at a dose of 500 mg four times a day for 2 weeks, was shown to prolong the time needed for cholesterol crystal formation significantly.[34] In an observational study of more than 2000 people, the prevalence of gallstones was half of what it was in study participants who did not supplement.[8] Good sources of vitamin C include red pepper, kiwi, broccoli, strawberries, and citrus.

▪ Dosage
The dose is 200 mg twice daily.

▪ Precautions
Gastrointestinal disturbance may occur, including diarrhea, nausea, vomiting, heartburn, and abdominal cramps. Other side effects include fatigue, flushing, headache, hyperoxaluria, and predisposition to urinary tract stones.[13]

Magnesium

People who consume sufficient magnesium have lower rates of gallstones.[10] Additionally, magnesium deficiency is a common mineral deficiency in people consuming the standard American diet, also a risk factor for gallstones. A diet rich in magnesium may be a factor in preventing gallstones. Magnesium is found in green leafy vegetables, nuts, and whole grains. A study showed that men consuming high amounts of magnesium through diet and supplements (average, 454 mg/day) were 28% less likely to have gallstone disease compared with men consuming low amounts (average, 262 mg/day).[35]

▪ Dosage
The dose is 300 mg daily.

▪ Precautions
Gastrointestinal discomfort such as diarrhea, nausea, and abdominal cramping may occur. Magnesium should be used with caution in patients with renal failure. Toxic levels cause muscle relaxation and loss of deep tendon reflexes.

Vitamin E

Animal studies showed that a cholesterol-free diet deficient in vitamin E can lead to cholesterol gallstones.[36] Moreover, when animals were given a high-fat diet along with vitamin E, they did not develop gallstones.[37] Therefore, supplementation with vitamin E may possibly help to prevent gallstones.

▪ Dosage
Vitamin E (mixed tocopherols): 400 units/day.

■ Precautions

Side effects are rare but include nausea, diarrhea, intestinal cramps, fatigue, weakness, headache blurred vision, rash, and creatinuria. Long-term use may increase cardiovascular risk in persons younger than 65 years old.

Calcium

Calcium preferentially binds secondary bile acids, such as deoxycholic and chenodeoxycholic acid, in the small intestine. These bile acids reduce the solubility of cholesterol, so once it is bound and excreted, the risk of gallstones is reduced. In a study that monitored the dietary intake of 860 men, calcium intake was inversely associated with gallstone disease.[23]

■ Dosage

Calcium gluconate or citrate: 1000 to 1500 mg/day with meals. Calcium citrate is better absorbed in older adults, but it costs more.

■ Precautions

Calcium can cause constipation and gastrointestinal irritation. It should not be taken with iron supplements because it decreases absorption of iron.

Lecithin

Phospholipids, such as lecithin, increase the solubility of biliary cholesterol, and one study suggested that they are just as important as bile acids in this process.[36] Supplementation of lecithin is associated with an increase in biliary phospholipids and a decrease in cholesterol. Studies also showed that supplementing causes higher concentrations in bile.[38] No strong evidence indicates that lecithin is effective in treating gallstones, but it may aid in prevention.

■ Dosage

Lecithin 500 to 1000 mg/day.

■ Precautions

Diarrhea, nausea, and abdominal pain or fullness may occur.

Olive Oil or Gallbladder "Flush"

The gallbladder flush (or liver flush) is a common remedy that is said to cause gallstone passage. Several versions of the treatment exist, including combinations of olive oil, lemon juice, and apple juice. Proponents of this treatment claim that it causes the passage of gallstones. However, when what is thought to be gallstones are chemically analyzed, they turn out to be saponified complexes of olive oil, minerals, and lemon juice.[39] Possibly, the monounsaturated fat in olive oil could stimulate the gallbladder to expel stones, but these stones could then become lodged in the common bile duct. Ideally, this approach would be avoided until ultrasound evaluation reveals the size and number of stones.

Botanicals: Choleretic Herbs

Herbal medicine has been used to treat gallbladder disease and is a good option for patients with small stones and mild symptoms. Choleretic herbs can stimulate bile production, flow, and solubility.[14,39] Their effects can be enhanced by combining them with terpenes (e.g., peppermint oil, discussed later) that can help with gallstone dissolution.

Milk Thistle (Silybum marianum)

The following list of choloretic herbs may be used individually, or an herbologist may mix a combination together in a tea. They can be combined with peppermint oil for synergistic effect.

■ Dosage

Standardized 70% silymarin extract, starting at 150 mg twice daily and increasing to three times daily if needed

■ Precautions

Milk thistle may have a laxative effect. It should be used with caution in patients allergic to plants in the Asteraceae/Compositae family (ragweed, daisies, marigolds).

Dandelion (Taraxacum officinalis)

The following list of choloretic herbs may be used individually, or an herbologist may mix a combination together in a tea. They can be combined with peppermint oil for synergistic effect.

■ Dosage

Give 4 to 10 g of dried leaf or 2 to 8 g of dried root, three times/day. Tea is made by steeping the same amount in 150 mL of boiling water for 10 to 15 minutes and then straining. One cup of tea should be consumed three times/day. The most convenient dosing is a 1:5 tincture, 5 to 10 mL three times/day.

■ Precautions

Dandelion can cause gastric hyperacidity. If used topically, it may cause contact dermatitis. Patients who are allergic to plants in Asteraceae/Compositae family (ragweed, daisies, marigolds) should be cautious. Dandelion also can have hypoglycemic effects.

Globe Artichoke (Cynara scolymus)

■ Dosage

The dose is 1 to 4 g of the leaf, stem, or root three times/day. Do not confuse this plant with Jerusalem artichoke.

■ Precautions

If used topically, may cause contact dermatitis. Again, caution in those allergic to Asteraceae/Compositae family (ragweed, daisies, marigold).

Turmeric (Curcuma longa)

An animal study demonstrated that mice fed a lithogenic diet had the incidence of gallstones reduced by 73% when these animals were supplemented with curcumin. Curcumin also reduces biliary cholesterol concentration.[40]

■ Dosage

The dose is 450 mg of curcumin capsule standardized extract or 3 g turmeric root daily in divided doses.

■ Precautions

Turmeric has blood thinning effects, so patients should be careful if they are taking other blood thinning medications. Turmeric should be used with caution in patients allergic to yellow food colorings or plants belonging to the Zingiberaceae (ginger) family.

Botanicals: Gallstone-Dissolving Herbs

Monoterpenes are a class of hydrocarbon molecules found in the essential oils of many plants. These compounds have choleretic properties and inhibit formation of cholesterol crystals.[16] A combination of monoterpenes, mainly consisting of menthol and pinene, is effective for stone dissolution.[41] A double-blind study concluded that the addition of menthol to ursodeoxycholic acid (UDCA) improved outcomes compared with UDCA alone, and that menthol was equally effective as the monoterpene combination.[42]

Peppermint Oil (Mentha Piperita)
Dosage
One or two enteric-coated capsules (0.2 mL/capsule) three times/day between meals

Precautions
Peppermint oil relaxes the lower esophageal sphincter, and this may lead to reflux or heartburn. (Enteric-coated capsules are used to avoid this effect.) It may also cause allergic reactions, flushing, and headache.

Pharmaceuticals

Treatment with bile acids can be used for gallstone dissolution. These acids work by inhibiting biliary secretion of cholesterol and increasing bile secretion from the liver. They may also improve gallbladder motility. They are most effective when used in patients with small stones, mild symptoms, and good gallbladder function. Patients with calcified or pigment stones are usually poor candidates for bile acid therapy. Incomplete dissolution and stone recurrence are both significant drawbacks to the therapy.

Ursodeoxycholic Acid (Ursodiol)
UDCA is a bile acid that lowers bile cholesterol saturation. Numerous studies have shown UDCA to prevent the formation of gallstones in obese patients undergoing rapid weight loss, either through calorie-restricted diets or bariatric surgery.[43] Maintenance therapy may also be effective for gallstone recurrence.[44]

Dosage
UDCA 300 mg twice daily.

Precautions
Possible adverse effects include hepatic impairment, elevation of liver enzymes, and gastrointestinal upset.

> Lifestyle is the key to treatment. Except for surgery, all treatments are associated with a high 5-year recurrence rate if lifestyle modifications are not made.

Estrogen Supplementation
A systematic review of multiple studies found that estrogen supplementation in postmenopausal women increased the likelihood of gallstones.[45] In addition, two randomized placebo-controlled studies also showed an increased risk of biliary disease with supplementation.[46] Both oral and transdermal estrogen supplements can increase biliary cholesterol saturation and decrease cholesterol nucleation time, which could raise the risk of gallstones.[47] The Heart and Estrogen/progestin Replacement Study revealed that supplementation in postmenopausal women with known coronary artery disease resulted in a significant increased risk for biliary surgery.[48] This additional risk should be considered when women elect hormone replacement therapy.

Surgery

Laparoscopic Cholecystectomy
Laparoscopic cholecystectomy is the recommended treatment for patients with symptomatic stones and gallbladder wall inflammation. However, it is not recommended for most patients with asymptomatic gallstones unless they are at risk for gallbladder carcinoma. A major advantage of surgical treatment is the avoidance of recurrence, but it must be weighed against other harms of surgery and anesthesia.

Extracorporeal Shock-Wave Lithotripsy
Lithotripsy can be an effective treatment for gallstones, especially when it is combined with bile acid therapy. Lithotripsy is rarely used for gallstones, however, despite its being a common treatment for renal stones.

Therapies to Consider

Homeopathy
Homeopathy has been used as a safe treatment for more than 2 centuries, despite a lack of scientific evidence. It may provide benefit when other treatment options have failed. After consultation, a professional homeopath may recommend various remedies, including Chelidonium, Colocynthis, or Lycopodium.

Acupuncture
Acupuncture, as part of traditional Chinese medicine treatment, can include addressing energy flow through the liver and gallbladder. This technique may be helpful for gallbladder function, as well as for alleviating discomfort caused by gallbladder disease.

Osteopathy
Although manual therapy is effective for treating musculoskeletal complaints, it is also used to treat other body systems. Osteopathy can help to regulate physiology and aid the body in establishing homeostasis. Viscerosomatic reflexes are changes in the musculoskeletal system that reflect visceral disorders. These reflexes are mediated by afferent neurons of the sympathetic nervous system. They are helpful in diagnosis, but they also can have treatment benefit by balancing the nervous system and influencing the viscera. Manual therapy does not replace others mentioned, but it may be a useful adjunct.

Percutaneous Solvent Dissolution Therapy
Organic solvents such as methyl-ter-butyl ether can be used to dissolve cholesterol gallstones when these agents are directly instilled into the gallbladder by percutaneous catheter through the liver.[14] This labor-intensive and invasive procedure is rarely performed.

Fatty Acid Bile Acid Conjugates

Fatty acid bile conjugates are novel synthetic lipid molecules made of fatty acids linked to cholic acid. They were developed after investigators noted that phospholipids are major cholesterol solubilizers in bile and possess anticrystallizing activity. When given orally, these conjugates are absorbed and secreted into bile. Animal studies showed that these substances can prevent cholesterol crystal formation and also dissolve existing ones.[36,49,50]

PREVENTION PRESCRIPTION

Preventing gallstones is easier than treating them. The same principles of prevention apply to many common chronic diseases (diabetes, heart disease) for an added benefit.

- Maintain a healthy weight, with slow gradual weight loss if body mass index is elevated.
- Exercise. Get moving in a way that is enjoyable and sustainable for you, at least 30 minutes five times weekly.
- Find a stress-reducing practice.
- Encourage a diet high in fiber, vegetables, fruit, nuts, and omega-3 fatty acids.
- Maintain a low intake of saturated fats, refined sugars, and high–glycemic load foods.
- Remember hydration. Drink at least 6 to 8 cups of clean water daily. Consider coffee if you enjoy it, 2 to 3 cups daily. A moderate intake of alcohol may be suitable for some patients.
- Consider an elimination diet.
- Consider supplementation: vitamin C, 200 mg twice daily; magnesium, 300 mg/day; vitamin E, 400 units/day with meals; calcium, 1000 to 1500 mg/day; and lecithin, 500 to 1000 mg/day.
- Avoid medications associated with gallstone risk: estrogen, ceftriaxone, octreotide, and fibrates. Take precautionary measures if taking these medications, have excessive weight loss, or are receiving total parental nutrition (TPN).

THERAPEUTIC REVIEW

Immediate surgical referral is warranted in the setting of severe recurring symptoms, elevation in liver enzymes, amylase, or white blood cell count. In patients with asymptomatic or mild cases and normal liver function, proceed with the therapies listed here.

Lifestyle

- Maintain a healthy weight.
- Exercise at least 30 minutes a day, five times a week.
- Participate in stress-reducing activity.

Nutrition

- Diet should be high in fiber, fruits, and vegetables.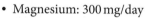
- Consider supplementing with fiber and flaxseed.
- Recommend diet low in saturated fat, rich in omega-3 fatty acids.
- Drink 6 to 8 cups of water daily.
- Avoid refined sugars.
- Avoid excess intake of legumes.
- Consider an elimination diet.

Supplements

- Vitamin C: 200 mg twice daily
- Calcium: 1000 to 1500 mg/day

- Magnesium: 300 mg/day
- Vitamin E: 400 units/day

Botanicals

- Milk thistle (*Silybum marianum*) standardized to 70% silymarin extract: starting at 150 mg twice a day and increasing to three times/day if needed
- Dandelion (*Taraxacum officinalis*): 1:5 tincture, 5 to 10 mL three times/day
- Artichoke (*Cynara scolymus*): 1 to 4 g of leaf, stem, or root three times/day
- Turmeric (*Curcuma longa*): 450-mg curcumin capsule, or 3 g root daily
- Peppermint oil (*Mentha piperita*): one to two enteric-coated capsules three times/day between meals

Pharmaceuticals

- Ursodiol (ursodeoxycholic acid): 300 mg twice daily with meals

Surgery

- Laparascopic cholecystectomy
- Patients with common bile duct obstruction (elevation of liver enzymes, lipase, and bilirubin, right upper quadrant pain, jaundice, and common bile duct dilation on ultrasound) may need either endoscopic retrograde cholangiopancreatography for stone removal or surgical exploration.

KEY WEB RESOURCES

National Center for Complementary and Alternative Medicine, National Institutes of Health: http://nccam.nih.gov.

National Digestive Diseases Information Clearinghouse, National Institutes of Health: http://digestive.niddk.nih.gov.

American Gastroenterological Association: www.gastro.org.

References

References are available online at expertconsult.com.

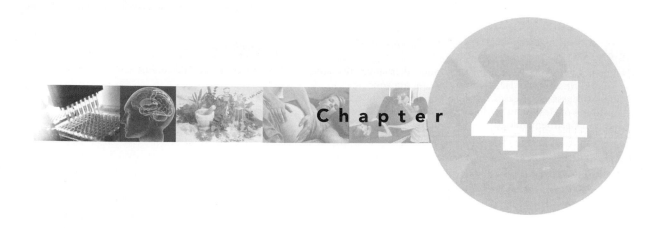

Recurring Abdominal Pain in Pediatrics

Joy A. Weydert, MD

Pathophysiology

Recurrent abdominal pain (RAP) in children was first defined by Apley and Naish in 1958 as consisting of least three episodes of pain over a 3-month period that is severe enough to interfere with normal activities. RAP is one of the most common reasons to seek medical attention.[1] It affects approximately 10% to 15% of all school-age children and is responsible for 2% to 4% of all pediatric outpatient visits.[2] Fewer than 10% of children with RAP are ever found to have an organic cause for pain; however, substantial morbidity, such as depression, anxiety, lifetime psychiatric disorders, social phobia, and somatic complaints, still occurs.[3] In addition, significant health care costs are associated with this disorder, not only from medical evaluations and medications, but also from missed work and productivity.[4] Children with RAP, on average, miss 26 days per year of school compared with only 5 days in children who do not have abdominal pain.[5] Absenteeism has been identified as a precursor to undesirable outcomes, including poor academic performance, increased rates of school dropout, substance abuse, and violence in adolescents.[6] Parents, teachers, and physicians frequently reinforce pain behavior by excusing these children from chores and other responsibilities, allowing absences from school, or providing medications.

We have traditionally recognized that the etiology and pathogenesis are multidimensional in that biologic, psychological, and social factors can all play significant roles in the presentation of RAP in children. With advances in our understanding of pain physiology, more mechanisms that explain the underlying processes will help how we approach the treatment of this condition.

A significant increase in the onset of new RAP cases in children occurs weeks to months after bacterial intestinal infections, and most of these children manifest symptoms consistent with irritable bowel syndrome (IBS).[7] Bacteria interact with intestinal epithelial cells and generate inflammatory mediators that stimulate the sensory nerve endings lying in the gut mucosa. Bacteria also affect intestinal permeability by allowing chemicals and antigens access from the gut lumen into and between the cell walls.[8] Knowing this, we may approach treatment to address lumen physiology and integrity, to decrease the inflammatory response that triggers neuronal sensitization and pain.

Imbalances of neurotransmitters may also contribute to RAP. In the brain-gut axis, which links together the neuroendocrine, immune, and enteric nervous systems, the brain and the gut share identical neurotransmitters because they both originated from the same cells embryologically. Low levels of serotonin have been associated not only with depression and headaches, but also with abdominal pain.[9] Along this line, dysregulation of the autonomic nervous system with an increased auditory startle reflex and low vagal tone has been demonstrated in children with RAP.[10,11] Therefore, therapies that decrease sympathetic arousal, normalize levels of circulating neurotransmitters, and balance the autonomic nervous system may be indicated.

Food sensitivity mediated immunologically by immunoglobulin G (IgG) antibodies has been identified as another trigger for RAP. Rather than the classic IgE food allergy response, which is more immediate, an IgG-mediated response is delayed following exposure to a particular antigen.[12] The most common IgG responses are to wheat, dairy, eggs, corn, and soy. This type of food sensitivity creates a low-level, chronic inflammatory response that triggers gut neuronal sensitivity and pain. This does not, however, trigger excessive calprotectin, a cytosolic protein in granulocytes produced in high levels in inflammatory bowel disease.[13]

Fructose malabsorption, a condition that causes gas, bloating, and cramping, has also been found to cause RAP in children who tested positive on breath hydrogen testing for fructose intolerance.[14]

Even obesity has been linked to a greater incidence of constipation, gastroesophageal reflux disease, IBS, encopresis, and functional abdominal pain. This association may be related to food choices (processed foods versus whole fruits and vegetables, higher intake of soda with high-fructose corn syrup), physical activity levels, hormonal status, or emotional state.[15] A thorough diet history is important in identifying possible triggers for RAP.

Another known factor relating to the incidence of RAP in children is the behavior profile of the patient and his or her genetic vulnerability. Some of these children exhibit anxiety, mild depression, withdrawal, and low self-esteem. Investigators have postulated that this behavior profile is frequently fostered within a family structure characterized by parental depression, enmeshment, overprotectiveness, rigidity, and lack of conflict resolution. These factors may influence the way in which the disorder is experienced and addressed.[16] Figure 44-1 nicely displays how all these factors contribute to the clinical expression of chronic pain.[17]

FIGURE 44-1

Pathogenesis of visceral hyperalgesia and clinical expression of chronic pain. Primary hyperalgesia develops when sensory neurons with cell bodies in dorsal root ganglia are recruited and sensitized after early or multiple pain experiences. Secondary hyperalgesia occurs when biochemical changes in pathways from the spinal cord to cerebral cortex result in increased pain perception. *Viscerosomatic convergence* refers to somatic and visceral afferent nerves terminating on the same spinal interneurons, so that the affected individual is unable to define a discrete pain location on the body. Psychological and developmental factors (within the brain) and psychosocial factors (*arrows* pointing to the brain) alter clinical expression of pain. (From Hyams JS, Hyman PE. Recurrent abdominal pain and the biopsychosocial model of medical practice. *J Pediatr.* 1998; 133:473–478.)

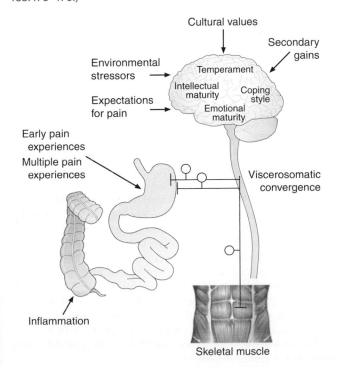

Children with RAP may demonstrate one of the classic presentations, as defined by the Rome Foundation's pediatric Rome III criteria, which may help guide the choice of therapies.[18]

1. Functional abdominal pain or syndrome; must include all the following:
- Episodic or continuous abdominal pain
- Insufficient criteria for the functional gastrointestinal disorders
- No evidence of an inflammatory, anatomic, metabolic, or neoplastic process
- Some loss of daily functioning
- Additional somatic symptoms such as headache, limb pain, or difficulty sleeping

2. IBS; must include all the following:
- Abdominal discomfort or pain associated with two or more of the following:
  - Improvement with defecation
  - Onset associated with a change in frequency or form of stool
- No evidence of an inflammatory, anatomic, metabolic, or neoplastic process

3. Functional dyspepsia; must include all the following:
- Persistent or recurrent pain or discomfort centered in the upper abdomen
- Pain not relieved by defecation or associated with change or form of stool
- No evidence of an inflammatory, anatomic, metabolic, or neoplastic process

4. Functional constipation; must include two or more of the following:
- Two or fewer defecations per week
- At least one episode of fecal incontinence per week
- History of retentive posturing or excessive volitional stool retention
- History of painful or hard bowel movements
- Presence of a large fecal mass in the rectum
- History of large-diameter stools that may obstruct the toilet

5. Abdominal migraine; must include all the following:
- Paroxysmal episodes of intense, acute periumbilical pain that lasts more than 1 hour
- Intervening periods of usual health lasting weeks to months
- Pain interfering with normal activities
- Pain associated with two or more of the following:
  - Anorexia
  - Vomiting
  - Photophobia
  - Nausea
  - Headache
  - Pallor
- No evidence of an inflammatory, anatomic, metabolic, or neoplastic process

6. Cyclic vomiting
- Two or more periods of intense nausea and unremitting vomiting or retching lasting hours to days
- Return to usual state of health lasting weeks to months

7. Aerophagia; must include two of the following:
- Air swallowing
- Abdominal distention because of intraluminal air
- Repetitive belching or increased flatus

Serious organic disease can be ruled out by a thorough history and physical examination and basic laboratory investigations. Pertinent positive results in this evaluation considered "red flags" include the following:

1. A family history of inflammatory bowel disease, ulcer disease, or significant psychosocial disorder
2. Pain that wakes the child from sleep
3. History of weight loss or growth delay
4. Blood in stool or bile-stained emesis
5. A history and physical examination revealing fevers, rashes, joint involvement, or perianal disease
6. Abnormal complete blood count, urinalysis, sedimentation rate, C-reactive protein, or stool for occult blood

If indicated by a positive history, the clinician may have to consider further testing (i.e., serologic testing for *Helicobacter pylori*, serum transaminases, amylase, lipase, stool for pathogens, and endoscopy).

> Rather than a diagnosis of exclusion, recurrent abdominal pain should be presented as a positive diagnosis identified as the most common cause of chronic abdominal pain in children. Parents can further be reassured that serious disease is unlikely if the history and physical examination are normal.

Integrative Therapy

Nutrition

Diet manipulation has been attempted for years as a treatment for RAP either through the elimination of certain foods (e.g., lactose-containing foods) or the addition of others (e.g., high-fiber foods). Research into these dietary interventions has had varying results.[19,20]

Fiber

Although fiber studies have been small and the evidence is weak, some investigators found that additional fiber may be beneficial to some children, especially those with constipation. This goal can be accomplished by increasing the amounts of fruit, vegetables, legumes, and whole grains in the diet. Breakfast cereals can also be a good source of fiber, especially cereals made with bran (Table 44-1).

If a child has difficulty obtaining adequate fiber through the diet, psyllium powder, 1 teaspoon (2 g) in 8 oz of cool water or juice, may be given up to three times a day. An increase in water intake is strongly recommended along with the increased fiber, to prevent constipation.

> Age of the child + 5 = recommended minimum daily grams of fiber. More fiber can be added as needed.

Food Elimination

If certain foods seem to exacerbate pain, the patient should certainly avoid them. If symptoms are suggestive or if the patient has a family history of lactose intolerance, initiate a 2- to 4-week trial of cessation of all dairy products (milk, cheese, yogurt, ice cream, and so forth). If no changes

TABLE 44-1. Fiber Content of Various Foods

FOODS	PORTION SIZE	FIBER (g)
High Fiber		
All-Bran cereal	½ cup	10
Figs, dried	3	10
Kidney beans	½ cup cooked	9
Baked beans	½ cup cooked	8
Broccoli	¾ cup cooked	7
Spinach	½ cup cooked	7
Yam baked in skin	1 medium	7
Whole wheat bread	2 slices	6
Baked potato with skin	1 medium	5
Blackberries	½ cup	5
Apple with skin	1 medium	3.5
Raspberries	½ cup	3.5
Lentils	½ cup cooked	3.5
Whole wheat spaghetti	1 cup	3.5
Wheaties cereal	1 oz	2.5
Low Fiber		
Bagel	1	Less than 1
Cornflakes	1 oz	Less than 1
Grapes	20	Less than 1
Watermelon	1 cup	Less than 1
Lettuce	1 cup	Less than 1

are noted after 2 weeks, then consumption of dairy products can be resumed. If some improvement was noted, then have the patient slowly reintroduce dairy in small quantities as tolerated. Reduce the intake of highly processed foods, especially those with refined carbohydrates (e.g., snacks, candy, cookies) because the fermentation of these sugars increases gas production. Studies showed that ingestion of various sugars, such as lactose, fructose, sorbitol, or fructose plus sorbitol, causes an increase in measured breath hydrogen and clinical symptoms in patients with RAP.[21,22] Subsequent reduction of these sugars caused a reduction in symptoms in 40% to 60% of the subjects studied. Fructose is readily available in sweetened soft drinks and juices. Sorbitol is the leading sweetener used in "sugar-free" foods.

Food allergy has been implicated in abdominal pain; however, attempts to test for this by the presence of IgE-mediated antibody responses has not been helpful. One study, however, focused on food elimination based on IgG antibodies detected by enzyme-linked immunosorbent assay. These antibodies may cause delayed sensitivity and irritation of the gastrointestinal tract. In a randomized, controlled trial, compliant patients who were placed on a food elimination diet that was based on high levels of IgG antibodies had a 26% greater reduction of symptoms compared with patients receiving a sham elimination diet[23] (see Chapter 84, Food Intolerance and Elimination Diet).

Behavior Modification

Reinforcing pain behavior is often done unknowingly but with good intentions toward the child. Help families recognize that special attention or treatment with pain episodes (i.e., staying home from school, being dismissed from chores or responsibilities, having one-on-one attention from a parent) may foster ongoing pain behavior and diminish the child's self-reliance. Encourage school attendance as well as completion of personal responsibilities. Physicians can also facilitate a return to a normal lifestyle by offering a thorough explanation of the diagnosis and pathophysiology, reassurance, and options for management and adaptation to the disorder.

Poor sleep can heighten the perception of pain; therefore, working on strategies to promote restorative sleep is important. Eliminate all stimulants in the evening before bedtime. This includes caffeine, decongestants, television, computer or video games, and arguments. Practice dusk simulation by dimming lights around the house 1 hour before bedtime and shifting to quieter activities. The child should take a warm bath with Epsom salt to relax tense muscles before bedtime. Make sure the bedroom environment is conducive to sleep—dark, quiet, and cool. If the child has difficulty falling asleep, have him or her practice the self-regulation techniques listed earlier. Also consider using calming herbs such as chamomile.

Botanicals

Chamomile (Matricaria recutita)

The active ingredients in chamomile include the volatile oils alpha-bisabolol and bisabolol oxide and the flavonoids apigenin, luteolin, and quercetin. These constituents have antiinflammatory effects that inhibit phospholipase A, cyclooxygenase, and lipoxygenase pathways.[24] Bisabolol has effects in the gastrointestinal tract receptors, thus causing relaxation of the smooth muscle. Apigenin works on the central nervous system benzodiazepine receptors with anxiolytic effects similar to those of diazepam (Valium) and alprazolam (Xanax) but without the sedative effects.[25,26] Chamomile can be given as a tea, as an extract, or by capsule in standardized preparations. Glyceride extracts of chamomile can be found for use in children to offset any concerns of preparations extracted with alcohol. One study done in infants with colic used an herbal tea preparation that included chamomile. This preparation was found effective in reducing colic episodes.[27]

■ Dosage

Adults weighing approximately 150 lb: 3 g three to five times per day
Children weighing approximately 75 lb: 1.5 g three to five times per day
Children weighing approximately 35 lb: 0.75 g three to five times per day

One heaping teaspoon of chamomile flowers steeped in hot water yields approximately 3 g. The extracts may come in 1 g/1 mL (1:1) dilution or 1 g/4 mL (1:4) dilution. Use the following doses as a guide:
150 lb
  1:1—15 to 30 drops three to five times per day
  1:4—2 teaspoons three to five times per day
75 lb
  1:1—8 to 15 drops three to five times per day
  1:4—1 teaspoon three to five times per day
35 lb
  1:1—4 to 8 drops three to five times per day
  1:4—½ teaspoon three to five times per day

■ Precaution

Chamomile is generally safe, although anyone allergic to ragweed, asters, or chrysanthemums should take it with caution. Chamomile is a member of this daisy family and has contributed to allergic reactions in rare cases.

Peppermint (Mentha piperita)

Analysis of peppermint oil typically shows more than 40 different compounds; however, the principal components are menthol, methone, and methyl acetate. The pharmacology focuses almost entirely on peppermint's menthol component, which has carminative effects (elimination of intestinal gas), antispasmodic effects, and choleretic effects (bile flow stimulant). The mechanism of action is thought to be inhibition of smooth muscle contractions by blocking calcium channels.[28] Many studies have been conducted using peppermint oil as a treatment for IBS, including one study in children.[29] Even though peppermint did not alter the associated symptoms of IBS, such as urgency of stool, stool patterns, or belching, it did reduce the pain. Peppermint is most widely used as a tea. Because of its calcium channel blockage effects, it may cause relaxation of the lower esophageal sphincter and lead to an increase in heartburn symptoms for some patients. An enteric-coated capsule is available for use in the treatment of IBS. With its delayed release in the small intestine, peppermint has little effect on the lower esophageal sphincter; therefore, it is less likely to cause heartburn.

■ Dosage

Tea: 1 to 2 teaspoons dried leaves steeped in 8 oz of hot water as needed
Enteric-coated capsules (200 mg or 0.2 mL):
  Two capsules three times a day for children weighing more than 100 lb
  One capsule three times a day for children weighing 60 to 100 lb

■ Precaution

Peppermint is generally regarded as safe; however, hypersensitivity reactions have been reported.

> Because of its smooth muscle–relaxing properties, peppermint has its greatest effect on pain related to abdominal spasm.

Ginger (Zingiber officinale)

Ginger contains many volatile oils (sesquesterpenes) and aromatic ketones (gingerols). Gingerols are believed to be the more pharmacologically active constituents. Historically, ginger has been used as far back as the fourth century BC for stomach aches, nausea, and diarrhea. It also has been used as a carminative, appetite stimulant, and choleretic. Ginger can simultaneously improve gastric motility and exert antispasmodic effects.[30] Studies have shown that ginger's antispasmodic effects on the visceral smooth muscle are likely the result of antagonism of serotonin receptor sites. One study, with a double-blind randomized crossover design, found that the use of ginger brought about a significant reduction of nausea and vomiting in women with hyperemesis gravidarum.[31] Because of its safety profile, ginger is regularly used in pregnancy, with no untoward fetal effects.

■ Dosage

Adults weighing approximately 150 lb: 1 to 2 g dry powdered ginger root per day (10 g fresh)

Children weighing approximately 75 lb: 0.5 to 1 g dry powdered ginger root per day (5 g fresh)

Children weighing approximately 35 lb: 0.25 to 0.5 g dry powdered ginger root per day (2.5 g fresh)

> Ginger can improve gastric motility while also exerting an antispasmodic effect. The pharmacist can dissolve ginger capsules in an 8.4% bicarbonate suspension with good stability and bioavailability for use in children unable to swallow pills.

A one-fourth inch slice of fresh ginger root is approximately 10 g. This is equivalent to 1 to 2 g of a dry powder form of ginger that is a more concentrated form found in capsules. Fresh ginger can be brewed as a tea sweetened with honey or can be chopped and added to foods, soups, or salads.

■ Precautions

Ginger is well tolerated when used in typical doses. At higher doses, side effects may include heartburn, abdominal discomfort, or diarrhea. Ginger may have antiplatelet effects and therefore may increase the risk of bleeding in some people.

> A general rule of thumb for estimating the amount of fresh ginger to use in children is to use the child's "pinky" finger (fifth finger) as the guide to the size of ginger to chop up and steep for tea.

Slippery Elm (Ulmus fulva)

Slippery elm has demulcent properties that can be used to protect the gastrointestinal tract from irritation. When used internally, slippery elm causes reflex stimulation of the nerve endings in the gastrointestinal tract that produces mucus secretion.[32] This effect may be particularly helpful in children with functional dyspepsia.

■ Dosage

A tea can be made with 1 cup boiling water and 1 tablespoon of powdered bark. Use 2 to 5 mL three times a day.

■ Precautions

No contraindications are associated with slippery elm. Spontaneous abortions have been reported with its use; therefore, it should not be used during pregnancy.

Lemon Balm (Melissa officinalis)

Lemon balm contains volatile oils and constituents that relax muscles, particularly in the bladder, stomach, and uterus, and thereby relieve cramps, gas, and nausea. This herb is generally regarded as safe and is one of the components of the product Iberogast, used widely for gastrointestinal problems. A meta-analysis of the double-blind randomized controlled trials conducted on Iberogast found significant improvements compared with placebo in patients with functional dyspepsia.[33]

■ Dosage

Capsules: 100 to 200 mg dried lemon balm three times daily or as needed

Tea: 0.5 to 1.5 g (¼ to 1 teaspoon) of dried lemon balm herb in hot water. Steep and drink up to four times daily.

Tincture: 0.5 to 1 mL (15 to 30 drops) three times daily

■ Precautions

Although no scientific evidence supports this, lemon balm may interact with sedatives and thyroid medications.

Supplements

Probiotics

The human intestinal tract is populated with various microbial species that are nonpathogenic and necessary for normal digestive functioning. The microorganisms, or probiotics, are now recognized as a way to fight disease and improve health. Studies in children showed a significant reduction of diarrhea symptoms, both from rotavirus infection and from antibiotic use, when these children were given probiotics.[34,35] Probiotics increase the number of rotavirus-specific IgA secreting cells and serum IgA levels. Probiotics are thought to be possibly helpful in treating RAP by degrading dietary antigens, restoring normal intestinal permeability, and alleviating intestinal inflammation that can trigger pain.[36] Two double-blind randomized placebo-controlled trials found that Lactobacillus GG reduced the frequency and intensity of pain in children with RAP/IBS when this probiotic was given over the course of 4 to 8 weeks.[37,38] One of these studies also demonstrated a decrease in the number of patients with abnormal intestinal permeability testing after treatment with Lactobacillus GG, but not with placebo.

■ Dosage

Use 10 to 100 billion colony-forming units (CFUs) per serving once or twice a day. These preparations can be of a single strain, such as Lactobacillus GG, or made of multiple strains such as Bifidobacterium bifidus, Lactobacillus acidophilus, or Lactobacillus reuteri, to treat both the small and the large intestine.

■ Precautions

Probiotics are considered safe for use. Lactobacillus sepsis associated with probiotic therapy was reported, but this adverse effect occurred in children who were considered immunocompromised and at high risk because of central line placement.

Pharmaceuticals

Despite a lack of controlled studies with established efficacy for many drugs used in functional bowel disorders,[39,40] these agents continue to be prescribed. For this reason, as well as worrisome side effects (for metoclopramide, irritability and dystonic reactions; for cisapride, arrhythmia and adverse outcomes in prolonged QT syndrome; for anticholinergics, constipation, blurred vision, tachycardia, and sedation; for tricyclic antidepressants, sedation, agitation, acute mental disturbance, and reduction in seizure threshold), these particular drugs cannot be safely recommended for use in children.

Histamine-2 (H₂) Receptor Antagonists and Proton Pump Inhibitors

For patients with dyspepsia as their primary symptom, histamine-2 (H₂) receptor antagonists and proton pump inhibitors can be used if other strategies are unsuccessful. Studies in children supporting such therapy are few, but these drugs may be beneficial and are relatively safe in the short term (6 to 8 weeks).[41]

■ Dosage
Cimetidine (Tagamet): 10 mg/kg/dose given four times daily; comes in 100-mg over-the-counter (OTC), 200-, 300-, 400-, and 800-mg tablets and 300-mg/5-mL suspension by prescription

Ranitidine (Zantac): 2 to 4 mg/kg/dose given twice daily; comes in 75-mg OTC, 150-, and 300-mg tablets, 150-mg granules, and 75-mg/5-mL suspension

Famotidine (Pepcid): 0.5 to 3.5 mg/kg/day divided two times a day; comes in 10-mg OTC, 20-, or 40-mg tablets and 40-mg/5-mL suspension

Omeprazole (Prilosec): 0.2 to 3.5 mg/kg/day daily or divided twice a day; comes in 10-, 20-, and 40-mg capsules

Lansoprazole (Prevacid): 1 to 2 mg/kg/day given daily; comes in 15- and 30-mg capsules

■ Precautions
Headaches, diarrhea, abdominal pain, and elevated liver function tests have been reported.

> Prolonged acid suppression can lead to malabsorption of key nutrients including vitamin B₁₂, iron, and calcium.

Cyproheptadine

This drug (also known by the brand name, Periactin), which has antihistamine effects, was studied through a double-blind randomized controlled trial conducted over 2 weeks in 29 children. The intensity and frequency of abdominal pain reported by the children were significantly improved in the treatment group compared with the control group.[42] This medication has historically been used as prophylactic treatment for migraine because of its effects on serotonin and histamine. These effects may have some benefit in children with abdominal migraines over a short period, although more studies need to be done.

■ Dosage
Children 7 to 14 years of age: 4 mg two or three times daily (maximum, 16 mg/day)

Children 2 to 6 years of age: 2 mg two or three times daily (maximum, 12 mg/day)

■ Precautions
The main side effects have been increased appetite and weight gain. Sedation and sleepiness have also been reported.

Biomechanical Therapy

Massage
Massage can ease pain by calming sympathetic arousal often found in children with RAP. With decreased sympathetic drive comes an improvement in gastrointestinal motility. Massage, either of the abdomen directly or indirectly by reflexology, is helpful in alleviating ileus and constipation and overall can be very comforting.[43]

Osteopathic Manipulative Therapy
Understanding somatovisceral pathways has led to the treatment of RAP with osteopathic manipulative therapy. Trigger points along the spine and in the large muscles of the back and trunk (e.g., external and internal oblique, rectus abdominis, iliocostalis thoracis and lumborum muscles) can cause referred pain to the abdominal region that mimics visceral disease. Release of these trigger points through manipulation decreases this reflex effect and therefore lessens the pain.[44]

Surgery

Exploratory surgery is not warranted unless strong indications are revealed through the history, physical examination, and laboratory investigations.

Bioenergetic Therapy

Traditional Chinese Medicine and Acupuncture
The philosophy of traditional Chinese medicine is that of restoring balance to the body through its flow of energy. Although large clinical trials have not been conducted using traditional Chinese medicine and acupuncture in children with RAP, one study measured the effects of hand acupuncture in reducing intermittent abdominal pain in 40 children. Pain intensity and medication use were considerably lower in the treatment group.[45] In a randomized double-blind placebo-controlled study using Chinese herbs, patients receiving herbs noted significant improvement in bowel symptoms, global well-being, and return to normal life activities compared with the group receiving placebo.[46] Although children may be fearful of needles, when acupuncture is performed by an experienced professional, many children have reported that it does not hurt. Acupressure or electroacupuncture may also be used as alternatives to needles.

Reiki and Healing Touch
Like traditional Chinese medicine, Reiki and healing touch are based on the concept of restoring normal energy flow through the body. In patients with disease or pain, this energy may be blocked or stagnant, thus disrupting its normal flow. Through energy work, this energy flow can be restored. Many randomized controlled studies have suggested that energy healing can be effective for pain, anxiety, depression, wound healing, and other problems.[47] Although no specific studies have been conducted in children with RAP, this therapy has no serious side effects and is considered safe (see Chapter 112, Human Energetic Therapies).

Mind-Body Therapy

Because of our knowledge of the brain-gut axis and the associated interactions, it is only logical that mind-body therapy be used in RAP. Studies published primarily in psychiatric journals supported the efficacy of interventions that teach stress management, progressive muscle relaxation, or coping behaviors or use cognitive-behavioral therapy.[48,49] One study showed that significant pain reduction occurred when biofeedback, cognitive-behavioral therapy, or parental support was added to fiber therapy in the multimodal treatment of RAP.[50]

Progressive Muscle Relaxation and Breathing Exercises

Both progressive muscle relaxation and breathing exercises, used alone or together, are forms of self-regulation that help decrease sympathetic arousal to promote comfort. Progressive muscle relaxation is a way for children to learn to feel the difference between tense and relaxed muscles and to use this knowledge to cope with abdominal pain. Progressive relaxation reduces anxiety associated with pain by demonstrating the mind-body phenomenon and patients' capacity for self-regulation. The benefits of these approaches are that they are easily taught, especially to school-age children, and they can be used anywhere. Scripts can be given to parents to use, or a tape can be made or purchased for home use (see Chapter 92, Self-Hypnosis Techniques and Chapter 93, Relaxation Techniques).

Biofeedback

Biofeedback is a form of relaxation using physiologic feedback instruments to reinforce behavior. As relaxation occurs, warmth can be brought to the fingertips, thus increasing the distal temperature. This temperature can be monitored by sensors placed on the fingers and can reinforce the positive behavior of relaxation as the temperature rises. Biofeedback may be beneficial for a person who is somewhat skeptical about the ability to control body functions with the mind. Someone trained in biofeedback who has the equipment readily available can best teach this modality.

In a study using heart rate variability biofeedback, children with functional abdominal pain were able to reduce their symptoms significantly in relation to increasing their autonomic balance, also significantly. The investigators believed that change in vagal tone was the potential mediator for this improvement.[51]

Hypnosis and Guided Imagery

With hypnosis and guided imagery, one achieves a state of focused attention in which the mind is more receptive to suggestion. The technique has been used successfully for all types of pain syndromes including RAP and is easily used in children older than 4 years of age (see Chapter 93, Self-Hypnosis Techniques, and Chapter 95, Guided Imagery).[52,53]

A randomized controlled trial on the use of therapist-directed guided imagery with progressive muscle relaxation found a significant decrease in the number of days with pain and missed activities compared with controls.[54] A similar study using audio-recorded guided imagery treatment also found benefit, with treatment effects maintained for over 6 months.[55] Gut-directed hypnosis therapy was found to be superior to standard medical therapy in reducing pain scores in children with long-standing abdominal pain in yet another randomized controlled trial.[56]

Psychotherapy

In children or families with significant psychosocial dysfunction, counseling by a child psychiatrist or clinical psychologist may be the best therapy. Cognitive-behavioral family intervention therapy, which often includes teaching specific coping skills, social skills, and relaxation, has been shown to be efficacious in studies of children with RAP.[57,58]

PREVENTION PRESCRIPTION

- Encourage liberal amounts of water and fiber, in the form of natural fruits and vegetables, to promote daily bowel movements.
- Promote probiotics if the patient has a history of antibiotic, steroid, or nonsteroidal antiinflammatory drug use.
- Ask the patient to practice breathing and relaxation exercises or other self-regulation techniques to reduce stress.
- Encourage healthy sleep habits to promote restorative sleep.
- Consider avoiding high amounts of processed foods and simple sugars including sorbitol.
- Encourage regular movement and exercise.

THERAPEUTIC REVIEW

Once a child has been thoroughly evaluated and organic disease has been ruled out, any of these therapies can be used in an age-appropriate manner.

■ Nutrition

- Avoid foods that have sorbitol and high-fructose corn syrup or are a source of refined carbohydrate because these are poorly digested.

- Prescribe a 2- to 4-wk trial of cessation of all dairy products if the history suggests lactose intolerance (see Chapter 84, Food Intolerance and Elimination Diet).

- Increase fiber by at least 10 g/day through the addition of fruits, vegetables, legumes, and whole grains or with psyllium, 1 teaspoon/8 oz cool water once to three times daily.

- Increase water intake along with the increase of fiber.

■ Behavior Modification

- Encourage attendance at school and other usual activities.
- Offer strategies to overcome the reinforcement of illness behavior at school and at home.
- Improve restorative sleep.

■ Botanicals

- Chamomile
  - 3 g three to five times/day (150-lb patient)
  - 1.5 g three to five times/day (75-lb patient)
  - 0.75 g three to five times/day (35-lb patient)
- Peppermint tea
  - 1 to 2 teaspoons dried leaves/8 oz hot water as needed
  - Enteric-coated capsules (200 mg)
  - Two capsules three times/day (approximately 100-lb patient)
  - One capsule three times/day (60- to 99-lb patient)
- Ginger
  - 10 g fresh (or 1 to 2 g dry powdered)/day (150-lb patient)
  - 5 g fresh (or 0.5 to 1 g dry powdered)/day (75-lb patient)
  - 2.5 g fresh (or 0.25 to 0.5 g dry powdered)/day (35-lb patient)
- Slippery elm
  - Make tea with 1 cup boiling water and 1 tablespoon powdered bark. Give 2 to 5 mL three times a day

- Lemon balm
  - 100- to 200-mg capsules three times/day
  - 0.5 to 1.5 g tea three times/day
  - 0.5 to 1 mL (15 to 30 drops) tincture three times/day

■ Supplements

- Probiotics: 10 to 100 billion CFUs once or twice/day

■ Pharmaceuticals

- Histamine-2 (H_2) receptor antagonists or proton pump inhibitors for maximum of 6 to 8 weeks if dyspepsia is the primary complaint (see text for dosing)
- Cyproheptadine: 2 to 4 mg two to three times/day for abdominal migraine

■ Biomechanical Therapy

- Massage
- Osteopathic manipulative therapy

■ Bioenergetic Therapy

- Traditional Chinese medicine and acupuncture
- Reiki and healing touch

■ Mind-Body Therapies

- Progressive muscle relaxation and breathing exercises (see Chapter 89, Breathing Exercises)
- Biofeedback
- Hypnosis and guided imagery (see Chapter 92, Self-Hypnosis Techniques, and Chapter 95, Guided Imagery)
- Psychotherapy

KEY WEB RESOURCES

YourChild: http://www.med.umich.edu/yourchild/topics/abpain.htm.

HeartMath: http://www.heartmath.com; StressEraser: http://stresseraser.com; and Wild Divine: http://www.wilddivine.com.

Health Journeys: http://www.healthjourneys.com; Kaiser Permanente Healthy Living to Go audio library: https://members.kaiserpermanente.org/redirects/listen/?kp_shortcut_referrer=kp.org/listen; and Guided Imagery: http://www.guidedimageryinc.com/store/children_teens_products.aspx.

This University of Michigan Web site provides information for parents on abdominal pain in children.

These Web sites offer biofeedback devices that can help stimulate parasympathetic activity toward a reduction in abdominal pain.

These Web sites are resources for guided-imagery recordings.

References

References are available online at expertconsult.com.

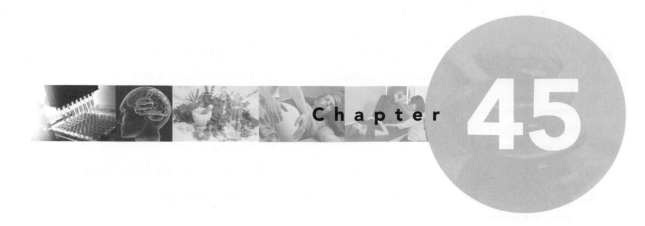

Chapter 45

Constipation

Tanmeet Sethi, MD

Pathophysiology

Constipation is estimated to affect up to 28% of the population, most commonly older adults, women, and children, and results in more than $6.9 billion in medical costs.[1] The symptom is usually intermittent and self-limiting, although some patients require intervention to achieve resolution. Table 45-1 demonstrates defining criteria for constipation,[2] but in practical clinical terms, the complaint of constipation and even the diagnosis are often made more subjectively. Asking what patients mean by the statement "I am constipated" may be the most important first step to management.[3] Most patients complaining of constipation describe a perception of difficulty with bowel movements or a discomfort related to bowel movements. The most common terms used by young healthy adults to define constipation are straining (52%), hard stools (44%), and the inability to have a bowel movement (34%).

> Routine diagnostic testing is not recommended for patients with no alarm symptoms and no signs of organic disorder.[4]

Functional constipation can most often be classified into three different categories:

1. Normal-transit constipation: Also known as functional constipation, this is the most common type. In functional constipation, stool passes through the colon at a normal rate, and bowel movement frequency is normal.[5] In this group of patients, constipation is likely the result of a perceived difficulty with evacuation or the presence of hard stools.[2]
2. Slow-transit constipation: This type is characterized by prolonged delay of transit of stool through the colon. Patients may complain of abdominal bloating and infrequent bowel movements.[6] The causes are unclear.
3. Pelvic floor dysfunction: These patients have uncoordinated evacuation of stool through the rectum. They are more likely to complain of a feeling of incomplete evacuation, a sense of obstruction, or a need for digital manipulation.[6]

Physicians should keep secondary causes of constipation (the most common being hypothyroidism) in mind, as well as medications that can cause constipation. In one study of more than 20,000 patients, certain drugs were found to have a two- to threefold increased risk of constipation.[7] Although the list of drugs that can cause constipation is quite lengthy, Table 45-2 [7,8] provides some of the most common offenders.

Integrative Therapy

Physical Activity

The generally accepted view is that increasing the amount of physical activity can be a preventive measure of constipation. In fact, a subset of the Nurses' Health Study showed that in more than 62,000 women, physical activity two to six times a week was associated with a 35% decrease in risk of constipation.[9] A previous National Health and Nutrition Examination Survey showed a twofold increased risk of constipation in persons with a low physical activity level. Despite these findings, data in support of exercise as an actual treatment for constipation have not been consistent. Nevertheless, many patients who comply with dietary and exercise recommendations have an improvement in symptoms.[10]

Nutrition

Fiber

Although dietary modification may not always succeed, all constipated patients should be advised initially to increase their dietary fiber intake as the simplest, most physiologic, and cheapest form of treatment.[1] Patients should be encouraged to ingest 20 to 25 g of fiber daily by eating whole grain breads, unrefined cereals, plenty of fruit and vegetables, or flax meal or bran. A careful meta-analysis showed that in 18 of 20 studies stool weight was increased by adequate fiber supplementation, and fecal transit was accelerated.[11,12] Dietary fiber appears to be less effective in severe constipation, especially of the slow-transit variant, in evacuation disorders, (fiber may actually worsen these two types), or

TABLE 45-1. Rome II Criteria for Functional Constipation

Adults*

- Two or more of the following six must be present:
  - Straining during at least 25% of defecations
  - Lumpy or hard stools in at least 25% of defecations
  - Sensation of incomplete evacuation for at least 25% of defecations
  - Sensation of anorectal obstruction/blockage for at least 25% of defecations
  - Manual maneuvers to facilitate at least 25% of defecations (e.g., digital evacuation, support of the pelvic floor)
  - Fewer than three defecations/wk

Infants and Children

- Pebble-like, hard stools for a majority of stools for at least 2 consecutive wk
- Firm stools up to twice/wk for at least 2 wk
- No evidence of structural, endocrine, or metabolic disease

From Lembo A, Camilleri M. Chronic constipation. *N Engl J Med.* 2003;349:1360–1368.
*Loose stools are rarely present without the use of laxatives; criteria for irritable bowel syndrome are not fulfilled.

TABLE 45-2. Medications Associated With Constipation

- Aluminum-containing antacids
- Diuretics
- Antidepressants
- Antihistamines
- Anticholinergics
- Nonsteroidal antiinflammatory agents
- Iron supplements
- Opioids
- Anticonvulsants
- Calcium channel blockers
- Beta blockers

in constipation secondary to medications.[13-15] In one study, women who engaged in regular physical exercise and who had a higher fiber intake (approximately 20 g/day) had a threefold lower prevalence of constipation compared with women who rarely exercised and had approximately 7 g of fiber a day.[9] If ensuring proper intake of fiber is difficult, a commercially packaged fiber supplement may also be used (discussed later under Supplements).

Increasing fiber intake too quickly can cause abdominal bloating or flatulence. To optimize compliance, increase fiber gradually over at least 2 to 3 weeks to 20 to 25 g/day and ensure increased fluid intake to avoid these symptoms.
An example of a 20-g fiber breakfast: ½ cup bran (10 g), three dried figs (10 g). Make palatable with 1 cup soy or almond milk (1 g fiber), 1 tablespoon brown sugar for taste, and 1 tablespoon of cinnamon (slows absorption of sugar).
Other high-fiber foods: 1 large apple or pear (5 g), ½ cup raspberries (9 g), 1 cup Raisin Bran (5 g), 2 Brazil nuts (2.5 g), 23 almonds (3.5 g), 1 cup peas (16 g), 1 cup black beans (15 g), 1 artichoke (10 g), 1 cup cooked broccoli (5 g)

In pediatric populations, decreased fiber intake has also been found to be a risk factor for chronic constipation.[16] One safe and effective dietary fiber recommendation for many children is the *age + 5 = daily grams of fiber* guideline.[17] According to this guideline, the amount of dietary fiber recommended daily is the sum of the child's year in age plus five.

In pregnant women, fiber supplements in the form of bran and wheat fiber were found to increase bowel frequency, soften stool, and be better tolerated than were stimulant laxatives.[18]

Food Triggers

A large body of evidence indicates that cow's milk and dairy products may be risk factors for chronic constipation in some children.[19-21]

Evidence supports a 4- to 6-week trial of elimination of dairy products as a component of the integrative treatment of childhood constipation.

Fluids

Although the generally accepted belief is to increase fluids both as a preventive measure and as treatment for constipation, supporting data are conflicting.[22] One study did show that increasing fluids with an increased fiber intake (25 g/day) led to greater stool frequency and decreased laxative use compared with increased fiber alone.[23] To date, no child studies have demonstrated the benefits of increasing fluid intake in states other than severe dehydration.[24] However, carbohydrates and especially sorbitol, found in some juices such as prune, pear, and apple, can cause increased frequency and water content of stools.[25]

Supplements

Commercially Packaged Fiber Supplements

These supplements include psyllium, methylcellulose, and polycarbophil and are bulking laxatives. More information, including dosing, is available in Table 45-3 and is provided later under Pharmaceuticals. Psyllium is an efficacious method to increase stool frequency and weight and improve stool consistency in idiopathic constipation.[26]

One double-blind multicenter study showed psyllium (5.1 g twice daily) to be superior to docusate sodium (100 mg twice daily) for softening stools by increasing stool water content and to have greater overall laxative efficacy in subjects with chronic idiopathic constipation.[27]

Probiotics

Lactobacillus reuteri, administered at a dose of 10^8 colony-forming units to infants older than 6 months of age, was found to increase bowel frequency.[28] A high-grade systematic review showed that use of probiotics in adults and children augmented the number of stools and reduced the number of hard stools.[29] These results were statistically significant but clinically only

TABLE 45-3. Agents for Treatment of Constipation in Adults

TYPE	GENERIC NAME	DOSAGE	ACG GRADE	COMMENTS
Bulking Laxatives				
	Psyllium (Metamucil)	Titrate up to 30 g/day in divided doses	B	Taken from the ground seed husk of the ispaghula plant; needs to be taken with plenty of water to avoid intestinal obstruction; undergoes bacterial degradation that may contribute to side effects of bloating and flatus; allergic reactions, such as anaphylaxis and asthma, reported but are rare
	Methylcellulose (Citrucel)	Titrate up to 6 g/day in divided doses	B	Semisynthetic cellulose fiber relatively resistant to colonic bacterial degradation; tends to cause less bloating and flatus than psyllium
	Polycarbophil (FiberCon)	Titrate up to 4 g/day in divided doses	B	Synthetic polymer of acrylic acid that is resistant to bacterial degradation
Osmotic Laxatives				
	Magnesium hydroxide (Milk of Magnesia)	30–60 mL/day	B	Small percentage actively absorbed in the small intestine; remainder draws water into the intestines along an osmotic gradient
	Polyethylene glycol (MiraLax)	17–34 g once to twice/day	A	Organic polymer that is poorly absorbed and not metabolized by colonic bacteria
	Lactulose	15–30 mL once to twice/day	A	Synthetic disaccharide consisting of galactose and fructose linked by a bond resistant to lactase and therefore not absorbed by the small intestine; undergoes bacterial fermentation in the colon resulting in formation of short-chain fatty acids; bacteria in the colon can metabolize up to 80 g of lactulose each day; gas and bloating common side effects
Stimulant Laxatives				
Anthraquinones	Sennosides (senna)	8.6–30 mg once to twice/day	B	Anthraquinones converted by colonic bacteria to their active form, which increases electrolyte transport into the bowel and stimulates intestinal motility; may cause melanosis coli, a benign condition usually reversible within 12 months; no definitive association established between anthraquinones and colon cancer or myenteric nerve damage
Diphenylmethane derivatives	Bisacodyl (Dulcolax)	10–15 mg/day orally 10-mg rectal suppository/day	B	Hydrolyzed by endogenous esterases; stimulates secretion and motility of small intestine and colon
Stool Softeners				
	Docusate sodium	50–100 mg once to twice/day	B	Ionic detergents that soften the stool by allowing water to interact more effectively with solid stool; may have modest effects on fluid absorption and secretion; efficacy in constipation not well established
	Docusate calcium	5–45 mL orally nightly	B	Alters stool by being emulsified into the stool mass and providing lubrication for passage of the stool; long-term use can cause malabsorption of fat-soluble vitamins, anal seepage, and lipoid pneumonia in patients predisposed to aspiration of liquids
Emollients				
	Mineral oil	5–45 mL orally nightly	B	Alters stool by being emulsified into the stool mass and providing lubrication for passage of the stool; long-term use can cause malabsorption of fat-soluble vitamins, anal seepage, and lipoid pneumonia in patients predisposed to aspiration of liquids

TABLE 45-3. Agents for Treatment of Constipation in Adults—cont'd

TYPE	GENERIC NAME	DOSAGE	ACG GRADE	COMMENTS
Chloride Channel Activator				
	Lubiprostone	8 mcg twice/day for IBS-C; 24 mcg twice/day for chronic constipation	Not graded	Activates ClC-2s in the intestine and causes fluid secretion and possible secondary effects on motility; nausea common; administer with food and water; approved for use in adults with chronic constipation and in women older than 18 yr old with IBS-C

From Eoff JC III, Lembo A. Optimal treatment of chronic constipation in managed care: review and roundtable discussion. *J Manag Care Pharm.* 2008;14(suppl A):1–15.
ACG, American College of Gastroenterology; bid, twice daily; ClC-2, type-2 chloride channel; IBS-C, irritable bowel syndrome with constipation; PEG, polyethylene glycol; po, by mouth; qd, every day; qhs, every night.

modest. The most thoroughly studied strains are *Bifidobacterium* and *Lactobacillus* (most specifically *Lactobacillus casei Shirota*). Probiotics may be useful to relieve constipation, but the effect may depend on the probiotic dose, the bacterial strain used, and the population studied.[12] More investigation is needed to evaluate specific recommendations on dosing and strain type (see Chapter 102, Prescribing Probiotics).

Mind-Body Therapy

Behavioral Training in Childhood Constipation

Education for parents and children is an important component of treatment of functional constipation.[30] The child's fear of a painful bowel movement is the most common motivating factor for fecal retention.

> In childhood constipation, explain the physiologic changes that occur as a consequence of chronic constipation, including a diminished ability to recognize the need to stool or that soiling has occurred.[31] Explain that this condition is common and is multifactorial in origin for most children and stress the need to avoid demeaning or embarrassing the child.

Biofeedback

In an instrument-based training program, patients receive auditory or visual feedback, or both, to help train the pelvic floor and relax the anal sphincter while simulating defecation. Biofeedback also improves rectal sensation to assist in proper evacuation.[10] Biofeedback is the preferred treatment for pelvic floor dysfunction, in which it has a success rate of 70% to 81% and is superior to standard treatment (laxatives, fiber, and education).[32-34] Randomized controlled trials (RCTs) showed that five biofeedback sessions are more effective than continuous polyethylene glycol (PEG) administration for treating pelvic floor dysfunction, and benefits last at least 2 years.[35] Although biofeedback is not an effective treatment for slow-transit constipation, it should be considered first-line treatment for pelvic floor dysfunction.

Hypnotherapy

Substantial evidence supports the use of hypnotherapy in constipation-dependent irritable bowel syndrome, which has considerable overlap with functional constipation.[36]

No specific data exist on hypnotherapy for the treatment of functional constipation, however. Until more evidence is available, it may at times be reasonable to try this noninvasive treatment, especially in patients who have difficulty relaxing the pelvic musculature.

Botanicals

Aloe

Dried latex (aloe latex) from the lining of the inner leaf has been used historically for laxative use. One double-blind RCT of an herbal preparation of aloe, psyllium, and celandin showed a statistically significant advantage of the herbal preparation over placebo.[37] Which part of the preparation was most responsible for the effect was unclear, however, and this preparation is not available in the United States.[37] The anthraquinones in aloe act as a stimulant laxative. A typical dose of aloe is 50 mg aloe extract taken at bedtime.

Traditional Chinese Medicine

Although numerous RCTs have reviewed the approaches of various components of traditional Chinese medicine to constipation, high-level systematic reviews showed that methodologic flaws limit their interpretation.[38-40] Further research is needed to support the potential use of these components: Chinese herbs, moxibustion, and auriculotherapy.

Abdominal Massage

Some evidence indicates that abdominal massage may be a helpful technique in the treatment of constipation. One small 8-week RCT demonstrated an increase in bowel movement frequency but no decrease in laxative use.[41] The study investigators concluded that this approach could be an adjunctive therapy to the treatment of constipation, but because of its delayed effect, which may first be noted after several weeks, abdominal massage is considered a long-term treatment.

Pharmaceuticals

A wide array of laxatives is available to patients. The clinician must understand how to counsel patients on the appropriate use, risks, and optimal dosing of these agents. Dosing and further information on all agents for adults are provided in Table 45-3,[42] and similar information for children is given in Table 45-4.[43]

TABLE 45-4. Agents for Treatment of Constipation in Children

TYPE OF MEDICATION	SELECTED MEDICATIONS	RECOMMENDED DOSAGE FOR MAINTENANCE THERAPY
Bulk-forming laxatives (OTC)	Methylcellulose (Citrucel) powder	Older than 6 yr: 1–1.5 g/dose Older than 12 yr: 4–6 g/dose
Dietary fiber (OTC) supplement (no systemic absorption)	Psyllium (Metamucil, Perdiem, Serutan, Fiberall, Konsyl)	6–11 yr: ½–1 rounded teaspoon in 8 oz liquid one to three times/day Older than 12 yr: 1–2 rounded teaspoons or one to two packets or one to two wafers one to four times/day or five capsules up to three times/day taken with 8 oz liquid
Osmotic laxative (OTC)	Magnesium hydroxide (Milk of Magnesia [MOM]); liquid, tablets	Younger than 2 yr: 0.5 mL/kg/day 2–5 yr: 5–15 mL/day or in divided doses one to two tablets before bedtime 6–12 yr: 15–30 mL/day in divided doses or three to four tablets before bedtime Older than 12 yr: 30–60 mL/day or in divided doses six to eight tablets before bedtime
	Magnesium citrate	Younger than 6 yr: 2–4 mL/kg/day 6–12 yr: 100–150 mL/day Older than 12 yr: 150–300 mL/day, in single or divided doses
	Magnesium citrate	Used only for bowel cleanout
Lubricants	Mineral oil (OTC)	5–11 yr: 5–20 mL every day or in divided doses Older than 12 yr: 15–45 mL/day every day or in divided doses or 1–4 mL/kg/day
Fiber supplement (OTC); powder, chewable tablets, caplets	Benefiber (partially hydrolyzed guar gum): 2 teaspoon = 3 g soluble fiber	7–11 yr: ½–1 tablespoon one to three times/day 12 yr–adult: 1–2 tablespoon one to three times/day
Stool softeners (emollients)	Docusate (Colace); liquid, capsule, gel cap (OTC)	Infants and children younger than 3 yr: 10–40 mg/day in one to four divided doses 3–6 yr: 20–60 mg/day in one to four divided doses 6–12 yr: 40–150 mg/day in one to four divided doses Older than 12 yr: 50–400 mg/day in one to four divided doses
Stimulants	Senna (Senokot, Senna-Gen, Senolax, Ex-Lax); granules, syrup, tablets (OTC)	1–5 yr: 5–10 mL/day 5–15 yr: 10–20 mL/day One tablet = 3 mL/granules = 5 mL/syrup
Osmotic enema	Phosphate enema (OTC)	Younger than 2 yr: not recommended 2–11 yr: 2.25-oz pediatric enema Older than 11 yr: 4.5-oz adult enema
Osmotic laxative	MiraLax (polyethylene glycol); GlycoLax	12 yr or older: 17 g (up to measuring line on cap) in 8 oz of water Older than 2–11 yr: 8.5 g (halfway to measuring line on cap) in 4 oz of water
Stimulant laxative	Bisacodyl (Dulcolax) Dulcolax: 5-mg tablet, 10-mg suppository	Older than 2 yr: one half to one suppository or one to three tablets per dose; no liquid form Adolescents: four tablets maximum
Miscellaneous	Glycerin suppository	Children: one infant suppository one to two times/day Children >6 yr: one adult suppository
	Glycerin enema; Enemeez Mini Enema (ingredients: docusate, polyethylene glycol, glycerin)	5–10 mL glycerin in 500 mL normal saline solution 5-mL tubes: one enema/day
Osmotic laxative	Lactulose (Cephulac, Cholac, Chronulac, Constilac, Duphalac, Enulose, Lactulox); crystals, syrup	Infants: 2.5–10 mL/day individual doses Children: 0.6–0.6 mL/kg/dose three to four times/day or 40–90 mL/day in divided doses or 1–3 mL/kg/day in divided doses (maximum, 3 oz/day) Adults: 15–30 mL/day (maximum, 60 mL/day)
	Sorbitol	1–3 mL/kg/day in divided doses, 70% solution

From Tobias N, Mason D, Lutkenhoff M, et al. Management principles of organic causes of childhood constipation. *J Pediatr Health Care.* 2008;22:12-23; with data from Guandalini S, 2005; *Mosby's Pediatric Drug Consult.* St. Louis: Mosby; 2006; and Pediatric Lexi-Drugs Online. http://lexi.com; 2006 available to subscribers.
OTC, Over the counter.

Bulk-forming Laxatives

Bulk-forming laxatives work naturally to add bulk and water to stools so that stools can pass more easily through the intestines. These laxatives are safe to take every day and include oat bran, psyllium (e.g., Metamucil), polycarbophil (e.g., FiberCon), and methylcellulose (e.g., Citrucel). They are most useful in patients with normal-transit constipation, and one study showed that 80% of this subgroup had resolution of symptoms compared with 35% in the other subgroups.[13]

Stimulant Laxatives

Stimulant laxatives work by stimulating intestinal motility and secretion of water into the bowel. They generally take 6 to 12 hours to take effect, and they may cause abdominal cramping and diarrhea.[5] Products in this class include senna and bisacodyl. Given the poor quality of study design, the lack of placebo-controlled trials, and inconclusive results, the American College of Gastroenterology Chronic Constipation Task Force stated that data were insufficient to make a recommendation about the efficacy of stimulant laxatives for the management of chronic constipation, and available data suggested minimal benefit with these products.[44] These agents can also cause melanosis coli, they may be habit forming, and they have unknown long-term effects on the colon.

Osmotic Laxatives

Saline or osmotic laxatives are hyperosmolar agents that cause secretion of water into the intestinal lumen by osmotic activity. Some of the most commonly used osmotic laxatives are oral magnesium hydroxide (Milk of Magnesia), oral magnesium citrate, sodium biphosphate (Phospho-Soda), PEG, and lactulose.[5]

Data on the commonly used osmotic laxative, magnesium, are sparse.[45] Despite a lack of evidence, patients and physicians find magnesium helpful and use it routinely.[46]

Using magnesium citrate, 150-mg capsules, to help with constipation: Start with two capsules at bedtime and two in the morning. If no stool occurs the next morning after 4 days, add one capsule (three) at bedtime. Add one capsule to the evening dose every 4 days until a soft stool is produced each morning. One of the first side effects of magnesium is diarrhea. This helps prevent toxicity from taking too much magnesium. Stop at eight capsules (total: six at bedtime and two in the morning). Use magnesium-containing laxatives cautiously in patients with congestive heart failure and chronic renal insufficiency because of the potential for electrolyte imbalances.

PEG is superior to lactulose in terms of stool frequency per week, form of stool, relief of abdominal pain, and the need for additional products, both in children and adults.[47] Evidence is sufficient to support PEG as first-line laxative treatment in children, both for efficacy and for palatability.[48]

Stool Softeners

These agents, which include docusate sodium, act by lowering surface tension, thus allowing water to enter the bowel more readily. Although stool softeners are generally well tolerated, their efficacy remains in question.[49]

Emollient Laxatives

Mineral oil, the most common example in this category, works by coating and softening the stool. Scant evidence supports the use of mineral oil, which also may lead to depletion of fat-soluble vitamins and runs the risk of aspiration in older adults and children.[50]

Chloride Channel Activators

Lubiprostone is the first agent in this class that has been approved by the Food and Drug Administration for treatment of chronic constipation. This agent works through chloride channels to increase intestinal fluid secretion. Because nausea is the most common complaint, lubiprostone should be taken orally with food and should be avoided in pregnant women and children. Its safety has been studied for up to 48 weeks of use.

PREVENTION PRESCRIPTION

- Eat high amounts of fiber-rich foods, including beans, vegetables, fruits, whole grain cereals, and bran.
- Minimize high-fat, low-fiber foods such as processed foods, dairy products, and meat products.
- Drink an adequate amount of fluid each day to stay hydrated, and increase the amount of water if using higher doses of fiber.
- Engage in regular physical activity to avoid constipation.
- Adopt a good self-care and stress management program to avoid the impact of stress on gut function.
- Stay tuned to the body's natural signals to pass stool.
- Take advantage of the gastrocolic reflex and allow elimination to occur after meals.
- In young children, ensure adequate fiber as they transition to solid foods.

THERAPEUTIC REVIEW

In this summary of therapeutic options for the treatment of constipation, the interventions are presented in a ladder approach from the least to the most invasive options. Although patients with more moderate to severe constipation may travel up the ladder more quickly, the initial approaches are critical for all patients.

■ Adults

- Removal of exacerbating factors
  - Review the patient's medication list, and eliminate any medications that may be causing or exacerbating the condition.
- Behavioral training
  - If patients experience difficulty in expulsion of stool, they should be advised to place a support approximately 6 inches in height under their feet when they are sitting on a toilet seat, to flex the hips toward a squatting posture.
- Nutrition
  - Include a *gradually* increasing amount of fiber in the diet up to 20 to 25 g a day through fruits, vegetables, whole grain breads and unrefined cereals, flax, or bran.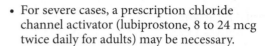
  - Encourage increased fluid intake, especially with the introduction of increased fiber in the diet.
- Movement
  - Encourage regular physical activity.
- Supplements
  - Consider adding a commercially packaged fiber supplement such as psyllium (Metamucil) or methylcellulose (Citrucel). Be sure to take it with at least 8 to 12 oz of liquid. Using less fluid can worsen constipation (see Table 45-3).
- Consider a probiotic strain of *Bifidobacterium* or *Lactobacillus* of at least 10^8 colony-forming units.
- Mind-body therapy
  - Address stress management skills.

- Biofeedback
  - In cases of pelvic floor dysfunction, this is a critical component of therapy.
- Pharmaceuticals
  - If the foregoing interventions do not resolve symptoms, consider osmotic laxatives with polyethylene glycol (17 to 34 g once or twice daily) as first-line therapy.
  - For severe cases, a prescription chloride channel activator (lubiprostone, 8 to 24 mcg twice daily for adults) may be necessary.

■ Children

- Behavioral training
  - Encourage daily sitting on the toilet, preferably after meals, and avoid embarrassing or punishing the child. Using a stool under the feet can also be used for children during toilet training.
- Removal of exacerbating factors
  - Consider a 4- to 6-week trial of elimination of dairy products.
- Nutrition
  - Ensure an adequate amount of fiber in the diet. Use the *age + 5 = daily grams of fiber* rule as a general guideline for dosing.
  - Increase fluid intake and, in particular, the amount of sorbitol-containing fruit juices (e.g., apple, pear) for osmotic effect.
- Movement
  - Encourage regular physical activity.
- Supplements
  - Consider adding a commercially packaged fiber supplement if necessary.
  - Consider a probiotic strain of *Bifidobacterium* or *Lactobacillus* of at least 10^8 colony-forming units.
- Pharmaceuticals
  - If these interventions do not resolve symptoms, consider osmotic laxatives with polyethylene glycol (0.5 to 4 teaspoons a day, depending on age) as first-line medical treatment (see Table 45-4).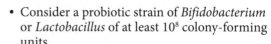

KEY WEB RESOURCES

The American College of Gastroenterology: http://www.acg.gi.org/
Patient Handout on Constipation: http://www.acg.gi.org/patients/pdfs/CommonGIProblems2.pdf
Mayo Clinic patient information on constipation in children: http://www.mayoclinic.com/health/constipation-in-children/DS01138

American Dietetic Association handout for Nutrition Therapy for Constipation: http://nutritioncaremanual.org/vault/editor/Docs/ConstipationNutritionTherapy_FINAL.pdf

References

References available online at expertconsult.com.

Section VIII Autoimmune Disorders

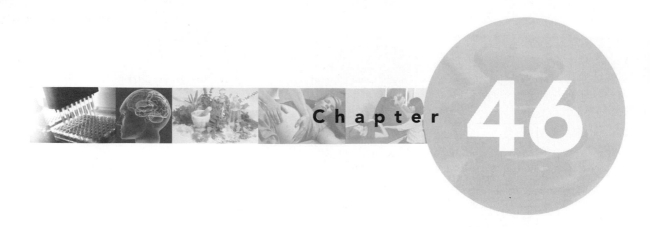

Chapter **46**

Fibromyalgia

Nancy J. Selfridge, MD, and Daniel Muller, MD, PhD

Pathophysiology

Diagnostic criteria for fibromyalgia syndrome (FM) have been reconsidered by Wolfe et al.[1] Chronic widespread pain of at least 3 months' duration remains a hallmark of the disease. However, tender points are no longer relevant. Rather, the number of painful areas reported by the patient in the past week is documented (Widespread Pain Index), and the severity of associated symptoms of fatigue, waking unrefreshed, and cognitive difficulties is assessed and scored (Symptom Severity Scale Score) (Fig. 46-1).[1] The previously noted increased prevalence in women may have been an artifact of using the tender point examination in the diagnostic criteria. When this criterion is eliminated, the difference in prevalence between women and men appears to be reduced.[2] This finding is further supported by previous research showing no impact of the menstrual cycle on symptoms of FM.[3] Increasing evidence supports the hypothesis that the pathophysiology of FM is the result of genetic and biologic factors, environmental triggers, and neurophysiologic abnormalities.[2,4]

Investigators generally agree that the increase in pain sensitivity that is typical of patients with FM is the result of central augmentation of sensory input and diminished central pain inhibitory function.[4,5] Among first-degree relatives of patients with FM, those who do not complain about any pain problems demonstrate increased pain sensitivity compared with healthy controls.[4] Careful history taking often reveals a stressful trigger event or period, such as an accident, a flulike illness, emotional stress, or overwork, preceding the onset of symptoms. Posttraumatic stress disorder often exists as a comorbidity.[6,7] Thus, the role of environment in the pathophysiology of FM cannot be downplayed and may help guide a clinician in creating treatment plans for patients with FM.

Functional magnetic imaging studies provide direct evidence of increased central pain sensitivity. In two similar studies, a nonpainful level of stimulation for control subjects was perceived as painful by patients with FM, and blood flow increased in specific brain areas shown to be associated with pain processing.[5,8]

Autonomic dysfunction is present in patients with FM and likely explains certain patient complaints, including worsening of symptoms with stress.[4] Several neuroendocrine and immune function alterations have been well documented. Cerebrospinal fluid levels of substance P are elevated, and additional abnormalities in the regulation of cortisol and in the adrenergic and serotonin systems have been noted.[9,10] Growth hormone secretion in response to exercise is impaired in patients with FM and appears to be linked to increases in proinflammatory cytokine levels after exercising.[11] The affinity and function of corticosteroid receptors on lymphocytes appear to be altered in FM, which changes the cellular response when lymphocytes are incubated with hormones in the laboratory.[12] Reports have noted decreased numbers of T cells expressing activation markers and a deficiency of interleukin-2 release.[13] Although these immunologic changes in FM do not meet criteria for an immunodeficiency or autoimmune disease, the lymphocyte abnormalities may reflect an altered response to hormone feedback, and altered patterns of cytokine release may contribute to fatigue and inflammatory-type symptoms. Although the foregoing alterations in immune and neuroendocrine function may not play a role in the etiology of FM, they may contribute to sustaining the symptoms.[14]

Alterations in the pituitary-adrenal axis in FM appear to be quite different from those seen in clinical depression; this finding is surprising given the frequent concurrence of the two conditions.[15] That comorbid depression in FM worsens both symptom severity and prognosis for FM sufferers has also become increasingly evident. Patients should be carefully screened for depression, and treatment for the depression should be aggressively pursued for optimum management of FM symptoms.[16]

In our practices, patients with FM often report having sensitive temperaments even before they developed physical symptoms. This quality of temperament is characterized by

FIGURE 46-1
Fibromyalgia clinical diagnostic criteria worksheet. (Data from Wolfe F, Clauw D, Fitzcharles M, et al. The American College of Rheumatology preliminary diagnostic criteria for fibromyalgia and measurement of symptoms severity. *Arthritis Care Res.* 2010;62:600–610.)

FIBROMYALGIA CLINICAL DIAGNOSTIC CRITERIA

1) Widespread Pain Index (WPI): Note the number areas in which the patient has had pain over the last week. In how many areas has the patient had pain? Score will be between 0 and 19.

- ☐ Shoulder girdle, Lt.
- ☐ Shoulder girdle, Rt.
- ☐ Hip (buttock, trochanter), Lt.
- ☐ Hip (buttock, trochanter), Rt.
- ☐ Jaw, Lt.
- ☐ Jaw, Rt.
- ☐ Upper Back
- ☐ Lower Back
- ☐ Upper Arm, Lt.
- ☐ Upper Arm, Rt.
- ☐ Upper Leg, Lt.
- ☐ Upper Leg, Rt.
- ☐ Chest
- ☐ Neck
- ☐ Abdomen
- ☐ Lower Arm, Lt.
- ☐ Lower Arm, Rt
- ☐ Lower Leg, Lt.
- ☐ Lower Leg, Rt.

Total WPI Score from above: __/19

2) Symptoms Severity Score (SS):
For the each of the three symptoms below, indicate the level of severity over the past week using the following scale:

0 = No problem
1 = Slight or mild problems; generally mild or intermittent
2 = Moderate; considerable problems; often present and/or at a moderate level
3 = Severe: pervasive, continuous, life-disturbing problems

Fatigue Score: __/3
Waking Unrefreshed Score: __/3
Cognitive Symptoms Score: __/3
Considering somatic symptoms* in general, indicate whether the patient has:
0 = No symptoms
1 = Few symptoms
2 = A moderate number
3 = A great deal of symptoms
Somatic Symptoms Score: __/3.
Total Symptom Severity Score: __/12 (Total of items under SS)

A patient satisfies clinical diagnostic criteria for fibromyalgia if the following 2 conditions are met:
1) WPU is =>7 and symptom severity score is =>5 OR WPI
   is between 3–6 and symptom severity score scale =>9.
2) Symptoms have been present for at least 3 months.

*Somatic symptoms for reference purposes: Muscle Pain, Irritable bowel syndrome, Fatigue/Tiredness, Thinking or remembering problem, Muscle Weakness, Headache, Pain/cramps in abdomen, Numbness/Tingling, Dizziness, Insomnia, Depression, Constipation, Pain in upper abdomen, Nausea, Nervousness, Chest pain, Blurred vision, Fever, Diarrhea, Dry mouth, Itching, Wheezing, Raynaud's, Hives/Welts, Ringing in ears, Vomiting, Heartburn, Oral ulcers, Loss/Change in taste, Seizures, Dry eyes, Shortness of breath, Loss of appetite, Rash, Sun sensitivity, Hearing difficulties, Easy bruising, Hair loss, Frequent urination, Painful urination, and Bladder spasms.

---

high levels of empathy, a tendency to be a caretaker, and a higher than normal sensitivity to environmental factors and emotional cues from others.[17,18] Such sensitivity may prove to be a genetically determined risk factor for FM. Thus, these patients may be the "canaries in the coal mine," by exhibiting FM symptoms not only in response to stressful physical and emotional trigger events but also as a consequence of living in a society that expects high productivity at the expense of self-care. High body mass index and reduced physical activity were found to be independent risk factors for FM.[19]

FM can coexist with and imitate various autoimmune diseases and some chronic infections such as Lyme disease and hepatitis C. Identification of such disorders as the cause of pain is important, to avoid treating these conditions as FM. For coexisting problems, the prudent approach is to pursue the difficult task of determining the contribution of FM to symptoms and thus avoid treating FM with escalating doses of immunosuppressive medications. Hypothyroidism must be ruled out as a treatable cause of similar symptoms. A thorough history should guide a clinician's evaluation. An exhaustive laboratory and imaging workup is seldom indicated.

Integrative Therapy

General Considerations

Patients with FM are often viewed as difficult and burdensome in busy practices. Our observation is that parallel syndromes (e.g., chronic chest wall pain, chronic abdominal pain of undetermined origin, irritable bowel syndrome, interstitial cystitis, chronic pelvic pain, dyspareunia, and vulvodynia) are found in many subspecialties. In our practice, patients with these problems often report experiences of feeling dismissed and disrespected in their encounters with physicians. FM is a syndrome diagnosis, and we have not yet pieced together from a large body of basic science and clinical research a pathophysiologic model to explain the onset and manifestations of FM unequivocally. Consequently, well-meaning physicians often tell patients that they "don't believe in fibromyalgia." We believe this is an error for two reasons. First, evidence of altered neurophysiology and immune function is clear, as previously mentioned, and some evidence indicates that at least one gene polymorphism may play a role.[4] Second, patients experience such statements as harmful and judgmental because they imply that the symptoms are not real or valid. Affirming the patient's experiences of what often appear to be bizarre symptoms, even when we cannot fully understand them, is important. Because allopathic interventions in FM demonstrate limited efficacy, we emphasize the importance of generous listening in the healing relationship. Patients experience this affirmation as therapeutic, and it is something that all of us can provide (see Chapter 3, The Healing Encounter). Until a sensible explanation for their symptoms is presented, many patients remain concerned that something is seriously wrong with them and that a diagnosis has been missed during evaluation. Explaining that current research points to a change in the way that the brain processes sensory information as the reason for physical symptoms can help patients significantly. The therapeutic benefit in this simple practice may be that listening to a patient's worry may help favorably alter the physiology of the stress response and thus help reduce autonomic dysfunction, pain sensitivity, and other symptoms.[20]

Nutrition

No specific diet has been shown to be effective for FM. An antiinflammatory diet, based on consumption of whole foods and avoidance of processed foods, may be helpful (see Chapter 86, The Antiinflammatory [Omega-3] Diet) and likely benefits the patient's health in a more general way. We emphasize complete avoidance of trans fats (partially hydrogenated oils, margarine, and shortening) and addressing a few common nutritional deficiencies in the standard U.S. diet. Increasing consumption of foods rich in omega-3 fatty acids, calcium, and antioxidants is strongly encouraged.

Exercise

A 2008 systematic review concluded that aerobic exercise has a beneficial effect on physical function and helps decrease some of the symptoms of FM.[21] Strength training may be helpful, but further study is needed. Adherence and attrition are problematic in many research studies on exercise in FM.

Many studies report a significant increase in symptoms of FM with exercise interventions.[21] In our experience, patients often report increased symptoms when they try to exercise. These symptoms are frequently severe and can lead to a cycle of muscle disuse. Not uncommonly, patients report feeling as though they "ran a marathon" after only a few minutes of exercise. Thus, though we support exercise prescriptions for all patients with FM, clinicians must think flexibly about exercise and be willing to revise recommendations based on patients' individual preferences and experiences. Pool exercise appears to provide as much physical fitness and symptom benefit as land exercise and may have additional benefit in improving psychological symptoms.[22] The Arthritis Foundation has information on exercise programs (1-800-283-7800). Tai chi proved beneficial in improving pain and quality of life in a randomized trial,[23] and a yoga intervention was similarly beneficial.[24] Even a cumulative daily 30 minutes of self-selected lifestyle physical activity provided clinically significant improvement in FM symptoms.[25]

Even though activation of the patient through exercise is a most desirable treatment goal, many patients demonstrate resistance. We have found it useful to explore with patients the reasons for resistance by asking, sometimes repeatedly over a long relationship, "What is hard about starting or sticking with an exercise program?" Severe postexercise pain is often cited, but many patients are similar to our usual primary care patients in that they have never embraced an active, exercise-oriented lifestyle. Exploring all the ways that one can move the body rather than selectively focusing on a structured exercise program can be useful. We often tell people to abandon the idea of "working out" and to think more in terms of "playing" or simply "moving." After all, who wants to have more work assigned to them? (See Chapter 90, Prescribing Movement Therapies.)

> Fibromyalgia research suggests that this is a disorder of central nervous system pain sensitization and augmentation associated with neuroendocrine and immune system abnormalities. Explaining this to patients may have some therapeutic benefit.

> Evidence suggests that Eastern movement practices such as tai chi, yoga, and qi gong, which contain strong meditative components, appear to be helpful for patients with fibromyalgia in reducing pain and improving function.

Bodywork

Physical therapy can restore muscle balance, and local therapy with stretching, heat, and cold can be beneficial. Massage therapy was shown to be more useful than transcutaneous nerve stimulation (TENS), but TENS was better than sham TENS and may be helpful in some cases.[26] Many patients with FM report that massage therapy is beneficial. Although strong evidence does not yet exist for bodywork as a treatment for FM symptoms, we believe that bodywork is generally safe and can be recommended as a modality to try as part of the self-caring that we wish to promote for our patients with FM.[27]

Mind-Body Therapy

Meditation

Meditation was shown to be helpful in FM in a few trials, although a randomized controlled trial showed dubious benefit.[28-31] Some of the studies documenting FM symptom improvement with Eastern movement therapies had a strong meditation component, which may contribute substantially to the efficacy of this type of exercise.[23,24,32] This training increases the ability to be comfortable in the present and thus can lessen the fear of future pain and, with practice, help transform the sensation of pain. Meditation may have additional, as yet undetermined benefits by favorably altering neurophysiology in patients with FM. Meditation is also useful for personal growth. We recommend training with a nondenominational teacher using a program such as Mindfulness Meditation, pioneered by Dr. Jon Kabat-Zinn.[33] If no teacher is available, tapes can be helpful. The focus on the present moment and the deep levels of personal inquiry cultivated in a meditation practice are actually quite useful to the practitioner working with patients with FM. Therefore, we also endorse this practice for people working with patients with FM.

Psychotherapeutic Interventions

One study found that 10 of 15 subjects responded to a 14-week cognitive-behavioral and relaxation training intervention; however, no patients remained improved on 4-year follow-up evaluation.[34] Electromyographic biofeedback, electroencephalographic biofeedback, and hypnotherapy have been helpful in controlled studies.[35-37] These modalities may be more acceptable for patients who reject meditation training and practice based on religious beliefs. A randomized, controlled study of an Affective Self-Awareness program involving a group intervention of emotional exploration through journaling and meditation demonstrated significant benefit for symptoms and perceived function in patients with FM.[38] Although more research is needed on mind-body interventions, we strongly believe that these generally low-risk and low-harm interventions should be part of every treatment plan for patients with FM. When patients are either not receptive to these interventions, or when patients experience increasing disability, it may be helpful to explore the following "four Rs."[39]

1. Roles: The patient's ability to maintain self-esteem through normal roles as spouse, parent, provider, and so on may be impaired. The work role requires careful evaluation and is often problematic in people who are becoming progressively more symptomatic and disabled. We focus on a simple question as a way of exploring where problems may exist: "In all your roles, are you living for your heart's desire?"
2. Reactions: The emotional reactions to events such as the diagnosis of FM or the events that trigger FM often follow a grieving process, as outlined by Kübler-Ross.[40] These stages are denial, anger, bargaining, depression, and acceptance. Patients are often stuck in anger and depression. In addition, the sensitive temperament of many of these patients is often associated with a greater physiologic reaction to all emotions.[17] Working with reactivity through a meditation practice and journaling can be uniquely helpful.
3. Relationships: The patient may often face seemingly insurmountable problems at home or in relationships at work that create repeated stress triggers for symptoms.
4. Resources: Psychotherapy, ministers, community programs, and self-help groups may each become a key for altering this progressive decrease in ability to function; guided imagery is particularly useful. Isolation and alienation clearly make patients symptomatically worse.

Emotional Awareness

Dr. John Sarno, a physiatrist at New York University, wrote a book that some patients may find useful.[41] Dr. Sarno referred to FM and many other chronic musculoskeletal pain disorders as "tension-myalgia syndromes." The short summary is that the patient may substitute physical pain for emotional pain. He believed that this simple realization can abrogate pain in certain persons. We have seen this happen in patients with FM and in those with chronic low back pain. Our experience suggests that a certain level of self-awareness and acceptance of the power of the mind are required to experience symptomatic improvement just with this insight. Selfridge wrote a book for patients that applied Dr. Sarno's principles to FM by using journaling, meditation, and other workbook format exercises.[42] Dr. Howard Schubiner and Dr. David Schechter produced excellent workbook programs around the same themes that can be very helpful and cost-effective ways for patients to pursue self-exploration (see Key Web Resources and Chapter 100, Emotional Awareness for Pain).

Acupuncture

One high-quality trial of electroacupuncture showed almost complete remission in 20%, satisfactory benefit in 40%, and no effects in 40% of patients with FM in a short-term study.[43] A review of several trials concluded that benefits were reduced over time.[44] A more recent study of acupuncture showed no significant effects compared with three sham acupuncture treatments.[45] However, a limitation of this more recent study was that it used directed acupuncture at fixed points. This study also pointed out the difficulty of blinding that may have affected the outcome of the original high-quality article on electroacupuncture.

Homeopathy

A controversial placebo-controlled trial of a homeopathic treatment (R toxicodendron 6c) decreased tender points.[46] A second study using individualized therapy for 3 months also showed modest positive effects compared with placebo.[47] We recommend referral to a homeopathic physician for evaluation and treatment. Homeopathic remedies are said not to work as well in the presence of certain pharmaceuticals (see Chapter 111, Therapeutic Homeopathy).

Supplements

Little evidence of efficacy exists for supplements and natural medicines in the treatment of FM. Further, some common supplement recommendations, such as the use of calcium supplements, selenium, and vitamin E, have come under scrutiny as possibly unsafe. Herbal and natural medicines potentially interact with one another and with prescription medication. Thus, we believe that a good peer-reviewed and frequently updated database (e.g., Natural Medicines Comprehensive Database; see Key Web Resources) be used by integrative clinicians to assess available evidence of efficacy and harm before recommending supplement and natural medicine therapy.

Omega-3 Fatty Acids
Use of omega-3 fatty acid supplementation in the form of pharmaceutical grade fish oil, 2 to 4 g daily in a single dose, may have a modest pain modulating effect for some patients and may help depression in some. In general, supplementation with omega-3 fatty acids may also lower cardiovascular risk and help to balance the predominance of proinflammatory omega-6 fatty acids in the typical U.S. diet.

Dosage
Give 2000 to 4000 mg daily in one dose.

Precautions
Omega-3 fatty acids inhibit platelet function and should be discontinued 2 weeks before elective surgical procedures. Use with caution along with anticoagulant therapy. Choose a pharmaceutical grade product to avoid heavy metal contamination.

Vitamin D
Low vitamin D levels appear to be epidemic in northern latitudes. Although the link between low vitamin D and the pain of FM remains unclear, evidence indicates that low vitamin D levels can be associated with widespread pain.[48] We have seen vitamin D–deficient patients eliminate all their FM-like pain when vitamin D levels become repleted. Thus, we recommend checking 25-(OH) vitamin D levels in patients at risk for vitamin D insufficiency and supplementing with vitamin D to keep blood levels optimal (40 to 100 ng/mL) year round. As a general rule, 1000 units of vitamin D will raise serum 25-(OH) vitamin D levels by approximately 10 ng/mL in adults. Although overdosing is unlikely, clinicians recommending vitamin D should be aware that vitamin D levels may be higher in our patients in the summer if they have sufficient skin exposure to sunlight.

Dosage
Cholecalciferol (vitamin D_3) oral supplements in capsule or liquid form are taken to attain a 25-(OH) vitamin D level of 40 to 100 ng/mL year round. Seasonal adjustment of dose may be necessary.

Precautions
Vitamin D is not to be used in patients who have primary hyperparathyroidism or granulomatous disease such as sarcoidosis because of the increased risk of hypercalcemia.

Magnesium
Magnesium may be helpful for some patients with FM, possibly through its muscle-relaxing properties, and it is quite safe.

Dosage
Give 400 to 750 mg of magnesium daily in a single dose.

Precautions
In higher doses, magnesium can cause abdominal cramping and increased frequency of stools.

S-Adenosylmethionine
S-adenosyl methionine (SAMe) was demonstrated to be safe and effective in alleviating depression in patients who failed to respond adequately to monotherapy with a selective serotonin reuptake inhibitor (SSRI), even though SAMe was given with the SSRI.[49] Although SAMe may have only a modest effect on other FM symptoms, this supplement can be helpful in patients who are reticent to use prescription pharmaceuticals to treat their FM and depressive symptoms.[50]

Dosage
The dose is 400 to 800 mg twice daily.

Precautions
SAMe can be activating and should not be taken close to bedtime because it can cause insomnia. It is expensive.

Botanicals

No adequate controlled trials of botanical treatments have been conducted. In anecdotal reports, many treatments lead to a benefit that wanes with time, a finding that may indicate a short-term placebo effect. Individual patients may benefit from trials of botanicals purported to be helpful for common symptoms of FM such as low energy, insomnia, and depressed mood.

Turmeric and Ginger
The use of turmeric and ginger in cooking with culinary doses may provide benefit for some patients. In these doses, these spices are likely safe and can be encouraged. When these agents are used in supplement doses, potential side effects and interactions must be considered.

Dosage
Ginger: As dried root, 1 g total per day, divided into two or three doses to start; increased to up to 4 g daily; as tea, 1 g of dried root steeped in 150 mL of boiling water for 5 to 10 minutes and strained; 1 cup up to four times daily
Turmeric: As powdered root, 0.5 to 1 g two or three times daily

Precautions
Because turmeric and ginger have platelet-inhibiting activities, they must be used with caution in people taking anticoagulant therapy and should be discontinued 2 weeks before elective surgical procedures. Both cause gallbladder contraction and may be problematic in patients with gallstones. Ginger may lower blood glucose levels.

Boswellia
Boswellia is an ayurvedic herb that has some documented antiinflammatory and analgesic effect. Although it has not been studied for FM, this herb may warrant a trial use in selected patients.

Dosage

The dose is 500 mg of standardized product three times daily.

Precautions

Platelet inhibition and increased bleeding risk are possibilities with this plant substance. Discontinue 2 weeks before elective surgical procedures.

St. John's Wort

For patients who need treatment for depression and do not wish to use prescription pharmaceuticals, St. John's wort may be helpful. It also has been shown to help with FM symptoms.

Dosage

As extract standardized to 0.3% hypericin content, use 300 mg up to three times daily; or as tea, steep 2 to 4 g of the dried herb in 150 mL of boiling water for 5 to 10 minutes and strain, and drink 1 cup up to three times daily.

Precautions

Multiple potential interactions with other drugs occur through stimulation of the cytochrome P-450 enzymes of the liver. The result is lower serum levels of drugs that are cleared by this mechanism.

Pharmaceuticals

Medications can be helpful for FM, although improvement in symptoms is seldom dramatic. Overall, 50% of patients will experience a 30% improvement in symptoms. Side effects are common and interfere with adherence.

Antidepressants

As previously stated, treating comorbid depression in patients with FM is in their best interest. Further, antidepressants can help improve sleep. Tricyclic antidepressants (TCAs) have been the gold standard of treatment because, in low doses, they tend to improve the sleep disturbance that is characteristic of FM. Side effects are often prohibitive in higher antidepressant doses. However, the newer dual serotonin and norepinephrine reuptake inhibitors (SNRIs) duloxetine and milnacipran compared quite favorably with amitriptyline in a meta-analysis, although the studies on amitriptyline were not of high quality.[51] All these drugs were better than placebo for mitigating FM pain and improving function, but the effect size for these improvements was not small. Thus, these newer agents may be good choices for patients with FM and depression because these drugs may help both problems.

Research on SSRIs for the pain of FM has shown mixed results.[52] When depression is present, these medications may be useful. Trazodone is a sedating antidepressant that we prefer when sleep disorder is present and when depressive symptoms are not prominent. One study demonstrated efficacy for FM, and in our practices, trazodone appears to be well tolerated by patients and often works in small doses.[53] Although cyclobenzaprine is not an antidepressant, it is closely related to the TCAs, and meta-analyses have supported its use in FM.[54] The practitioner should develop a familiarity with several different antidepressants to feel comfortable managing the myriad side effects. In addition, patients sometimes add St. John's wort to their regimens, because St. John's wort

has been shown to be beneficial for mild to moderate depression. Serotonin syndrome is a distinct risk when this natural medicine is taken with SSRIs or with SNRIs. Be sure to ask specifically about the use of St. John's wort in patients who are taking these prescription antidepressants.

Tricyclic Antidepressant Dosage

Amitriptyline: 5 to 10 mg nightly initially, titrating upward as needed

Nortriptyline: 50 mg nightly initially, titrating upward as needed

Tricyclic Antidepressant Precautions

Excessive sedation, anticholinergic effects, and hypotension may occur.

Selective Serotonin Reuptake Inhibitor Dosage

Fluoxetine: 5 to 20 mg initially, titrating upward as needed

Paroxetine: 10 to 20 mg daily initially, titrating upward as needed

Selective Serotonin Reuptake Inhibitor Precautions

Activation or sedation, induction of mania, hot flushes and sweating, weight gain, sexual dysfunction, and multiple potential drug interactions are possible. Paroxetine has been associated with discontinuation syndrome (withdrawal).

Trazodone Dosage

Give 25 to 50 mg nightly, titrating upward to 300 mg or until patient reports good sleep and no excess morning grogginess.

Trazodone Precautions

Oversedation, orthostatic hypotension, morning grogginess, and vivid dreams may occur.

Cyclobenzaprine Dosage

Give 2.5 to 10 mg initially, up to 40 daily, in divided doses.

Cyclobenzaprine Precautions

Excessive sedation and an increase in "mental fogging" may occur.

Dual Norepinephrine and Serotonin Reuptake Inhibitor Dosage

Duloxetine: 30 mg once daily for 1 week, then increasing to 60 mg daily

Milnacipran: started at 12.5 mg once daily on the first day, and increased by 12.5 to 25 mg daily for the first week until 50 mg twice daily dosing attained (100 mg twice daily may ultimately be necessary for symptom relief)

Dual Norepinephrine and Serotonin Reuptake Inhibitor Precautions

Precautions are potentially the same as for TCAs and SSRIs.

Nonsteroidal Antiinflammatory Drugs

Nonsteroidal antiinflammatory drugs (NSAIDs) had a poor showing in a controlled trial testing their analgesic efficiency in FM.[55] Because of the limited evidence of efficacy and the potential for adverse effects, particularly with long-term use, the wise approach may be to discourage NSAID use in FM and instead to suggest supplements or botanicals such as omega-3 fatty acids, ginger, turmeric, or Boswellia for their modest analgesic effects.

Anticonvulsants

Gabapentin has been used off-label for FM because of its indication for use in chronic pain. This agent appears safe and efficacious for FM.[56] A similar pharmaceutical, pregabalin, appeared to be effective compared with other newer drugs for FM in a meta-analysis.[57] Both drugs often cause somnolence and dizziness. Significant weight gain with pregabalin is not uncommon and can interfere with adherence. Because significant weight gain may also increase the risk of other chronic diseases such as type 2 diabetes, this side effect cannot be considered trivial.

◼ Dosage

Gabapentin: started 300 mg once daily and increased by one tablet to twice per day, then three times per day as tolerated; maximum dose, 3600 mg daily

Pregabalin: started with 50 mg three times daily, then increased over 7 days to the maximum of 600 mg per day

◼ Precautions

Gabapentin may cause sedation, dizziness, cognitive impairment, and leukopenia, whereas pregabalin may cause sedation, dizziness, weight gain, and thrombocytopenia.

Analgesics: Tramadol

One controlled trial showed a beneficial effect of tramadol.[58] The use of tramadol with antidepressants can cause serotonin syndrome. Tramadol can also cause excessive sedation. Tramadol may be useful in allowing a 4-week drug holiday from antidepressant therapy, to reset neural receptors, and in intermittent therapy for exacerbations. In general, we avoid the long-term use of benzodiazepines and narcotics because of a lack of evidence of efficacy and because of potential safety and addiction issues.

◼ Dosage

Tramadol: 50 to 400 mg daily in divided doses.

◼ Precautions

Sedation, habituation, and serotonin syndrome with antidepressants may occur.

Soft Tissue Injection

The use of subcutaneous tender point injections may be helpful, particularly if these injections are given into palpable areas of muscle spasm. We rarely feel the need to do this procedure, given all the other potential tools that can help patients. These injections are often given as 0.5 to 1 mL of 1% lidocaine per site, although dry needling or saline may work as well. The use of corticosteroids for injection should be avoided.

Therapies to Consider

Adequate studies have not been conducted on the roles of traditional Chinese, Ayurvedic, or spiritual medicine in the management of FM. We counsel our patients to learn about several different modalities and then record in a journal their feelings about these modalities. Then, after discussion, patients can visit

practitioners of the selected therapies to explore the approaches further. If the economic burden is not too great, addition of the therapeutic modality may be in order. Another area of potential benefit for patients with FM is emerging from the growing field of energy psychology. Emotional Freedom Techniques (EFT), or tapping, as it is sometimes called, and Eye Movement Desensitization and Reprocessing (EMDR) are showing anecdotal evidence of value in alleviating physical and psychological symptoms in patients with FM (see Chapter 101, Energy Psychology). How these therapies work remains to be determined, but they are simple and quite harmless, and EFT can be taught to the patient to use at home for self-treatment. A good description and several anecdotes about EFT can be reviewed on the Web site www.emofree.com. Patients may similarly benefit from reading about FM, sensitivity, and EFT.[59] Descriptions of EMDR, its history, and evidence of efficacy can be reviewed at www.emdr.com. These therapies may bypass cognitive level processes to diminish or eliminate the central nervous system connection between the neurophysiology of traumatic memory and emotions and the physiology of bodily felt symptoms. We hope the future will bring research directed at examining in depth the efficacy and possible mechanisms of these therapies.

> Mainstays of a treatment plan for fibromyalgia include an exercise prescription, mind-body types of interventions, treatment of comorbid depression, and judicious trials of other complementary and alternative medicine modalities and allopathic pharmaceuticals. However, *every* treatment plan should be individualized and flexible.

PREVENTION PRESCRIPTION

No proven preventive strategy exists for FM, but the following may help to fortify a susceptible individual against the "slings and arrows of outrageous fortune":

- ◼ Exercise and maintain a normal body weight. Combine aerobics, strength training, and stretching. Consider tai chi and yoga. Make exercise a time to play.
- ◼ Eat a healthy whole foods diet, rich in plant sources of antioxidants. Avoid trans fats and excess caffeine, alcohol, and sugars.
- ◼ Honor your temperament and sensitivity. Learn more about yourself and your unique needs and values in work and relationships.[59,60]
- ◼ Journal to stay in touch with your inner feelings and to give voice to negative feelings and stressful events when they arise.
- ◼ Put yourself high on the list of things to take care of each day. Consider regular massage therapy or other bodywork to this end.
- ◼ Learn to meditate, and practice daily. We recommend a mindfulness-based stress reduction course.
- ◼ Allow yourself creative outlets such as art, music, dancing, or creative writing.
- ◼ Live for your own heart's desires, and allow yourself time and space to figure out what these are.
- ◼ If you get stuck in life, find a good psychotherapist.

THERAPEUTIC REVIEW

This summary provides the most helpful options for treating FM symptoms. FM has no documented "cure." Studies have reported an improvement in 5% to 53% of patients, although 47% to 100% of patients continue to meet criteria for FM 2 to 5 years after diagnosis.[61] Only a few patients experience complete resolution of symptoms. Despite these dismal statistics, we cannot emphasize enough the therapeutic benefit of generous listening and affirming the patient's felt experience. In our practices, approximately 75% of patients will report "some" relief of symptoms with treatment. Better response to treatment is seen in younger patients and in those with continued employment, supportive families, and an absence of litigation or affective disorders.[62]

Nutrition

- Encourage a whole foods antiinflammatory diet with ample plant antioxidants, omega-3 fatty acids, and minerals.

- Counsel avoidance of trans fats and simple sugars.

Exercise

- Write an exercise prescription tailored to the patient's individual preferences and fitness starting point.

- Encourage aerobic exercise, strength training, and stretching.

- Suggest warm-water exercise classes, tai chi, yoga, and qi gong.

- Even 30 minutes of daily cumulative lifestyle activity is beneficial.

Mind-Body Therapy

- Encourage mindfulness meditation training and daily practice.

- Suggest reading *The Mindbody Prescription*[41] and working through one of the available mind-body workbook programs.

- Suggest journaling about emotions and stressors to help increase affective self-awareness.

- Refer for cognitive-behavioral therapy if roles and relationships are problematic or if the patient feels "stuck."

- Consider biofeedback and hypnotherapy as alternatives.

Acupuncture

- If the patient can afford treatments, encourage a five-session trial.

Bodywork

- Suggest regular massage therapy or other bodywork as a way of endorsing self-care.

Supplements

- Omega-3 fatty acids (fish oil): 2000 to 4000 mg daily
- Magnesium: 400 to 750 mg daily
- Vitamin D_3 (cholecalciferol) to maintain 25-(OH) vitamin D levels higher than 40 ng/mL and lower than 100 ng/mL year round
- S-adenosylmethionine: 800 mg twice daily

Botanicals

- Turmeric, ground root: 500 to 1000 mg two to three times daily
- Ginger, ground root: 1 g to 4 g total daily divided into two to three doses
- Boswellia: 250 to 500 mg three times daily
- St. John's wort: 300 mg three times daily

Pharmaceuticals

- Amitriptyline: 5 to 50 mg nightly as tolerated
- Nortriptyline: 25 to 100 mg daily
- Fluoxetine: 10 to 20 mg daily
- Paroxetine: 10 to 30 mg daily
- Duloxetine: 30 mg for 1 week, increasing to 60 mg thereafter
- Milnacipran: 12.5 mg daily to start, increasing to 50 mg twice daily by the end of the first week; 100 mg twice daily may be needed
- Cyclobenzaprine: 2.5 mg daily, titrating to 40 mg daily in divided doses as needed
- Trazodone: 25 to 300 mg nightly as needed
- Gabapentin: 300 mg initially, increasing slowly to a maximum of 3600 mg daily as tolerated
- Pregabalin: 50 mg three times daily, increasing to total of 600 mg per day over 7 days
- Tramadol: 50 to 400 mg daily in divided doses

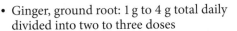
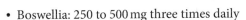

KEY WEB RESOURCES

http://www.unlearnyourpain.com	Dr. Howard Schubiner's Mind Body Program (workbook on emotional awareness and mind-body syndrome for patients with fibromyalgia)
http://www.mindbodymedicine.com	Dr. David Schechter's Mind Body Medicine (workbook on emotional awareness and mind-body syndrome for patients with fibromyalgia)
http://www.emofree.com	Emotional Freedom Therapy (tapping) for fibromyalgia
http://www.emdr.com	Eye movement desensitization and deprocessing for fibromyalgia
http://www.med.ufl.edu/rheum/FMSarticles/article25.htm	Diagnostic summary of fibromyalgia from the University of Florida
http://naturaldatabase.therapeuticresearch.com	Natural Medicines Comprehensive Database

References

References are available online at expertconsult.com.

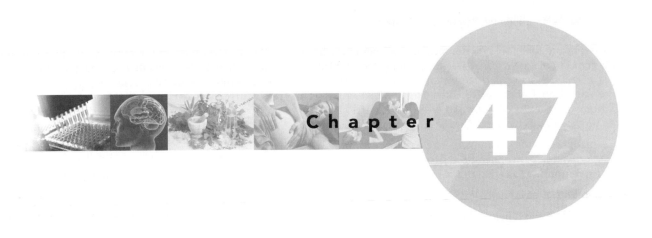

Chapter 47

Chronic Fatigue Spectrum

Jacob Teitelbaum, MD

Pathophysiology

Chronic fatigue syndrome (CFS) and fibromyalgia syndrome (FMS) are two common names for an overlapping spectrum of disabling syndromes. FMS alone is estimated to affect more than 3 to 6 million people in the United States, and it causes more disability than rheumatoid arthritis.[1] The prevalence of these disorders has also increased dramatically from 2% of the population to 4% to 8% worldwide since 2000.[2-4] Myofascial pain syndrome (MPS) affects many millions more. Although we still have much to learn, effective treatment is now available for most of these patients.[5,6]

CFS, FMS, and MPS represent a syndrome, a spectrum of processes with a common end point. Because the syndromes affect major control systems in the body, myriad symptoms do not seem to be related initially. Research suggests mitochondrial and hypothalamic dysfunction as common denominators in these syndromes.[7-10] Dysfunction of hormonal, sleep, and autonomic control (all centered in the hypothalamus) and energy production centers can explain the many symptoms and the reason that most patients have a similar set of complaints.

To make it easier to explain to patients, I use the model of a circuit breaker in a house: "If the energy demands on the body are more than it can meet, the body trips the circuit breaker. The ensuing fatigue forces the person to use less energy and thus protects him or her from harm. Conversely, although a circuit breaker may protect the circuitry in the home, it does little good if you do not know how to turn it back on or that it even exists."

This analogy actually reflects what occurs. Research in genetic mitochondrial diseases shows not simply myopathic changes, but also marked hypothalamic disruption. Because the hypothalamus controls sleep, the hormonal and autonomic systems, and temperature regulation, it has higher energy needs for its size than other areas. Therefore, as energy stores are depleted, hypothalamic dysfunction occurs early and results in the disordered sleep, autonomic dysfunction, low body temperatures, and hormonal dysfunctions commonly seen in these syndromes. In addition, inadequate energy stores in muscle result in muscle shortening (think of rigor mortis) and pain, which are further accentuated by the loss of deep sleep. Reduction in stages 3 to 4 of deep sleep results in secondary drops in growth hormone and tissue repair. As discussed later, disrupted sleep causes pain. Therefore, restoring adequate energy production through nutritional, hormonal, and sleep support and eliminating the stresses that overuse energy (e.g., infections, situational stresses) restore function in the hypothalamic "circuit breaker" and also allow muscles to release, thus allowing pain to resolve. Our placebo-controlled study showed that when this was done, 91% of patients improved, with an average 90% improvement in quality of life, and most patients no longer qualified as having FMS by the end of 3 months ($P < .0001$ versus placebo).[6]

> Chronic fatigue syndrome, fibromyalgia, and to some degree myofascial pain syndrome reflect an energy crisis in the body. It is similar to blowing a fuse in your home. These disorders can have many causes, they protect the body from further harm, but they dramatically reduce function. Causes include infections, disrupted sleep, pregnancy, hormonal deficiencies, toxins, and other physical or situational stresses. The "blown fuse" is the hypothalamus—resulting in poor sleep and in hormonal, autonomic, and temperature dysregulation.

Diagnosis

The criteria for diagnosing CFS are readily available elsewhere. What is important is that these criteria were meant to be used for research and therefore have stringent exclusion criteria to create a "pure" research cohort. These exclusionary criteria eliminate approximately 80% to 90% of patients who clinically have CFS, and therefore I do not recommend them for clinical use. For example, anyone who was significantly depressed in the past, even 30 years earlier, can technically never develop CFS. The American College of Rheumatology (ACR) criteria for FMS are more useful clinically. According to the ACR, a person can be classified as having FMS if he or she has the following:

- A history of widespread pain. The patient must have been experiencing pain or achiness, steady or intermittent, for at least 3 months. At times, the pain must have been present

  - On both the right and left sides of the body

  - Both above and below the waist

  - At the midbody (e.g., for example, in the neck, midchest, or midback, including a headache)

- Pain on pressing at least 11 of the 18 spots on the body that are known as tender points

The presence of another clinical disorder, such as arthritis, does not rule out a diagnosis of FMS.[11] Although the tender point examination takes time to master, it clinically adds little and is in the process of being eliminated in the newer 2010 ACR diagnostic criteria.[12]

A simpler approach is available that is very effective clinically. If the patient has the paradox of severe fatigue combined with insomnia (someone who is exhausted should sleep all night) and does not have severe primary depression, and if these symptoms do not go away with vacation, he or she will have a CFS-related process. If the patient also has widespread pain, FMS is probably present as well. Both disorders respond well to proper treatment, as discussed later. Alternatively, clinicians may wish to ask the patient whether he or she has the symptoms described in Table 47-1. In addition to strengthening the diagnosis of CFS and FMS, asking about the symptoms summarized in Table 47-1 shows the patient that the health care provider understands this illness.

Although a matter of disagreement in the classical ACR criteria, clinically it is clear that FMS may be secondary to other causes. Secondary causes may be suggested by laboratory findings such as elevations in erythrocyte sedimentation rate, alkaline phosphatase, creatine kinase, rheumatoid factor, antinuclear antibody (1:640 or higher), or thyroid-stimulating hormone (TSH). Depression is less likely to be a secondary cause of FMS and CFS symptoms in patients who express frustration over not having the energy to do the things, as opposed to a lack of interest. These patients likely are simply frustrated by their illness and are not depressed. MPS shares many of the metabolic features seen in FMS and

TABLE 47-1. Symptoms of Chronic Fatigue

- Severe fatigue lasting over 4 months
- Feeling worse the day after exercise
- Diffuse, often migratory, achiness
- Disordered sleep
- Difficulty with word finding and substitution, poor short-term memory, and poor concentration, often described as "brain fog"
- Bowel dysfunction (Many people with irritable bowel syndrome [IBS] or spastic colon have chronic fatigue syndrome or fibromyalgia syndrome, and their IBS also resolves with treatment.)
- Recurrent infections such as sore throats, nasal congestion, or sinusitis

often resolves with the treatments discussed in this chapter, but evaluation for structural problems should also be done for this more localized process.

Current research and clinical experience show that these patients have a mix of disordered sleep, hormonal insufficiencies, low body temperature, and autonomic dysfunction with low blood pressure and neurally mediated hypotension. This mix makes sense because the hypothalamus is the major control center for all four of these functions.

> *Simple diagnostic approach:* If the patient has the paradox of severe fatigue combined with insomnia (if someone is exhausted, he or she should sleep all night), and these symptoms do not go away during a vacation, the likely diagnosis is chronic fatigue syndrome–related process. If the patient also has widespread pain, fibromyalgia is probably present as well. Both conditions respond well to proper treatment, as discussed in this chapter.

Anything that results in inadequate energy production or energy needs greater than the body's production ability can trigger hypothalamic dysfunction. This includes infections, disrupted sleep, pregnancy, hormonal deficiencies, and other physical or situational stresses. Although still controversial, a large body of research also strongly suggests mitochondrial dysfunction as a unifying theory in CFS and FMS.[10] Some viral infections have been shown to suppress both mitochondrial function and hypothalamic function. As noted earlier, in several genetic mitochondrial diseases, severe hypothalamic damage is seen. This is likely because the hypothalamus has high energy needs.

Integrative Therapy

Fortunately, two studies (including our recent randomized controlled trial)[5,6] showed an average 90% improvement rate with the SHINE protocol. The acronym SHINE stands for treating Sleep, Hormonal dysfunction, Infections, Nutritional support, and Exercise as able. Patients with fatigue and insomnia coupled with widespread pain can be seen as having a body-wide "energy crisis." Treating with the SHINE approach may help them.

> Two studies (including our randomized controlled study) showed an average 90% improvement rate when the SHINE protocol was used to treat chronic fatigue syndrome and fibromyalgia. SHINE stands for Sleep, Hormonal support, Infections, Nutritional support, and Exercise as able.

As discussed earlier, using the acronym SHINE simplifies treatment of these patients. Therefore, the treatment recommendations in this chapter are structured using this model.

Sleep

SHINE has been editorialized as "an excellent and powerfully effective part of the standard of practice for treatment of people who suffer from FMS and MPS."[13] A foundation of CFS and FMS is sleep disorder.[14] Many patients can sleep solidly only for 3 to 5 hours a night and have multiple awakenings. Even more problematic is the loss of deep stage 3 and 4 "restorative" sleep. Using natural therapies or medications that increase deep restorative sleep, so that the patient has 7 to 9 hours of solid sleep without waking or hangover, is critical. Continue to adjust the treatments each night until the patient is sleeping 8 hours a night without a hangover.

Most addictive sleep remedies, except for clonazepam (Klonopin) and alprazolam (Xanax), actually decrease the time that is spent in deep sleep and can worsen FMS. Therefore, they are not recommended. More than 20 natural and prescription sleep aids can be tried safely and effectively in FMS and CFS. For a more detailed list, see my free "long form" treatment protocol (discussed in the next subsection).

Natural Sleep Remedies
I recommend you begin with the following:

- Valerian: 200 mg
- Passionflower: 90 mg
- L-Theanine: 50 mg
- Hops: 30 mg
- Wild lettuce: 18 mg
- Jamaican dogwood: 12 mg

These are all combined in a product called the Revitalizing Sleep Formula by Integrative Therapeutics (see Key Web Resources). Patients (and anyone with poor sleep) can take one to four capsules at bedtime. These six botanicals can help muscle pain and libido, as well as improving sleep.[15-19] The effectiveness of valerian increases with continued use, but approximately 5% to 10% of patients will actually find it stimulating and not be able to use it for sleep. Although I am discriminating about the products I recommend, I have a policy of not taking money from any natural or pharmaceutical companies, and 100% of the royalties for my products also go to charity.

- The dose of melatonin is 0.5 to 1 mg at bedtime.
- The dose of 5-hydroxytryptophan (5-HTP) is 200 to 400 mg, taken at night. This naturally stimulates serotonin, but it may take 6 to 12 weeks to be fully effective. Do not give more than 200 mg a day if the patient is taking antidepressants, because 5-HTP theoretically could drive serotonin too high. 5-HTP can also help with pain and weight loss, at 300 mg a day for at least 3 months.
- Give calcium and magnesium at bedtime because these help sleep.
- The smell of lavender helps sleep, so place two to three sprays on the pillow at bedtime.

Pharmaceutical Sleep Aids
If natural remedies are not adequate to result in at least 8 hours a night of sleep, consider these medications:

- Zolpidem (Ambien): 5 or 10 mg at bedtime. This medication is very helpful for most patients and is my first choice among the sleep medications. Patients can take an extra 5 to 10 mg in the middle of the night if they wake.

- Gabapentin (Neurontin): 100 to 900 mg at bedtime can help sleep, pain, and restless legs syndrome.
- Cyclobenzaprine (Flexeril): 5 to 10 mg
- Trazodone: 50 mg. Use one half to six tablets at bedtime. Use this medication first if anxiety is a major problem.
- Amitriptyline (Elavil) or doxepin: 10 mg. Use one half to five tablets at bedtime. Amitriptyline can cause weight gain and can exacerbate restless legs syndrome.

Some patients will sleep well with the Revitalizing Sleep Formula herbal preparation or 5 to 10 mg of zolpidem, whereas others will require all the foregoing treatments combined. Because the malfunctioning hypothalamus controls sleep and the muscle pain also interferes with sleep, it is often necessary and appropriate to use multiple sleep aids. Tizanidine (Zanaflex), pregabalin (Lyrica), and many other nonbenzodiazepines can also help sleep. Because of next-day sedation and the independent half-life of each medication, patients with CFS and FMS do better by combining low doses of several medications than by taking a high dose of one.

> These patients must have at least 8 hours of deep sleep a night. Because of the hypothalamic dysfunction, they often need aggressive assistance to treat their insomnia. Begin with herbal mixes such as the Revitalizing Sleep Formula, and then add in magnesium, 5-hydroxytryptophan, and melatonin at bedtime as needed. If additional pharmaceutical support is needed, I recommend beginning with zolpidem, trazodone, or gabapentin.

Although less common, three other sleep disturbances must be considered and, if present, treated. The first is sleep apnea. This condition should especially be suspected if the patient snores and is overweight or hypertensive. If two of these three conditions are present and the patient does not improve with treatment, I would consider a sleep apnea study. Ask the sleep laboratory also to look for upper airway resistance syndrome. Preapproval from the patient's insurance company is recommended because the test usually costs $1500 to $2600. Some patients prefer to do their own inexpensive screening by videotaping themselves for one night during sleep.

Sleep apnea is treated with weight loss and nasal continuous positive airway pressure. A sleep study or a videotape or DVD of the patient while sleeping will also detect restless legs syndrome, which is also fairly common in FMS.[20] It is treated with supplemental magnesium, by keeping ferritin levels higher than 60 ng/mL,[21] and with zolpidem, clonazepam, or gabapentin.

Hormonal Dysfunction

Hormonal imbalance is associated with FMS. Sources of this dysfunction include hypothalamic dysfunction and autoimmune processes such as Hashimoto thyroiditis. When the hypothalamus is not able to regulate hormone balance efficiently, medical management can do so until hypothalamic function is restored. When focusing on achieving hormonal balance, standard laboratory testing aimed at identifying a single hormone deficiency is less effective. For example, increased hormone binding to carrier proteins is often present in CFS and FMS. Therefore, total hormone levels are often normal, whereas the active hormone levels are low. This situation creates a functional deficiency in the patient. In addition, most blood tests use 2 standard deviations to define blood test norms. By definition, only the lowest or highest 2.5% of the population is in the abnormal (treatment) range. This does not work well if more than 2.5% of the population has a problem. For example, as many as 20% of women older than 60 years are estimated to have antithyroid peroxidase antibodies and may be hypothyroid. Other tests use late signs of deficiency such as anemia for iron or vitamin B_{12} levels to define an abnormal laboratory value.

The goal in the management of CFS and FMS is to restore optimal function while keeping laboratory values in the normal range for safety. One way to convey the difference between the "normal" range based on 2 standard deviations and the optimal range that the patient would maintain if he or she did not have CFS or FMS is as follows:

"Pretend your laboratory test uses 2 standard deviations to diagnose a 'shoe problem.' If you accidentally put on someone else's shoes and had on a size 12 when you wore a size 5, the normal range derived from the standard deviation would indicate you had absolutely no problem. You would insist the shoes did not fit, although your shoe size would be in the normal range. Similarly, if you lost your shoes, the doctor would pick any shoes out of the normal range pile and expect them to fit you."

Thyroid Function

Suboptimal thyroid function is very common and very important. Because thyroid-binding globulin function and conversion of thyroxine (T_4) to triiodothyronine (T_3) may be altered in CFS and FMS, checking a free T_4 level is important. Treating *all* patients with chronic myalgia with thyroid hormone replacement is also important if their T_4 blood levels are lower than even the 50th percentile of normal (Janet Travell, personal communication). Many patients with CFS or FMS also have difficulty in converting T_4, which is fairly inactive, to T_3, the active hormone. Additionally, T_3 receptor resistance may be present, thus requiring higher levels.[22,23]

Synthroid has only inactive T_4, whereas desiccated thyroid (Armour Thyroid), or a compounded combination of T_4 and T_3, has both inactive T_4 and active T_3. Many clinicians give an empirical trial of desiccated thyroid, or T_4 plus T_3, 0.5 to 3 grains every morning, adjusted to the dose that feels best to the patient as long as the free T_4 is not higher than the upper limit of normal. I am likely to recommend an empirical trial of thyroid hormone therapy in most patients with CFS or FMS.

Physicians generally interpret a low-normal TSH (i.e., 0.5 to 0.95) as a confirmation of euthyroidism. The rules are different in CFS and FMS, however. In this setting, hypothalamic hypothyroidism is common, and the patient's TSH can be low, normal, or high.[24] This is why I recommend an empirical therapeutic trial of thyroid hormone treatment in the presence of chronic fatigue or myalgias despite normal laboratory test results. The inadequacy of thyroid testing is further suggested by studies that show the following:

- Most patients with suspected thyroid problems have normal blood study results.[25,26]

- When patients with symptoms of hypothyroidism and normal laboratory values were treated with thyroid (in this study, levothyroxine at an average dose of 120 mcg every day), many improved significantly.[25]

- Having a TSH level of 0.5 to 1.4 is associated with a 69% lower risk of myocardial infarction–related death than is having a TSH of 2.5 to 3.5 (to put this in perspective, statins for primary prevention decrease heart attack death by only approximately 1%).[26]

Additional recommendations are as follows:

- Adjust the thyroid dose clinically by using the dose that feels the best to the patient, as long as the free T_4 test does not show hyperthyroidism. Do *not* use TSH or T_3 levels to monitor thyroid replacement.[27] Because of the hypothalamic suppression, TSH levels may be low despite inadequate hormonal dosing. Because T_3 is largely produced and functions intracellularly, we do not have normal ranges for exogenously given T_3. Therefore, I predominantly use clinical signs and symptoms and free T_4 levels to monitor therapy.

- Make sure that the patient does not take any iron supplements within 6 hours or calcium supplements within 2 hours of the morning thyroid dose or the thyroid hormone will not be absorbed. Have the patient take the iron between 2:00 and 6:00 PM on an empty stomach and away from any hormone treatments.

- Thyroid supplementation can increase a patient's cortisol metabolism and unmask a case of subclinical adrenal insufficiency. A patient who feels worse while taking low-dose thyroid replacement may need adrenal support as well.

> Because of the hypothalamic dysfunction, hormonal deficiencies are common despite normal blood test results. If symptoms suggest deficiencies, treat hypothyroidism with thyroid replacement (a therapeutic trial is warranted in most of these patients), treat adrenal insufficiency (suggested by low blood pressure, irritability when hungry or hypoglycemic, and recurrent respiratory infections and sore throats) with hydrocortisone and natural adrenal support, and low estrogen or testosterone levels with natural hormones.

Adrenal Insufficiency

The hypothalamic-pituitary-adrenal axis does not function well in CFS and FMS.[7,28,29] This dysfunction and adrenal exhaustion from chronic or severe stress are two key causes of inadequate adrenal function. Because early researchers studying adrenal insufficiency and cortisol were not aware of the physiologic doses for cortisol, they used high doses, and their patients developed severe complications. These side effects are *not* seen with adrenal glandular, herbal, or nutritional support or with physiologic doses of hydrocortisone (Cortef), that is, up to 20 mg a day.[30] A 20-mg dose of hydrocortisone is approximately equivalent in potency to 4 to 5 mg of prednisone. Unfortunately, many hypoadrenal patients are treated only when they are ready to develop an addisonian crisis. Research and clinical experience show that this approach misses many hypoadrenal patients.[5,6,30,31]

Symptoms of an underactive adrenal gland include weakness, hypotension, dizziness, sugar cravings with irritability when hungry, and recurrent infections, all of which are common in CFS and FMS. I recommend natural adrenal support for most patients with CFS or FMS, especially if they have any of the foregoing symptoms. The needed natural therapies include the following:

- Adrenal glandulars. These contain most of the "building blocks" needed for adrenal repair.

- Licorice extract, which contains glycyrrhizin, a compound that raises adrenal hormone levels. Licorice also protects against stomach irritation, which can occur with hydrocortisone and occasionally even with glandulars.

- Pantothenic acid, vitamin C, vitamin B_6, betaine, and tyrosine: These nutrients are critical for adrenal function and energy, and high doses are often needed.

All these elements are present in a glandular and herbal preparation for adrenal support called Adrenal Stress End (from Integrative Therapeutics; see Key Web Resources), which is very safe and effective. I usually prescribe one to two capsules each morning (or one to two in the morning and one at noon), and the capsules can be taken along with hydrocortisone. This approach helps both symptoms and adrenal repair.

I also consider a therapeutic trial of 5 to 15 mg hydrocortisone in the morning, 2.5 to 10 mg at lunchtime, and 0 to 2.5 mg at 4:00 PM (maximum of 20 mg a day). Most patients find that 5 to 7.5 mg of hydrocortisone each morning plus 2.5 to 5 mg at noon to be optimal (the equivalent of 1.5 to 3 mg prednisone daily). Alternatively, sustained-release compounded hydrocortisone can be used. After keeping the patient on the initial dose for 2 to 4 weeks, adjust the dose up to a maximum of 20 mg daily or, if no benefit has been evident, taper it off. Adjust the hydrocortisone to the lowest dose that feels the best. Give most of the hydrocortisone in the morning and at lunchtime. I often tell my patients to take the last dose, 2.5 to 5 mg, no later than 4:00 PM. Otherwise, the hydrocortisone may keep the patient up at night. After 9 to 18 months, taper the hydrocortisone off over a period of 1 to 4 months. If symptoms recur after the hydrocortisone is stopped, continue treatment with the lowest optimal dose.

Different approaches to treatment are possible, and more is not better. High-dose cortisol taken at night worsens already disrupted sleep patterns. In a study by McKenzie et al,[32] patients received a very high dose of approximately 25 to 35 mg of hydrocortisone daily, which disrupted patients' sleep ($P \le .02$).[32] Although the investigators did not treat the disrupted sleep, most patients still felt somewhat better while taking the treatment. A small percentage of the patients had significantly suppressed posttreatment cosyntropin (Cortrosyn) test results, without complications, and the investigators therefore, I believe incorrectly, recommended against using any dose of hydrocortisone in CFS and FMS.[33] Our study did not show adrenal suppression with lower hydrocortisone dosing.[6] Dr. Jefferies,[30,31] with thousands of patient-years' experience in using low-dose hydrocortisone, recommended an empirical trial of 20 mg a day in all patients with severe, unexplained fatigue and found this to be quite safe for long-term use. Research and clinical experience suggest that using hydrocortisone at 20 mg a day or less in patients with CFS or FMS is safe and often very helpful.[34] An extensive review of the safety of long-term prednisone in doses lower than 5 mg a day in patients with rheumatoid arthritis patients also supported the safety of this approach.[35]

Dehydroepiandrosterone

Dehydroepiandrosterone (DHEA) is a major adrenal hormone that has been dubbed a "fountain of youth" hormone.[36] DHEA is stored as DHEA-sulfate (DHEA-S), and levels of free DHEA fluctuate markedly throughout the day. Therefore, I recommend checking DHEA-S levels and not DHEA levels. Many patients with CFS or FMS have suboptimal DHEA-S levels, and the benefit of treatment is sometimes dramatic. Most women need 5 to 25 mg a day, and most men need 25 to 50 mg a day. I use the middle of the normal range for a 29-year-old patient and keep the DHEA-S level at 150 to 180 mcg/dL in women and 350 to 480 mcg/dL in men. Too high a dose in women can cause elevated testosterone and can result in acne, darkening of facial hair, and insulin resistance.

Estrogen Deficiency

Although we are trained to diagnose menopause by cessation of menstrual periods, hot flashes, and elevated follicle-stimulating hormone and luteinizing hormone, these are late findings. Estrogen deficiency often begins many years before and may coincide with the onset of FMS.[37] To compound the problem, research done by Sarrel showed that most women who have a hysterectomy, even with the ovaries left intact, develop estrogen deficiency within 6 months to 2 years after the surgical procedure.[37]

To summarize, the initial symptoms of estrogen deficiency are poor sleep, poor libido, brain fog, achiness, premenstrual syndrome, and decreased neurotransmitter function. If a woman's symptoms of CFS and FMS are worse at ovulation and the 10 days before her period (times when estrogen levels are dropping), then a trial of estrogen is warranted. Although a birth control pill can be used, side effects of bleeding and fluid retention are common for the first 3 to 4 months. Bio-identical hormones are better tolerated and are likely safer. Therefore, natural 17-beta-estradiol as (Estrace, Climara) patches may be preferable. The usual dose of estradiol patch (Climara) is one 0.05- to 0.1-mg patch a week, and the usual dose of oral estradiol (Estrace) is 0.5 to 1 mg a day, adjusted to what feels best to the patient. I prefer to use Biest, a compounded natural estrogen that combines estriol with estradiol, at a dose of 0.1 to 0.5 mg a day.

Unlike estradiol, early data on estriol suggest that it does not raise breast cancer risk and may actually lower it (Jonathan Wright, MD, personal communication). In addition, estriol also has immune-modulating and other properties that can be beneficial in FMS. In the absence of a hysterectomy, progesterone should be added to prevent uterine cancer. If you are prescribing the Biest cream, have the pharmacist make a combination of Biest plus progesterone 30 to 50 mg, in addition to testosterone 0.5 to 1 mg all in 0.2 mL of cream (which can be applied to the mucosal surface of the labia each evening). When the creams are applied to the skin instead of to the mucosal surfaces, patients often stop absorbing the cream after a few years of use. Clinical experience is suggesting that the lower doses of testosterone and Biest recommended here may be preferable to the higher doses used in the past.

Testosterone Deficiency

Testosterone deficiency is important in both men and women. Clinicians should check a free testosterone level rather than total testosterone, because free testosterone is a better measure of testosterone function. If the age-adjusted free testosterone is low or low normal (lowest quartile), a trial of treatment is often very helpful. Among my patients with CFS or FMS, 70% of men and many women have free testosterone levels in the lowest quartile, whereas their total testosterone levels are usually normal. One study found that treating low testosterone in women decreased FMS pain. Only natural testosterone should be used for treatment. In men, topical testosterone (AndroGel) works fairly well. Applying 25 to 50 mg once daily is a good dose in men, and 0.5 to 1 mg is recommended in women.

Despite the concerns about athletes who use very high levels of synthetic testosterone, research shows that raising low testosterone levels in men by using natural testosterone actually results in lower cholesterol, decreased angina and depression, and improved diabetes.[38]

Immune Dysfunction and Infections

Immune dysfunction is part of the process. In fact, the other name for CFS is chronic fatigue and *immune dysfunction* syndrome (CFIDS). Literally dozens of infections are present in CFIDS and FMS, including viral, parasitic, *Candida*, and antibiotic-sensitive infections. Most of these infections seem to resolve on their own as the immune system recovers with the SHINE protocol.

Some infections do require treatment. I treat all patients with CFS for *Candida* and treat all parasites based on testing stool for ova and parasites. Dysbiosis may also need to be treated.

Chronic sinusitis responds poorly to antibiotics but responds well to antifungals. Conservative measures such as saline nasal rinsing and avoiding refined carbohydrates are more appropriate than are long-term antibiotics.[39] Our experience has shown, and research at the Mayo Clinic in Rochester, Minnesota also suggests, that chronic sinusitis is predominantly caused by a sensitivity reaction to yeast, with secondary bacterial infections resulting from swelling and obstruction. Most of our patients find that their chronic sinusitis goes away on the yeast protocol discussed here. Avoiding antibiotics also decreases the risk of secondary fungal overgrowth in the sinuses and gastrointestinal tract.

When initially treating sinusitis and for acute flares, our patients find that a compounded nose spray containing a combination of itraconazole, xylitol, mupirocin, very-low-dose bismuth, and cortisone can be very helpful. This nose spray is available from the ITC Compounding and Natural Wellness Pharmacy (888-349-5453). Ask for the Sinusitis Spray, which ITC can mail to the patient after the prescription is called into the pharmacy. The dose is one to two sprays in each nostril twice a day for 2 to 6 weeks. Ordering the one bottle is adequate for most patients. Although the chronic sinusitis often resolves after 6 weeks of fluconazole (Diflucan) and the sinus spray, the patient can use the spray as needed if symptoms recur. If sinusitis or spastic colon symptoms recur, however, the patient likely is also having regrowth of *Candida* in the gut, and if other CFS symptoms are recurring, I consider a 6-week retreatment with fluconazole. I treat all patients with CFS or FMS for *Candida* and do not find additional *Candida* testing to be necessary, reliable, or helpful.

Yeast Infection

Treatment of yeast infection in patients with CFS or FMS consists of the following:

1. *Acidophilus* bacteria, 4 to 8 billion colony-forming units per day, can help to restore normal bowel flora. In addition, patients must avoid sugar because yeast grows by fermenting sugar. This includes food juices, which have as much sugar as sodas. To improve compliance (and show compassion), I do allow patients to have chocolate.
2. Anti-Yeast (a mix of natural antifungals by Nutri Elements) is taken for 5 months. This contains coconut oil powder (50% caprylic acid), 240 mg; oregano powder extract, 200 mg; *Uva ursi* extract, 120 mg; garlic powder (deodorized), 240 mg; grapefruit seed extract, 160 mg; berberine sulfate, 80 mg; and olive leaf extract, 200 mg.
3. After 4 weeks on the Anti-Yeast, add 200 mg of fluconazole (Diflucan) each day for 6 weeks, and repeat the 200 mg per day for another 6 weeks if needed.

> Because of the immune suppression, most of these patients must be treated empirically for yeast/fungal/*Candida* overgrowth. Nasal congestion or sinusitis and spastic colon are often caused by *Candida* and resolve with the treatments discussed earlier.

In patients with low-grade fevers or chronic lung congestion, occult infections such as with *Chlamydia* and *Mycoplasma fermentans* incognitus are being found. Empirical therapy with doxycycline 100 mg twice daily for 6 months to 2 years, during nystatin therapy, can be helpful in unique cases. Research is showing that human herpesvirus 6, cytomegalovirus, and Epstein-Barr virus are also sometimes active in CFS and FMS.

Nutritional Support

Patients with CFS or FMS are often nutritionally deficient. This occurs because of (1) malabsorption from bowel infections, (2) increased needs because of the illness, and (3) inadequate diet. B-complex vitamins, ribose, magnesium, iron, coenzyme Q10, malic acid, and carnitine are essential for mitochondrial function.[10,40] These nutrients are also critical for many other processes. Although blood testing is not reliable or necessary for most nutrients, I do recommend checking vitamin B_{12}, iron, total iron-binding capacity, and ferritin levels.

I begin patients with CFS or FMS on the nutritional regimen described next.

Multivitamin

A high-quality multivitamin suited for their needs should contain at least 50 mg of B-complex vitamins, 150 mg of magnesium glycinate, 900 mg of malic acid, 600 units of vitamin

D, 500 mg of vitamin C, 15 mg of zinc, 50 mcg of selenium, 200 mcg of chromium, and amino acids. A powdered vitamin is generally better tolerated, better absorbed, and less expensive than tablets.

D-Ribose

Because CFS and FMS represent an energy crisis, patients must have what is needed for optimal mitochondrial function. If you remember your biochemistry training on the Krebs citric acid cycle, the key energy molecules are adenosine triphosphate, reduced flavin adenine dinucleotide, and reduced nicotinamide-adenine dinucleotide. These molecules are made up predominantly of ribose in addition to B-complex vitamins and adenosine. Some of my patients improved markedly with improved energy and decreased pain when they were given one scoop (5 g) of ribose three times a day for 3 weeks, followed by one scoop twice a day (Corvalen, Bioenergy Life Science; see Key Web Resources). Two studies with a total of 298 patients with CFS or FMS that were conducted by 53 health practitioners showed an average 61% increase in energy at 3 weeks.[41,42] If ribose is going to help, improvement is usually seen within 1 month (a 280-g container is a fair therapeutic trial). Ribose is a very powerful new addition to our therapeutic armamentarium for treating fatigue, pain, and cardiac dysfunction.

■ Dosage

Give 5 g (one scoop of Corvalen) of ribose three times a day for 3 weeks, followed by 5 g twice a day.

■ Precautions

D-Ribose is natural, quite safe, tastes good (sweet like sugar), and is very low in side effects. Rarely, it can cause a mild drop in blood glucose as it stimulates energy production. If patients feel overenergized or hyperactive when they take ribose, simply have them take it with a meal or lower the dose. This response also suggests the need for adrenal support.

> Widespread nutritional deficiencies are common, and no single tablet will address them all. Patients should consider a good multiple vitamin, with the addition of ribose at 5 g two to three times daily, coenzyme Q10 at 200 mg daily, and acetyl-L-carnitine at 1000 mg daily for approximately 4 to 9 months, then PRN.

Iron

If the patient's iron percent saturation is less than 22% or the ferritin is less than 60 mg/mL, supplement with iron (taken on an empty stomach because food markedly decreases iron absorption). Iron should not be taken within 6 hours of thyroid hormone because iron blocks thyroid absorption. Continue treatment until the ferritin level is greater than 60 mg/mL and the iron percent saturation is higher than 22%.

Vitamin B₁₂

If the vitamin B_{12} level is less than 540 pg/mL, I recommend vitamin B_{12} injections, 3000 mcg intramuscularly three times a week for 15 weeks, then as needed based on the patient's clinical response. Studies of CFS are showing absent or near-absent cerebrospinal fluid vitamin B_{12} levels despite normal serum vitamin B_{12} levels.[43] Metabolic evidence of vitamin B_{12} deficiency is seen even at levels of 540 pg/mL or more.[44] Severe neuropsychiatric changes are also seen in vitamin B_{12} deficiency even at levels of 300 pg/mL (a level higher than 209 is technically normal).[45] As an editorial in the *New England Journal of Medicine* suggested, the old-time doctors may have been right about giving vitamin B_{12} shots.[46] Compounding pharmacies can make vitamin B_{12} at 3000 mcg/mL concentrations. I use hydroxycobalamin, although methylcobalamin may be more effective, albeit more expensive.

Coenzyme Q10

The dose of coenzyme Q10 is 200 mg a day. This conditionally essential nutrient improves energy production in patients with CFS or FMS. It is especially critical in patients taking statin-family cholesterol treatments (which can actually cause FMS pain and which I avoid using in patients with FMS).

Acetyl-L-Carnitine

Treating with acetyl-L-carnitine, at 500 mg twice daily for 4 months, is strongly recommended. Biopsies show that intracellular levels are routinely low in patients with CFS. This not only causes weakness, but also contributes to the average 32-lb weight gain seen in CFS or FMS.

Diet

No one diet is best for everyone. I recommend that patients eat those things that leave them feeling the best (which is not always the same as what they crave). Having said this, however, most patients with CFS find that they do best with a high-protein, low-carbohydrate diet. They should avoid sugar, as well as excessive caffeine (which is a loan shark for energy) and excess alcohol. Warn the patient about a possible 7- to 10-day withdrawal period when eliminating sugar and caffeine. If patients have low blood pressure or orthostatic dizziness, increasing salt intake markedly should also be considered.

Exercise as Able

Patients must prevent deconditioning. Conversely, because of decreased energy production, too much exercise will result in postexertional fatigue, often leaving patients bedridden for a day or so afterward. Therefore, I recommend that patients see how far they can comfortably walk each day and initially walk that amount. After 2 to 3 months on the SHINE protocol, patients will find they can usually begin conditioning and increase the walk by a minute every 1 to 2 days, as able. Using a pedometer is helpful, and the goal is reaching 10,000 steps a day. Patients should increase the exercise level only as is comfortable to them.

Mind-Body Therapy

Psychological Well-Being

Many illnesses are associated with various psychological profiles. In CFS and FMS, a common profile is a "mega-type-A" overachiever who, because of childhood low self-esteem, overachieves to gain approval. These patients tend to be perfectionists and have difficulties protecting their boundaries—that is, they say yes to requests when they feel like saying no. Instead of responding to their bodies' signal of fatigue by resting, they redouble their efforts. Taking time to rest and getting and staying out of abusive personal and work environments are critical. As they start to feel better, these patients need to be instructed to take it slowly and not go back to the toxic environment or level of overfunctioning that made them sick in the first place. A simplified approach is for patients to learn to say no to things that feel bad.

> Although the metabolic problems require treatment, most chronic illnesses will not fully resolve unless mind-body issues are also treated. In chronic fatigue syndrome and fibromyalgia, this means that the patients must stop seeking approval and must learn to say no when they feel like it. Teach patients to do and keep their attention on what feels good from a centered place. In summary, follow your bliss!

PREVENTION PRESCRIPTION

- Nutrition: Avoid excess sugar and receive optimal nutritional support. Patients usually feel best with a high-protein, low-carbohydrate diet.
- Sleep: Encourage 8 hours of sleep a night.
- Exercise by doing things that are fun and feel good.
- Follow your bliss! If you are chronically doing things that feel bad to you, your body is unlikely to support you in the long term. Develop the habit of only doing, and keep your attention on, things that feel good from a centered place (e.g., the heart or solar plexus center).

THERAPEUTIC REVIEW

Treat chronic fatigue syndrome, fibromyalgia syndrome, and myofascial pain by restoring energy levels metabolically. Do this by using the SHINE protocol summarized here:

■ Sleep

- Adjust the dose of sleeping aids as needed to obtain 8 to 9 hours of solid sleep without waking or hangover.
- Supplements
  - Consider the following botanicals to help with sleep: valerian, 200 mg; passionflower, 90 mg; L-theanine, 50 mg; hops, 30 mg; piscidia, 12 mg; and wild lettuce, 28 mg. A product that contains these ingredients is the Revitalizing Sleep Formula (by Integrative Therapeutics): Take two to four capsules each night 30 to 90 minutes before bedtime. This formula can also be used during the day for anxiety.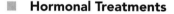
  - 5-Hydroxytryptophan: 200 to 400 mg at night
  - Melatonin: 0.5 mg at bedtime
- Pharmaceuticals
  - Zolpidem: 10 mg, one half to one at bedtime
  - Trazodone: 50 mg, one half to six at bedtime
  - Clonazepam: 0.5 to 1 mg
  - Gabapentin: 300 mg, one to two capsules at bedtime. It also helps relieve pain and restless legs syndrome.

■ Hormonal Treatments

- Desiccated thyroid (triiodothyronine [T_3] plus thyroxine [T_4]): Follow free T_4 to make sure of appropriate dosing and be careful not to overtreat. Otherwise, dose for clinical effect. For Armour Thyroid, 30 mg = 0.5 grains. Adjust dose based on clinical signs and symptoms.
- Hydrocortisone, 5-mg tablets: one half to two and one half tablet(s) at breakfast, one half to one tablet at lunch, and 0 to one half tablet at 4 PM. Use the lowest dose that feels the best to the patient.
- Dehydroepiandrosterone (DHEA): Keep DHEA-sulfate levels between 140 and 180 mcg/dL for female patients and between 300 and 500 mcg/dL for male patients. A common dose for women is 5 to 25 mg, and a common dose for men is 25 to 50 mg daily.
- Biest (female patients), 0.1 to 0.5 mg; plus progesterone, 30 to 50 mg; plus testosterone, 0.5 to 1.0 mg, all in 0.2 mL of cream. Apply 0.2 mL of cream to inner labia at bedtime.
- Testosterone (male patients): topical patch or compounded, 25 to 50 mg every morning

▪ Infections: Anti-Yeast Treatments

- Avoidance of sweets: This includes sucrose, glucose, fructose, and corn syrup. Encourage whole fruits with fiber and avoid sweetened fruit juices. Consider stevia as a sugar substitute.

- Probiotics: Consider a *Lactobacillus acidophilus*–containing probiotic twice daily for 5 months and then consider taking one daily to maintain a healthy bowel.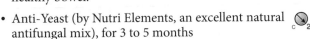

- Anti-Yeast (by Nutri Elements, an excellent natural antifungal mix), for 3 to 5 months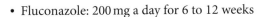

- Fluconazole: 200 mg a day for 6 to 12 weeks

▪ Nutritional Treatments

- Encourage a high-protein, low-carbohydrate diet rich in fruits and vegetables.

- Recommend a high-quality multiple vitamin that contains at least:

  - B-complex vitamin: 50 mg
  - Magnesium: 150 mg combined with malic acid, 900 mg
  - Vitamin D: 600 units
  - Vitamin C: 500 mg

- Zinc: 15 mg

- Selenium, 50 mcg

- One product that contains these ingredients is Energy Revitalization System Powder, made by Integrative Therapeutics: one half to one scoop a day (as feels best). If diarrhea occurs, mix the powder with milk or start with a lower dose and work your way up to the dose that feels best, or divide the daily dose into smaller doses and take two to three times a day.

- Mitochondrial energy treatments: Use these for 3 to 9 months.

- D-Ribose (Corvalen, from 1-866-267-8253; www.Corvalen.com): one scoop of powder three times a day for 3 weeks, then twice a day

- Coenzyme Q10: 200 mg a day

- Acetyl-L-carnitine: 500 mg twice a day for 3 months

▪ Exercise

- Encourage the use of a pedometer, with a goal of 10,000 steps a day. The patient should increase the exercise level only as is comfortable, and increasing it too quickly can cause a flare of fatigue.

KEY WEB RESOURCES

Integrative Therapeutics, Inc.: http://www.integrativeinc.com/Home.aspx.	This is the company that I respect most in the natural supplements industry. They carry the Energy Revitalization System vitamin powder and B-complex vitamins and the Revitalizing Sleep Formula.*
Bioenergy Life Science: http://www.douglaslabs.com/corvalen	This is a good resource for Corvalen D-ribose. ITC Compounding and Natural Wellness Pharmacy: http://www.itcpharmacy.com/. This company (888-663-4224) is an excellent compounding pharmacy that ships worldwide and is a good source for natural hormones, pain creams, and the sinusitis nose spray.
Vitality 101!: www.endfatigue.com	This is my Web site, and I invite you to use the free "Symptom and Lab Analysis" program. E-mail me at endfatigue@aol.com for the free "Treatment Tools" file. These will dramatically simplify patient care.

---

*Editor's Note: Dr. Teitelbaum is an unpaid member of medical board of Integrative Therapeutics. Although he promotes a number of products in this chapter that can be obtained on his Web site, he claims to donate all proceeds to charity.

References

References are available online at expertconsult.com.

Chapter 48

Rheumatoid Arthritis

Daniel Muller, MD, PhD

Pathophysiology

Rheumatoid arthritis (RA) is likely caused by a pathologic immune response in a genetically predisposed person to an environmental insult, probably a viral or bacterial infection.[1] Epidemiologic studies show that genes encoding the class II major histocompatibility antigens are linked to clinical features of RA. The HLA-DR4 and DR1 proteins present foreign and self-antigens to T cells. These molecules are presumed to play a direct role in the etiology of this autoimmune disease by presenting an "arthritogenic" viral or bacterial antigen to T cells. However, no organism has been definitively linked to the etiology of RA. Antibiotic therapy with minocycline is helpful in mild disease, although minocycline may act through direct immunomodulatory or antiinflammatory effects rather than through antibacterial activity. Other genes of the immune, endocrine, and neural systems may contribute to the pathogenesis of RA. The precise pathophysiologic cascade is not yet defined. RA is an autoimmune inflammatory disease in which immunosuppressive drugs constitute the mainstay of therapy. Certain cytokines, such as tumor necrosis factor (TNF), interleukin (IL)-1 and IL-6, appear to play important roles because inhibitors of these molecules decrease disease activity.[2-5] Similarly, the importance of the roles of cell surface molecules on B and T cells can be shown when these molecules are used as targets for immunomodulatory therapy.[6,7]

Nonsteroidal antiinflammatory drugs (NSAIDs) act to inhibit the enzymes that produce inflammatory prostaglandins, particularly thromboxanes and leukotrienes. The newer NSAIDs preferentially inhibit the cyclooxygenase (COX)-2 enzyme that produces certain of these inflammatory molecules. Unfortunately, these COX-2 inhibitors may have increased thrombotic and hence cardiovascular risks, and they may not offer any increased gastroprotection.[8,9] Celecoxib (Celebrex) is still on the market, albeit with increased warnings; other COX-2 inhibitors have been withdrawn from the market. Omega-3 fatty acids and certain botanicals such as ginger and turmeric also may act through decreasing the production or activity of inflammatory prostaglandins.[10-14]

The neural, endocrine, and immune systems all share communication molecules that interact extensively. Molecules from the hypothalamic-pituitary-adrenal axis, particularly cortisol and corticotropin-releasing factor, and from the sympathetic-adrenal-medullary system are linked to disease activity in RA.[15] Corticosteroid drugs have powerful disease-suppressing activity, with equally powerful adverse side effects such as osteoporosis.[16,17] Prolactin and the estrogenic and androgenic sex hormones have been postulated to play roles as well. Other environmental factors such as nutrition, coffee, and tobacco also may contribute to the increased risk of RA.[18,19]

Stress and psychological factors have been linked to the etiology of RA and to disease exacerbations.[20] In one study, psychological factors and depression accounted for at least 20% of disability in patients with RA, greater than the 14% attributable to articular signs and symptoms.[21] In another study, helplessness had a direct effect on disease activity.[22]

Data point to an increased risk for cardiovascular disease in patients with inflammatory and autoimmune diseases. Current recommendations include controlling underlying disease, monitoring the ratio of total cholesterol to high-density lipoprotein, use of statins and angiotensin-converting enzyme inhibitors for antiinflammatory activity, and caution with the use of COX-2 inhibitors and steroids.[23]

Diagnosis

In 2010, new criteria for diagnosing RA were approved by the American College of Rheumatology and the European League against Rheumatism (ACR/EULAR) (Fig 48-1).[24] Definite RA is confirmed by the presence of synovitis in at least one joint, the absence of a better alternative diagnosis, and a score of 6 or greater (out of a possible 10) from four domains: number and site of involved joints (0 to 5), rheumatoid factor or anticyclic citrullinated peptide (0 to 3), elevated sedimentation rate or C-reactive protein (0 to 1), and duration greater than 6 weeks (0 to 1). Prior criteria had been

FIGURE 48-1
American College of Rheumatology and European League against Rheumatism (ACR/EULAR) diagnostic criteria for rheumatoid arthritis (RA): 6 out of 10 points or more suggest the diagnosis of RA. ACPA, anticyclic citrullinated peptide; CRP, C-reactive protein; ESR, erythrocyte sedimentation rate; Rf, rheumatoid factor. From Aletaha D, Neogi T, Silman AJ, et al. 2010 Rheumatoid arthritis classification criteria: an American College of Rheumatology/European League against Rheumatism collaborative initiative. *Arthritis Rheum.* 2010;62:2569–2581.

Joint involvement (0–5)	
1 med/large joint	0
2–10 med/large joints	1
1–3 small joints	2
4–10 small joints	3
>10 joints (at least 1 small)	5
Serology (0–3)	
Neither Rf nor ACPA positive	0
At least one test low positive	2
At least one test high positive	3
Duration of synovitis (0–1)	
<6 weeks	0
>6 weeks	1
Acute phase reactants (0–1)	
Neither CRP nor ESR abnormal	0
Abnormal CRP or abnormal ESR	1

criticized for insensitivity to early RA disease. The newer criteria are directed toward instituting more aggressive therapy sooner. Official diagnostic criteria are used for inclusion into studies and do not always reflect diagnoses made in the clinic. In practice, a diagnosis of RA may include findings included in earlier diagnostic criteria, such as duration of morning stiffness greater than 1 hour, subcutaneous nodules, x-ray changes, and histologic changes in biopsies of synovial tissue. Further, these ACR/EULAR diagnostic criteria do not include newer methods of diagnosis such as ultrasound and magnetic resonance imaging. Earlier treatment of RA results in better long-term outcomes. These criteria will be used to test whether more aggressive treatment will be helpful in disease in which joint damage has not yet taken place.

Integrative Therapy

Exercise

Joint pain can inhibit activity and lead to muscle disuse and atrophy. In turn, muscle atrophy can lead to decreased stability of joints. Light weight training can maintain or even increase muscle strength around joints and can lead to increased joint stability. Stretching muscles can help decrease flexion contractures. Aerobic exercise improves mood, decreases fatigue, and helps control weight gain. Water exercise can be helpful because it is less stressful on joints, but weight training and walking work better to decrease bone loss (osteoporosis). The Arthritis Foundation has information on programs (see Key Web Resources). Asian exercise disciplines such as tai

chi and yoga can also be beneficial. A form of tai chi called the range of motion (ROM) dance is particularly suited to persons with disabilities (see Key Web Resources).

Physical and Occupational Therapy

Physical therapy and occupational therapy programs can be invaluable in the treatment of RA. Goals are to improve range of motion and strengthen muscles. Joint protection from deformities can be aided by education and use of splints, orthotics, ambulatory aids, and other devices. Massage and local heat and cold applications can decrease inflammation, increase circulation, and relax muscles.

Mind-Body Therapy

Self-help courses given through the Arthritis Foundation provide information about diseases and medication and can help in developing coping skills. Simply writing in a journal about positive and negative emotions for 15 minutes a day can be powerful medicine that relieves symptoms by 25% or more (see Chapter 96, Journaling for Health).[25]

The benefit of psychological interventions for RA was reviewed in a meta-analysis of 27 studies. Comparisons showed benefit in increasing physical activity and in decreasing pain, disability, depression, and anxiety. Self-regulation techniques, such as goal setting, planning, self-monitoring, feedback, and relapse prevention, were particularly helpful in reducing depression and anxiety.[26]

Meditation has been shown to be helpful for chronic pain.[27] A study of meditation in psoriasis, an autoimmune inflammatory skin disease, showed decreased time to clearing the skin disease.[28] Two studies investigated the role of meditation in RA. Pradhan et al[29] found reductions in psychological stress and increases in measures of well-being at 6 months, but no effects on the progression or activity of RA disease. Zatura et al[30] reported that both cognitive therapy and meditation were helpful in RA, with better responses in subjects with depression. I continue to recommend this modality for RA (see Chapter 98, Recommending Meditation). The effects of mind-body therapies on depression are important because depression is correlated with pain levels and measures of inflammatory markers.[31]

Nutrition

Food Triggers

Fasting clearly decreases symptoms in RA; however, symptoms rapidly recur with the resumption of food intake.[32] A few people with RA appear to have a food intolerance that exacerbates their disease. Many more people believe that certain foods exacerbate symptoms, but this effect was not shown in blind trials of food exposure. The offending foods are usually dairy products, wheat, citrus, or nuts. An elimination diet for 2 weeks with the reintroduction of the suspected food can be done with or without the supervision of a physician or a nutritionist (see Chapter 84, Food Intolerance and Elimination Diet).

Omega-3 and Omega-9 Fatty Acids

Increased intake of omega-3 fatty acids from cold-water fish, such as salmon, and from nuts, such as walnuts, as well as from flaxseed or hempseed, can provide modest improvement in the control of RA.[10,11,32] The role of saturated fatty acids and trans fats in increasing symptoms is unproved. In view of the association of these saturated and trans fats with cardiovascular disease, however, reduction in intake is worthwhile (see Chapter 86, The Antiinflammatory Diet).

Cooked vegetables and olive oil have been found to be independently protective for the development of RA. Omega-9 fatty acids in olive oil may confer anti-RA activity.[33]

Coffee
A high intake of coffee (4 or more cups a day) has been linked to an increased risk of RA.[18,19] Intake should be decreased to less than this level, or the patient can switch to green tea, for the possible benefit from its antioxidant polyphenols.

Elimination of Tobacco Use
Smoking causes oxidant stress on connective tissue, as evident from the increased wrinkles seen in long-term smokers. One study showed a clear association between smoking and increased risk of RA. In this Swedish population, more than 50% of RA cases could be attributable to smoking in association with certain HLA-DR genes.[34] Patients with RA should be counseled to avoid tobacco.

Supplements
Essential Fatty Acids
Omega-3 fatty acids can be increased by dietary means or through supplementation. Approximate doses for supplementation are eicosapentaenoic acid, 30 mg/kg/day, and docosahexaenoic acid, 50 mg/kg/day.[10,32]

Gamma-linolenic acid, 1.4 to 2.8 g/day, the equivalent of 6 to 11 g of borage oil daily, also has been shown to be helpful.[11] Effects may not be felt for 6 weeks or more, and continued improvement may occur after many months.

Conjugated Linoleic Acids
One study showed that 3-month supplementation with conjugated linoleic acids (CLAs) showed reductions in standard measures of RA activity (DAS28), morning stiffness, and erythrocyte sedimentation rate. This study provided 2.5 g CLA daily in two capsules containing equal amounts of *cis*-9, *trans*-11 CLA and *cis*-12, *trans*-10 CLA.[35]

Antioxidants
Antioxidant vitamins may be helpful in RA, as they seem to be in osteoarthritis. Additionally, vitamin E has some analgesic effects.[12] Vitamin E should be taken at 800 units daily as mixed tocopherols, and vitamin C at 250 mg twice per day. Selenium can be found in many foods, including nuts; intake should be at least 100 mcg daily, not to exceed 400 mcg daily.

The recommended intake of calcium to prevent osteoporosis is 1000 to 1200 mg daily. Adding magnesium, at 400 to 750 mg daily, and a vitamin D supplement, at 2000 units per day, is probably a prudent approach.[36]

Echinacea should be avoided by patients with rheumatoid arthritis because of anecdotal reports of increased symptoms in persons with autoimmune disease.

Botanicals
Ginger
Ginger (*Zingiber officinale*) may have efficacy in RA by inhibiting inflammatory prostaglandins.[13]

Dosage
As the dried root, 1 g two or three times per day to start, increase up to 4 g daily. As a tea, 1 g of dried root steeped in 150 mL of boiling water for 5 to 10 minutes and strained, 1 cup up to four times daily. It can also be taken in 500-mg capsules for a dose of 1 g two or three times a day.

Precautions
The stimulation of increased bile flow can cause pain in the presence of cholelithiasis. Other risks include bleeding, hypertension or hypotension, and hypoglycemia.

Turmeric
Turmeric (curcumin) in an open trial was shown to be similar to NSAIDs in efficacy.[13]

Dosage
As powdered root, 0.5 to 1 g two or three times daily.

Precautions
Risks include bleeding, gastrointestinal intolerance, and impaired fertility.

Pharmaceuticals
Nonsteroidal Antiinflammatory Drugs
NSAIDs can be used on a short-term basis with minor risk of gastrointestinal toxicity. The long-term use of NSAIDs, particularly in older adults, poses significant risks for gastrointestinal bleeding. Many NSAIDs are available, and many of the newer ones are restricted on some formularies. The classic NSAIDs are ibuprofen (Motrin), in a dose of 800 mg three times daily, and naproxen (Naprosyn), in a dose of 500 mg twice daily. Both have antiplatelet activity. The advantage of using the COX-2 inhibitor celecoxib for possible decreased gastrointestinal toxicity has been called into question.[9] Celecoxib shares a lack of antiplatelet effects with other newer NSAIDs. These drugs also have the potential for renal toxicity and are no more effective than older NSAIDs. Data point to the risk of increased thrombosis in patients taking COX-2 inhibitors who have a preexisting increased risk of thrombosis or cardiovascular disease.[8] Two other COX-2 inhibitors have been withdrawn from the market. Celecoxib is used in a dose of 200 mg twice daily.

Corticosteroids
Corticosteroids can rapidly decrease RA symptoms, often within a few hours at high doses. However, both short-term and long-term toxic effects are well known. High and even moderate doses can lead to avascular necrosis of joints such as the hip, knee, or shoulder; fortunately, this is a rare occurrence. With proper care and early diagnosis of avascular necrosis, disability and joint replacement may be avoided. With long-term corticosteroid use, osteoporosis is a significant risk when doses of prednisone or equivalent are higher 7.5 mg daily. Other risks include atherosclerosis, diabetes

mellitus, cushingoid features, acne, and infection. Often a minor disease flare can be treated with a moderately high dose such as 30 to 40 mg of prednisone orally and a rapid taper over the course of 1 to 2 weeks. In some patients, a low dose of corticosteroids appears necessary for optional function; prednisone, 5 to 7.5 mg daily, is often used for this purpose.[16,17] A common method of treating a flare is to give a long-acting depot preparation such as triamcinolone acetonide (Kenalog), 80 mg intramuscularly. This approach can often control disease for 1 to 2 months, long enough for the slower-acting disease-modifying antirheumatic drugs (DMARDs) to start working. For disease flares in isolated joints, once infection is ruled out, an intra-articular injection of triamcinolone, 2.5 to 40 mg, can be given to control local disease.

> A single joint with severely decreased range of motion and increased pain is presumed to be infected until proven otherwise. The patient should be hospitalized overnight for joint aspiration to obtain culture specimens. Blood should also be drawn for cultures, followed by administration of intravenous antibiotics until results of culture are known.

Antibiotics

Antibiotics, particularly minocycline (Minocin) in a twice-daily dose of 100 mg, may be useful in patients with less severe disease.[37] Side effects include gastrointestinal intolerance, dizziness, photosensitivity rash, vaginitis, skin and gingival discoloration, and, rarely, hepatic, lung, and kidney injury. The salutary effects of these agents may not be caused by their antibacterial activity, because the tetracyclines also show immunomodulatory and antiinflammatory activities.

Disease-Modifying Antirheumatic Drugs: Overview

DMARDs are also referred to as slow-acting antirheumatic drugs (SAARDs) because they usually take 6 weeks to 3 months to show activity. The use of most U.S. Food and Drug Administration (FDA)–approved DMARDs is supported by Cochrane Reviews, including low-dose steroids, hydroxychloroquine, sulfasalazine, methotrexate (with folic acid), azathioprine, leflunomide, cyclophosphamide, etanercept, adalimumab, and infliximab (Fig. 48-2).

Hydroxychloroquine and Sulfasalazine

Hydroxychloroquine (Plaquenil) and sulfasalazine (Azulfidine-EN) are used early in disease when a diagnosis may not be clear or in patients with no characteristic erosive disease. Both drugs have little short-term and long-term toxicity.

■ Dosage

The current accepted dose of hydroxychloroquine is 200 mg twice daily, which carries little risk of toxicity; nevertheless, an ophthalmologic examination to test for retinal toxicity is recommended every 6 to 12 months. To reduce gastrointestinal intolerance, sulfasalazine is usually used in an enteric-coated form; dosing is started at 500 mg a day and raised by one tablet every few days until a dose of 1 g twice daily is reached.

■ Precautions

When used in high doses, hydroxychloroquine carries a risk of retinal toxicity resulting from deposition of the drug into the retina. Sulfasalazine can uncommonly cause rash, hepatotoxicity, and leukopenia.

Methotrexate

Of all of the DMARDs, methotrexate (Rheumatrex) has been shown to be tolerated for longer periods of treatment than any other drug.[3,38] Methotrexate is a folate antagonist and has a multitude of immunomodulatory activities, but its exact mechanism of action in RA is unknown. Doses of methotrexate for RA are usually between 5 and 25 mg given once a week. The dose is usually given orally in tablet form; however, the liquid form can be used orally and is sometimes less expensive. A common practice is to start with 7.5 mg orally once per week, although many practitioners, including myself, recommend starting higher doses such as 15 mg/week. With use of higher doses of 20 mg and more, patients are often taught to self-administer the dose subcutaneously once per week to avoid possible problems with gastrointestinal absorption. To decrease side effects, I always prescribe folic acid, 1 to 2 mg, to be taken each day. A decision to start methotrexate therapy or to raise or decrease the dose should be placed in the hands of a practitioner with extensive experience. Methotrexate is the standard by which all other drugs are judged, yet few patients achieve remission, and less than a majority will achieve a 50% improvement on composite scores.

Contraindications to use of methotrexate include the following: preexisting hepatic, renal, or pulmonary disease; unwillingness to discontinue alcoholic beverages; and recent malignant disease. Methotrexate has many side effects, the most prominent being hepatitis, bone marrow suppression, pneumonitis, mouth sores, nausea, and headache. A complete blood count, platelet count, and determination of aspartate transaminase, albumin, and creatinine levels are done initially and then every 2 weeks for 6 weeks after methotrexate therapy is begun. Thereafter, monitoring can be done every 4 to 8 weeks. A baseline hepatitis screen and chest radiography are recommended. Tuberculosis skin testing is reserved for patients with strong risk factors or an abnormal appearance on chest radiograph.

Other Immunosuppressive Drugs

Many other immunosuppressive drugs are used in RA. Leflunomide (Arava) is a newer drug that is similar in efficacy to methotrexate.[39] Leflunomide interferes with pyrimidine synthesis, whereas methotrexate interferes with purine synthesis. Leflunomide has fewer hepatotoxic effects and possibly little bone marrow toxicity but is much more likely to cause diarrhea. Azathioprine (Imuran) is metabolized to 6-mercaptopurine and interferes with inosinic acid synthesis. It is often substituted for methotrexate; however, its use is associated with gastrointestinal and bone marrow toxicity. Other immunosuppressive drugs less commonly used are mycophenolate mofetil (CellCept), cyclosporine (Neoral), tacrolimus (Prograf), and chlorambucil (Leukeran). Cyclophosphamide (Cytoxan) is often used to treat rheumatoid vasculitis.

FIGURE 48-2

Treatment algorithm for rheumatoid arthritis (RA) in adults.

*When starting methotrexate (MTX), add 1 mg of folic acid by mouth daily to decrease side effects, warn patients to avoid alcohol, and schedule laboratory studies (complete blood count, differential, platelets, aspartate aminotransaminase, albumin, creatinine) before starting, then every 2 weeks for 6 weeks, then every 2 months if results are normal.

†When adding another disease-modifying antirheumatic drug (DMARD) to MTX, decrease the dose of MTX to 10 to 15 mg once per week. Ca, calcium; FA, fatty acid; HCQ, hydroxychloroquine; IM, intramuscular; Mg, magnesium; Se, selenium; SQ, subcutaneous; SSZ, sulfasalazine; TB, tuberculosis; vits, vitamins.

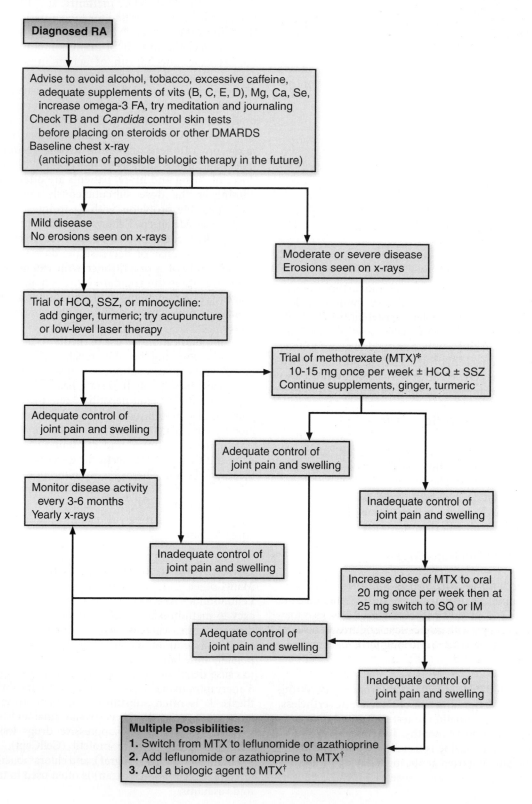

Recombinant Biologics

Advances in the therapy of RA have targeted cytokines and cell surface molecules used to communicate between cells of the immune system.[3-7] Etanercept (Enbrel), adalimumab (Humira), and infliximab (Remicade) are TNF inhibitors.[40-42] Etanercept is given subcutaneously once or twice per week, adalimumab is given subcutaneously once every 2 weeks, whereas infliximab is usually given intravenously once every 2 months. Two newer TNF inhibitors, certolizumab (Cimzia) and golimumab (Simponi), have been approved for use and can be given subcutaneously once per month.[43] These drugs are most often used with another DMARD, usually methotrexate, to reduce the development of autoantibodies. Short-term safety is very high, with little toxicity. As many as 30% of patients may show almost complete remission of symptoms with the combination of methotrexate and an anti-TNF agent. Currently, approximately 10 years of data are available on long-term safety and efficacy.[3] Use of these agents carries a risk of life-threatening exacerbations of severe infections, especially sepsis. Patients should temporarily discontinue the anti-TNF therapy during presumed infections and restart the therapy when the infection has resolved. All patients must be tested for latent tuberculosis with the purified protein derivative (PPD) skin test before they begin therapy. These drugs also may exacerbate demyelinating disorders; therefore, they should be avoided in patients with suspected or proven multiple sclerosis or optic neuritis.

An IL-1 receptor antagonist, anakinra (Kineret), is approved for the treatment of RA. It is given subcutaneously daily and also increases the risk of serious infection. Anakinra is generally thought to have lower efficacy in RA than other biologics. Agents directed toward a cell surface molecule on B cells (rituximab [Rituxan]),[6] and a costimulatory molecule on T cells (abatacept [Orencia]),[7] have been approved for use in RA. The latest biologic (tocilizumab [Actemra]) is directed toward another cytokine, IL-6, and has been approved for use in RA, but it has risks of neutropenia and increased cholesterol and liver function values. Thus, tocilizumab will require additional laboratory monitoring compared with the other biologics.[5]

Acupuncture

Several small controlled trials of acupuncture in RA showed decreased knee pain for an average of 1 to 3 months.[44]

Low-Level Laser Therapy

Low-level laser therapy uses a single-wavelength laser source that likely has photochemical, not thermal, effects on cells. A Cochrane Review suggests that this therapy may be considered for short-term relief of pain and morning stiffness for patients with RA, particularly because it has few side effects.[45]

Surgery

Loss of joint function and intractable pain may be indications for surgical intervention. Synovectomy can be helpful when systemic therapy and intra-articular corticosteroids are ineffective. Joint replacement can help restore function and increase independent activity. Patients with RA have an increased risk of surgical and postoperative complications. Cervical spine disease can lead to spinal instability and risk of neurologic injury. Replacement of one joint can result in increased stress on other joints during recovery and rehabilitation. Long-term corticosteroid use can cause fragility of vessels and connective tissue and thus increase the risks of surgery.

Therapies to Consider

The roles of traditional Chinese medicine or Ayurvedic, homeopathy, or spiritual therapies in the management of RA have not been adequately studied. Patients should learn about several different modalities and then record their feelings about these approaches in a journal. They may then choose to visit a practitioner of a selected modality for a trial of the techniques. If the economic burden is not too great, further exploration of that therapeutic technique may be appropriate.

PREVENTION PRESCRIPTION

No proven methods of preventing rheumatoid arthritis exist. However, the following can be recommended:

- Laugh as much as possible. Watch funny movies, read funny books, get up every morning and force yourself to laugh. You'll find it is awkward at first, but it works anyway!
- Journal about stressful events. Make a list of 25 things for which you are grateful.
- Be creative. Do art, dance, play an instrument, beat a drum, write poetry or prose.
- Meditate; I recommend mindfulness meditation.
- Find meaning in life. Ask what gives you the energy to get up in the morning.
- Investigate your personality.[46] Try new things that you are afraid to do.
- If you feel stuck, find a good psychotherapist.
- Exercise. Combine aerobics, strength training, and stretching. Make it a time to play!
- Love people. Hang out with "positive people," make sure they outweigh the "negative" people in your life. Find "positive" support groups.
- Eat well. Try a vegetarian diet. Make sure to balance your protein intake, and make sure you have adequate vitamin intake.
- Eliminate coffee, smoking, and alcohol. Make high-sugar desserts a small, rare treat.

THERAPEUTIC REVIEW

Evidence is accumulating that current allopathic treatments are successful in slowing joint destruction and in decreasing the mortality associated with rheumatoid arthritis (RA).[38,40–42,47] In addition, the rates of extra-articular manifestations of RA, such as Felty syndrome and rheumatoid vasculitis, seem to be decreasing. Therefore, in any but the mildest cases of RA, an integrated approach should include the disease-modifying antirheumatic drugs (DMARDs), usually starting with methotrexate.

■ Exercise

- Muscle strengthening and stretching can be invaluable for maintaining function. Physical therapy can be used initially for instruction; tai chi in the form of the range-of-motion dance can be helpful.

■ Mind-Body Techniques

- Meditation is highly recommended for patients with RA who are willing to devote the daily time to looking more closely at the connections among body, mind, and spirit. Also recommended are relaxation exercises and the development of methods to cope with stress. Tai chi and yoga also may include a meditative component to the training.

- Journaling should be encouraged (see Chapter 96, Journaling for Health).

■ Removal of Exacerbating Factors

- Use of coffee, tobacco, and alcohol should be eliminated.

- If intolerance to dairy products, wheat, citrus, or nuts is suspected, a trial of an elimination diet for 2 weeks with the reintroduction of the suspected food can be undertaken (see Chapter 84, Food Intolerance and Elimination Diet).

■ Nutrition

- A diet rich in omega-3 fatty acids is achieved by increasing intake of cold-water fish or adding flaxseed meal or flaxseed oil. Olive oil should be increased in the diet as well. An antiinflammatory diet is also recommended (see Chapter 86, The Antiinflammatory Diet).

■ Supplements

- Omega-3 fatty acids are recommended; doses for supplementation are eicosapentaenoic acid, 30 mg/kg/day, and docosahexaenoic acid, 50 mg/kg/day, along with gamma-linolenic acid, 1.4 to 2.8 g/day, the equivalent of 6 to 11 g of borage oil daily.

- Conjugated linoleic acid (borage oil, evening primrose oil) can be tried, at 2.5 g/day.

- Vitamin E should be taken in a dose of 800 units daily as mixed tocopherols, and vitamin C can be taken in a dose of 250 mg twice daily. Selenium intake, as nuts or supplements, should be at least 100 mcg daily, not to exceed 400 mcg daily. Recommended intake of calcium is 1.5 g daily; magnesium, 400 to 750 mg daily, and a vitamin D supplement of 2000 units/day are also recommended.

■ Botanicals

- Start with ginger, at 1 g twice daily to a maximum of 4 g daily.

- If no effect is seen after 6 to 8 weeks, turmeric 0.5 to 1 g two to three times daily can be tried.

■ Pharmaceuticals

- NSAIDs are used as little as possible owing to gastrointestinal toxicity. The classic NSAIDs are ibuprofen, 800 mg three times daily, and naproxen, 500 mg twice daily.

- The COX-2 inhibitors decrease but do not eliminate the risk of gastrointestinal bleeding. The dose of celecoxib is 200 mg twice daily.

- Most patients with RA are receiving combinations of drugs. Most patients are given methotrexate therapy unless they have contraindications or side effects.

- A common combination is methotrexate and hydroxychloroquine. Corticosteroids in moderately high doses with a rapid taper are often used for exacerbations.

- Commonly, a TNF inhibitor such as etanercept, adalimumab, infliximab, certolizumab, or golimumab is added if methotrexate is only partially effective. If one to two TNF inhibitors are unsuccessful, try rituximab, abatacept, or tocilizumab.

- Leflunomide or azathioprine is often substituted for methotrexate if side effects of methotrexate are intolerable.

- Methotrexate and leflunomide can be used together with only a modest increase in risk of side effects. The DMARDs and the recombinant biologics have many varied side effects, some of which are only now being defined. New biologics are being developed, including oral formulations. The immunosuppressive pharmaceuticals should be used only with input from a subspecialist rheumatologist.

■ Acupuncture

- Acupuncture can be tried for any patient with RA. This modality may be less effective in patients taking corticosteroids.

Low-Level Laser Therapy

- Low-level laser therapy can be tried with little risk of side effects.

Surgery

- Loss of joint function and intractable pain may be indications for surgical intervention. Synovectomy can be helpful when systemic therapy and intra-articular corticosteroids are ineffective. Joint replacement can help restore function and increase independent activity.

Caution

Studies have not been done on the possible additive effects of ginger, turmeric, vitamin E, and an NSAID for increased risk of hemorrhage. Other commonly used supplements or botanicals such as ginkgo may add further risk. Particular care must be used in patients taking other antiplatelet agents or warfarin sodium (Coumadin). In addition, the interactions of supplements and botanicals with allopathic pharmaceuticals are not fully understood. All health care professionals involved in the patient's care must be aware of all therapies being used. The addition of any new treatment should prompt increased laboratory monitoring for patients receiving immunosuppressive pharmaceuticals.

KEY WEB RESOURCES

Arthritis Foundation. www.arthritis.org.	Information on all aspects of rheumatoid arthritis, treatment, self-help, and other resources from the Arthritis Foundation (800-283-7800)
National Center for Complementary and Alternative Medicine. www.nccam.nih.gov/health/RA	Information on integrative therapies
Tai Chi Health. www.taichihealth.com; http://www.taichihealth.com/indexrom.html	A range-of-motion dance from Tai Chi Health (800-488-4940) that is particularly suited to persons with disabilities

References

References are available online at expertconsult.com.

Chapter 49

Inflammatory Bowel Disease

Leo Galland, MD

Pathophysiology

Crohn's disease (CD) and ulcerative colitis (UC) are thought to result from inappropriate activation of the mucosal immune system, facilitated by regulatory defects in the mucosal immune response and failure of the mucosal barrier that separates immune response cells from the contents of the intestinal lumen. The normal gut flora act as a trigger for the inflammatory response and appear to play a central role in pathogenesis.[1] In both diseases, increased numbers of surface-adherent and intracellular bacteria have been observed in mucosal biopsies.[2,3] Patients with UC and CD share immunologic abnormalities that are common among patients with other types of autoimmune disorders, including up-regulation of subtype 17 helper T-cell (Th17)–positive lymphocytes and the proinflammatory cytokines tumor necrosis factor-alpha (TNF-alpha) and interleukin-1 (IL-1), IL-6, and IL-23, accompanied by down-regulation of regulatory T cells and the antiinflammatory cytokine IL-1 receptor antagonist (IL1ra).[4-7]

Despite these similarities, CD and UC have distinct differences in pathophysiology. The immune response underlying the pathologic features of CD, as in other granulomatous diseases, is driven by lymphocytes with a Th1 phenotype and their cytokines: IL-2 and interferon-gamma (IFN-gamma). The lymphocytes that organize the inflammatory response in UC demonstrate an atypical type 2 helper T-cell (Th2) phenotype, with IL-5 as a distinctive cytokine mediator.[8] Another interesting but unexplained difference between CD and UC is the effect of cigarette smoking, which increases the risk and decreases therapeutic responsiveness of patients with CD but has the opposite effect in patients with UC.[9] Response to diet and probiotics is often different for the two disorders, as discussed later.

The current consensus is that the development of inflammatory bowel disease (IBD) requires the combined effects of four basic components: (1) the input of multiple genetic variations that govern intestinal barrier function, repair, and immunity; (2) alterations in the intestinal microflora; (3) acquired aberrations of innate and adaptive immune responses; and (4) global changes in environment and hygiene. Most researchers believe that none of these four components can by itself trigger or maintain IBD, but that a combination of various factors is probably needed to bring about CD or UC in individual patients. This model implies that different and diverse mechanisms underlie IBD in different patients and that each patient may have a distinctive illness with his or her own clinical manifestations and a personalized response to therapy.[10] This model is well suited to the patient-centered diagnostic and therapeutic perspective of integrative medicine, in which the specific antecedents, triggers, and mediators of disease in each patient, rather than the disease entity, form the basis for therapy.[11]

Malnutrition is a major reversible complication of IBD. The mechanisms of malnutrition include anorexia resulting from the systemic effects of IL-1, a catabolic state induced by TNF-alpha, malabsorption secondary to disease or surgical resection, nutrient losses through the inflamed and ulcerated gut, small bowel bacterial overgrowth resulting from strictures or fistulas, and the side effects of drug therapy.[12] Inflammation increases oxidative stress in the bowel mucosa and decreases levels of antioxidants.[13] Nutritional deficiencies described in mucosal biopsies of patients with IBD include vitamin C,[14] zinc, copper, and the zinc- and copper-dependent enzyme superoxide dismutase (Cu-Zn SOD).[15] Plasma levels of vitamins A and E are lower and plasma levels of the oxidative stress marker 8-hydroxy-deoxy-guanosine (8-OHdG) are higher in patients with IBD than in controls.[16] Compared with controls, children and adults with IBD have lower blood levels of zinc and selenium, mineral cofactors of antioxidant enzymes,[17-19] and adults with UC may show lower levels of beta-carotene, magnesium, selenium, and zinc.[20] Micronutrient deficits may favor self-perpetuation of IBD by causing defects in the mechanisms of tissue repair.[21] Micronutrient deficiencies may also contribute to some complications of IBD, such as growth retardation, osteopenia, urolithiasis, and thromboembolic phenomena.[12]

In CD, abnormal mucosal barrier function may play a primary role in pathogenesis. Small intestinal permeability is increased among healthy first-degree relatives of patients with CD[22] and is increased in noninflamed enteric tissue obtained from patients.[23] Aspirin, a drug that increases intestinal permeability of healthy controls, causes an exaggerated increase in intestinal permeability of first-degree relatives of patients with CD.[24] The rate of relapse among patients who have entered remission is directly proportional to the degree of small intestinal hyperpermeability measured with chemical probes.[25] Hyperpermeability is associated with polymorphism of genes associated with regulation of epithelial barrier function,[4] and it increases exposure of the intestinal immune system to luminal antigens. Intestinal epithelial lymphocytes of patients with CD are abnormally sensitive to antigens derived from Enterobacteriaceae and *Candida albicans,* both normally present in the small intestine.[26]

Integrative Therapy

General Principles

No single diet or set of supplements is right for every patient with CD or UC. Any intervention, even if supported by clinical trial data, may cause exacerbation of IBD in an individual patient. Each patient should serve as his or her own control, with symptoms, signs, and laboratory parameters followed closely. The evidence-based information presented in this chapter is at best a guide to help practitioners apply therapeutic options to individual patients. The only thing that matters is what works for this patient.

Enteral Feeding

Defined formula diets, either elemental or polymeric, are successful in improving the nutritional status of patients with IBD and preventing complications of surgery.[11] In CD, but not in UC, enteral feeding of defined formula diets as primary therapy has been shown to induce remission of active disease in 30% to 80% of patients.[11] Although enteral feeding is most commonly used in pediatric patients because of growth-enhancing and steroid-sparing effects,[27] it is equally effective in adults,[28] and it appears to have a direct antiinflammatory effect on the bowel mucosa.[29] Theories to explain the antiinflammatory effect of enteral feeding in CD include alteration in intestinal microbial flora,[30] diminution of intestinal synthesis of inflammatory mediators, and nonspecific nutritional repletion or provision of important micronutrients to heal the diseased intestine.[11] Decreased dietary antigen uptake, an early concept, is not a likely mechanism; polymeric diets, composed of whole protein, are as effective as elemental diets, in which nitrogen is supplied as free amino acids.[31,32] Results are conflicting concerning the effect of supplemental food on the response to enteral feedings.[33,34]

Part of the benefit derived from enteral feeding may reflect dietary fat content.[11] Those liquid diets that are most effective in inducing remission of active CD are either very low in fat or supply one third of their dietary fat in the form of medium-chain triglycerides (MCTs) from coconut oil.[35,36] The addition of long-chain triglycerides derived from vegetable oils attenuates benefit,[37] whereas diets enriched with MCT oil are as effective as very-low-fat diets.[38] MCT oil may have a direct antiinflammatory effect, by modulating expression of adhesion molecules and cytokines.[11] The potential role of omega-3 fatty acids in treatment of IBD is discussed later in the section on supplements.

The main advantage of enteral feeding as primary therapy for CD is avoidance of medication side effects, especially in children.[39] Although no clear clinical predictors of response have been established, clinicians believe that patients treated early in the course of CD are more likely to respond than are patients with long-standing disease.[11] Small studies have indicated that remission may be more likely in patients with ileal involvement than colonic involvement only[40] and with perforating or fistulating disease than with more superficial disease.[41] The main disadvantages of enteral feedings is poor compliance because of the lack of palatability and the high rate of relapse (more than 60%) following the discontinuation of these feedings. The use of exclusion diets (discussed later) may significantly extend the benefit of enteral feeding regimens.

Specific Carbohydrate Diet

The Specific Carbohydrate Diet (see Key Web Resources) is a food-based approach to enteral nutrition for patients with IBD and many anecdotal reports have noted long-term remission without medication.[42] The alleged mechanisms of action of this diet are improvement of nutritional status and alteration in ileocecal flora by the proper choice of nutritious carbohydrate sources.[43] The diet is far more effective for patients with CD than UC (Elaine Gottschall, personal communication, 1994). In practice, the diet consists of meat, poultry, fish, eggs, most vegetables and fruits, nut flours, aged cheese, homemade yogurt, and honey. Forbidden foods include all cereal grains and their derivatives (including sweeteners other than honey), legumes, potatoes, lactose-containing dairy products, and sucrose. Early studies found that high sucrose intake predisposed to CD[44-47] and that control of disease was enhanced by its avoidance.[48]

I have used the Specific Carbohydrate Diet as primary treatment for patients with CD since the 1990s and have observed an overall response rate of 55%, unrelated to duration of illness but most pronounced in patients with ileitis or perianal fistula.[49] Improvement occurred in symptoms and laboratory parameters, such as serum albumin and erythrocyte sedimentation rate (ESR), and permitted decreased use of glucocorticoids.

Diets that induce remission of CD do not usually induce remission of UC, although they improve patients' nutritional status and prevent complications related to surgery.[11] Although I have occasionally seen a patient with UC who responded very well to the Specific Carbohydrate Diet, research suggests that modification in dietary sources of fat and protein, rather than carbohydrates, may be therapeutic for patients with UC. A role for dietary fat in the pathogenesis of UC is suggested by the association between incident UC and high consumption of vegetable oils rich in linoleic acid (18:2n6).[50] These individuals also show increased levels of arachidonic acid (20:4n6), a metabolite of linoleic acid, in fat biopsies, before development of UC.[51] In contrast, dietary omega-3 fatty acids, especially docosahexaenoic acid (DHA, 22:6n3) may exert a preventive effect on development of UC.[52]

Nutritional approaches to treatment of UC have examined the therapeutic potential of short-chain fatty acids, in particular butyric acid.[11] Not only do short-chain fatty acids nourish the colonic epithelium, but also they lower intraluminal pH, thus favoring growth of *Lactobacillus* and *Bifidobacterium* (considered to be beneficial organisms, or probiotics) and inhibiting the growth of *Clostridium, Bacteroides,* and *Escherichia coli,* which are potential pathogens. In addition to serving as the preferred energy substrate for colonic epithelial cells, butyrate has a true antiinflammatory effect, preventing activation of the proinflammatory nuclear transcription factor NF-kappaB.[53] When added to 5-aminosalicylic acid (5-ASA) enemas, butyrate (80 mmol/L) induces remission in ulcerative proctitis that is resistant to combined 5-ASA–hydrocortisone enemas.[54] Because butyrate is normally produced by bacterial fermentation of indigestible carbohydrate in the colon, studies have examined the effect of fiber supplementation on the course of UC. These studies are described later in the section on prebiotics.

Patients with UC are not deficient in butyrate, but they appear unable to use it, perhaps because organic sulfides produced by their enteric flora inhibit the epithelial effects of butyrate.[55,56] Protein consumption is a major determinant of sulfide production in the human colon.[57] Higher intake of protein, especially from animal sources, is associated with an increased risk of developing UC.[58]

For patients with UC in remission, the risk of relapse is directly influenced by higher consumption of protein, especially meat protein, and by total dietary sulfur and sulfates.[59] An interesting effect of 5-ASA derivatives, drugs proven to help prevent relapse of UC, is inhibition of sulfide production by gut bacteria, with sulfasalazine having the strongest effect.[60] Levels of sulfate-reducing bacteria, required for production of sulfides from dietary sulfate, are higher in fresh fecal samples of patients with UC and active pouchitis than in patients with UC and normal ileoanal pouches or in postcolectomy patients with familial polyposis who have ileoanal pouches.[61] Based on these findings, a reasonable if unproven dietary approach to help patients with UC maintain remission would be one high in fiber and omega-3 fatty acids and low in meat, eggs, dairy fat, and vegetable oils.

Exclusion Diets

Exclusion diets eliminate specific symptom-producing foods and have been used to maintain remission of IBD. Although self-reported food intolerance is common among patients with IBD,[62] most of the data from controlled studies have been gathered from patients with CD. In the East Anglia Multicentre Controlled Trial, 84% of patients with active CD entered clinical remission after 2 weeks of a liquid elemental diet,[63] which produced a significant decrease in ESR and C-reactive protein (CRP) and an increase in serum albumin. Patients were then randomized to receive treatment either with prednisolone or with a specific food exclusion diet. To determine which foods each patient needed to avoid, a structured series of dietary challenges was conducted. Patients would introduce foods of their choice, one at a time. Any food that appeared to provoke symptoms was excluded from further consumption; foods that did not provoke symptoms were included in a maintenance diet. At 6 months, 70% of

patients treated with diet were still in remission, compared with 34% of patients treated with prednisolone. After 2 years, 38% of patients treated with specific food exclusion were still in remission, compared with 21% of steroid-treated patients. In previous uncontrolled studies, some of the same investigators had used a diet consisting of one or two meats (usually lamb or chicken), one starch (usually rice or potatoes), one fruit, and one vegetable, instead of the elemental diet, to induce remission. Structured food challenges were then used to construct a maintenance diet free of symptom-provoking foods. Compliance with the specific food elimination diet was associated with a rate of relapse that was less than 10% per year.[64] Individual foods found most likely to provoke symptoms in this study were wheat, cow's milk and its derivatives, cruciferous vegetables, corn, yeast, tomatoes, citrus fruit, and eggs.

Many patients with CD develop antibodies to baker's and brewer's yeast, *Saccharomyces cerevisiae* (ASCA).[65] Lymphocytes of ASCA-positive patients proliferate after stimulation with mannan, a lectin common to most types of yeast. For these patients, lymphocyte proliferation is associated with increased production of TNF-alpha.[66] A small placebo-controlled study found that patients with stable, chronic CD experienced a significant reduction in the CD activity index (CDAI) during 30 days of dietary yeast elimination and a return to baseline disease activity when capsules of *S.cerevisiae* were added to their diets.[67]

An observational study of patients with UC suggested that dietary practices based on food avoidance did not appear to modify the risk of relapse,[68] but a small experimental study from South Africa found that diarrhea, rectal bleeding, and the appearance of the colon on sigmoidoscopy improved significantly more for patients receiving a diet that systematically eliminated symptom-provoking foods than for those assigned only to monitor their diets.[69] The potential value of this study is reduced by the small number of patients and the maintenance of remission despite a return to an unrestricted diet after 6 months. Earlier reports from dietary trials led to an estimate that 15% to 20% of patients with UC have specific food intolerance that affects severity of illness, with cow's milk protein the leading offender.[70] This estimate is consistent with my clinical experience (see Chapter 84, Food Intolerance and Elimination Diet).

Supplements

Nutritional supplements may be used to correct or prevent the deficiencies that are common among patients with IBD or to achieve an antiinflammatory effect.

Folates

5-ASA derivatives, sulfasalazine in particular, impair folic acid transport.[71] Reduced folic acid in patients with IBD is associated with hyperhomocysteinemia,[72] a risk factor for deep vein thrombosis,[73] which is an extraintestinal complication of IBD. Concurrent administration of folic acid with 5-ASA derivatives prevents folic acid depletion and has been shown to reduce the incidence of colon cancer in patients with UC.[74,75] One study found that a high dose of folic acid (15 mg/day) reversed sulfasalazine-induced pancytopenia in two patients.[76]

Vitamin B_{12}

Because vitamin B_{12} absorption may be impaired by ileal inflammation and by small bowel bacterial overgrowth, deficiency of vitamin B_{12} has long been described as a potential complication of CD.[77] Although frank vitamin B_{12} deficiency is unusual, lower vitamin B_{12} levels are associated with increased serum homocysteine in patients with CD.[78] Ischemic strokes in a woman with CD were associated with vitamin B_{12}–reversible hyperhomocysteinemia.[79] A single dose of 1000 mcg of cobalamin by injection corrects the megaloblastic anemia associated with CD.[80]

Vitamin B_6

Median vitamin B_6 levels are significantly lower in patients with IBD than in controls; low levels are associated with active inflammation and hyperhomocysteinemia.[81] Although some homocysteine is removed by folate-vitamin B_{12}–dependent remethylation, the bulk of homocysteine is converted to cystathionine in a reaction catalyzed by vitamin B_6. Ischemic stroke and high-grade carotid obstruction in a young woman with CD were attributed to hyperhomocysteinemia, vitamin B_6 deficiency, and a heterozygous methylene-tetrahydrofolate reductase gene mutation. The investigators believed that vitamin B_6 deficiency was the principal cause of hyperhomocysteinemia in this patient.[82]

Vitamins E and C

Blood levels of vitamins E and C are often reduced in patients with IBD.[83] Administration of alpha-tocopherol, 800 units per day, and vitamin C, 1000 mg per day, to patients with stable, active CD decreased markers of oxidative stress but had no effect on the CDAI.[84] A small study of patients with ulcerative proctitis demonstrated significant improvement after 2 weeks of vitamin E administered as a rectal suppository.[85]

Vitamin A

Although levels of carotenoids[86] and retinol[87] are diminished in patients with active CD, low levels appear to be related not to malabsorption but to inflammation,[88,89] as well as a reduction in circulating retinol binding protein.[90] Supplementation with vitamin A at doses of 100,000 to 150,000 units per day had no effect on symptoms or CDAI.[91,92]

Vitamin D

Reduced blood levels of 25-OH cholecalciferol, the major vitamin D metabolite, are common in patients with CD and are related to malnutrition and lack of sun exposure.[93,94] One study found that patients with CD who received 1200 units of vitamin D_3 daily for 12 months had less than half the risk of relapse than those treated with placebo.[95] Administration of vitamin D, 1000 units per day for 1 year, prevented bone loss in patients with active disease.[96] The major causes of bone loss in IBD, however, are the effects of inflammatory cytokines and glucocorticoid therapy,[97] not vitamin D status. Calcitriol (1,25-dihydroxycholecalciferol), the most active metabolite of vitamin D, may actually be increased in patients with IBD because activated intestinal macrophages increase calcitriol synthesis; elevated calcitriol is associated with increased risk of osteoporosis and may serve as a marker of disease activity.[98] Hypercalcemia is a rare complication of excess calcitriol, and serum calcium should be monitored in patients with IBD receiving vitamin D supplements.[99]

Vitamin K

Biochemical evidence of vitamin K deficiency has been found in patients with ileitis and in patients with colitis who were treated with sulfasalazine or antibiotics.[100] Serum vitamin K levels in CD are significantly decreased compared with normal controls and are associated with increased levels of undercarboxylated osteocalcin, a finding indicating low vitamin K status in bone. In patients with CD, undercarboxylated osteocalcin is inversely related to lumbar spine bone density.[101] Furthermore, the rate of bone resorption in CD is inversely correlated with vitamin K status, a finding suggesting that vitamin K deficiency may be another etiologic factor in osteopenia of IBD.[102] The optimal dose of vitamin K for correction of deficiency is not known. Patients with active disease may not absorb oral vitamin K, even at high dosage.[103]

Calcium

Although calcium supplementation is recommended for maintaining bone density in patients with IBD, especially those receiving glucocorticoids, calcium supplementation (1000 mg per day) with 250 units of vitamin D per day, conferred no significant benefit to bone density at 1 year in patients with corticosteroid-dependent IBD and osteoporosis.[104] Nonetheless, calcium supplementation should be given to patients with low dietary calcium intake. In experimental animals, low dietary calcium increases severity of IBD.[105]

Zinc

Low plasma zinc is common in patients with CD and may be associated with clinical manifestations such as acrodermatitis, decreased activity of zinc-dependent enzymes such as thymulin and metallothionein, reduction in muscle zinc concentration, and poor taste acuity.[11] Zinc absorption is impaired and fecal zinc losses are inappropriately high.[18] Zinc-deficient adolescents with CD grow and mature more normally when zinc deficiency is treated. Anecdotally, correction of zinc deficiency as a specific intervention has been associated with global clinical improvement, a finding suggesting that zinc replacement may have beneficial effects on disease activity.[106] A small study of patients in remission from CD found that high-dose supplementation with zinc sulfate, 110 mg three times a day for 8 weeks, significantly decreased small intestinal permeability for a period of 12 months.[107] In patients with active disease, zinc sulfate, 200 mg per day (but not 60 mg per day) significantly increased plasma zinc and thymulin activity.[108]

> Zinc competes with copper, iron, calcium, and magnesium for absorption. When administering high doses of zinc, consider administering a multimineral at a separate time of day. Zinc is absorbed best if not taken at the same time as copper, magnesium, or iron.

Selenium

Low selenium levels in patients with CD are associated with increased levels of TNF-alpha and decreased levels of the antioxidant enzyme glutathione peroxidase (GSHPx).[109] In one study, although selenium supplementation raised plasma selenium to the level of a control population, it did not significantly increase activity of GSHPx.[110] Patients with small bowel resection are at risk for severe selenium deficiency; monitoring of selenium status and selenium supplementation has been recommended for this group in particular.[111] Patients receiving enteral feeding with liquid formula diets experience decreased selenium concentrations proportional to the duration of feeding, a finding suggesting that additional selenium supplementation is also needed by these patients.[112]

Magnesium

Magnesium deficiency is a potential complication of IBD, a result of decreased oral intake, malabsorption, and increased intestinal losses from diarrhea. Urinary magnesium is a better predictor of magnesium status than is serum magnesium in this setting.[113] Reduced urinary magnesium excretion is a significant risk factor for urolithiasis, one of the extraintestinal manifestations of IBD.[114] For patients with IBD, the urinary ratio of magnesium and citrate to calcium is a better predictor of lithogenic potential than is urinary oxalate excretion.[115] Supplementation with magnesium and citrate may decrease urinary stone formation, but diarrhea is a dose-related, limiting side effect.

Chromium

Glucocorticoid therapy increases urinary chromium excretion, and chromium picolinate, 600 mcg per day, can reverse steroid-induced diabetes in humans, with a decrease in mean blood glucose from 250 to 150 mg/dL. Chromium supplementation may be of benefit for patients receiving glucocorticoids who have impaired glucose tolerance.[116]

Iron

Anemia occurs in approximately 30% of patients with IBD.[117] The causes of anemia in these patients include iron deficiency from blood loss, cytokine-induced suppression of erythropoiesis, and side effects of medication. Some investigators have speculated that iron deficiency actually increases the IFN-gamma response in Th1-driven inflammation and may contribute to aggravation of CD.[118] Most clinicians, however, avoid oral iron supplements, however, because they believe that iron can increase oxidative stress in the gut, given that very-high-dose iron supplementation consistently aggravates experimental colitis in rodents.[118] The doses used in rodent studies are orders of magnitude greater than the doses given to patients, however. The relative risks and benefits of oral iron supplementation for patients with IBD are uncertain.

Fish Oils

Biochemical studies indicate that 25% of patients with IBD show evidence of essential fatty acid deficiency.[119] In experimental animals, fish oil feeding ameliorated the intestinal mucosal injury produced by methotrexate.[120] In tissue culture, omega-3 fatty acids stimulated wound healing of intestinal epithelial cells.[121] As mentioned earlier,[52] high dietary intake of omega-3 fatty acids is associated with a reduced incidence of UC. For patients with active UC, a fish oil preparation supplying 3200 mg of eicosapentaenoic acid (EPA) and 2400 mg of DHA per day decreased symptoms and lowered the levels of leukotriene B_4 (LTB_4) in rectal dialysates, with improvement demonstrated after 12 weeks of therapy.[122] A similar preparation improved histologic score and symptoms of patients with proctocolitis.[123] At a dose of 4200 mg of omega-3 fatty acids per day, fish oils were shown to reduce dose requirements for antiinflammatory drug therapy of UC.[124] At a dose of 5100 mg of omega-3 fatty acids per day, fish oils combined

with 5-ASA derivatives prevented early relapse of UC better than 5-ASA derivatives plus placebo, but fish oils alone did not maintain remission.[125] In all studies of UC, the fish oil preparations consisted of triacylglycerols. In vitro, fish oil has a more pronounced antiinflammatory effect on tissue culture of colonic specimens from patients with UC than from patients with CD.[126] Controlled trials of omega-3 therapy for CD have been generally disappointing,[127] although an early study from Italy using a delayed-release preparation supplying free EPA (1800 mg per day) and free DHA (800 mg per day) was much more effective than placebo in preventing relapse of CD in patients not taking 5-ASA derivatives.[128] The main side effect of fish oils is diarrhea.

Glutamine

Glutamine appears to have a special role in restoring normal small bowel permeability and immune function. Patients with intestinal mucosal injury secondary to chemotherapy or radiation benefit from glutamine supplementation with less villous atrophy, increased mucosal healing, and decreased passage of endotoxin through the gut wall.[129] Although integrative practitioners often advocate glutamine therapy for treatment of IBD, controlled studies have shown no benefit from glutamine supplementation at doses as high as 20 g per day in patients with CD.[130,131] Glutamine excess aggravates experimental colitis in rodents[132] and increases oxidative stress,[133] so high-dose glutamine supplements may be contraindicated in patients with colitis.

N-Acetylglucosamine

N-Acetylglucosamine (NAG) is a substrate for synthesis of glycosaminoglycans, glycoproteins that protect the bowel mucosa from toxic damage. Synthesis of NAG by N-acetylation of glucosamine is impaired in patients with IBD.[134] In explants of bowel tissue from patients, incorporation of added NAG was depressed in patients with inactive UC and increased to control levels in those with active colitis, a finding probably indicating the response of gut tissue to inflammation.[135] In a pilot study, NAG (3 to 6 g per day for more than 2 years) given orally to children with refractory IBD produced symptomatic improvement in most patients and an improvement in histopathologic features.[136] In children with distal colitis or proctitis, the same dose of NAG was administered by enema with similar effects.[134]

N-Acetylcysteine

N-Acetylcysteine is needed for synthesis of glutathione, has antioxidant and antiinflammatory effects, and has been shown to ameliorate experimental colitis. In a small, short-term clinical trial, N-acetylcysteine (800 mg per day), when added to mesalamine therapy of patients with active UC, produced a significant improvement in clinical response compared with mesalamine plus placebo.[137]

Phosphatidylcholine

Phosphatidylcholine (PC) is a component of cell membranes that is secreted into the intestinal mucus barrier, where it down-regulates TNF-alpha signaling.[138] PC concentration of ileal and colonic mucus of patients with UC is approximately one sixth the concentration found in healthy controls or patients with CD, a finding suggesting that this deficit may play a specific pathogenetic role in UC.[139] A clinical trial of delayed-release PC, 500 mg four times a day, allowed 80% of patients with steroid-dependent UC to withdraw from steroids without disease exacerbation; the response rate in the placebo arm of the trial was only 10%.[140] In other placebo-controlled studies by the same group, 6000 mg per day of delayed-release PC added to 5-ASA inhibitors effected significant reductions in clinical, endoscopic, and histologic disease activity and improved quality of life when compared with placebo.[141] Response to delayed-release PC takes a median of 5 weeks and occurs at doses as low as 1000 mg per day.[142]

Melatonin

Although some researchers have advocated melatonin as a therapy for IBD, melatonin is a potent inducer of Th1 lymphocytes, and aggravation of UC and CD with melatonin supplementation has been reported.[143-145]

> Some supplements may be strongly contraindicated because of potential toxicity: the strongest evidence exists for melatonin in Crohn disease, glutamine in ulcerative colitis, and *Echinacea* in patients taking immunosuppressants.

Probiotics

Probiotic therapy of IBD is attracting considerable attention because of the recognition that alteration of intestinal microflora may modulate intestinal immune responses[146] and act as triggers for inflammation in patients with IBD.[147] Because of the large numbers of probiotic preparations available, this section discusses only those preparations that are commercially available in the United States and that have been studied in clinical trials of patients with IBD. More data exist for their benefits in UC than in CD.

VSL-3

VSL-3 is a proprietary mixture of *Lactobacillus acidophilus, Lactobacillus bulgaricus, Lactobacillus casei, Lactobacillus plantarum, Bifidobacterium brevis, Bifidobacterium infantis, Bifidobacterium longum,* and *Streptococcus salivarius* ssp *thermophilus,* supplied in sachets containing 900 billion colony-forming units (CFUs) each. When added to therapy with the 5-ASA derivative balsalazide, VSL-3 (one sachet twice a day) induced faster remission of active UC than balsalazide or mesalamine alone.[148] Induction of remission with VSL-3 alone has been attained in 42%[149] to 54%[150] of adults with mild to moderate UC. VSL-3 also prevents relapse of pouchitis (postcolectomy inflammation of the ileal pouch).[151] Two sachets once a day produced remission rates far better than placebo over a 1-year period.[152] A clinical trial in children who were receiving steroid and mesalamine induction therapy for UC found that VSL-3, when compared with placebo, increased the rate of remission induction from 36.4% to 92.8% and reduced the rate of relapse within 12 months from 73.3% to 21.4%.[153] A possible problem with VSL-3 is poor compliance among patients not participating in clinical trials, perhaps because of the cost or inconvenience of administration.[154]

Lactobacillus GG

Lactobacillus rhamnosus var GG, at a dose of 10 to 20 billion CFUs per day, was found to prevent the onset of pouchitis in patients with ileal pouch–anal anastomosis during the first 3 years after surgery in a placebo-controlled trial.[155] *Lactobacillus* GG has been ineffective in inducing or maintaining remission of patients with CD[156] or in preventing relapse of CD after surgical resection.[157]

Saccharomyces boulardii

This plant-derived yeast demonstrated multiple antiinflammatory effects when it was administered to laboratory animals, including interference with the activity of NF-kappaB, a critical promoter of inflammatory cytokine transcription, and promotion of peroxisome proliferator-activated receptor-gamma (PPAR-gamma) activity, which protects the gut mucosa from inflammation.[158] *S. boulardii* has shown benefit in both UC and CD. The addition of *S. boulardii* (250 mg three times a day) to maintenance mesalamine therapy of patients with chronic, active UC was associated with induction of remission within 4 weeks in 17 of 25 patients.[159] This trial was uncontrolled. In a placebo-controlled trial, the same dose was given to patients with stable, active CD and mild to moderate diarrhea. *S. boulardii* reduced the frequency of diarrhea and the CDAI when it was given over a 10-week period, with benefits apparent within 2 weeks.[160] When added to mesalamine therapy of patients with CD in remission, *S. boulardii* (1000 mg per day) reduced the frequency of relapse from 37% to 6.25% during 6 months, when compared with mesalamine alone,[161] and it also decreased the pathologic elevation of small intestinal permeability.[162]

Although *S. boulardii* is considered nonpathogenic, case reports of *S. boulardii* fungemia have been described in critically ill or immunocompromised patients exposed to this yeast. At least 18 reports of this complication have been published, including a report in which airborne spread of *S. boulardii* occurred in an intensive care unit.[163]

Prebiotics

Prebiotics are nondigestible food ingredients that stimulate the growth or modify the metabolic activity of intestinal bacterial species that have the potential to improve the health of their human host. Criteria for classification of a food ingredient as a prebiotic are that it remain undigested and unabsorbed as it passes through the upper part of the gastrointestinal tract and is a selective substrate for the growth of specific strains of beneficial bacteria (usually *Lactobacillus* or *Bifidobacterium*), rather than for all colonic bacteria. Prebiotic food ingredients include bran, psyllium husk, resistant (high-amylose) starch, inulin (a polymer of fructofuranose), lactulose, and various natural or synthetic oligosaccharides that consist of short-chain complexes of sucrose, galactose, fructose, glucose, maltose, or xylose. The best-known effect of prebiotics is to increase fecal water content, thus relieving constipation.

Bacterial fermentation of prebiotics yields short-chain fatty acids such as butyrate. Fructooligosaccharides (FOSs) have been shown to alter fecal biomarkers (pH and the concentration of bacterial enzymes such as nitroreductase and beta-glucuronidase) in a direction that may convey protection against the development of colon cancer.[164] FOSs have also been shown to reduce fecal concentration of hydrogen sulfide in healthy volunteers,[165] an effect that may decrease colonic inflammation in patients with UC. In fact, several studies suggested benefits of various prebiotics for the treatment of UC. Oat bran, 60 g per day (supplying 20 g of dietary fiber), increased fecal butyrate by 36% in patients with UC and diminished abdominal pain.[166] A dietary supplement containing fish oil and two types of indigestible carbohydrate, FOS and xanthum gum, allowed reduction of glucocorticoid dosage when compared with a placebo in patients with steroid-dependent UC.[167] A Japanese germinated barley foodstuff (GBF) containing hemicellulose-rich fiber, at a dose of 20 to 30 g per day, increased stool butyrate concentration,[168] decreased the clinical activity index of patients with active UC,[169] and prolonged remission in patients with inactive UC.[170] Wheat grass juice, 100 mL twice daily for 1 month, tested in a small placebo-controlled trial of patients with distal UC,[171] produced a significant reduction in rectal bleeding, abdominal pain, and disease activity as measured by sigmoidoscopy.

Synbiotics

Synbiotics are combinations of probiotics and prebiotics. A mixture of *B. longum* and inulin-derived FOSs administered for 1 month as monotherapy to patients with UC produced improvement in sigmoidoscopic appearance, histologic features, and several biochemical indices of tissue inflammation when compared with a placebo control.[172] A Japanese study found that the administration of *B. longum*, 20 billion CFUs per day, with psyllium powder, 8 g per day for 4 weeks, to patients with UC reduced CRP by 76% and improved quality of life, whereas neither agent alone was effective.[173]

Bovine Colostrum

Colostrum is the first milk produced after birth and is particularly rich in immunoglobulins, antimicrobial peptides (e.g., lactoferrin and lactoperoxidase), and other bioactive molecules, including growth factors. Peptide growth factors in colostrum may provide novel treatment options for various gastrointestinal conditions.[174] Colostrum enemas, 100 mL of a 10% solution, administered twice a day by patients with distal UC, proved superior to a control enema in promoting healing; all patients were also taking a fixed dose of mesalamine.[175] Studies of oral colostrum in IBD have not been reported, but 125 mL three times a day fed to healthy human volunteers was shown to prevent the increase in intestinal permeability produced by indomethacin.[176] This finding suggests that peptide growth factors survive passage through the stomach and upper small bowel.

Dehydroepiandrosterone

Dehydroepiandrosterone (DHEA) is the steroid hormone produced in greatest quantity by the human adrenal cortex and is circulating primarily in the sulfated form, DHEA-S. DHEA inhibits activation of NF-kappaB, which is activated in inflammatory lesions. Patients with IBD have lower levels of DHEA-S in serum and intestinal tissue than do controls.[177] This finding is partially associated with prior treatment with glucocorticoids.[178] In men with IBD, low DHEA-S is associated with increased risk of osteoporosis.[179] In a pilot study, 6 of 7 patients with refractory CD and 8 of 13 patients with refractory UC responded to DHEA (200 mg per day for 56 days), with decrease in the clinical activity index.[180] A case report demonstrated benefit of the same dose of DHEA in a woman with severe refractory pouchitis, with relapse occurring 8 weeks after discontinuation of DHEA.[181]

Botanicals

In traditional Chinese medicine and Ayurveda, herbal extracts are the mainstay of treatment for IBD and appear to be effective when used by practitioners trained in those systems. Botanicals commonly taken by patients with IBD include slippery elm, fenugreek, devil's claw, *Gingko biloba*, *Angelica sinensis* (Dong quai), and licorice. Although these botanicals all express antioxidant or antiinflammatory activity in vitro,[182–184] data from clinical trials are lacking. Four botanical therapies with high safety profiles and that are readily available in the United States have been studied in clinical trials and are discussed here.

Curcumin

A complex of flavonoids derived from the spice turmeric *(Curcuma longa)*, curcumin has potent antiinflammatory effects in vitro.[185,186] Despite its poor solubility, stability, and systemic bioavailability, curcumin showed benefits in two small clinical trials of patients with CD and UC. In a placebo-controlled trial of patients with UC in remission, curcumin, 1000 mg twice a day, was administered with meals for 6 months along with maintenance sulfasalazine or mesalamine. The relapse rate in the curcumin group was 4.65%, compared with 20.51% in the placebo group. In an uncontrolled study, four of five patients with CD demonstrated reduction of the ESR and CDAI, and four of five patients with ulcerative proctitis were able to reduce concomitant medication dosage while they were taking a pure curcumin preparation.[187] A study of patients with colorectal cancer demonstrated that a dose of 3600 mg per day of curcumin orally yielded only trace levels in peripheral blood but reached a pharmacologically active concentration in neoplastic and normal colonic mucosa, thus inhibiting a key step in carcinogenesis.[188] Because IBD is a major risk factor for colon cancer, this finding makes curcumin an attractive therapeutic agent.

Boswellia serrata

The Ayurvedic herb *Boswellia serrata* (Indian frankincense) contains boswellic acids, which inhibit leukotriene biosynthesis in neutrophilic granulocytes by noncompetitive inhibition of 5-lipoxygenase.[189] During a small 6-week trial, 350 mg three times a day of *Boswellia* gum resin was as effective as sulfasalazine, 1000 mg three times a day, in reducing symptoms or laboratory abnormalities of patients with active UC.[190] The rate of remission was 82% with *Boswellia* and 75% with sulfasalazine.[191] A proprietary *Boswellia* extract, H15, was found as effective as mesalamine in improving symptoms of active CD in a randomized double-blind study from Germany.[192]

Aloe Vera

Aloe vera gel has a dose-dependent inhibitory effect on production of reactive oxygen metabolites, prostaglandin E_2, and (at high doses) IL-8, by human colonic epithelial cells grown in tissue culture.[193] Oral aloe vera gel, 100 mL twice a day for 4 weeks, produced a clinical response significantly more often than placebo (response ratio, 5.6) in patients with UC.[194] Remission occurred in 30% of patients taking aloe vera gel and in 7% of patients receiving placebo. Aloe also reduced histologic disease activity, whereas placebo did not. No significant side effects were described, although aloe vera gel is often used as a laxative. Acemannan, an extract of *Aloe vera*, concentrated to a mucopolysaccharide concentration of 30% of solid weight, was demonstrated to reduce symptoms and indices of inflammation in controlled studies of patients with UC.[195]

Pistacia lentiscus *Resin (Mastic Gum)*

In the Mediterranean region, mastic gum has a long history of use as a food and herbal remedy for gastrointestinal complaints. A pilot study of 10 patients with mild to moderate active CD who were given 2220 mg per day of mastic gum over 4 weeks demonstrated reduction in the CDAI and circulating levels of CRP and IL-6.[196] These findings were associated with a reduction in TNF-alpha production by peripheral blood mononuclear cells.[197]

Mind-Body Therapy

Although investigators widely believe that stress aggravates IBD, a prospective study did not validate the notion that stressful life events can trigger relapse.[198] A significant relationship between stress and inflammation has been found only when UC and CD are studied independently, but studies of mixed samples of patients with CD or UC have mostly had negative results. The results of five studies of psychological interventions in IBD were negative or only modestly supportive of benefit.[199] Three prospective studies of different types of psychotherapy for patients with IBD failed to show any improvement in medical outcome compared with standard care.[200-202] Counseling by a trained IBD counselor focusing primarily on illness-related concerns, however, resulted in decreased rates of relapse and outpatient visits, but not of hospitalization, over a 2-year period.[203] Higher levels of social support are associated with improved outcomes among patients with CD, especially patients with low body mass index.[204]

Self-Management Training

Knowledge, skill, and confidence in self-health management are highly correlated with health-related quality of life in patients with IBD.[205] A patient-centered educational approach developed at the University of Manchester in the United Kingdom was shown to have a significant impact on health care use by patients with UC. When compared with a control group that received customary care, the intervention group required one third as many physician visits and one third as many hospitalizations. The difference in outcome was not related to specific treatments employed, but rather to the empowerment of patients to be actively involved in managing their own care.[206] The method used was as follows: During a 15- to 30-minute consultation, physicians specifically asked patients about the symptoms they had experienced during past relapses and reviewed past and current treatments used to control symptoms, with an emphasis on the specific effectiveness of each treatment and its acceptability to the patient. Physician and patient then design a personalized self-management strategy based on the patient's recognition of symptoms and a mutually acceptable treatment protocol for the patient to initiate at the onset of a relapse.

Acupuncture

Acupuncture and moxibustion are commonly employed by practitioners of Chinese medicine for treatment of UC. Uncontrolled studies from China claimed excellent results.[207,208] A review of studies from both the Chinese and Western literature supported the efficacy of acupuncture in the regulation of gastrointestinal motor activity and secretion through opioid and other neural pathways.[209] A review of clinical trials of acupuncture for gastrointestinal disorders found one clinical trial of UC and one of CD with robust research designs. In each trial, true acupuncture was superior to sham acupuncture with regard to effect on disease activity indices.[210] A meta-analysis from Korea of five clinical trials of moxibustion for UC found favorable results when compared with conventional drug therapy, but all studies were deemed of poor quality and subject to bias.[211]

Pharmaceuticals and Helminths

Antimicrobial Drugs

Antibiotics are sometimes helpful for exacerbations of IBD, especially for CD and for draining fistula.[212,213] Metronidazole is the most commonly used agent; it is the first-line drug for treatment of pseudomembranous colitis caused by *Clostridium difficile* toxin, a complication of IBD that, in patients with active colitis, may occur spontaneously without prior antibiotic exposure. *S. boulardii* (1000 mg per day) enhances the therapeutic efficacy of metronidazole in the treatment of recurrent *C. difficile* colitis.[214] Some other natural products may interfere with the efficacy of metronidazole: Silymarin, a group of flavonoids extracted from milk thistle, at a dose of 140 mg per day for 9 days, decreased the peak plasma concentration and bioavailability of metronidazole and its major metabolite by 30% in healthy volunteers.[215] Vitamin E (400 units per day) with vitamin C (500 mg per day) reduced the effectiveness of metronidazole against metronidazole-sensitive *Helicobacter pylori* infection by 40%.[216]

A discussion of antibiotic protocols for IBD is outside the scope of this chapter. Commonly employed agents include ciprofloxacin, clarithromycin, and rifaximin.[217,218]

Antifungal therapy is sometimes embraced by integrative practitioners. Its use was supported by a study from Poland.[219] Quantitative stool cultures revealed high levels of colonization with *Candida* species (primarily *Candida albicans*) in 37% of patients with active UC of at least 5 years' duration and 20% of those with shorter duration but in only 1% of controls with irritable bowel syndrome. Patients with high yeast levels who were treated with fluconazole for 4 weeks in addition to conventional therapy had a significant improvement in clinical and endoscopic disease activity compared with similar patients treated with placebo plus conventional therapy.

> Always ask patients about the effect of antibiotics, including those drugs used for unrelated illnesses, on their gastrointestinal symptoms. Improvement of symptoms during antibiotic therapy may be an indication to use that antibiotic empirically during an exacerbation of symptoms. Aggravation of symptoms during antibiotic therapy may be an indication to avoid the specific antibiotic and employ probiotics.

Naltrexone

The opioid antagonist naltrexone has been described as an immune modulator when it is used at low doses.[220] In an open study of 17 patients with active CD who were receiving 4.5 mg per day of naltrexone for 12 weeks, 89% exhibited improvement in CDAI, and 67% achieved clinical remission. The benefits persisted for 4 weeks after therapy was discontinued. The most common side effect was sleep disturbance.[221]

Helminths

An application of the hygiene hypothesis to IBD reasons that loss of indigenous colonization with helminths is responsible for dysregulated immune responses.[222,223] Pork whipworm (*Trichuris suis*) and hookworm (*Necator americanus*) have been administered to patients with IBD in an effort to induce remission.[224] Clinical trials have demonstrated significant effects of oral administration of *T. suis* ova in both UC and CD. In patients with UC who received 2500 ova every 2 weeks for 12 weeks, the disease activity index was significantly reduced in 43.3% of patients receiving *T. suis* and 16.7% of those receiving placebo.[225] In an uncontrolled study of patients with active CD who received 2500 ova every 3 weeks for 24 weeks, the rate of clinical disease remission was 72.4%.[226]

5-Acetylsalicylic Acid Derivatives

Mesalamine, sulfasalazine, balsalazide, and olsalazine are used for inducing remission in mild cases of UC or CD and for maintenance of remission. The value of continuous therapy with 5-ASA derivatives at relatively high doses for maintenance of remission in UC is now well established. Side effects may include folate deficiency (discussed earlier), exacerbation of diarrhea, hair loss, and rash.

> The efficacy of 5-aminosalicylic acid (5-ASA) derivatives in inducing remission of inflammatory bowel disease can be enhanced by fish oils supplying 4000 mg of eicosapentaenoic acid plus docosahexaenoic acid per day and by probiotics (VSL-3, two packets a day, or *Saccharomyces boulardii*, 250 mg three times a day).

Glucocorticoids

Steroids are used to induce remission of IBD, but they have shown no benefit in maintaining remission. Not only do glucocorticoids suppress adrenal function, cause a decline in release of DHEA (discussed earlier), and impair immune function, but also their side effects include cataracts, growth failure, hypogonadism, and osteopenia. These agents decrease intestinal calcium absorption, increase renal calcium excretion, and induce parathyroid hormone secretion.

Immunosuppressants

6-Mercaptopurine and its derivative, azathioprine, are used for induction and maintenance of remission in IBD. Although usually well tolerated at low doses, these agents may cause leukopenia, anemia, and hepatic dysfunction and promote opportunistic infection. Immune-stimulating herbs, such as *Echinacea* and *Astragalus* species, may reverse the benefits of immune suppressants in the treatment of autoimmune disorders.[227,228] Concomitant use should be avoided.

Cyclosporine is occasionally used for inducing remission in refractory UC. Its absorption is drastically reduced by St. John's wort[229] and may be dangerously increased by peppermint oil.[230] Cyclosporine nephrotoxicity is diminished by administration of fish oil supplying 3000 to 4000 mg of omega-3 fatty acids per day[231,232] and by vitamin E (D-alpha tocopherol, 500 units per day).[233] Ipriflavone, a semisynthetic

isoflavonoid used for prevention of bone loss, may produce lymphopenia.[234] Patients receiving immunosuppressants should avoid this agent.

Tumor Necrosis Factor-alpha Blockade

TNF-alpha blockade with infliximab (Remicade) is a major advance in drug therapy for inducing remission of IBD. Adverse events reported in patients treated with anti-TNF agents include acute infusion reactions, delayed hypersensitivity–type reactions, autoimmune diseases such as drug-induced lupus and demyelination, and infection.[235] Cigarette smoking interferes with response to infliximab in patients with CD.[236]

Surgery

Surgical resection of inflamed bowel is considered a last resort in the management of patients with IBD. Correction of malnutrition and the use of probiotics (discussed earlier) may enhance responses to surgery for IBD.

PREVENTION PRESCRIPTION

- Observational studies suggest that diet influences the risk of developing IBD. The following dietary changes are associated with reduced risk:
  - High-fiber diet (at least 25 g per day)
  - Limited use of foods with added sugar or fat and avoidance of vegetable oils except olive oil
  - Limited consumption of beef or poultry (UC)
  - Omega-3 fatty acids from animal and vegetable sources should supply at least 1% of calories, and omega-6 fatty acids should supply no more than 7% of calories.
- For patients with IBD in remission, prevention of relapse may benefit from the following interventions:
  - Prolonged use of 5-aminosalicylic acid (5-ASA) derivatives plus folate, typically 1 mg/day
  - Along with a 5-ASA derivative, also prescribe *Saccharomyces boulardii*, 1000 mg per day. Constipation is a significant side effect.
- Additional evidence-based interventions for relapse prevention include the following:
  - Vitamin D_3: 1200 units per day for CD
  - Curcumin: 1000 to 1800 mg twice a day with meals for patients with UC. These interventions not only reduce the risk of relapse but also may reduce the risk of colon cancer.
  - For maintenance of remission in patients with UC, a high-fiber, low-meat diet with limited alcohol, supplemented with fish oils supplying approximately 5000 mg/day of omega-3 fatty acids (main side effect is diarrhea) and the probiotic VSL-3
  - A specific food exclusion diet, individually tailored, avoidance of tobacco exposure, and reduced consumption of sucrose for maintenance of remission in patients with CD
  - Folic acid, vitamin B_6, and vitamin B_{12} at doses that keep circulating homocysteine low, to prevent thrombotic complications
  - Vitamin D: 1200 units/day, to prevent bone loss and perhaps relapse

THERAPEUTIC REVIEW

All patients with inflammatory bowel disease (IBD) should be under the care of a gastroenterologist for regular endoscopic examination and prescription of appropriate drug therapy. The main role of the integrative practitioner is to help patients develop effective self-management strategies and enhance conventional treatment with an individualized nutritional prescription and the use of nutritional and botanical supplements.

Laboratory Tests

Certain laboratory tests are useful for fulfilling this role effectively. Commonly used tests include complete blood count, erythrocyte sedimentation rate, C-reactive protein, and serum albumin. Useful markers of nutritional status in IBD also include plasma zinc and homocysteine, serum and urine magnesium, serum iron, ferritin and transferrin, and 25-OH vitamin D. In steroid-treated patients with refractory disease, serum dehydroepiandrosterone sulfate (DHEA-S) may be useful. Patients with recent onset, relapse, or exacerbation of IBD—especially those with diarrhea—should undergo stool testing for parasites, pathogenic bacteria, *Clostridium difficile* toxins, and yeast.

Self-Management

- Spend an office visit ensuring that patients can recognize the symptoms of relapse and have a plan for controlling them.

- Use a mutually acceptable treatment protocol for the patient to initiate at the onset of a relapse.

Nutrition

- Avoid sucrose and symptom-provoking foods.

- As described earlier, the Specific Carbohydrate Diet, an exclusion diet, or a defined formula diet may help relieve symptoms and may help induce or maintain remission, especially in patients with Crohn's disease (CD).

- Balance dietary restrictions with the need for adequate macronutrient intake.

- Replace vegetable oils with olive, flaxseed oil, or coconut oil (1 to 2 tablespoons/day).

- Recommend oat bran, 60 g/day, for patients with mild-to-moderate ulcerative colitis (UC).

Supplements

- Folate: 1 mg/day or more especially for patients with high homocysteine or taking 5-ASA derivatives

- Vitamin B$_{12}$: 1 mg/month for patients with ileitis or previous ileal resection, receiving folic acid, or with high homocysteine

- Vitamin B$_6$: 10 to 20 mg/day, especially for patients with high homocysteine or taking high-dose folic acid or with urolithiasis

- Vitamin D$_3$: 1000 units/day or more to maintain levels of 25-OH vitamin D at 40 ng/mL

- Zinc: 25 to 200 mg/day to maintain plasma zinc at more than 800 mg/L

- Calcium: 1000 mg/day for patients taking steroids or with low dietary calcium

- Selenium: 200 mcg/day for patients with ileal resection or on liquid formula diets

- Magnesium citrate: 150 to 900 mg/day for patients with urolithiasis. Watch out for magnesium's laxative effect.

- Chromium: 600 mcg/day for patients with steroid-induced glycemia

- Fish oils supplying 4000 to 5000 mg/day of omega-3 fatty acids (eicosapentaenoic acid and docosahexaenoic acid) for patients with UC. Fish oils may cause diarrhea. Most fish oil capsules are only 50% omega-3 fatty acids.

- *N*-Acetylglucosamine (NAG): 3000 to 6000 mg/day

- Prebiotic oligosaccharides: approximately 10 g per day for UC. They can cause distention and flatulence.

Biologic Agents

- VSL-3: one sachet twice a day for patients with mild-to-moderate UC who are not sensitive to corn, the growth medium used. Any probiotic may aggravate bowel symptoms in patients with IBD.

- *Saccharomyces boulardii*: 250 mg three times daily or 500 mg twice daily for patients with chronic stable disease or to help maintenance of remission in patients not shown to be sensitive to yeast. *S. boulardii* may cause constipation.

- DHEA: 200 mg/day for patients with refractory disease and low DHEA-S

Botanicals

- *Boswellia serrata* gum resin: 350 mg three times daily for patients with UC who are intolerant of 5-ASA derivatives

- Curcumin: 1000 mg twice daily with meals

- Mastic gum: 1000 mg twice daily for patients with CD

Continued

- Aloe vera gel: 100 mL bid for patients with UC. Aloe may cause diarrhea.

Pharmaceuticals

- 5-ASA derivatives for induction of remission in mild-to-moderate colitis and for maintenance of remission

- Antibiotics for acute exacerbations of CD or UC or perianal disease

- Glucocorticoids for induction of remission in severe disease

- 6-Mercaptopurine or azathioprine for steroid-dependent IBD or for maintenance of remission when 5-ASA derivatives fail

- TNF-alpha blockers. For patients with severe CD, initiating pharmaceutical therapy with immunosuppressants and TNF-alpha blockers (step-down therapy) produces superior long-term results to initiating therapy with steroids and 5-ASA derivatives (step-up therapy) . None of these studies included dietary interventions, which are of proven value in CD.

Surgical Resection

- For patients with colonic dysplasia or for those who fail to respond to medical management

- Postsurgical recurrence rate is high for CD, and pouchitis is a frequent complication of ileal pouch–anal anastomosis for UC.

KEY WEB RESOURCES

PillAdvised.com: http://www.nutritionworkshop.com/medication-sandsupplementsinteractions/login.php	This free database details interactions involving drugs, nutrients, and supplements.
Crohn's and Colitis Foundation: www.ccfa.org	This Web site provides information about improving quality of life and ongoing research into inflammatory bowel disease (IBD).
Specific Carbohydrate Diet: www.breakingtheviciouscycle.info	This site contains a description of the Specific Carbohydrate Diet (SCD) and details about its implementation.
Digestive Wellness: http://www.digestivewellness.com	This online store is for patients using the SCD.
Imix Naturals: http://www.imixnaturals.com/index.aspm	This company supplies Absorb Plus, a palatable enteral feeding for patients with active Crohn's disease.
Ovamed: www.ovamed.org	This Web site is a source of information related to helminth therapy of IBD.

References

References are available online at expertconsult.com.

Section IX Obstetrics/Gynecology

Chapter 50

Postdates Pregnancy

D. Jill Mallory, MD

Pathophysiology

Postdates or postterm pregnancy is defined as a pregnancy that extends to or beyond 42 weeks of gestation (294 days or estimated date of delivery [EDD] plus 14 days). A normal pregnancy lasts approximately 40 weeks from the start of a woman's last menstrual period, but any pregnancy that lasts between 37 and 42 weeks is considered normal. Approximately 4% to 7% of all singleton pregnancies extend to 42 weeks, or 14 days beyond the EDD.[1]

Postterm pregnancy is associated with a higher perinatal mortality rate (stillbirth and newborn death within the first week) and a higher risk of complications during delivery, such as an emergency cesarean delivery, shoulder dystocia, postpartum hemorrhage, birth asphyxia, meconium aspiration syndrome, and neonatal birth injury.[2] Current research suggests that the lowest infant mortality rate is achieved when pregnant women have completed at least 41 weeks of gestation before labor is induced and when induction occurs before or at 42 weeks of gestation, although the absolute risk of problems from delivering beyond 42 weeks is low.[2] The overall risk of perinatal death is estimated at 0.4% in women who deliver beyond 42 weeks of gestation and 0.3% for women who deliver between 37 and 42 weeks of gestation.[3]

Because of this small increase in perinatal mortality, the induction of labor is widely practiced at or before 42 weeks of gestation, and postterm pregnancy has become the most common reason for induction.[4] Unfortunately, labor induction itself is not without risks. Obstetric problems associated with induction of labor in postterm pregnancy include cesarean section, prolonged labor, postpartum hemorrhage, and traumatic birth. These problems are more likely to result from induction when the uterus and cervix are not ready for labor.[2] Furthermore, induction of labor brings with it an increased risk of uterine rupture, uterine hyperstimulation, fetal distress, and instrumentation.[5]

Very few studies have taken into consideration women's experiences and opinions when it comes to the timing of induction of labor, and for women seeking a natural, unmedicated labor and birth, induction poses many philosophic challenges.

Accurate dating is obviously important in reducing the need for induction, and studies have shown that early ultrasound is associated with a reduced incidence of pregnancies misclassified as postterm.[6] When women have accurate pregnancy dating and are approaching 41 weeks of gestation, many may seek nonpharmaceutical measures of cervical ripening and labor induction. One small study of 50 women showed that many were opposed to medical induction of labor, and yet they used self-help measures to stimulate labor at home.[7] More research is needed in the realm of nonpharmaceutical cervical ripening and labor induction options for women who have postdate pregnancies.

Integrative Therapy

Nutrition

Pineapple

Pineapple *(Ananas ananas),* which contains the compound bromelain, has historical medicinal use both as a whole food and in extract form. Bromelain has been proposed as the active ingredient, and it is present only in the fresh fruit because the canning process destroys it. Bromelain has been used to elicit uterine contractions as a means of shortening labor. Some animal model research suggests that instead of increasing cervical prostaglandins, bromelain may actually inhibit them.[8] No research is available on the possible effectiveness of bromelain for induction of human uterine contractions, although this use is widely suggested in lay pregnancy resources. Some investigators suggest that pineapple's effects on labor may result from gastrointestinal stimulation by fiber and sugar, thus affecting local neural pathways.[9] No known risks are associated with pineapple use in pregnancy.

Supplements

Castor Oil

Castor oil, derived from the bean of the castor plant, has a very rich history of use for labor stimulation that dates back to ancient Egypt. One survey completed in 1999 found that 93% of U.S. midwives reported using castor oil to induce labor.[10] Despite this prevalence, research into the use of castor oil has been minimal. Only one study looking at safety was included in a Cochrane Review, and unfortunately, the study was small and of poor methodologic quality.[11] It included 100 women at term and compared ingestion of castor oil with no treatment. Outcomes evaluated included cesarean section rate, meconium staining of amniotic fluid, and Apgar scores. All women who ingested castor oil had nausea; otherwise, outcomes were no different from those in women who did not ingest castor oil. A retrospective observational study done in Thailand of 612 women looked at timing of delivery, fetal distress, meconium-stained amniotic fluid, tachysystole of the uterus, uterine rupture, abnormal maternal blood pressure during labor, Apgar scores, neonatal resuscitation, stillbirth, postpartum hemorrhage, severe diarrhea, and maternal death.[12] No differences were seen in outcomes between the women who ingested castor oil and the women who did not. This finding suggests that castor oil is safe to use but may not be helpful. Prospective randomized controlled trials are needed.

Evening Primrose Oil

Evening primrose oil (*Oenothera biennis*), a rich source of gamma-linoleic acid (GLA), is often used for several women's health conditions, including breast pain (mastalgia), menopausal and premenstrual symptoms, and labor induction or augmentation. This supplement is used widely during the last month of pregnancy by midwives in the United States for cervical ripening and to decrease the incidence of postdates pregnancy.[10] Evening primrose oil is typically administered as two capsules intravaginally at bedtime, starting after 38 completed weeks of pregnancy. When used as a cervical ripening agent, evening primrose oil has been shown to reduce the risk of postdates presentation.[10] Five studies, three of which were small randomized controlled trials, indicated the safety of vaginal evening primrose oil. One study investigated oral administration and showed that this route was not effective.[13] Furthermore, the oral use of evening primrose oil during pregnancy may also be associated with more prolonged labor and an increased risk of premature rupture of membranes, arrest of descent, oxytocin use, and vacuum extraction.[13] This finding is not surprising because oral administration during pregnancy was never a traditional use. Larger trials assessing efficacy are needed.

Homeopathy

Homeopathy is a safe choice for pregnant women and babies because the remedies used in this system of healing have no pharmacologic action.[14] In the United States, the use of homeopathic remedies has increased, and a survey among nurse-midwives in North Carolina reported that 30% recommend homeopathic substances for use during pregnancy.

The two most common homeopathic remedies used for labor induction are cimicifuga (homeopathic black cohosh) and caulophyllum (homeopathic blue cohosh), which are believed to act directly on the uterus and cervix. These remedies have been used around the world for labor stimulation, especially in Europe and India. Caulophyllum is used either to induce labor or to augment labor if uterine contractions are short and irregular or when uterine contractions stop.

Caulophyllum and cimicifuga are both indicated for dysfunctional uterine contractions and are thought to help initiate a coordinated and effective contraction pattern. Cimicifuga is used specifically to ease the fear of labor and delivery in women who have a history of traumatic childbirth, miscarriage, or abortion.[15] Cimicifuga alone is administered as a single dose of 30 C or 200 C potency every 30 minutes for at least 2 hours, or together with caulophyllum 200 C, alternating doses of the two remedies for a total of six doses in 24 hours. Other remedies that are commonly used for labor induction include aconite, arsenicum, gelsemium, phosphorus, and pulsatilla. These are all given in 200 C potency, as a single dose (two pellets).[16]

A 2003 Cochrane Review examined the use of caulophyllum, cimicifuga, and some of these other homeopathic remedies.[14] The review looked at only two studies comparing homeopathy and placebo for cervical ripening or labor induction and found that small sample sizes and insufficient detail in the research made it impossible to draw any meaningful clinical conclusions. More research needs to be done to determine whether homeopathy is a potentially viable alternative to oxytocin and prostaglandins for labor induction. Furthermore, studies should be designed to incorporate individualized homeopathic treatments, prescribed by a trained homeopath, to account for the individualized nature of this modality.

> For labor induction, caulophyllum and cimicifuga homeopathic remedies are as follows: 30 C or 200 C given every 30 minutes alternating, for a total of six doses in 24 hours. No remedy is given the next day. Repeat the same protocol on day 3 if needed. Other remedies to consider are gelsemium, for fear of birth, and pulsatilla, for when contractions come and go, but labor never becomes established.

Botanicals

Red Raspberry Leaf

Red raspberry leaf (*Rubus idaeus, Rubus occidentalis*) has been used as a uterine tonic and general pregnancy tea for at least 2 centuries. Although this botanical is often mistakenly recommended to induce labor, its actual role is to increase blood flow to the uterus and aid the uterine muscle fibers in more organized contraction. Studies indicate that some of the plant components, such as fragrine, an alkaloid, do act directly on smooth muscle.[17] Historical uses include prevention of miscarriage, prevention of postdates pregnancy, decrease of discomfort in prodromal labor, and decrease of morning sickness. Red raspberry leaf was probably also consumed for nutritional support because the plant contains many nutrients, including vitamins A, C, and E, as well as calcium, iron, and potassium. It is most commonly consumed as a tea, taken as 1 to 3 cups daily. Many studies have documented the safety of this botanical. One randomized controlled trial of 192 women showed no adverse effects to mother or baby, a shorter second stage of labor (a mean difference of 10 minutes), and a lower rate of forceps use.[16] One retrospective, observational study of more than 150 women also found that red raspberry leaf reduced the risk of postdates pregnancy, but more conclusive data are needed.[14]

Black Cohosh

This herb (*Cimicifuga racemosa)* also has a long history of use. Native Americans mixed it with chamomile, ginger, and raspberry tea to induce menses and labor. The active compounds in black cohosh include terpene glycoside fractions, such as actein and cimifugoside, which have been associated with an estrogenic effect and are thought to reduce levels of pituitary luteinizing hormone, thus decreasing ovarian production of progesterone.[15] This effect may contribute to the initiation of uterine contractions because the relaxing effect of the high levels of progesterone on the uterine muscle decreases before the initiation of labor. The plant also contains formononetin, which is thought to have a uterine-stimulating effect.[18] At least one case report has been published of toxicity in an infant whose mother was given an unknown dose of black cohosh at term.[19] At this time, the German Commission E, an expert committee established by the German Ministry of Health that evaluates herbal products, does not recommend the use of black cohosh in pregnancy.[20]

Blue Cohosh

The herb blue cohosh *(Caulophyllum thalictroides)* also has a long tradition of use as a uterine tonic. It was traditionally used by Native Americans during the 2 to 3 weeks before the onset of labor.[18] Between 1882 and 1905, blue cohosh was listed in the *United States Pharmacopoeia* for labor induction.[18] The plant contains the glycosides caulosaponin and caulophyllosaponin, which have documented oxytocic effects.[21]

Blue cohosh has some reported adverse neonatal effects, such as fetal hypoxia, myocardial infarction, and congestive cardiac failure.[22] Whether these effects resulted from the herb itself is not known, given that herbs are often used in combination with other plants, and adulteration and contamination problems can occur. Until further research on this plant is done, it is best avoided for labor induction.

> At this time, the use of blue and black cohosh is best avoided in pregnant women, out of safety concerns.

Biomechanical Therapy

Breast Stimulation

Breast stimulation has historically been used to induce or augment labor since as early as the eighteenth century.[23] Stimulation of the breast is thought to increase the production of endogenous oxytocin in pregnant and nonpregnant women. The most commonly used protocol for breast stimulation involves using either a manual or electric breast pump or manual massage around the areola of the nipple for 1 hour a day, for 3 consecutive days.

The Cochrane Collaboration performed a systematic review of 6 trials, with a total of 719 participants, that compared breast stimulation with no intervention to induce labor in women at term.[24] The review found that breast stimulation significantly reduced the number of women who had not gone into labor at 72 hours compared with no intervention.[24] Breast stimulation also reduced the risk of postpartum hemorrhage by 84%.[24]

Breast stimulation for labor induction allows women participation in the induction process and has the advantage of being a low-cost and nonpharmaceutical means of labor induction. Observational studies have shown a link between bilateral breast stimulation and uterine hyperstimulation.[25] For this reason, unilateral stimulation is typically recommended. Until safety issues have been more thoroughly evaluated, this technique should not be used in high-risk populations.

Shiatsu

Shiatsu is an ancient form of massage based on Chinese acupuncture theory that often includes the use of breathing and stretching. Shiatsu can be done through the clothes or on bare skin and uses static pressure, which can vary from light holding to deep physical pressure applied with the palm of the hand or thumb. Shiatsu lends itself well to maternity settings because specific shiatsu techniques can be taught to birth partners or practitioners. It has historically been used in midwifery practices to induce or augment labor.[26]

One small pilot study evaluated shiatsu for induction and augmentation of postterm labor.[27] Sixty-six women with postterm pregnancies were studied in a hospital-based midwifery practice. Pregnant women were taught to massage three acupuncture points in conjunction with breathing techniques and exercises. The controls attended the same clinic, but they were not taught the techniques. The investigators found that the women with postterm pregnancies who used shiatsu were significantly more likely to have spontaneous labor than were the study participants who did not use shiatsu.

Bioenergetics

Acupuncture

As part of the ancient system of medicine known as traditional Chinese medicine, acupuncture has been used in pregnancy for thousands of years. Modern studies have evaluated the insertion of fine needles into specific points on the body, as well as the use of mild electrical currents through these needles, known as electroacupuncture. A 2004 Cochrane Systematic Review evaluated acupuncture for inducing labor.[28] The investigators identified 3 trials, including 212 women, for review. The first case series used electroacupuncture at 38 to 42 weeks of gestation to induce labor successfully in 21 of 31 women. The second series used acupuncture with and without electrical stimulation to induce labor in 10 of 12 women at 19 to 43 weeks of gestation. The third study induced labor with electroacupuncture in 78% of 41 women.[28] The overall conclusion was that fewer women using acupuncture required induction of labor by other methods.

Several studies have been published since the foregoing Cochrane Review. One randomized controlled trial of 45 women found that acupuncture at points LI4 and SP6 shortened cervical length at term and reduced the time between the EDD and delivery.[29] A larger double-blind randomized controlled trial of 181 women in Denmark did not show any benefit of induction of labor in women with postdates pregnancies who were treated with acupuncture.[30] No adverse effects were seen. Another smaller trial of 67 women in Brazil showed effects similar to those with misoprostol for cervical ripening, with a higher frequency of vaginal delivery and no obstetric complications.[31] The inherent difficulties in blinding for acupuncture treatment make the study of this

TABLE 50-1. Acupressure Points for Induction
of Labor

1. Midway along the top of the trapezius muscles, if you were to draw a line from the acromion to C7
2. The motion sickness point at the angle between the first and second metacarpals
3. In the semicircle around the distal medial and lateral malleoli
4. The little toe, all over

Massage these points for at least 2 to 3 minutes each.

From Mallory J. Integrative care of the mother-infant dyad. *Prim Care.* 2010;37:149–163.

technique challenging. Certainly, the studies do agree that acupuncture is safe in pregnancy, and it may be worth trying in patients who wish to avoid pharmaceutical induction of labor. Table 50-1 provides acupuncture points that patients can massage at home to stimulate labor.

Lifestyle

Sexual Intercourse

Unprotected sexual intercourse is thought to encourage the onset of labor by two means. One is the release of endogenous oxytocin in the mother, and the other is cervical ripening caused by seminal prostaglandins. A Cochrane Review looked at an observational study of 28 women at term. Unprotected intercourse for 3 consecutive nights did not significantly change Bishop scores (1.0 with coitus versus 0.5 controls; $P > .05$), nor did it increase the number of women who went into labor at the end of 3 days (relative risk, 0.99; 95% confidence interval, 0.45 to 2.20).[32] Larger studies are needed to determine whether sexual intercourse has any significant effect on reducing the risk of postdates pregnancy.

Pharmaceuticals

Misoprostol

Misoprostol is a prostaglandin E_1 analogue widely used for off-label indications such as induction of labor in postdates pregnancy. This hormone is given by insertion through the vagina or rectum, or by mouth, to ripen the cervix and elicit uterine contractions. A Cochrane Review looked at 121 trials and found that small doses of misoprostol were as effective as other methods of labor induction.[33] Larger doses of misoprostol were found to be more effective than prostaglandins for induction, and larger doses also reduced the need for additional oxytocin. Another Cochrane Review showed that the oral route of administration is preferable to the vaginal route. The main risk of misoprostol use is hyperstimulation of the uterus. At this time, misoprostol is not approved by the Food and Drug Administration for induction of labor.

▪ Dosage

The most common dose used in the United States is 25 mcg intravaginally every 4 hours (maximum, 50 mcg). Wait for more than 4 hours after last dose before adding oxytocin. Misoprostol comes in 100- and 200-mcg formulations.

▪ Precautions

Uterine hyperstimulation, uterine rupture, diarrhea, nausea, vomiting, headache.

Although misoprostol is commonly used for labor induction in the United States, it has not been approved by the Food and Drug Administration for this use.

Oxytocin

Oxytocin is the most common induction agent used worldwide. It is used alone, in combination with amniotomy or following cervical ripening with other pharmacologic or nonpharmacologic methods. Oxytocin is a synthetic analogue of the natural labor hormone by the same name. It binds to oxytocin receptors in the uterine myometrium, increases intracellular calcium, and stimulates uterine contractions. A Cochrane Review of more than 61 studies concluded that it is safe and effective.[34] A black box warning placed on the drug by the FDA states that oxytocin is not to be used for elective labor induction.

▪ Dosage

Start with 0.5 to 2 milliunits/minute, and increase by 1 to 2 milliunits/minute every 15 to 40 minutes until the uterine contraction pattern is established. The maximum for induction is 40 milliunits/minute. Oxytocin is available in intravenous and intramuscular preparations.

▪ Precautions

Increased use of epidural anesthesia, uterine hyperstimulation, uterine rupture, abruptio placentae, fetal distress, nausea, vomiting.

Vaginal Prostaglandins (PGE$_2$ and PGF$_{2alpha}$)

Prostaglandins have been used for the induction of labor since the 1960s. These drugs are synthetic analogues of the body's naturally occurring prostaglandins, which function to ripen the cervix and bring about contractions. A Cochrane Review looked at 63 randomized controlled studies of various forms of prostaglandins and found them to be a safe and effective means of labor induction.[35] Prostaglandin E_2 is the most commonly used type, and it increases the likelihood of vaginal birth in 24 hours without increasing the risk of cesarean section.[35]

▪ Dosage

The dose is one 10-mg pessary intravaginally. The insert releases 0.3 mg/hour over 12 hours. Remove at 12 hours, at the onset of active labor, or if uterine hyperstimulation occurs. The agent is available as a 10-mg sustained-release insert. It is also available as an intravaginal tablet or gel.

▪ Precautions

Uterine hyperstimulation, fetal distress, uterine rupture, bronchospasm, abdominal cramps, headache, nausea, diarrhea.

Mechanical Methods

Potential advantages of mechanical methods, compared with pharmacologic methods, for the induction of labor in postdates pregnancy include simplicity of use, lower cost, and reduction of side effects, such as uterine hyperstimulation and fetal distress. However, special attention should be paid to contraindications such as a low-lying placenta, risk of infection, and maternal discomfort.

Amniotomy

The deliberate rupture of membranes may be sufficient to bring about labor without the use of pharmaceuticals. This approach has the advantage of being cheap, but it may be uncomfortable for some women. If the time between amniotomy and delivery of the baby is long, infection may occur. The risk of umbilical cord prolapse is also increased, especially if the fetal head is ballotable at the time of membrane rupture. Anecdotal reports note that amniotomy may be less beneficial in nulliparous women. More evidence is needed regarding effectiveness compared with placebo or compared with other methods of induction of labor.[36]

Membrane Sweeping

Sweeping of the membranes, also known as membrane stripping, is a simple manual technique usually done in the outpatient setting. The technique involves inserting a finger into the cervical os during a sterile vaginal examination and sweeping the finger in a circular motion to detach the membranes from the lower uterine segment. This method sometimes works to initiate labor by increasing the local production of prostaglandins. A Cochrane Review of 72 studies found that sweeping of the membranes, performed routinely for women at term, was associated with a reduced frequency of pregnancy extending beyond 41 weeks.[37] This method is considered safe and reduces the need for pharmaceutical means of induction of labor in postdates pregnancy.[37] Adverse effects include maternal discomfort, vaginal bleeding, and irregular contractions.

Transcervical Foley Catheter Insertion

This approach involves placing a 30-mL Foley catheter bulb transcervically, inflating it with sterile saline solution, and applying maintenance traction. One randomized controlled trial found this technique equivalent to intravaginal misoprostol for cervical ripening, without the risk of uterine hyperstimulation.[38] Complications include acute febrile reaction, pain, vaginal bleeding, and altered fetal presentation.

PREVENTION PRESCRIPTION

■ Women can be encouraged in the preconception period to track their menstrual cycles and sexual activity closely to aid in accurate pregnancy dating. When women are unsure of their pregnancy dates, first trimester ultrasound reduces the number of women later incorrectly classified as having postdates pregnancies.

■ Good self-care in pregnancy, including aromatherapy, good nutrition, massage, sexual intercourse, spiritual practices, chiropractic, and yoga during the latter weeks of pregnancy may serve to relax the mother and allow the natural rise of oxytocin and reduction of stress hormones, thus resulting in a greater likelihood of spontaneous onset of labor.[39-41]

■ Membrane sweeping, done routinely at 38 weeks, may also reduce the risk of a pregnancy that continues beyond 41 weeks.

THERAPEUTIC REVIEW

These therapeutic options for prevention of postdates pregnancy and induction of labor in postdates pregnancy may be considered in the healthy, term patient, with no medical complications that would make delivery urgent.

◼ Nutrition

• Pineapple consumption is commonly recommended for labor induction. Although pineapple has no proven benefit, the risks of this intervention are low.

◼ Supplements

• Castor oil has a long history of use for labor induction. It is considered safe, but it has not been proven effective. Side effects include nausea. Doses are not standardized.

• Evening primrose oil is possibly effective as a cervical ripening agent when it is used to reduce the risk of postdates pregnancy. The dose is two capsules intravaginally at bedtime, starting at 38 weeks of pregnancy. This supplement should not be used orally in pregnancy.

• The homeopathic remedies caulophyllum and cimicifuga can be dosed at 200 C potency, by alternating the two remedies every 30 minutes, for a total of six doses in 24 hours to help stimulate labor. The benefit is unknown, and risks are minimal.

◼ Botanicals

• Red raspberry leaf, taken as 1 to 3 cups of tea daily during the third trimester, may reduce the risk of postdates pregnancy.

• Despite a strong history of use, black cohosh and blue cohosh should be avoided in pregnancy because of safety concerns until more data are available.

◼ Biomechanical Therapy

• Unilateral breast stimulation can be done for 1 hour per day for 3 consecutive days to induce labor at term.

• Shiatsu may reduce the risk of postdates pregnancy.

◼ Acupuncture

• Evidence is mixed on the effectiveness of acupuncture to reduce the risk of postdates pregnancy, for cervical ripening, and for labor induction. Acupuncture is considered safe.

Lifestyle

- Sexual intercourse may not be effective for reducing the risk of postdates pregnancy.

Pharmaceuticals

- Misoprostol is commonly used for cervical ripening and labor induction, despite a lack of approval by the Food and Drug Administration for this indication. See the doses and precautions discussed in the text.

- Oxytocin may be used to induce uterine contractions in postdates pregnancy, when cervical conditions are favorable. See the doses and precautions discussed in the text.

- Vaginal prostaglandins may be used for cervical ripening and labor induction, and they are a good choice in postdates pregnancy in patients with unfavorable cervical conditions. See the doses and precautions discussed in the text.

Mechanical Therapy

- Amniotomy may be used to induce or augment labor, and it may be more beneficial in multiparous women.

- Membrane sweeping can be considered routinely at 38 weeks to reduce the risk of postdates pregnancy.

- Transcervical Foley catheter insertion can be done for cervical ripening in postdates pregnancy, and it may have lower risks than pharmaceutical ripening agents.

KEY WEB RESOURCES

American College of Obstetricians and Gynecologists: http://www.acog.org/publications/patient_education/bp069.cfm	Patient handout on postdates pregnancy
American College of Nurse-Midwives: http://www.mymidwife.org/	Consumer information on pregnancy and midwifery

References

References are available online at expertconsult.com.

Chapter 51

Labor Pain Management

Michelle J. Mertz, MD, and Connie J. Earl, DO

We have the pleasure of discussing the only topic in this section of the book that is not a pathologic condition. Childbirth is uncomplicated in most women, and it typically results in a joyful outcome. To many, birth is considered a rite of passage, a sacred experience that should be honored. Birth experiences are widely variable in length of labor, severity of pain, and emotions surrounding the event. Women's preferences regarding birth are equally variable. For this reason, labor management is best when individualized and when options and preferences are discussed before the onset of labor. One systematic review noted that women's satisfaction with their childbirth experience was less affected by pain control than by personal expectations, the amount of support they received from caregivers, the quality of the caregiver-patient relationship, and their own involvement in decision making.[1]

After a period of heavily medicated birth in the United States during the midtwentieth century, a backlash against the medical model arose, and women began to demand the right to choose their own childbirth experience. Today, women are much more at liberty to influence these experiences. This chapter explores the birthing woman's many options for pain management.

Physiology

Labor is separated into three stages. The first stage involves dilation of the cervix and the beginning descent of the fetus into the pelvis. The second stage is full dilation and birthing of the fetus, and the third stage is passage of the placenta.

Pain in the first stage is primarily visceral, resulting from the mechanical dilation of the cervix and lower uterus. Nociceptive information is carried back on sympathetic fibers to the posterior nerve root ganglia at T10 through L1, as well as on parasympathetic fibers from the pelvic splanchnic nerves (S2 through S4).[2] The T10-L1 segmental levels also receive nociceptive information from the skin of the back.[2] This last mechanism may explain why many women feel contractions in their back. Pressure on the pelvic nerves may explain why labor pain can radiate to the thighs

or buttocks as well. In some cases of fetal malposition, such as occiput posterior or occiput transverse, the woman may experience more severe back labor resulting from a relative increase in diameter of the head passing through the pelvis in these positions. Back labor is not isolated to the occiput posterior or occiput transverse position, however.

During the second stage of labor, pain primarily stems from mechanical stretching and distention of the perineum and pelvic floor musculature. This is somatic pain, carried to the central nervous system on the pudendal nerve fibers (S2 through S4).[2] It is often described as sharp. Many women report a sensation of rectal pressure during descent of the fetus. As the presenting part begins to stretch the perineum, many women describe a classic "ring of fire" sensation.

Pain Relief in Labor

Any acute pain, including labor pain, has two main physiologic components: the transmission of the physical pain stimulus to the brain and the interpretation of the information that is filtered through the hypothalamic and limbic systems. Thus, the experience of pain is influenced by emotions and memories.[3] Whereas pharmaceutical agents are typically geared toward relief of physical pain, many of the nonpharmacologic methods do not attempt to remove the sensation, but instead target the perception of the pain stimulus. One mechanism proposed for many of the therapies discussed in this chapter is the *gate control theory:* sensations such as pressure, vibration, pain, or temperature stimulate superficial tactile nerve endings, and this stimulation leads to inhibition of the pain signal transmission from the organs and deeper tissues at that segmental level.[4]

Integrative Therapy

Continuous Labor Support or Doula

Historically, women have long provided continuous labor support to other women in labor. In the twentieth century, a break in that tradition occurred as birth moved from an out-of-hospital midwifery model of care to a more institutionalized model. Since the 1980s, a resurgence in labor support has attempted to integrate the two models. Research in this area typically focuses on the labor "doula," a person present solely to support the birthing woman and her family.[5] Doulas have no medical role in the labor or birth and are often hired in the second or third trimester of pregnancy to form a relationship with the birthing family before labor begins.

A large Cochrane Review demonstrated a significant decrease in pain medication required, length of labor, and incidence of cesarean delivery and operative delivery with continuous labor support by a doula.[6] This benefit was most pronounced when doula support was begun in early labor.[6] The most important factor appears to be the continuous presence of labor support.[7] An earlier study demonstrated that even the continuous presence of a silent female observer had a positive effect on the foregoing outcomes, although the greatest benefit was observed when a trained doula was present.[8] Continuous support is most efficacious when the provider is not a member of the hospital staff.[9,10] Given the benefits, all women in labor should be offered a doula.

Childbirth Preparation

Half of the women in the United States are estimated to attend some sort of childbirth education class during pregnancy.[11] Many approaches are used, but most classes aim to prepare women and their partners for childbirth and parenthood. Some of these classes introduce women and their partners to various pain relief techniques reviewed in this chapter. Data on pain in labor in relation to childbirth education are sparse. Although individual studies have demonstrated benefits of prenatal education besides pain relief, a review of the literature found the study methods too diverse to comment on benefits clearly.[12] A large randomized controlled trial (RCT) found no difference in epidural rate or pain level rated retrospectively with one form of childbirth education.[13] Given the popularity of antenatal education, more research is needed to determine its best use.

Lifestyle

Exercise
Research suggests that regular aerobic exercise during pregnancy is associated with decreased pain scores in labor.[14] Moderate-intensity exercise in labor has also been observed to lower pain scores, even after the exercise ends.[15] No known risks to the fetus are associated with moderate exercise, though some increased uterine activity occurs with exercise at term.[15,16] Women should be encouraged to exercise regularly during pregnancy.

Biomechanical Therapy

Positions During Labor and Ambulation
Western medicine long ago adopted the lithotomy position as the position of choice for childbirth, mostly for ease of the practitioner. In contrast, historically around the world, women have employed an upright position in the first and second stages of labor.[17]

Ambulation and an upright position during the first stage of labor is associated with a decreased length of the first stage, a decreased use of epidural anesthesia, and no difference in adverse maternal or neonatal outcomes.[18] Additionally, in women with a fetal malpresentation associated with back labor, the hand and knees position during labor appears to decrease back pain.[19]

The use of an upright or side-lying position in the second stage of labor is associated with a decreased length of the second stage. It was also associated with a decreased report of severe pain in a systematic review of 23 RCTs.[20] A small but significant increase in the incidence of blood loss greater than 500 mL was reported, but without adverse maternal or fetal outcomes. Unless medically contraindicated, all women should be allowed to ambulate and choose the positions they assume in labor and birth.

Water Immersion
Originally relegated to home birth and out-of-hospital birthing centers, water birth and water immersion in labor are now options in many hospital labor and delivery units. Laboring in water has many purported advantages, including ease of position change with the decreased effects of gravity, relaxation, decreased sensation of pain, and greater control for the laboring woman over her personal space.

A Cochrane Review of water immersion demonstrated a significant reduction in use of pain medication with water immersion in the first stage of labor and no difference in adverse maternal or neonatal outcomes.[21] Two of these RCTs also demonstrated increased maternal satisfaction with water immersion in the second stage of labor,[21] with no difference in mode of delivery or adverse maternal or neonatal outcomes.[21,22] A small RCT found increased normal vaginal delivery in water birth compared with land birth.[23] More research is needed to evaluate water birth. Water immersion in labor does not appear to increase the risk of chorioamnionitis or endometritis, even in women with ruptured membranes.[24]

> The temperature of the water should be no more than 99°F to avoid raising maternal core temperature in labor.[21]

Chiropractic, Osteopathic, and Manual Therapy
Back pain is a common phenomenon in pregnancy because the body changes shape, joints relax from hormonal effects, and the spine and frame are required to support added weight. Some data suggest that back pain in pregnancy may be associated with increased back pain in labor.[25] One small retrospective study demonstrated that women who received prenatal chiropractic manual therapy reported less pain in labor than those who did not.[25] Manual therapy is an option for the management of musculoskeletal back pain in pregnancy, and it may lead to less pain in labor for women who receive regular treatments during pregnancy. Further study in this area is needed. No adverse events have been reported with the use of manual therapy in pregnancy.[26]

Massage

Although research is limited, intrapartum massage has been shown to reduce pain perception[27-31] and decrease anxiety[27-29] in early labor. No evidence indicates that it decreases the use of pain medication in labor. Regardless of the paucity of research on this topic, clinicians generally accept that massage can promote relaxation and enhance the quality of women's birth experiences.

Sterile Water Injections

Nearly 30% of women have severe continuous back pain in labor that persists between contractions. Sterile water injections in the low back can be used to relieve this pain. In contrast to isotonic saline, the salt-free water causes irritation as well as physical distention of the skin. The underlying mechanism of pain inhibition is not fully understood. Many investigators refer to the process of counterirritation,[32,33] in which one type of pain masks another, or to the gate control theory.

Several studies demonstrated that intracutaneous or subcutaneous sterile water injections provided good pain relief in the first stage of labor, particularly for low back pain.[34-40] The effect remained for up to 2 hours.[34-39] These injections are simple to administer, inexpensive, and carry no known risks. They were not shown to reduce the use of pain medication in these studies. Administration can be quite painful, but the pain is transient, and subcutaneous injection may be less painful than the intracutaneous route.[41] The precise location of the points does not appear critical to the success of the procedure.[42]

Technique

Palpate the posterior superior iliac spines, and mark them with a pen. From these sites, measure 3 cm inferiorly and 2 cm medially. Mark these two spots, and swab all four spots (two on the left and two on the right) with alcohol.[42] During a contraction, inject 0.1 to 0.5 mL of sterile water subcutaneously or intracutaneously with a fine needle, thus forming a small white bleb, as during a tuberculin skin test. Repeat at the remaining three sites as quickly as possible. It may help for two providers to inject simultaneously. Repeat as necessary.

Bioenergetics

Transcutaneous Electrical Nerve Stimulation

Transcutaneous electrical nerve stimulation (TENS) emits low-voltage electrical impulses through electrodes, with operator-controlled variation in frequency and intensity. TENS units are portable, battery operated, and relatively inexpensive. TENS has typically been used to treat musculoskeletal and neuropathic pain, although its efficacy is controversial. The mechanism of action most often proposed is the gate control theory. Application of the electrodes is not standardized in labor. Although electrodes are typically applied paraspinally at T10 and S2, many studies also describe acupoints and cranial placement.[42]

FIGURE 51-1
Acupressure to SP6.

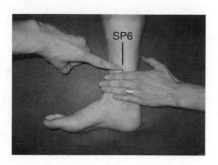

A Cochrane Review of studies with notably heterogeneous methods demonstrated little evidence of significant pain relief in labor from the use of TENS. Despite this finding, fewer women reported severe pain with the use of TENS, and women who had true TENS were more likely to want to use it in a future labor than those who received sham TENS.[43] The trials that applied TENS to known acupoints more consistently demonstrated pain relief.[44,45] Application can be intermittent or continuous, although continuous TENS may be more effective in active labor.[45]

> The application of transcutaneous electrical nerve stimulation may interfere with electronic fetal monitoring.

Acupuncture

In obstetrics, acupuncture has been used to promote version in a breech presentation, decrease nausea, induce or augment contractions, and provide pain relief.[46] It has also been used for pain management during perineal suture repair. Spleen 6 (SP6) and large intestine 4 (LI4) are the most commonly used acupoints in labor (Figs. 51-1 and 51-2).

Early data were quite hopeful,[47] but the most comprehensive meta-analysis to date found fewer optimistic results among more recent, well-designed trials.[48-51] The considerable heterogeneity among the study designs and outcomes evaluated makes it challenging to draw conclusions comfortably. When acupuncture was compared with minimal acupuncture (superficial needling), research remained equivocal regarding the efficacy of acupuncture for pain relief in labor.[49-51] Compared with no acupuncture, however, both manual acupuncture[51] and electoacupuncture[48,52] demonstrated decreased pain for 30 minutes after treatment. Additionally, women receiving acupuncture used fewer pharmacologic and invasive methods of analgesia,[53-55] were more satisfied with their pain relief,[48,50,52] and were more relaxed.[55] No adverse events have been demonstrated.[48-50,53-55]

> SP6 and LI4 are purported to cause uterine contractions and should therefore not be used if labor is not desired.[56]

FIGURE 51-2
A and B, Acupressure to LI4.

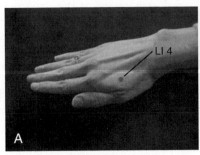 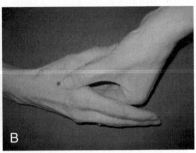

Acupressure

Acupressure is a variation of acupuncture involving the application of constant pressure on specific acupoints. Like acupuncture, acupressure is frequently used to enhance labor, manage labor pain, and shorten the time to delivery.[57] Because the needles are replaced by pressure, this technique is noninvasive, requires no equipment, and can easily be taught to partners or support staff. Several RCTs have demonstrated reduction in labor pain with 30 minutes of acupressure at SP6.[57-59] One study found similar results with acupressure at LI4 and bladder 67 (BL67).[60] Pain relief has generally been found to last 1 to 2 hours after treatment. No study to date has found acupressure to replace the use of epidural or other pharmacologic analgesia.

> *Find SP6:* Located one hand breadth (four finger widths based on the proximal interphalangeal joints) above the prominence of the medial malleus, in a depression just medial to the border of the tibia (see Fig. 51-1).[56]
>
> *Find LI4:* Ask the patient to squeeze the thumb against the base of the index finger (see Fig. 51-2A). LI4 is on the dorsum of the hand, at the height of the muscle bulge, level with the end of the crease. It is between the first and second metacarpal bones (see Fig. 51-2B).[56]

Mind-Body Therapy

Hypnotherapy

Hypnosis is a state of focused concentration in which the patient is relatively unaware, but not completely blind to her surroundings.[46] *Hypnotherapy* refers to the clinical use of suggestions under hypnosis to achieve specific therapeutic goals.[64] During labor, these suggestions focus on the diminished awareness of pain, fear, and anxiety, thus leading to a decreased perception of each. Generally, this technique requires practice before the onset of labor.

A comprehensive review[61] included studies that demonstrated decreased use of pain medication,[62] higher pain thresholds,[62] shorter hospital stays,[63] less surgical intervention,[63] fewer complications,[63] and a more satisfying birth experience[64] in hypnotized women. Despite heterogeneity among trials, outcomes consistently favored hypnosis.[61] Hypnosis is relatively contraindicated in patients who are vulnerable to psychotic decompensation.

Yoga

Yoga uses the breath to focus on the interconnectedness between the mind and the body. It is thought to bring the individual toward a state of greater relaxation, increased self-awareness, and increased emotional well-being. Yoga also promotes muscle strength and flexibility.[65] Although yoga has been linked to improved birth weight[66,67] and decreases in labor duration,[66] preterm labor, intrauterine growth restriction, and emergency cesarean rate,[67] only two studies have focused on maternal comfort in labor. They demonstrated that regular yoga practice in pregnancy was associated with higher levels of maternal comfort during labor and 2 hours afterward and shorter duration of first stage and total time of labor.[65,68] Neither study demonstrated a decrease in use of pain medication, but investigators noted that the yoga group remained "in control" despite intensifying labor. The nonrandomized controlled trial demonstrated[68] that women who participated in a prenatal yoga program had significantly fewer pregnancy discomforts and increased childbirth self-efficacy. Participants also felt more in control and had lower pain levels that allowed them to be more active in their childbirth experience. Yoga is considered safe in pregnancy because all poses can be modified for the pregnant woman.

Music and Audioanalgesia

The use of music as adjunct therapy has been shown to reduce pain significantly in patients with chronic, postoperative, and cancer pain. Music has also been shown to decrease anxiety during colposcopy and in cardiac patients.[69-71] Many people have extrapolated the analgesic effects of music to labor as well. In the limited available studies, music therapy indeed appears to be mildly effective in reducing both labor pain and distress from that pain.[75,76] Music should be offered to women in labor if they desire.

Biofeedback

With biofeedback, physiologic information such as pulse or blood pressure is recorded through electrodes and shown in real time on a monitor while the patient adjusts her behavior or thoughts to control physiologic functions that were previously considered involuntary. Patients like biofeedback because it puts them in control and allows them to learn by trial and error.[46] Results are equivocal regarding the efficacy of biofeedback in labor.[74-76] The technique is risk free; however, it does require practice to master during pregnancy.

Biochemical Therapy: Aromatherapy

Aromatherapy is a natural healing art that uses essential oils extracted from aromatic botanical sources. These oils can also be used in the bath water, rubbed on clothing or towels for use as a compress, mixed with oil and applied, or kept available in small vials to open and smell. Examples of essential oils used in labor are lavender, chamomile, mandarin, clary sage, ginger, frankincense, eucalyptus, jasmine, lemon, and peppermint. In one large observational study, women consistently reported aromatherapy to be a helpful adjunct to their labor experience. Incidentally, a substantial overall reduction was noted in the use of systemic opioids in the hospital during the 8 years of the study. Frankincense was rated most highly for pain relief, followed by lavender. Rose and lavender were rated most highly for anxiety reduction. One percent of patients noted mild adverse reactions, such as nausea, itchy rash, and headache.[77] One small underpowered RCT demonstrated a positive trend for decreased pain perception with aromatherapy.[78]

Botanicals

Raspberry Leaf

Raspberry leaf is commonly used as a uterine tonic.[79] As many as 25% of women in the United States use raspberry leaf in pregnancy,[80,81] and up to one third of U.S. nurse midwives use raspberry leaf to stimulate labor.[81] A review of the existing studies demonstrated a positive trend toward decreases in length of first and second stage of labor and operative vaginal delivery.[82] No data are available on pain in labor with prenatal raspberry leaf. None of the studies have evaluated raspberry leaf tea, although this is typically how it is used.

◼ Dose

The dose is 1.2 g orally twice daily,[83] starting in the third trimester.

Motherwort, Cramp Bark, and Black Cohosh

These botanicals are used by some herbalists to relieve back pain and spastic uterine contractions during labor.[79] No human studies have evaluated the efficacy of these botanicals. Black cohosh may be linked to hepatotoxicity and should be used with caution until more data are available.[79]

Skullcap

Skullcap is traditionally used for relief of anxiety during labor. No human trial has evaluated these claims, but rodent studies demonstrated an anxiolytic effect in vivo and a mild tocolytic effect in vitro.[84,85]

Pharmaceuticals

Maternal discomfort in labor is multifactorial. A few common combinations of pharmaceuticals are often given together in labor to address the pain, nausea, anxiety, and extreme fatigue that often accompany this process. Pharmaceuticals can be divided into two main categories: systemic and regional.

Systemic Agents

Essentially all analgesic agents cross the placenta.[86-89] Because of the complexity of fetal circulation, only a small percentage of the drug may reach the fetal brain.[90] Therefore, the mother may be affected by a certain concentration of drug without affecting the fetus. Providers should anticipate that beat-to-beat variability of the fetal heart rate may be reduced markedly with the use of these agents, but this may not necessarily affect the clinical status of the newborn. Systemic agents can be divided into three types: opioids, sedatives, and antiemetics (the last two are not fully discussed here).

◼ Opioid Analgesia

Parenteral opioids are frequently used for pain relief in labor, although a large meta-analysis demonstrated that the efficacy is mild to moderate at best, and maternal satisfaction is moderate as well.[91] Whether one opioid is superior to the others remains unclear.[91] Institutional preference often dictates the choice. All opioids are associated with maternal and neonatal respiratory depression, delayed gastric emptying, and nausea and vomiting, which may increase the risk of aspiration if general anesthesia becomes necessary. Some centers use patient-controlled intravenous infusion pumps programmed to give a predetermined amount of drug at the patient's request. Please see Table 51-1 for a comprehensive list of parenteral opioids and their profiles.

◼ Sedatives

Sedatives do not possess any analgesic qualities. They are often used in early labor to reduce anxiety, augment the analgesic effects of narcotics, and decrease the nausea often associated with narcotics. Barbiturates, phenothiazines, and benzodiazepines are examples. The last two classes are not commonly used because of their many maternal and neonatal risks.[92,93] Promethazine (Phenergan) is an antiemetic and is the most widely used sedative in labor. It rapidly crosses the placenta and has no known antagonist. In large doses or small doses combined with opioids, promethazine can depress the fetus for long periods of time. When used carefully with an opioid such as morphine in prodromal labor, however, promethazine may promote therapeutic rest for the patient. In some institutions, zolpidem, a sleep aid, is alternately given for therapeutic rest.

Local and Regional Anesthesia

Because local and regional analgesia methods do not depress the central nervous system, the birthing woman remains awake and able to participate actively, and the neonate is alert on delivery. Regional anesthesia provides the most effective form of pain relief in obstetrics, and the term refers to partial or complete loss of sensation below the T8 to T10 level.[94] Depending on the agent used, motor blockade may also be present. Examples of regional anesthesia include spinal anesthesia and epidural anesthesia. Several options for more localized anesthesia also are available, such as the pudendal block, paracervical block, and perineal block. Please refer to Tables 51-2 and 51-3 for detailed information regarding local and regional blocks, respectively.[95,96]

TABLE 51-1. Parenteral Analgesia

DRUG	DOSE	PROS	CONS	COMMENTS
Morphine Opioid	2–5 mg IV Onset less than 5 min Lasts 1.5–2 hr 10 mg IM Onset 10–20 min Lasts 2.5–4 hr	Long-acting when given IM	Nausea and vomiting[90] Urinary retention[90] Orthostatic hypotension[90]	Used primarily for therapeutic rest during early prodromal labor[90]
Meperidine (Demerol) Opioid agonist	25–50 mg IV every 1–2 hr Onset 5 min 50–100 mg IM every 2–4 hr Onset 30–45 min	Less respiratory depression than with morphine[90] Slightly less urinary retention than with morphine[90]	Active metabolites accumulate in fetal tissue after first hr[90] Active metabolites may cause dose-dependent neurobehavioral depression demonstrated up to 3 days[94] Neonatal risk if delivery occurs within 1–4 hr Nausea and vomiting[90] Delay in gastric emptying	Losing favor in pain management
Fentanyl Opioid	50–100 mcg IV every hr Onset 1 min Can load up to 200 mcg	Rapid pharmacokinetics No active metabolites Less neonatal neurobehavioral depression[90]	Requires frequent redosing May cause transient benign sinusoidal fetal heart tracing[94]	
Butorphanol (Stadol) Opioid agonist- antagonist	1–2 mg IV every 4 hr Onset 1–2 min 1–2 mg IM every 4 hr Onset 10–30 min	Ceiling effect for respiratory depression[90] Nausea and vomiting less common[90]	Somnolence[90] Dysphoria[90] Dizziness[90]	May cause increased blood pressure; avoided in hypertension or preeclampsia[94] Opioid antagonist effect may promote opioid withdrawal in opioid- dependent women[90]
Nalbuphine (Nubain) Opioid agonist- antagonist	10 mg IV Onset 2–3 min 10 mg IM every 3 hr Onset 15 min Maximum dose 160 mg over 24 hr	Ceiling effect for respiratory depression[94] Nausea and vomiting less common than with meperidine[94]	Maternal sedation[94] Dizziness[90] May cause benign transient sinusoidal fetal heart tracing[94]	Potency similar to morphine[90] Opioid antagonist effect may promote opioid withdrawal in opioid- dependent women[90]

75 mg meperidine = 10 mg morphine = 0.1 mg fentanyl = 10 mg nalbuphine.[95]
IM, intramuscularly; IV, intravenously.

TABLE 51-2. Other Analgesia

TYPE	DESCRIPTION	PRECAUTIONS	INDICATIONS	TECHNIQUE
Local Perineal Analgesia	Direct perineal infiltration with rapidly acting agent Local analgesia lasting 20–40 min[90]	Intravascular injection can rarely cause seizures, hypotension, and cardiac arrhythmias. Avoid injecting into the fetal scalp.	Used before episiotomies, outlet forceps, and laceration repair	Use 1%–2% lidocaine without epinephrine or 2-chloroprocaine. Aspirate for blood before injecting. Use as little as possible to avoid toxicity.
Paracervical Block	Simple, effective Duration of analgesia dependent on type of anesthesia used	Fetal bradycardia, which can be associated with fetal acidosis.[94] Do not use in mothers with fetuses with acute or chronic distress.[90]	Pain relief for cervical dilation Administration limited to first stage of labor	Inject 5–6 mL of local anesthetic without epinephrine into lateral fornices of cervix (4 and 8 o'clock or 3 and 9 o'clock).
Pudendal Nerve Block	Safe Variably effective	Risk of injecting directly into large vessels that lie in close proximity to injection site Hematoma[94] Infection[94]	Pain relief in second stage Spontaneous vaginal delivery, episiotomy, some outlet and low forceps, or to supplement epidural block	Inject 5–10 mL of local anesthetic slightly below the ischial spines bilaterally. Aspirate before injection to reduce the risk of local anesthetic toxicity.

TABLE 51-3. Regional Blocks

TYPE	DESCRIPTION	INDICATIONS/EFFECTS	PRECAUTIONS
Spinal Block	A single-shot long-acting local anesthetic is often used with or without an opioid agonist.	This is used for the second stage of labor and short procedures such as cesarean delivery.	Hypotension, which may lead to decreased uterine perfusion[94] Pruritus (when opioids are added)[94] Blunting of the pressure sensation during the second stage of labor
Combined Spinal-Epidural Block	This combines the rapid onset of spinal analgesia with the ability for continuous infusion of analgesic though the epidural catheter.*	This widely used block provides immediate pain relief during the second stage of labor. It can convert to anesthesia adequate for cesarean section. It continues to provide postcesarean pain relief.	Impaired ability to push if the motor block is too dense Increased risk for operative vaginal delivery[94] Prolongation of labor[94] Fever,[97] periodically leading to suspicion of infection and subsequent interventions
Epidural Anesthesia	Local anesthetic and opioid are injected through a catheter into epidural space, to allow for continuous infusion. The dose can be titrated over the course of labor.	The same catheter can be used for labor, vaginal delivery, and cesarean section. The block is usually not initiated until active labor is established.	Transient fetal heart rate deceleration[94] Increased need for oxytocin (Pitocin) augmentation[94] Headache[94] Transient painful sensation in legs or buttocks (with spinal)[94] Epidural or spinal hematoma (rare)[94] Abscess (rare)[94]
"Walking" Epidural Anesthesia	This epidural block preserves motor strength for more effective pushing. Most women are not able to walk or support their weight.		High spinal anesthesia, resulting in paralysis of the respiratory muscles (rare)[94] Neurotoxicity (rare)[94]

*Maternal satisfaction, obstetric outcomes, and neonatal outcomes do not appear to differ between the combined spinal-epidural block and the epidural block.[96]

Therapies to Consider

Hot or Cold Application

Although the use of hot or cold application for pain relief in labor is common practice among doulas and labor support staff, no RCTs have evaluated this therapy. Easy to initiate, the use of heat or ice should depend on the desires of the laboring woman. Typically, heat is applied to the back, neck, shoulders, or abdomen by using warm compresses, microwaveable rice-filled pillows, or electric heating pads. Caution should be taken to avoid burns; the heat should never be painful. Cold is typically applied to the forehead, back, or neck with a cool washcloth, ice-filled sac or glove, or ice pack. Cold soda cans, which can double as massage tools on the lower back, can also be used. One study demonstrated a decrease in pain scores with ice massage to the acupoint LI4 during contractions.[97]

Homeopathy

Although many birth attendants administer homeopathy for pain, anxiety, and labor management, the use of remedies is largely driven by traditional homeopathic literature. Currently, no data are available on homeopathy in labor and birth; however, research indicates that homeopathy is a very safe form of therapy with minimal side effects.[98] If a woman is interested in using homeopathy, consult a homeopath or homeopathic literature to find appropriate remedies.

Reflexology

Reflexology focuses on zones in the hands and feet that are believed to correspond to specific areas of the body.[99] The practitioner applies manual pressure in these zones to achieve therapeutic benefits in the target organ, gland, or body part. No studies to date have evaluated reflexology in labor, but reflexology can be assumed to help promote relaxation. The uterine point is located between the medial malleolus and the heel pad, and the cervical point is on the heel pad.[46] One proposed technique is to massage or hold the first three toes during a contraction.[100]

PREVENTION PRESCRIPTION

■ Cultivate the patient-provider relationship prenatally when possible.
■ Discuss the woman's expectations about labor prenatally.
■ Discuss preferences for labor pain management before labor begins.
■ Involve the laboring woman in decision making.
■ Recommend that women arrange for continuous labor support.
■ Recommend regular moderate exercise or yoga practice during pregnancy.

THERAPEUTIC REVIEW

The laboring woman has many options for pain control. Individually, many of these therapies are quite effective in reducing pain, but nearly all may be used in combination. No research has evaluated the synergistic effect, but we recommend offering women multiple options.

- Plan for continuous labor support. Consider hiring a trained doula.

- Consider childbirth education classes to prepare for labor and birth.

Lifestyle

- Regular prenatal exercise
- Moderate exercise or movement during labor

Biomechanical Therapy

- Ambulation or upright position during first stage of labor
- Upright or side-lying position during second stage of labor
- Hands and knees position for back labor
- Water immersion
  - First stage
  - Second stage
- Massage during labor
- Regular chiropractic, osteopathic, or manual treatment in pregnancy
- Sterile water injections for back labor
- Hot or cold application

Bioenergetics

- Transcutaneous electrical nerve stimulation in labor, with possible focus on acupoints
- Acupuncture during labor

- Acupressure during labor
- Homeopathy

Mind-Body Therapy

- Regular yoga practice in pregnancy
- Hypnotherapy techniques prenatally to prepare for labor
- Music/audioanalgesia during labor
- Biofeedback techniques during pregnancy to prepare for labor

Biochemical: Aromatherapy

- Aromatherapy during labor (e.g., frankincense, lavender, rose)

Botanicals

- Raspberry leaf to shorten labor: 1.2 mg twice daily in the last trimester
- Motherwort or skullcap. This can have a calming effect for anxiety.
- Black cohosh

Pharmaceuticals

- Parenteral opioids for mild to moderate pain relief
  - Choice of medication and dose institutionally driven
  - See Table 51-1 for options and doses
- Promethazine: 12.5 to 25 mg orally or intravenously every 4 to 6 hours as needed for sedation and nausea
- Local anesthesia
  - See Table 51-2 for technique and details
- Regional anesthesia or epidural anesthesia
  - See Table 51-3 for options and details

DONA International: www.dona.org	Find a doula, and learn about doulas.
Betts D. Natural Pain Relief Techniques for Childbirth Using Acupressure: http://acupuncture.rhizome.net.nz/downloads/Acupressure.pdf	Locate acupressure points, and find further information on acupressure in labor.
Hypnobabies: http://www.hypnobabies.com; and Hypnobirthing: http://hypnobirthing.com	Locate resources for using hypnosis during labor and childbirth.
Kaiser Permanente guided imagery: https://members.kaiserpermanente.org/redirects/listen	Listen to a free downloadable guided imagery session to help prepare for labor. This Web site also includes other guided imagery downloads for pregnancy and childbirth.

References

References are available online at expertconsult.com.

Chapter 52

Nausea and Vomiting in Pregnancy

Andrea Gordon, MD, and Judy Platt, MD

Pathophysiology

Nausea and vomiting in pregnancy (NVP) represent a conundrum for the pregnant woman. On the positive side, NVP are correlated with better fetal outcomes than the absence of these symptoms,[1] but at the extreme NVP can interfere with nutrition and hydration for the mother and developing fetus. Symptoms may range from occasional mild nausea to multiple episodes of daily vomiting resulting in weight loss and electrolyte abnormalities. This severe manifestation is often referred to as hyperemesis gravidarum. Definitions of hyperemesis gravidarum vary, but commonly accepted criteria include weight loss (often more than 5% of prepregnancy weight), electrolyte disturbances, and ketonuria.

Usually appearing before the ninth week of pregnancy, NVP will affect up to 85% of normal pregnancies, with symptoms generally remitting by the fourteenth week. Initial presentation of symptoms after the ninth week should prompt a workup to determine an alternative cause. NVP may be mild, but up to 20% of women find their symptoms so significant that they cannot continue to work.[2] The reported incidence of hyperemesis gravidarum, the most severe end of the spectrum, varies from 0.5% to 2%. This severely debilitating condition is the most common reason for hospital admission in the first trimester and the second most common problem for which pregnant women are admitted to the hospital, after preterm labor.[3]

Even at the milder end of the symptom continuum, NVP can lead to decreased quality of life and missed time from work. The aptly named Motherisk Pregnancy-Unique Quantification of Emesis and Nausea (PUQE) index has been shown to demonstrate a significant correlation between the presence and severity of NVP and poorer quality of life.[4,5] This effect on quality of life and the economic impact of missed work emphasize the need to control these symptoms. Mild or moderate vomiting does not appear to have

any significant effects on the fetus. Among women with severe hyperemesis, the reported incidence of low birth weight is higher, but increased reporting of birth defects has not been noted.[6] In fact, several investigators suggested that NVP represent an evolutionary adaptation that helps protect the developing fetus from exposure to foods that may contain potential toxins.[7,8]

The cause of NVP is unknown. Both biologic and psychological factors have been proposed. Human chorionic gonadotropin (HCG) and estrogen have been studied as triggers for these symptoms. Suggestive evidence includes the finding that pregnant women with higher levels of HCG, which occur in molar pregnancies and multiple gestations, have significantly more episodes of vomiting and higher rates of hyperemesis gravidarum. This theory is also supported by the observations that nonpregnant women who experience nausea and vomiting after exposure to estrogens are more likely to experience NVP, cigarette smoking is known to reduce both estrogen and HCG levels, and pregnant smokers are less likely to experience hyperemesis gravidarum.[9]

No controlled studies support the theory that NVP comprise a conversion disorder or an inability to respond to life stress.[10,11] The association of high levels of HCG and estradiol with increasingly severe episodes of vomiting in pregnancy indicates a physiologic origin, as do epidemiologic factors. Daughters and sisters of women who had hyperemesis are more likely to have NVP as well. Other risk factors include a previous pregnancy affected by hyperemesis, a female fetus, and a history of motion sickness or migraines.[12]

Integrative Therapy

When treatment is considered, risks and benefits must be clearly explained to the pregnant woman. Minimizing the risks of any treatment is desirable, but the presence of a developing fetus makes it more urgent to decrease any unnecessary exposures. This is an ideal time to use integrative approaches because drugs generally represent more risk than do other modalities. In addition, some of the behavior modifications such as exercise are beneficial in and of themselves.

Lifestyle

Although lifestyle modifications have not been studied to determine their efficacy, these interventions are safe and have been anecdotally reported to be useful.[13]

Avoid Odors

Some women report that NVP are triggered by strong odors such as foods, cigarette smoke, or perfume. Avoiding these stimuli may be helpful. Women should be supported in doing so, for example, by passing off cooking duties to someone else, avoiding tasks with strong odors such as feeding the dog, or politely asking coworkers not to wear perfume for a few weeks.

Increase Rest

Sleep requirements increase in early pregnancy.[14] Women frequently report nausea in association with feelings of exhaustion. Caregivers should educate pregnant patients that fatigue is common and support them in trying to obtain the additional rest they need.

Exercise

Light to moderate aerobic exercise may help decrease NVP symptoms. Additional benefits may include improved sleep and lessened constipation and fatigue. If patients were active before the pregnancy, they can continue at their previous level (avoiding overheating), but even if they were not, becoming gently active can be beneficial.

Nutrition

Low blood glucose levels seem to trigger nausea and then vomiting in many women, so small, frequent, high-protein, high-fiber meals are often recommended.[15] A potentially helpful approach is to decrease simple carbohydrates that rapidly raise blood glucose and thus stimulate insulin secretion, which can cause rapidly falling blood glucose (see Chapter 85, The Glycemic Index/Load). However, this includes food such as pasta, white rice, potatoes, and white bread, whose blandness seems desirable when patients are nauseated, so education is key. Some patients find that eating something as soon as they wake up and then every 2 hours can suppresses nausea. Each pregnant woman may have specific foods she avoids because of a taste or smell that triggers nausea, but it may also be necessary to avoid spicy or fatty foods because they can exacerbate symptoms. Little published evidence exists on the efficacy of dietary changes, but benefit clearly outweighs harm. In one international survey, dietary interventions seemed to help 22% of women with hyperemesis gravidarum.[16]

Two studies found that taking a multivitamin before pregnancy or before 6 weeks of gestation was associated with a decreased incidence of NVP. Although this approach would not help a woman already suffering with symptoms, it could be helpful for women at risk for symptoms in their next pregnancy.[17,18]

Botanicals

Ginger Root (Zingiber officinale)

Historically, ginger has been effectively and safely used to treat nausea, including that of pregnancy. Randomized controlled trials have shown that ginger is effective for treating NVP,[19] and it is the most thoroughly studied herb for this indication. Some trials have shown ginger to be not only more effective than placebo,[20] but also comparable to or better than vitamin B$_6$[21,22] and comparable to dimenhydramate.[23] Patients should be advised that it may take longer for ginger to work: up to 3 days, rather than 1 day for the dimenhydrate. The U.S. Food and Drug Administration (FDA) has listed ginger as a food supplement that is generally recognized as safe,[24] and studies have not shown any increased incidence of malformations in children of mothers using ginger.[25]

Ginger seems to work primarily in the gastrointestinal tract on serotonin receptors in the ileum, the same receptors affected by some antiemetics, such as ondansetron. Some evidence indicates that ginger constituents may also have some action in the central nervous system.[26] No toxicity has been demonstrated, although ginger can cause abdominal discomfort or heartburn when it is taken in large doses, especially on an empty stomach.

■ Dosage

Most of the studies have used 250 mg powdered ginger in capsules four times daily, or 500 mg twice daily has been used.[20,23,24,27] A higher dose of 650 mg three times daily has also been used.[28] However, ginger can be consumed in many forms, including as a food, candied, or an infusion (tea). To make a tea, use 1 teaspoon of grated fresh ginger root in 1 cup of hot water, and drink approximately 3 cups a day; dried leaves can also be used. One study showed that eating five cookies a day, each containing 0.5 g of ginger, was also effective.[29]

■ Precautions

In theory, doses greater than 2 g daily may have an anticoagulant effect.

> Using ginger throughout the day is helpful. Patients can incorporate ginger into their diet by sprinkling dried or candied ginger in oatmeal, having some ginger tea, and adding fresh ginger to soup or stir-fries.

Chamomile (Matricaria chamomilla)

Chamomile is a flowering plant that is often used for various types of gastrointestinal upset, including travel sickness, colic, and inflammatory diseases of the bowel. It is commonly used for NVP,[30–32] although no research on this application has been published. Chamomile appears to be safe and well tolerated, however, and the FDA labels it as safe.[33]

■ Dosage

Prepare it as a tea, and sip as needed.

■ Precautions

Chamomile should be used with caution in patients who are allergic to the Asteraceae/Compositae family, which includes ragweed, daisies, and many other flowers. Some erroneous concern exists about teratogenicity, but that concern is based on a study with alpha-bisabolol at high doses that could not be achieved by someone drinking tea.[34]

Peppermint Leaf (Mentha piperita)

Peppermint is another herb often used in pregnancy.[35,36] The active parts are the stems, leaves, and flowers, as well as the peppermint oil that is distilled from these plant parts. Studies have shown peppermint oil to be effective for reducing bowel spasms in irritable bowel syndrome and for patients receiving barium enemas, but peppermint oil has not been studied in pregnancy.[37] Its mechanism of action is by reduction of spasm in smooth muscle, and it may help with NVP by reducing esophageal dysmotility. This effect can also reduce lower esophageal sphincter pressure, however, and result in reflux. Theoretical concerns exist with using the essential oil in pregnancy because it may cross the placental barrier, but the amount of peppermint ingested in teas or foods seems to be safe.[34] Peppermint has been rated as safe by the FDA.[33]

■ Dosage

The dose is 2 to 3 cups of tea daily. Many women find peppermint candies or gum to be effective in squelching nausea. A dose of 0.2 mL in 2 mL of isotonic saline solution has been used for postoperative nausea and can be tried if teas or foods containing peppermint are not tolerated.[38]

■ Precautions

Peppermint can aggravate reflux by decreasing lower esophageal sphincter tone.

Bioenergetics

Acupressure: Stimulation of the P6 Neiguan Point

Acupressure of the pericardium 6 (P6) Neiguan (meridian) point, which is located on the inner wrist, may be beneficial. A Cochrane analysis noted equivocal results, based on limited evidence, for all forms of stimulation of the point, including acupuncture and acoustic stimulation.[39] A study conducted in Korea found significantly less NVP in a group of women with hyperemesis gravidarum.[40] Other studies using a crossover design, which were not included in the Cochrane analysis, also showed benefit to using acupressure at the P6 point,[40,41] and another trial found decreased nausea with P6 stimulation but no change in the frequency of vomiting.[42] Many patients are willing to try acupressure because it costs little and has no significant side effects.

Patients can be taught to find the P6 point and treat themselves with either manual pressure or the application of "Sea-Bands" (Fig. 52-1). These elastic bands with attached plastic disks were originally used for motion sickness. Patients can create their own version of such bands by placing a small, round object such as a bead over the point and securing it

---

FIGURE 52-1
A, The P6 Neiguan acupressure point is located on the volar aspect of the forearm by placing the examining hand three fingerbreadths below the wrist crease. The patient's finger widths should be used for measurement. The P6 point is essentially in the midline between the tendons of the palmaris longus and flexor radialis muscles. **B,** Location of this point. PC, pericardium.

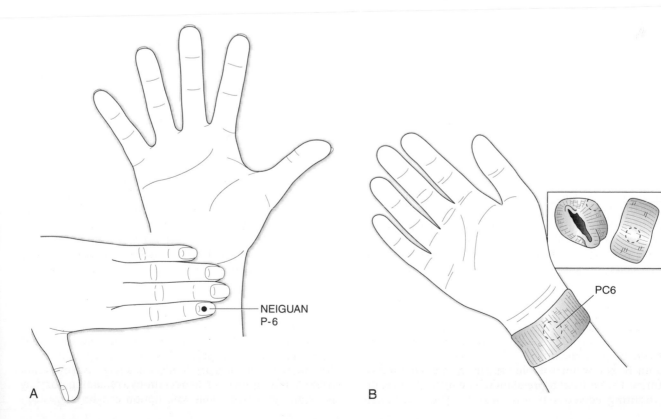

NEIGUAN P-6

PC6

A   B

with tape and then massaging the bead. This therapy has no known negative side effects.

To have a patient accurately locate the P6 point, have her lay one hand palm up, with the other hand placed palm down at right angles to the upturned arm. The first three fingers of the palm-down hand are held close together, and the edge of the ring finger is placed at the crease of the wrist closest to the palm in alignment with the middle finger of the upturned hand. The P6 point, between the palmaris longus and flexor radialis tendons, is now readily palpable under the tip of the index finger of the examining hand (see Fig. 52-1A). This point is often tender, a characteristic that aids in its location. Many patients use this acupressure in conjunction with other interventions because it has no known side effects or interactions.

> Patients can stimulate the P6 point at any time, but they should be cautioned against using any other acupressure points without consulting a trained practitioner. Some commonly used points, such as the Ho-Ku point between first and second metacarpals (often used for headaches), can stimulate contractions.

Mind-Body Therapy

Hypnosis

Hypnosis has been studied as a treatment for hyperemesis gravidarum. A review of six studies showed encouraging effects, but methodologic problems did not allow a definitive recommendation.[43] This intervention is safe, however, and some women may want to try it for all levels of NVP. One approach has been to suggest to a woman that the "nausea center" in her brain is very sensitive to the hormones of pregnancy and to suggest that she is able to "turn down" that sensitivity as one would a thermostat.[44] This imagery may be helpful for some patients.

NVP may have an element of conditioned response, as noted with chemotherapy-associated vomiting. Some uncontrolled studies showed that hypnosis can reduce vomiting and anticipatory vomiting in patients undergoing chemotherapy,[10] so the potential exists for hypnosis to work for NVP. Because this treatment may require several sessions of training, the time and expense may be prohibitive for some patients.

Counseling and Psychotherapy

Although the general consensus is that NVP does not represent a conversion disorder and is not caused by emotional responses to the pregnancy,[10] evidence indicates that women with NVP may be under more stress. Two investigators stated that NVP "could subject any normal expectant mother to stress sufficient to trigger adjustment disorders, generalized anxiety or even depressive episodes."[10] In recognition of this extraordinary stress, counseling or psychotherapy may be helpful in coping with the symptoms and their effects on a woman's life.

Supplements

Vitamin B₆ (Pyridoxine)

Vitamin B_6 is a water-soluble vitamin that is an effective treatment for nausea in pregnancy. The benefit in reducing vomiting episodes is less clear.[45,46] The mechanism

of action of pyridoxine remains unknown, but extensive analysis for teratogenicity shows no negative effect on pregnancy outcome.[47] A popular medication for nausea and vomiting, known as Bendectin in the United States and Diclectin in Canada, contained pyridoxine and doxylamine. Bendectin was withdrawn from the United States market in 1983 out of safety concerns about teratogenicity, but no studies validated this possibility. Diclectin remains available in Canada and is one of the most widely studied and used medications in pregnancy today. Following removal of Bendectin from the market, no reduction in birth defects was reported, but hospitalization rates for NVP doubled.[48]

> Diclectin, a combination of doxylamine 10 mg and pyridoxine 10 mg, is available in Canada and can be purchased online (canadadrugs.com). It is expensive, at more than a dollar a pill. A less expensive alternative is to combine Unisom (contains 25 mg doxylamine), one half tablet at bedtime, with 50 mg of pyridoxine.

Patients can expect significant reduction of nausea with few side effects if they take vitamin B_6.

■ Dosage

The most effective dosage appears to be 30 to 75 mg daily in three divided doses. Studies performed with the higher end of the dosing range have shown effectiveness against vomiting as well as nausea.[45,46] When vitamin B_6 alone is not effective, many pregnant women combine it with doxylamine to obtain relief from NVP.

■ Precautions

Pyridoxine can cause sensory neuropathy, which is related to the daily dose and duration of intake. Doses exceeding 1000 mg daily or total doses of 1000 g or more pose the most risk, so the doses that have been used for NVP appear generally to be safe.[49]

Pharmaceuticals

Antihistamines

Several histamine (H_1) receptor antagonists have been studied for the treatment of NVP. The most frequently studied and used is doxylamine (Unisom, an over-the-counter sleep aid). An extensive review of safety data revealed no adverse pregnancy outcomes from doxylamine alone or in combination with pyridoxine.[50] Other drugs in this group, which all have shown some evidence of efficacy and safety for controlling NVP, are dimenhydrinate (Dramamine), cetirizine (Zyrtec), meclizine (Antivert), hydroxyzine (Vistaril), and diphenhydramine (Benadryl).[51]

■ Dosage

Most patients should use 12.5 mg of doxylamine, the amount in one half of a scored tablet. This is the amount of doxylamine that was contained in Bendectin. Indeed, many women try to "make" a form of Bendectin by combining doxylamine with vitamin B_6. This safe option can be suggested if vitamin B_6 alone or with ginger or P6 point stimulation is not working adequately. Diphenhydramine, given in 25- to 50-mg doses up to every 6 hours, is also safe and easily obtained.

■ Precautions
All antihistamines can cause drowsiness.

Phenothiazines
The phenothiazines used to treat NVP include promethazine (Phenergan), prochlorperazine (Compazine), chlorpromazine (Thorazine), and perphenazine (Trilafon). Only promethazine has randomized, controlled study data supporting its efficacy and safety.[39,51] However, some evidence indicates that all medications in this group have some efficacy in the treatment of NVP.[47] These medications may be used in the outpatient setting, but therapy is often not started until hospital admission for treatment of dehydration or intractable vomiting. The variable dosing forms are advantageous for NVP: these drugs can be self-administered orally or rectally or given intramuscularly by medical personnel if needed.

■ Dosage
For promethazine, begin with 12.5 mg rectally or orally and progress to 25 mg every 4 hours as needed.

■ Precautions
Side effects of promethazine include sedation, hypotension, dystonia, and extrapyramidal symptoms. If needed, diphenhydramine, 25 mg, can be given orally every 6 hours to treat dystonia or extrapyramidal side effects.

Dopamine Antagonists
Two dopamine antagonists have been studied for treatment of NVP: trimethobenzamide (Tigan) and metoclopramide (Reglan). Trimethobenzamide has been shown to be safe,[52] but it has been largely studied for nausea in other settings such as chemotherapy.[53] Only one double-blind trial focused on the effectiveness of trimethobenzamide in treating NVP.[54] This study showed that trimethobenzamide alone or in combination with pyridoxine significantly improved symptoms of nausea and vomiting compared with placebo.[54]

Metoclopramide is not associated with malformation risk,[55,56] and it has been shown to be effective in hyperemesis gravidarum, with or without promethazine.[57,58] A combination of vitamin B_6 and metoclopramide was shown to be better than prochlorperazine or promethazine in improving the subjective symptoms of patients with NVP.[59]

■ Dosage
Metoclopramide can be given orally in 5- to 10-mg doses three times daily before meals.

■ Precautions
The side effects of metoclopramide are similar to those of the phenothiazines but occur less frequently.

5-Hydroxytryptamine₃ Receptor Agonists
Ondansetron (Zofran), a 5-hydroxytryptamine₃ receptor agonist, is a potent antiemetic originally used for treatment of chemotherapy-induced nausea and vomiting. Data on NVP are very limited, but a study of hospitalized patients who received intravenous ondansetron or promethazine showed that these medications were equally effective and had no negative effects on the fetus.[60]

■ Dosage
Ondansetron is given orally or intravenously, 2 to 8 mg up to every 8 to 12 hours.

■ Precautions
Adverse reactions to ondansetron include headache, fever, and bowel dysfunction, although this agent is reported to be better tolerated by patients than promethazine, with no dystonic or extrapyramidal side effects.

> Ondansetron is available in an orally disintegrating tablet. This can be useful if someone feels too nauseated to swallow any medication.

Corticosteroids
Several small studies evaluated corticosteroids, primarily methylprednisolone, for efficacy in reducing NVP and hyperemesis. Methylprednisolone reduced symptoms of NVP along with hospital readmission rates for hyperemesis.[61] Another trial found that promethazine worked more rapidly than prednisolone, but after a week both medications worked equally well, and the prednisolone group had fewer side effects.[62] Various oral and intravenous dosages have been studied, but the most common regimen is an oral 2-week course of 48 mg daily. Most patients respond within 3 days, so if no improvement has been seen by that time, longer treatment is generally not indicated. Methylprednisolone may be continued for up to 6 weeks, but longer use may result in adverse maternal effects related to prolonged steroid exposure.[61,63] Evidence also indicates that a shorter course of hydrocortisone is effective for treating intractable hyperemesis.[64] A meta-analysis found an increased risk of oral clefts associated with prednisone use.[65]

■ Dosage
The dose of methylprednisolone is 16 mg orally or intravenously every 8 hours for up to 2 weeks (tapered course to avoid adrenal suppression). The dose of hydrocortisone is 300 mg intravenously daily for 3 days.

■ Precautions
Avoid corticosteroid use before 10 weeks of gestation if possible. Avoid prolonged use for more than 6 weeks to reduce risk of maternal side effects.

Intravenous Fluids
Intravenous fluids have not been specifically studied for the treatment of hyperemesis, but they are often coadministered with other medications in the hospital setting for the treatment of dehydration. Intravenous fluid is generally recommended when patients fail to tolerate oral fluids for a prolonged period or show electrolyte abnormalities indicating dehydration. Dextrose and intravenous thiamine can be added to fluids when vomiting has been prolonged and persistent.[12]

Extreme Measures for Intractable Nausea and Vomiting in Pregnancy

Enteral or Parenteral Feedings

Evidence to support enteral or parenteral feedings comes from case reports and small series.[66,67] In general, the prudent approach is to start with enteral feedings and move on to peripheral parental nutrition and finally to total parental nutrition if all other methods fail. Serious and even life-threatening complications have been reported with parenteral nutrition, so it is used only as a last resort.[68]

Therapeutic Abortion

With current medical interventions such as intravenous hydration and medications, it is rare for NVP to be so severe as to be life-threatening. This was not the case in the early twentieth century, when severe NVP represented an important cause of maternal deaths.[69] However, maternal morbidity in the form of Wernicke encephalopathy caused by vitamin B_1 deficiency, esophageal rupture, acute tubular necrosis, and splenic avulsion have all been reported to be caused by intractable vomiting of pregnancy.[1] When the maternal condition is deteriorating as a consequence of hyperemesis gravidarum despite aggressive medical intervention, pregnancy termination may be indicated (Fig. 52-2). Fortunately, symptoms usually subside rapidly as HCG levels fall.

Therapies to Consider

Homeopathy

No studies have evaluated the efficacy of homeopathic remedies in the treatment of NVP. Practitioners cite anecdotal evidence of homeopathy use, but choosing the correct remedy can be complex because many subtle differences in symptoms are taken into account. Some of the remedies commonly used include nux vomica, sepia, and ipecac.[70] Because homeopathic preparations are extensively diluted, they should be safe for pregnant women and would likely have no adverse effects if they are not helpful. Some investigators recommend avoiding any remedies with potencies (dilutions) greater than 12 C, however.[71]

Traditional Chinese Medicine

Practitioners of traditional Chinese medicine (TCM) may recommend acupuncture, acupressure, and herbs, but they also use certain foods such as umeboshi plums (a very salty preserved fruit) to combat nausea. In addition, these clinicians may use practices such as moxibustion, cupping, or massage. Because the TCM views of health and the body's function are different from those in Western medicine, a certified TCM practitioner should advise on the use of these approaches.[72] Different patterns of symptoms lead to different treatments.[73] Information about training and accreditation of TCM practitioners can be found at the National Certification Center for Acupuncture and Oriental Medicine (www.nccaom.org).

> Umeboshi plums can be found in most Asian grocery stores. If the plum itself is too salty, some women obtain relief of nausea by sucking on the pit only. Another option is to use one fourth to one half a plum at a time.

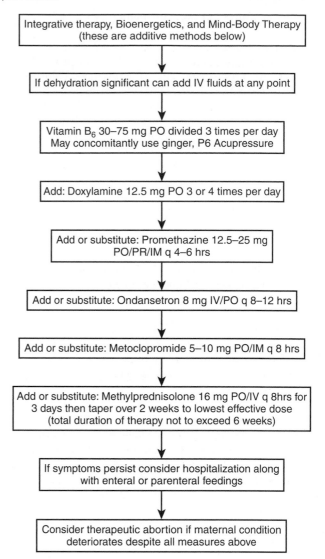

FIGURE 52-2
Integrative therapy, bioenergetics, and mind-body therapy algorithm. IM, intramuscularly; IV, intravenous; PO, orally; q, every; PR, per rectum.

Integrative therapy, Bioenergetics, and Mind-Body Therapy (these are additive methods below)

↓

If dehydration significant can add IV fluids at any point

↓

Vitamin B_6 30–75 mg PO divided 3 times per day
May concomitantly use ginger, P6 Acupressure

↓

Add: Doxylamine 12.5 mg PO 3 or 4 times per day

↓

Add or substitute: Promethazine 12.5–25 mg PO/PR/IM q 4–6 hrs

↓

Add or substitute: Ondansetron 8 mg IV/PO q 8–12 hrs

↓

Add or substitute: Metoclopromide 5–10 mg PO/IM q 8 hrs

↓

Add or substitute: Methylprednisolone 16 mg PO/IV q 8hrs for 3 days then taper over 2 weeks to lowest effective dose (total duration of therapy not to exceed 6 weeks)

↓

If symptoms persist consider hospitalization along with enteral or parenteral feedings

↓

Consider therapeutic abortion if maternal condition deteriorates despite all measures above

PREVENTION PRESCRIPTION

- Eat frequent, small meals that are high in protein to avoid low blood glucose levels.
- Avoid overconsumption of simple carbohydrates such as cakes, candy, and starchy foods because they may lead to low glucose levels, which could stimulate more nausea.
- Consider trying more salty foods and tart liquids because these are reported by some women to be better tolerated.
- Avoid triggers such as pungent odors or unpleasant visual stimuli that may worsen nausea.

THERAPEUTIC REVIEW

Lifestyle, botanical, bioenergetic, and mind-body therapies are additive to all the other methods listed here. If dehydration is significant, add intravenous fluids at any point. C 2

Bioenergetics

- Acupuncture (P6) B 1

Mind-Body Therapy

- Hypnotherapy B 1

Supplements

- Vitamin B_6: 30 to 75 mg PO divided three times per day A 1

- Ginger: 250 mg powdered in capsules four times daily, or 500 mg twice daily; can increase to 650 mg three times daily as needed B 1

Pharmaceuticals

- Doxylamine: 12.5 mg orally three or four times daily A 1

- Add or substitute promethazine: 12.5 to 25 mg orally, rectally, or intramuscularly every 4 to 6 hours B 2

- Add or substitute ondansetron: 8 mg intravenously or orally every 8 to 12 hours B 2

- Add or substitute metoclopramide: 5 to 10 mg orally or intramuscularly every 8 hours B 2

- Add methylprednisolone: 16 mg orally or intravenously every 8 hours for 3 days then taper over 2 weeks to the lowest effective dose (total duration of therapy not to exceed 6 weeks) B 2

- If symptoms persist, consider hospitalization along with enteral or parenteral feedings. C 3

Surgery

- Consider therapeutic abortion if the maternal condition deteriorates despite all the measures described here and in Figure 52-2. C 3

KEY WEB RESOURCES

Motherisk morning sickness information: http://www.motherisk.org/prof/morningSickness.jsp	This Web site contains a treatment algorithm for hyperemesis gravidarum.
Merck Manual: http://www.merckmanuals.com/professional/gynecology_and_obstetrics/symptoms_during_pregnancy/nausea_and_vomiting_during_early_pregnancy.html?qt=pregnancy&alt=sh	This Web site provides a brief overview of diagnosis and treatment of nausea and vomiting in pregnancy.
BMJ Clinical Evidence: http://clinicalevidence.bmj.com/ceweb/conditions/pac/1405/1405.jsp	This article describes the effects of treatment for nausea and vomiting in pregnancy and the effects of treatments for hyperemesis gravidarum. Registration is required to access this Web site.
Motherisk Pregnancy-Unique Quantification of Emesis and Nausea (PUQE) index: http://www.medscape.com/viewarticle/712662_3	This index can be used as a way for patients to quantify and track symptoms and may be helpful when comparing treatments. This index can also be found at Koren G, Boskovic R, Hard M, et al. Motherisk-PUQE (pregnancy-unique quantification of emesis and nausea) scoring system for nausea and vomiting of pregnancy. *Am J Obstet Gynecol.* 2002 May;186(5 Suppl Understanding):S228-S231.

References

References are available online at expertconsult.com.

Chapter 53

Premenstrual Syndrome

Tieraona Low Dog, MD

Pathophysiology

Premenstrual syndrome (PMS) is defined as a recurrent, cyclic set of physical and behavioral symptoms that occurs 7 to 14 days before the menstrual cycle and is troublesome enough to interfere with some aspects of a woman's life. PMS is estimated to affect up to 40% of menstruating women, and the most severe cases occur in 2% to 5% of women who are between 26 and 35 years of age.[1] Although PMS has been recognized as a medical disorder for many years, the cause remains a mystery (Table 53-1). The complex relationships that exist among hormones may offer insight into why some women suffer more than others. For instance, mild elevations of prolactin, a hormone that is primarily involved in regulating the development of the breast during pregnancy, have been associated with PMS, menstrual irregularities, and breast tenderness, whereas low levels of thyroid hormone can contribute to depression, fatigue, and heavy menses.

Hormonal Influences

A deficiency of progesterone or an abnormally high estrogen-to-progesterone ratio during the luteal phase has been a popular theory of the origin of PMS for many years, although studies comparing hormone levels in women with PMS with those in women without the disorder have failed to support this hypothesis.[2] In the 1950s, Dr. Katherina Dalton was one of the first to postulate this theory. Dr. Dalton administered natural progesterone in the form of injection, suppositories, or subcutaneous pellets; 83% of women in the study reported complete relief of PMS symptoms.[3] Because of the strict inclusion criteria of the study, however, only 18% of women with PMS appeared to be suitable candidates for this therapy. A 1985 study using oral micronized progesterone (100 mg in the morning and 200 mg before bedtime), starting 3 days after ovulation and continuing for 10 days, found progesterone to be clearly superior to placebo for the symptoms of anxiety, stress, and poor concentration.[4]

Prolactin

Prolactin levels peak at ovulation and generally remain elevated during the luteal phase of the menstrual cycle. Prolactin excess is associated with menstrual irregularities, diminished libido, depression, and hostility.[5] Some authorities suggested that up to 62% of women with menstrual disorders have some elevation of prolactin.[6] Prolactin plays a role in breast stimulation and may be related to premenstrual breast tenderness. However, no consistent abnormalities have been found in women with PMS.[2]

Aldosterone

Aldosterone levels normally rise at ovulation and remain elevated during the luteal phase of the menstrual cycle. This elevation of aldosterone may be responsible for the congestive symptoms of PMS, such as edema, breast swelling, abdominal bloating, weight gain, and headaches. However, differences in absolute levels of aldosterone between symptomatic and asymptomatic women are not noted in the literature.[7]

Endogenous Opiates

Some researchers, who observed an increase in beta-endorphin levels after ovulation, hypothesized that women with PMS may have a lower level of these circulating endogenous opiates or a more sudden withdrawal that causes them to experience greater sensitivity to pain and depression in the luteal phase of the menstrual cycle.[8]

Vitamin B_6 and Magnesium

Vitamin B_6 (pyridoxine) is required for the metabolism of amino acids, carbohydrates, and lipids. The active forms of this vitamin are necessary coenzymes for the decarboxylation of 5-hydroxytryptophan to 5-hydroxytryptamine (5-HT) and of dopa to dopamine. Pyridoxine deficiency is associated with elevations of prolactin and low levels of serotonin and dopamine.[9] Pyridoxine deficiency can lead to depression, peripheral neuropathy, and mood changes.

TABLE 53-1. Proposed Causes of Premenstrual Syndrome

Hormonal Factors	Estrogen deficiency Estrogen excess High estrogen-to-progesterone ratio Progesterone deficiency Prolactin excess Beta-endorphin deficiency
Fluid and Electrolytes	Aldosterone excess Vasopressin excess High sodium-to-potassium ratio Renin-angiotensin abnormalities
Neurotransmitters	Serotonin deficiency Cortisol excess Hypoglycemia Reduced glucose tolerance Thyroid abnormalities Adrenal insufficiency
Prostaglandins	Prostaglandin excess Prostaglandin deficiency Essential fatty acid deficiencies
Vitamins and Minerals	Pyridoxine deficiency Vitamin A deficiency Vitamin E deficiency Magnesium deficiency Calcium excess Calcium deficiency Potassium deficiency Trace mineral deficiency Zinc deficiency Dopamine deficiency Norepinephrine deficiency Low platelet monoamine oxidase activity
Hereditary	Genetic risk
Psychological Factors	Beliefs about menstrual cycle Coexisting psychiatric disorders Poor coping skills Poor self-esteem
Social Factors	Current marital and sexual relationships Former marital and sexual relationships Social stress Psychosexual experiences Cultural attitudes about PMS Societal attitudes about PMS Poor social network

PMS, premenstrual syndrome.

Although serum levels of magnesium are often normal in women with PMS, researchers have noted lowered red blood cell magnesium levels in women with the disorder.[10] Calcium and dairy products may interfere with absorption, whereas refined sugar increases urinary excretion of magnesium. Magnesium deficiency can reduce dopamine and thyroid activity (with resultant increase in prolactin) and lead to depression, mood changes, and muscle cramping.

TABLE 53-2. Symptoms of Premenstrual Syndrome

Abdominal bloating	Insomnia
Acne	Irritability
Anxiety	Joint pain
Back pain	Lethargy
Change in appetite	Low libido
Clumsiness	Low self-esteem
Constipation	Mood swings
Depression	Nervousness
Diarrhea	Social isolation
Dizziness	Sugar cravings
Fatigue	Tender breasts
Headache	Water retention

Hypoglycemia

The body appears to be more sensitive to insulin in the luteal phase of the menstrual cycle, a finding that led some researchers to hypothesize that transient hypoglycemia may account for some PMS symptoms.

Prostaglandins

Prostaglandins are associated with breast pain, fluid retention, abdominal cramping, headaches, irritability, and depression.[11] Patients with physical premenstrual complaints and dysmenorrhea have been shown to respond to prostaglandin inhibitors.

Psychosocial Theory

Emotional and physical stressors have been found to influence the menstrual cycle. Travel, illness, stress, weather changes, and other environmental factors may affect ovulation, length of menstrual cycle, and severity of PMS.[12] Cultural, societal, and personal attitudes toward menstruation also appear to play a role in the presence and severity of PMS. The dynamic interplay of environment, spirit, and physiology demands an integrated biopsychosocial approach to treatment.

Symptoms

More than 150 symptoms have been associated with PMS. The most common are listed in Table 53-2.

The American Psychiatric Association (APA) defined the diagnostic criteria for premenstrual dysphoric disorder (PMDD), a more severe form of PMS. To be diagnosed with PMDD, a woman must have at least five of the following symptoms, and they must occur cyclically and be serious enough to interfere with her normal activities:

1. Feeling of sadness or hopelessness; possible suicidal thoughts
2. Feelings of tension or anxiety
3. Mood swings marked by periods of teariness
4. Persistent irritability or anger

5. Disinterest in daily activities and relationships
6. Trouble concentrating
7. Fatigue or low energy
8. Food cravings or binging
9. Sleep disturbances
10. Feeling out of control
11. Physical symptoms such as bloating, breast tenderness, headaches, and joint or muscle pain

Although this addition to the fourth edition of the APA's *Diagnostic and Statistical Manual of Mental Disorders,* published in 1994 (DSM-IV), is useful for recognizing PMDD as a valid disorder, that behavioral aspects comprise the primary focus is disturbing. With the vast numbers of physiologic and hormonal interactions taking place in a woman's body, a multitude of explanations would seem to exist for the variety of symptoms. Thus, assuming that numerous therapies may help and that not all remedies are universally effective is reasonable.

Classifications

Dr. Guy Abraham developed a system for categorizing PMS into four distinct subgroups.[13] They can be summarized as follows:

PMS-A (anxiety) is believed to be related to high levels of estrogen and deficiency of progesterone. Women experience irritability, anxiety, and emotional lability.

PMS-C (carbohydrate craving) is of unclear origin but may be caused by enhanced intracellular binding of insulin. Women with this subtype experience increased appetite, sugar and carbohydrate craving, headache, and heart palpitations.

PMS-D (depression) is most likely caused by low levels of estrogen that lead to excessive breakdown of neurotransmitters. Low estrogen levels may be caused by enhanced adrenal androgen or progesterone secretion.

PMS-H (hyperhydration) is the result of increased water retention secondary to elevations of aldosterone. Elevations of aldosterone in the premenstrual period may be the result of excess estrogen, excessive salt intake, stress, or magnesium deficiency. Women with this subtype report weight gain, breast tenderness and fullness, swelling of the hands and feet, and abdominal bloating.

Although used by many practitioners, these categories should be considered only guidelines, because the basis for their separation has not been adequately confirmed by current research, and most women do not neatly fit into just one of the groups.

Clinical Evaluation

A complete physical examination, including pelvic evaluation and laboratory tests, should be performed to rule out anemia and hypothyroidism. A prolactin test may be included. An extremely useful approach is for a woman to record her symptoms on a daily basis for at least two complete menstrual cycles to allow the clinician to see just what her symptoms are and how they are related to her menses.

The clinician must address any other underlying medical conditions that may masquerade as PMS. One report found that 75% of women receiving care for PMS at specialized clinics had another diagnosis that accounted for many of their symptoms, primarily major depression and other mood disorders.[14]

Integrative Therapy

Once the diagnosis has been established, an integrative approach should be considered. Therapies to be explored include exercise, dietary manipulation, dietary supplements, mind-body approaches, acupuncture, traditional Chinese medicine, counseling, and conventional medications.

Exercise

Exercise remains understudied in the scientific world because it does not fit well into the double-blind placebo-controlled study design. The few studies that have been conducted on the role of exercise in PMS have clearly shown that women who engage in regular physical exercise have fewer symptoms of PMS than women who do not. Women who exercise regularly note improvement in all symptoms of PMS.[15] The frequency, rather than the intensity, of exercise appears to diminish the negative mood and physical symptoms that occur during the premenstrual period.[16] Exercise may reduce symptoms by reducing estrogen levels, decreasing circulating catecholamines, improving glucose tolerance, and raising endorphin levels.[17] Aerobic activity appears to be most beneficial; however, yoga and tai chi are probably equally effective if they are performed at least three times per week.

Diet and Nutrition

Many people in the United States fail to eat a healthy diet, but some researchers have found this observation to be even more accurate for women with PMS. A 1983 report noted that women with PMS consumed 275% more refined sugar, 79% more dairy products, 78% more sodium, 62% more refined carbohydrates, 77% less manganese, and 53% less iron than women without PMS.[18] These dietary excesses and deficiencies may explain some of the symptoms women experience in the premenstrual period. Dairy products are high in sodium and interfere with magnesium absorption. Refined sugars increase the urinary excretion of magnesium.[19] Heavy intake of sugar also increases sodium and water retention owing to the rapid release of insulin. Dietary salt may exacerbate swelling. Consumption of caffeine-containing beverages was associated with increases in both the prevalence and severity of PMS in college students.[19] A study of Chinese women found that increasing tea consumption was linked to a rising prevalence of PMS.[20] Women experiencing irritability or difficulty sleeping during the premenstrual period should be encouraged to reduce or limit their intake of caffeine (Table 53-3).

> Fiber-rich, low-fat diets suppress the ability of fecal bacteria to deconjugate estrogen and thereby enhance fecal estrogen excretion.

Dietary Fat

Fiber-rich, low-fat diets may be beneficial for women with PMS because these diets reduce blood levels of estrogen. Estrogen is conjugated in the liver and sent to the small intestine for elimination in the feces. Intestinal bacteria can deconjugate estrogen and allow it to be reabsorbed into the body.

TABLE 53-3. Caffeine Amounts in Common Foods and Beverages

SERVING SIZE (oz)	CAFFEINE (mg)
Coffee, instant (6–8)	65–100
Coffee, percolated (6–8)	85–135
Coffee, filtered (6–8)	115–175
Coffee, decaffeinated (6–8)	1–5
Tea, instant (6–8)	35–70
Tea, brewed (6–8)	28–150 .
Tea, iced (6–8)	40–45
Chocolate, dark semisweet (1)	5–35
Chocolate, milk (1)	1–15
Cola beverage (8)	25–30

From Thys-Jacobs S, Starkey P, Bernstein D, et al. Calcium carbonate and the premenstrual syndrome: effects on premenstrual and menstrual symptoms. Premenstrual Syndrome Study Group. *Am J Obstet Gynecol.* 1998;179:444–452.

Several studies showed that reducing fat (less than 20% of total calories) and increasing fiber for only 3 months can lower a woman's serum estrogen level.[20] If one accepts the theory that elevations of estrogen can worsen PMS symptoms, then consuming a diet high in fruits, vegetables, and whole grains and low in saturated fat may be wise. Four to six small meals should be consumed throughout the day to ease both food cravings and mood swings. Alcohol consumption should be limited because it can worsen PMS symptoms.

No food-based strategy has been adequately tested to determine its effects on PMS. However, recommendations such as eating a high-fiber diet, limiting caffeine, and cutting back on high-sugar foods have few drawbacks and numerous health benefits.

Supplements

Calcium

Ovarian hormones influence calcium, magnesium, and vitamin D metabolism. Estrogen is involved in calcium metabolism, calcium absorption, and parathyroid gene expression and secretion. Clinical trials in women with PMS found that calcium supplementation improves several mood and somatic symptoms.

A prospective randomized double-blind placebo-controlled parallel-group multicenter clinical trial was conducted to evaluate the effectiveness of calcium carbonate for PMS. Healthy premenopausal women were recruited nationally at 12 outpatient centers and screened for moderate to severe, cyclically recurring premenstrual symptoms. Symptoms were prospectively documented over 2 menstrual cycles with a daily rating scale that included 17 core symptoms and 4 symptom factors (negative affect, water retention, food cravings, and pain). Of the 720 women screened for the trial, 497 were enrolled, and results for 466 were valid for the efficacy analysis. Women were randomly allocated to receive

1200 mg calcium carbonate or placebo daily for 3 menstrual cycles. Routine blood chemistry analysis, complete blood cell count, and urinalysis data were obtained for all participants. Each participant kept a daily diary to document symptoms, adverse effects, and compliance with therapy. The primary outcome measure was a 17-parameter symptom complex score. No differences in age, weight, height, use of oral contraceptives, or menstrual cycle length were reported between the treatment and control groups. No differences existed between the groups in the mean screening symptom complex score of the luteal phase ($P = .659$), menstrual phase ($P = .818$), or intermenstrual phase ($P = .726$) of the menstrual cycle. During the luteal phase of the treatment cycle, a significantly lower mean symptom complex score was noted in the calcium-treated group by the third month ($P < .001$). The researchers concluded that "calcium supplementation is a simple and effective treatment in premenstrual syndrome, resulting in a major reduction in overall luteal phase symptoms."[21]

A review of studies focusing on calcium for the management of premenstrual symptoms was published in the *Annals of Pharmacotherapy*.[22] On the basis of the medical literature, the reviewer concluded that "calcium supplementation of 1200 to 1600 mg/day, unless contraindicated, should be considered a sound treatment option in women who experience premenstrual syndrome."

▣ Dosage
The dose is 500 to 600 mg twice per day elemental calcium as carbonate or citrate.

▣ Precautions
Calcium products made from oyster shell, dolomite, or bone meal occasionally contain lead.[23] Labels containing the letters "USP" indicate that the product meets the purity and dissolution standards established by the U.S. Pharmacopeia; however, this is a voluntary standard, and many products do not bear USP on their labels. Calcium supplements should not be taken at the same time as tetracycline, iron supplements, thyroid hormones, or corticosteroids because calcium binds to these substances and interferes with their effectiveness and its own absorption. Iron absorption can be reduced by as much as 50% by many forms of calcium supplementation.

Magnesium

Women with PMS have been shown to have low levels of magnesium in their red blood cells. Magnesium deficiency produces fatigue, irritability, mental confusion, PMS, menstrual cramps, insomnia, muscle cramps, and symptoms of heart disturbances. A 2002 Cochrane Review found that magnesium was superior to placebo for relieving dysmenorrhea, likely through inhibition of prostaglandin $F_{2\alpha}$.[24] Whether magnesium would be helpful for women with PMS who do not experience menstrual pain is unclear, although some integrative practitioners empirically use magnesium as part of a treatment strategy for PMS, particularly in women with menstrual migraine or a tendency to constipation. Dietary sources of magnesium include green leafy vegetables, tofu, legumes, nuts, seeds, and whole grains.

▣ Dosage
The dose is 200 to 600 mg/day of magnesium as chelate, citrate, or glycinate.

Precautions

Adverse effects of magnesium excess include abdominal cramping and diarrhea. Signs of magnesium toxicity are hypotension, irregular heartbeat, muscle weakness, nausea, diarrhea, and change in mental status. The kidneys excrete magnesium, so women with renal insufficiency must be cautious with magnesium supplementation.

Vitamin B$_6$

Pyridoxine is a water-soluble B vitamin that serves as a cofactor in more than 100 enzyme reactions, many of which are related to the production and metabolism of neurotransmitters. The use of pyridoxine (vitamin B$_6$) to alleviate PMS symptoms has been evaluated in more than 28 trials since 1975. This research was inspired by the work of Adams et al,[25] who first reported that vitamin B$_6$ successfully alleviated the depression associated with use of oral contraceptives. Wyatt and associates[26] performed a systematic review of these studies. Ten randomized placebo-controlled double-blind parallel or crossover studies were examined. Studies of cyclic mastalgia and multivitamin preparations with at least 50 mg of vitamin B$_6$ were also included. Only 3 of these trials scored higher than 3 on the Jadad scale for methodologic quality. Most trials were small (fewer than 60 women). One of the largest studies included women who were also taking oral contraceptives, analgesics, diuretics, and psychotropic medications, thus making the effects of vitamin B$_6$ difficult to ascertain. None of the trials included power calculations. Using a random effects model, Wyatt et al[26] found the overall odds ratio in favor of pyridoxine to be 1.57 (95% confidence interval [CI], 1.40 to 1.77). When the researchers looked at the effects on depressive symptoms in 5 trials, they found the overall odds ratio in favor of pyridoxine to be 2.12 (95% CI, 1.80 to 2.48).

Current thinking postulates that pyridoxine may ease symptoms of PMS through its ability to increase the synthesis of serotonin, dopamine, norepinephrine, histamine, and taurine.[27] Serotonin is important for the regulation of sleep and appetite and the prevention of depression. Low levels of serotonin and dopamine may play a role in premenstrual symptoms.[28] Trials used doses ranging from 50 to 500 mg/day. For most women, the prudent approach is probably to limit single doses of vitamin B$_6$ to 50 mg and not to exceed 100 mg/day. Research suggests that the liver cannot process more than a 50-mg dose of pyridoxine at one time.[29] Conversion of pyridoxine to its active form depends on other nutrients, such as magnesium and riboflavin. Taking vitamin B$_6$ as part of a multiple-vitamin supplement or using the active form, pyridoxal-5-phosphate, may be advisable.

Dosage

The dose is 50 to 100 mg/day of pyridoxine or pyridoxal-5-phosphate.

Precautions

Although pyridoxine is a water-soluble vitamin, it can be associated with toxicity when it is taken in moderate to large doses over time. A few reports have noted nerve damage occurring with prolonged ingestion of 150 mg/day.[30] Toxicity may occur if large doses of pyridoxine overwhelm the liver's ability to add a phosphate group to form pyridoxal-5-phosphate, the active form of vitamin B$_6$.

> Combining chaste tree with vitamin B$_6$ may be a beneficial first step in the treatment of premenstrual syndrome.

Botanicals

Chaste Tree (Vitex agnus-castus)

Dioscorides, the Greek physician, described the dried ripe fruits of the chaste tree (Vitex agnus-castus) some 2000 years ago. The Latin name agnus castus means "chaste lamb," in reference to the belief that the seeds reduce sexual desire. From this belief stemmed the other common name of the herb, monk's pepper. Many herbalists consider V. agnus-castus one of the primary herbs for alleviating PMS, a use that is supported by randomized human trials. The most rigorous study to date of chaste tree for PMS was a 3-month double-blind placebo-controlled trial by Schellenberg[31] that randomized 170 women diagnosed with PMS to receive 20 mg of fruit extract (Ze 440: 60% ethanol mass/mass [m/m], extract ratio, 6 to 12:1; standardized for casticin) or placebo. Five of six self-assessment items indicated significant superiority for chaste tree (irritability, mood alteration, anger, headache, and breast fullness). Other symptoms, including bloating, were unaffected by treatment. Overall, the reduction in symptoms was 52% for the active versus 24% for placebo ($P < .001$). The trial investigators concluded: "Agnus castus is a well tolerated and effective treatment for premenstrual syndrome, the effects being confirmed by physicians and patients alike."

Two studies conducted in Chinese women also reported favorable results. A randomized double-blind placebo controlled multicenter 16-week study of 217 women with moderate to severe PMS found that 40 mg of chaste tree extract was superior to placebo, as measured by the PMS diary 17-item daily rating scale ($P < .0001$).[32] No serious adverse events were reported. A smaller randomized placebo-controlled 3-month study of 64 Chinese women with moderate to severe PMS also found that 40 mg per day chaste tree extract significantly reduced symptoms in the PMS diary 17-item daily rating scale ($P < .05$).[33]

One study evaluated the use of chaste tree in PMDD. A single-blind rater-blinded study of 41 women (ages 25 to 45 years) who were diagnosed with PMDD and who had regular menstrual cycles failed to note any significant difference between fluoxetine and chaste tree with respect to the Hamilton Depression Rating Scale (HAM-D), the Clinical Global Impression Scale-Severity of Illness (CGI-SI), or the Clinical Global Impression-Improvement (CGI-I).[34] Unfortunately, the investigators did not provide any details regarding the chaste tree product (e.g., extraction method, extract strength).

One comparative trial found chaste tree to be as effective as pyridoxine for relieving PMS symptoms,[35] whereas a pilot study using the combination of St. John's wort (Hypericum perforatum) and chaste tree found the combination highly effective for relieving PMS symptoms in perimenopausal women.[36]

A chaste tree preparation is known to act, in part, by reducing prolactin, increasing progesterone, and binding opiate receptors.[37] Binding of opioid receptors may be the primary mechanism involved in PMS, given that symptoms such as anxiety, food cravings, and physical discomfort are directly and inversely proportional to the decline of beta-endorphin levels. *Vitex* has an inhibitory action on prolactin because of its dopamine agonist properties. Women with hyperprolactinemia often experience menstrual dysfunction. Some researchers postulate that the correction of hyperprolactinemia causes the reversal of luteinizing hormone suppression and results in full development of the corpus luteum during the luteal phase of the cycle.[38] Studies in both animals and humans have demonstrated prolactin inhibition with *Vitex*. The German health authorities approved the use of chaste tree fruit for irregularities of the menstrual cycle, premenstrual complaints, and mastodynia.[39]

Dosage
The dose varies according to the preparation used in trials. Generally, practitioners recommend 250 to 500 mg/day of dried fruit or 20 to 40 mg daily of chaste berry extract.

Precautions
Chaste tree has been rarely associated with gastrointestinal reactions, alopecia, headaches, tiredness, dry mouth, and increased menstrual flow.

> Binding of opioid receptors may be the primary mechanism of action of chaste tree. As beta-endorphin levels decline, so do common premenstrual syndrome symptoms such as anxiety, food cravings, and physical discomfort.

Black Cohosh (Actaea racemosa, Cimicifuga racemosa)
The Eclectics (early physicians who used botanical medicines extensively) used black cohosh for restlessness, nervous excitement, breast pain, and menstrual headaches.[40] Although most research has focused on black cohosh for the alleviation of menopausal complaints, a study of 135 women found a standardized extract of black cohosh to be effective in reducing the symptoms of anxiety, tension, and depression in women with PMS.[41] Researchers found that compounds in black cohosh bind 5-HT7 receptors, a characteristic that could partially explain the positive effects of this botanical on mood.[42] The German health authorities endorsed the use of black cohosh for premenstrual discomfort and dysmenorrhea.[43]

Dosage
The dose is 20 to 40 mg of the standardized extract twice daily (generally standardized to triterpene glycosides as a marker compound).

Precautions
The most common complaint is gastrointestinal disturbance. Other potential adverse effects are headache, heaviness of the legs, and weight gain. Two safety reviews concluded that black cohosh is relatively safe when it is used appropriately; since these reviews, however, case reports suggesting a possible link between black cohosh use and liver damage were published in the medical literature. After an extensive review of the literature, the U.S. Pharmacopeia Dietary Supplements Expert Information Committee recommended that women who have, or who are at risk for, liver disease check with their health care provider before they use black cohosh.[44]

Ginkgo (Ginkgo biloba)
If women experience primarily congestive symptoms in the premenstrual period (fluid retention, breast tenderness, weight gain), a trial of ginkgo may offer some relief. A double-blind placebo-controlled trial of ginkgo was conducted with 165 women complaining of premenstrual symptoms. Participants received placebo or a standardized extract of ginkgo (EGb761 24% ginkgo flavones and 6% terpenes; Dr. Willmar Schwabe GmbH & Co, Karlsruhe, Germany), 80 mg twice daily, from day 16 of one menstrual cycle through day 5 of the next cycle. Evaluation by patient and physician found ginkgo to be effective for alleviation of breast pain and tenderness and fluid retention.[45] Ginkgo is known to augment venous tone and reduce capillary fragility.

Dosage
The dose is 80 mg of a standardized extract twice daily from day 16 of one menstrual cycle through day 5 of the next cycle.

Precautions
Ginkgo may cause gastrointestinal symptoms, headache, dizziness, palpitations, and allergic skin reactions.

Caution
Patients should be carefully supervised if ginkgo is used with anticoagulant medications; however, bleeding risk is probably quite low in otherwise healthy individuals taking ginkgo. A randomized double-blind placebo-controlled crossover study found no change in coagulation factors, platelet aggregation, or bleeding times in 50 healthy male volunteers who took 240 mg ginkgo extract (EGb761).[46]

Evening Primrose Oil (Oenothera biennis)
Evening primrose oil is extracted from the seeds of the evening primrose plant, a wildflower native to North America and introduced to Europe in the early 1600s. The seed oil has been studied for medicinal effects for decades because it is a rich source of linoleic acid and gamma-linolenic acid. Some researchers reported that women with PMS have impaired conversion of linoleic acid to gamma-linolenic acid, thus leading to the investigation of gamma-linolenic supplementation for symptom alleviation. However, a systematic review identified seven placebo-controlled trials of evening primrose oil and reported that all suffered from methodologic flaws.[47] The two highest-quality studies failed to show any beneficial effects of evening primrose oil in PMS, although the sample sizes were small in both trials.

Dosage
Evening primrose oil products are generally standardized to specific amounts of gamma-linoleic acid. Capsules typically contain 320 to 360 mg linoleic acid and 40 mg gamma-linolenic, although levels vary among manufacturers. Vitamin E is often added to prevent

rancidity. The range of doses used in clinical studies is 1 to 6 g/day.

■ Precautions

Evening primrose oil is extremely well tolerated. Minor gastrointestinal symptoms are sometimes reported in the literature.

St. John's Wort (Hypericum perforatum)

Clinical trials using selective serotonin reuptake inhibitor (SSRI) medications have shown that approximately 60% of women with severe PMS obtain significant relief with use of these drugs. This finding is interesting, given that some herbalists recommend the popular herbal antidepressant St. John's wort (Hypericum perforatum) for women reporting depression and irritability in the premenstrual period.

The only trial located addressing the question of St. John's wort and PMS was a prospective, open uncontrolled observational study. Nineteen physically and mentally healthy women with PMS completed a daily symptom ratings diary for one cycle and attended a medical screening interview before they were given the diagnosis of PMS. Participants were then given 300 mg/day St. John's wort extract standardized to 900 mcg hypericin. Symptoms were rated daily with the use of validated measures. The Hospital Anxiety and Depression Scale and the Social Adjustment Scale were administered at baseline and after one and two menstrual cycles. The researchers report a reduction of PMS symptom scores between baseline and the end of the trial of 51%. More than two thirds of participants noted a 50% decrease in symptom severity. The researchers concluded: "The results of this pilot study suggest that there is scope for conducting a randomized, placebo-controlled, double-blind trial to investigate the value of *Hypericum* as a treatment for premenstrual syndrome."[48]

■ Dosage

The dose generally used for depression is 300 to 600 mg of St. John's wort standardized to contain 3% to 5% hyperforin or 0.3% hypericin three times per day.

■ Precautions

Women taking medications that increase photosensitivity, protease inhibitors (for human immunodeficiency virus), cyclosporine, or other medications that are metabolized by the cytochrome P-450 CYP3A4 system or P-glycoprotein should avoid St. John's wort.

Kava (Piper methysticum)

Physicians sometimes prescribe alprazolam, a benzodiazepine, for the treatment of PMS. Because of the risk of habituation and side effects, practitioners have looked for other anxiolytics that could be of benefit. Numerous practitioners have recommended the South Pacific herb kava for this purpose. A meta-analysis concluded that kava is an effective treatment for anxiety when compared with placebo, although no studies of kava in PMS are available for review.

Concerns have been raised about the safety of kava, however. Approximately 30 cases of hepatotoxicity potentially related to the use of kava products have been reported in the literature. Numerous countries have banned the sale of kava, including Germany, Switzerland, Ireland, Canada,

Australia, and the United Kingdom. The U.S. Food and Drug Administration (FDA) issued a cautionary statement, but the herb is still sold in the United States. Until the safety issue is further elucidated, looking for other approaches to help alleviate troublesome symptoms of PMS seems wise. A better option for women reporting irritability and difficulty sleeping during the premenstrual period may be valerian (discussed next).

Valerian (Valeriana officinalis)

Valerian is a common ingredient in over-the-counter relaxants and sleep aid products in both Europe and the United States. It is often included in herbal formulations for PMS with a dominant profile of anxiety or irritability. The herb is sold as a single ingredient but is often found in combination with other relaxant herbs such as hops (Humulus lupulus), passionflower (Passiflora incarnata), or lemon balm (Melissa officinalis). The German Commission E endorses valerian for restlessness and sleeping disorders caused by nervous conditions,[49] and the World Health Organization recognizes it as a "mild sedative, sleep-promoting agent, milder alternative to or possible substitute for stronger sedatives (e.g., benzodiazepines), and for treatment of nervous excitation and sleep disturbances induced by anxiety."[50] No clinical trials have evaluated the use of valerian for PMS, but this botanical is often included in formulations on the basis of its mild anxiolytic effects and ability to promote sleep.

■ Dosage

The crude herb is usually taken at a dose of 2 to 3 g (equivalent to 10 to 15 mL of tincture [1:5 strength]) approximately 1 hour before bedtime. Smaller doses are often used during the day for relieving mild irritability and anxiety. Standardized extracts are also widely available and should be taken as directed on the label.

■ Precautions

Valerian is generally safe when taken appropriately and is not considered habit-forming. The World Health Organization noted that the use of valerian is contraindicated during pregnancy and lactation because of the lack of studies in this area.

Mind-Body Therapy

Mind-body therapies are approaches grounded in the emerging scientific understanding that thoughts and feelings affect physiology and physical health. Mind-body therapies for PMS include psychotherapy (cognitive-behavioral therapy and group therapy), relaxation techniques and training, body work (massage and reflexology), hypnotherapy, biofeedback, guided imagery, yoga, and qi gong. Most studies are preliminary, but practitioners should not be dissuaded from recommending them if they are deemed beneficial for a particular patient.

Acupuncture

Acupuncture is only one tool used in traditional Chinese medicine (TCM) for the treatment of disease and promotion of health. traditional Chinese medicine uses a different system for diagnosis and has a long history of treating what would be called PMS in conventional medicine. Although many women report benefit, a systematic review of clinical trials using acupuncture for the relief of PMS found the data inconclusive.[51] Given the overall safety of acupuncture, clinicians should not dissuade women who choose to explore traditional Chinese medicine or acupuncture for relief of their symptoms.

Pharmaceuticals

Selective Serotonin Reuptake Inhibitors
In addition to numerous lifestyle recommendations already mentioned, growing numbers of physicians are prescribing SSRIs for the treatment of PMS and PMDD. A Cochrane Review of 15 trials that evaluated the efficacy of SSRIs in the management of PMS reported that these medications are very effective for improving both behavioral and physical symptoms. However, withdrawals related to side effects were 2.5 times more likely to occur in treatment groups, particularly at higher doses.[52] SSRIs should be considered for women with severe forms of PMS (PMDD) that do not respond to lifestyle, mind-body, or supplement approaches.

THERAPEUTIC REVIEW

Lifestyle
- Learn strategies for effective stress management, obtain adequate sleep, and maintain a regular exercise routine. Consider mind-body approaches such as breathing techniques and yoga.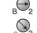

Nutrition
- Eat a well-balanced diet rich in fiber and low in fat.
- Limit intake of alcohol, salt, caffeine, and refined sugar products.

Supplements
- Calcium: 500 to 600 mg twice daily
- Vitamin B6: 50 to 100 mg/day
- Magnesium: 200 to 600 mg/day

Botanicals
- Chaste tree (Vitex): 250 to 1000 mg crude herb or 20 to 40 mg daily of a standardized extract

Treatment for Specific Symptoms
- Breast tenderness
  - Caffeine restriction
  - Chaste tree (Vitex): 250 to 500 mg crude herb or 20 to 40 mg daily of a standardized extract
  - Evening primrose oil: 1.5 g twice daily (continuous)

- Ginkgo biloba: 80 mg standardized extract twice daily (ovulation through menses)
- Anxiety and mood swings
  - Black cohosh: 20 to 40 mg standardized extract twice daily (continuous therapy)
  - Calcium: 500 to 600 mg twice daily
  - Chaste tree (Vitex): 250 to 500 mg crude herb or standardized extract daily
  - Valerian root: 2 to 3 g crude herb or standardized extract 45 minutes before bed
  - Kava root: up to 210 mg kavalactones in standardized extract per day
- Depression
  - St. John's wort: 300 to 600 mg standardized extract three times daily (continuous therapy)
  - Vitamin B6: 50 mg once or twice daily
- Cramps
  - Magnesium: 200 to 600 mg/day
  - Black haw: 1 to 6 g/day
- Insomnia
  - Valerian root: 2 to 3 g crude herb or standardized extract before bed
- Severe PMS or PMDD
  - Chaste tree (Vitex): 250 to 1000 mg crude herb or 20 to 40 mg daily of a standardized extract
  - Serotonin reuptake inhibitors

KEY WEB RESOURCES

U.S. Department of Health and Human Services Office on Women's Health: www.womenshealth.gov	This Web site has numerous resources on women's health, including premenstrual disorder.
PMS Symptom Tracker: http://www.womenshealth.gov/faq/pms-ymptracker45.pdf	This form allows patients to record their symptoms throughout the month.
American College of Obstetrics and Gynecology handout on premenstrual syndrome: http://www.acog.org/publications/patient_education/bp057.cfm#premenstrual	This handout also contains a symptom record.
National Women's Health Network: www.nwhn.org	This Web site is an online resource on women's health issues.

References

References are available online at expertconsult.com.

Chapter 54

Dysmenorrhea

Greta J. Kuphal, MD

Dysmenorrhea refers to painful uterine cramping associated with menses. In addition to lower pelvic discomfort, women may also experience low back pain, radiation of pain to the anterior thighs, nausea, vomiting, diarrhea, headache, and various other symptoms starting 1 to 3 days before the onset of menses and typically lasting through the first few days of bleeding. *Primary dysmenorrhea* refers to pain that is not associated with other, obvious pelvic disease and typically begins with the onset of ovulatory cycles just after menarche. *Secondary dysmenorrhea* is associated with another diagnosis (e.g., cervical stenosis, endometriosis) and typically has a later onset, usually after age 20 years. This discussion focuses on primary dysmenorrhea because treatment for secondary dysmenorrhea is determined by the underlying cause.

Estimates of the percentage of women affected by dysmenorrhea range from 16% to 90%. Some investigators claim the most reliable estimate to be approximately 75%, based on a large Swedish study of 19-year-old women. Most of these women's symptoms were mild, but 23% and 15% reported suffering from moderate and severe pain, respectively.[1] In addition to the discomfort endured by affected women, dysmenorrhea also results in significant missed school and work and in decreased quality of life.[2]

Dysmenorrhea seems to be more significant in women with earlier age at menarche and in those with longer episodes of bleeding. Being overweight appears to affect the likelihood of painful cramping, as well as the duration, significantly. Smoking has been associated with prolonged pain, and although alcohol consumption does not increase the probability of painful cramping, it seems to increase the duration and severity of cramping in women with dysmenorrhea.[3] Other predisposing factors include age less than 30 years, low body mass index, longer menstrual cycles, heavy menstrual bleeding, nulliparity, clinically suspected pelvic inflammatory disease, history of sexual abuse, psychological symptoms, chronic exposure to stress, and exposure to secondhand smoke.[4-7]

Pathophysiology

The pathogenesis of primary dysmenorrhea seems to involve elevated levels of prostaglandins in response to the rise and fall of progesterone that occur after ovulation. As progesterone production decreases by the corpus luteum, lysosomes in the endometrial cells break down and release phospholipase A_2, which converts cell membrane fatty acids into arachidonic acid, the precursor to prostaglandins. In women with dysmenorrhea, excessive elevation of prostaglandins, specifically prostaglandin $F_{2\alpha}$ and prostaglandin $E_{2\alpha}$, leads to uterine hypercontractility, painful cramping, and other prostaglandin-related symptoms such as nausea, vomiting, and diarrhea. These contractions decrease blood flow to the uterus and cause ischemia, which sensitizes nerve fibers to the inflammatory prostaglandins and endoperoxides.[8,9] Elevated levels of vasopressin have also been found in women with dysmenorrhea. This hormone increases uterine contractility, thereby contributing to cramping and ischemia.[10]

Integrative Therapy

Lifestyle

Exercise

Evidence for exercise as a treatment modality for dysmenorrhea has been mixed and limited in quality.[11] Early studies indicated that the type of exercise was less important than the desire to alleviate symptoms with exercise.[12] However, chronic stress seems to increase perimenstrual symptoms,[5] and exercise is certainly a valid tool for managing stress. Given that exercise is important for overall health and weight management (and being overweight is a risk factor for dysmenorrhea, as mentioned earlier), discussing regular exercise with patients suffering from dysmenorrhea certainly has a place.

Substance Use

Tobacco and alcohol use have been associated with worse symptoms of dysmenorrhea. Patients should be counseled on this and supported in addressing unhealthy use of these substances.

Nutrition

Omega-3 Fatty Acids

The release of arachidonic acid from the membranes of cells of the endometrium leads to an increase in proinflammatory prostaglandins. Omega-6 fatty acids are precursors to arachidonic acid, and our consumption of omega-6 compared with omega-3 fatty acids has greatly increased over the past century. The antiinflammatory diet (see Chapter 86, The Antiinflammatory Diet) can change the ratio of omega-6 to omega-3 polyunsaturated fatty acids in our bodies and may thereby modulate the levels of prostaglandins, inflammation, and painful uterine contractions produced. Studies have shown that higher consumption of omega-3 polyunsaturated fatty acids (either through supplementation or diet) leads to a decrease in painful menses.[13–15]

Table 54-1 lists dietary sources of omega-3 polyunsaturated fatty acids, as well as other nutrients described in the next section that have been found to be helpful in the treatment of primary dysmenorrhea.[16,17]

■ Dosage

If supplementing with omega-3 fish oil capsules, the dose is 1500 to 2000 mg daily of docosahexaenoic acid and eicosapentaenoic acid or two to three servings of cold-water fish per week.

Supplements

Magnesium

Magnesium has been found to be beneficial in the treatment of arrhythmias, severe asthma, migraine, dyspepsia, and constipation. Its role in dysmenorrhea may be related to its effect on intracellular calcium concentration,[18] a reduction in prostaglandin synthesis,[19] or its muscle relaxant properties. A Cochrane Review found three studies showing that magnesium was more effective than placebo in decreasing menstrual pain and the use of analgesic medications. The studies were small, but the results encouraging.[20a]

The form of magnesium is important because some forms are more likely to cause diarrhea (see the section on

dosage). Foods rich in magnesium include fish, nuts, leafy greens, whole grain cereals, and baked potatoes with the skin.[17] Magnesium is a largely intracellular cation, so red blood cell magnesium may be a more accurate measure of nutrient status than the typically used serum magnesium.

■ Dosage

Unless constipation is present, consider doses of 200 to 600 mg daily of forms of magnesium less likely to cause loose stools: magnesium glycinate (chelated magnesium), magnesium gluconate, or magnesium chloride. See Table 54-1 for dietary sources of magnesium.

■ Precautions

Use magnesium with caution in individuals with impaired renal function. If diarrhea develops, decrease the dose until this condition is relieved because diarrhea is one of the first signs of magnesium toxicity.

Vitamin B_6 (Pyridoxine)

A series of small studies ($N = 21$ to 24) in 1988 compared various permutations of vitamin B_6 versus magnesium versus vitamin B_6 and magnesium versus placebo and found that vitamin B_6 was better than placebo and better than a combination of vitamin B_6 and magnesium at decreasing visual analogue pain scores and tablets of ibuprofen used.[20a] A mechanism offered to explain the possible beneficial effect of vitamin B_6 is its role in increasing the influx of magnesium into the cell, thereby supporting the effects of magnesium described earlier.

■ Dosage

The dose is 100 mg daily. If a higher dose is used, close monitoring is needed. See Table 54-1 for dietary sources of vitamin B_6.

■ Precautions

Vitamin B_6 toxicity typically manifests as neuropathy that reverses with decreased intake.[17] Doses described were 100 mg twice daily; however, the Institute of Medicine established the upper tolerable intake level for vitamin B_6 as 100 mg daily for adults.

> Vitamin B_6 and magnesium may work synergistically because vitamin B_6 increases the influx of magnesium into the muscle cell.[20b]

TABLE. 54-1. Dietary Sources of Nutrients Found to Decrease Pain of Dysmenorrhea

OMEGA-3 FATTY ACIDS	MAGNESIUM	VITAMIN B_1	VITAMIN B_6	VITAMIN E
Cold-water fish (e.g., salmon, herring, sardines)	Halibut	Fortified grains (breads, cereals, pasta, wheat germ)	Fortified cereals	Vegetable oils (wheat germ, sunflower, safflower)
Leafy green vegetables	Almonds, dry roasted		Potatoes with skin	Almonds
Flaxseeds (ground)	Cashews, dry roasted	Lean pork	Bananas	Sunflower seeds
Walnuts	Soybeans	Fish	Garbanzo beans (chickpeas)	Spinach
	Spinach	Dried beans	Chicken breast	Broccoli
		Peas	Pork loin, lean only	Fortified cereals, juices, and spreads
		Soybeans		

Data from MedlinePlus. *Thiamin.* http://www.nlm.nih.gov/medlineplus/ency/article/002401.htm Accessed 24.02.11; and Office of Dietary Supplements, National Institutes of Health. *Dietary Supplement Fact Sheets.* http://ods.od.nih.gov/factsheets/ Accessed 20.02.11.

Vitamin B₁ (Thiamine)

One of the largest double-blind placebo-controlled studies investigating the effect of a nutritional supplement on dysmenorrhea was a trial of vitamin B_1. This crossover trial involved 556 Indian adolescents who were randomized to receive 100 mg of vitamin B_1 daily for 90 days, followed by placebo for 60 days or placebo for 60 days, followed by 100 mg daily of vitamin B_1. In both groups, complete resolution or significant improvement in pain did not occur until the participants had received thiamine for at least 30 days. "Cure" rates by the end of the trial were approximately 90% in both groups.[21] This overwhelming success at "curing" dysmenorrhea certainly raises the question of whether the results could be confirmed with another study in a different population. The mechanism by which this treatment works may simply be reversal of a deficiency that can manifest with decreased pain tolerance, muscle cramping, and fatigue, which are symptoms similar to those of premenstrual syndrome.[19]

■ Dosage

The dose is 100 mg daily for 90 days. Consider continuing treatment if symptoms recur after initial improvement. See Table 54-1 for dietary sources of thiamine.

■ Precautions

Orally, thiamine is usually well tolerated. It rarely can cause dermatitis or a hypersensitivity reaction.[22]

Vitamin E

Vitamin E has been proposed to provide relief from dysmenorrhea through antiinflammatory action and through induction of a marked rise in beta-endorphin level.[23,24] Several randomized placebo-controlled studies including a total of 383 women 15 to 21 years old, showed a significant decrease in the severity and duration of pain with vitamin E compared with placebo. Doses used varied from 150 to 500 units daily for either 2 days before and 3 days after or for 10 days before and 4 days after the onset of menses.[25-27] The tolerable upper intake level in healthy people is 1000 mg/day, equivalent to 1100 units of synthetic vitamin E (D-L-alpha-tocopherol or alpha-tocopherol or SRR-tocopherol) or 1500 units of natural vitamin E (D-alpha tocopherol or RRR-tocopherol).[28,29]

■ Dosage

The dose is 400 units daily for a few days before and a few days after the onset of menses. See Table 54-1 for dietary sources of vitamin E.

■ Precautions

Doses higher than 400 units of vitamin E have higher potential for adverse effects in unhealthy individuals.

Botanicals

French Maritime Pine Bark Extract (Pinus pinaster)

Pycnogenol is the trade name for this extract of French maritime pine bark. It has numerous active constituents such as flavonoids, procyanidins, and phenolic acids, and the list of indications ranges from asthma, chronic venous insufficiency, and hypertension to coronary artery disease and diabetes. In dysmenorrhea, it may have antispasmodic effects and inhibit uterine contractions through its components ferulic acid and caffeic acid. A study of 116 women with low menstrual pain (did not require analgesic medication) or dysmenorrhea were monitored for two cycles and then treated with either 30 mg twice daily of Pycnogenol or placebo through another two menstrual cycles. Although no difference was noted in the treatment group compared with placebo in the women with low menstrual pain, a significant decrease in pain scores and in analgesic use was reported in women with dysmenorrhea, and the effect seemed to persist for at least 1 month after cessation of the extract.[30]

■ Dosage

The dose is 30 mg twice daily for 2 months. The effect may last for at least 1 month after cessation.

■ Precautions

Pycnogenol is generally well tolerated. Side effects may be limited to gastrointestinal problems, dizziness, and vertigo but have possibly included headache and mouth ulceration.[31]

Fennel (Foeniculum vulgare)

Fennel essential oil has been found to be comparable to the nonsteroidal antiinflammatory (NSAID) medication mefenamic acid.[32,33] The mechanism seems to involve the inhibition of uterine contraction induced by prostaglandin E_2 and oxytocin.[34]

■ Dosage

The dose is 30 drops of fennel extract at the onset of menses and then continuously every 6 hours for the first 3 days of menses.

■ Precautions

Fennel has a Generally Recognized as Safe (GRAS) status in the United States, but case reports exist of neurotoxicity in two breastfeeding infants whose mothers drank an herbal combination tea containing fennel.[35] Fennel supplements should be avoided during pregnancy because in vitro studies have shown some toxic effects on fetal cells.[36]

SCA by Gol Daro Herbal Medicine (Saffron [Crocus sativus], Celery Seed [Apium graveolens], Anise or Fennel [Foeniculum vulgare])

An Iranian blend of highly purified extracts of saffron, celery seed, and anise (SCA by Gol Daro Herbal Medicine) was compared with mefenamic acid and placebo for effectiveness in alleviating symptoms of dysmenorrhea in 163 women 18 to 30 years old. SCA, at 500 mg three times daily, was found to be more effective than placebo and the NSAID, at 250 mg three times daily, in decreasing menstrual pain intensity and duration. All agents were taken for 3 days at the start of the menstrual cycle. No side effects were noted.[37]

■ Dosage

The dose is 500 mg of SCA three times daily for three days starting with onset of pain or bleeding.

■ Precautions

Saffron is generally well tolerated and has a GRAS rating unless it is taken at high doses. Taking 5 g or more of saffron can cause severe side effects, and doses of 12 to 20 g can be lethal.[38] Celery seed also has a GRAS rating but may cause allergic reaction (especially in individuals sensitive to mugwort, birch, dandelion, or wild carrot); large amounts should be avoided in pregnancy because of potential abortifacient effects.[39]

Willow Bark Extract (Salix cortex)

The major active ingredient of willow bark, salicin, was the original source of aspirin. It appears to inhibit the cyclooxygenase-2 pathway. Other components of willow bark may have other antiinflammatory properties. Willow bark does seem to inhibit platelet aggregation, but not as much as aspirin.

■ Dosage

The dosage is 240 mg daily of salicin, in divided doses. This is roughly equivalent to 87 mg of aspirin. Willow bark extract may work better if it is started the day before expected symptoms.[40]

■ Precautions

Willow bark extract is generally safe, but avoid it in children with viral infections, given theoretical risk of Reye syndrome. It can cause gastrointestinal side effects but less than those seen with NSAIDs. Avoid in kidney disease and in patients allergic to aspirin.

Cramp Bark (Viburnum opulus) and Black Haw (Viburnum prunifolium)

Traditionally, these herbs have been used as uterine relaxants. Very few data are available regarding their efficacy. The root bark and stem bark of black haw contain certain active ingredients, including scopoletin and oxalic acid. Scopoletin may be a uterine relaxant. Because of the presence of oxalic acid, black haw should be avoided in patients with a history of renal stones. Black haw also contains salicylates that could trigger an allergic reaction in patients sensitive to aspirin.[41]

■ Dosage

The dose is 2 to 3 mL of a tincture made in 1:3 proportion every 2 hours or as needed; or 4 to 8 mL of fluid extract (1:1) three or four times daily; or simmer 1 tablespoon of bark in 12 oz of water for 15 minutes, and drink one third cup every 2 to 3 hours as needed.[42]

■ Precautions

Avoid black haw in persons with a history of renal stones or aspirin allergy.

Pharmaceuticals

Nonsteroidal Antiinflammatory Drugs

As inhibitors of prostaglandin formation, NSAIDs such as naproxen, ibuprofen, and mefenamic acid have been shown to be quite effective for the treatment of dysmenorrhea when compared with placebo or acetaminophen. These medications are used and tolerated by a great many women and bring relief from painful menstrual cramping. NSAIDs are not effective in approximately 20% of cases, however, and they can be associated with significant side effects.

Gastrointestinal symptoms such as nausea and indigestion seem to be especially common with naproxen. Overall, NSAIDs are associated with a higher risk than placebo of such mild neurologic adverse effects as headache, drowsiness, dizziness, and dryness of the mouth. Naproxen and indomethacin seem to be especially more likely to produce these types of symptoms.[43]

Hormonal Treatments

Combined oral contraceptive pills have been shown to reduce menstrual pain significantly. A meta-analysis of nearly 500 women showed decreased pain with both low-dose and medium-dose estrogen formulations. The type of progesterone does not seem to matter. Side effects noted were nausea, headache, and weight gain.[44] More serious side effects of oral contraceptive pills include thromboembolic and cardiovascular events, and the risks of these adverse effects rise greatly with age and cigarette smoking.

Levonorgestrel-containing intrauterine devices have been reported to decrease menstrual cramping,[45] perhaps by inhibiting buildup of the endometrium and thus reducing total prostaglandin load. Such devices also frequently reduce menstrual flow, which may be desirable in some cases. Uterine perforation, one of the more serious risks of placement of an intrauterine device, occurs at a rate of approximately 2 in 1000. The expulsion rate is approximately 5% in the first year. These devices have the advantage of providing contraception for up to 5 years before they must be replaced.

Mind-Body Therapy

A comprehensive health plan for any individual with chronic pain often involves recognition of the component of the experience of the pain that is influenced by perception of that experience. Chronic pain is frequently accompanied by mood disturbances such as depression and anxiety. At times, distinguishing whether mood affects pain or the other way around may be difficult; the relationship is likely bidirectional. Given the risk factors listed earlier of a history of sexual abuse and psychological symptoms, it is easy to see that a significant mind-body relationship may play a role in some cases of dysmenorrhea.

A 2007 Cochrane Review (reprinted in 2010) included five studies that looked at behavioral interventions such as biofeedback, relaxation techniques, and pain management training. An overall benefit was apparent, but the studies were small, and some had relatively poor methodology.[46] In areas such as this, the relationship between the provider and the individual is so important. Listening to and understanding the individual on a deeper level allow the provider to determine more appropriately whether, for example, referral to a counselor or health psychologist may be beneficial. Providers skilled in relaxation techniques or guided imagery may be able to strengthen their therapeutic relationship with patients by employing those skills for symptoms of dysmenorrhea.

Bioenergetic Therapy

Heat Therapy

Patients may report that they have tried using heating pads or microwavable bean bags, with some relief of symptoms. Studies have shown that heat does indeed decrease pain and, when combined with NSAIDs, reduces the time until noticeable pain relief is achieved.[47,48] Recommend heat of approximately 39°C (102°F) for up to 8 to 12 hours on the lower abdomen or back.

Precautions
Ensure that the heat is not so high that it causes burns or is applied to areas of decreased sensation because injury may not be recognized.

Magnet Therapy
A study of 35 women in London found a significant decrease in pain over one menstrual cycle by using a 2700-gauss magnet that attached to the underwear over the suprapubic area. The noncompletion rate in this study was significant, but the investigators reported that this was a pilot study for a much larger study using the same device. The manufacturer of the device was involved in funding of the study.[49] The device is sold in England and on the Internet for approximately $40 U.S. A Korean study using 800- to 1299-gauss magnets over the suprapubic area, lower back, and medial lower leg had similar results.[50]

Transcutaneous Electrical Nerve Stimulation
By delivering electrical currents and various frequencies through the skin, transcutaneous electrical nerve stimulation (TENS) machines appear to affect the body's ability to receive and understand pain signals. TENS devices are used quite commonly for musculoskeletal pain, including low back pain, and are portable, thus making them available for home and clinic use. A 2010 Cochrane Review found 7 small studies covering a total of 164 women suffering with dysmenorrhea that compared high- or low-frequency TENS therapy or TENS therapy with placebo TENS, placebo pill, or medical treatment (NSAIDs). The results of the meta-analysis showed that high-frequency TENS (using 50 to 100 Hz) was significantly more effective than placebo for relief of dysmenorrhea. The effect of low-frequency TENS (1 to 4 Hz) was not significant but trended toward benefit over placebo. Neither was as effective as medical therapy.[51] Consideration of the long-term effects of electromagnetic radiation to the pelvis, especially in young women, may be wise.

Acupuncture
Acupuncture is becoming more and more widely accepted in the Western world as a treatment modality for various indications, pain among the most common. Investigating efficacy can be difficult, however, in that control arms for acupuncture studies are challenging to design because even sham acupuncture may indeed have some therapeutic benefit. A 2009 systematic review of 27 trials showed that only 9 trial groups adequately described their randomization methods, and none described their allocation concealment methods. However, the results of the studies included did support significant benefit of acupuncture over pharmaceutical or herbal interventions. Two of the studies did not show benefit of acupuncture over sham acupuncture.[52] A 2011 Cochrane Review found 34 trials studying acupuncture and acupressure for dysmenorrhea.[53] Ten trials were included in the review: 6 involving acupuncture and 4 involving acupressure. Of the 24 trials not used, nearly all were excluded because of either details around randomization or the use of multiple interventions (e.g., Chinese herbs, moxibustion).

Meta-analysis of the 6 included acupuncture trials ($N = 673$) did indeed show significant benefit of acupuncture for dysmenorrhea compared with control, NSAIDs, and Chinese herbs. Acupuncture also was shown to have a positive impact on other menstrual symptoms (e.g., headache, nausea) and quality of life.[53]

Several reviews[54,55] pointed to a methodologically sound trial of 48 women randomized to acupuncture, sham acupuncture, no treatment control, or visitation control (office visits only without treatment). This study found a significant decrease in the number of patients who had "improved" symptoms (greater than 50% reduction in pain scores) with true acupuncture compared with controls.[56] A larger study of similar design would certainly be beneficial in securing acupuncture's role in the treatment of dysmenorrhea.

The World Health Organization lists primary dysmenorrhea as one of the indications "for which acupuncture has been proved—through controlled trials—to be an effective treatment."[57] Dysmenorrhea was also on the National Institute of Health's 1997 list of indications for which acupuncture was deemed potentially useful.[58]

Acupressure
Acupressure has an advantage over acupuncture in that it can be performed on oneself or with simple devices and is therefore practically and financially more accessible to greater numbers of women with primary dysmenorrhea.

A 2010 review of randomized controlled trials of acupressure alone as treatment for primary dysmenorrhea, trials that used outcome measures of pain relief and adverse effects, found four that met inclusion criteria (total $N = 458$; range, 61 to 216). Although considerable deficits were noted in descriptions of randomization and allocation concealment methods, acupressure treatments did seem to bring about an overall significant reduction in menstrual pain.[59] Points used varied in each study. One study that showed benefit used a "cotton Lycra panty brief with a fixed number of lower abdominal and lower back latex foam 'acupads' that provide pressure" on specific acupressure points and that was worn for as long as comfortable.[60] The 2011 Cochrane Review of acupuncture and acupressure for primary dysmenorrhea also included four acupressure studies ($N = 271$).[53] Meta-analysis of these studies did show a significant decrease in pain with acupressure compared with placebo. Two of the four studies in this review used auricular acupressure,[61,62] which may decrease the accessibility of treatment.

> Simple regimens described have used the acupressure points spleen 6 (SP6) and large intestine 4 (LI4).[63,64] Figures 54-1 and 54-2 illustrate the locations of these points. Consider alternating between 6 seconds of pressure and 2 seconds off for a total of approximately 5 minutes. Pressure should initially be relatively light (just shy of "really hurting") but increase as the treatment continues. Work on each point on both sides of the body for a total treatment of approximately 20 minutes. To decrease time if performing on oneself, consider acupressure on the right SP6 with the left hand while pressing on the left LI4 with the right hand for 5 minutes and then reversing for another 5 minutes.

FIGURE 54-1
Spleen 6 (Sanyinjiao): Four finger widths superior to the prominence of the medial malleolus posterior to the medial margin of the tibia. When a patient is experiencing dysmenorrhea, the point may be very tender.

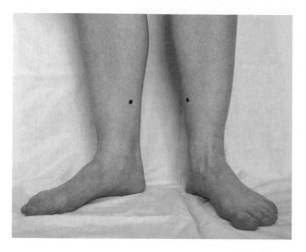

FIGURE 54-2
Large intestine 4 (Hegu): On the dorsum of the hand midway between the first and second metacarpals at the level of the midpoint of the shaft of the second metacarpal. When a patient is experiencing dysmenorrhea, the point may be very tender.

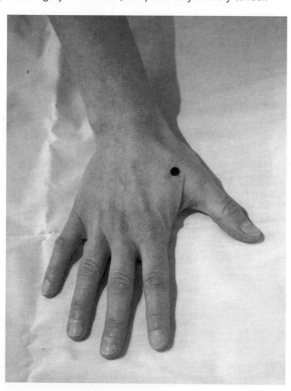

Biomechanical Therapy

Spinal Manipulation Therapy
Therapies such as osteopathic or chiropractic manipulation of the spine may increase spinal mobility and blood flow to the pelvis and lead to improvement in symptoms of dysmenorrhea. A 2006 Cochrane Review concluded that spinal manipulation therapy showed no benefit over sham manipulation in improvement of symptoms of dysmenorrhea, although both interventions decreased pain.[59] The investigators acknowledged, however, that significant challenges exist with the control arm in such studies in that, similar to acupuncture, sham manipulation may actually have some clinical benefit.[65] One of the studies included in the review also measured pretreatment and posttreatment serum levels of a prostaglandin $F_{2\alpha}$ metabolite. Pain and the metabolite were decreased in both spinal manipulation therapy and sham manipulation groups.[66] This finding may indicate that spinal manipulative therapies do indeed have a role in the treatment of dysmenorrhea, but the evidence is challenged by the inability to find a true placebo.

Surgery
Laparoscopic presacral neurectomy and laparoscopic uterine nerve ablation (LUNA) are surgical approaches to relieving dysmenorrhea. A 2010 update of a 2005 Cochrane Review found 2 studies with a total of 68 women that showed decreased menstrual pain after LUNA compared with diagnostic laparoscopy at 12 months but not at 6 months postoperatively. A third trial in the review found that laparoscopic presacral neurectomy resulted in significantly better relief scores compared with LUNA at 12 months but not at 3 months after surgery.[67]

Therapies to Consider

Aromatherapy With Massage
A study of 57 Korean college women with dysmenorrhea compared abdominal massage with aromatherapy (a mix of 2 drops of lavender, 1 drop of clary sage, and 1 drop of rose in 5 mL of almond oil), abdominal massage with almond oil only, and no intervention. The aromatherapy group showed a significant decrease in menstrual discomfort based on scoring using a visual analogue scale compared with massage alone or no treatment. Massages in the study took place for approximately 15 minutes daily for 1 week before the start of menses. No side effects were reported.[68]

Aromatherapy Massage for Dysmenorrhea
Use slow, smooth, and continuous strokes with mild to moderate pressure and a mixture of lavender, clary sage, and rose oils in almond oil (see earlier). The strokes should start with the masseur's left hand on top of the right in the right lower quadrant of the abdomen, go up to the ribs, and then across the abdomen to the left lower quadrant. The masseur can then provide gentle kneading of the left and right lower abdomen, followed by stroking across the abdomen. This sequence can be repeated for a total of 15 minutes and done daily for one week before the expected onset of menses.

PREVENTION PRESCRIPTION

- Maintain a healthy weight.
- Follow an anti-inflammatory diet.
- Participate in regular, moderate-intensity aerobic exercise.

- Avoid use of tobacco.
- Avoid alcohol in excess.
- Employ effective stress management techniques.

THERAPEUTIC REVIEW

Exercise

- The benefits of exercise on stress reduction and maintenance of a healthy weight may reduce risk factors for dysmenorrhea. C 1

Nutrition

- Diets rich in omega-3 fatty acids can reduce menstrual pain. Supplement with 1500 to 2000 mg daily of docosahexaenoic acid and eicosapentaenoic acid. Through diet, omega-3 fatty acids can be obtained with two to three servings of cold-water fish weekly and other, plant-based sources. B 1

Supplements

- Magnesium (glycinate, gluconate, or chloride): 600 mg daily, decreased if diarrhea develops. Use with caution in patients with kidney disease. B 2

- Vitamin B_6 (pyridoxine): 100 mg daily (may work better with magnesium) B 2

- Vitamin B_1 (thiamine): 100 mg daily for 90 days, or longer if symptoms recur after cessation B 1

- Vitamin E: 400 units daily B 1

Botanicals

- French maritime pine bark extract/Pycnogenol: 30 mg twice daily. The effect may last for at least 1 month after cessation. B 1

- Fennel: 30 drops of extract at the onset of menses, then every 6 hours for the first 3 days of menses. Avoid during pregnancy or lactation. B 1

- SCA (saffron, celery, and anise, by Gol Daro Herbal Medicine): 500 mg three times daily for three days starting with onset of pain or bleeding. B 2

- Willow bark extract: 240 mg daily of salicin in divided doses, started the day before expected symptoms. C 2

- Cramp bark and black haw: 2 to 3 mL of a tincture made in 1:3 proportion every 2 hours or as needed; or 4 to 8 mL of fluid extract (1:1) three or four times daily; C 2

or simmer 1 tablespoon of bark in 12 oz of water for 15 minutes, one third cup consumed every 2 to 3 hours as needed

Pharmaceuticals

- Nonsteroidal antiinflammatory drugs such as ibuprofen, 400 to 600 mg with food every 6 hours, starting the day before symptoms expected to occur until symptoms cease A 2

- Combined contraceptive pills B 2

- Levonorgestrel-containing intrauterine device C 3

Mind-Body Therapy

- Consider counseling or health psychology referral for relaxation techniques, biofeedback, or pain management training, for example, if determined relevant given the individual's history. C 1

Bioenergetic Therapy

- Use a heating pad or microwavable bean bag on the low back or abdomen for up to 8 to 12 hours. B 1

- Consider purchasing a magnet therapy device (e.g., mn8; see Key Web Resources). B 1

- Consider using a transcutaneous electrical nerve stimulation unit. B 2

- Consider acupuncture. B 2

- Consider acupressure. B 1

Biomechanical Therapy

- Consider spinal manipulation therapy (chiropractic or osteopathic treatment). B 2

- As a last resort, laparoscopic presacral neurectomy may be more effective than laparoscopic uterine nerve ablation. B 3

Other Therapies to Consider

- Aromatherapy with abdominal massage using 2 drops of lavender, 1 drop of clary sage, and 1 drop of rose in 5 mL of almond oil B 1

KEY WEB RESOURCES	
mn8: http://www.mn8.uk.com/about.php	Web site for purchase of magnet devices for dysmenorrhea that insert into underwear
Environmental Defense Fund Seafood Selector: http://www.edf.org/page.cfm?tagID=1521	Guide for safe fish consumption
Office of Dietary Supplements, National Institutes of Health: http://ods.od.nih.gov/	Health information for nutritional supplements
AcuMedico: http://www.acumedico.com/acupoints.htm	Acupuncture points database describing how to locate acupuncture points
Young Living Essential Oils: http://www.youngliving.com/essential-and-massage-oils	Organic essential oils for combining with olive oil for uterine massage for dysmenorrhea

References

References are available online at expertconsult.com.

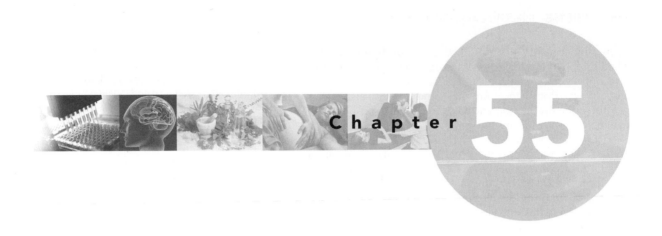

Chapter 55

Uterine Fibroids (Leiomyomata)

Allan Warshowsky, MD

Pathophysiology

Prevalence and Etiology of Uterine Fibroids

Prevalence estimates for uterine fibroids indicate that they affect 5.4% to 77% of women, depending on the method of diagnosis.[1] A fibroid tumor can be very small and difficult to feel, especially in obese women. These tumors have also been known to grow as large as a watermelon. Most gynecologists do not consider fibroid tumors a problem until they reach the size of a 12-week pregnancy. At that size, it becomes difficult to feel small ovarian tumors. Newer imaging techniques make this issue less of a concern because even large fibroid tumors allow for evaluation of ovaries through sonography and other imaging techniques. Other reasons for considering surgery would be symptoms such as bleeding and painful menstruation or dysmenorrhea. Historically, hysterectomy has been the procedure of choice for patients with large fibroid tumors. Approximately 300,000 hysterectomies are performed per year for these benign tumors. Hysterectomy is an invasive procedure; in 1975, 1700 deaths occurred among the 787,000 hysterectomies performed.[2] More recent studies have confirmed the morbidity of these invasive procedures.[3,4] Conventional medicine has little else to offer other than a "watch and wait" attitude to women who suffer from small fibroids. If these small fibroids are approached from an integrative holistic perspective when they are initially observed, much of the disability and many invasive surgical procedures can be avoided.

The second edition of the American College of Obstetrics and Gynecology's *Guideline for Women's Health Care* suggests the following: "As benign neoplasms, uterine leiomyomata (fibroids) usually require treatment only when they cause symptoms."[5] If we can use an integrative, holistic approach that eliminates symptoms and stops growth of these benign fibroid tumors, women can avoid invasive surgery and disability.

Hormonal Changes in the Normal Ovulatory Menstrual Cycle

The healthy menstrual cycle is a marvel of nature. In the first part of the cycle, the follicular cells of the ovary produce estradiol. This follicular phase lasts from 7 to 21 days. During this part of the cycle, follicle-stimulating hormone (FSH) and luteinizing hormone (LH) are produced and secreted by the anterior pituitary gland in the brain.

The necessary midfollicular phase peak of estradiol affects an LH surge during this part of the cycle. Ovulation occurs after the LH surge. Only after ovulation is progesterone produced and secreted by the corpus luteum of the ovary.

LH and FSH are in a feedback loop inhibition relationship with the main ovarian hormone, estradiol. The anterior pituitary gland is also under the control of the hypothalamus through the secretion of gonadotropin-releasing hormone (GnRH). The limbic system, which contains the amygdala and hippocampus, encircles the hypothalamus and the pituitary gland and is known to be the repository of emotions in the body. The limbic system and thus our emotions and perceptions affect the production and secretion of GnRH. The physiology of this is not clear, but clinicians all know of women who become menopausal after a significant stressor in their lives.

We must also consider the association of ovarian hormones with the thyroid and adrenal glands. Alterations of thyroid function are invariably associated with menstrual irregularities of all kinds. Low progesterone-to-estradiol (P/E_2) ratios are associated with reduced conversion of less

515

active thyroxin (T_4) to more active triiodothyronine (T_3). Therefore, hypothyroidism with normal levels of T_4 and low levels of T_3 can be an indicator of sex hormone imbalance and estrogen dominance. Adrenal gland function also affects sex hormone production and metabolism and must be evaluated along with the thyroid and ovarian hormones.

The origin of fibroids is not well understood. Some evidence indicates that chromosomal abnormalities may play a role. Chromosomal translocations, deletions, inversions, and breakpoints have been shown to be associated with familial patterns of fibroid growth.[6] Some of the fibroids in affected families tend to be quite large.

The incidence of uterine fibroids is higher in African American, obese, nonsmoking, and perimenopausal women than in other women. Fibroid tumors are associated with high estrogen levels, or estrogen dominance. Obesity and the perimenopausal state are often associated with higher estrogen levels. Studies have shown that estrogen levels are actually higher in perimenopausal women, and adipocytes are endocrine organs capable of producing estrone, a strong estrogen. The inflammatory mediators interleukin-2 (IL-2), IL-6, tumor necrosis factor-alpha (TNF-alpha), and leukotriene B_4 (LTB_4) are also produced in the adipocyte and contribute to fibroid formation.[7]

Vitamin D research has begun to shed some light on the higher incidence of fibroids in African American and other dark-skinned women.[8] Low vitamin D (measured as 25-hydroxyvitamin D_3) levels are associated with increased inflammatory cytokines and have been shown to be associated with higher incidence of epithelial cancers such as those of breast, colon, and prostate. Vitamin D is necessary for healthy cell apoptosis, or regulated cell death, and also has profound effects on glucose metabolism. Later discussion explains how unhealthy glucose metabolism can contribute to fibroid growth through the development of insulin resistance.[9] Measuring 25-hydroxyvitamin D_3 is important because this form of the vitamin circulates to all cells of the body and is a good measure of total body reserve of vitamin D_3. The optimal range of 25-hydroxyvitamin D_3 is between 40 and 100 ng/mL.[10] Replenishment is with vitamin D_3 at the range of 50,000 units/week for 12 weeks, at which time the measurement should be repeated.[11]

Studies by Dr. Elizabeth Stewart et al[12] in Boston supported the connection between systemic inflammation and fibroid growth. She proved that various growth factors, such as fibroblast growth factor, vascular endothelial growth factor, and transforming growth factor, which are concentrated in fibroid cells, are responsive to inflammatory mediators. These stimulated growth factors increase blood vessel growth or angiogenesis in the fibroid and thereby stimulate and support growth. All successful tumors increase their own blood supply and enable growth. Controlling vascularity with antiangiogenesis factors, as shown by the work of Dr. Judah Folkmann,[13] can then reduce the growth of the tumor or fibroid by decreasing its blood supply.

The theorized gut connection to fibroid growth concerns bacterial imbalance or dysbiosis. A dysbiotic intestinal environment creates gut-associated inflammatory mediators. These inflammatory mediators include IL-2, IL-6, TNF-alpha, and other leukotrienes and cytokines. These substances bathe the pelvis, where nature's fertilizer, estradiol, stimulates the growth of atypical cells that develop into autonomously

FIGURE 55-1
The fibroid that can be felt and measured is the physical manifestation of estrogen dominance and inflammation. Estrogen dominance and inflammation in the body are created and supported by the underlying sugar dysregulation, intestinal dysbiosis, detoxification errors, environmental factors, and genetics.

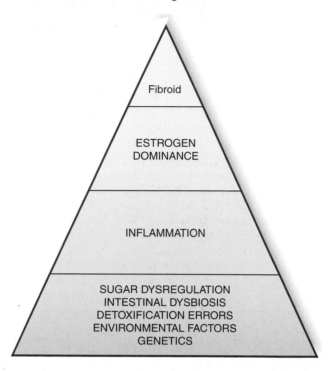

growing leiomyomata, or fibroids. Intestinal dysbiosis with associated bacterial and yeast overgrowth also contributes to estrogen dominance through the estrogenic effects of bacterial toxins and yeast mycotoxins.

Estrogen Dominance

Estrogen dominance is a term coined by the late Dr. John Lee (Fig. 55-1).[14] It applies to conditions associated with stronger estrogen effects than can be balanced with existing progesterone. Estrogen dominance can also manifest through imbalanced estrogen metabolism, as discussed later. Fibroids are just one condition associated with estrogen dominance (Table 55-1). Others are as follows:

- Autoimmune diseases: Hashimoto thyroiditis, systemic lupus erythematosus, rheumatoid arthritis, multiple sclerosis, ulcerative colitis, scleroderma, Sjögren syndrome, and others
- Fibrocystic breast problems
- Gallbladder disease
- Cervical dysplasias and other hormone-dependent cancers (breast, uterine, and ovarian)
- Endometriosis
- Infertility
- Menstrual irregularities of all kinds
- Polycystic ovary syndrome
- Premenstrual syndrome

TABLE 55-1. Factors That Promote Estrogen Dominance and Subsequent Fibroid Growth

Poor Dietary Choices*	Low-isoflavone, low-fiber foods (constipation) High–glycemic index foods Hormone-rich meats, poultry, and dairy Excessive inflammation-causing saturated fats Excessive-gluten grains
Intestinal Dysbiosis	High beta-glucuronidase levels[†] Estrogen-like mycotoxins Intestinal parasites
Sugar Dysregulation	Insulin resistance Low sex hormone–binding globulin Anovulation with low progesterone-to-estradiol ratios
Environmental Issues[‡]	Xenobiotics Polychlorinated biphenyls, dioxins, heavy metals Birth control pills and hormone replacement therapy[§] Violence and sex effects on limbic system
Stress	High cortisol levels contributing to low progesterone
Reduced Estrogen Detoxification	Leading to estrogen dominance

*Data from Goldin BR, Adlercreutz H, Gorbach SL, et al. Estrogen excretion patterns and plasma levels in vegetarian and omnivorous women. *N Engl J Med.* 1982;307:1542–1547.
[†]Data from Minton JP, Walaszek Z, Hanausek-Walaszek M, Webb TE. β-Glucuronidase levels in patients with fibrocystic breast disease. *Breast Cancer Res Treat.* 1986;8:217–222.
[‡]Data from Wolff MS, Toniolo PG, Lee EW, et al. Blood levels of organochlorine residues and risk of breast cancer. *J Natl Cancer Inst.* 1993;85:648–652.
[§]Data from Gruber CJ, Tschugguel W, Schneeberger C, Huber JC. Production and actions of estrogens. *N Engl J Med.* 2002;346:340–352.

Effects of Diet, Digestion, Absorption, and the Intestinal Environment on Hormone Balance

Hormone imbalance and estrogen dominance are often associated with intestinal dysbiosis. Intestinal dysbiosis designates an unhealthy gut environment often associated with greater intestinal permeability or "leaky gut." Signs and symptoms of dysbiosis include digestive issues, such as bad breath, body odor, bloating, gas, nausea, and constipation. The concept of leaky gut describes a condition in which, instead of protein disassembly into amino acids that are transported through the intestinal cells, large peptides and proteins are absorbed intact into the body and stimulate inflammatory reactions, as well as immune and hormonal imbalance.

Intestinal dysbiosis can be caused by antacid abuse and resultant hypochlorhydria, antibiotics, chronic stress, eating practices that do not enhance digestion and absorption (eating on the run), intestinal infection, and birth control pills.

Intestinal dysbiosis can contribute to estrogen dominance through several mechanisms. beta-Glucuronidase is an enzyme produced by pathogenic gut bacteria.[15] It cleaves the glucuronic acid molecule conjugated to estradiol that would enable its excretion and thus allows the estradiol to

reenter the body. The result is an elevation of total body estrogen that puts more stress on the liver and its detoxification capacities. Pathogenic intestinal bacteria and pathogenic yeasts can also produce bacterial and mycotoxins that have strong estrogenic effects. Concomitant inflammation can increase estrogen production and the growth factors that reside in the fibroid tissue and support angiogenesis.

Intestinal dysbiosis can be diagnosed with the proprietary Comprehensive Digestive Stool Analysis (Genova Diagnostics; see Key Web Resources). Elevations of the organic acid indican can indicate poor protein digestion and suggest intestinal dysbiosis (Organix test, Metametrix Clinical Laboratory; see Key Web Resources). Greater intestinal permeability is evaluated using the lactulose-mannitol test. In this test, the variable absorption of the two sugars lactulose and mannitol determines whether permeability in the intestines is increased. The larger sugar lactulose should not find its way into the urine, unlike the smaller sugar mannitol. Finding abnormal ratios of these two sugars in the urine after oral ingestion indicates increased intestinal permeability or dysbiosis.

Intestinal dysbiosis is treated with an intestinal restoration program such as the 4-R program described by Jeffrey Bland.[16] The four Rs are as follows:

- Remove irritants affecting the gut. This includes microorganisms, food allergens, and other toxins.

- Replace betaine hydrochloride, enzymes, bile salts, and fiber.

- Reinoculate with prebiotics (inulin) and probiotics.

- Repair, which is done with gut restorative nutrients, including zinc, glutamine, *N*-acetylcysteine, *N*-acetylglucosamine, *Boswellia*, cat's claw, licorice root, and curcumin.

For further information, see Chapter 84, Food Intolerance and Elimination Diet.

For a woman to have symptomatic fibroids and not to have functional intestinal dysfunction and associated dysbiosis is uncommon.

Effects of Insulin Resistance on Hormone Balance and Estrogen Dominance

Elevations of insulin and insulin-like growth factor-I can also contribute to estrogen dominance and fibroid growth. Metabolic syndrome (prediabetes) is a disorder of elevated insulin related to increasing insulin resistance.[17] The syndrome is defined by a constellation of signs and symptoms including abdominal obesity with a waist-to-hip ratio greater than 0.8:1 (waist circumference larger than 35 inches in women), a high level of triglycerides with a low level of high-density lipoprotein cholesterol and a high level of low-density lipoprotein cholesterol, hypertension, impaired glucose tolerance, increasing hypoglycemia, and a higher incidence of adult-onset diabetes. Metabolic syndrome is associated with these laboratory markers:

- Elevation of fasting insulin and blood glucose

- Elevation of fasting fructosamine

- High hemoglobin A1c measurement (greater than 6%)

- Increased inflammatory mediators: IL-2, IL-6, TNF-alpha, LTB_4

- Increased levels of prostaglandin 2 series, thus increasing inflammation

- Greater estrogen production in adipocytes in the form of estrone (E_1)

- Estrogen dominance, most apparent in polycystic ovary syndrome, which is highly associated with insulin resistance

- Decreased sex hormone–binding globulin (SHBG) that increases the amount of free estradiol available at the cellular level[18]

- Increased aromatase enzyme levels, which increase conversion of testosterone and androstenedione (testosterone precursor) to estradiol and estrone and also increase estrogen dominance

Insulin sensitivity can be improved by various methods, all thoroughly discussed in Chapter 31, Insulin Resistance and the Metabolic Syndrome.

Liver Detoxification and Estrogen Dominance

Systemic detoxification consists of two phases that need to be in balance. In phase 1, lipid-soluble substances—toxins, hormones, or drugs—are transformed into intermediate substances by the cytochrome P-450 set of enzymes.[19] This enzyme system can be up-regulated or down-regulated by various drugs, stressors (e.g., alcohol, cigarette smoke, smoke from charred meat), and herbs. An example in the world of estrogen dominance and uterine fibroids is the effect of gluten grains on estrogen metabolism. Gluten, the active protein in the wheat, rye, and barley reduces the cytochrome P-450 isoenzyme 3A4 and leads to reduced estrogen metabolism and subsequent estrogen dominance.

The intermediate substances that are formed in phase 1 must then be made water soluble. In phase 2 of the detoxification process, the intermediates are conjugated with amino acids and peptides such as glucuronic acid, glutathione, and glycine, or they undergo conjugation processes such as methylation, sulfation, acetylation, and sulfoxidation.[20] These now water-soluble substances can be excreted in stool, urine, or sweat or as water vapor through the lungs.

The ready for excretion estradiol–glucuronic acid molecule previously discussed is cleaved in the dysbiotic gut by elevated amounts of the enzyme beta-glucuronidase, which is produced by imbalanced gut bacteria.

Phase 1 and phase 2 detoxification errors cannot be determined by conventional aspartate aminotransferase and alanine aminotransferase enzyme levels, which are indicators only of hepatocyte breakdown. More integrative and functional assessments of detoxification can be made through organic acid testing or functional detoxification tests that evaluate the phase 1 cytochrome P-450 enzyme system and phase 2 conjugation factors. Estrogen metabolites and their intermediaries consist of the catechol (hydroxy) estrogens and the methylestrogens. The anticarcinogenic estrogen modulator 2-hydroxyestrone ($2OH-E_1$) comes from naturally produced ovarian estrogens; high levels of this substance as 2-methoxyestrone reduce the risk of breast cancer. Higher amounts of 4-hydroxyestrone ($4OH-E_1$) occur with

metabolism of conjugated estrogens (Premarin) to form DNA-damaging quinones. Epigallocatechin gallates (a catechin in green tea) and other antioxidants such as vitamins A and C and E, selenium, *N*-acetylcysteine, and lipoic acid convert quinones to mercapturates. This process occurs through the production of glutathione. 16alpha-Hydroxyestrone ($16OH-E_1$) forms a very strong bond with the estrogen receptor, is a strong estrogen, and has carcinogenic potential. These estrogen metabolites are not all good or bad. Like everything else in nature, they need to be in balance.

Appropriate levels of 16alpha-hydroxyestrone support good bone density. The ratio of the three hydroxyestrogens and their methylated end products, which can be measured in urine (Metametrix Clinical Laboratory) or blood (Genova Diagnostics), can help evaluate risk in estrogen dominance conditions. In menstruating women, the ratio of $2OH-E_1$ to $16OH-E_1$ should be evaluated during the luteal (late) phase of the cycle. The following factors increase either this ratio or the level of $2OH-E_1$:

- A diet rich in the cruciferous vegetables (broccoli, Brussels sprouts, kale, cabbage, cauliflower)

- Indole-3-carbinol (I-3-C), which comes from cruciferous vegetables (broccoli, Brussels sprouts, cabbage, kale): 200 to 800 mg/day

  - Diindolylmethane (I-3-C activated by stomach acid), used alone or in conjunction with I-3-C

- Epigallocatechin gallates (green tea extract)

- Isoflavones, including soy, flaxseed, and kudzu[21]

- Omega-3 fatty acids

- Vigorous exercise, a minimum of 30 minutes three times/ week

The ratio of $2OH-E_1$ to $16OH-E_1$ can be reduced, with an increased proportion of $16OH-E_1$, by the following conditions:

- Obesity

- Hypothyroidism

- Xenoestrogens: any estrogenic substances, including dioxins and polychlorinated biphenyls

- Cimetidine (Tagamet) and other drugs that interfere with the cytochrome P-450 system[22]

- Estriol: Although in most people estriol is a metabolic end product, concern exists that as a stereoisomer it can revert to the $16alphaOH-E_1$ from which it was formed; this is more of a concern when estriol is prescribed as part of a bio-identical hormone replacement therapy program.

Most of the studies of hormone imbalance and fibroid tumors of the uterus have concerned themselves with estrogen dominance, although mifepristone studies create some controversy and doubt.[23] Mifepristone is better known as RU-486, the "abortion pill." It functions as a progesterone receptor antagonist. Long-term use of mifepristone has been associated with fibroid regression.[23] As a progesterone receptor antagonist, mifepristone's action would suggest that progesterone also stimulates fibroid growth. The answer may not be that simple because progesterone also increases blood vessel support of the endometrium in anticipation of a fertilized egg. My opinion is that some fibroids may take advantage of the increased progesterone-supported blood supply and increase in size because of it. The negative effects associated with long-term mifepristone use are bone loss and endometrial hyperplasia, conditions indicating that more complicated mechanisms may be at work. Mifepristone may also affect estrogen receptors. More studies are needed.

Determining Whether a Fibroid Has Malignant Potential

The malignant potential (sarcomatous change) of fibroids or leiomyomata is less than 1%. Whether a fibroid changes from benign to malignant or is malignant to begin with is not well established. One sign that can indicate a malignant fibroid or leiomyosarcoma is rapid growth. Unfortunately, the only conventional way to evaluate malignancy is to remove the fibroid and examine a sample for the number of mitotic events per high-power field; more than 20 mitoses per high-power field would indicate sarcomatous change. Table 55-2 lists tests that should be considered in evaluating a patient with fibroid tumors of the uterus.

Complementary and Alternative Medicine Studies on Fibroid Tumors of the Uterus

To date, few complementary and alternative medicine studies on holistic approaches to fibroids have been conducted.[24] Most studies are concerned with comparisons of the various invasive treatments.

Zhongli and Shurong conducted a study in 223 women with fibroids who were treated with acupuncture and Chinese botanicals. Effectiveness in reducing symptoms was rated at more than 90%.

The U.S. herbal literature describes treatments for fibroids with the herbs gossypium, *Hydrastis, Phytolacca, Rubus,* the viburnums, *Achillea,* and trillium. One study combined visualization, imagery, body therapy, and Chinese botanicals to treat symptoms and reduce growth of fibroids in 37 women.[25] The age-matched controls used progestins, birth control pills, and nonsteroidal antiinflammatory drugs (NSAIDs). Outcome measures were reduced growth, fewer symptoms, and patient satisfaction. At the end of the 6-month study period, a statistically significant benefit of the complementary and alternative medicine approach over the conventional medical treatment was found in each of the outcome measures.

Integrative Therapy

Nutrition

The patient should begin a hormone-balancing diet involving foods with low inflammation effects, low acidity, and a low glycemic load.

Foods That Increase Estrogen Dominance

Acidic and inflammatory foods, such as red meats, poultry, and dairy products, are sources of arachidonic acid, which increase inflammatory prostaglandins and other inflammatory mediators that help to support fibroid growth through the process of angiogenesis. Avoiding commercial meat products also reduces exposure to the added hormones in these products.[26] Small amounts of range-fed meats can be added back as inflammation subsides (see Chapter 86, The Antiinflammatory Diet).

Sweets and other foods with a high glycemic index are potentially stressful and can raise insulin levels, increase estrogen dominance, and also support fibroid growth. Eating a breakfast containing good-quality protein, fats, and carbohydrates in combination is imperative to avoid hypoglycemic stress–induced cortisol and epinephrine elevations, which deplete lean muscle and increase the tendency for insulin resistance through gluconeogenesis (see Chapter 85, The Glycemic Index/Load).

TABLE 55-2. Tests to Consider for Evaluation of a Patient With Fibroid Tumors of the Uterus

25-Hydroxyvitamin D measurement*	Low levels increasing fibroid growth by several mechanisms (see text)
Vitamin A measurement†	Low levels shown to increase menorrhagia
Iron or total iron-binding capacity measurement, ferritin measurement	Low iron stores reducing myometrial contractility and increasing menstrual blood loss
Progesterone/estradiol ratio (100–300:1) Luteal phase progesterone measurement	Low luteal phase progesterone level support estrogen dominance and fibroid growth
Thyroid function testing	Hypothyroidism associated with menstrual dysfunction
MTHFR polymorphism	35% weakness in methylation, increased estrogen dominance
Comprehensive digestive stool analysis	Intestinal dysbiosis a cause of estrogen dominance through several mechanisms (see text)
Phase 1 and phase 2 detoxification evaluation	Unhealthy estrogen metabolism contributing to estrogen dominance
Transvaginal and abdominal ultrasonography	To determine the size and location of fibroids and rule out ovarian tumors
Testing for celiac disease (antigliadin antibodies)	Gluten grain sensitivity common in fibroid tumor sufferers and can lead to further estrogen dominance

*Data from Chiu KC, Chu A, Vay LWG, Saad MF. Hypovitaminosis D is associated with insulin resistance and beta cell dysfunction. *Am J Clin Nutr.* 2004;79:820–825.
†Data from Lithgow DM, Politzer WM. Vitamin A in the treatment of menorrhagia. *S Afr Med J.* 1977;51:191–199.

Gluten grains, especially wheat, rye, and barley, contain genetically engineered gluten that is much stronger than what was found in the more ancient gluten grains such as spelt. These newer grains can increase estrogens by inhibition of the cytochrome P-450 3A4 enzyme system and can also affect thyroid hormone. All people with chronic estrogen dominance must be tested for gluten sensitivity by antigliadin antibody testing.

Alcohol is not a problem if it is consumed in moderation. Studies show that women consuming more than five alcoholic drinks per week have a higher risk of breast cancer. This increase probably results from the effect of alcohol on the detoxification of estrogens. Organic coffee in moderation (1 to 2 cups per day) is also safe. Artificial ingredients, colorings, flavorings, and preservatives should be eliminated. Margarines and other sources of trans fatty acids and hydrogenated oils are also unhealthy and must be avoided.

Foods That Reduce Estrogen Dominance

Deep sea, cold-water fish, such as wild Pacific salmon, sardines, mackerel, and cod, have large quantities of the omega-3 oils (eicosapentaenoic acid [EPA] and docosahexaenoic acid [DHA]).[27] Because heavy metals such as mercury contribute to estrogen dominance, I recommend eating fish with lower levels of mercury. These are fish at the lower end of the food chain. The larger game fish such as swordfish, tuna, and bass concentrate the contaminants from eating the smaller fish. The small crustaceans, krill, are a good source of noncontaminated EPA and DHA. Algae sources of DHA are also available.

Seeds and nuts, especially flaxseed, hemp seed, and chia seed, contain isoflavones much like soy.[28] They tend to be hormone balancing. I recommend 2 to 4 tablespoons per day added to a soy- or kudzu-containing protein powder shake first thing in the morning. Seeds and nuts such as pumpkin seeds, sunflower seeds, and walnuts are also good sources of omega-3 oils.[29]

Cruciferous vegetables such as broccoli, Brussels sprouts, cabbage, and cauliflower support healthy estrogen metabolism (Fig. 55-2). Legumes such as adzuki beans, peas, lentils, and edamame all have hormone-modulating flavonoids and can safely be eaten.[30]

> A head of cabbage contains approximately 1200 mg of indole-3-carbinol. Eating one fourth of a cabbage daily would provide 300 mg of indole-3-carbinol daily.

I have been consistently impressed by the reduction of symptoms related to estrogen dominance by the elimination of milk casein, high-glycemic carbohydrates, and gluten grains. The symptoms that seem to be most affected are gastrointestinal symptoms, headache, dermatologic rashes, fatigue, insomnia, and mood issues.

Lifestyle

Exercise

Aerobic exercise consumes oxygen and helps to "burn" carbohydrates. Oxygen-consuming exercises are exemplified by running, fast walking, and swimming. Because carbohydrates are consumed during aerobic exercise, this form of

FIGURE 55-2
Metabolism of selected estrogens. DHEA, dehydroepiandrosterone.

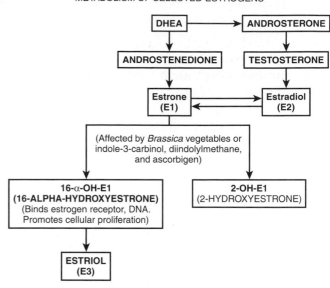

METABOLISM OF SELECTED ESTROGENS

exercise is associated with improvement in insulin resistance and sugar use.

Anaerobic exercise classically uses fats as an energy source. That is why weight trainers consume medium-chain triglycerides during their workouts. Weight training also helps stabilize hormones such as growth hormone and testosterone. Because fat cells (adipocytes) are known to produce inflammatory mediators and estrogens, limiting adipose tissue also reduces estrogen dominance. A regimen of 30 minutes of regular exercise three times per week has also been shown to lower the incidence of breast cancer and colon cancer.

Botanicals: Overview

Botanical therapies can be very useful in reducing fibroid growth and in decreasing fibroid symptoms.[31] Not much is available in the way of scientific study, but many of these herbs have been used by naturopaths and herbalists for many years.

Botanicals for Liver and Detoxification Support

Healthy estrogen metabolism must be reestablished to reverse estrogen dominance. By obtaining functional liver detoxification studies performed by laboratories such as Genova Diagnostics, Metametrix, and Doctor's Data, the clinician can determine which specific aspects of the detoxification pathway the patient is lacking and give the appropriate nutritional support. Many botanicals and nutraceuticals can be helpful in restoring and maintaining healthy detoxification.

Epigallocatechin Gallates From Green Tea

Epigallocatechin gallates reduce the DNA-damaging effects of $4OH-E_1$. They may also be antiangiogenesis factors.

Dosage
The dose is 3 cups/day (240 to 320 mg of polyphenols).

Precautions
These agents can cause insomnia if they are consumed in large amounts.

Indole-3-Carbinol or the Stomach-Activated Diindolylmethane
I-3-C increases the production of estrogen-modulating $2OH-E_1$.[32]

Dosage
The dose is 200 to 400 mg/day.

Precautions
I-3-C is generally free of side effects.

Milk Thistle (Silybum marianum)
Milk thistle is a general liver antioxidant that supports healthy detoxification and estrogen metabolism.

Dosage
The dose is 280 to 420 mg of milk thistle per day standardized to 70% to 80% silymarin content.

Precautions
This agent is virtually devoid of negative effects.

Botanicals to Modulate Pelvic Lymphatic Drainage

These botanical formulas are used in combination to modulate pelvic lymphatic drainage. Scudder's alterative (a combination herbal product containing corydalis, alder root, mayapple root, figwort, and yellow dock) modulates cellular metabolism. Echinacea/Red Root compound modulates toxin elimination, immune system, and inflammatory mediators.

Dosage
The dose is 30 drops of Scudder's alterative combined with Echinacea/Red Root compound as a tea twice/day for 3 months. This is followed by 2-weeks without this treatment.

Precautions
This combination of formulas has no known negative effects.

Botanicals and Herbal Combinations Shown to Reduce the Growth of Fibroids

Fraxinus
Fraxinus is also known as white ash or *Ceanothus* compound.

Dosage
The dose is 30 to 40 drops of tincture in hot water twice/day for 3 months, followed by a 2-week break; repeat.

Precautions
Fraxinus has no known toxicity.

Turska's Formula
Turska's formula (aconite, phytolacca, gelsemium, bryonia) is used by naturopaths and U.S. herbalists to reduce size of growths. It contains some potentially toxic herbs (aconite and phytolacca). Bryonia has been classified by the U.S. government as an endangered species, so the formula has been increasingly difficult to obtain, and variations have also been developed with different herbal combinations.

Dosage
The dose is 5 to 10 drops/day in hot water. Use only under the care of a knowledgeable herbalist.

Precautions
This formula should be used in small amounts. It can be toxic at higher dosage and can cause gastrointestinal distress, peripheral blood cell changes, cardiac toxicity, headache, and double vision.

Chaste Berry (Vitex agnus-castus)
Chaste berry, or *Vitex*, is an herb with a long reputation for balancing progesterone production.[33] It has dopaminergic effects and modulates prolactin secretion from the pituitary gland. Evidence also indicates that it helps reduce growth and shrink small fibroids.

Dosage
The dose is 200 to 500 mg/day.[34]

Precautions
Minor gastrointestinal distress is a rare side effect.

Myomin
Another herbal combination that has a long history of use is Myomin, which contains the following herbs:
200 mg *Smilax glabra* Roxb. (sarsaparilla), a progesterone modulator
160 mg *Curcuma zedaoria*, which has antiinflammatory effects
160 mg *Cyperus rotundus*
160 mg *Aralia dasyphylla* Mig.
120 mg *Pericarpium arecae*

Dosage
The dose is two to three capsules three times/day after meals.

Precautions
Myomin has no significant side effects.

Herbal Therapies for Specific Symptoms

Menorrhagia
Heavy bleeding from fibroids tends to be the symptom that brings most women to the operating room. Menorrhagia is defined as loss of more than 80 mL per menses. Controlling heavy bleeding, or menorrhagia, is probably the most important first step in the fibroid healing program. Severe iron deficiency anemia is one of the most common reasons for surgery. Combinations of herbs that act differently within the uterus can be very effective in reducing blood loss and keeping women out of the operating room. Use of a combination of the following herbal types can significantly reduce menstrual bleeding.

Uterine-toning herbs: These include red raspberry, false unicorn root, and black cohosh.

Astringent herbs: These include yarrow, lady's mantle, beth root, and cinnamon.

Oxytocic herbs: I have only used shepherd's purse for oxytotic effect. It has a long history of use among midwives to help control postpartum bleeding.

These herbs are also used in combination. A combination botanical preparation consisting of tinctures of a tonic herb such as red raspberry and an astringent herb such as yarrow can be used at a dose of 30 drops each twice a day for 2 weeks before the period. This protocol helps the uterus prepare for healthy uterine contractions both to expel the menstrual flow and to optimize effective and nonspasmodic uterine contractions. When bleeding begins, add 30 drops of an oxytotic herbal tincture such as shepherd's purse. The combination of all three herbal tinctures can be taken every 30 minutes for up to 6 doses. No scientific reason exists for using 6 doses as an arbitrary cutoff. I believe that if the patient is still hemorrhaging after 3 hours of using these herbs, something else needs to be considered. However, this protocol has been extremely useful in reducing menorrhagia and reversing iron deficiency anemia. Other herbs in the same categories can be substituted if the patient has a reaction to one of the herbs or if the effect is less than desired. Several botanical companies such as Gaia and Herbpharm standardized herbal tinctures (see Key Web Resources below).

Dosage
See the preceding protocol.

Precautions
These herbs have minor gastrointestinal effects. Yarrow rarely causes rash or sun sensitivity. Shepherd's purse in large doses may interfere with thyroid function. Follow-up with thyroid function testing is suggested.

Antiinflammatory Botanicals
Inflammatory prostanoids, cytokines, and leukotrienes increase the cellular growth factors that support vascularization of the fibroid. Specific botanicals can reduce this inflammation. Botanicals are often found in combination products, such as one containing *Boswellia* (400 mg), ginger (200 mg), turmeric (300 mg), and cayenne (50 mg) in every two tablets.

Dosage
One to two tablets are taken three times/day. The patient may take one to two tablets every 2 hours as needed.

Precautions
Taking such a combination product on an empty stomach can cause abdominal pain in sensitive individuals. These herbal preparations can be taken with food.

Systemic Enzymes
Elimination of excessive inflammation with potent systemic enzyme formulations may reduce the size of fibroids by limiting vascularization of fibroids and by enzymatic myolysis of the fibroid.[35] Such systemic enzymes are Neprinol, Wobenzym, Vitalzyme, and bromelain (from pineapple stems).[36] Other preparations of proteases can also be used. Neprinol[37] has the following ingredients:

- SEBkinase
- Peptizyme SP
- Serrapeptase
- Lipase
- Protease
- Amla
- Papain
- NattoSEB
- Nattokinase
- Bromelain
- Rutin
- Coenzyme Q10
- Magnesium

Dosage
These enzyme formulations should be taken on an empty stomach to avoid action on food rather than on the protein of the fibroid. The dose is gradually built up from 1 tablet three times/day to 15 tablets per day in divided doses.

Precautions
As with any antiinflammatory agent taken on an empty stomach, the clinician must caution the patient about stomach pain. Such enzyme preparations must be used with caution in patients with gastritis and history of gastric ulcer, as well as in patients who take blood thinners.

Antiangiogenesis Factors
The work by Judah Folkman[13] in cancer therapy illustrates the effect of antiangiogenesis on reducing tumor growth. The convolvulus product and other antiangiogenesis factors are used to reduce blood flow to the fibroids.[38] *Convolvulus arvensis* (bindweed) works as an antiangiogenesis factor.[39] Green tea catechins and polyphenols also have antiangiogenic effects.

Dosage
The dose is two tablets three times/day, slowly increased from one tablet twice/day.

Precautions
Headaches are a side effect if the dosage is increased too rapidly. Increase slowly to avoid headaches.

Nutraceuticals

Vitamin C and the Citrus Bioflavonoids (Rutin and Hesperidin)
Vitamin C strengthens capillary desmosomes and can also be helpful in reducing menorrhagia.[40] The citrus bioflavonoids rutin and hesperidin enhance this vitamin C effect and are also mildly estrogenic and as such can have a tonic effect, by reducing the effects of estrogen dominance.

Dosage
The dose is 1000 to 2000 mg/day, but the dosage can be increased up to 75% of bowel tolerance.

■ Precautions

Vitamin C has been known to cause diarrhea. This is what has been referred to as bowel tolerance. Reducing the dosage to 75% of the amount that causes diarrhea may be the most appropriate individualized approach to that patient. Some question exists about the use of vitamin C in patients with a history of kidney stones.

B Vitamins

Vitamins B_1, B_2, B_3, B_5, and B_6 are important for sugar, fat, and neurotransmitter metabolism, hormone balance, and healthy cortisol production from the adrenal gland.[41] Vitamin B_3 in the form of niacinamide is also a potent antiinflammatory agent. Niacin can be used to reduce menstrual cramping often associated with fibroids.[42] Other B vitamins, such as choline and inositol, support healthy liver function. Vitamins B_2, B_6, B_{12}, and folic acid support the process of methylation, which is necessary for healthy hormone metabolism and for DNA repair. Vitamins B_5 and B_6 also support adrenal function, which is important in healthy hormone balance.

■ Dosage

A 50-mg B-complex vitamin can supply basic vitamin B needs. Separate additional B vitamins may be necessary. The recommended dose of vitamin B_{12} is 2000 units/day.

The dose of folic acid is 800 mcg or more per day. Doses up to 5 to 10 mg/day have been used for cervical dysplasias. Approximately 35% of the population is estimated to have a mutation of the *MTHFR* gene that decreases their ability to methylate. Most laboratories check for the *MTHFR* C677T gene mutation. I recommend this test, and if a patient is heterozygous or homozygous for the mutation, supplementation, at least in part, with methylfolate seems wise. A reasonable dose of methylfolic acid is 1 to 2 mg/day.

■ Precautions

When high doses of folic acid are used, attention must be taken to supplying vitamin B_{12} in addition, to avoid masking the signs of pernicious anemia. Peripheral neuropathies have been reported with vitamin B_6 dosages larger than 200 mg/day. Practicing caution when dosing and educating patients to report any tingling in their fingers and toes are important.

> For treatment of menstrual cramps, consider having the patient take niacin, 100 mg twice/day throughout the month, then 100 mg every 2 hours while having cramps.

Vitamin D

Vitamin D is very important for the healthy functioning of every cell in the body. It has been found to be useful for the following functions:

- Sugar metabolism
- Programmed cell death (apoptosis)
- Balanced inflammatory reactions
- Reduction in incidence of epithelial cancers
- Bone health
- Healthy thyroid function
- Healthy calcium metabolism

Because of fear of sun exposure and resultant skin cancer, most people use ultraviolet B–blocking, sun protective factor (SPF) 30 or higher sun block.[43] This situation has created almost an epidemic of low levels of vitamin D. Measuring 25-hydroxyvitamin D levels and restoring them to at least 40 ng/dL are imperative. Investigators have estimated that 32 ng/dL will be required to prevent rickets in children. Restoration of vitamin D levels can be accomplished by using 50,000 units/week of vitamin D_2 for 12 weeks and then remeasuring. Supplying at least 1200 mg/day of calcium to a patient being treated with vitamin D is important.[44]

■ Dosage

If the 25-hydroxyvitamin D blood level is low, give 50,000 units of vitamin D_2 once a week for 12 weeks; then recheck the 25-hydroxyvitamin D level.

■ Precautions

As with any fat-soluble vitamin, excessive amounts of vitamin D can be toxic. Measuring blood levels again after 12 weeks of supplementation is necessary. Supplying at least 1200 mg/day of calcium in the diet and as a supplement can prevent loss of calcium from bone. Evaluation of parathyroid hormone levels screens for hyperparathyroidism and is important before supplementing. Evidence indicates that supplementation with the other fat-soluble vitamins A, E, and K may be necessary for optimal absorption.

Calcium D Glucarate

Calcium D glucarate reduces the activity of the enzyme beta-glucuronidase, which is produced in patients with intestinal dysbiosis. This enzyme, which is produced by dysbiotic intestinal bacteria, cleaves the glucuronic acid–estrogen bond on estrogens meant to be excreted and instead puts them back into circulation. By the action of beta-glucuronidase, estrogen dominance increases and adds more stress to the already stressed detoxification system.

■ Dosage

The dose is 500 mg twice/day.

■ Precautions

No precautions are reported.

Iron

Women with fibroids tend to have heavy menses, or menorrhagia, which is defined as losing more than 80 mL of blood during menstruation. This greater iron loss associated with the blood loss sets up a vicious circle.[45] The lower the iron level becomes, the more weakly the myometrial muscle cells contract, thus contributing to more menstrual blood loss. Evaluation and treatment of low iron stores by measurement of iron levels, total iron-binding capacity, and serum ferritin levels help guide restoration of iron levels and maintain healthy myometrial contractility. A boggy, noncontractile uterus bleeds more than a healthy, well-toned one.

■ Dosage

The dose is 325 mg/day of ferrous sulfate or its equivalent. Higher doses may be needed during menses.

Precautions

Measuring serum iron levels during supplementation prevents iron overload. Some iron formulas can be constipating.

Selenium

Selenium is a potent antioxidant that supports the action of vitamin E. It also is used in the production of the antioxidant glutathione. Selenium is necessary for the action of thyroid hormone.

Dosages

The dose is 200 to 500 mcg/day.

Precautions

Dosages exceeding 1000 mcg/day can precipitate skin and nail changes. "Garlic breath" may be an early sign of too much selenium.

Magnesium and Zinc

Important for hormone support, magnesium and zinc are responsible for catalyzing approximately 500 different reactions in the body. These minerals are estimated to be deficient in 50% to 75% of the population. One theory for the craving of chocolate in the premenstrual period is the need for magnesium[46]; chocolate is rich in this mineral.

Dosages

The dose of magnesium is 400 to 600 mg/day, and the dose of zinc is 15 to 30 mg/day.

Precautions

Taking too much magnesium can increase diarrhea. Magnesium can also compete with calcium for absorption; if this problem is suspected, magnesium should be taken separately from calcium. Zinc may interfere with copper absorption, and supplementation requires that 2 mg copper be added to the protocol. Red blood cell levels should be checked.

> Women who crave chocolate (a rich source of magnesium) before their period may benefit from magnesium replacement therapy.

Omega-3 Fatty Acids (Eicosapentaenoic Acid and Docosahexaenoic Acid)

The omega-3 essential fatty acids (EPA and DHA) help maintain the fluidity of all cell membranes, reduce inflammatory mediators, and are building blocks for hormones. These essential fatty acids are not made in the body and must therefore be consumed. Clinicians have seen time and again how increased and unbalanced inflammation contributes to fibroid tumor problems.

Dosage

The dose is 3 to 6 g/day of EPA and DHA (fish oil).

Precautions

Caution is recommended when prescribing more than 3 to 4 g/day of omega-3 acids to diabetic patients. Reports have noted elevations of blood glucose.

Mind-Body Therapy

Encourage patients to create emotional flexibility by "staying in the moment." Stretching and yoga exercises not only help maintain physical flexibility, but also promote emotional flexibility. Living in the present moment,[47] we modulate stress effects that come from worrying about a possible future that may never come and from fretting about a past that cannot be changed. This chronic stress, which raises cortisol levels and lowers dehydroepiandrosterone (DHEA) levels, contributes to estrogen dominance by "stealing" or shunting progesterone to produce more cortisol.

Body awareness exercises, such as tai chi and qi gong, and meditation and visualization exercises help to reduce blood flow to fibroids and lessen their impact and their growth. Moving and other meditation exercises help to mobilize stagnated energy, as do acupuncture, deep tissue massage, craniosacral work, and psychotherapeutic techniques such as bioenergetics.

Exercise of all kinds has been shown to reduce the harmful effects of stress. Meditation also helps reduce cortisol levels.[48] Many of these techniques focus on chakras or energy centers that correspond to anatomic nerve plexuses or glands of the endocrine system. One such technique is the Freeze Frame technique, developed by The HeartMath Institute: The patient is taught to focus on heart energy or the fourth chakra while breathing into the heart. Thoughts that are stressful are not internalized but instead are blown out with the exhale. This is a simple but powerful way to stay in the moment and reduce the inflammatory effects of stress on the body (see Chapter 94, Enhancing Heart Rate Variability).

Journaling is a technique for ridding the body of stored emotional energy. Removing this stagnating energy is like cleaning out the closet and getting rid of all the clutter in your life. Energy moves again.

While meditating and performing visualization exercises, the patient is instructed to be aware of second chakra issues—relationships, creative blocks, and abuse issues. Journaling has been shown to help reduce the negative effect of these stored emotions (see Chapter 96, Journaling for Health).

Another powerful technique that supports meditation and stress reduction and thereby alleviates symptoms of fibroids and reduces their growth is visualization of the desired results and the intent of bringing healing energy into the area to be healed.

Pharmaceuticals: Gonadotropin Receptor Agonists

The following gonadotropin-releasing hormone (GnRH) receptor agonists may be used.

Leuprolide Acetate

Leuprolide acetate (Lupron) is used to shrink fibroids before surgery to make the tumors easier to remove.[49] This agent can effect a 30% to 60% reduction in fibroid size. Surgeons sometimes complain that using leuprolide decreases their ability to enucleate fibroids easily during myomectomy.

Dosage

The dose is 3.75 to 7.5 mg/month given intramuscularly for 1 to 6 months.

Precautions

Unfortunately, if nothing else is done to prevent regrowth, many fibroids rapidly achieve the same size they were before treatment. This agent causes chemical castration, menopausal symptoms, and osteoporosis.

Danazol

Danazol (Danocrine), which suppresses LH and FSH, can also be used to shrink fibroids.

Dosage

The dose is 600 to 800 mg/day.

Precautions

Precautions are the same as those listed for leuprolide acetate, but they are more intense.

Agents for Menorrhagia Associated With Fibroids

Norethindrone Acetate

Norethindrone acetate is used for menorrhagia associated with fibroids.

Dosage

A dose of 5 to 15 mg/day has been effective in slowing bleeding.

Precautions

The risk of blood clots, fluid retention, breast tenderness, nausea, insomnia, and depression is increased.

Progesterone-Containing Intrauterine Device

Studies have shown that progesterone-containing intrauterine devices (Mirena, Progestasert) reduce menstrual flow.[50]

Precautions

An intrauterine device may be difficult to insert in a woman who has not experienced vaginal delivery, and it may not be effective for a submucous fibroid.

Birth Control Pills

Birth control pills have been shown to reduce menstrual flow.

Dosage

Either daily dosing or the newer 3-month (Seasonal) dosing is effective.

Precautions

All the precautions considered when the pill is prescribed for contraception are relevant here.

Nonsteroidal Antiinflammatory Drugs

Studies have shown that NSAIDs, such as ibuprofen and naproxen (Aleve), reduce menorrhagia by 20% to 50%.

Dosage

The dose of naproxen is one to two 220-mg tablets or capsules every 12 hours. The dose of ibuprofen is 400 mg every 4 to 6 hours.

Precautions

All NSAIDs can increase gastric discomfort and raise the risk of gastrointestinal bleeding.

Tranexamic Acid (an Antifibrinolytic Agent)

Tranexamic acid has been approved for treatment of menorrhagia at doses of 650 mg three times daily during menses. It is very effective and is without serious negative effects.

Natural Hormones

Natural Progesterone

The optimal ratio for progesterone to estradiol during the reproductive years ranges from 100:1 to 300:1. Estrogens are measured in picograms (a trillionth of a gram), and progesterone is measured in nanograms (a billionth of a gram), so the progesterone levels in nanograms per deciliter should be multiplied by 1000 to calculate the ratio.

Preparations of 3% progesterone cream[51] supply 400 mg of progesterone per 2-oz. jar. Vaginal suppositories can contain 100 to 400 mg progesterone per suppository. For heavy menstrual bleeding, vaginal applications of progesterone may be more helpful.[52]

Dosage

The dose of 3% progesterone cream is approximately ¼ teaspoon twice/day for the 2 weeks of the luteal part of the cycle, to supply 20 to 40 mg/day. A 10% cream supplies approximately 100 mg per application and may be necessary to balance estrogens in a patient receiving bioidentical hormone therapy or in cases of severe progesterone need.

Precautions

If excessive amounts of cream are applied to adipose tissue rather than thin skin, sadness or depression may result. Stimulating estrogen receptors can lead to short-term breast cysts or tenderness. Progesterone can exacerbate intestinal yeast problems. In the presence of sugar dysregulation, progesterone can raise insulin-like growth factor-I levels in the breast and may increase atypical breast cell formation. Studies of mifepristone (RU-486), the progesterone receptor antagonist, suggest a role for progesterone in fibroid growth. Clinically, I have witnessed fibroid growth in progesterone-deficient women when progesterone was used therapeutically. This seems to be more of a problem with larger fibroids. High body burdens of lead can also interfere with progesterone effect.

Dehydroepiandrosterone

DHEA reduces IL-6, a potent inflammatory cytokine that can promote the production of estrogens in the body. DHEA stimulates the peroxisome proliferator-activated receptor-gamma receptor, thus reducing inflammation, increasing insulin sensitivity, and reducing estrogen levels by maintaining healthy sugar metabolism and normal insulin levels. It also helps balance the effects of stress on the body by being in equilibrium with cortisol.

Dosage

The dose of DHEA is 5 to 10 mg one or twice/day. The dose of 7-keto DHEA is 25 to 50 mg/day.

■ Precautions

DHEA can convert to estradiol. Use of the 7-keto form may obviate this issue. Following hormone levels is always necessary when supplementing.

Surgical Treatment

The conventional approach to dealing with uterine fibroids remains largely surgical.[1] Total abdominal hysterectomy—removal of the uterus with cervix, ovaries, and fallopian tubes—is the most common procedure recommended. Subtotal procedures are also performed. These procedures may leave the cervix (supracervical hysterectomy) or the ovaries and fallopian tubes. Hysterectomy can also be performed by the vaginal or laparoscopic route. Robotic laparoscopies are now performed at some centers.

Hysterectomy and other invasive procedures are not without consequence. Postoperative recovery can take up to 4 to 6 weeks. Infectious complications can affect 10% of women. Major injuries to bladder, bowel, ovaries, and ureters happen approximately 1% of the time.

Myomectomy involves removal of the fibroid only, thereby preserving the uterus. Myomectomy can also be performed abdominally or through the laparoscope.

Myolysis techniques require the use of an energy source, which is applied to the fibroid through various instrumentation methods. The energy used may be ultrasound, laser, or electrical. The interior of the fibroid is destroyed, and the fibroid shrinks. The U.S. Food and Drug Administration has approved a myolysis[53] procedure using magnetic resonance imaging guidance and ultrasound as an energy source (ExAblate).

Uterine artery embolization is another procedure that effectively reduces blood flow to the fibroid and hastens shrinkage. Inert polyvinyl alcohol particles are placed in the uterine artery through an artery in the upper thigh.

Except for total hysterectomy, all these procedures have one thing in common: the fibroids grow back. Complications of the procedures include infections, pain, and injuries to major organs in the area, such as ureters, bowel, and bladder.

Other Therapies to Consider

Unblocking the energy of the second chakra is an approach to treatment of uterine fibroids.

Castor Oil Packs

Castor oil packs are hot packs made with wool flannel and hexane-free castor oil. Evidence suggests that they work through the lymphatic system and reduce inflammation. The castor oil pack is applied over the fibroid for 20 to 60 minutes per session. This device is a very effective meditation and visualization tool. The patient meditates on her uterus and visualizes the fibroid shrinking. She also visualizes the blood supply to the fibroids as pipes with turnoff valves and, while doing the meditation, visualizes turning off the valves, thus shutting down the blood supply to the fibroids. The spiritual aspects of healing come into play here.[54]

Through meditation and visualizing the healing of their fibroids, patients are instructed to be aware of any thoughts, feelings, or memories that can be associated with stagnation of second chakra energy and subsequent growth of the fibroid. The classic second chakra issues include relationship issues, not only with people but also with jobs, money, control, and the outside world. Creativity issues may also be expressed here. Abuse issues may come up also and can be related to physical, emotional, or sexual abuse. The idea is to remove these blockages to the healthy flow of energy from the pelvis, where they are creating stagnation and the growth of the fibroid. The release of these issues can be ritualized by having the patient journal everything that comes up and then put the pages into a bowl and burn them—letting them go.

Acupuncture and Deep Pelvic Massage

Acupuncture and deep pelvic massage (Mayan massage is one technique) are other ways of moving or restoring pelvic energy. These modalities are all complementary with the other approaches presented here.

Homeopathy

The following homeopathic remedies can be quite effective in reducing symptoms, as specified:

- Aurum muriaticum: to reduce size of fibroids
- Belladonna: for heavy, red bleeding
- Hydrastinum muriaticum: for large anterior wall fibroids with bladder symptoms
- Ignatia: for grief associated with fibroids
- Medorrhinum 200 C: fibroid: for benign tumors
- Phosphorus 6 C, 200 C: for bright red bleeding with no clots
- Sabina: for bright red bleeding with clots and for severe cramps
- Secale: for almost black blood and for profuse bleeding
- Sepia: for pressure and anger
- Silicea 6 C: for heavy bleeding; for cold, thin, and fatigued patients
- Thlaspi bursa pastoris 6 C (shepherd's purse): for frequent, heavy dark bleeding

See Chapter 111, Therapeutic Homeopathy.

PREVENTION PRESCRIPTION

- ■ Consume a hormone-balancing, vegetarian-style, low–saturated fat diet, including soy, green tea, ground flaxseed, omega-3 fatty acid, and cruciferous vegetables.
- ■ Follow a moderate-exercise program (4 to 5 hours/week).
- ■ Reduce xenobiotic (hormone-like) exposures such as pesticides, atrazine (herbicide), and polycyclic aromatic hydrocarbons (found in diesel exhaust), and avoid petroleum-based cosmetics.
- ■ Maintain an appropriate weight.
- ■ Practice stress modification techniques.
- ■ Take a high-potency multivitamin and multimineral supplement.
- ■ Foster healthy digestion and elimination.
- ■ Maintain healthy relationships and have a sense of purpose in life.

THERAPEUTIC REVIEW

This integrative, holistic approach to healing fibroid tumors of the uterus can help avoid some of the more invasive therapies offered. It is very effective in reducing the symptoms associated with these benign tumors. I initially ask patients to commit to a 3-month trial period, during which they will do as much of the program as possible.

At the end of these first 3 months, we assess symptoms, such as menorrhagia and dysmenorrhea, and any growth or shrinkage of the fibroids. The program is considered successful if the patient perceives a reduction in symptoms and no further fibroid growth has occurred. We then continue the program for 3-month periods while continuing to monitor symptoms and uterine size. If at any time symptoms recur or worsen or the fibroids begin to grow, other more aggressive measures must be considered, including surgery.

Lifestyle

- Maintain an appropriate weight.
- Avoid xenoestrogens (dioxins, polychlorinated biphenyls) by eating organic foods.
- Obtain regular aerobic exercise.

Nutrition

- Follow a hormone-balancing diet. The patient should consume a diet that reduces inflammation, acidity, and hormone, pesticide, and antibiotic residues; these foods may encourage the growth of fibroids. High–glycemic index foods similarly should be avoided because of their effects on insulin and sex hormones. Gluten grains also increase estrogens through action of the phase 1 cytochrome P-450 enzyme 3A4 and must be limited. The patient should add foods that will be hormone balancing, such as soy and flaxseed. She should approximate the Asian diet, with 30 to 70 mg/day of isoflavones and 2 tablespoons of ground flaxseed per day. Omega-3 fatty acids, found in foods such as wild Pacific salmon and sardines, should be consumed at approximately 2 to 4 g/day and are also antiinflammatory.
- Reduce intake of saturated fats and trans fatty acids (red meat, dairy, fried foods)
- Increase intake of omega-3 fatty acids (vegetables, nuts, flaxseed, cold-water fish)
- Eat a low–glycemic index diet.
- Avoid gluten as much as possible and completely if gluten sensitive.
- Eat cruciferous vegetables (broccoli, cabbage, cauliflower, Brussels sprouts).
- Drink 3 cups of green tea daily.

Gut and Detoxification Restoration

- The clinician should restore hormone balance and remove sources of inflammation by looking for and healing intestinal dysbiosis and supporting liver detoxification.
- Search for and treat hidden sources of gut dysbiosis, such as heavy metal overload, parasites, and food sensitivities.

Supplements

Add nutrients to support hormone metabolism:

- B-50 complex vitamin daily.
- Magnesium salts are taken at 400 to 600 mg/day.
- Maintain vitamin D₃ levels in the range of 40 to 100 ng/mL.
- Support normal levels of vitamin A to reduce menorrhagia.
- Citrus bioflavonoids, 1000 mg once or twice/day, can also reduce menorrhagia.
- Zinc needs to be at optimal level; consider supplementing if low.
- Indole-3-carbinol or diindolylmethane are taken at 200 to 800 mg/day to reduce estrogen dominance.
- Calcium D glucarate is taken at 500 mg twice/day to reduce increased enterohepatic recirculation of estrogens.

Hormones

- Natural progesterone cream 3% can help restore hormone balance. Use ¼ teaspoon twice/day from day 14 to day 28 of the cycle. If this is not enough, increase to 10% cream, add progesterone as a vaginal suppository, or place a progesterone-containing intrauterine device (IUD). Submucous fibroids may preclude the use of an IUD.
- Insufficiencies in adrenal or thyroid hormones can and have been shown to increase symptoms related to fibroids. Assess and treat low thyroid levels and adrenal insufficiency.
- DHEA has important implications related to the immune system, sugar metabolism, and stress modification. If the DHEA level is low, add 5 to 20 mg of DHEA/day. Watch for conversion to estrogens.

Botanicals

- Add botanicals to reduce heavy bleeding:
  - Red raspberry leaf and yarrow are used for 2 weeks before the period at 30 drops each; once the period starts, add 30 drops of shepherd's purse.
  - Botanicals to support lymphatic drainage from the pelvis are also added. These consist of Gaia herbal combinations such as Scudder's alterative and Echinacea/Red Root formulas. They are taken twice/day at 30 drops each.

Continued

- antiangiogenesis factors such as Convolvulus and green tea extract may reduce blood flow to the fibroids.

- To reduce inflammation, add antiinflammatory systemic enzymes (Wobenzyme, Vitalzyme, Neprinol) up to 15 tablets/day in divided doses taken on an empty stomach.

■ Mind-Body Therapies

- Meditation and visualization exercises using castor oil packs help restore health to the pelvic organs by allowing for the free flow of energy in the second chakra through the corresponding meridians. These activities also help identify stored emotional issues in these energy areas of the body and their impact on the fibroid.

■ Conventional Therapies

- Should the less invasive and more natural approaches fail to reduce the symptoms or growth of the fibroid, one can resort to the time-tested, more invasive conventional approaches. These powerful tools should be considered when necessary. The integrative holistic approach can still be used to help prevent any further growth of fibroids after the conventional treatment is performed.

- Surgery (hysterectomy)

- Strong pharmaceuticals: Leuprolide acetate (Lupron), 3.75 mg intramuscularly once a month for up to 6 months

- Interventional radiographic procedures

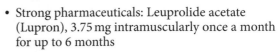
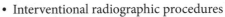

KEY WEB RESOURCES

Genova Diagnostics: www.gdx.net Gaia Herb: www.gaiaherbs.com Herbpharm: www.herb-pharm.com	Source for the Comprehensive Digestive Stool Analysis used to diagnose intestinal dysbiosis
Metametrix Clinical Laboratory: www.metametrix.com	Source for the Organix test of protein digestion
Doctor's Data: www.doctorsdata.com	Source for essential and toxic elemental testing. Source for standardized herbal tinctures

---

References

References are available online at expertconsult.com.

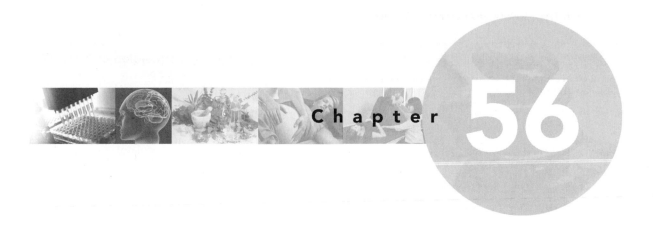

Chapter 56

Vaginal Dryness

Myrtle Wilhite, MD

Pathophysiology and Epidemiology

Vaginal dryness is defined as a reduction in lubrication of the luminal surface of the female vagina. It can occur at any age.

- Dryness alone may cause discomfort; other symptoms may include itch or dyspareunia. See Table 56-1 for risk factors.

- Often, a change in serum estrogen levels is a precipitating factor in vaginal dryness, as can happen with the use of oral contraceptives or loss or blockade of ovarian estrogen production.

- Vaginal dryness prevalence ranges from 13% to 31%,[1] although rates are significantly higher for postmenopausal women (50%),[2] as well as in women treated for breast cancer (63%).[3]

- Vaginal atrophy (also known as atrophic vaginitis or urogenital atrophy) is an inflammation of the vagina (and the outer urinary tract) associated with thinning and shrinking of the tissues, as well as decreased lubrication. The prevalence of vaginal atrophy in postmenopausal women is 43% in the United States, but it varies by nation.[4]

  Vaginal dryness can be further classified as *simple* or *complex.*

- Simple vaginal dryness suggests that the vagina and neurovasculature are healthy and functional, and resolution of the dryness solves the problem.

- Complex vaginal dryness indicates multiple factors, and the additional components often interfere with therapeutic resolution of the condition. Complex issues such as diabetes, hypertension, vaginal atrophy, or high-tone pelvic floor dysfunction may complicate therapy. Vaginal stenosis or inflexible pelvic floor muscles may prevent internal massage of the vagina and must be addressed before remediation of vaginal dryness can progress.

Physiology of Vaginal Lubrication

Vaginal lubrication consists of ultrafiltered blood, and thus is reliant on healthy blood flow.

- The vagina contains no glands.

- Blood pressure pushes fluid from the capillaries through intercellular gap junctions between vaginal epithelial cells.[5] The resultant vaginal transudate is mainly composed of water and very small proteins that combine at the vaginal surface with dead epithelial cells.

- Sufficient pelvic blood flow depends on the bioavailability of nitric oxide (NO). Gaseous NO is produced in capillary endothelia in response to shear stress or in response to sexual arousal through parasympathetic nitrergic nerves.[6] Once produced, NO induces vasodilation through a cyclic guanosine monophosphate cascade, which diminishes as phosphodiesterase enzymes break down the cascade.

- Therefore, vaginal lubrication production depends on the synthesis, enzymatic facilitation, and bioavailability of NO (Box 56-1). The enzymatic function of NO synthase is enhanced by steroid hormones, most notably estrogen in a rapid-action nongenomic effect.[7]

- The presence of NO is not sufficient for its effect. Many biologic feedback mechanisms suppress the production of NO, because high production of NO in an inflammatory environment can lead to irreversible free radical production.[8] Metabolic conditions of low inflammation support the bioavailability of NO in facilitating vaginal lubrication.

> The vagina's lubrication comes not from glands but from a transudative fluid expressed through vaginal epithelial cells. Transudation requires adequate perfusion and nitric oxide.

TABLE 56-1. Risk Factors for Vaginal Dryness

Reduced Estrogen Availability	Postpartum status, breast-feeding Menopausal transition Premature ovarian failure Oophorectomy Pelvic radiotherapy
Other Medical Conditions	Untreated hypertension Diabetes (types 1 and 2), metabolic syndrome Pituitary disorders Neuropathies, especially autonomic neuropathy Dermatoses (psoriasis, lichen sclerosis, Sjögren syndrome)
Prescription Medications	Antihistamines and decongestants Antidepressants (SSRIs, atypical, TCAs) Antiestrogen therapy for chemoprophylaxis Antiestrogen therapy for endometriosis or fibroids Chemotherapy Diuretics Progesterone predominant oral contraceptives
Unwise Behaviors	Dehydration, including alcohol use Use of douches, extremely hot baths, or strong detergents and dehydrating soaps Use of highly absorptive tampons Use of male condoms with insufficient external lubricant Lack of sufficient arousal before vaginal penetration Smoking

SSRIs, selective serotonin reuptake inhibitors; TCAs, tricyclic antidepressants.

BOX 56-1. Manipulation of Nitric Oxide Function

Production of Nitric Oxide
Sufficient L-arginine from Mediterranean diet
   Nuts (peanuts, almonds, walnuts, hazelnuts)
   Fruits (berries, chocolate)
   Beans
   Some meats (fish, chicken)
   Some seeds (sunflower, flaxseed)
Sufficient dietary calcium

Facilitation of the Activity of Nitric Oxide Synthase
Hormones
   Estrogen: rapid nongenomic effect
   Estrogen, soy phytoestrogens, testosterone: genomic effect
Medications and supplements
   Niacin (recouples nitric oxide synthase)
   Angiotensin converting-enzyme inhibitors
   Angiotensin II receptor blockers
   Ginseng
Other
   Presence of high-density lipoprotein
   Reduction of hyperglycemia

Prolonged Activity of Nitric Oxide and Cyclic Guanosine Monophosphate
Phosphodiesterase-5 inhibitors (sildenafil, tadalafil, vardenafil)

Bioactivity of Nitric Oxide
Medications/supplements
   Aspirin
   Vitamin D (decreases inducible nitric oxide synthase)
   Ginkgo (decreases inducible nitric oxide synthase and nitric oxide scavenger)
   Red wine, plant polyphenols and flavanoids

Other
Routine moderate exercise

Pathophysiology of Vaginal Epithelium

Mature vaginal epithelial cells produce and store glycogen, which is released during normal cell death and provides nutritional support for *Lactobacillus* species. *Lactobacillus* uniquely releases hydrogen peroxide during metabolism and thereby acidifies the luminal vaginal pH. The vaginal maturation index[9] correlates strongly with noninfected, noninflamed vaginal pH, and both values can be used to assess the health of vaginal tissue.

Changes in the tissue and function of the vagina during the menopausal transition (perimenopause) are highly influenced by declining levels of sex hormones. Waning estrogen levels cause decreased cellular maturation (vaginal maturation index decreases; pH increases), decreased mitotic activity of the basement membrane (reduced cellular renewal), decreased collagen synthesis (weaker dermal structure), and thickened dermoepidermal junctions (making it more difficult for capillary fluid to move through to the surface).[11] All these factors lead to a dry, immature, weakened cellular structure, which is more susceptible to friction damage and decreased repair capacity.

Antiestrogen therapy can lead to moderate to severe vaginal atrophy.[12] Selective estrogen receptor modulators, such as tamoxifen, increase mucin production and maturity of vaginal epithelium[13] while simultaneously reducing blood flow to vaginal tissues in experimental models.[14] Aromatase inhibitors cause severe vaginal dryness resulting from estrogen production suppression.[15]

Integrative Therapy

Topical Vaginal Lubricants

Topical lubricants are inexpensive, easy to use, and highly effective for addressing vaginal dryness.[16] Although all sexual lubricants should reduce friction, some lubricants also increase the *moisture* content of the vaginal surface, whereas others excel at *sealing* the surface effectively and thus holding moisture in place. A successful outcome lies in knowing how to choose the right lubricant, and experimentation is highly encouraged because the specific needs of an individual may not be easily ascertained without home trials. Both the chemical properties and the comfort in use determine the degree of client acceptance and long-term compliance.

TABLE 56-2. Features of Commercially Available Lubricants

PRODUCT	BASE	pH	MOISTURE	SEALS	THICK/THIN	COMMENTS
Astroglide	Water	6.5	No	No	Thin	Glycerin/high osmolality
Astroglide X	Silicone	N/A	No	Yes	Thin	
Carrageenan	Water	4.4	Yes	No	Thick	Normal osmolality
KY Intrigue	Silicone	4.4	No	Yes	Thin	
KY Silk-E	Water	3.8	Yes	Yes	Thin	Aloe
Liquid Silk	Water and silicone	5.2	Yes	Yes	Thin	Medium to high osmolality
Maximus	Water and silicone	5.0	Yes	Yes	Thick	High osmolality
Pre~	Water	7.0	Yes	No	Thin	Normal osmolality
Pink (aka Gun Oil)	Silicone	4.6	Yes	Yes	Thick	Aloe
Replens	Petroleum oil	2.8	Yes	Yes	Thick	Medium to high osmolality
Sliquid Organics Silk	Water and silicone	6.5	Yes	Yes	Thin	Aloe
Surgilube	Water	N/A	No	No	Thick	Glycerin/high osmolality

N/A, not available.

Base ingredients determine function and acceptability of genital lubricants. The two main base ingredients are water or polymers (silicone or oil). In general, the most effective lubricants have the following properties:

1. They incorporate both moisturizing and moisture-sealing qualities.
2. They have a pH compatible with vaginal pH (4.4-6.5).
3. They do not have allergenic or contact irritant components.
4. They meet the physical slip and cushion needs of the user.

Water-based lubricants: Water-based lubricants tend to be the most moisturizing; however, some are formulated at such high osmolality that they actually dehydrate the skin after use. Examples of lubricants that increase skin dehydration include Astroglide17, Surgilube, and KY Jelly.

- Ingredients are often added to increase slip or cushion. Examples include: glycerin, hydroxymethylcellulose, and propylene glycol. Glycols, glycerin, and cellulose are digestible by vaginal bacteria (primarily *Lactobacillus*) and may lead to unwanted bacterial or yeast overgrowth.

Polymer-based lubricants: Silicone-based (inorganic polymers) and oil-based (organic polymers) lubricants have the capacity to seal in moisture, but they are much more difficult to remove from skin. In addition, they can cause falls if they are spilled on tile or smooth surfaces, and they may stain fabrics.

- The type of oil matters. Petroleum-based (aliphatic) oils are strong solvents, highly effective at dissolving latex (an elastic hydrocarbon polymer of *cis*-1,4-polyisoprene), and are not easily cleared from the vaginal lumen. Oils composed of fatty acids (olive, avocado, and coconut) are relatively weak bipolar solvents and do not appear to degrade latex products.[18] However, olive oil goes rancid easily, avocado may stain sheets a green tint, and coconut is difficult to clear over time from the intravaginal lumen.

Preservatives deserve special mention.

- Preservatives are compounds that inhibit or kill unwanted contaminants in solutions. They can be classified into four main categories: detergents (nonoxynol 9, phenoxyethanol), oxidants, chelating (parabens) and metabolic inhibitors (quaternary ammoniums, and organomercurials).

- No perfect preservative for vaginal use exists. Some detergents (nonoxynol 9) have been shown to increase human immunodeficiency virus transmission,[19] whereas others are known to be mild to severe contact allergens (parabens, phenoxyethanol, quaternium compounds).

- Of the available preservatives, methylparaben (which acts as a chelating agent useful against molds and yeasts) has the lowest toxicity. Although parabens are very weakly estrogenic (1000 times less effective at binding estrogen receptors than estrogen),[20] the use of methylparaben has far less impact than using other more harmful preservatives or topical hormonal (estrodiol or estriol) options.

No topical botanical formulation has met utility criteria for vaginal application. Because of the possibility for contact dermatitis, no topical herbal or botanical extract can be recommended at this time.

Table 56-2 gives relevant properties of commonly available sexual lubricants. Although no one lubricant will meet the needs of every person or couple, suggested over-the-counter lubricants with different properties are listed below. Formulations and availability change quickly, however, so check for availability locally or on the Internet.

Liquid Silk Lubricant

Liquid Silk has both moisturizing (water-based) and moisture-sealing (dimethicone) features without glycerin or aloe. It is available in 10-mL sample packets, the pH is 5.2, and it is comfortable for most premenopausal and postmenopausal women.

Dosage

Massage Liquid Silk into the vulva and vagina as needed or after a shower or bath, up to three times daily. Press-release (rather than stroke) is used when skin is fragile or easily torn. This agent is very useful for vulvar dermatoses such as lichen sclerosis and psoriasis.

Precautions

Nonglycerin Liquid Silk is formulated with propylene glycol and parabens, both of which can be skin irritants. Paraben levels are lower in this European product than in U.S. formulations.

Pink Silicone Lubricant

Pink Silicone Lubricant is a combination product, but contains more silicone proportionally than the aloe and water base. It is more useful as a moisture sealer than as a moisturizer, adding cushion during sexual intimacy for premenopausal or postmenopausal women. The pH is 4.5, and it is available in 5-mL sample packets.

Dosage

Pink is more useful than water-based lubricants for reducing friction during vaginal penetration. Some couples massage this onto the partner before penetration.

Precautions

Pink contains aloe, which can cause dermatitis. The pH is fairly acidic, and some women report a burning sensation.

Sliquid Organic Silk Lubricant

Sliquid Organic Silk is a combination product that incorporates a water base with silicone (dimethicone) without glycerin. It is preserved with phenoxyethanol. This partly organic formulation is available in 5-mL sample packets. The pH is 6.5, which is comfortable for some women but irritatingly high for others.

Dosage

This agent is massaged into the vulva and vagina as needed, up to three times daily. Press-release (rather than stroke) when skin is fragile or easily torn.

Precautions

This agent contains aloe, which can cause dermatitis.

Vaginal Renewal Program

Regular vaginal penetration through sexual activity has been associated with enhanced sexual function in postmenopausal women.[21] However, some women lose sexual function rapidly, and experience sudden-onset dyspareunia, which prohibits sexual activity. The Vaginal Renewal (VR) program helps women recondition the health and flexibility of the skin of the vulva and vagina by reducing friction tearing of vulvar skin, as well as increasing blood flow to the vulva and vaginal canal. VR is indicated for women just beginning to feel the effects of hormonal changes, women who have completed pelvic radiation therapy,[22] and women with vaginal atrophy who experience skin tearing and pain when they attempt vaginal penetration.

Dilation is not the goal; blood flow is. During the development of the VR program, we found that vibrating wands were more effective in improving function than static (nonvibrating) dilators. Hard plastic vibrating wands caused less tissue trauma than dilators with soft, textured, or adhesive surfaces tore fragile vaginal epithelium too easily.

VR is completely compatible with topical estrogen therapies, and the combination can be more effective and faster-acting than estrogen or VR alone. Many women experience enough improvement from the combination of estrogen therapy and VR that they are able to discontinue the use of estrogen completely. The VR program does not require the use of estrogen, however, and is preferred by clients and clinicians when topical estrogen is contraindicated.

Precaution

Because comfortable penetration depends on the flexibility of both the skin and the pelvic floor muscles, some women recondition their vaginal skin only to experience uncomfortable or painful penetration because their pelvic floor muscles are inflexible. Referral to a pelvic floor physical therapist is indicated before continuing VR, and no further vaginal penetration should be attempted until a pelvic floor muscle evaluation is completed. VR is contraindicated for persons with vaginismus or an aversion to touching their own genitals.

Specific Situations

Vaginal Dryness Causing Daily Discomfort

1. Choose a moisturizing lubricant, and place it by toilet or use after shower.
2. Dispense a nickel- to quarter-sized amount on the fingers.
3. Use a press-release motion over the entire vulva. Apply additional lubricant as needed if it soaks into skin.
4. Dispense another nickel- to quarter-sized amount on the fingers.
5. Use a press-release motion and a rolling motion and apply to the inner labia, introitus, and perineum.
6. Repeat one or twice daily as needed.
7. If dryness is felt internally, insert 1 mL lubricant using a vaginal applicator at night.

Rehabilitation of Vaginal Dryness With Atrophy

1. Follow the instructions for daily moisturizing.
2. In the clinic, help the client choose an appropriately sized vibrating wand.
   a. The diameter of wand is the most important criterion; choose one that can be inserted comfortably at pelvic examination. A smaller diameter is always better. The client can graduate to a larger size when a finger can be placed beside the wand comfortably during vaginal penetration.
   b. Low-Hertz vibration is more effective than high-Hertz vibration.
3. Instruct the client to do the following:
   a. At home, lubricate the wand.
   b. Turn on the massage wand.
   c. In a reclining position, insert the wand into the vagina to the deepest comfortable depth.
   d. Lie back and let the wand vibrate for 5 to 10 minutes.
   e. Remove the wand and clean with soap and water.
   f. Repeat daily to three times weekly, as needed.

■ Dryness-Related Dyspareunia

1. Follow the earlier instructions for moisturizing and rehabilitation. Only proceed with sexual intimacy when no pain or discomfort is felt with largest massage wand size.
2. Lubricate penetration object (penis, fingers, glass or steel dildo) with a silicone-based lubricant before penetration.
3. If the penetration object is made of silicone, cover the object with a nonlubricated condom, and apply silicone lubricant to the outside of the condom.

Other Behaviors

Smoking Cessation

Smoking causes functional changes in endothelial health that enhance oxidative stresses.[23] Because smoking is a known risk factor for vaginal dryness,[24] smoking cessation strategies should be pursued as a part of a comprehensive strategy.

Habitual Physical Exercise

Exercise is an effective way to combat vascular aging and enhance the function of small vessel blood flow,[25] including vaginal perfusion.[26] Aerobic exercise positively affects NO (Fig. 56-1),[27] and it is linked to improved endothelial and cardiovascular health.[28]

■ Dosage

Walk once per day, for 30 to 60 minutes to the level of a gentle sweat. Walking before anticipated sexual activity improves vaginal lubrication as well as subjective symptoms of arousal[29] (see Chapter 88, Writing an Exercise Prescription).

■ Precautions

Vigorous exercise is not indicated, but exercising to the level of a gentle sweat is sufficient. Walking is ideal.

Nutrition

Dietary reduction in inflammation assists NO-dependent blood flow. For example, despite the increased incidence of sexual dysfunction in women with diabetes,[30] adherence to a Mediterranean diet is associated with a lower prevalence of sexual dysfunction in this patient population.[31]

Mediterranean Diet

A low-glycemic, low-carbohydrate, Mediterranean diet positively manipulates endothelial health and NO bioavailability. Increasing NO bioavailability *before* NO production is beneficial because increasing NO in the presence of inflammatory or oxidized conditions worsens NO bioavailability and damages endothelia directly.

- First, focus consumption on initially increasing both lipid-based and water-based antioxidants, and reduce high-glycemic index foods that spike blood glucose levels and increase insulin resistance (see Chapter 85, The Glycemic Index/Load).

- Second, increase food consumption that targets protein levels of L-arginine (see Box 56-1). Fortunately, these foods are beneficial to satiety, and many incorporate both antioxidants and L-arginine simultaneously.

- Finally, consider whether soy phytoestrogens may be of benefit. Experimentally, fermented soy may also function as a free radical scavenger.[32]

■ Dosage

Adhere strictly to a Mediterranean diet, with small meal portions and between-meal grazing on nuts and dried berries or cherries (see Chapter 86, The Antiinflammatory Diet).

■ Precautions

Soy consumption (90 mg isoflavone/day) has shown positive effects on vaginal dryness,[33] but safety is in question,[34] particularly for Western populations.[35]

FIGURE 56-1

Nitric oxide interventions. ACE-I, angiotensin-converting enzyme inhibitor; ARB, angiotensin II receptor blocker; eNOS, endothelial nitric oxide synthase; iNOS, inducible nitric oxide synthase; nNOS, neuronal nitric oxide synthase; PDE5, phosphodiesterase-5.

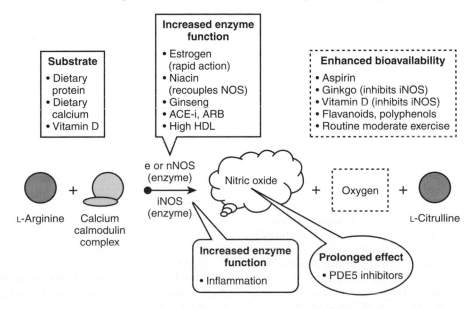

Supplements

Vitamin D₃

Vitamin D_3 plays an important role in assisting dietary calcium, manipulating calcium at neural membranes, and in formation of the calmodulin cofactor required for NO production. Vitamin D also independently acts as a free radical scavenger, so increases the bioavailability of NO after production.

◼ Dosage

The initial dose is vitamin D_3, 2000 units orally per day. It is taken with fish oil and calcium citrate. After 1 month, check blood levels of 25(OH)D, and aim for a serum level of 50 ng/mL. For women with more pronounced menopausal symptoms, aim for a serum level of 60 ng/mL.

◼ Precautions

Calcium metabolism and kidney disorders, as well as some inflammatory disorders (sarcoidosis, tuberculosis), are worsened with vitamin D therapy.

Fish Oil (Highly Purified Omega-3 Fatty Acid)

Omega-3 fatty acids assist in the absorption of vitamin D and act as lipid-based antioxidants helping neural function.

◼ Dosage

The dose is 2 to 4 g orally per day. It is taken with vitamin D and calcium. It may be stored in the freezer to reduce "fish burps."

◼ Precautions

Fish oil and omega-3 fatty acids act as anticoagulants, so the dosage must be modified in women taking heparin, warfarin (Coumadin), selective serotonin reuptake inhibitors, aspirin, ginkgo, high-dose garlic, or other potentially blood-thinning regimens.

◼ Calcium Citrate

Sufficient extracellular calcium is required for NO production.

◼ Dosage

The dose is 250 mg orally per day. It is taken with vitamin D and fish oil.

◼ Precautions

Adherence to the Mediterranean diet provides the remainder of calcium needed for vitamin D to use. However, high-dose calcium supplementation (more than 1000 mg/day) is associated with adverse effects,[36] and it is not recommended. Calcium carbonate is not easily absorbable.

Niacin

Reversal of endothelial dysfunction is well addressed with niacin therapy.[37]

◼ Dosage

The dose is 1000 mg two to three times per day.

◼ Precautions

Warn about a flushing reaction. A prolonged incremental increase beginning at 100 mg/day is most successful. Initially, niacin may exacerbate vulvar dermatoses because recoupling of NO production temporarily enhances inflammation.[38]

L-Arginine (as Supplement)

This acts as the protein substrate for NO production.

◼ Dosage

The dose is 500 to 1000 mg daily.

◼ Precautions

Dietary supplementation is more strongly suggested than direct supplementation. L-Arginine may cause hyperglycemia, hypotension, and nausea. It is contraindicated in kidney disease. High serum levels of L-arginine and L-citrulline (byproduct) also act as feedback inhibitors of NO production.

Botanicals

Ginkgo (Ginkgo biloba)

Ginkgo acts on nitric oxide vasodilation in several different ways.[39] It modulates NO second messenger action, scavenges excess NO, inhibits NO production under inflammatory conditions, and inhibits platelet activation.

◼ Dosage

The dose of *Ginkgo biloba* extract 50:1 is 60 mg twice daily. The dose may be increased to 120 mg twice daily.

◼ Precautions

Use ginkgo cautiously with anticoagulants, nonsteroidal antiinflammatory drugs, including aspirin, or high dietary intake of garlic.

Ginseng (Panax ginseng)

Ginseng facilitates endothelial NO release and is a potent antioxidant.

◼ Dosage

The dose is 1 to 2 g root tea infusion three times daily.

◼ Precautions

Ginseng has potential phytoestrogenic activity.[40] It may cause agitation and insomnia.

Not Recommended

Attempts to reverse vaginal dryness with oral black cohosh[41] and topical genistein[42] have been unsuccessful. Damiana (*Turnera diffusa*) blocks progesterone receptors without receptor activation but may boost unopposed estrogen activity.[43]

Pharmaceuticals

Estriol

A 2-week regimen of vaginal daily estriol cream improves vaginal dryness,[44] and it may be indicated as initial therapy in severe cases of vaginal atrophy.[45]

◼ Dosage

The dose of estriol cream is 1 mg intravaginally per day for 2 weeks. It is tapered to three times per week for 2 months, then discontinued. Concurrent use of the VR program may allow earlier taper and prevent recurrence.

◼ Precautions

In breast cancer survivors taking aromatase inhibitors, estriol causes measurable systemic changes suggestive of an estrogen effect.[46]

Estriol is the main estrogen of pregnancy that helps prepare the vagina for delivery. However, estriol does stimulate breast cell proliferation (although less than estradiol) and should be used only as very short-term therapy in cases of severe dysfunction (see the earlier discussion of vaginal renewal for nonhormonal therapy).

Phosphodiesterase-5 Inhibitors

Physiologically, phosphodiesterase-5 inhibitors reduce insulin resistance in endothelial capillaries,[47] in addition to prolonging vasodilation. This produces a beneficial genital perfusion effect in women.[48]

Dosage

Phosphodiesterase-5 inhibitors can be utilized in two different ways. They can be used at a very low dose nightly to increase sleep-related genital perfusion.[49] Alternatively, they can be tried for on-demand sexual activity, taken 30-60 minutes prior to sexual activity. The dose is 12.5 to 100 mg daily. It may be taken at night to reduce symptoms of nausea or hypotension and assist sleep-related perfusion. The client should experiment to determine whether timing before sexual intimacy improves vaginal lubrication.[50]

Precautions

Sildenafil may cause nausea, headache, nasal congestion, renal or hepatic impairment, hypotension, change in vision, and ototoxicity. It is contraindicated with nitrates and $alpha_1$ blockers.

Not Recommended

Oral raloxifene is not recommended for vaginal dryness.[51]

Prevention Prescription

- Maintain regular exercise and movement to enhance blood perfusion to the perineum.
- Consume a Mediterranean diet that is rich in berry fruits, nuts, vegetables, and whole grains, and low in red meat and processed carbohydrates. Focus on foods with high L-arginine levels.
- Favor beverage choices of tea (black, green, red, or white), coffee, or water.
- Maintain therapeutic or sexual vaginal penetration (once a week) to stimulate vaginal lubrication and elasticity.
- Experiment to find a topical sexual lubricant that is comfortable and moisturizes the vulva and vagina.
- Check vitamin D levels and supplement to keep the level higher than 50 ng/mL.
- Take calcium citrate, 250 mg daily with vitamin D.
- Take 2 to 4 g daily of an omega-3 fish oil.
- Avoid tobacco products.

Therapeutic Review

Three main strategies are used for resolving vaginal dryness without hormones, and they are most effective when combined. The first two strategies use the Vaginal Renewal program.

- Use a client-matched topical lubricant (see Table 56-2).
- Use massage and vibration to create shear stress on the endothelial capillaries, thus increasing blood flow and vaginal lubrication.
- Holistically address diet and lifestyle issues that help facilitate the production and bioavailability of nitric oxide (NO; see Box 56-1 and Fig. 56-1).

Nutrition

- First, reduce overall metabolic inflammation with strict adherence to a Mediterranean diet with daily exercise. This approach enhances NO bioavailability and reduces the potential for increasing inflammatory free radical production.
- Then, focus the diet more specifically on foods high in L-arginine, and selectively strip high-glycemic foods from the diet. Address satiety with proteins.

Supplements

- Consider adding L-arginine, 500 mg daily, to enhance NO production.
- Calcium citrate: 250 mg daily,
- Vitamin D: 2000 units daily
- Omega-3 fish oil: 2 to 4 g daily

Botanicals

- *Ginkgo biloba* extract 50:1: 60 mg twice daily
- *Panax ginseng:* 1-2 g root tea infusion three times daily

Pharmaceuticals

- Use an angiotensin-converting enzyme inhibitor or angiotensin II receptor blocker for treatment of hypertension (instead of a beta blocker or diuretic).
- To increase high-density lipoprotein and recouple NO production, consider niacin, starting at a very low dose and gradually increasing to 1000 mg two to three times a day.
- Consider whether phosphodiesterase-5 inhibitors (sildenafil, 12.5 to 100 mg daily) may facilitate daily genital perfusion to increase genital blood flow and vaginal lubrication.
- For severe cases, have estriol cream compounded at 1 mg/g of cream, and apply to the vulva and intravaginally daily for 2 weeks. Then reduce to three times per week for 2 months and discontinue. Utilize the Vaginal Renewal program concurrently for faster recovery.

KEY WEB RESOURCES

Dietary Fiber Food: http://www.dietaryfiberfood.com/larginine-high.php	List of foods high in L-arginine
A Woman's Touch: http://www.sexualityresources.com	Information on the Vaginal Renewal program (Dr. Wilhite is an owner of this Web site and business.)
University of Michigan Healing Foods Pyramid: http://www.med.umich.edu/umim/food-pyramid/index.htm	Food pyramid of the Mediterranean Diet

References

References are available online at expertconsult.com.

Section X Urology

Benign Prostatic Hyperplasia

David Rakel, MD

Pathophysiology

Even though benign prostatic hyperplasia (BPH) is one of the most common diseases of aging men, its etiology remains relatively unknown. From our current understanding, BPH appears to be related to age, androgens (dihydrotestosterone [DHT]), estrogens, and detrusor dysfunction of the bladder neck. An accumulation of DHT inhibits prostatic cell death, promotes cell proliferation, and thus increases the size of the gland (Fig. 57-1).

As a man passes his fifth decade, serum testosterone levels decrease, and estrogen (as well as prolactin, luteinizing hormone, and follicle-stimulating hormone) levels rise. Estrogen increases the number of androgen (DHT) receptors in the prostate and inhibits androgen metabolism by interfering with hydroxylation. As urinary outflow obstruction develops, the detrusor muscles of the bladder try to compensate by increasing pressure to expel urine, a process that leads to instability of the muscle and worsening symptoms. In summary, factors that promote the accumulation of DHT and estrogens lead to symptoms of BPH and obstruction of the lower urinary tract that, in turn, cause detrusor muscle dysfunction. Stimulation of the alpha-adrenergic system leads to contraction of the smooth muscle fiber that further restricts flow in an enlarged prostate gland. Finally, reason exists to believe that prostaglandins, leukotrienes, and insulin resistance play roles in the inflammatory process of the prostate.

Components of the metabolic syndrome have been shown to cause prostatic enlargement.[1,2] Insulin resistance and truncal obesity appear to be the main culprits.[3] Elevated insulin levels increase sympathetic nerve activity and also bind to insulin-like growth factor (IGF) receptors that stimulate prostate cell growth.[4] Excessive amounts of visceral fat also increase the circulation of estradiol and further stimulate prostate cell growth by increasing DHT levels (Fig. 57-2). Obesity, metabolic syndrome, and insulin resistance also increase systemic inflammation, which is also correlated with the incidence of BPH.[5]

Light to moderate alcohol consumption has been associated with a protective effect on BPH and lower urinary tract symptoms. The association of light to moderate alcohol consumption with an improvement in insulin sensitivity[6] and a decrease in testosterone concentrations[7] may help explain the beneficial influence of alcohol. This positive effect is not seen in men with high alcohol consumption, however.[8] Consuming seven or more alcoholic drinks per week is associated with worsening symptoms.[9]

Integrative Therapy

Table 57-1 gives the mechanism of action of common pharmaceuticals, botanicals, and supplements used for BPH, and Table 57-2 gives information on botanicals and hormones that can worsen symptoms of BPH.

Nutrition

Soy

Soy is thought to work in two ways. It is an inhibitor of 5-alpha-reductase, and it is a low-potency estrogen. Soy may block the receptor sites that the stronger estrogens use to increase the accumulation of DHT. Consumption of nonfermented soy products (tofu, soy milk, edamame) has also been found to result in a decreased incidence of prostate cancer.[10,11]

Beta-sitosterol (a major phytosterol found in soy) was found to increase urinary flow and decrease residual volume in the bladder in a double-blind placebo-controlled study using a 20-mg dose.[12] A 3.5-oz serving of soybeans, tofu, or another soy food preparation provides approximately 90 mg of beta-sitosterol.[13] A 1-oz preparation (which is a portion approximately the size of the palm of the hand) equals approximately 25 mg.

Cholesterol

Cholesterol has been associated not only with BPH but also with prostate cancer. Cholesterol metabolites (epoxycholesterols) have been found to accumulate in the hyperplastic

FIGURE 57-1
Inhibitors of aromatase, 5-alpha-reductase, and hydroxylation. BPH, benign prostatic hyperplasia; DHT, dihydrotestosterone.

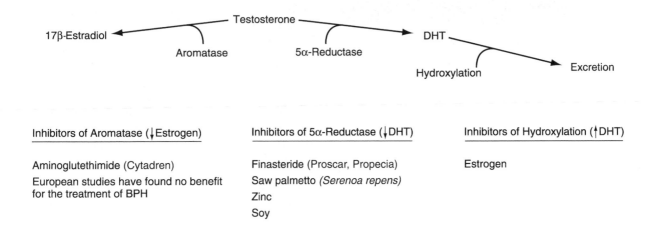

Inhibitors of Aromatase (↓Estrogen)

Aminoglutethimide (Cytadren)
European studies have found no benefit
for the treatment of BPH

Inhibitors of 5α-Reductase (↓DHT)

Finasteride (Proscar, Propecia)
Saw palmetto (Serenoa repens)
Zinc
Soy

Inhibitors of Hydroxylation (↑DHT)

Estrogen

FIGURE 57-2
Influences affecting the promotion and prevention of benign prostatic hypertrophy (BPH) and lower urinary tract symptoms (LUTS). DHT, dihydrotestosterone; IGF, insulin-like growth factor.

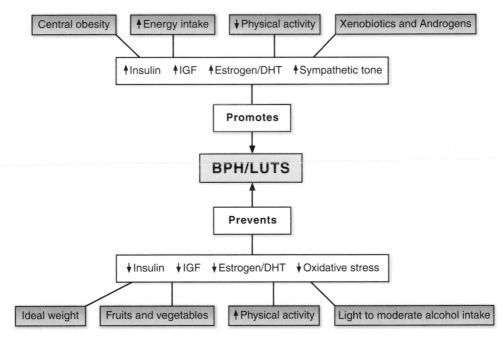

and cancerous prostate gland. For this reason, hypocholesterolemic drugs (3-hydroxy-3-methylglutaryl–coenzyme A reductase inhibitors or "statins") have been associated with a lower risk of BPH and prostate cancer.[14] In addition, treating the dyslipidemia of metabolic syndrome (high triglycerides, low high-density lipoprotein) with exercise and a low–glycemic index/load diet (see Chapter 85, The Glycemic Index/Load) may also prove beneficial because of the association of BPH with metabolic syndrome. Foods high in cholesterol and saturated fat are also rich in arachidonic acid, which is the main precursor of inflammation. Reducing consumption of these foods can benefit BPH by reducing inflammatory triggers.

Omega-3 Fatty Acids
A diet rich in omega-3 fatty acids helps reduce the influence of prostaglandins and leukotrienes on the inflammatory component of BPH (see Chapter 86, The Antiinflammatory Diet). Recommend foods rich in omega-3 fatty acids such as cold-water fish (salmon, mackerel, and sardines), vegetables, and ground flaxseed or flaxseed oil. Flaxseed oil can be taken in capsule form. Recommend lignan-rich flaxseed oil, two to four 500-mg capsules twice a day. Patients can also buy whole flaxseeds, grind 2 tablespoons (approximately 30 g) of the seeds, and sprinkle the ground flaxseed on salads or yogurt or add it to a smoothie. Flaxseed has the added benefit of lignan fiber, which helps bind estrogen in the gut and thus promotes estrogen removal.

TABLE 57-1. Mechanism of Action of Common Pharmaceuticals, Botanicals, and Supplements Used for Benign Prostatic Hyperplasia

MECHANISM OF ACTION	THERAPY
Alpha₁-Adrenergic Blockade	Alfuzosin (Uroxatral) Doxazosin (Cardura) Prazosin (Minipress) Tamsulosin (Flomax) Terazosin (Hytrin)
5-Alpha-Reductase Inhibition	Finasteride (Proscar) Dutasteride (Avodart) Saw palmetto (*Serenoa repens*)
Antiproliferative Action	African wild potato (*Hypoxis hemerocallidea*) Beta-Sitosterol Lycopene Pumpkin seed (*Cucurbita pepo*) Pygeum (*Prunus africana*) Red clover (*Trifolium pratense*) Soy Stinging nettle root (*Urtica dioica*)
Antiinflammatory Action	Rye grass pollen (*Secale cereale*) (Cernilton)

Modified from http://naturaldatabase.com.

TABLE 57-2. Products That Can Worsen Symptoms of Benign Prostatic Hyperplasia

MECHANISM OF ACTION	PRODUCT
Sympathetic stimulation: Increases tone of prostatic stroma, causes constriction of urethra, and can also stimulate bladder spasm	Bitter orange Ephedra Country mallow Yohimbe
Anticholinergic stimulation: Makes urination more difficult by inhibiting bladder contraction and causing urinary retention	Henbane Scopolia Jimson weed Wild lettuce
Hormonal stimulation: Accelerates growth of the prostate	Androstenediol Dehydroepiandrosterone (DHEA) Androstenedione Pregnenolone

Adapted from Lee M. Management of benign prostatic hyperplasia. In: *Pharmacotherapy: A Pathophysiological Approach.* 5th ed. New York: McGraw-Hill; 1999.

Supplements

Beta-Sitosterol

Beta-sitosterol is a sterol found in almost all plants. It is one of the main subcomponents of a group of plant sterols known as phytosterols that are very similar in composition to cholesterol. These plant sterols are the active ingredients in popular margarine spreads (Take Control, Benecol) used to lower cholesterol. Beta-sitosterol is found in rice bran, wheat germ, peanuts, corn oils, and soybeans. High levels are also found in botanicals such as saw palmetto, rye grass pollen, pygeum, and stinging nettles, which have been found to be beneficial for BPH. Unlike cholesterol, beta-sitosterol cannot be converted to testosterone. It is also inhibits aromatase and 5-alpha-reductase. Beta-sitosterol is likely one of the many reasons that eating vegetables is good for health. Encourage adequate consumption of these plants in the diet.

Two randomized studies showed a benefit of beta-sitosterol in treating BPH, with little potential harm.[15,16] This benefit persisted for up to 18 months of use.[17] A Cochrane Review found beta-sitosterol to improve urinary symptoms and flow measures. This supplement does not appear to reduce the size of the prostate gland.[18]

■ Dosage
The dose is 60 mg twice daily. This dose can be reduced to 30 mg twice daily after symptoms improve.

■ Precautions
Beta-sitosterol is well tolerated. Gastrointestinal side effects are the most common. This supplement can enhance the cholesterol-lowering effects of antihyperlipidemic medications.

Zinc

Intestinal uptake of zinc is inhibited by estrogen. Because estrogen levels increase in aging men, men with BPH may have low zinc levels. In fact, marginal zinc deficiency is common in older adults, and in men it may worsen the symptoms of BPH. In the 1970s, research showed that supplementing with zinc resulted in a reduction in the size of the prostate gland and in symptoms of BPH.[19] Further research showed that zinc inhibits 5-alpha-reductase,[20] and it also inhibits the binding of androgens to their receptors in the prostate.[21] This effect on androgens is thought to result from zinc's ability to inhibit prolactin, which, like estrogen, increases the receptors for DHT in the prostate. Therefore, zinc not only decreases the production of DHT, but it also inhibits DHT binding to its receptors.

Coffee can decrease zinc absorption by 50%. Because caffeine stimulates the adrenergic nervous system (smooth muscle of the prostate), encourage patients with BPH to limit their intake.

Prescription drugs that can result in low serum zinc levels include thiazide diuretics, steroids, methotrexate, tetracyclines, and fluoroquinolones. Consider zinc supplementation in those patients with BPH who are taking these medications. Do not give zinc to patients taking tetracycline or fluoroquinolone antibiotics, however, because zinc can affect the absorption of these drugs. Pumpkin seeds are a rich source of zinc, and this may explain their potential therapeutic benefit for BPH.

■ Dosage
The dose of zinc is 30 mg per day.

In prescribing zinc supplementation, be aware that zinc competes with copper, calcium, and iron absorption. Make sure that the patient does not take more than the recommended dose and does not take calcium and iron supplements with zinc.

Botanicals

Saw Palmetto (Serenoa repens)

Saw palmetto has been found to be a weak inhibitor of 5-alpha-reductase, but it may have a more active role in reducing the number of estrogen and androgen (DHT) receptors, as well as an antiinflammatory effect on the prostate. Saw palmetto inhibits fibroblast growth factor and epidermal growth factor and stimulates apoptosis, thus further slowing prostate cell proliferation. Its principal ingredient, the sterol beta-sitosterol, is also found in soy products (see earlier), as well as in other herbs used to treat diseases of the prostate including pygeum bark, stinging nettle root, and pumpkin seed extract.

Saw palmetto reduces the inner prostatic epithelium but does not reduce the size of the gland. Nonetheless, saw palmetto has been found to improve symptom scores, nocturia, residual urine volume, and urinary flow in patients with BPH. It does not affect prostate-specific antigen (PSA) levels.[22] In a large randomized study, saw palmetto was found to be as effective as finasteride (Proscar) but without the drug's side effects, and the International Prostate Symptom Score (IPSS) was reduced by 37%.[23] However, a more complete evaluation of 30 randomized trials by a 2009 Cochrane Review of 5222 subjects concluded that no significant difference existed between *Serenoa repens* (saw palmetto) and placebo for the treatment of urinary symptoms related to BPH.[24]

Although the evidence for BPH improvement is marginal, saw palmetto has three positive influences on the prostate gland: it is antiandrogenic, antiproliferative, and antiinflammatory.

■ Dosage

The dose is 160 mg twice daily. Allow 8 weeks before seeing therapeutic benefit.

■ Precautions

Mild adverse effects have included headache, nausea, diarrhea, and dizziness. Saw palmetto does not influence the cytochrome P-450 enzyme system of the liver, and drug interactions are rare.

> The most beneficial saw palmetto extract is composed of at least 85% fatty acids and 0.2% sterols. For example, a 160-mg pill should have a minimum of 136 mg fatty acids and 0.32 mg sterols.

Product lines that have been proven to be composed of at least 85% fatty acids and 0.2% sterols include the following: Nature's Way, CVS, Centrum, Natrol, Bayer, Quanterra, Sundown Herbals, NaturPharma (Walmart), and Walgreens.

Rye Grass Pollen (Secale cereale)

Rye grass pollen is also known as grass pollen and grass pollen extract. Clinical studies used a form called Cernilton (flower pollen), a brand manufactured by Cernitin. This has been bought by the company Graminex and is now marketed under the name of PollenAid.

This extract has been used in Europe for BPH since the 1970s. Double-blind clinical studies found it to be effective, with an overall response rate near 70%.[25] Rye grass contains a substance that has been found to inhibit prostatic cell growth[26] and reduce inflammation of the prostate by inhibiting prostaglandins and leukotrienes.[27]

Studies have shown the greatest improvement in nocturia, urinary frequency, and residual urine volume.[28] Rye grass and flower pollen are also used for symptomatic relief of prostatitis and prostatodynia.

■ Dosage

The typical dose of rye grass pollen is 126 mg three times daily. A standardized extract 20:1 of *Secale cereale* can be obtained through the following companies: Graminex PollenAid, 500 mg three times daily, or Pure Encapsulations ProstaFlo, 320 mg three to five capsules per day in divided doses.

■ Precautions

Abdominal distention, heartburn, and nausea may occur. This product is not likely to cause allergy because allergenic proteins are removed in the manufacturing process.

Pygeum africanum (synonym: Prunus africana)

Pygeum is obtained from the bark of the African plum tree. As with saw palmetto, its benefits are thought to come from fatty acids (sterols) that reduce inflammation through the inhibition of prostaglandins, as well as prostatic cholesterol levels that are precursors to testosterone production. Pygeum also increases prostatic and seminal fluid secretions.

A meta-analysis revealed that men taking pygeum had a 19% reduction in nocturia and a 24% reduction in residual urine volume. Peak urine flow was increased by 23%, and side effects were mild and similar to those reported with placebo.[29] The TRIUMPH study included treatment outcomes of BPH from six European countries. After 1 year of therapy, participants who received either *Pygeum africanum* or *Serenoa repens* (saw palmetto) showed a 43% improvement in IPSS scores and improvement in quality of life compared with no treatment.[30]

Pygeum is more expensive than saw palmetto, and overharvesting of the bark is threatening the survival of the species.

■ Dosage

The dose is 100 to 200 mg each day.

■ Precautions

Nausea and abdominal pain may occur.

Pharmaceuticals

Alpha-Adrenergic Blocking Agents

The TRIUMPH study mentioned earlier followed 2351 men with BPH.[30] After 1 year, those therapies that showed the most benefit in IPSS scores were, in descending order; alpha blockers (68%), finasteride (57%), and *Serenoa repens* or *Pygeum africanum* (43%) compared with watchful waiting. Of the therapies discussed, the alpha blockers are likely to give the most subjective improvement. Blocking the alpha-adrenergic system results in relaxation of the smooth muscle fibers of the prostate gland, with reduction of symptoms and improved urinary flow. The response is rapid (within hours), and studies have shown long-term efficacy.

The most commonly used drugs, terazosin (Hytrin) and doxazosin (Cardura), require dose titration to avoid postural hypotension. The newer and more expensive alpha$_1$-adrenergic antagonist tamsulosin (Flomax) is more specific for the prostatic tissue, thus reducing the incidence of hypotension and the need to titrate the dose.

Dosage
For terazosin (Hytrin), start at 1 mg nightly and titrate every week to effect, up to a maximum of 20 mg. Terazosin is available in 1-, 2-, 5-, and 10-mg formulations. For doxazosin (Cardura), start at 1 mg nightly and titrate every week to effect, up to a maximum of 8 mg. Doxazosin comes in 1-, 2-, 4-, and 8-mg formulations. The dose of tamsulosin (Flomax) is 0.4 mg 30 minutes after a meal every day, up to a maximum of 0.8 mg per day. Tamsulosin is available in a 0.4-mg formulation.

Precautions
Postural hypotension, dizziness, fatigue, headache, nasal stuffiness, and retrograde ejaculation may occur.

5-Alpha-Reductase Inhibition
Finasteride prevents the conversion of testosterone to DHT and lowers DHT serum levels. This drug can take as long as 6 months to work, but it appears to halt the progression of prostate growth. In terms of patient satisfaction and symptom reduction, finasteride is not a great drug unless the goal includes treatment of male-pattern baldness. Finasteride causes a 50% reduction of PSA.

Dosage
The dose of finasteride is 5 mg once a day, and it comes in 5-mg tablets. The dose of dutasteride is 0.5 mg once daily, and it is available in 0.5-mg tablets.

Precautions
Decreased ejaculatory volume (2.8%), impotence (3.7%), and decreased libido (3.3%) have been reported. These drugs can take up to 6 months to show benefit.

Surgery

When severe symptoms are not controlled with the previously discussed therapies, consider urologic referral for minimally invasive therapy or surgical resection, as follows:

- Transurethral microwave thermotherapy (TUMT) uses a microwave antenna that generates heat in the transition zone and results in coagulation necrosis. This procedure is performed on an outpatient basis.
- Transurethral needle ablation (TUNA) involves the placement of small needles in the prostate via cystoscopy that emit radiofrequency energy resulting in necrosis of prostatic tissue.

The minimally invasive procedures described here have decreased morbidity compared with transurethral resection of the prostate but are not as effective in reducing symptoms, and no tissue is obtained for pathologic evaluation.

- Transurethral resection of the prostate (TURP) is the gold standard and will likely result in the greatest symptomatic improvement (95% of patients have improved symptoms). Complications such as incontinence (1%), blood transfusion (3% to 5%), retrograde ejaculation (20% to 75%), and stricture formation (5%) are becoming less severe with the use of laser prostatectomy that reduces bleeding. TURP is the most invasive procedure (except for open prostatectomy) and requires a hospital stay.
- Transurethral incision of the prostate (TUIP) involves endoscopic placement of one to two incisions along the prostatic capsule to reduce urethral constriction. This procedure has been found to be effective (83% of patients have improved symptoms) and safe for men with smaller glands (smaller than 30 g) who may not need TURP.

PREVENTION PRESCRIPTION

- Avoid excessive amounts of saturated fat, such as those found in red meet, fried foods, and dairy.
- Replace vegetable oils with olive or canola oil for cooking.
- Consume omega-3–rich fats found in cold-water fish, nuts, greens, and ground flaxseed.
- Consider light to moderate (1 glass or less daily) alcohol consumption.
- Eat plenty of natural plants, particularly those rich in beta-sitosterol, such as green leafy vegetables, rice bran, wheat germ, peanuts, corn oils, nuts, and soybeans.
- Encourage soy-based foods such as soy milk, edamame, soy nuts, and tofu. Try to eat 1 to 2 oz per day, and consider substituting soy milk for dairy milk.
- Avoid dietary supplements or environmental exposures that may increase circulating hormone levels such as pesticides, herbicides, and recombinant bovine growth hormone (rBGH)-rich dairy products. Also avoid drugs that include dehydroepiandrosterone (DHEA), androstenedione, testosterone, and human growth hormone.
- Maintain appropriate weight, and perform regular aerobic exercise.
- Treat metabolic syndrome with exercise, weight loss, and a low–glycemic index/load diet to reduce inflammation of the prostate (see Chapter 85, The Glycemic Index/Load, and Chapter 31, Insulin Resistance and the Metabolic Syndrome).

THERAPEUTIC REVIEW

This is a summary of therapeutic options for benign prostatic hyperplasia (BPH). A patient presenting with severe symptoms (BPH Symptom Index Score or International Prostate Symptom Score [IPSS] greater than 19) will benefit by jumping ahead to a more aggressive therapy such as alpha blockers or referral to a surgeon. For the patient who has mild to moderate symptoms, however, this ladder approach is appropriate (see Tables 57–1 and 57–2).

■ Removal of Exacerbating Factors

- Ask the patient to stop taking over-the-counter cold remedies or diet aids (phenylpropanolamine [PPA]), nasal decongestants (pseudoephedrine), herbs (ma huang, Ephedra), or caffeinated products that contain sympathomimetics, which increase prostatic muscle tone.

- Consider asking the patient to stop taking pharmaceutical products that have anticholinergic effects leading to urinary retention. These agents include antihistamines, bowel antispasmodics, bladder antispasmodics, tricyclic antidepressants, and antipsychotics.

■ Nutrition

- Increase soy-rich foods in diet. A 1-oz serving each day (approximately the size of the palm of the hand) provides approximately 25 mg.

- Encourage a low-fat and cholesterol-free diet.

- Encourage foods rich in omega-3 fatty acids (salmon, nuts, or flax), or take 1 tablespoon of lignan-rich flaxseed oil twice daily or 1 to 2 tablespoons of ground flaxseed twice daily.

■ Supplements

- Beta-sitosterol: 60 mg twice daily
- Zinc: 30–40 mg daily

■ Botanicals

- Start with Saw palmetto: 160 mg twice daily
- Or pygeum: 100 to 200 mg daily
- If no improvement occurs after 8 weeks, consider adding the following:
  - Rye grass pollen: 126 mg three times daily
    - Rye grass pollen has more of an antiinflammatory effect, which may act synergistically with saw palmetto or pygeum.
  - Other herbal products that have potential benefit include stinging nettles and pumpkin seed extract.

■ Pharmaceuticals

- If no improvement occurs with the use of botanicals, discontinue them and start an alpha-adrenergic blocker (see text for doses).
- If the patient is unable to tolerate an alpha blocker, consider finasteride, at 5 mg daily.

■ Surgical Therapy

- If the patient's symptoms persist or worsen despite the foregoing measures, refer for urologic evaluation and treatment, with the following options:
  - Transurethral microwave thermotherapy (TUMT)
  - Transurethral incision of the prostate (TUIP)
  - Transurethral resection of the prostate (TURP)

KEY WEB RESOURCES

American College of Physicians: BPH Symptom Index Calculator: http://cpsc.acponline.org/enhancements/238BPHSymptomCalc.html	Tool for calculating the BPH (Benign Pprostatic Hyperplasia) Symptom Index Score (also known as the International Prostate Symptom Score [IPSS])
AUA (American Urological Association) Foundation: Management of Benign Prostatic Hyperplasia: http://www.urologyhealth.org/urology/index.cfm?article=144	Patient Education on BPH
Mayo Clinic: Benign Prostatic Hyperplasia: http://www.mayoclinic.org/bph/treatment.html	Surgical Options for BPH

References

References are available online at expertconsult.com.

Chapter 58

Urolithiasis

Jimmy Wu, MD

Pathophysiology

Over the past few decades, an increasing percentage of the U.S. population has had the misfortune of experiencing the disabling pain that accompanies urolithiasis. The National Health and Nutrition Examination Survey (NHANES) reported that approximately 5% of persons in the United States will have experienced at least one symptomatic stone in their lifetime.[1] Notable epidemiologic risks include being white, male, and living in hot, arid regions.[2] As evidenced by Hippocrates' reference to "…persons laboring under the stone,…" in his famous oath, this common medical problem has challenged even history's most renowned healers.[3]

In addition to being responsible for so much morbidity in individual patients, kidney stones were estimated by a retrospective study to cost more than $5.3 billion in lost work hours and direct health care expenses in the year 2000.[4] Because most patients with idiopathic kidney stones have some underlying urine metabolic abnormality, the risk of recurrence is 40% at 5 years and 75% at 20 years.[5] This tendency for urologic stones to reemerge within the same people presents an opportunity for health care providers to promote a preventive and integrative approach in protecting against stone recurrence.

Data demonstrate certain epidemiologic disparities in gender, location, and race. For reasons that are still unclear, men consistently have a higher risk of developing kidney stones than do women. Geographically, the "stone belt," consisting of the southeastern U.S. region, also tends to have higher prevalence of renal lithiasis, likely because of its hotter climate. Finally, black U.S. residents appear to suffer less from this disease than do their white counterparts.[6]

To provide the most appropriate counseling, the clinician must understand how kidney stones form and what elements are commonly present in stones. Kidney stones are a product of normally soluble material (e.g., calcium, oxalate) supersaturating in urine to a level that facilitates crystallization of that very material (Fig. 58-1).[7] With this origin in mind, any approach that discourages urinary crystallization or promotes crystallization inhibition forms the basis for the preventive recommendations described in this chapter.

More than 80% of kidney stones primarily consist of calcium, usually calcium oxalate. These oxalate stones may also contain phosphate or uric acid. The remainder of kidney stones can be divided into stones that have uric acid, struvite (magnesium ammonium phosphate or infection stone), or cystine as their primary constituents. Most calcium stone formers possess some sort of urinary metabolic abnormality that can be detected with a 24-hour urine sample[7] (Table 58-1).

> Patients with recurring stones or with a stone manifesting before they are 30 years old should have a 24-hour urine test to check for high levels of calcium, oxalate, and uric acid or low levels of citrate.

Many patients (33% to 66%) who suffer from calcium-based kidney stones have hypercalciuria, which is mostly idiopathic but can be familial. The urine is supersaturated with a high enough level of calcium that calcium renal calculi begin to form. When patients also have accompanying hypercalcemia, other disorders must be ruled out (e.g., hyperparathyroidism, sarcoidosis, cancer).[8]

Similarly, patients who are found to have high urinary oxalate levels are predisposed to passing calcium oxalate stones. Hyperoxaluria has two main causes. A rare primary form is inherited as an autosomal recessive trait. The more common acquired form involves increased oxalate absorption secondary to ileal compromise and fat malabsorption (enteric fat does not absorb but rather binds to dietary calcium and thus allows for higher levels of absorbed oxalate).[9]

FIGURE 58-1
Kidney stones in the kidney, ureter, and bladder. (From National Kidney and Urologic Diseases Information Clearinghouse: <http://kidney.niddk.nih.gov/kudiseases/pubs/stonesadults/index.htm>; Accessed 26.09.11.)

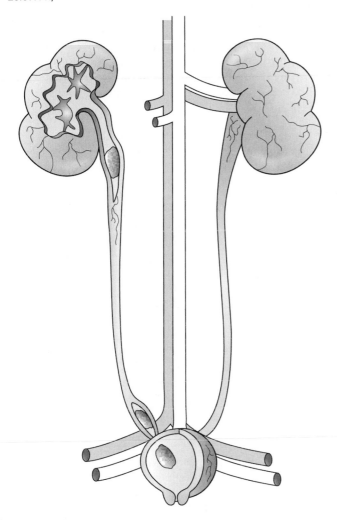

TABLE 58-1. Lithogenic Values of Urinary Biochemical Factors With Dietary Prescription

URINE FACTOR	24-HR URINE VALUE	DIETARY PRESCRIPTION
Fluid volume	Less than 2 L	Maintain total fluid intake at more than 2 L/day Reduce caffeine Stay more hydrated if strenuous physical activity
Calcium	Female: more than 250 mg Male: more than 300 mg	Maintain adequate dietary calcium intake Reduce sodium and animal protein intake Reduce calcium supplements Reduce carbohydrate intake
Oxalate	More than 40 mg	Maintain adequate dietary calcium intake Reduce dietary oxalate intake Avoid vitamin C supplements Increase magnesium-rich foods
Citrate	Female: less than 550 mg Male: less than 450 mg	Increase fruit and vegetable intake Reduce sodium and animal protein
Uric acid	Female: more than 600 mg Male: more than 800 mg	Reduce purine-high foods Reduce animal protein intake Reduce alcohol intake

Data from Graces F, Costa-Bauza A, Prieto RM. Renal lithiasis and nutrition. *Nutr J.* 2006;5:1-7; and Taylor EN, Curhan GC. Diet and fluid prescription in stone disease. *Kidney Int.* 2006;70:835-839.

The third metabolic disorder found in patients with calcium stones is hypocitraturia. Citrate serves as a protective factor against calcium stone formation because it can chelate calcium in urine, thereby forming a soluble complex that is harmlessly excreted. Therefore, people with low levels of citrate in their urine are at risk for calcium stone formation.[9]

Of the disorders related to stones that are not composed of calcium, primary uric acid nephrolithiasis is the next most common (10%). Any factor that acidifies the urine pH (e.g., protein intake, insulin resistance) creates an environment more susceptible to stone formation. The other two factors that contribute to uric acid stone formation include low urinary volume (e.g., dehydration, diarrhea) and hyperuricosuria (e.g., enzymatic deficiency syndromes, drugs, gout).[10]

Struvite stones typically form in patients who have chronic urinary tract infections with urease-producing bacteria such as *Proteus* or *Klebsiella*. These patients classically develop staghorn calculi found in the renal pelvis. The stones consist of multiple magnesium ammonium phosphate crystals and calcium carbonate-apatite.[11]

Finally, cystine stones (1%) are the result of cystinuria, which is a rare genetic autosomal recessive metabolic disorder. Cystine stones should be considered in patients who have their first stone during childhood (median age, 12 years).[12]

Integrative Therapy

Nutrition and Supplementation

Any recommendation that limits lithogenic ingredients and promotes lithoprotective factors serves as the basis for the nutritional and supplemental suggestions given here (see Table 58-1; Table 58-2). The literature on the role of nutrition and supplements in kidney stone prevention is abundant, but solid evidence to support the dietary recommendations given here is lacking.

In general, people who have unhealthy lifestyles and develop qualities of the increasingly common metabolic syndrome are at increased risk for stone formation. A study that used NHANES data found strong associations between people who had various features of metabolic syndrome

TABLE 58-2. Foods High in Bioelements Related to Kidney Stone Formation

Lithoprotective		
CALCIUM (DIETARY)	**MAGNESIUM**	**CITRATE**
Milk	Almonds	Orange
Yogurt	Cashews	Lemon
Cheese	Soybean	Cranberry
Broccoli	Potato	Pineapple
Salmon	Nuts	High-citrate juices and sodas

Lithogenic		
SODIUM	**OXALATE**	**PURINE**
Potato chips	Rhubarb	Legumes
Canned foods	Spinach	Spinach
Frozen dinners	Chocolate	Red meat
Soy sauce	Peanuts	Alcohol
Table salt	Cashews	Sardines

Data from Office of Dietary Supplements, National institutes of Health: http://ods.od.nih.gov/factsheets/list-all/; Accessed 26.09.11; and Graces F, Costa-Bauza A, Prieto RM. Renal lithiasis and nutrition. *Nutr J.* 2006;5:1–7.

(e.g., obesity, hypertension, diabetes, hyperlipidemia) and stone formation. This finding underlines the overall importance of promoting healthy nutrition and physical activity in the prevention of kidney stones.[13–15]

Water

The dietary recommendation to increase fluid intake has strong scientific support for preventing recurrent renal lithiasis. Several observational studies dating to 1966 postulated that increased fluid intake is beneficial, and one randomized controlled trial in 1996 actually showed that fluid intake achieving a urinary volume of 2 L reduced the stone recurrence rate from 27% to 12%.[13,14,16,17]

A safe recommendation is to ask patients to drink 2 to 3 L of water per day. One approach is to tailor the fluid recommendation to the calculated urine volume from the 24-hour urine test. For example, if the 24-hour urine volume is 1.5 L, it will be best to advise the patient to drink two more 8-ounce $(2 \times 240 = 480 \, mL)$ cups of water to achieve 2 L total.[18] Although no evidence exists for the following, some practitioners recommend that their patients maintain urine at a very light color. Some clinicians have also advocated drinking water at bedtime because urinary concentration usually occurs during sleep.[19] Endurance athletes with stones must be especially aware of their fluid loss through sweat. Furthermore, caution should be used when ingesting mineral water because it may contain calcium or other lithogenic material.

Beverages

A few studies examined the efficacy of encouraging or discouraging different types of beverages for the prevention of stones. In particular, fruit-based juices were studied because of their citrate (lithoprotective) content. However, vitamin C was shown to increase urine oxalate (lithogenic); not surprisingly, evidence for fruit-based juices remains ambiguous.[13]

Several studies showed that grapefruit juice increases the risk for stones; conversely, lemon juice, orange juice, and cranberry juice have mostly been viewed as protective against renal stones.[6,13,20–23]

Not much is discussed about the role of soft drinks in stone formation, but the general recommendation is to limit soda consumption, possibly because of the caffeine content.[23,24] Caffeine, through a dilution effect, can increase the risk of calcium oxalate stone formation.[23] However, sodas with higher citrate content may theoretically neutralize any lithogenic effect.[21] Other caffeinated beverages such as coffee and tea (especially black tea) should also be avoided.[13]

Calcium (Dietary and Supplement)

Contrary to conventional wisdom, limiting dietary intake of calcium is not recommended. This conclusion was proven several times with strong evidence. Two prospective observational studies from the 1990s concluded that kidney stone formation was inversely associated with dietary calcium intake.[25–27] In addition, a 5-year randomized controlled trial comparing groups that differed by the calcium load in their diet proved that decreasing dietary calcium was a risk factor for symptomatic stone recurrence.[25,28]

The theory behind this conclusion is that dietary calcium protects against stone formation by binding with oxalate and thereby reducing urinary oxalate levels. It takes a smaller increase of urinary oxalate than of urinary calcium to precipitate stone formation. Therefore, a high urinary oxalate level is a larger risk factor in calcium oxalate stone formation. This finding explains why dietary calcium is actually lithoprotective.[26]

In contrast, investigators have suggested that the effect of calcium supplements is different. A 1997 study showed that calcium supplements in women resulted in a higher risk of calcium stone formation. The rationale for this finding was that the supplements were not taken with food, and calcium's function in reducing dietary oxalate absorption was thereby nullified. However, other data showed a neutral effect of calcium supplements in men and younger women.[18,25,27,29]

Oxalate

Despite several studies, no consensus exists regarding the effect of dietary oxalate on stone formation, even in patients with hyperoxaluria.[13] Because of its low bioavailability, dietary oxalate may not be readily absorbed.[6,18] Therefore, no firm recommendation can be made about limiting dietary oxalate, although such advice is not harmful. Oxalate-rich foods include nuts (almonds, peanuts, pecans, walnuts, cashews), vegetables (rhubarb, spinach), and chocolate.[13,18]

Vitamin C

Vitamin C can be metabolized to oxalate and therefore could increase risk of stone formation. One trial showed that supplemental vitamin C increased urinary oxalate excretion; however, no evidence indicates that vitamin C actually causes an increase in symptomatic stone formation. Therefore, recurrent stone formers should not be instructed to limit their dietary vitamin C intake, especially because foods high in vitamin C are also high in citrate. A reasonable approach is to suggest limiting supplemental vitamin C.[6,13,18,30]

Sodium

Studies showed that increased dietary sodium results in elevated calcium in the urine and reduced urinary excretion of citrate. This combination effect makes high sodium intake a potential risk factor for higher stone recurrence. One recommendation is that, especially for patients with hypercalciuria, sodium intake should be restricted to less than 3 to 6 g per day.[6,13,18]

Protein

An increase in dietary protein intake appears to raise urinary calcium and uric acid levels and decreases urinary citrate levels.[6,13,18] Therefore, reducing protein intake can also benefit patients with calcium and uric acid stones. Some studies examined combination diets, and participants who followed diets with a low-protein component had a lower stone recurrence rate.[31]

Carbohydrates

Some investigators postulated that a possible relationship between higher intake of carbohydrates or refined sugar and increased urinary calcium may be partially responsible for the higher rates of kidney stones in wealthier countries.[6] However, the association is too weak to recommend carbohydrate cessation to protect against stone recurrence.

Omega-3 Fatty Acid

Increased intake of dietary omega-3 fatty acids does not reduce the risk of kidney stone formation. However, using fish oil supplements as prevention is promising because small studies showed that these supplements reduced urinary excretion of calcium and oxalate.[25,32,33]

Purines

People with uric acid stones are generally advised to avoid a high-purine diet. Purine-containing foods include organ meats, legumes, mushrooms, spinach, alcohol, sardines, and poultry.[10]

Magnesium

In theory, magnesium binds to oxalate and thus potentially decreases the risk of calcium oxalate stones. Sparse data suggest that dietary and supplemental magnesium can lower the risk of stone formation in men.[25,20,34] Dietary magnesium can be mostly found in dairy products, meat, seafood, avocados, dark green vegetables, and cocoa.[13]

Botanicals and Other Herbal Medicines

Many studies have examined the potential use of various botanicals and herbs for prevention of stone formation. However, most studies have used in vitro or animal models. Only a few trials have demonstrated some promise within human models.[35]

Phyllanthus niruri (e.g., stonebreaker, chanca piedra) is a plant that has been studied and used in Brazil; it has been studied in the human population and has shown efficacy in preventing stone recurrence.[35] Other studied herbals include Andrographis paniculata, Hibiscus sabdariffa, and Orthosiphon grandiflorus.[35] Most of these are frequently taken as teas.

> Phyllanthus niruri may potentiate insulin and other antidiabetic medications, as well as antihypertensive medications. Do not take during pregnancy.

Probiotics

Oxalobacter formigenes is an anaerobic bacterium responsible for degrading oxalate in the body. Investigators have postulated that a probiotic containing this species would be useful for preventing stone formation in patients with hyperoxaluria. There have not been many studies that have shown actual benefit in decreasing symptomatic stone incidents, but several have demonstrated the physiologic significance of this bacterium in decreasing urinary oxalate levels.[36,37]

Traditional Chinese Medicine

Acupuncture

Although data on acupuncture as a preventive measure for kidney stones are scant, this technique has been used extensively as an analgesic for both the acute renal colic presentation and for patients receiving a planned extracorporeal shock wave lithotripsy (ESWL) procedure.[38]

> Some anecdotal evidence indicates that acupuncture using techniques that facilitate energy manipulation of the kidney and bladder can help with acute stone-related pain and with stone recurrence.[39]

Herbals

Limited data from the Kampo traditional Japanese herbal medicine tradition indicate that some herbal mixtures, including Chorei-to, Wullingsan, Jin Qian Cao, and Niao Shi mixture, have been helpful, mostly as diuretics, in stone prevention.[38,40]

Ayurvedic Medicine

Including P. niruri as described earlier, several Ayurvedic medicines are commonly used for nephrolithiasis management. These include Tribulus terrestris, Orthospihon stamineus/grandiflorus (Java tea), and Dolichos biflorus (horse gram).[40]

Pharmaceuticals

This discussion includes medications that have demonstrated efficacy for the prevention of stone recurrence. Management of acute nephrolithiasis-related symptoms (e.g., pain, nausea) is not discussed in this chapter.

Alkalinizers

This drug class primarily works to increase urine pH. Because uric acid stones tend to supersaturate in acidic urine, alkalinizers such as potassium citrate and sodium bicarbonate are mostly used to prevent documented uric acid stones. Potassium citrate is preferred because it can also reduce urinary calcium, and it provides citrate as a lithoprotective element.[41]

■ Dosage

The dose of potassium citrate is 10 mEq three times a day (if $U_{citrate}$ is greater than 150 mg/day) or 20 mEq three times a day (if $U_{citrate}$ is less than 150 mg/day) with meals, up to 100 mEq/day. It comes in 5- and 10-mEq pills.

The dose of sodium bicarbonate is 650 mg three times a day. It is available in 325-and 650-mg tablets, as well as in powder form.

■ Precautions
Potassium citrate may cause nausea or hyperkalemia (especially when it is taken with other medications that may cause hyperkalemia). Sodium bicarbonate may cause bloating.

Calcium Channel Blockers
This drug class has some data supporting its use as an "expulsive" medication that assists with stone passage. Nifedipine has as an antispasmodic effect on the ureter and eliminates the fast uncoordinated component of ureteral smooth muscle contraction. Most studies have examined its use with a steroid (25 mg/day of methylprednisolone), which has demonstrated a higher stone-expulsion rate, shorter expulsion time, and reduced need for analgesia.[41]

■ Dosage
The dose of nifedipine is 30 mg daily extended release (ER) for 20 to 30 days. It comes in 30-mg ER tablets.

■ Precautions
Nifedipine may cause flushing, peripheral edema, lightheadedness/dizziness, headache, and gastrointestinal upset.

Alpha₁ Channel Blockers
Alpha$_1$ channel blockers also work as antispasmodics, especially on the distal ureter. Several studies, especially of distal ureteral stones, demonstrated efficacy, with a higher stone-expulsion rate.[41]

■ Dosage
For doxazosin, start 1 mg at night and titrate every week to effect, to a maximum of 8 mg/day. It comes in 1-, 2-, 4-, and 8-mg tablets.

The dose of tamsulosin is 0.4 mg, taken 30 minutes after a meal daily, to a maximum of 0.8 mg daily. It comes in 0.4-mg tablets.

The dose of alfuzosin is 10 mg ER daily. It is available in 10-mg ER tablets only.

■ Precautions
Postural hypotension, dizziness, fatigue, headache, nasal stuffiness, and retrograde ejaculation may occur.

> Medical expulsive therapy is recommended for stones up to 10 mm. Alpha blockers appear to perform better with stones 5 to 10 mm.[42]

Thiazide Diuretics
Because thiazides can lower calcium excretion by as much as 50%, they benefit patients with recurrent stones resulting from hypercalciuria. This drug class should be considered if recurrence persists despite appropriate dietary changes. Studies showed a 90% reduction in the incidence of new stones with thiazide therapy. Chlorthalidone can be given just once a day because of its lower half-life.

However, the clinician should be wary of hypokalemia because low potassium can reduce urinary citrate excretion. To avoid hypokalemia, adding potassium citrate is advisable.[41]

■ Dosage
Hydrochlorothiazide is taken at 25 mg daily, but higher doses may be needed to achieve an adequate calcium-lowering effect. It comes in 12.5-, 25-, and 50-mg tablets.

Chlorthalidone is taken at 25 mg daily. It comes in 25-mg tablets.

■ Precautions
Hypokalemia, hyperuricemia, hyponatremia, dizziness, and headache may occur.

Xanthine Inhibitors
Frequently used in patients with gout, these medications can also be used for stone formers with hyperuricosuria (with either uric acid or calcium stones). Xanthine inhibitors interfere with the conversion of xanthine into uric acid.[10]

■ Dosage
The dose of allopurinol is 200 to 300 mg per day in divided doses once to three times a day.

■ Precautions
Be cautious in patients with renal failure.

Surgery

Most stones smaller than 4 mm are generally watched conservatively and are believed to have a 90% chance of passing by themselves, especially if they are found in the distal ureter. Stones between 4 and 6 mm have a dramatically smaller chance of passing (50%), whereas stones between 7 and 10 mm have only a 20% chance of passing spontaneously. Besides larger stones, stones that are located more proximally in the ureter have greater difficulty for spontaneous resolution.[42]

Surgery is considered for kidney stones that are believed to have a low chance of self-resolution. Surgical treatment includes lithotripsy, ureteroscopy, and percutaneous nephrostomy, and the choice of therapy depends on several factors, including position and size.

Extracorporeal Shock Wave Lithotripsy
Of the three surgical options, ESWL is the least invasive and considered to be first-line therapy in the appropriate context. Lithotripsy has been considered to be just as effective as ureteroscopy for stones that are smaller than 10 mm (86% versus 90% stone-free rate), regardless of location in the ureter. If the stone is larger, lithotripsy may have to be performed several times (Fig. 58-2).[43]

Serious complications of ESWL are not common, but the procedure can cause transient pain, hematuria, nausea, and vomiting. More life-threatening complications have been common in patients who have required multiple treatments for larger stones. Pregnancy, uncontrolled hypertension, uncontrolled coagulopathy, and distal obstruction to the stone are absolute contraindications.[43]

FIGURE 58-2
Extracorporeal shockwave lithotripsy. (From National Kidney and Urologic Diseases Information Clearinghouse: <http://kidney.niddk.nih.gov/kudiseases/pubs/stonesadults/index.htm>; Accessed 26.09.11.)

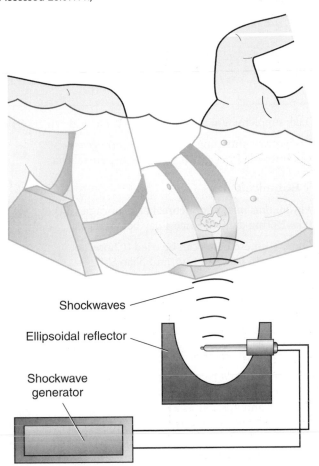

FIGURE 58-3
Ureteroscopic stone removal. (From National Kidney and Urologic Diseases Information Clearinghouse: <http://kidney.niddk.nih.gov/kudiseases/pubs/stonesadults/index.htm>; Accessed 26.09.11.)

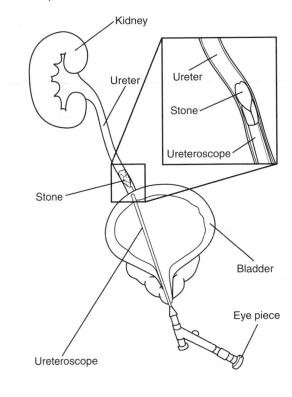

Rigid and Flexible Ureteroscopy

Although ESWL can be considered for stones that are larger than 10 mm, ureteroscopy has greater success (73% versus 67%). Ureteroscopy involves passing a scope through the ureter to remove the stone physically, sometimes with the help of laser (Fig. 58-3). Especially with larger, proximal, and impacted stones, this technique is preferred. In patients who have absolute contraindications to ESWL therapy, ureteroscopy is an acceptable alternative.[43,44] With the development of more advanced technology (flexible and smaller-caliber scopes) and techniques, complications such as ureteral perforation or stricture formation have become much less common.[43,44]

Percutaneous Nephrolithotomy

Because of a larger side effect profile, percutaneous nephrolithotomy is reserved for patients with renal calculi (especially staghorn struvite stones) and large impacted proximal ureteral stones. Patients in whom ureteroscopy fails are also candidates for percutaneous nephrolithotomy. This technique involves inserting a needle through the skin into the kidney's collecting system and dilating the tract to 1 cm, to allow the urologist to break up and remove the stones (Fig. 58-4).[43,44] Just like any other invasive procedure, percutaneous nephrolithotomy has complications such as bleeding, injury to other organs, and infection.[44,45]

FIGURE 58-4
Percutaneous nephrolithotomy. (From National Kidney and Urologic Diseases Information Clearinghouse: <http://kidney.niddk.nih.gov/kudiseases/pubs/stonesadults/index.htm>; Accessed 26.09.11.)

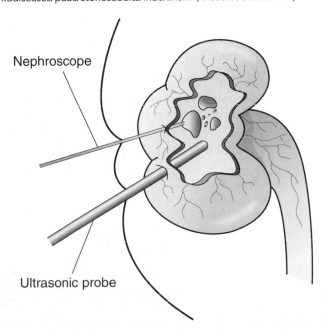

PREVENTION PRESCRIPTION

- Maintain a daily fluid intake of 2 to 3 L (approximately 8 to 10 glasses of water). Try to limit situations that exacerbate dehydration (e.g., hot weather, endurance exercise).
- Do *not* limit your dietary calcium intake. A low-sodium, low-protein diet can be helpful.
- Drink lemonade, orange juice, and cranberry juice, but limit grapefruit juice and sodas.
- Develop a healthy lifestyle that maintains a normal body mass index.
- For patients with hyperoxaluria, limit intake of foods with high oxalate levels, including nuts (almonds, peanuts, pecans, walnuts, cashews), vegetables (rhubarb, spinach), and chocolate.

THERAPEUTIC REVIEW

The purpose behind these suggested therapeutic options for kidney stones is to prevent recurrence of symptomatic stones. Regardless of stone composition, all patients with kidney stones should be advised to increase their water intake. Depending on the type of stone and results of metabolic evaluation, additional dietary, supplemental, and medical recommendations can also be made. Surgery is reserved for patients with large stones, recalcitrant disease, obstructing disease, and stones located in certain positions along the urologic tract that are difficult to access.

■ Removal of Exacerbating Factors

- Avoid excessive exposure to any environment or activity that promotes dehydration (warmer climates or strenuous physical activity).
- Maintain general healthy eating and physical activity habits that prevent development of metabolic syndrome conditions (e.g., obesity, hypertension, hyperlipidemia).

■ Nutrition

- Drink lots of water, with 2 to 3 L per day recommended (8 to 10 glasses of water).
- Do not limit dietary calcium intake.
- Limit caffeine, soda, grapefruit juice, protein, carbohydrate, and salt intake (less than 2.5 g daily).
- Drink lemonade, orange juice, and cranberry juice.
- Decrease consumption of oxalate-containing foods, especially if you have hyperoxaluria.
- Decrease intake of purine-rich foods, especially if you have uric acid stones.
- Tailor your diet based on the type of metabolic abnormality.

■ Supplements

- Limit supplemental calcium, but if needed for bone fortification, take with food.
- Limit supplemental vitamin C.
- Take supplemental omega-3 fatty acids.
- Take supplemental magnesium.
- Probiotics containing *Oxalobacter formigenes* can be used, especially if you have hyperoxaluria.

■ Botanicals

- *Phyllanthus niruri* (stonebreaker, chanca piedra): take 250 mg daily to twice a day before meals.
- Other Chinese herbs can be tried (Chorei-to, Wullingsan, Jin Qian Cao, and Niao Shi).
- Other herbs frequently used in Ayurvedic medicine (*Tribulus terrestris, Orthospihon stamineus/grandiflorus* [Java tea], and *Dolichos biflorus)* can be considered.

■ Energy Medicine

- Acupuncture can be used for pain after extracorporeal shock wave lithotripsy (ESWL) and possibly as a kidney or bladder energy-modifying treatment.

■ Pharmaceuticals

- Diuretics, especially thiazides (hydrochlorothiazide, 25 mg daily) can be used for their hypocalciuric effect.
- Potassium citrate is useful as an alkalinizer and citrate promoter, at 10 mEq three times a day (if $U_{citrate}$ greater than 150 mg/day) or 20 mEq three times a day (if $U_{citrate}$ less than 150 mg/day) with meals, up to 100 mEq/day.
- Alpha$_1$ blockers (tamsulosin, 0.4 mg 30 minutes after a meal daily; maximum, 0.8 mg daily) and calcium channel blockers (nifedipine, 30 mg daily extended release) can facilitate stone expulsion.
- Allopurinol, at 200 to 300 mg daily, can help prevent uric acid stones.

■ Surgical Therapy

- ESWL is very successful for smaller stones (less than 1 cm) located in the distal ureter.
- Ureteroscopy can be used for larger stones that are located more proximally or are impacted.
- Percutaneous nephrolithotomy is reserved for recalcitrant stones and for staghorn calculi.

References

References are available online at expertconsult.com.

Chapter 59

Chronic Prostatitis

Mark W. McClure, MD

Pathophysiology

Prostatitis is the most common reason that men younger than age 50 years, and the third most common reason that men older than age 50 years, see a urologist. Nevertheless, most new diagnoses of prostatitis are made by primary care physicians.[1] Investigators estimate that one in every two men will experience prostatitis symptoms during their lifetime.[2] Although the term prostatitis literally means prostatic inflammation, inflammation is not always present, and neither is infection. In fact, patients are often diagnosed with prostatitis simply because they experience pain during a rectal examination.[3] In an effort to standardize the terminology used to describe the different types of prostatitis, the National Institutes of Health proposed the four categories listed in Table 59-1.[4]

Only 5% of men with prostatitis have bacterial prostatitis.[5]

Bacterial prostatitis is usually caused by manipulation of the urinary tract, unsafe sexual practices, and spasms of the muscular tissue in the bladder neck, prostatic urethra, and external urethral sphincter. Muscular spasms induce prostatitis by interrupting the smooth flow of urine and thereby causing reflux of urine into ducts that permeate the prostate. Chronic bacterial prostatitis, which is characterized by prostatic calculi, ductal obstruction, and chronic inflammation, is more common than acute bacterial prostatitis.[6]

One reason that bacterial prostatitis is rare can be traced to a substance called antibacterial factor. Secreted by cells that line the prostatic ducts, antibacterial factor kills bacteria on contact. In the 1970s, researchers discovered that zinc was the active component of antibacterial factor. Although the prostate has the highest zinc concentration of any tissue in the body, men with chronic bacterial prostatitis have extremely low concentrations of zinc within their prostates, even though their blood zinc levels are usually normal.

Most men (95%) have nonbacterial prostatitis.[7] Chronic abacterial prostatitis is subdivided into two categories, depending on the number of inflammatory white blood cells (WBCs) in the expressed prostatic secretions (EPS): An amount of 10 or more WBCs per high-power field in the EPS is labeled chronic inflammatory abacterial prostatitis (category IIIa); a lesser amount is labeled chronic noninflammatory abacterial prostatitis (category IIIb). From a practical standpoint, however, commonly measured parameters such as WBCs in EPS, WBCs in urine, and urine cultures fail to distinguish patients with chronic prostatitis from controls.[1]

Although controversial, the origin of chronic inflammatory abacterial prostatitis has been linked with occult bacterial infection, nanobacteria, genetic factors, hormonal imbalance, aging, chemical irritants, fungal infections, and autoimmunity.[2,8,9] Researchers theorize that noninflammatory abacterial prostatitis is caused by spasms of the pelvic floor musculature, stress, and intraprostatic urinary reflux.[2,10] Cytokines produced by leukocytes and prostate epithelial cells can also produce prostatic inflammation in the absence of bacteria.[7] Although provocative, none of these theories provides a unified mechanism for the cause of chronic prostatitis.

In contrast to the inflammation or infection theory, current research suggests that chronic prostatitis is an aspect of chronic pelvic pain resulting from a complex, interrelated cascade of events unique to each individual.[11] The condition is initiated by a trigger such as trauma, infection, irritation, or dysfunctional voiding. The condition may abate spontaneously or in response to therapeutic interventions. Conversely, if the condition persists, especially in an individual who is anatomically or genetically susceptible, it can lead to local tissue damage and inflammation, as well as peripheral and central nervous system sensitization. With continued stimulation, the nervous system becomes up-regulated, and the response to pain becomes extenuated locally and in adjacent areas even if the involved tissue response remains stable or lessens.[12] In addition, persistent pelvic and perineal

TABLE 59-1. Categories of Prostatitis

I	Acute bacterial prostatitis
II	Chronic bacterial prostatitis
III	Chronic abacterial prostatitis
	IIIa: Inflammatory (more than 10 WBC/hpf in expressed secretions)
	IIIb: Noninflammatory (less than 10 WBC/hpf in expressed secretions)
IV	Asymptomatic inflammatory prostatitis

Data from Krieger JN, Nyberg LJ, Nickel JC. NIH consensus definition and classification of prostatitis. *JAMA.* 1999;282:236–237.
WBC/hpf, white blood cells per high-power field.

pain induces chronic pelvic muscle tension, which begets more pain in a feed-forward cycle. Anxiety, depression, fear, and maladaptive coping mechanisms can further exacerbate the situation.[8]

Although treatment guidelines can help steer physicians in the right direction, physicians in clinical practice use a process of elimination, based on the results of trial-and-error therapies, to diagnose and treat patients with prostatitis.[13] For both the patient and the physician, the hallmark of successful treatment is the resolution of symptoms. Fortunately, according to data from the Chronic Prostatitis Collaborative Research Network, after 2 years of follow-up, men with chronic prostatitis or chronic pelvic pain rarely experienced clinically significant progression of symptoms, and nearly one third considered themselves significantly improved.[14]

Integrative Therapy

Physicians routinely treat prostatitis with a combination of art and science. Just the same, before integrative therapies are instituted, proper medical evaluation is mandatory because other conditions (e.g., bladder cancer, prostate cancer, and interstitial cystitis) can mimic prostatitis symptoms. Once a proper diagnosis has been established, it is safe to proceed with the measures described here.

Lifestyle

Lifestyle—daily choices that are under our control—can either improve or worsen prostatitis symptoms. Healthful choices such as regular exercise, sufficient rest, nutritious food, and stress reduction improve symptoms.[6,15] Unhealthful choices have the opposite effect.

Nutrition

Although foods are taken for granted, they are potent medicine that can either increase or decrease prostatitis symptoms.

Do's

The following measures, which can improve prostatitis symptoms, should be encouraged:

- Fruits and vegetables: Five to nine daily servings of brightly colored fruits and vegetables should be eaten. Rich in antioxidant vitamins and minerals, fruits and vegetables may improve prostatitis symptoms by reducing inflammation.[16]

- Flaxseed: Flaxseeds are a rich source of antiinflammatory omega-3 essential fatty acids and a nutritious phytoestrogen-containing fiber called lignan. Flaxseeds should be ground in a coffee grinder, and 1 teaspoon should be sprinkled over cereal or vegetables twice daily. The unused portion should be stored in the refrigerator.

- Soy: Encourage two servings of soy protein daily. Soy protein reduces not only prostatic inflammation, but also the risk of prostate cancer.[17]

- Water: Drink at least 64 oz of water daily. Water dilutes noxious urinary irritants.

Don'ts

The following substances can worsen prostatitis symptoms. Therefore, patients should be encouraged to avoid them.

- Hot spicy foods
- Alcohol or caffeinated beverages
- Refined sugar
- Junk food or foods high in saturated fat

Sugar and saturated fats aggravate prostatitis by inducing the production of arachidonic acid and associated inflammatory prostaglandin and leukotriene molecules.

Supplements

Zinc

Zinc is essential for proper immune function, and this may explain why men with depressed prostate zinc concentrations are more susceptible to chronic bacterial prostatitis. Unfortunately, supplemental zinc is unable to normalize depressed prostate zinc concentrations. However, taking oral zinc supplements can normalize seminal fluid zinc levels and reverse prostatitis-induced infertility.

▪ Dosage
The dose is 40 mg zinc gluconate (less expensive) or zinc picolinate (better absorbed) daily.

▪ Precautions
Taking more than 40 mg of zinc daily can depress serum copper levels and impair immunity. Zinc supplements should be taken 2 hours before or 4 to 6 hours after taking quinolone antibiotics.[18]

Quercetin

A naturally occurring plant flavonoid, quercetin reduces prostatic inflammation and inhibits bacterial infection.[19] Onions, parsley, sage, tomatoes, and citrus fruits are rich natural sources of quercetin.

▪ Dosage
Fruit and vegetable consumption can provide between 15 and 40 mg of quercetin daily. Quercetin is available in capsules (250, 300, and 500 mg) and tablets (50, 250, and 500 mg).

Take between 250 and 500 mg of quercetin 20 minutes before meals three times daily. Bromelain derived from the stem of pineapple plants *(Ananas comosus)* improves the absorption of quercetin; therefore, an equivalent amount of bromelain should be taken daily along with quercetin three times daily.

Precautions

Quercetin may increase the blood level of digoxin, felodipine, cyclosporine, estrogen, and doxorubicin, and it can theoretically interfere with the activity of quinolone antibiotics. Patients taking cisplatin chemotherapy should not take quercetin.[20]

Botanicals: Overview

Although herbs are effective for various prostate disorders, in contrast to prescription drugs, herbs take 4 to 6 weeks to achieve their maximum effect. Just the same, herbs are less expensive, have fewer adverse effects, and often work when prescription drugs have failed. Herbs can be taken singly or in combination.

Herbs That Decrease Prostatic Inflammation

Prostatic inflammation causes pain and swelling. Referred pain radiates along the nerves that supply the prostate. The herbs discussed here can reduce prostatic inflammation.

Saw Palmetto (Serenoa repens)

Derived from the berries of the dwarf palmetto palm tree, saw palmetto induces apoptosis in prostate epithelial cells and inhibits two enzymes that convert arachidonic acid to prostaglandin E_2 and leukotriene molecules, thus inhibiting the inflammatory cascade.[21]

Dosage

Take two capsules of a solid extract containing 160 mg of saw palmetto standardized to contain 85% to 95% fatty acids and sterols once daily or in divided doses.

Precautions

Occasional upset stomach may occur.

Rye Grass Pollen (Secale cereale)

European and Scandinavian physicians routinely use a proprietary brand of rye pollen extract (Cernilton, now marketed as PollenAid) to treat men with nonbacterial prostatitis successfully. Rich in phytosterols, *Secale cereale* blocks the formation of inflammatory prostaglandin and leukotriene molecules.[22]

Dosage

The typical dose of PollenAid is one capsule or two tablets three times daily before meals with a glass of water.

Precautions

Occasional upset stomach may occur.

South African Star Grass (Hypoxis rooperi)

Commonly used by European physicians to treat benign prostatic hyperplasia, South African star grass is rich in phytosterols, especially beta-sitosterol.[23] Beta-sitosterol not only reduces prostatic inflammation, but it also lowers serum cholesterol.

Dosage

Dosage depends on the formulation. Select a product that contains at least 50% beta-sitosterol and take as directed.

Precautions

Occasional gastrointestinal adverse effects can occur.

Clivers (Galium aparine)

Rich in antioxidant flavonoids, clivers is a nonirritating diuretic herb that reduces prostatic inflammation.

Dosage

Drink 1 glass of water containing 30 to 40 drops of liquid extract three times daily.

Precautions

None are noted.

Agrimony (Agrimonia eupatoria)

The flowering portion of agrimony is rich in antioxidants known as catechins that can inhibit inflammation.

Dosage

The daily dose is 3 g of herb. Drink 1 glass of water containing 30 drops of liquid extract three times daily.

Precautions

None are noted.

Stinging Nettle (Urtica dioica)

Nettle root is packed with polysaccharides that inhibit inflammatory prostaglandin and leukotriene molecules, thereby reducing prostatic pain and swelling and improving urinary flow.[24]

Dosage

The normal daily dose is 4 to 6 g. For tea, add 1.5 g of coarse powdered herb (1 teaspoon = 1.3 g) to cold water, heat to boiling for 1 minute, steep covered for 10 minutes, and then strain. For dry extract, take one 120-mg capsule twice daily.

Precautions

Occasional stomach upset can occur.

Herbs That Decrease Painful Urination

In addition to drinking plenty of water and avoiding urinary tract irritants, the patient seeking to alleviate dysuria can use the herbs discussed in this section.

Marshmallow Root (Althaea officinalis)

Marshmallow root soothes inflamed mucous membranes and stimulates immune function.[25]

Dosage

Marshmallow root is available as a tea, liquid tincture, or capsule. Drink several cups of tea daily, drink 1 glass of water containing 30 to 40 drops of tincture daily, or take capsules containing an equivalent of 6 g of powdered root daily in divided doses.

Precautions

Marshmallow root can delay the absorption of drugs taken simultaneously.

Eryngo (Eryngium campestre)
The dried leaves, flowers, and roots of eryngo are used to make an herbal tincture that assuages dysuria.

■ Dosage
Drink 1 glass of water containing 60 drops of liquid tincture three or four times daily.

■ Precautions
None are noted.

Herbs That Prevent Recurrent Urinary Tract Infections

A urinary tract infection can cause bacterial prostatitis because urine can reflux into prostatic ducts during voiding.[5] Scientific research suggests that the herbs discussed in this section may help prevent recurrent urinary tract infections.

Cranberry (Vaccinium macrocarpon)
Although not specific for prostatitis, proanthocyanidins contained in cranberries can prevent *Escherichia coli*, *Klebsiella pneumonia*, *Proteus* species, *Pseudomonas aeruginosa*, and *Staphylococcus aureus* from adhering to urothelial mucosa.[26] This finding is relevant because *Escherichia coli* is the most common cause of bacterial prostatitis.

■ Dosage
Drink 8 oz of *unsweetened* cranberry juice daily, or take a standardized solid cranberry extract, one capsule three times daily for prevention or two capsules three times daily if infection is present.

■ Precautions
None are noted.

Uva ursi (Arctostaphylos uva-ursi)
Approved by the German Commission E for inflammatory disorders of the urinary tract, uva ursi leaves contain a potent urinary antiseptic called arbutin. Arbutin is hydrolyzed in alkaline urine to hydroquinone. Hydroquinone inhibits bacteria that commonly cause prostatitis.

> Owing to its high tannin content, uva ursi should not be taken for more than 1 week. Uva ursi is contraindicated in pregnant women, patients with renal disease, nursing mothers, and children younger than 12 years old.

■ *Dosage*
Uva ursi is available as a tea (steep 3 g of ground herb [1 heaping teaspoon] in 150 mL cold water for 12 to 24 hours and then strain; drink 1 cup four times daily), as a solid extract (the hydroquinone derivative, calculated as water-free arbutin, is dosed at 100 to 210 mg four times daily), and as a 1:1 fluid extract (drink 1.5 to 4 mL in water three times daily).[27]

■ Precautions
Uva ursi is safe when taken as directed. Avoid medications or foods that acidify the urine (e.g., cranberries) while taking uva ursi because it works best in alkaline urine.

Pharmaceuticals
Antiinflammatory Medications
Although antiinflammatory medications cannot cure prostatitis, they can reduce prostatic inflammation and pain.[5]

■ Dosage
One can prescribe 200 mg of celecoxib daily for 2 to 4 weeks.

■ Precautions
If taken long term, most nonsteroidal antiinflammatory drugs can cause gastrointestinal bleeding and renal impairment. Selective cyclooxygenase-2 inhibitors may increase the risk of heart attack and stroke, especially at higher doses.

Alpha-Adrenergic Blockers
Routinely used to treat benign prostatic hyperplasia, alpha-adrenergic blockers relax smooth muscle tissue in the prostatic urethra and bladder neck. Although data are conflicting, alpha-adrenergic blockers may improve prostatitis symptoms, especially in men without long-standing disease and in men with symptomatic bladder outlet obstruction.[28]

■ Dosage
Doxazosin and terazosin must be titrated to the maximum effective dosage. Alfuzosin, silodosin, and tamsulosin do not require titration. Take 10 mg of alfuzosin or 8 mg of silodosin with the same meal daily or 0.4 mg of tamsulosin 30 minutes after the same meal daily. If the medication has not improved prostatitis symptoms within 4 to 6 weeks, further medication is rarely helpful.

■ Caution
Patients planning cataract surgery should inform their ophthalmologist that they are taking an alpha-adrenergic blocker.

■ Precautions
Alpha-adrenergic blockers can cause postural hypotension, asthenia, dizziness, nasal congestion, and delayed or retrograde ejaculation. Alfuzosin and silodosin should not be taken in patients with moderate or severe hepatic insufficiency or severe renal insufficiency. The potential exists for syncope with all alpha-adrenergic blockers.

Antibiotics
Ideally, antibiotics should be reserved for culture-proven bacterial infection. Nevertheless, clinical investigators at the National Institutes of Health reported that clinicians routinely prescribe antibiotics in more than 95% of patients with prostatitis.[13] Researchers found that bacterial count, leukocyte count, and antibiotic levels could not predict a favorable response to antibiotics.[29] Furthermore, antibiotics may improve prostatitis symptoms because they suppress inflammation caused by cytokines, not because they eradicate infection.[7]

> Approximately one third of patients with nonbacterial prostatitis respond to antibiotics, the same proportion that responds to placebo.[30,31]

Pending the results of a post–prostatic massage urine culture, prescribing quinolone antibiotics is a reasonable approach. If patients are allergic to quinolone antibiotics, alternate choices include trimethoprim-sulfamethoxazole, tetracycline, macrolide (azithromycin or clarithromycin), or erythromycin. If the culture results are negative, the antibiotics may be stopped. Conversely, if the patient shows clinical improvement, antibiotic therapy may be continued.

■ Dosage

A 1-month course of antibiotics usually suffices; however, men with chronic bacterial prostatitis may require protracted antibiotic therapy.

■ Precautions

Probiotics should be taken in addition to antibiotics, but separate from them, to minimize antibiotic-related gastrointestinal adverse effects.

Biomechanical Techniques

Sitz Bath

Taking a hot sitz bath for 15 minutes twice daily increases blood flow to the prostate, reduces prostatic inflammation, and enhances immune function.

Prostatic Massage

A time-honored treatment for prostatitis, prostate massage forces secretions laden with dead bacteria and cellular debris into the prostatic urethra. To perform prostate massage, insert the dominant gloved index finger into the patient's rectum to the base (deepest aspect) of the prostate (Fig. 59-1). Next, slide the pad of the index finger to the lateral aspect of the prostate. Inform the patient that the following procedure may be uncomfortable. Maintain constant firm pressure against the surface of the prostate while sweeping the finger horizontally to the midline. Continue this process in a stepwise fashion by moving from the base of the prostate to the apex (closest aspect) of the prostate. Repeat the same maneuver on the opposite side of the prostate. If fluid is discharged from the tip of urethra, a drop can be dabbed on a glass slide for microscopic examination. To obtain a specimen for culture, instruct the patient to wipe the tip of the penis with an antiseptic wipe and then void directly into a culture container (not the toilet). Prostate massage works best in combination with antibiotic therapy for treating chronic bacterial prostatitis.[32]

Physical Therapy

Research has shown that men with chronic pelvic pain syndrome often develop guarding behavior in their pelvic musculature that results in a feed-forward pain cycle in which repeated tensing of pelvic muscles causes an accumulation of noxious chemicals producing pain that causes additional muscle contractions. Techniques that decrease muscle tension (e.g., trigger point release, pelvic floor reeducation, biofeedback, and relaxation techniques) can improve symptoms of chronic pelvic pain syndrome.[33]

FIGURE 59-1
Digital rectal examination. BPH, benign prostatic hyperplasia.

DIGITAL RECTAL EXAMINATION

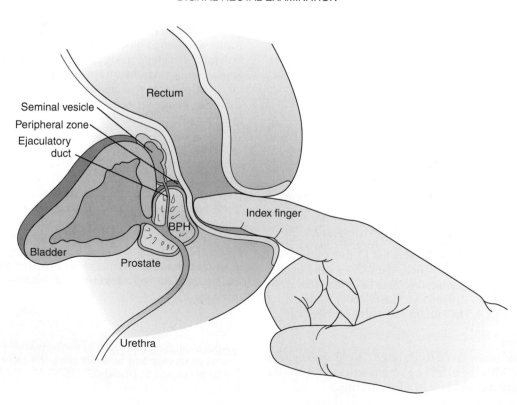

Transurethral Microwave Therapy

Three sham-controlled trials showed that transurethral microwave therapy is an effective, safe, and durable treatment for resistant nonbacterial prostatitis. This technique can also kill bacteria that cause chronic bacterial prostatitis.[5]

Mind-Body Therapy

Chronic prostatitis exacts a heavy emotional toll on men. According to one survey, the quality of life for these men was on par with men suffering from chronic low back pain, heart disease, or inflammatory bowel disease.[34] Furthermore, the mental consequences of chronic prostatitis were deemed worse than those associated with congestive heart failure and diabetes.[35] The following mind-body modalities can help alleviate the pain and suffering that accompany chronic prostatitis by providing men with new coping skills:

- Relaxation Techniques (see Chapter 93, Relaxation Techniques)
- Guided imagery (see Chapter 95, Guided Imagery)
- Meditation (see Chapter 98, Recommending Meditation)
- Yoga
- Psychological counseling

Stress Reduction

Although stress is a part of everyday life, heightened levels of stress worsen the symptoms of prostatitis. Mediated through the sympathetic nervous system, prolonged stress increases the incidence of urinary tract infections, depresses the immune system, and increases spasms of the bladder, urethra, and pelvic musculature. Although stress cannot be eliminated, it can be controlled (see Chapter 93, Relaxation Techniques).

Therapies to Consider

Homeopathy

Safe and effective homeopathic remedies for nonbacterial prostatitis deserve further consideration. Consult a licensed homeopathic physician, if one is available. Otherwise, the authors of *Everybody's Guide to Homeopathic Medicines* recommended trying one of the following homeopathic medications, according to the predominant symptom[36]:

- Pulsatilla: Pain in the prostate after urination
- Chimaphila umbellata: Prostate soreness made worse with pressure, especially sitting
- Kali bichromium: Prostate pain worsened by walking and improved by standing
- Causticum: Pressure and pulsations in the prostate with pain radiation into the urethra and bladder after voiding a few drops
- Sabal serrulata: Prostatism symptoms and dysuria
- Lycopodium: Pressure in the prostate accentuated during and after voiding

Dosage

These remedies are available at many health food stores. A common starting dose is a 1:100 dilution with 30 cycles of succussion that is known as 30 C, taken two to three times daily for up to 5 days during acute symptoms and less frequently as the symptoms improve. For chronic cases, take a low potency twice daily for up to 2 weeks (see Chapter 111, Therapeutic Homeopathy, for additional information).

Traditional Chinese Medicine

Chinese herbal therapies and acupuncture can improve annoying prostatitis symptoms.[37] Consult a qualified traditional Chinese medicine practitioner. For a list of certified practitioners, contact the National Certification Commission for Acupuncture and Oriental Medicine (see Key Web Resources box).

PREVENTION PRESCRIPTION

- Exercise at least 30 minutes three times weekly.
- Obtain at least 7 hours of sleep daily.
- Practice stress reduction and relaxation techniques daily.
- Eat two servings of soy products and at least five to nine servings of fruits and vegetables daily.
- Drink at least 64 oz of water daily.
- Avoid junk food, hot and spicy foods, alcohol, and caffeine.

THERAPEUTIC REVIEW

Unless symptomatic patients are allergic, start them on a quinolone antibiotic pending results of a post–prostatic massage urine culture. If the culture result is positive, further treatment should be based on culture results. If the culture result is negative, the antibiotics can be stopped unless symptoms improve, in which case antibiotic therapy may be continued. Antibiotics should be taken for 1 month along with a probiotic (but not at the same time of day). Patients who fail to respond, and those who have recurrent prostatitis, should be referred to a urologist for further evaluation. Other measures that are helpful for bacterial and nonbacterial prostatitis are listed here.

Nutrition

- Eat fresh fruits and vegetables.
- Add soy and ground flaxseed to the diet.
- Drink plenty of water.
- Avoid urinary irritants such as caffeinated beverages, junk food, tobacco products, alcohol, and spicy food.

Continued

Mind-Body Therapy

- Encourage stress reduction techniques.

- Consider meditation, counseling, and biofeedback.

Supplements

- Take a high-potency multivitamin daily.

- Also take additional zinc gluconate or picolinate 40 mg daily, plus quercetin 250 to 500 mg and an equal amount of bromelain 20 minutes before meals three times daily.

Botanicals

- Depending on symptoms, a 6-week trial of one or more of the following herbs should be tried:

  - Saw palmetto (*Serenoa repens*): 160 mg twice daily

  - PollenAid (*Secale cereale*): one capsule or two tablets three times daily before meals

  - Stinging nettle (*Urtica dioica*): dry extract, 120 mg twice daily

- If no improvement occurs, consider trying a different herbal combination.

Pharmaceuticals

- Try a 2- to 4-week course of a cyclooxygenase-2 inhibitor to alleviate painful prostatitis symptoms.

- If muscle spasms are suspected, try a 4- to 6-week trial of an alpha-adrenergic blocker.

- If improvement occurs, continue the medication; otherwise, stop.

Biomechanical Techniques

- Recommend daily sitz baths as needed.

- Consider physical therapy and regular prostatic massage.

Prostatitis Symptom Index

- Monitor therapeutic response by asking patients to fill out a prostate symptom index form before initiating therapy and monthly thereafter as long as symptoms persist (Fig. 59-2).[38]

FIGURE 59-2

National Institutes of Health prostatitis symptom index. (From Litwin MW, McNaughton-Collins M, Fowler FJ Jr, et al. The National Institutes of Health chronic prostatitis symptom index: development and validation of a new outcome measure. *J Urol.* 1999;162:374)

Pain or Discomfort

1. In the last week, have you experienced any pain or discomfort in the following areas:

	Yes	No
a. Areas between rectum and testicles (perineum)	○ 1	○ 0
b. Testicles	○ 1	○ 0
c. Tip of the penis (not related to urination)	○ 1	○ 0
d. Below your waist (in your pubic or bladder area)	○ 1	○ 0

2. In the last week, have you experienced:

	Yes	No
a. Pain or burning during urination	○ 1	○ 0
b. Pain or discomfort during or after ejaculation	○ 1	○ 0

3. How often have you had pain or discomfort in any of these areas over the last week?
   - ○ 0 Never
   - ○ 1 Rarely
   - ○ 2 Sometimes
   - ○ 3 Often
   - ○ 4 Usually
   - ○ 5 Always

4. Which number best describes your AVERAGE pain or discomfort on the days that you have had it over the past week?

   ○ 0 (No pain)   ○ 1   ○ 2   ○ 3   ○ 4   ○ 5

   ○ 6   ○ 7   ○ 8   ○ 9   ○ 10 (Extreme pain)

Urination

5. How often have you had a sensation of not emptying your bladder completely after you finished urinating, over the last week?
   - ○ 0 Not at all
   - ○ 1 Less than 1 time in 5
   - ○ 2 Less than half the time
   - ○ 3 About half the time
   - ○ 4 More than half the time
   - ○ 5 Almost always

6. How often have you had to urinate less than two hours after you finished urinating, over the last week?
   - ○ 0 Not at all
   - ○ 1 Less than 1 time in 5
   - ○ 2 Less than half the time
   - ○ 3 About half the time
   - ○ 4 More than half the time
   - ○ 5 Almost always

Impact of symptoms

7. How much have your symptoms kept you from doing the kinds of things you would usually do, over the last week?
   - ○ 0 None
   - ○ 1 Only a little
   - ○ 2 Some
   - ○ 3 A lot

8. How much did you think about your symptoms, over the last week?
   - ○ 0 None
   - ○ 1 Only a little
   - ○ 2 Some
   - ○ 3 A lot

Quality of life

9. If you were to spend the rest of your life with your symptoms just the way they have been over the last week, how would you feel about it?
   - ○ 0 Delighted
   - ○ 1 Pleased
   - ○ 2 Mostly satisfied
   - ○ 3 Mixed (about equally satisfied and dissatisfied)
   - ○ 4 Mostly dissatisfied
   - ○ 5 Unhappy
   - ○ 6 Terrible

Scoring the NIH-Chronic Prostatitis Symptom Index Domains

Pain: Total of items 1a, 1b, 1c, 1d, 2a, 2b, 3 and 4 _____

Urinary symptoms: Total of items 5 and 6 _____

Quality of Life Impact: Total of items 7, 8 and 9 _____

References

References are available online at expertconsult.com.

Chapter 60

Erectile Dysfunction

Luke Fortney, MD

Pathophysiology

Erectile dysfunction (ED), the most common sexual problem in men, affects up to one third of men at some point in their lives. ED is defined as the inability to achieve or maintain a sufficient erection for satisfactory sex. The prevalence of ED increases with age,[1] and ED is associated with poor cardiovascular health, psychosocial factors, hormonal disorders, recreational drug abuse, and adverse effects from prescribed medications. Less common are anatomic, traumatic, or infectious causes.[2] Normally, an erection is stimulated by a combination of neurovascular, hormonal, and environmental factors beginning with sexual interest and desire. Through parasympathetic activation, endothelial cells are directly activated to produce nitric oxide (NO), which is the major hormonal mediator needed to initiate and maintain an erection. With NO present, the corpus cavernosum is engorged with arterial blood as a result of smooth muscle endothelial relaxation while venous return is simultaneously restricted.[3]

Evaluation

The World Health Organization and the American Urological Association recommend a limited ED evaluation,[4] starting with the five-item International Index of Erectile Function Questionnaire (IIEF-5) (Table 60-1).[5] A careful review of medications that contribute to ED (Table 60-2) is recommended, as is substance abuse screening for alcohol, tobacco, or marijuana.[6] Risk factors should be assessed in all patients presenting with ED (Box 60-1).[7,8] Blood pressure and weight or abdominal girth measurements are useful initial assessments of cardiovascular health, which is the main risk factor for ED. Testicular, prostate, penis, and breast inspection should also be considered, to rule out hypogonadism, hypertrophy or mass, Peyronie's disease, and gynecomastia, respectively.[9] Nocturnal penile tumescence can be assessed by patient self-report or use of the "stamp test,"[10] Rigiscan, or Snap-Gauge cuff testing.[7,11] The presence of nocturnal erections in a patient with ED suggests a psychogenic origin such as stress, fatigue, or mood disorders.[7,12] Advanced imaging such as penile duplex ultrasonography is not recommended for the diagnosis of ED.[7,13]

Further workup includes laboratory fasting glucose and lipids, thyroid-stimulating hormone, complete blood count, prostate-specific antigen, urinalysis, creatinine, and electrolytes.[4,7] Serum total testosterone levels should be considered for men older than 50 years or men with signs of hypogonadism who are younger than 50 years old. In addition to positive physical examination findings, hypogonadism is defined as a morning serum total testosterone level less than 300 ng/dL (10.4 nmol/L).[2,4,7,14]

> Presentation of erectile dysfunction is a window of opportunity to improve health and reverse the development of cardiovascular disease.

Integrative Therapy

Pharmaceuticals

Phosphodiesterase Inhibitors

Phosphodiesterase type 5 (PDE5) inhibitors (Table 60-3) such as sildenafil, vardenafil, and tadalafil remain first-line therapy options for ED.[7,15] These drugs are very effective, are used as needed, and are generally well tolerated and safe.[16,17] Common side effects include headache, nasal congestion, flushing, abnormal vision, and dyspepsia. Evidence supports equal effectiveness of these agents.[18–20] However, approximately one third of men do not respond to PDE5 inhibitors, and these agents are not considered effective for improving libido.[21] PDE5 activity is testosterone dependent, and the prevalence of hypogonadism in men is 5% to 15%.[22,23]

■ Dosage

Doses are provided in Table 60-3.

TABLE 60-1. International Index of Erectile Function Questionnaire (IIEF-5)

Over the Past 6 Months:	SCORE				
	1	2	3	4	5
1. How do you rate your **confidence** that you could get and keep an erection?	Very low	Low	Moderate	High	Very high
2. When you had erections with sexual stimulation, **how often** were your erections hard enough for penetration?	Almost never/never	A few times (much less than half the time)	Sometimes (about half the time)	Most times (much more than half the time)	Almost always/always
3. During sexual intercourse, **how often** were you able to maintain your erection after you had penetrated (entered) your partner?	Almost never/never	A few times (much less than half the time)	Sometimes (about half the time)	Most times (much more than half the time)	Almost always/always
4. During sexual intercourse, **how difficult** was it to maintain your erection to completion of intercourse?	Extremely difficult	Very difficult	Difficult	Slightly difficult	Not difficult
5. When you attempted sexual intercourse, **how often** was it satisfactory for you?	Almost never/never	A few times (much less than half the time)	Sometimes (about half the time)	Most times (much more than half the time)	Almost always/always

IIEF-5 Scoring:
The IIEF-5 score is the sum of the ordinal responses to the five items.
22–25: No erectile dysfunction
17–21: Mild erectile dysfunction
12–16: Mild to moderate erectile dysfunction
8–11: Moderate erectile dysfunction
5–7: Severe erectile dysfunction

From Rosen RC, Cappelleri JC, Smith MD, et al. Development and evaluation of an abridged, 5-item version of the International Index of Erectile Function (IIEF-5) as a diagnostic tool for erectile dysfunction. *Int J Impot Res.* 1999;11:319–326.

Testosterone

Testosterone supplementation in hypogonadism is superior to placebo in improving erections, sexual function, and libido.[22,24] Testosterone supplementation with either compounded bio-identical testosterone or pharmaceutical brands should be monitored regularly with complete blood count, liver function tests, and annual prostate-specific antigen with digital rectal examination.[25]

Dosage

Pharmaceutical testosterone (e.g., Androderm, AndroGel, Striant, Testim) is prescribed at 12.5 to 100 mg applied topically every morning and titrated to normal serum total testosterone laboratory levels that are checked monthly.[25] Compounded bio-identical testosterone preparations are available through reputable compounding pharmacies[26] (see Chapter 34, Hormone Replacement in Men).

Prostaglandin E₁ Injection

In comparison, the prostaglandin E₁ agent alprostadil is self-administered as an intracavernosal injection (e.g., Caverject, Edex) or urethral suppository (e.g., Muse). Alprostadil is considered the gold standard of ED therapy, but is still second-line therapy to oral PDE5 inhibitors.[7,27,28] However, alprostadil is expensive, requires training and comfort with self-administration, may rely on urology consultation, and can be uncomfortable or inconvenient. Dosing for alprostadil intracavernosal injection ranges from 2.5 to 7.5 mcg three times a week as needed. Alprostadil intraurethral suppository treatment ranges from 125 to 1000 mcg daily as needed.

Gene Therapy

Gene therapy involves local injection of a plasmid containing the Maxi-K protein gene *(MKPG)*, which is expressed through cellular transcription and translation into a potassium channel needed for an erection. Although *MKPG* injection therapy appears safe, it is invasive, relatively new, expensive, often not covered by insurance, and unavailable in most locations, and the long-term effects have not been established. Advantages include enabling sexual spontaneity, twice-yearly injection therapy, and synergistic activity with PDE5 inhibitor medications, and it can be used by men taking nitrates.[7,29–31]

Vacuum Erection or Constriction Device

For those men who are comfortable, motivated, and open-minded, vacuum erection or constriction devices (e.g., Erec-Tech, Firma) have shown promise for postsurgical, structural (e.g., Peyronie's disease), and prostate cancer radiation rehabilitation.[32–34] Satisfaction rates are higher than 80%, but these devices should be avoided in men with sickle cell disease or other bleeding disorders.[35,36] Patients should be counseled by a health care worker experienced with these devices.

Surgery

Penile prosthesis surgery (e.g., Coloplast) emerged in the 1970s, and many men who are managed with medication or supplements are likely to require penile prosthesis implantation as ED progresses.[7,37] However, this surgical procedure is invasive, has increased risk for complications, is expensive, and is not typically covered by insurance.

> Pharmaceutical medications work better and do not share the risk of contaminated or adulterated products. Dependable nutraceuticals should be considered in appropriate patients who are intolerant of pharmaceuticals or who are more philosophically in line with nonpharmaceutical agents.

Nutraceuticals

In general, supplements are much less effective than pharmaceuticals for treating ED.[38] In 2007, the U.S. Food and Drug Administration issued a statement warning

TABLE 60-2. Medications That May Contribute to Erectile Dysfunction

MEDICATION CLASS	EXAMPLES
Alcohol and Drugs of Abuse	Alcohol, amphetamines, barbiturates, cocaine, heroin, marijuana, tobacco
Analgesics	Opiates
Anticholinergics	Tricyclic antidepressants
Anticonvulsants	Phenytoin, phenobarbital
Antidepressants	Lithium, monoamine oxidase inhibitors, selective serotonin reuptake inhibitors, tricyclic antidepressants
Antihistamines	Dimenhydrinate, diphenhydramine, hydroxyzine, meclizine, promethazine
Antihypertensives	Alpha blockers, beta blockers, calcium channel blockers, clonidine, methyldopa, reserpine
Antiparkinsonian agents	Bromocriptine, levodopa, trihexyphenidyl
Cardiovascular agents	Digoxin, disopyramide, gemfibrozil
Cytotoxic agents	Methotrexate
Diuretics	Spironolactone, thiazides
Hormones	5-Alpha-reductase inhibitors, corticosteroids, estrogens, LH-releasing hormone agonists, progesterone
Immunomodulators	Interferon-alfa
Sedatives	Benzodiazepines, butyrophenones, phenothiazines

Data from references 2, 6, and 7.

BOX 60-1. Risk Factors for Erectile Dysfunction

- Advancing age
- Alcohol abuse or alcoholism
- Cardiovascular disease
- Diabetes mellitus
- Drug abuse (e.g., marijuana, cocaine, methamphetamine)
- Dyslipidemia or hypercholesterolemia
- History of pelvic/prostate irradiation or surgery
- Hormonal disorders (e.g., hypogonadism, hypothyroidism, hyperprolactinemia)
- Hypertension
- Medications (e.g., antihistamines, benzodiazepines, selective serotonin reuptake inhibitors)
- Neurologic disorders (e.g., dementia, multiple sclerosis, parkinsonism, paraplegia or quadriplegia, stroke)
- Obesity
- Penile venous leakage
- Peyronie's disease
- Psychological conditions (e.g., anxiety, depression, guilt, history of sexual abuse, marital or relationship strain, stress)
- Sedentary lifestyle
- Tobacco use

Data from references 2, 4, and 7.

TABLE 60-3. First-line Pharmaceutical Phosphodiesterase Type 5 Inhibitors for Erectile Dysfunction

MEDICATION	DOSE	ONSET	DURATION	PRECAUTIONS	SOR/HARM
Sildenafil (Viagra)	25–100 mg	15–60 min	4 hr	Avoid with nitrates and alpha blockers	A ⬆₁
Vardenafil (Levitra)	5–20 mg	30 min	4 hr	Avoid with nitrates and alpha blockers	A ⬆₁
Tadalafil (Cialis)	5–20 mg	15–45 min	36 hr	Avoid with nitrates and alpha blockers	A ⬆₁

Data from Brant WO, Bella AJ, Lue TF. Treatment options for erectile dysfunction. *Endocrinol Metab Clin North Am.* 2007;36:465–479; and Palit V, Eardley I. An update on new oral PDE5 inhibitors for the treatment of erectile dysfunction. *Nat Rev Urol.* 2010;7:603–609.
SOR, strength of recommendation.

BOX 60-2. Products That Are Not Safe or Reliable for Use According to the Food and Drug Administration[39,40]

- Aziffa
- Enzyte
- Erex
- Erexis
- Eyeful
- Hard Drive
- Libidinal
- Man Up
- Maxyte
- Mojo
- Monster Excyte
- OMG/OMG45
- Prolatis
- Red Magic
- Rockhard Weekend
- Size Matters
- Stiff Nights
- Straight Up
- Stud Capsules
- Verect
- WOW
- Xaitrex
- Xytamax
- Zilex
- Zotrex

Data from U.S. Food and Drug Administration (FDA). FDA Warns Consumers Not to Use Super Shangai, Strong Testis, Shangai Ultra, Shangai Ultra X, Lady Shangai, and Shangai Regular (also known as Shangai Chaojimengnan). <www.fda.gov/NewsEvents/Newsroom/PressAnnouncements/2007/default.htm>; Accessed 22.03.11; Natural Standard. Erectile Dysfunction Products Recalled. <http://naturalstandard.com/news/news201008010.asp>; 2010 Accessed 22.03.11.

BOX 60-3. Supplements With Insufficient Evidence

- 5-Hydroxytryptophan (5-HTP)
- Ambra grisea (ambrein)
- Androstenediol
- Ashwagandha
- Brazilian wandering spider venom (peptide Tx2-6)
- *Bufo* toad (bufotenine, Chan Su)
- *Butea superba*
- Chaste tree berry
- Clove
- Coleus
- Creatine
- Deer velvet
- Ephedra
- Maca *(Lepidium meyenii)*
- Melatonin
- *Muira puama* (potency wood)
- Niacin
- Pomegranate
- Pygeum
- Rhinoceros horn
- Rhodiola
- Saw palmetto
- Spanish fly (cantharides)
- *Tribulus terrestris* (TT)
- Wild yam

Data from references 38, 42, and 43.

consumers to avoid use of impotence supplements.[39,40] Patients should be counseled to avoid email promotions and Internet advertisements for these and other products that falsely claim to enhance male libido and sexual function. Further, many of these products are contaminated or adulterated,[41] and they are not considered reliable or safe for use (Box 60-2). Other products may be commonly used but are ineffective (Box 60-3).[38,42,43] However, some evidence indicates that the judicious use of high-quality nutraceuticals may be considered in appropriate situations (Table 60-4).[44-65]

Bioenergetics

Evidence is generally lacking for acupuncture and massage in treating ED.[66] Further, massage therapy may be socially inappropriate in this context. Evidence is also lacking for osteopathic and chiropractic manipulation.[42] Further, evidence for yoga, energy medicine, physical therapy, and the Alexander technique for the specific treatment of ED is insufficient.[42] However, these and other methods should be individually adapted and encouraged as part of overall health management as appropriate.[67]

Mind-Body Therapy

Sexual desire, arousal, and climax are mediated through complex psychoneurological mechanisms. Psychological interventions are recommended as a strength of recommendation taxonomy category 1B for ED resulting from anxiety, depression, posttraumatic stress disorder, guilt, sex abuse history, relationship strain, performance anxiety, postsurgical adjustment disorder, and general stress.[7,42,68-73] Evidence is insufficient to recommend art therapy, hypnosis, aromatherapy, meditation, or guided imagery.[42] However, appropriate relaxation methods should be individually adapted and encouraged as needed.[67,72]

Lifestyle

A strong association exists between chronic diseases of lifestyle and ED (see Box 60-1), and treatment must include weight loss, healthy nutrition, and regular exercise.[2,6,7,74,75] First-line therapy also involves a review of medications that can contribute to ED (see Table 60-2). Research shows that men with ED are at significant risk for cardiovascular disease.[75-77] One study found that ED symptoms manifest on average 3 years earlier than symptoms of CAD.[78] Conversely, blood pressure control is associated with a lower prevalence of ED, particularly in older patients.[79] Similarly, metabolic syndrome seems to play an important role in the etiopathogenesis of ED.[74,80,81] For men diagnosed with diabetes mellitus, the prevalence of ED is as high as 89%.[78,79] Further, obesity nearly doubles the risk of ED.[1,80] Investigators have also noted a possible association between

TABLE 60-4. Common Supplements for Erectile Dysfunction

SUPPLEMENT/HERB	MECHANISM	DOSE	PRECAUTIONS	TIP	SOR/HARM
Panax ginseng[38,45-47]	Ginsenosides, increased NO	900 mg tid	Insomnia, mania, dysrhythmias	SS-cream[46] may help premature ejaculation	B / 1
Dehydroepiandrosterone[48,49]	Testosterone precursor, increased NO	50 mg daily	Insomnia, mania, acne, gynecomastia	May take up to 24 wk; best in HTN, least helpful in DM	B / 2
Yohimbine[38,50-53] (Yocon)	MAO inhibition, calcium and alpha blockade, NO	5-10 mg tid	HTN, CAD, DM, mood disorders, renal/liver disease, BPH	Use very cautiously, monitor closely	A / 2
L-Arginine[54,55] (Prelox, Sargenor, R-Gene-10 Solution)	Precursor to NO	1000-2000 mg tid	Gout, asthma, GI upset	Additive effect with pycnogenol[54]	B / 1
Pycnogenol[54,56] (Prelox, Sargenor)	Pine bark extract, activates NO synthase	40 mg tid	GI upset, vertigo, warfarin use	Alone may take up to 12 wk; additive effect with 500 mg L-arginine tid	B / 1
Propionyl-L-carnitine[57,58]	Antiinflammatory, mediates NO	1000 mg bid	GI upset	Improves sildenafil effectiveness after prostate surgery and DM	C / 1
Horny goat weed/*Epimedium*[59-61] (Etana)	Icariin, PDE5 inhibition	2000 mg daily/200 mg daily	Prolonged QT, HTN, GI upset, mania	May also help osteoporosis	C / 2
Ginkgo biloba[62,63]	Flavonoids, terpenoids	60-120 mg bid	ASA, warfarin use, GI upset	May help ED due to SSRIs	B / 2
Saffron[64,65]	Crocins increase plasma oxygen	200 mg daily	Dry mouth, allergy (rare)	May help ED due to depression; expensive	C / 1

From Natural Medicines Comprehensive Database. *Erectile Dysfunction.* <http://naturaldatabase.therapeuticresearch.com/nd/Search.aspx?cs=&s=ND&pt=&sh=6&fs=ND&id=331&r=3&searchid=26261145&txt=erectile+dysfunction#selected>; Accessed 22.03.11 (subscription required).
ASA, acetylsalicylic acid; bid, twice daily; BPH, benign prostatic hyperplasia; CAD, coronary artery disease; DM, diabetes mellitus; ED, erectile dysfunction; GI, gastrointestinal; HTN, hypertension; MAO, monoamine oxidase; NO, nitric oxide; PDE5, phosphodiesterase type 5; SOR, strength of recommendation; SSRIs, selective serotonin reuptake inhibitors; tid, three times daily.

ED and periodontal disease.[82] The risk of ED is nearly double in men who smoke,[83] and alcoholism is known to affect sexual function in men.[83] ED therefore presents a window of opportunity to motivate lifestyle changes toward greater health.[80] One study found that men who seek treatment for ED may prefer alternatives to pharmaceutical intervention, such as lifestyle change.[70]

The most important recommendation to prevent erectile dysfunction is to encourage overall healthy behaviors to improve well-being and reduce the incidence of chronic disease.

No exercise or nutrition regimen is specifically favored for treatment of ED. However, exercise and nutrition should be tailored to each patient's specific needs. Other lifestyle recommendations include regular dental care such as flossing, which may be beneficial for cardiovascular disease and ED.[84] In addition, prolonged or frequent bicycle riding may inhibit neurovascular flow to the perineum and thereby negatively influence ED. In these patients, a trial of rest, change in exercise routine, or cycling adaptations (e.g., split seat or recumbent posture) can be tried.

Therapies to Consider

Comprehensive treatment plans based in Ayurveda, traditional Chinese medicine, and homeopathy may have value in facilitating greater overall health in the context of ED. However, evidence is insufficient to recommend specific treatments within these traditions for ED. Detoxification may be a beneficial jump-start to a healthy lifestyle and can be considered for some patients (see Chapter 104, Detoxification).

PREVENTION PRESCRIPTION

- Obtain regular vigorous exercise most days of the week for 30 to 60 continuous minutes.
- Follow a healthy calorie-controlled antiinflammatory or Mediterranean diet rich in phytonutrients and antioxidants (organic fruits and vegetables), omega-3 fatty acids, whole grains, nuts, seeds, legumes, filtered water, green or rooibos tea, and lean or organic meats.
- Reduce stress through rest, vacation, meditation, breathing exercises, yoga, journaling, sauna, and selected manual therapies.
- Maintain healthy sexual relationships, good communication, and regular erections and ejaculations (three times/week).
- Avoid tobacco, marijuana, and other illegal or recreational drugs.
- Be moderate with alcohol consumption (2 drinks or less per day on average).
- Avoid antinutrients such as high-fructose corn syrup, trans fats, artificial sweeteners, colors, or preservatives, and processed foods.
- Avoid pesticides, herbicides, and overuse of chemical or cleaning products.
- Avoid heating or storing food in plastics (e.g., bisphenol-A endocrine and hormone disruptor).

THERAPEUTIC REVIEW

Workup and Evaluation

- History with International Index of Erectile Function-5 (IIEF-5) short survey and medication review
- Physical examination with blood pressure, body mass index, and genitourinary examination
- Laboratory tests (complete blood count, fasting glucose and lipids, electrolytes, creatinine, liver function tests, thyroid-stimulating hormone, prostate-specific antigen, morning total serum testosterone)

Lifestyle

- Antiinflammatory diet
- Weight loss
- Regular exercise 30 to 60 minutes daily
- Stress reduction
- Smoking cessation[83]
- Alcohol reduction

First-Line Pharmaceuticals

- Trial of phosphodiesterase type 5 inhibitor

  - Sildenafil (Viagra): 25 to 100 mg orally daily as needed or
  - Vardenafil (Levitra): 5 to 20 mg orally daily as needed or
  - Tadalafil (Cialis): 5 to 20 mg orally every 72 hours as needed

Nutraceuticals

- Yohimbine: 5 to 10 mg three times daily
- *Panax ginseng*: 900 mg three times daily
- Pycnogenol: 40 mg three times daily with or without 500 to 1000 mg of L-arginine three times daily
- L-Arginine: 1000 to 2000 mg three times daily
- Saffron: 200 mg daily (particularly in erectile dysfunction with depression)
- Propionyl-L-carnitine: 1000 mg twice daily (to improve sildenafil response)
- Avoidance of proprietary or low-quality brands

Mind-Body Therapy

- Psychotherapy for patients with mood disorder, posttraumatic stress disorder, sex abuse history, relationship strain, or performance anxiety
- Stress reduction through yoga, meditation, breathing, massage, journaling, psychotherapy, and rest

Second- and Third-Line Therapies

- Vacuum erection or constriction devices with training or
- Alprostadil (Muse) urethral suppositories: 125- to 1000-mcg pellet intraurethrally daily as needed or
- Alprostadil (Caverject) injections: 2.5 to 7.5 mcg intracavernosal injection three times weekly as needed or
- Surgery with urology referral

Continued

■ **Hormone Replacement**

- Hypogonadism or testosterone deficiency diagnosis, low total serum testosterone less than 300 ng/dL.

- Topical testosterone: 12.5 to 100 mg every morning 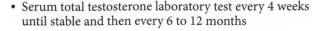 titrated to normal laboratory levels checked every 4 weeks until stable

- Compounded bioidentical testosterone

- Serum total testosterone laboratory test every 4 weeks until stable and then every 6 to 12 months

- Initial and annual serum total testosterone, complete blood count, liver function tests, and prostate-specific antigen laboratory tests with genitourinary examination

KEY WEB RESOURCES

Cornell University Medical College: http://www.cornellurology.com/sexualmedicine/ed	Academic resource for the evaluation of erectile dysfunction (ED)
Titan Healthcare: http://www.titanhealthcare.co.uk/index.cfm/go/home	Information on vacuum erection devices and options for purchase
MedlinePlus, National Institutes of Health: http://www.nlm.nih.gov/medlineplus/erectiledysfunction.html	Patient education tutorial on ED
American Association of Sexuality Educators, Counselors, and Therapists: http://www.aasect.org	Information and resource to help find a certified therapist
Mayo Clinic: http://www.mayoclinic.com/health/erectile-dysfunction-herbs/MC00064/METHOD=print	Patient handout on herbs for ED
Penn Medicine, University of Pennsylvania: http://www.pennmedicine.org/encyclopedia/em_PrintArticle.aspx?gcid=003339&ptid=1	Information about the ED stamp test

References

References are available online at expertconsult.com.

Section XI Musculoskeletal Disorders

Osteoarthritis

Adam I. Perlman, MD, MPH; Lisa Rosenberger, ND, LAc; and
Ather Ali, ND, MPH

Osteoarthritis (OA) is a slowly progressive degenerative disease of the joints that afflicts approximately 27 million people in the United States.[1-6] OA is already the most frequently reported chronic condition in older adults, and with the aging of the baby boom population and increased rates of obesity, investigators estimate that by 2030, more than 67 million people in the United States (25% of the population) will have OA.[6-8] The costs of OA in terms of human suffering are extremely high.

Because conventional therapies for OA have limited effectiveness, and toxicities associated with suitable drugs often limit use, many patients are left to face surgery or chronic pain, muscle weakness, lack of stamina, or loss of function.[2,9-15] OA of the hip or knee is particularly disabling because it limits ambulation, but OA also strikes the hands, spine, feet, and other joints with the same destructive process (Fig. 61-1).[1,3,11-13] The end point of the OA disease process is total loss of joint cartilage in the affected area with the need for joint replacement.[12,13]

OA is a disease with multiple causes. It should be considered not a consequence of wear and tear but, rather, a breakdown of normal physiologic pathways. The whole joint is affected in OA, with pathologic changes in bone, cartilage, and synovium.[16,17] Imbalances within the joint occur between metabolic and degradative processes facilitated by cytokines, inflammatory mediators, and chondrocyte activity.[16-18] OA is broadly broken down into two categories: primary OA, in which no specific risk factors, except for age, can be identified; and secondary OA, in which changes can be related to systemic or local factors. Figure 61-2 shows the systemic and local factors that increase susceptibility to OA.

Pathophysiology

Normal Joints

The major constituents of cartilage are water, proteoglycans (composed of protein cores in addition to chondroitin sulfate and keratin sulfate side chains), and collagen (predominantly type II). Collectively, these constituents form the extracellular matrix (ECM). Chondrocytes are metabolically active cells that are responsible for synthesis of the ECM. Proteoglycans provide elasticity of cartilage, and collagen supplies tensile strength. Muscles and ligaments provide support and protection, whereas nerve endings supply proprioceptive information. Cartilage health and function depend on compression (pumping fluid from the cartilage into the joint space and into capillaries and venules) and release (allowing cartilage to reexpand, hyperhydrate, and absorb nutrients).

Early Changes of Osteoarthritis

Early in OA, the articular cartilage surface becomes irregular, with superficial clefts in the tissue and increased chondrocyte proliferation and cluster formation.[17] Increased hydration of the ECM leads to a failure of the elastic restraint of collagen (i.e., weakening of the collagen network); in addition, proteoglycan distribution becomes altered.[16,17] Progression of OA leads to a net decrease in proteoglycans and an increase in the permeability of water. Loss of elasticity and greater permeability of water lead to higher chondrocyte stress and more exposure to degradative enzymes. As the process continues, the articular cartilage undergoes deepening of the clefts and irregularities that eventually result in ulceration and exposure of the bone.[16-18]

Late Changes of Osteoarthritis

In late OA, subchondral osteoblasts increase bone formation, thus leading to stiffer and less compliant bones. This process, in turn, results in microfractures, followed by callus formation, more stiffness, and more microfractures. The osteophytes (outgrowths of bone) that form are the hallmarks of OA. They ultimately restrict motion. Subchondral cysts are formed in an attempt to equalize pressure. Gross ulceration of articular cartilage produces focal and then diffuse areas of complete loss of cartilage. In later stages, ECM levels of proteoglycans and keratan sulfate decrease, as does the length of chondroitin

FIGURE 61-1

Degenerative joint disease. Anteroposterior (**A**) and lateral (**B**) views of the knee show the characteristic finding of osteoarthritis. Joint space narrowing and osteophyte formation at the medial and patellofemoral compartments with varus alignment at the knee are visible. A large suprapatellar joint effusion is also apparent. (From Scott NW. *Insall and Scott Surgery of the Knee.* 4th ed. Philadelphia: Churchill Livingstone; 2005.)

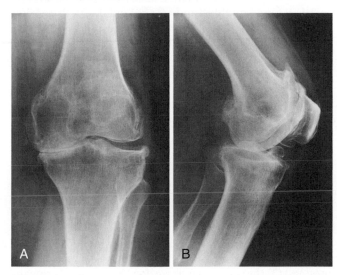

FIGURE 61-2

Systemic and local factors that increase susceptibility to arthritis. (Modified from Dieppe P. The classification and diagnosis of arthritis. In: Kuettner K, Goldberg V, eds. *Osteoarthritic Disorders.* Rosemont, IL: American Academy of Orthopaedic Surgeons; 1995:7.)

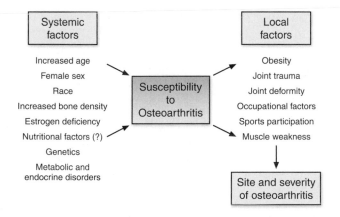

sulfate chains. These changes in concentrations of components within the ECM lead to cartilage resembling the composition of immature cartilage.[17] Soft tissues around the joint are also affected, leading to inflammatory infiltrates in the synovium, greater laxity of ligaments, and weakened muscles.

Other factors in the inflammatory and destructive processes in the joint include the matrix metalloproteinase (MMP) family of proteinases, which degrade proteoglycans and collagen,[17,18] and the cytokines interleukin-1 (IL-1) and tumor necrosis factor-alpha (TNF-alpha), which upregulate MMP gene expression, facilitate damage to the joint, and inhibit reparative pathways that would restore joint

integrity.[19] Other cytokines involved in OA processes include the proinflammatory cytokines IL-6, IL-8, IL-11, IL-17, and leukemia inhibitory factor (LIF), as well as the antiinflammatory cytokines IL-4, IL-10, and IL-13.[19]

Integrative Therapy

Integrative therapy in OA is aimed at reducing pain, improving joint functionality, and reducing further progression of the disease. Some complementary therapies have potential disease-modifying effects, such as glucosamine and chondroitin sulfates, whereas other treatments provide symptomatic relief.

Nutrition

Antiinflammatory Diet

An antiinflammatory diet is characterized by emphasizing omega-3 fatty acids (found primarily in deep-water fish), minimizing omega-6 fatty acids, and emphasizing unprocessed whole grains, beans, and fruits and vegetables. Fish oil, especially eicosapentaenoic acid, is often added as a supplementary measure. Significant overlap exists between the antiinflammatory diet and the Mediterranean diet that can reduce risk of cardiovascular disease.[20,21]

Antiinflammatory diets have demonstrated clinical benefits in persons with inflammatory diseases such as rheumatoid arthritis.[20,22] More extensive antiinflammatory dietary measures such as a gluten-free vegan diet have been shown to reduce inflammatory markers in patients with rheumatoid arthritis,[23] as well as improving symptoms.[24]

Williams et al[25] found that a diet high in fruits and vegetables, independent of lifestyle effects and body mass index, was likely protective against radiographic hip OA (see Chapter 86, The Antiinflammatory Diet).

Weight Loss

Weight is directly related to the development of OA; overweight persons are at a higher risk.[26] In patients who already have symptomatic OA, weight loss may decrease pain and slow progression of the disease.[27] In one study, a 10% reduction in weight led to a 28% improvement in function.[28] Messier et al[29] found that a combination of moderate exercise with modest weight loss provided better overall improvements in self-reported measures of function and pain, as well as in performance measures of mobility in a population of older overweight and obese adults with OA of the knee, than did either intervention alone. In a 2010 study,[30] investigators found that a 10% weight loss in obese and overweight patients with OA was associated with a reduction in biomechanical pathologic features of OA of the knee by decreasing knee joint compressive loads during walking compared with low to no weight loss (see Chapter 38, An Integrative Approach to Obesity).

A 10% reduction in weight in obese individuals can lead to a 28% improvement in function.

Exercise

Three types of exercise should be incorporated into a program for OA sufferers: aerobic training, resistance training and muscle strengthening, and flexibility and range of motion. Because both group-based and home-based programs may be effective, the patient's preference is an important consideration.[31]

The Fitness and Arthritis in Seniors Trial (FAST) assessed the effectiveness of aerobic and resistance exercise on pain, disability, and disease progress in patients with knee OA. Positive effects were found for both types of exercise.[32,33] In addition, aerobic training can reduce risk factors associated with disease states, such as heart disease and diabetes, and thereby improve overall health status. Recommended exercises are walking, biking, swimming, aerobic dance, and aerobic pool exercises. For patients with symptomatic hip OA, aquatic exercises can be effective.[33]

> Exercise is the most effective nonpharmacologic treatment for reducing pain and improving function. Some form of physical activity should be done on most days, with a more formal exercise routine at least three days per week.

Muscles are important shock absorbers and help stabilize the joint. Therefore, periarticular muscle weakness may result in progression of structural damage to the joint in OA. In addition, insufficient loading of a joint leads to atrophy of both articular cartilage and subchondral bone.[34] Strength training generally helps offset the loss of muscle mass and strength typically associated with normal aging. Strength training has been found beneficial for older adults, especially those with OA because it not only improves muscle strength but also increases function and reduces pain.[35] Clinicians should reassure patients with OA that strengthening exercises will not exacerbate their symptoms if the exercises are done in the appropriate manner and dose.[35]

Flexibility is a general term that encompasses the range of motion of single or multiple joints and the ability to perform certain tasks. The range of motion of a given joint depends primarily on the structure and function of bone, muscle, and connective tissue. Cartilage needs regular compression and decompression to enable it to remodel and repair damage, as well as to receive appropriate nutrients. OA affects the structure of these tissues such that range of motion and flexibility are reduced. The basis of exercise interventions to improve flexibility is that the muscle and connective tissue properties can be improved, thereby enhancing function.[36]

General Recommendations

Although doses vary, patients should consider 20 minutes of exercise, three times a week, building up to at least 180 minutes of mild to moderate exercise per week. The exercise recommendations given here are based on studies assessing exercise for the treatment of OA. The regimens are only guidelines and should be modified according to a patient's current health status and severity of OA. These regimens can also be appropriate for those attempting a weight loss program.

Aerobic Exercise

This form of exercise has three phases: (1) the warmup phase (slow walking, calisthenics: arm circles, trunk rotation, shoulder and chest stretches and side stretches), for 10 minutes; (2) the stimulus phase (walking at 50% to 70% of heart rate reserve), for 40 minutes; and (3) the cool down phase (slow walking and flexibility exercises: shoulder stretch, hamstring and lower back stretch), for 10 minutes.

■ Dosage

Patients should exercise for 1 hour per session, three times weekly.[32]

Resistance Training and Muscle Strengthening

A strength training program that provides progressive overload to maintain intensity throughout the exercise program has been found to be most beneficial for improvements in strength, function, and pain reduction in older adults with OA.[35]

A resistance program also has three phases: (1) the warmup phase, for 10 minutes; (2) the stimulus phase, for 40 minutes; and (3) the cool down phase, for 10 minutes. During the stimulus phase, exercises should improve the overall muscular fitness of the person and strengthen the major muscle groups of both the upper and lower extremities. Each exercise should be done in 2 sets of 12 repetitions. Exercises can include leg extension, leg curl, step-up, heel raise, chest fly, upright row, military press, biceps curl, and pelvic tilt. These exercises can be performed with dumbbells, cuff weights, or resistance machines.[32]

■ Dosage

Patients should exercise for 1 hour per session, three times weekly.

Flexibility and Range of Motion

Exercises that develop and improve range of motion also aid in maintaining flexibility. These exercises involve static movements and maintained stretching of the major muscle groups. The exercises should be performed two to three times/week and be of moderate intensity (5 to 6 out of 10, with 10 the most intense).[36,37]

■ General Precautions

Two precautions should be considered before implementation of an exercise program in patients with OA: (1) exercise of an acutely inflamed or swollen joint should be deferred until the acute process subsides and (2) an exercise stress test should be performed to identify cardiac disease in those at risk.[38]

■ Precautions With Resistance and Strength Training

When beginning a resistance and strength training program, patients should start with the lowest possible resistance (1.3 kg for upper body and 1.1 kg for lower body). Weight should be increased in a stepwise fashion guided by the patient's tolerance. If a patient is able to complete 2 sets of 10 repetitions, then the weight is tolerable. If a patient establishes a plateau in weight tolerance, then it is appropriate to increase the weight when the patient is able to perform 2 sets of 12 repetitions for 3 consecutive days.[32]

Mind-Body Therapy

Telephone Interventions

Telephone-based strategies can be an integral part of the management of chronic disease. A randomized controlled trial evaluated whether telephone-based or office-based interventions, or both, improved the functional status of patients with OA.[39] Subjects in the intervention groups were contacted monthly by telephone or scheduled clinic visits by trained people who were not health care professionals. At each contact, the following items were discussed: (1) joint pain, (2) medications, (3) gastrointestinal and other medication-related symptoms, (4) date of the next scheduled outpatient visit, (5) an established mechanism by which patients could telephone a physician during weekends and evenings, and (6) barriers to keeping appointments. At 1 year, in comparison with the control group, persons receiving telephone calls reported less physical disability and pain and tended to have better psychological status.[40] The Internet may be used in the future to improve patient outcomes.

■ Dosage

Telephone calls are made to patients twice weekly for 6 months[39] or monthly.[40]

■ Precautions

A good patient-provider relationship ensuring effective communication and the ability to understand and implement medical guidance over the telephone should exist before patients are counseled by telephone.

Group Programs

The Arthritis Self-Management Program (ASMP) is a community-taught, peer-led intervention in which patients gain the confidence and the necessary tools to manage their disease. Participants attend 2-hour weekly sessions for 6 weeks. These sessions include education about pathophysiology and pharmacotherapy, as well as the design of individualized exercise and relaxation programs, appropriate use of injured joints, aspects of patient-physician communications, and methods for solving problems that arise from illness. The sessions are taught from an interactive model, which promotes individual participation and self-management techniques.[41] A 4-year follow-up study found that participants had reduced pain and fewer physician visits, and they spent fewer days in the hospital.[41]

■ Dosage

Patients attend a group course with an experienced teacher twice weekly for at least 12 weeks.

■ Precautions

This approach may not work for patients who need more attention or individual face-to-face education.

Yoga

One small randomized controlled trial demonstrated that weekly yoga for 8 weeks, in addition to patient education, group discussion, and support, improved pain and tenderness symptoms in patients with OA of the hand.[42] Yoga may also help patients in pain to become more aware of pain, as well as cognitive and behavioral responses associated with pain.[43,44]

■ Dosage

Although the dose is variable, patients should consider Hatha yoga, at 1 hour per week for 8 weeks.

■ Precautions

Several types of yoga practices exist; it is important to begin with gentle, easy exercises.

Physical Modalities

Reduction of Joint Loading

Patients with OA of the knee or hip should avoid prolonged periods of standing, kneeling, or squatting. In patients with unilateral OA of the hip or knee, a cane, when held in the contralateral hand, may diminish joint pain by reducing joint contact force. Bilateral disease may necessitate the use of crutches or a walker.[45] A Cochrane Review on the use of braces or orthoses for knee OA indicated only limited evidence to support the effectiveness of these devices.[46] However, the trials that have been undertaken indicate good symptom relief from the use of wedged insoles in patients with OA of the medial knee compartment.[47] The 2008 Osteoarthritis Research Society International (OARSI) guidelines indicated that patients with knee OA and mild to moderate varus or valgus instability may benefit from knee bracing because bracing can reduce pain, improve stability, and reduce the risk of falling.[33]

Heat Therapy

Application of heat can raise the pain threshold and produce muscle relaxation. Moist heat produces greater elevation of the subcutaneous temperature than dry heat and is often preferable for relief of pain. A randomized placebo-controlled double-blind clinical trial examining the effects of local hyperthermia induced by 433.92-MHz microwave diathermy in OA of the knee found that three 30-minutes sessions per week for 4 weeks produced significant improvements in pain reduction and physical function.[48]

Superficial heat penetrates the skin only a few millimeters and does not reach deeper joints such as the hip and knee. In contrast, a heat mitten may raise the temperature of the small joints of the hand.[49]

■ Dosage

For commercial hot packs (temperature, 165°F to 170°F), treatment time is 15 to 30 minutes, and the temperature is adjusted to the patient's tolerance by using commercial covers or increasing towel thickness between the patient and the hot pack. For diathermy, patients undergo 30-minute sessions three times weekly for 4 weeks.

Precautions

The risk of thermal injury is higher in patients with poor circulation or impaired sensation.[45] Use heat therapy with caution in patients who have reduced peripheral circulation or severe cardiac insufficiency. Be aware of superficial metal implants and open or closed wounds in skin.

Cold Therapy

Cold applications are often recommended after strenuous exercise to relieve muscle aching. They may be delivered by ice packs, ice massage, or local spray. Superficial cooling can decrease muscle spasm and raise the pain threshold. A Cochrane Review of three randomized controlled trials showed that ice treatment may improve range of motion and reduce edema in knee OA.[50]

Dosage

Most cold applications are for 20 to 30 minutes and are reapplied in 2 hours. Rewarming times should be at least twice as long as cooling times, to avoid excessive cooling.

A classic ice pack (23°F to 32°F) is a mixture of crushed ice and cold water wrapped in terry cloth or enclosed in a plastic bag. These packs usually maintain a surface temperature above freezing and thus do not require an insulator between the patient's skin and the pack.

Cold packs (33°F to 50°F) are a mixture of water and antifreeze that forms a gel mixture in a vinyl cover. These gel packs may induce frostbite because of their low temperature, so a layer between the skin and the pack is warranted. Treatment should be limited to less than 30 minutes with these cold packs.

Precautions

Cold applications should not be used in patients with Raynaud's phenomenon, cold hypersensitivity, cryoglobulinemia, or paroxysmal cold hemoglobinuria.[45]

Transcutaneous Electrical Nerve Stimulation

Transcutaneous electrical nerve stimulation (TENS) has been considered as a treatment modality for OA of the knee or hip. It can help with short-term pain relief, and no serious side effects have been reported.[33]

Dosage

For conventional TENS, the frequency is 85 pps, the pulse width is 75 μsec. The intensity is sensory, with placement of pads over the target tissue, dermatome, or nerve distribution. The duration of application is 15 to 30 minutes to 4 hours (until relief is obtained). The frequency of application is one to six times daily, depending on the patient's response and the intensity of pain.

Precautions

Use TENS with caution in patients who have cardiac pacemakers, implanted cardioverter defibrillators, ECG monitors, other electronic implants, skin allergic reactions, and impaired skin sensation, as well as in patients who drive or operate hazardous machinery and are currently taking pain medications.

Stimulation over the intercostal muscles should be avoided or closely monitored because, in one case report of a patient with cardiac disease, this stimulation led to respiratory failure. In addition, caffeine intake higher than 200 mg/day (approximately 3 cups of coffee/day) decreased the ability of the TENS to modulate pain.[51]

Massage

Massage may lead to improvement in pain and function. A randomized control trial of Swedish massage therapy in patients with OA found significant improvements in pain, stiffness and physical function, pain perception, knee range of motion, and time to walk 50 ft.[52] Research to replicate these findings and further define the role of massage in the treatment of OA of the knee is ongoing. Research evaluating the role of massage in the treatment of other joints afflicted with OA is also needed.

Dosage

The dose of Swedish massage is 60 minutes per week.

Precautions

Although the risk of local pain from excessive pressure or bruising does exist, massage is commonly performed and is generally not harmful. Massage likely has no serious risks.

Acupuncture

Acupuncture-associated analgesia is believed to work through the release of opioid peptides.[53] Numerous randomized controlled trials have been undertaken to assess the efficacy of acupuncture for treatment of pain associated with OA. In a 1975 study, 40 patients were randomly allocated to receive acupuncture either at standard points or at placebo or sham points.[18] Analysis before and after treatment showed a statistically significant improvement in tenderness and subjective report of pain in both groups.[54] In a 1982 study, 32 patients with OA of the hip, knee, or humeroscapular joint were randomly allocated either to receive weekly acupuncture or to take piroxicam, with checkup visits at 2, 4, 6, 12, and 16 weeks. The extent of improvement was equal in both groups at 2 weeks (30%); after that, however, the acupuncture group showed greater pain relief than the piroxicam group.[55] A systematic review of 11 randomized controlled trials of acupuncture for OA concluded that the most rigorously conducted studies showed that acupuncture is not superior to sham needling in reducing pain from OA.[56] The most recent Cochrane Review of acupuncture reported that although sham-controlled trials do have statistically significant benefits, the benefits do not meet the predefined thresholds for clinical relevance, and the benefits are small.[57] The investigators also noted that the benefits are likely the result of placebo effect or participant expectations.[57]

Another randomized controlled trial, however, suggested that acupuncture may indeed provide relief for OA pain, unlike sham acupuncture.[58] In this trial, 570 patients with knee OA were randomly allocated to receive 23 sessions of either true or sham acupuncture over 26 weeks or to participate in 6 2-hour education sessions over 12 weeks (control). Persons in the true acupuncture group showed an improvement in function at 8 weeks and a significant improvement in pain at 26 weeks compared with the sham and control groups, as evidenced by scores on the Western Ontario and McMaster Universities Arthritis Index (WOMAC).[58]

Acupuncture may serve as an adjunct to a conventional medical regimen by allowing a reduction in dosage of non-steroidal antiinflammatory drugs (NSAIDs) and therefore potentially reducing the side effects occasionally seen with long-term NSAID use.[59] Each state has its own requirements for acupuncture licensure and certification. Patients should be referred only to a licensed or certified practitioner.

The 2008 OARSI recommendations for managing OA of the knee noted that acupuncture may be of symptomatic benefit in patients with knee OA.[33] In addition, although multiple sham-controlled trials showed minimal benefit over sham, acupuncture may still provide symptomatic relief for patients with OA who are wary of or unable to use pharmaceutical interventions.[60]

■ Dosage

Acupuncture treatments vary depending on the patient's underlining conditions, the severity and location of pain, and the practitioner's assessment. However, most acupuncture treatments last between 15 and 30 minutes with needles inserted. A common acupuncture regimen consists of treatment once to three times weekly.

■ Precautions

Acupuncture may cause bleeding or bruising at the site of needle insertion. Therefore, patients taking blood thinning medications may have a higher incidence of this side effect.

> Acupuncture has been shown to improve both pain and function in osteoarthritis of the knee. Six or more treatments are often required before efficacy can truly be assessed.

Supplements

Glucosamine Sulfate and Chondroitin Sulfate

Glucosamine's primary role is as a substrate for glycosaminoglycans and the hyaluronic acid backbone used in the formation of proteoglycans found in the structural matrix of joints.[61] Chondroitins are the main glycosaminoglycans in human joints and connective tissue, and they play a role in cartilage formation through the stimulation of chondrocyte metabolism and synthesis of collagen and proteoglycans.[62] Destructive synovial enzymes are inhibited by chondroitin.[63] Unlike other therapies used as symptom modifiers, such as NSAIDs, these supplements are potentially structure modifying.[33] Glucosamine sulfate and chondroitin sulfate are sulfate derivatives of glucosamine and chondroitin, and doubts regarding their absorption and metabolic fate have fueled skepticism about their therapeutic potential.[64] This dilemma has stimulated numerous studies.

In a 2001 double-blind randomized controlled trial,[65] 212 patients with knee OA were randomly assigned to receive either 1500 mg of glucosamine sulfate or placebo once daily for 3 years. Seventy-one of 106 patients receiving placebo completed the trial, and radiographs of their knees showed progressive joint space narrowing. Sixty-eight of 106 patients receiving glucosamine sulfate completed the trial, and they had no radiographic evidence of joint space narrowing. This study concluded that oral administration of glucosamine sulfate over the long term could prevent joint structure changes in patients with OA of the knee, as well as improve symptoms.[65]

Two randomized controlled trials looked at the effectiveness of chondroitin sulfate in OA.[66,67] In one trial, 300 patients with knee OA were randomly assigned to receive either 800 mg of chondroitin or placebo once daily for 2 years.[66] Although the study found no significant symptomatic effect, results suggested that long-term chondroitin sulfate use may retard radiographic progression of the disease. A 2004 study of 120 patients receiving either the same dosage of chondroitin sulfate or placebo for 1 year provided some evidence that chondroitin sulfate may reduce pain and improve function associated with knee OA.[67]

To evaluate the benefit of glucosamine sulfate and chondroitin sulfate for OA, a meta-analysis combined with systematic quality assessment was performed.[68] Fifteen double-blind randomized placebo-controlled trials were included in the analysis. The knee was the joint studied in all the trials, and in one study the hip was also evaluated. Glucosamine or chondroitin sulfate was taken orally in 12 of the studies, intramuscularly in 2 of the studies, and intra-arterially in 1 of the studies. Glucosamine sulfate or chondroitin sulfate demonstrated a moderate to large effect on OA symptoms. However, methodologic problems may have led to exaggerated estimates of benefit. Overall, these compounds do appear to have efficacy in treating OA symptoms, and they are safe.[68] Glucosamine may not be as effective in patients who are obese compared with patients of normal weight.

The Glucosamine/Chondroitin Arthritis Intervention Trial (GAIT) compared 1500 mg of glucosamine hydrochloride alone and in combination with chondroitin in 1500 people with mild knee pain from OA. Using an end point of 20% reduction in pain, no significant benefit of each supplement individually or in combination was noted. Those individuals with more severe symptoms (moderate to severe OA) reported a 22% reduction in pain. Glucosamine hydrochloride was used in this trial. Most over-the-counter products contain glucosamine sulfate.[69]

Glucosamine and chondroitin are sold as dietary supplements in most health food stores, as well as in many pharmacies. They are often sold in combination; however, it is unclear whether the combination is superior to either treatment alone.[70] In December 1999 and January 2000, a health consultant firm purchased 25 brands of glucosamine, chondroitin, and combination products to test whether the products contained the amounts listed on their respective labels. Nearly one third of the products did not contain the stated amounts of the supplements.[71] According to Vangsness et al,[72] glucosamine and chondroitin sulfate have shown inconsistent but overall positive efficacy in decreasing OA pain and improving joint function. The safety of these compounds was equivalent to that of placebo. In addition, although the literature suggests that individual use of glucosamine sulfate, chondroitin sulfate, or glucosamine hydrochloride has therapeutic value, the effectiveness of monotherapy with these agents has not been proven.[72]

Dosage

The dose of glucosamine sulfate is 500 mg three times daily, and the dose of chondroitin sulfate is 300 mg three times daily, both for a minimum of 6 weeks.

Precautions

Potential adverse effects include dyspepsia, nausea, and headache.

S-Adenosylmethionine

S-Adenosylmethionine (SAMe) is a physiologic molecule formed in the body from the essential amino acid methionine. It functions in a wide variety of anabolic and catabolic reactions in all living cells. Although the mechanism of action on the symptoms of OA is not fully understood, it may be related to the agent's ability to stimulate proteoglycan synthesis in OA cartilage.[73] The U.S. Food and Drug Administration approved SAMe for sale as a dietary supplement in 1999; however, it has been used since the mid-1970s, primarily in Europe to treat depression and arthritis.[74]

> To encourage production of S-adenosylmethionine in the body, patients with osteoarthritis who have low folic acid levels should consider increasing these levels through higher consumption of dark green leafy vegetables or supplementation.

A 1987 double-blind randomized controlled trial compared 1200 mg of SAMe with 1200 mg of ibuprofen taken by 36 patients with OA of the knee, hip, or spine, or a combination, for 4 weeks.[75] Morning stiffness, pain at rest and during motion, crepitus, swelling, and limitation of motion in the affected joints were assessed before and after treatment. The study found that both treatments were well tolerated and equally effective in lessening symptoms. The investigators thus concluded that SAMe exerted a beneficial effect on the symptoms of OA.[75] Similar results were found in a trial comparing 1200 mg of SAMe and 150 mg of indomethacin; SAMe was better tolerated.[76] A later randomized double-blind crossover study comparing celecoxib with SAMe in 56 patients with knee OA suggested that SAMe may be as effective as celecoxib at reducing symptoms but may have a slower onset of action.[77] *The Arthritis Foundation's Guide to Alternative Therapies* noted that SAMe is a promising treatment worth trying for pain relief, but that more scientific evidence is needed to prove that it supports cartilage repair.[78]

Dosage

The dose is 400 to 1600 mg daily; a common regimen is 600 mg twice daily.

Precautions

Watch for nausea and gastrointestinal distress. Ensure adequate intake of vitamin B_{12} and folate through diet (green leafy vegetables) or supplementation to optimize SAMe supplementation.[79,80] Do not take close to bedtime because of the risk of insomnia.

Methylsulfonylmethane

Methylsulfonylmethane (MSM) is a dietary supplement commonly sold for the treatment of OA. The MSM metabolite dimethyl sulfoxide is found naturally in the human body. Because sulfur is necessary for the formation of connective tissue, MSM is thought to be useful in the treatment of OA. Animal studies have suggested that MSM may help decrease inflammatory joint disease,[81] but unfortunately, no published human trials are available. Overall, the literature on the sulfur-containing compounds SAMe and MSM, in OA appears to be limited. However, the literature shows trends toward decreased pain and increased function with consistent use of these compounds. The therapeutic benefit and safety of these compounds for long- and short-term use needs to be further researched, especially through randomized clinical trials.[72,82]

Dosage

The dose is 1000 to 3000 mg three times daily.

Precautions

Watch for nausea, diarrhea, and headache. Although MSM is promoted as being nontoxic, clinical data are lacking, and further scientific study is needed to define the efficacy and safety of this supplement.

Pharmaceuticals: Nonopioid Analgesics

Acetaminophen

Acetaminophen acts by inhibiting prostaglandin synthesis in the central nervous system. It may relieve mild to moderate joint pain and may be used as initial therapy on the basis of its overall cost, efficacy, and toxicity profile.[83]

Dosage

The dose is 325 to 1000 mg every 4 to 6 hours, up to a maximum of 4 g/day.

Precautions

Reactions are uncommon with normal therapeutic doses of acetaminophen but include nausea, rash, and minor allergic reactions, transient drop in white blood cell count, liver toxicity, and prolongation of the half-life of warfarin. Patients with hepatic impairment or active hepatic disease must be monitored when acetaminophen is prescribed for the long term. Patients with viral hepatitis, alcoholism, or alcoholic hepatic disease are at greater risk for acetaminophen-induced hepatotoxicity.[84] Long-term acetaminophen use should be avoided in patients with underlying renal disease. Tobacco smoking may also potentially increase the risk for acetaminophen-induced hepatotoxicity.[84]

Tramadol

Tramadol is a synthetic opioid agonist that inhibits reuptake of norepinephrine and serotonin. It should be considered for patients with moderate to severe pain in whom acetaminophen therapy has failed and who have contraindications to NSAIDs.[75]

Dosage

The dose is 50 to 100 mg every 4 to 6 hours, up to a maximum of 400 mg/day.

■ Precautions
Watch for nausea, constipation, drowsiness, and, rarely, seizures.

Pharmaceuticals: Nonsteroidal Antiinflammatory Drugs

Nonselective Cyclooxygenase Inhibitors
Nonselective NSAIDs are a group of chemically dissimilar agents that act primarily by inhibiting the cyclooxygenase (COX) enzymes and thus inhibit the production of prostaglandins in peripheral tissues. Examples are aspirin, ibuprofen, naproxen, indomethacin, sulindac, and piroxicam.

■ Dosage
- Aspirin: 2.6 to 5.4 g in divided doses daily
- Ibuprofen: 300 to 800 mg three or four times daily; maximum, 3200 mg/day
- Naproxen: 250 to 500 mg twice daily; maximum, 1500 mg/day
- Indomethacin: 25 mg two or three times daily; maximum, 200 mg/day
- Sulindac: 150 to 200 mg twice daily; maximum, 400 mg/day
- Piroxicam: 20 mg daily or 10 mg twice daily

Cyclooxygenase-2 Inhibitor
COX-2–specific inhibitors act in the same manner as nonselective COX inhibitors, but their action is confined to inflamed tissues. Celecoxib (Celebrex) is the only COX-2 inhibitor currently available on the market.

■ Dosage
The dose of celecoxib (Celebrex) is 200 mg daily or 100 mg twice daily.

■ Precautions for All Nonsteroidal Antiinflammatory Drugs
Precautions vary with specific agent and include epigastric distress, nausea, vomiting, gastrointestinal bleeding (nonselective NSAIDs more than COX-2 inhibitors), prolonged bleeding (aspirin), headache, dizziness, and renal toxicity. Epidemiologic studies have shown that COX-2 inhibitors may increase the risk of myocardial infarction.[85]

The choice between nonselective NSAIDs and COX-2–specific NSAIDs should be based on the risk of upper gastrointestinal bleeding.

> Data from epidemiologic studies demonstrate that among persons 65 years old and older, 20% to 30% of all hospitalizations and deaths resulting from peptic ulcer disease are attributable to NSAID use.[86]

Persons at increased risk of gastrointestinal bleeding are those 65 years of age or older, as well as those with a history of peptic ulcer disease, previous upper gastrointestinal bleeding, concomitant use of oral corticosteroids or anticoagulants, and, possibly, smoking and alcohol consumption.[87] Patients in this category may benefit from a COX-2–specific inhibitor or a nonselective NSAID with gastroprotective therapy (e.g., misoprostol, omeprazole, or high-dose famotidine).

Pharmaceuticals: Opioid Analgesics

Patients with OA who have tried acetaminophen, tramadol, and NSAIDs without success may consider opiates. Opiates bind to receptors in the central nervous system to produce effects that mimic the action of endogenous peptide neurotransmitters—specifically, the relief of intense pain. These agents should usually be avoided for long-term use, but their short-term use helps in the treatment of acute exacerbations of pain.[88] Commonly used opiates are fentanyl, meperidine, propoxyphene, acetaminophen plus propoxyphene, hydromorphone, long-acting morphine, oxycodone plus acetaminophen, and acetaminophen plus hydrocodone.

■ Dosage
Doses and routes vary.

■ Precautions
In addition to the potential for addiction to these agents, side effects include constipation, nausea, vomiting, sedation, urinary retention, and respiratory depression.

Pharmaceuticals: Topical Analgesics

In patients with OA of the hands or knees, topical analgesics may relieve mild to moderate pain.[89] A cream may be used alone or in combination with an oral agent.

Capsaicin Cream
Capsaicin cream (Zostrix) is a commonly used topical agent. It exerts its pharmacologic effect by depleting local sensory nerve endings of substance P, a neuropeptide mediator of pain.

■ Dosage
A thin film of capsaicin cream (0.025%, 0.075%) should be applied to the symptomatic joint four times daily.

■ Precautions
A local burning sensation is common but rarely leads to the discontinuation of therapy.

Diclofenac
Aside from capsaicin cream, diclofenac sodium is available as a topical solution. This product (Pennsaid) combines diclofenac with dimethylsulfoxide (DMSO). Pennsaid is indicated for the treatment of signs and symptoms of OA of the knee. Most studies have shown topical diclofenac to be equivalent to oral diclofenac in the treatment of OA of the knee.[90-94] Pennsaid, in particular, has also shown similar effectiveness in treatment of OA of the knee, although further studies to compare Pennsaid with other formulations of diclofenac have yet to be done.[90]

■ Dosage
Diclofenac topical (Pennsaid 1.5% topical solution plus DMSO, Solaraze 3% gel, Voltaren topical 1% gel) is applied to the knee four times daily. It may also be used for other areas of body or joint pain. The Flector patch is applied directly to the area of pain. The skin patch can be worn for up to

12 hours and then removed. Apply a new patch at that time if pain continues. Do not wear a skin patch while taking a bath or shower or while swimming.

■ Precautions
Although diclofenac is applied topically, it is absorbed systemically and has possible side effects. Aside from local irritation at the site of application, diclofenac topical solutions, like other NSAIDS, may the increase risk of serious cardiovascular thrombotic events, myocardial infarction, and stroke or increased gastrointestinal events such as bleeding, ulceration, and perforation of stomach or intestines.

Intra-Articular Steroid Injections

Injections are useful in treating a joint effusion or local inflammation that is limited to a few joints. Injections should be limited to three or four per year because of concern about the possible development of progressive cartilage damage through repeated injections in weight-bearing joints.[95]

Other Pharmaceuticals: Diacerein

Diacerein (INN), also known as diacetylrhein, is a drug used in the treatment of OA. It works by inhibiting IL-1. A 2006 Cochrane Review found no significant difference between diacerein and NSAIDS.[96] Although diacerein may have a better risk-to-benefit ratio compared with NSAIDS, it also has an important side effect of diarrhea. In addition, diacerein may have a mild effect on the symptoms of OA and structure-modifying effects in patients with symptomatic OA of the hip, and further research is necessary to confirm the short- and long-term effectiveness and toxicity.[33,96]

■ Dosage
The dose is 50 mg twice daily.

■ Precautions
Diacerein may cause diarrhea. It is also a long-acting drug with symptomatic effects appearing 4 weeks after beginning treatment.[96]

Surgery

Surgical treatment is usually considered only after failure of nonsurgical treatments. The two categories of surgery are nonbiologic and biologic.[89]

Nonbiologic Approaches

- *Osteotomy:* This conservative approach may provide effective pain relief and slow disease progression. Its greatest benefit is in patients with only moderately advanced disease.

- *Arthroscopy:* Removal of loose cartilage fragments can prevent locking and relieve pain. When joint space narrowing is substantial, this type of surgical procedure is of limited benefit.

- *Arthrodesis or joint fusion:* This alleviates pain and is most commonly performed in the spine and in small joints of the hand and foot. In the hip and knee, it is reserved for very young patients with unilateral disease.

- *Arthroplasty or total joint replacement:* This is the mainstay of surgical treatment of the hip, knee, and shoulder. It is the most effective of all medical interventions and can restore patients to near-normal function. It is limited in durability in persons with life expectancies exceeding 20 years and in those who wish to participate in high-demand activities.

Biologic Approaches

- Biologic restoration of articular cartilage uses resident hyaline cartilage, which is stimulated to repair its own defects.

- Biologic restoration of articular cartilage is performed using one of three types of cartilage transplantation: osteochondral autografting, osteochondral allografting, and tissue engineering.

Therapies to Consider

Omega-3 Fatty Acids
Omega-3 fatty acids, the precursors for antiinflammatory prostaglandin production in the body, can be very supportive in the treatment of patients with OA. Multiple studies have shown efficacy of increased omega-3 fatty acids in the diet or by supplementation for reducing or alleviating symptoms of rheumatoid arthritis.[97-100] In different animal (dog) studies, investigators found that dietary supplementation with omega-3 fatty acids from fish oil led to an increase in weight-bearing tolerance and a reduction in the need for the NSAID carprofen.[101,102] An in vitro study showed that omega-3 fatty acids caused a reduction in the levels of mRNA for a disintegrin and metalloproteinase with thrombospondin motifs (ADAMTS)-4, ADAMTS-5, matrix MMP-3, MMP-13, COX-2 (but not COX-1), IL-1alpha, IL-1beta and TNF-alpha, which are key contributors to the pathologic process of OA. Investigators also found in this study that eicosapentaenoic acid was most effective, followed by docosahexaenoic acid, and finally by alpha-linoleic acid. Arachidonic acid, an omega-6 fatty acid, had no effect.[103]

Curcumin
Curcumin is the active ingredient in the spice tumeric. It has been used in various cultures around the world, particularly in India and Asia. Research on curcumin has found that it has many properties, which may explain the diversity of it's traditional uses. These properties include anticancer, antiinflammatory, antioxidant, and hypolipidemic effects.[104] Curcumin has been researched for benefits in the treatment and management of cardiovascular disease, hypercholesterolemia, diabetes mellitus, insulin resistance, weight loss, and inflammatory conditions.[104] This supplement may be most beneficial for those with OA with other concomitant conditions, such as obesity, diabetes, heart disease, or autoimmune conditions.

In 2009, an in vitro study using articular chondrocytes found that curcumin acted as a strong inhibitor of inflammatory and catabolic mediators, nitric oxide stimulated by IL-1beta, prostaglandin E_2, IL-6, IL-8, and MMP-3, produced by chondrocytes.[105]

Avocado Soybean Unsaponifiables
Avocado soybean unsaponifiables (ASU) are extracts of unsaponifiable fractions from one-third avocado oil and two-thirds soybean oil.[106] In multiple animal and human in vitro studies, investigators been found that ASU extract has an effect on various cytokines in articular chondrocytes and monocyte/

macrophages.[107] In a multicenter randomized controlled trial, persons taking ASU had slightly lower need for NSAIDs and an improvement in functional disability. Improvement was greatest in patients with hip OA.[106] Most of the in vitro and in vivo studies have used an ASU product that is patented and sold in Europe (Piascledine 1300, Laboratoires Expanscience, France). Because this formulation is unique, the data obtained from its use cannot be extrapolated to all ASU extracts, and thus further studies examining various ASU extracts from multiple manufacturers and processes of extraction are needed.[107]

Boswellia serrata

Boswellia serrata, also known as H15 or indish incense, is a botanical used in traditional Ayurvedic medicine; in vitro, it decreases leukotriene synthesis.[108] A double-blind pilot study evaluated the efficacy of H15 in 37 patients with rheumatoid arthritis. Treatment with H15 showed no measurable efficacy.[108] A double-blind randomized controlled trial found that *Boswellia* improved symptoms of knee OA. Treatment included a combination of herbs, rather than *Boswellia* alone.[109] A single-blind randomized controlled trial in which *Boswellia* was taken along with *Withania, Curcuma,* and a zinc complex found that this combination led to improvement in pain and disability in OA.[110]

Although the literature on this agent is promising, it is insufficient to support the use of *B. serrata* for OA. Taken in combination with other herbs, *Boswellia* may improve pain and function.

Ginger

Ginger root is an herb used extensively as a spice in many world cuisines. More recently, attention has focused on the possible medical benefits of ginger, including reduction of nausea and analgesic effects. One study suggested that ginger may be moderately effective in reducing pain from knee OA.[111] This 6-week multicenter randomized controlled trial evaluated the effect of a highly concentrated standardized ginger extract in 261 patients in comparison with placebo. A moderate reduction of pain was observed in the ginger-treated group. Some mild adverse gastrointestinal effects were also observed in the ginger group, but the overall safety profile was good.

Magnet Therapy

A popular therapy for the treatment of various medical conditions is the application of a magnetic field. The biologic effects of low-level magnetic fields have been studied since the 1500s. Explanations of these effects include increased circulation and decreased inflammation.[112] One double-blind randomized controlled study[113] evaluated bipolar magnets for the treatment of chronic low back pain. The researchers concluded that the application of magnets had no effect on patients' pain.[113] However, a later randomized controlled trial suggested that standard-strength magnetic bracelets may be effective in decreasing pain from OA of the knee and hip.[114] Although magnet therapy does appear to be harmless, its therapeutic use remains questionable. According to the OARSI guidelines for the management of hip and knee OA, five placebo-controlled randomized controlled trials showed that improvement in function was small and efficacy for reduction in pain was not significant with pulsed electromagnetic field therapy.[115]

Therapeutic Touch

In a 6-week single-blinded, randomized controlled trial, therapeutic touch was evaluated for effectiveness in the treatment of OA of the knee. Thirty-one participants were enrolled and randomized to therapeutic touch, mock therapeutic touch, or standard care. The main outcome measures were pain and its impact, general well-being, and health status measured by standardized validated instruments, as well as the qualitative measurement of a depth interview. Twenty-five participants completed the study. The findings were that participants receiving therapeutic touch had significant improvements in pain, function, and general health status compared with both placebo and control groups.[116] Further studies with a larger sample size and further evaluation into treatment time and time for course of treatment are needed.

PREVENTION PRESCRIPTION

- Maintain appropriate weight.
- Exercise regularly with a combination of aerobics, resistance training, and stretching.
- Consider glucosamine and chondroitin sulfate if at high risk for osteoarthritis.
- Avoid excessive trauma to the joints.

THERAPEUTIC REVIEW

▪ Nutrition

- Antiinflammatory diet: individualized

- Weight loss: individualized program

▪ Exercise

- Aerobic exercise: 1-hour sessions, three times weekly

- Resistance training/muscle strengthening: 1-hour sessions, three times weekly

- Flexibility exercise: two to three times weekly

▪ Mind-Body Therapy

- Telephone interventions: twice weekly for 6 months

- Group programs: group course with experienced teacher twice weekly for at least 12 weeks

- Yoga: 1 hour weekly for 8 weeks

Continued

Physical Modalities

- Knee bracing: as needed   B⊘₁
- Heat applications: as needed   B⊘₂
- Cold applications: 20 to 30 minutes, reapplied every 2 hours   C⊘₁
- Transcutaneous electrical nerve stimulation: 15-minute to 4-hour session, daily to six times daily   B⊘₂
- Swedish massage therapy: 60 minutes weekly   B⊘₁
- Acupuncture: 15- to 30-minute sessions, weekly to three times weekly   B⊘₁

Supplements

- Glucosamine sulfate and chondroitin sulfate: glucosamine sulfate, 500 mg three times daily; and chondroitin sulfate, 400 mg three times daily, both for a minimum of 6 weeks   B⊘₁
- S-Adenosylmethionine: 400 to 1600 mg daily; common regimen, 600 mg twice daily   B⊘₂
- Methylsulfonylmethane: 1000 to 3000 mg three times daily   C⊘₁

Pharmaceuticals

- Acetaminophen: 325 to 1000 mg every 4 to 6 hours; maximum, 4 g/day   A⊘₂
- Tramadol: 50 to 100 mg every 4 to 6 hours; maximum, 400 mg/day   A⊘₂
- Nonsteroidal antiinflammatory drugs: dose variable by drug   A⊘₃
- Opioid analgesics: doses and routes variable   A⊘₃
- Capsaicin cream (topical): thin film of cream (0.025%, 0.075%) applied to the symptomatic joint four times daily   B⊘₂
- Diacerein: 50 mg twice daily   B⊘₂

Injections

- Intra-articular steroid injections   B⊘₃

Surgery

- Knee replacement   A⊘₃

KEY WEB RESOURCES

Johns Hopkins University Arthritis Center: http://www.hopkins-arthritis.org/patient-corner/disease-management/exercise.html	Information for clinicians on exercise in osteoarthritis
Johns Hopkins University Arthritis Center: http://www.hopkins-arthritis.org/patient-corner/disease-management/yoga.html	Information for clinicians on yoga for arthritis
Arthritis Today: http://www.arthritistoday.org/index.php	Online magazine with information on arthritis for patients
National Center for Complementary and Alternative Medicine: http://nccam.nih.gov/health/acupuncture/	Information for clinicians and patients on acupuncture
The Brace Shop: http://www.braceshop.com/	Resource for braces for arthritis

---

References

References are available online at expertconsult.com.

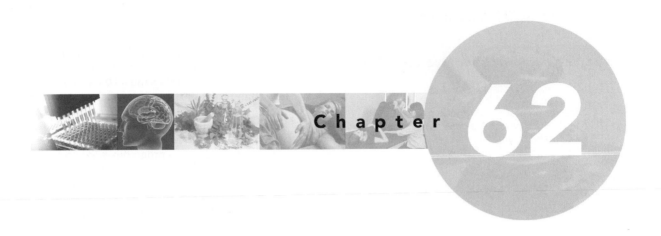

Chapter 62

Myofascial Pain Syndrome

Robert Alan Bonakdar, MD

Pathophysiology and Epidemiology

Myofascial pain syndrome (MPS) and similar terms (Box 62-1) refer to pain and associated sequelae developing from and aggravated by myofascial trigger points (TrPs). The actual prevalence of MPS varies, based on terminology and diagnostic criteria. Myofascial pain is considered to be the leading cause of musculoskeletal pain, however, and it affects up to 85% of the population at some point during their lives.[1] The prevalence of MPS also appears to be related to age and gender. Persons 30 to 60 years of age appear to a have a 37% (male) and 65% (female) prevalence, whereas those older than 65 years of age have a rate higher than 80%.[2,3] Although MPS is highly prevalent, because of its varied presentation and complex comorbidities, no widely accepted treatment guidelines currently exist, and physicians often characterize available individual treatment options as insufficient.[4]

The actual mechanism for initiation of a TrP is not well understood but it likely arises from leakage of acetylcholine in dysfunctional motor end plates and thereby causes shortening of sarcomeres and formation of precursor taut muscular bands. These bands, which are found commonly in the latent state in asymptomatic individuals, may become activated in response to predisposing factors (Table 62-1). These factors are believed to be the exclusive causes of active TrPs (thereby making MPS a secondary phenomenon). Once activated, TrPs are associated with multisystem, especially vascular and neurologic, dysfunction. Doppler ultrasound examination of active TrPs demonstrates constricted vascular beds and enlarged vascular volumes that create higher peak systolic velocities and negative diastolic velocities as compared with latent myofascial TrPs and normal muscle sites.[5]

Subsequent to sensitization of motor end plates, TrP activation appears to be further propagated neurologically by activation of mechanosensitive afferents, as well as their connection at the dorsal horn of the spinal cord. Once established, this process may have cortical ramifications such as thalamic asymmetry, which may create spontaneous or stimuli-generated tissue hypersensitivity in a progressive process known as central sensitization. Because of cortical sensitization, patients with MPS may exhibit phenomena including allodynia and spontaneous contralateral sensitivity initiated from a unilateral TrP.[6] The hypothesized mechanism for MPS generation is illustrated in Figure 62-1.

Once initiated, MPS has classic features, typically linked to active TrPs, that allow physical and electrophysiologic identification and differentiation from other pain conditions, including fibromyalgia (Box 62-2).[7] In addition to physical signs, differentiation is sometimes possible between MPS and fibromyalgia on the basis of comorbidities seen in patients with fibromyalgia, including greater fatigue, sleep dysfunction, mood disturbance, headaches, and irritable bowel syndrome.[8] Although differentiating between these two entities is advantageous, coexistence of MPS with fibromyalgia is quite common, thus making distinct classification often difficult and in some cases not possible.[9] MPS is believed to be a secondary phenomenon, so in addition to proper diagnosis, initiating and propagating factors must be investigated and, if possible, corrected. Of key importance is the appreciation by the treating clinician of the possible and likely psychological and lifestyle triggers of MPS. Therefore, the contributing factors in MPS are quite broad and require a biopsychosocial assessment to determine proper treatment. Some of the more common medical and psychological triggers of MPS are listed in Table 62-1.

Integrative Therapy

Lifestyle

Exercise

Low physical activity level has been linked to the development and progression of MPS. Conversely, exercise is essential in myofascial rehabilitation through its physiologic effect on tissue including improvement in tissue oxygenation,

BOX 62-1. Synonyms for Myofascial Pain Syndrome

- Myofascial pain and dysfunction
- Trigger points syndrome
- Localized fibromyalgia
- Fibromyositis
- Muscular rheumatism
- Soft tissue syndrome
- Somatic dysfunction
- Tension myalgia

TABLE 62-1.   Predisposing and Coexisting Conditions Requiring Identification in Myofascial Pain Syndrome

Skeletal and Soft Tissue Abnormalities	Trauma Repetitive stress injury Muscular strain or tear Ligamentous sprains Joint instability (spondylolisthesis) Osteoarthritis Facet joint abnormality Local inflammatory conditions (e.g., tendinitis or bursitis, epicondylitis, costochondritis) Craniofacial or temporomandibular joint (TMJ) dysfunction (e.g., TMJ syndrome, headaches of various origin) Leg-length discrepancies
Functional Asymmetry	Postural and ergonomic dysfunction Pelvic girdle dysfunction? Prolonged immobility
Neurologically Mediated Reflex Sympathetic Dystrophy Syndrome	Neurologically mediated reflex sympathetic dystrophy Spinal and peripheral nerve entrapment: Cervical and lumbar radiculopathy Sciatic nerve, median nerve (carpal tunnel syndrome), others
Other Rheumatologic Disorders	Polymyalgia rheumatica Polymyositis
Metabolic Deficiencies	Calcium Magnesium Potassium Iron Vitamins C, B_1, B_6, and B_{12}
Medical Conditions	Anemia Hypothyroidism Hyperuricemia Hypoglycemia Celiac disease Chronic infections Visceral diseases
Psychological Disorders	Chronic stress Sleep deprivation and dysfunction Depression Anxiety Somatization disorders

sensitivity, and range of motion, as well as cortical effects including modulation of neurochemicals such as endorphins and serotonin. Exercises must be chosen carefully to diminish significant postexertional flaring (typically defined as more pain 2 hours after activity than at baseline). Flaring can be detrimental by potentially promoting both central sensitization and activity avoidance. To maximize the benefit of an activity regimen, a progressive and preferably guided program of active and passive movement, especially when combined with posture correction, is recommended. This type of exercise program, especially when combined with relaxation techniques, has demonstrated significant success in improving pain and functional status in patients with MPS[10] (see Chapter 88, Writing an Exercise Prescription).

> Exercise should be introduced or intensified slowly to reduce the risk of a postexercise flare in pain, which is defined as having more pain 2 hours after exercise than at baseline.

Sleep

Sleep regulation is an important factor in the progression of MPS. Several comparative studies found significantly reduced sleep quality in patients with MPS than in patients with other pain disorders.[11] In addition, poorer sleep quality predicts higher comorbidity and poorer response to planned therapy. Even in patients without a pain condition who are placed in an experimental setting of frequently disrupted sleep for several nights, investigators report a significant drop in pain threshold and a rise in musculoskeletal discomfort and fatigue.[12] The clinician should discuss sleep difficulties with patients who have MPS and describe strategies to correct sleep as a paramount goal in the treatment plan, such as stress management, sleep hygiene, and biochemical interventions (see Chapter 8, Insomnia).

Mind-Body Therapy

The clinician should assess past or ongoing psychosocial stresses or traumas that may be related to MPS. Several questionnaires (e.g., Millon Behavioral Health Inventory) can help identify stresses or psychogenic attitudes that may be higher in MPS, including premorbid pessimism, future despair, and somatic anxiety.[13] Treatment approaches can be effectively based on the symptoms and patient's preference. Several choices of mind-body therapy are described here.

Relaxation and Awareness Techniques

Relaxation techniques—breathing techniques (see Chapter 89, Breathing Exercises), guided imagery (see Chapter 95, Guided Imagery), mindfulness-based stress reduction, and meditation (see Chapter 98, Recommending Meditation)—are believed to be helpful in pain alleviation and, specifically, the stress-mediated component of myofascial pain through a decrease in autonomic arousal. A reduction in sympathetic arousal specifically and an improvement in parasympathetic tone diminish several key physiologic influences on myofascial pain, including vasospasm, muscle spasm, and adrenal gland–mediated dysfunction in tissue inflammation and nutrient uptake. In addition, techniques such as biofeedback and mindfulness-based stress reduction have an awareness component that can be highly effective in reducing predisposing factors, including

FIGURE 62-1
Integrated mechanism for development of myofascial pain syndrome.

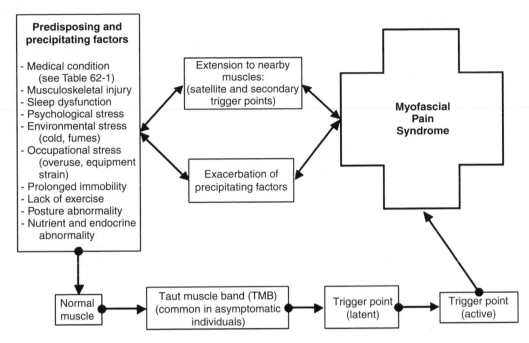

<table>
<tr><td colspan="2">

BOX 62-2. Classic and Confirmatory Signs of Active Trigger Points in Myofascial Pain Syndrome

</td></tr>
</table>

- Palpable, taut muscular band containing a nodular structure
- Tenderness to palpation locally or in referred pattern replicating patient complaints
- Visual or tactile identification of local twitch response produced with needling or snapping ("guitar string") palpation
- Decreased range of movement of the involved muscle
- Increased spontaneous electrical activity on electromyography
- Low skin resistance points found over trigger points, unlike in surrounding tissue (skin resistance may normalize after treatment of trigger points)
- Imaging of local twitch response induced by needle penetration of tender nodule
- Characteristic referred pattern of pain for specific muscles involved (as described by Simmons and Travell[7])

A useful question to ask patients with myofascial pain syndrome is where in the body they carry their stress (neck, back, stomach, head). Have patients use this sign of stress as a "red flag" that, when it appears, encourages them to step back and see what in their life may be exacerbating their pain. Once the subconscious stressor enters the consciousness, the pain often improves because the body no longer needs to sympathize.

poor posture, shallow breathing, and repetitive stress. Several studies have pointed out this benefit.

In one study, a randomized program of physical self-regulation with training in breathing, postural relaxation, and proprioceptive reeducation was taught to 44 patients with myofascial facial pain and compared with standard care. At 26-week follow-up, the two-time, 50-minute intervention demonstrated a significant reduction in pain ($P < .04$); as well as affective distress, somatization, obsessive-compulsive symptoms, tender point sensitivity, and sleep dysfunction.[14]

In addition to being highly effective in decreasing the pain and sequelae of MPS, mind-body techniques can also be cost effective. In another study, a biofeedback-based program implemented in a primary care setting for functional disorders including MPS was measured against standard care ($N = 70$). Implementation of the program brought about significantly lower frequency and severity of symptoms, as well as lower medical costs, for the 6 months after the intervention ($P < .001$).[15] The clinician should reinforce the importance of mind-body techniques in overcoming MPS, a condition that the patient may understand on mainly physical terms. In addition, various techniques should be reviewed to locate those most suitable for the particular patient's needs (see Chapter 93, Relaxation Techniques, and Chapter 100, Emotional Awareness for Pain).

Biomechanical Therapy

Posture Correction
Any active treatment regimen must discuss, train for, and reinforce the need for active postural correction.[16] Dysfunctional posture both at rest and during work activities increases tissue strain and asymmetry. If not corrected, poor posture is theorized as a leading factor in the development and

maintenance of MPS. Evaluation by a well-trained clinician (physical or occupational therapist or body mechanics specialist such as a Feldenkrais or yoga practitioner) can provide invaluable information on the presence and severity of such dysfunction. Baseline and follow-up evaluations by a biofeedback therapist can also be helpful in demonstrating physiologic progress to the patient. Ongoing correction and monitoring can help patients with MPS realize the preventive capabilities of this often overlooked intervention. Several trials demonstrated that postural correction, especially when combined with behavioral therapies, can be successful in decreasing MPS.[17]

Massage Therapy, Manual Therapy, and Myofascial Release Techniques

Massage therapy and manual therapy (MT) have been shown to change several important components of MPS. In general, MT has demonstrated up-regulation of modulatory neurochemicals, including oxytocin, serotonin, and dopamine. Locally, MT has been shown to cause alteration in circulation and range of motion. The efficacy of practitioner-provided MT in MPS was demonstrated in several trials. Specifically, several schools of myofascial release techniques were developed to address the key features of MPS. Many of these techniques are based on Simmons and Travell's foundational work, *Myofascial Pain and Dysfunction: The Trigger Point Manual*[7]. Myofascial release, as well as spray and stretch techniques, should be considered as a first-line approach to MPS[18] (see Chapter 106, Strain/Counterstrain). Providing instructions on identification and home MT of TrPs has been shown to have added benefit in improving TrP sensitivity and pain intensity. Providing passive and active MT works well with other active treatments (thermotherapy and topical therapy) in improving awareness and self-management of MPS.[19]

Low-Level Laser Therapy

Low-level laser therapy (LLLT) has been used for several decades in Europe for pain management, and soft tissue conditions are among the conditions most effectively treated with this technique. The mechanism of action of LLLT is not completely elucidated, but it may be related to improvements in microcirculation, inflammatory response, and adenosine triphosphate production.[20,21] In addition, direct laser treatment of TrPs is believed to increase serotonin production, and trials demonstrated increased excretion of serotonin byproducts after treatment.[22] One 4-week trial (N = 60) comparing LLLT with dry needling and placebo laser demonstrated a significant improvement in pain at rest and with activity, as well as a rise in pain threshold in the laser-treated group.[23] LLLT has the advantage of being noninvasive and thus well tolerated, especially in patients with high tissue sensitivity. The treatment regimen and device specifications vary widely; clinicians should review the available research on the efficacy of the lasers they are considering incorporating into their practices.

Biostimulation

Similar to LLLT, more conventional avenues of biostimulation (e.g., electrical stimulation, ultrasound) have been applied to MPS because of their ability to increase tissue microcirculation and help correct the myofascial contraction-relaxation cycle. The mechanism of action of such techniques is related to correction of electrical disturbances found in TrP areas. Namely,

TrPs typically demonstrate lower resistance and microvoltage abnormalities compared with surrounding tissue. In addition, electrostimulation has been shown to be partially inhibited by the use of naloxone, and thus, its benefit is likely related in part to endorphin up-regulation at the spinal cord and higher centers. Use of these techniques, including transcutaneous electrical nerve stimulation (TENS) and interferential and neuromuscular stimulation (NMS), has provided patient-dependent improvements in pain threshold and range of motion.[18,24] Point-specific devices such as electrotherapeutic point stimulation (ETPS) are also available to help identify and locally address TrPs. Response to these treatments is variable, so several modalities should be tried in the clinic setting to assess response. If one technique is successful, the patient should be taught to use it at home. Figure 62-2 demonstrates the application of various types of biostimulation.

Hydrotherapy and Thermotherapy

As discussed earlier, the tissue of patients with MPS tends to have abnormal microcirculation, which can have negative ramifications, including buildup of inflammatory markers and a drop in tissue temperature and effective range of motion. The application of short-term intense heat (heating pad, diathermy, warm hydrotherapy) and long-term use of low-intensity heat pads can help alter the thermal dysregulation and muscle spasm seen in MPS. Similarly, water immersion, by removing weight from the joints, facilitates reduction in muscle spasm and joint stiffness and thereby facilitates functional mobility. Because of the benign nature of these interventions, patients with MPS should undergo thermotherapy and hydrotherapy when available and, if possible, in combination with other therapies.[18]

Biochemical Therapy

Topical and Transdermal Applications

Topical medications can be a useful adjunct because of their ability to disrupt hypersensitive signaling from the myofascial focus to the spinal cord and higher centers. Lidocaine in various topical formulations (cream, transdermal patch) is believed to block sodium channels that may increase pain signaling. Lidocaine 5% patches were tested in a 1-month open-label trial in 27 patients with myofascial pain.[25] By trial's end, several key parameters, including average pain intensity, mood, sleep, walking ability, and enjoyment of life, were significantly improved ($P < .05$). Antiinflammatory preparations (e.g., transdermal ketoprofen) have been shown to be helpful in related conditions, such as delayed-onset muscle soreness.[26] Moreover, in patients with temporomandibular joint dysfunction, topical applications of diclofenac have demonstrated efficacy similar to that of oral administration, with fewer adverse effects.[27]

Botanical and nonprescription applications, including capsaicin and menthol, appear to have intrinsic local pain modulatory activity.[28,29] Specifically, capsaicin can deplete sensory C-fibers of substance P, the principal neurotransmitter of nociceptive impulses, and can thus potentially decrease central sensitization. Application of topical agents also provides active patient feedback on the location and sensitivity of myofascial pain. Clinicians should become familiar with local compounding pharmacies that can provide topical options for patients with myofascial pain.

FIGURE 62-2
Application of various types of biostimulation in myofascial pain syndrome. **A,** Interferential and neuromuscular stimulation. (RS 4i unit courtesy of RS Medical, Vancouver, Wash.) **B,** Individual trigger point electrostimulation. (Electrotherapeutic point stimulation unit courtesy of Acumed Medical Supplies, Toronto.) **C** and **D,** Low-level laser therapy. (**C,** Courtesy of Theralase, Markham, Ontario, Canada; **D,** Courtesy of Meditech International, Toronto.)

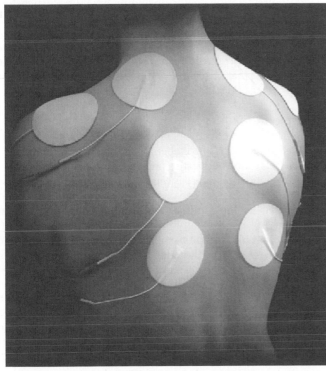

A

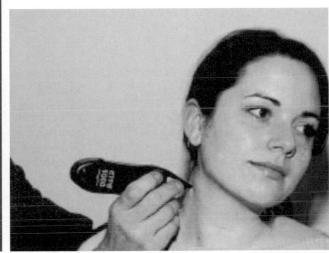

B

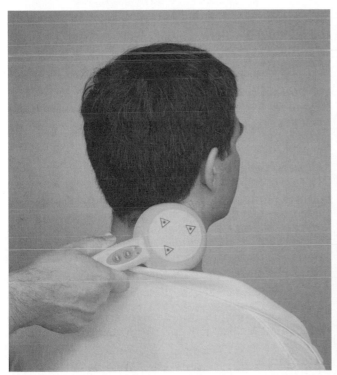

C

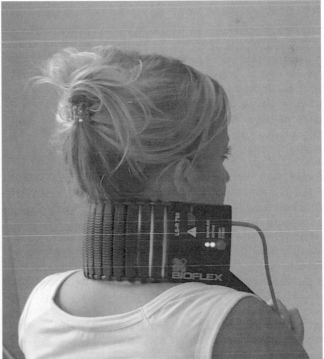

D

■ Dosage

Patients can apply up to three lidocaine 5% (Lidoderm) patches for up to 12 hours. Patches can be cut to size, and they come in a carton of 30 patches.

Patients can apply the capsaicin 0.025% patch (which also comes in 0.025%, 0.035%, 0.05%, 0.075%, 0.1, and 0.25% cream, gel, and lotion formulation) to the painful area three to four times daily for 3 to 4 consecutive weeks to reduce pain sensitivity. Patients should wash their hands and avoid their eyes after applying capsaicin.

Each diclofenac (Flector Patch) patch contains 180 mg of diclofenac, and one box contains five patches. One patch is applied to the painful areas twice daily.

Compounding pharmacies can prepare creams and gels with ketoprofen (the preferred compounded nonsteroidal antiinflammatory drug [NSAID]) combined with other agents (e.g., lidocaine, cyclobenzaprine, capsaicin). A dime-sized amount of gel (start with 10% to 20%) is rubbed into the painful area every 8 hours as needed.

Trigger Point Needling or Injection

Various needling and injection techniques have been endorsed for treatment of myofascial pain. The mechanistic rationale for the use of these techniques is based on several lines of evidence. The simplest technique, dry needling of primary TrPs, has demonstrated reversal of spontaneous electrical activity, one of the hallmark abnormalities noted in MPS.[30] Dry needle-evoked inactivation of a primary TrP in the shoulder region also improves pain sensitivity of satellite TrPs, as well as range of motion in the zone of pain referral.[31] Additionally, certain types of dry needling may activate muscle afferents more effectively than superficial needling to produce segmental analgesia.[32–36]

Injection techniques that involve introduction of sterile water, saline solution, or various pharmaceutical agents are conjectured to provide adjunctive benefit to needling, based on both the properties of the injected agent and the tissue pressure effects created by the volume of agent introduced. The appropriateness and superiority of various techniques, including dry needling and the injection of saline, anesthetics, corticosteroids, and botulinum toxin type A have not been clarified in clinical trials and systematic reviews because of variation in trial size and methodology.[37,38] Several trials found no distinct advantage for TrP injection over dry needling.[39, 40] Further, studies have both demonstrated and refuted the advantage of injection of active drug (e.g., lidocaine, botulinum toxin) over saline injection.[41,42]

Without a clear advantage of needling interventions, dry needling and acupuncture (see later) are initially recommended to evaluate their efficacy and patient tolerance. Injection of saline and other active agents should be reserved for more advanced or refractory cases and administered by clinicians with the proper understanding of the role of these agents in comprehensive management. Although injection therapy is potentially effective in short-term TrP management, it is often pursued without regard to the global needs of patients with MPS. To minimize a repetitive cycle of passive interventions, clinicians are admonished to address triggers and active treatment options for MPS (e.g., posture correction, home stretching, mind-body therapies) that are pursued in conjunction with injection therapy. All needle interventions with potential benefit are based on the experience of the practitioner in isolating TrPs. Adverse effects may be related to incorrect needle placement, reaction to the injected agent, or improper use of the aseptic technique.

Pharmaceuticals

Certain prescription agents, including NSAIDs, corticosteroids, muscle relaxants, antidepressants (especially tricyclic), anxiolytics, and opiates are mentioned in the treatment of MPS. Unfortunately, when looking at their efficacy in the setting of temporomandibular disorder–associated MPS, one review noted that "… evidence in support of the effectiveness of these drugs is lacking."[43]

Muscle Relaxants

Evidence for the effectiveness of muscle relaxants (e.g., tizanidine hydrochloride, cyclobenzaprine) and medication with muscle relaxation properties, including benzodiazepines and tricyclic antidepressants, is variable in MPS.[44] A Cochrane Review examining the use of cyclobenzaprine in MPS found that, based on the minimal available published research in this area and the difficulty in estimating risk versus benefit, evidence was insufficient to support the use of this drug in the treatment of MPS.[45] Although not routinely endorsed, muscle relaxants may be worth a short-term trial to assess improvement while initiating a multimodality program. In a randomized trial of temporomandibular disorder, cyclobenzaprine (10 mg/night) was compared with clonazepam (0.5 mg/night). Cyclobenzaprine was better than placebo and clonazepam when incorporated into a program of self-care and education for the management of jaw pain. Unfortunately, no significant improvement in sleep was noted.[46]

■ Dosage

Cyclobenzaprine, 10 mg at bedtime taken for a limited course, may provide some pain relief for temporomandibular disorder.

■ Precautions

This drug is structurally related to tricyclic antidepressants. Caution should be used when cyclobenzaprine is taken with this class of drugs.

Nonsteroidal Antiinflammatory Drugs

The use of NSAIDs may be justified in the short-term treatment of acute myofascial strain. In one study, ibuprofen appeared to work as well without the addition of a muscle relaxant (800 mg of ibuprofen three times/day, with or without the use of cyclobenzaprine 10 mg three times/day).[47] However, less evidence is available on the long-term use of NSAIDs in the setting of MPS.

■ Dosage

Ibuprofen, 800 mg three times daily with meals for short periods of time, can help reduce the pain of myofascial strain.

Antidepressants

Antidepressants are often considered in the setting MPS because of potential benefit in common mood and sleep comorbidities. The benefit of these agents for primary MPS in nondepressed individuals may not be significant, however, with the possible exception of amitriptyline, which was tested (at 75 mg/day) in a small ($N = 31$), 32-week placebo-controlled double-blind three-way crossover study trial versus the highly selective serotonin reuptake inhibitor citalopram (at 20 mg/day). Study participants taking amitriptyline had significantly reduced myofascial tenderness and headache intensity than participants taking placebo ($P = .01$ and $P = .04$, respectively). The researchers concluded that amitriptyline may elicit its analgesic effect in myofascial pain by reducing transmission of painful stimuli from myofascial tissue, as opposed to reducing overall pain sensitivity: "We suggest that this effect is caused by a segmental reduction of central sensitization in combination with a peripheral anti-nociceptive action."[48]

Dosage

Amitriptyline, 75 mg at bedtime, can reduce myofascial pain and headaches.

Diet and Dietary Supplements

Myofascial pain has been attributed to abnormalities (typically, functional or intracellular deficiencies) of several nutrients, although no consensus exists about individual nutrients. Specifically, deficiencies of minerals (e.g., magnesium, calcium, and zinc) and vitamins or enzymes (e.g., vitamin D, vitamin B_{12}, and coenzyme Q10) have been reported in patients with MPS.[49] The level and type of deficiency, however, have not been consistent. In one trial, significant deficiencies in zinc levels in patients with MPS versus controls were noted without similar deficiencies in other nutrients such as magnesium or folic acid. These results may have reflected the type of testing done, including traditional extracellular versus intracellular testing. Although typical electrolyte analyses ("panels") may rule out gross abnormalities, levels of these electrolytes are usually normal in MPS. Clinicians should be aware of ionized or intracellular testing methods (e.g., SpectraCell, SpectraCell Laboratories, Houston) that may identify more occult deficiencies. The response to replacement of nutrients (e.g., magnesium in the setting of migraine) appears to be more highly correlated with intracellular or ionized fraction level, but not total serum levels.[50-52] On the basis of identified or suspected nutrient abnormalities, clinicians should use focused dietary and nutrient supplementation with careful patient monitoring of symptoms, to note any possible improvement.

> Consider checking serum levels of vitamin B_{12}, 25-hydroxyvitamin D, coenzyme Q10, and electrolytes, as well as red blood cell magnesium levels in patients with myofascial pain syndrome.

Recommendations on the use of dietary supplements in MPS suffer from inconsistencies, as noted earlier.[53] Especially in patients with refractory cases of MPS unresponsive to lifestyle change, clinicians should proceed with supplements that may possess properties beneficial for pain and comorbid symptoms. A stepwise approach in which dietary supplements are incorporated and evaluated on a 2- to 3-month trial basis (i.e., a therapeutic trial) is suggested. These supplements may include those helpful for muscle function (e.g., magnesium, malic acid, calcium, vitamin D, coenzyme Q10), antiinflammatory action (e.g., essential fatty acids, white willow bark, *Boswellia*), or comorbidities such as sleep or mood dysfunction (e.g., St. John's wort, *S*-adenyl-L-methionine [SAMe], valerian, melatonin). As with prescription medications, the use of dietary supplements should be monitored on a regular basis to ensure benefit and to minimize adverse reactions.

Bioenergetics

Traditional Chinese Medicine

The use of traditional Chinese medicine, specifically acupuncture, was one of the earliest attempted treatments of MPS. More recently, investigators have speculated about the correlation between acupuncture and myofascial TrPs. In 1977, Melzack et al[54] postulated an approximately 70% correlation between these two entities, although this correlation has been disputed.[55] Because of the likely coexistence of these entities, a separate discussion of dry needling and localized acupuncture appears somewhat arbitrary. However, acupuncture offers treatment avenues based on meridian and energetic dysfunction, which may entail treatment at distal or reflex points (auricular therapy) and thereby provide additional therapeutic options.[56] The global assessment of the patient that is undertaken in Chinese medicine is especially helpful in MPS because of likely comorbidities that must be considered in the formulation of a treatment plan.

The specific type of acupuncture pursued for MPS is somewhat controversial. Several reports argue that deep needling may be more effective in decreasing MPS than superficial needling, although the two terms have not been well defined.[34,35] Conversely, Japanese acupuncture treatment, which typically uses superficial needling, was also shown to be effective in MPS in controlled trials.[57] The depth, frequency, and duration of treatments should be tailored to the patient; treatments typically should take place one or more times per week initially, followed by a gradual decrease with functional improvement.

PREVENTION PRESCRIPTION

- Encourage posture awareness with frequent repositioning and adaptive stretching to reduce strain.
- Consider an ergonomic evaluation if patients remain in one position for prolonged periods at work.
- Incorporate stress management techniques to identify and reduce stress buildup. Ask patients to pay attention to where they carry stress in the body and use this to learn from the body's symptoms.
- Incorporate a regular exercise and movement program. At a minimum, patients should exercise three times/week for 30 minutes each session while stimulating movement, range of motion, and tone in all muscle groups.
- Encourage adequate quantity and quality of sleep.
- Encourage the consumption of a healthy diet rich in fruits and vegetables with adequate fluid content to ensure perfusion to muscles.
- Encourage maintenance of an ideal weight.

THERAPEUTIC REVIEW

Myofascial pain syndrome (MPS) is a disorder that affects up to 85% of the general population at some point and is primarily characterized by local and referred pain, as well as comorbidities affecting mood, sleep, energy, and functional status. Although numerous treatment options are available, no widely accepted treatment guidelines exist. Clinically, MPS is a condition that is often difficult to treat, and physicians often characterize available treatments as insufficient.[4] Based on its complex nature, MPS is a condition that requires a biopsychosocial evaluation and incorporation of individualized, preferably active, treatments option geared at underlying propagating factors with a focus on long-term neurobehavioral and functional rehabilitation.

◼ Exclusion and Treatment of Conditions That Mimic or Contribute to Myofascial Pain Syndrome

- See Table 62-1.
- Symptom-focused laboratory testing should be considered, including 25-OH vitamin D_3, coenzyme Q10, carnitine, vitamin B_{12}, folate, methylmalonic acid, and, as appropriate, baseline thyroid-stimulating hormone, creatine phosphokinase, alkaline phosphatase, and complete blood count and electrolytes with intracellular magnesium to rule out modifiable causes of MPS and associated symptoms.

◼ Removal of Exacerbating Factors

- Take measures to correct sleep dysfunction, including sleep hygiene and other interventions.
- Increase awareness of stress and environmental triggers (poor posture, repetitive stress) by using periodic daily cues.

◼ Lifestyle Measures

- Incorporate stress management techniques
- Biofeedback, preferred for baseline myofascial and autonomic measures and retraining efforts
- Guided imagery
- Meditation
- Exercise to decrease deconditioning and improve myofascial biomechanics. Mindful exercise (e.g., yoga, tai chi) is especially helpful in improving MPS.

◼ Biomechanical Interventions

- Posture evaluation and correction: Consider ongoing optimization with yoga, Feldenkrais, and physical therapy.

- Manual and manipulative techniques, including massage, myofascial release, and spray and stretch: These should be considered in areas of distinct trigger points. Osteopathic manipulation is desired when functional skeletal asymmetry is provoking MPS. Refer to Simmons and Travell[7] for detailed instructions. Several techniques can be taught to and successfully incorporated by the patient (e.g., compression massage with stretch).
- Biostimulation: Low-level laser therapy, electrostimulation, hydrotherapy, and thermotherapy are recommended on a regular basis to assess reduction in symptoms, especially pain, with transition to home therapy.

◼ Bioenergetic Interventions

- Acupuncture is used to release trigger points and decrease autonomic arousal.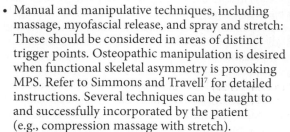
- Other energetic treatments (e.g., healing touch, Reiki) should be used to assess for and treat energy imbalance.

◼ Nutrition

- Have patients increase their intake of fruits and vegetables, with a focus on appropriate levels of vitamins and minerals essential for musculoskeletal function.
- Consider a trial of an antiinflammatory diet or elimination diet (see Chapter 86, The Antiinflammatory [Omega-3] Diet, and Chapter 84, Food Intolerance and Elimination Diet).

◼ Supplements

- Consider an 8- to 12-week trial of supplements for correction of myofascial pain and comorbid conditions (including identified deficiencies):
  - Magnesium: starting with a chelated form if available for increased gastrointestinal tolerance; magnesium glycinate, 100 to 200 mg twice daily, advance as tolerated (other formulation doses vary; typically, starting at a low dose and advanced based on gastrointestinal tolerance)
  - Malic acid: 600 mg, one to two capsules daily
  - Carnitine: 2000 mg/day
  - D-Ribose: 5 g twice daily
  - Coenzyme Q10: 100 to 300 mg/day (dose increased based on response and serum levels)
  - B vitamins typically used: 50 to 100 mg of thiamine (vitamin B_1) and pyridoxine (vitamin B_6), 0.5 to 2 mg of folic acid and vitamin B_{12}
  - Vitamin D_3: 800 to 1000 units/day (higher levels in deficiency states)

■ Pharmaceuticals

- Topical pharmaceuticals

  - Compounded creams with ingredients based on patient presentation are applied to affected areas three times/day. Patients should be warned that some topical agents cause localized burning or rare allergic reactions. Systemic absorption negligible if these agents are used as directed.

  - Ketoprofen 10% to 20%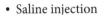

  - Lidocaine 5%

  - Capsaicin 0.025% to 0.075%

  - Cyclobenzaprine 5%

  - Oral pharmaceutical

- If the response to other interventions is unsatisfactory, consider a trial of amitriptyline (up to 75 mg/day) for long-term treatment, as well as a trial of short-term antiinflammatory agents for acute exacerbations.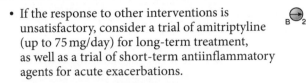

- Needle-based injection therapy

  - If the patient's symptoms persist or worsen despite the preceding measures, consider needle-based intervention in a stepwise approach.

  - Acupuncture or dry needling

  - Saline injection

  - Anesthetic injection (e.g., a combination of 2% lidocaine and 0.05% bupivacaine in a 1:3 ratio up to 8 mL total)

  - Botox injection

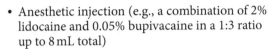
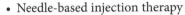

All treatments should be well integrated, with the goal of improving patient awareness of biomechanical and stress triggers. Treatments should gradually move from passive (practitioner directed and supervised) to active (patient initiated), with improving awareness of the patient's ability to address and diminish the myofascial pain cycle.

KEY WEB RESOURCES

Mayo Clinic: Myofascial Pain Syndrome: http://www.mayoclinic.com/health/myofascial-painsyndrome/DS01042/METHOD=print	Handout on myofascial pain syndrome for patients
ReliefInsite: www.reliefinsite.com American Chronic Pain Association: http://www.theacpa.org Pain log: http://www.theacpa.org/painlog/painlog.aspx	Web sites that offer pain tracking tools to enhance communication with the health care provider
Mayo Clinic: Stress Management: http://www.mayoclinic.com/health/relaxation-technique/SR00007 University of Wisconsin Health Services: Stress and Sleep: http://www.uhs.wisc.edu/services/wellness/stress.shtml	Stress management and relaxation tools Resources for stress and sleep management
UCLA Ergonomics: http://ergonomics.ucla.edu/exercises.html	Exercise and stretching guides that can be done at home
Arthritis Foundation: http://www.arthritis.org YMCA: http://www.ymca.net/	Organizations offering exercise and stretching classes, including aquatic therapy

References

References are available online at expertconsult.com.

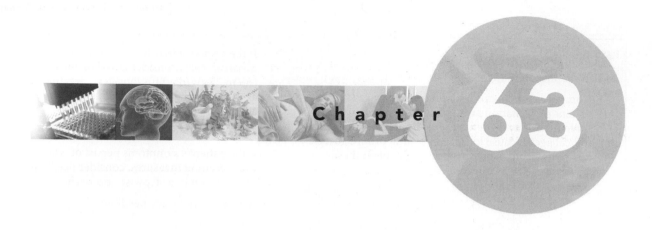

Chapter 63

Chronic Low Back Pain

Joel M. Stevans, DC, and Robert B. Saper, MD, MPH

Low back pain (LBP), the most common type of pain in the United States, results in substantial morbidity, disability, and cost to society.[1-6] Annual direct costs associated with this condition are more than $50 billion in the United States, and indirect costs (e.g., productivity) are estimated to be even greater.[6,7]

The lifetime prevalence of LBP ranges between 60% and 85%; therefore, most adults will experience an episode of LBP at least once during their lifetime.[8] LBP is the fifth most common reason for visits to primary care physicians, and it is the single most common reason that U.S. adults use complementary and alternative medicine.[9] Of these alternative therapies, manipulation, massage, acupuncture, and mind-body approaches such as yoga are frequently used.[10] The prognosis for acute LBP (ALBP) is very good. Most episodes resolve within 6 weeks, regardless of treatment given. Recurrence rates are high (20% to 35%), however, and approximately 5% to 20% of patients will go on to develop chronic LBP (CLBP).[11-13]

Despite its high prevalence and substantial impact on patients, the medical system, and society, back pain remains poorly understood, with relatively little consensus on optimal treatment. An integrative approach, in which the evidence for various conventional and complementary and alternative medicine therapies is considered in the context of the patient's clinical picture, preferences, and values, is therefore ideally suited to address this costly and complex condition.

Pathophysiology

LBP is a vexing clinical problem. Two conceptual frameworks have emerged for the evaluation and treatment of this condition. The first is the biomedical model, which characterizes signs and symptoms to identify the causative agent and thereby allows delivery of targeted biologically oriented interventions.[14] This model is necessary and best suited for initial evaluation and for ruling out serious disorders. The second conceptual framework is the biopsychosocial model.[15] This paradigm requires the clinician to expand on the biomedical model and accept the nonspecific nature of

LBP. The purpose of the biopsychosocial evaluation shifts from the characterization of a causative agent to the identification of inappropriate attitudes and beliefs, high levels of distress, and fear avoidance behaviors that can impede recovery of function and place the patient at higher risk for developing CLBP. To manage patients with back pain effectively, providers must use both approaches.

ALBP is defined as pain in the lumbosacral region, with or without leg pain, that has been present for less than 6 weeks.[14] The condition is considered subacute when it has been present for 6 to 12 weeks. By extension, CLBP is defined as pain persisting for more than 12 weeks. Patients with ALBP and CLBP are challenging because a definitive pathoanatomic cause of the condition can be identified only in approximately 15% of cases. Definitive causes of LBP include disk herniation with suspected radiculopathy or spinal stenosis (5%), osteoporotic compression fracture (4%), and inflammatory arthropathies (3%) (Fig. 63-1). Other specific organic causes of LBP are cancer and infection (1%), cauda equina syndrome (less than 1%) and visceral disorders (less than 2%) such as aortic aneurysm and pelvic, gastrointestinal, and renal disease.[1,14,16] These definitive causes are uncommon, and most patients presenting with back pain have nonspecific LBP. Nonspecific back pain may emanate from ligaments, facet joints, muscle, fascia, nerve roots, the vertebral periosteum, or the outer portion of the disk.[1] However, precise identification of a specific diagnosis is not necessary to manage these patients effectively. In fact, far too often patients with nonspecific back pain see multiple providers and pursue a biomedical model by undergoing numerous tests and imaging procedures in a futile attempt to identify an exact cause of the pain. This exhaustive effort to identify the precise cause of the pain is time consuming and costly, and it can lead to frustration for both patient and provider. The prognosis for most patients with ALBP is good, and most patients are effectively managed with a brief assessment, patient education, judicious use of analgesics, and reassurance.

FIGURE 63-1

Specific pathoanatomic conditions causing low back pain. **A,** Lateral view of the lumbosacral spine illustrating spondylolysis of the L5 vertebra with associated spondylolisthesis at L5-S1. *Spondylolysis* refers to a defect in the pars interarticularis of the vertebra, which may be congenital or a result of stress fracture. *Spondylolisthesis* refers to the anterior displacement of a vertebra on the one beneath it. This may occur as a result of spondylolysis, as shown, or as a result of degenerative disk disease, usually in older adults. This process may contribute to narrowing of the spinal canal in spinal stenosis. **B,** The lumbar spinal canal in health and disease. *Left,* The normal spinal canal. *Center,* The spinal canal in central spinal and nerve root canal stenosis in the neutral position. *Right,* The effect of lumbar extension on the spinal canal. (From Deyo RA, Weinstein JN. Low back pain. *N Engl J Med.* 2001;344:363–370.)

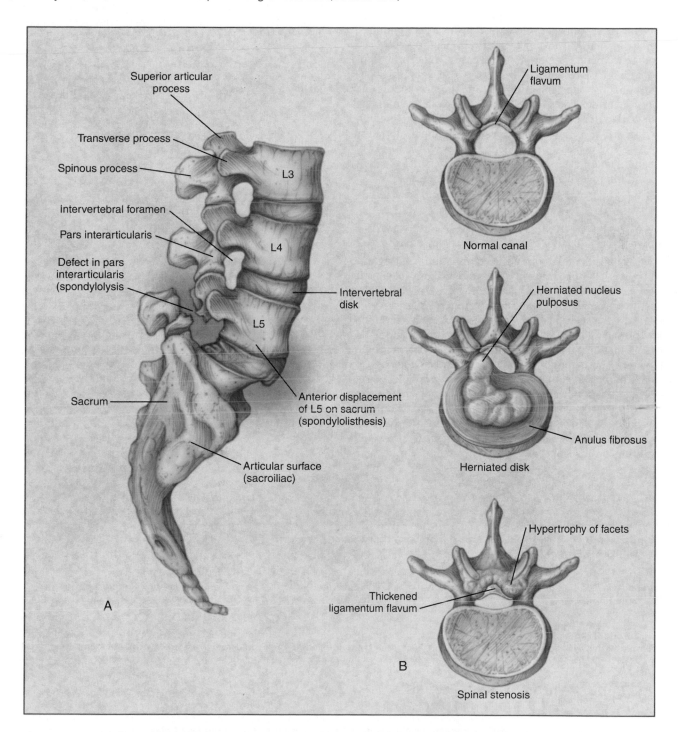

Applying a biopsychosocial model to patients with LBP is particularly appropriate to identify factors that may predispose a patient with ALBP to CLBP or that may perpetuate the chronicity of a preexisting back problem. In fact, many of the most important predictors of ongoing disabling low back problems are fear avoidance and inappropriate pain coping behaviors, nonorganic signs on physical examination (Table 63-1), and psychiatric comorbidities.[17] Therefore, clinicians must recognize that the patient's experience of LBP can be positively or negatively shaped by his or her attitudes, beliefs (e.g., fear of movement and reinjury), psychosocial factors (e.g., mood, support systems, employment and occupation, financial resources), behaviors (e.g., coping skills, catastrophizing, substance abuse), and family, social, and cultural environments[18-20] (Fig. 63-2). Often, a self-reinforcing downward cycle of avoidance and disuse can lead to increasing distress and functional and occupational disability (Fig. 63-3). In contrast, motivated patients with less fear of movement and greater self-efficacy can better manage their pain and improve their function over the long term.

Evaluation

History
Patients with ALBP or CLBP should be evaluated with a comprehensive history and physical examination. During the workup, it is helpful to think in terms of three basic diagnostic categories: nonspecific LBP, back pain with suspected radiculopathy or spinal stenosis, or back pain that is a result of a specific disease.[16] The history should begin with a description of the primary complaint, to identify pain severity and functional limitations. The patient should be questioned about the pattern and nature of any lower extremity symptoms, as well as the presence of significant neurologic deficits, gait abnormalities, or bowel or bladder dysfunction. Attention to any history of trauma, immunosuppression, constitutional symptoms, substance use, comorbidities, and previous history of back troubles including spinal surgery is important. In addition, postures or spinal loading strategies (e.g., flexion, extension) that aggravate or palliate the patient's lumbar spine or extremity symptoms should be explored.

Physical Examination
Emphasis in the examination should be placed on back inspection, palpation, range-of-motion testing, orthopedic maneuvers, and a comprehensive neurologic evaluation. The clinician should observe the patient for antalgic posture, the Gower sign (using hands to "walk" up the thighs from a flexed

FIGURE 63-2
Biopsychosocial model of pain. (From Main CJ, Williams AC. ABC of psychological medicine: musculoskeletal pain. *BMJ.* 2002;325:534–537)

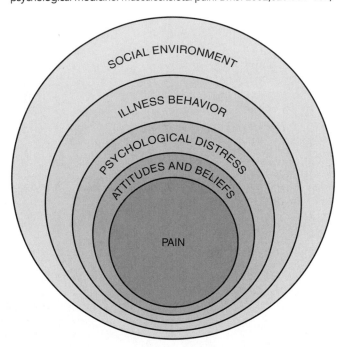

TABLE 63-1. Waddell's Nonorganic Signs*	
SIGN	**DESCRIPTION**
Superficial or Nonanatomic Tenderness	Pain with light or superficial palpation of the skin, or widespread deep tenderness that is not localized to one skeletal or neuromuscular structure, does not follow an anatomic distribution, and often extends to the thoracic spine, sacrum, or pelvis
Pain on Axial Loading or Simulated Rotation	Pain with downward pressure applied to the top of the patient's head when standing, or back pain when the shoulders and pelvis are passively rotated as a unit with the patient standing relaxed with the feet together
Nonreproducibility of Pain When Patient Is Distracted	A positive physical finding elicited during the examination that is not present later in the examination when the patient is distracted and the finding is checked again (e.g., pain with a standard straight leg raise test, but not when the examiner passively extends the leg of a seated patient)
Regional Weakness or Sensory Change	Regional, nonanatomic sensory change (stocking sensory loss, or sensory loss in an entire extremity or side of the body) or regional weakness (weakness that is jerky, with intermittent resistance such as cogwheeling or catching)
Overreaction	An exaggerated painful response to a stimulus that is not reproduced when the same stimulus is given later, or an exaggerated response to a stimulus that should not cause back pain (e.g., gently pinching the skin on the back in the area of pain)

*Elicitation of one or more of these signs on physical examination suggests a nonorganic or psychological component to the patient's back pain.
Adapted from Chou R, Shekelle P. Will this patient develop persistent disabling low back pain? *JAMA.* 2010;303:1295–1302.

position because of proximal leg weakness), or reverse lumbopelvic rhythm (bending knees to return from flexed position).[21,22] Range-of-motion testing, especially repetitive flexion and extension, is informative. Particular attention should be paid to repetitive movements that centralize the pain or cause it to move from a more peripheral location (e.g., buttocks) to a more central location (midline of the lumbar spine). Orthopedic tests such as the straight leg raise and slump test (the seated Lasègue test) may be useful in identifying nerve root tension.[23] The neurologic examination should focus on the L4, L5, and S1 myotomes (heel and toe walking), dermatomes (light touch or pin prick sensation), and deep tendon reflexes (knee and ankle)[16,24–28] (Table 63-2).

The presence or absence of *red flags* (signs or symptoms suggestive of serious definitive but less common causes of back pain including cauda equina syndrome, cancer, fracture, infection, severe disk disease or spinal stenosis with radiculopathy, and progressive neurologic deficits) must be determined first.[16,24–27] Table 63-3 lists constellations of red flags concerning for specific disorders causing LBP and recommendations for prompt further evaluation and referral.[16,24–26,28–30] For patients with suspected radiculopathy or spinal stenosis, a combination of watchful waiting and conservative treatment measures aimed at alleviating pain and improving function is appropriate. If these patients demonstrate persistent leg pain or neurologic findings after 4 to 6 weeks of conservative care, however, orthopedic or neurosurgical referral is indicated.[1]

Imaging

The consensus across major international LBP practice guidelines is that plain radiographs, computed tomography (CT), and magnetic resonance imaging (MRI) are of limited benefit in most patients with back pain. These recommendations are based on the knowledge that abnormal imaging findings are common in asymptomatic individuals, and such findings are poorly correlated with symptom severity and clinical outcomes.[31–33] Despite these facts, the use of imaging procedures continues to rise.[31] For many patients, these findings are irrelevant and may foster detrimental beliefs about their condition. A meta-analysis concluded that "immediate, routine lumbar-spine imaging in patients with low back pain and no features suggesting serious underlying conditions did not improve clinical outcomes."[34] Lumbar imaging should be primarily reserved for the investigation of definitive causes of back pain in patients with *red flags*, such as substantial or progressive neurologic involvement.[16,24,35,36]

Subgrouping

Clinicians increasingly appreciate that the broadly defined category of nonspecific back pain does not represent a uniform population of patients. Many clinicians argue that nonspecific LBP is in fact a heterogeneous condition, and therefore, a "one size fits all" treatment approach leads to unsatisfactory results.[37] This situation has led to several attempts to subgroup patients, by linking each subgroup to a specific treatment with the goal of identifying best management strategies.[38–40] Two of the better-studied methods of subgrouping patients with back pain are the Treatment-Based Classification (TBC) system and the McKenzie Method of Mechanical Treatment and Diagnosis (MTD). The TBC uses specific clusters of signs and symptoms to classify patients into one of three main categories: specific exercises (flexion, extension, and lateral shift patterns), stabilization exercises, and manipulation. A specific set of therapeutic interventions is suggested for each of these categories. The MTD classifies patients by evaluating the cause and effect relationship

FIGURE 63-3

Downward cycle of fear avoidance, disuse, and disability. (Adapted from Main CJ, Williams AC. ABC of psychological medicine: musculoskeletal pain. *BMJ* 2002;325:534–537.)

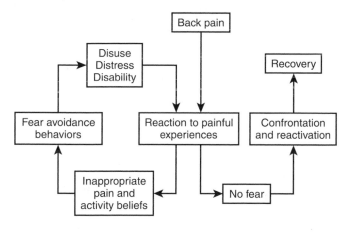

TABLE 63-2. Lumbosacral Nerve Root Syndromes

NERVE ROOT	SYMPTOMS	SIGNS
L2-4	Acute back pain radiating around the anterior leg into the knee and possibly the foot	Decreased hip flexion, knee extension, leg abduction; decreased sensation in the anterior thigh down to the medial aspect of the lower leg; diminished knee reflex in severe cases
L5	Back pain radiating down the lateral leg to the foot	Decreased foot dorsiflexion, toe extension, foot inversion and eversion; mild weakness of leg abduction in severe cases
S1	Pain radiating down the posterior leg to the foot; leg pain greater than back pain	Decreased leg extension, foot inversion, plantar flexion, and toe flexion; decreased sensation in the posterior leg and lateral foot; loss of ankle reflex
S2-4	Sacral or buttock pain radiating down the posterior leg or into the perineum	Leg weakness; saddle anesthesia; bowel and bladder dysfunction

Adapted from Rutkove SB. Overview of lower extremity peripheral nerve syndromes. In: Basow DS, ed. *UpToDate*. Waltham, MA: UpToDate; 2010.

TABLE 63-3. Specific Conditions Causing Low Back Pain

SYNDROME	RED FLAGS	FURTHER EVALUATION
Cauda Equina Syndrome	• Widespread neurologic symptoms • Fecal incontinence or urinary retention • Weakness in limbs and/or gait abnormality • Saddle numbness	• Medical Emergency: immediate magnetic resonance imaging and neurosurgical referral
Lumbar Radiculopathy	• Severe lower extremity pain • Significant neurologic deficits indicative of nerve root compression • Sensory impairment, weakness, or diminished deep tendon reflexes consistent with nerve root distribution	• If no improvement with conservative treatment after 6 weeks, magnetic resonance imaging considered
Spinal Canal Stenosis	• Pain, sensory loss, or weakness in one or both legs • Pain worse with walking or standing • Pain relieved with sitting or lumbar flexion	• Magnetic resonance imaging
Spondyloarthropathy	Presence of four or more of the following: • Age younger than 40 years • Insidious onset • Improvement with exercise • No improvement with rest • Pain at night (with improvement on arising or walking)	• HLA-B27 • Erythrocyte sedimentation rate • C-reactive protein
Cancer	• History of cancer • Age older than 50 years • Failure to improve with treatment • Worsening pain especially at night, at rest, or when lying down • Urinary retention	• Erythrocyte sedimentation rate • Plain film radiographs • Magnetic resonance imaging
Fracture	• Age older than 50 years • Osteoporosis • Significant trauma • Steroid use • Structural deformity	• Plain film radiographs (cannot distinguish new from old compression fractures) • Computed tomography • Magnetic resonance imaging
Infection	• Fever • Immunosuppression • Intravenous drug use • Multiple comorbidities • Trauma	• Complete blood count • Erythrocyte sedimentation rate • C-reactive protein • Magnetic resonance imaging

between a patient's historical pain behavior and the pain response to repeated test movements, positions, and activities. The MTD describes three syndromes: postural (end-range stress of normal structures), dysfunction (end-range stress of shortened structures possibly resulting from scarring, fibrosis, or nerve root adhesion), and derangement (anatomic disruption or displacement within the spinal segment). Each distinct syndrome is addressed with specific static physical postures and repetitive movements.[41]

Yellow Flags

Screening for *yellow flags* (factors associated with a poor prognosis for LBP) is also critical (Table 63-4).[14,18,19,36] Clinicians must uncover unhelpful beliefs that a patient may hold about his or her back pain. For example, beliefs that back pain is the result of a progressive disorder, or that passive treatment rather than active self-management is most beneficial, must be identified and corrected. Questioning patients about their beliefs regarding what can cause and help their pain, and observing for guarded movements and avoidance patterns during the examination, can

help identify patients with *fear avoidance beliefs*. Identifying and correcting beliefs that physical activity and the resultant discomfort can be harmful for the back is important because these beliefs can perpetuate a vicious cycle of disuse and disability.[16,18,25] Depression, anxiety, maladaptive responses to stress, and social withdrawal should be explored and addressed as necessary.[16,25,42] Patients' economic circumstances and workplace factors such as low job satisfaction, high physical job demands, inability to modify work demands, high levels of job stress, low workplace social support, or dysfunctional workplace relationships may also perpetuate LBP.[14,18]

Integrative Therapy

The goals of LBP treatment should be to enhance coping skills, restructure inappropriate beliefs, and improve functional ability and activity tolerance. Therapeutic interventions need to be coordinated in an effort to achieve this end, and special emphasis should be placed on active patient participation, rather than passive treatments.

TABLE 63-4. Yellow Flags: Risk Factors for Disability and Chronic Low Back Pain

PSYCHOSOCIAL FACTORS	OCCUPATIONAL FACTORS	INTERVIEW QUESTIONS
• Inappropriate attitudes and beliefs • Poor or maladaptive coping strategies • High levels of emotional distress • Fear avoidance behavior • Depressed mood and social isolation • Resistance to change • Family reinforcement of illness behavior	• Work status • Low job satisfaction • High physical job demands • Inability to modify work • High levels of job stress • Working conditions • Worker's compensation claim or litigation • Health benefits and insurance	• What do you believe is causing your back pain? • What do you think will help your back pain? • Do you think your pain will ever get better? • How do you deal or cope with your back pain? • Have you been feeling worried, down, or blue? • How do your family, friends, and coworkers respond when you have pain? • Have you had time off work because of your back pain? • When do you think you will return to work?

Education and Self-Care

Education concerning the benign nature of most back pain, recovery goals, and appropriate self-care should be provided to all patients with ALBP or CLBP.[16,24,25] Brief educational interventions can be effective in reducing disability by reassuring the patient, dispelling inappropriate beliefs regarding back pain, promoting self-management, and encouraging a return to normal activities.[16,24-27] Examples of useful educational messages and self-management strategies include the following:

• Stay active and carry on as normally as possible.

• Staying active may "hurt" but will not cause "harm."

• Perform physical activities in manageable, graded stages.

• Track your own functional progress, and do more each day.

Working with the patient to correct misunderstandings, identify barriers to recovery, instill healthy coping strategies, and empower the individual to take responsibility for the long-term management of the condition is particularly important.[14,18]

> Identify and correct beliefs that physical activity will worsen back pain.

Mind-Body Therapy

Behavioral Therapy

Behavioral therapy refers to various approaches that include cognitive-behavioral, operant, and respondent methods. Cognitive-behavioral therapy is based on the premise that an individual's thoughts (as opposed to external factors such as injury, people, or environmental circumstances) trigger his or her feelings and behaviors.[43] The benefit of this approach is that a positive change in thoughts and beliefs can lead to positive changes in feelings and behaviors even if the back pain remains unchanged.[43] Operant therapy uses reinforcement to change behavior. This reinforcement may be a reward for attainment of a goal or certain behavior. Alternatively, operant therapy can use a lack of reinforcement for certain maladaptive behaviors such as activity avoidance or catastrophizing. Respondent therapies, such as progressive muscle relaxation, aim to modify physiologic responses through self-training.[44,45] Evidence shows that behavioral therapy is more effective than usual care for short-term pain relief and behavioral outcomes.[46,47] Additionally, rates of return to work are better for patients receiving behavioral therapy when compared with rest, analgesics, physical therapy, or back exercises.[46] Specifically, operant conditioning has been shown to be more effective than wait list controls for short-term pain relief. Cognitive-behavioral therapy has also been shown to improve pain and disability outcomes compared with wait list controls.[46,47] When different behavioral techniques have been compared with one another, no significant differences have been found.[46] Behavioral therapies may be considered as treatment options for patients with CLBP[16,24-27] (see Chapter 100, Emotional Awareness for Pain).

Yoga

Yoga is an increasingly popular practice consisting of three major components: physical postures (asanas), breathing techniques (pranayama), and meditation. The numerous popular yoga styles vary in intensity, pace, and balance of asana, pranayama, and meditation. Several published randomized controlled trials for CLBP support the use of standardized yoga sequences for decreasing pain, improving function, and reducing analgesic use.[48-51] Given this evidence, two international guidelines recommend yoga as a treatment option for CLBP.[16,24] Patients with CLBP who pursue yoga should ideally use a program specifically tailored for back pain. Yoga styles particularly suited for restoration from CLBP include, but are not limited to, Hatha, Viniyoga, Iyengar, Kripalu, and Anusara. Instructors should have experience working with patients with chronic pain. Yoga has not been studied in ALBP, nor is recommended for this condition. Although yoga has not been studied for the prevention of ALBP or recurrent LBP, anecdotal reports and observation suggest that it may be helpful and reasonable for this purpose.

Multidisciplinary Functional Restoration

Multidisciplinary functional restoration programs are typically intensive (more than 100 hours) biopsychosocial interventions combining cognitive-behavioral therapy with physical rehabilitation. These programs are often offered by a team that may include physicians, exercise instructors, physical and occupational therapists, and mental health professionals. Moderate to strong evidence indicates that these programs reduce pain and improve function in patients with CLBP, as well as improve readiness and return to work. Less intensive programs and those without a behavioral component are less effective.[16,46,52] Multidisciplinary functional restoration programs can be considered for patients in whom less intensive treatment options have failed and who continue to exhibit high levels of physical and psychological distress and disability.[16,24,25]

First-Line Pharmaceuticals

Oral pharmacotherapy is the most commonly used intervention for CLBP. Most international guidelines recommend the use of acetaminophen and nonsteroidal antiinflammatory drugs (NSAIDs) as initial pharmacologic interventions for pain control.[16,24–26]

Acetaminophen

Acetaminophen is recommended as a first-line medication for ALBP or CLBP. It has a favorable safety profile and has been found to be beneficial in multiple musculoskeletal conditions.[53]

■ Dosage

The recommended dose of acetaminophen is 500 mg, one to two tablets three to four times a day.

■ Precautions

Hepatotoxicity can occur with doses at or higher than the recommended maximum daily dose of 4 g/day, particularly in patients with preexisting liver disease or heavy alcohol use.[53]

Nonsteroidal Antiinflammatory Drugs

NSAIDs such as ibuprofen and naproxen can also be used as first-line analgesics either alone or in combination with acetaminophen. NSAIDs have moderate to strong evidence for short-term pain control in ALBP and CLBP.[16,24,25,46,53,54] Given that no single NSAID has been found to be superior to others, the choice should be based on cost, dosing schedule, and patient preference. The potential benefits associated with these medications should be weighed against possible risks. NSAIDs can cause dyspepsia, gastritis, peptic ulcer, and gastrointestinal bleeding. Prolonged high levels of NSAID use are associated with worsening renal function. Each patient should be individually assessed for the risk of these potential adverse events and counseled accordingly. As with all analgesic medications, the minimal dose that is effective should be recommended, and long-term use should be avoided if possible.

■ Dosage

For ibuprofen, the dose is 400 to 800 mg three times per day. The dose of naproxen is 375 to 500 mg twice daily.

■ Precautions

Patients taking NSAIDs on a long-term basis should undergo regular monitoring of renal function. Cyclooxygenase-2 inhibitors such as celecoxib are newer NSAIDs marketed for their gastroprotective effects. However, these drugs have been associated with an increase in cardiovascular risk, and their use should be discouraged in lieu of acetaminophen and traditional NSAIDs.[16,24,25,46,53,54]

Second-Line Pharmaceuticals

Weak Opioids

Analgesics such as codeine (15 to 30 mg up to four times daily), hydrocodone (5 to 10 mg up to four times daily), and tramadol (50 to 100 mg up to four times daily) may be considered when acetaminophen and NSAIDs are ineffective or patients have contraindications to their use.[16,24,25,53] Moderate to strong evidence indicates effectiveness of weak opioids in reducing pain and disability associated with ALBP and CLBP.[16,24,25,53] However, this benefit must be balanced by the potential for adverse effects, dependence, and abuse. The most reliable predictor of abuse is a personal or family history of substance abuse.[53]

■ Dosage

Doses are as follows: codeine, 15 to 30 mg up to four times daily; hydrocodone, 5 to 10 mg up to four times daily; and tramadol, 50 to 100 mg up to four times daily.

■ Precautions

Side effects of opioids are common and can include constipation, nausea, somnolence, pruritus, dysphoria, and sexual dysfunction.[25,53] Even though stronger opioid analgesics are often prescribed for ALBP (e.g., short-acting oxycodone) and CLBP (e.g., long-acting morphine and oxycodone), evidence supporting their use is limited, and they have a greater potential for dependence and abuse.[16,24,35,53] Stronger opioids should be considered only for short-term use in patients with severe pain who are at low risk for abuse. Rarely long-acting opioids in CLBP can be considered if all other therapeutic options have been exhausted, evidence indicates poor function related to back pain, and the patient has no personal or family history of abuse. A referral to a pain specialist may be indicated for patients requiring prolonged opioid use. All patients requiring prolonged opioids should be required to sign a narcotic pain medication agreement with the provider.

Muscle Relaxants

Muscle relaxants have antispasmodic properties and include benzodiazepines (e.g., diazepam) and nonbenzodiazepines (e.g., cyclobenzaprine, carisoprodol). Benzodiazepines are effective for short-term pain relief in ALBP or acute exacerbations of CLBP and can be used sparingly off-label for this purpose.[35,46,53] Benzodiazepine use is best restricted to bedtime only, given the strong sedating effects of these drugs. In addition, benzodiazepines have a great potential for dependence and abuse. Therefore, they should be used only on a short-term basis and should not be prescribed to patients with a history of abuse.[16,25,46,53] Nonbenzodiazepines are also effective for ALBP but are not recommended for CLBP.[16,35,46,53]

Tricyclic Antidepressants

Low-dose tricyclic antidepressants (e.g., amitriptyline, 10 to 25 mg at bedtime) can be effective adjuncts for pain relief in CLBP.[16,25,46,53] Medications in this class should not be used as first-line therapy. Selective serotonin reuptake inhibitors are not recommended for CLBP.[16,25,46,53]

Botanicals and Supplements

Devil's Claw

Devil's claw (*Harpagophytum procumbens*; see Table 64-3 in Chapter 64, Neck Pain) belongs to the Pedaliaceae family and is also known as grapple plant, wood spider, and harpago.[55,56] A Cochrane Review found two high-quality trials that examined the analgesic effects of devil's claw for back pain and showed strong evidence that this botanical was better than placebo for short-term improvements in pain.[16,56]

Dosage

Daily use of 2400 mg, divided three times per day and ingested by tablet or capsule standardized to 2% harpagosides and 3% total iridoid glycosides, is recommended.[55,56]

■ Precautions

Devil's claw extract may inhibit certain cytochrome P-450 enzymes, and therefore, appropriate monitoring of patients taking medications such as statins, imidazoles, and protease inhibitors is recommended. As with many botanicals and supplements, prothrombin time levels in warfarin users should be carefully monitored.

Willow Bark

Willow bark comes from a family of deciduous trees and shrubs commonly known as white willow or European willow (Salix alba) and purple willow (Salix purpurea). Willow bark contains salicylates and is the botanical precursor to aspirin. Willow bark has been shown to be better than placebo for short-term improvements in pain.[16,56]

■ Dosage

The three routes of administration of willow bark are tea, capsule, and tincture.[57] Willow bark containing 240 mg of salicin taken once daily is recommended.

■ Precautions

Willow bark should be avoided in patients who are allergic or sensitive to salicylates. Willow bark can cause dyspepsia but usually less than seen with NSAIDs. Concomitant use of willow bark and anticoagulants and antiplatelet drugs should be avoided.[57]

Other Remedies

Several other herbal formulations and natural medicines have been investigated as treatment for ALBP and CLBP. Two of the better-known therapies are topical capsicum and glucosamine sulfate. Some evidence indicates that capsicum may be beneficial, but glucosamine sulfate is not recommended.[16,56,58,59]

Biomechanical Interventions

Spinal Manipulation

Spinal manipulation involves the application of high-velocity, low-amplitude forces to the joints of the spine through long or short levers. Spinal manipulation is primarily performed by chiropractors, but it also can be provided by osteopaths, physical therapists, and physicians. Specific manipulative techniques differ slightly within and among professions, but a unifying element is the use of a high-velocity thrust or impulse to apply the manipulative force. The exact mechanism of action of spinal manipulation has yet to be determined, but it is believed that the thrust procedure normalizes joint biomechanics, acts on the nervous system through the stimulation of afferent joint receptors, or both.

Spinal manipulation is effective in improving function and pain in both ALBP and CLBP compared with sham manipulation, analgesic medications, or exercise therapy.[60-62] Serious adverse events (e.g., disk herniation, cauda equina syndrome) associated with lumbar spine manipulation are rare, with an estimated risk of less than 1 in 1,000,000 manipulations.[63] Additionally, all major international guidelines recommend spinal manipulation as a treatment option for ALBP and CLBP.[16,24-27]

The TBC uses a clinical prediction rule to identify patients who are likely to respond to spinal manipulation. The prediction rule has been validated for use in patients with ALBP or acute exacerbation of CLBP.[64,65] The five criteria in the prediction rule are (1) duration of the current episode is less than 16 days, (2) extremity symptoms not distal to the knee, (3) low fear avoidance (less than 19) as determined by the Fear Avoidance Beliefs Questionnaire Work Subscale, (4) palpation of one or more hypomobile lumbar segments, and (5) one or both hips with internal rotation range of motion greater than 35 degrees.[64] In one report, patients who met four out of five criteria and who received manipulation had more than a 90% likelihood of a successful outcome, as defined by a 50% improvement in Oswestry Disability Questionnaire scores at 1 week.[64] In this subpopulation, the clinical benefit was also maintained at 4 weeks and at 6 months.[64]

Patients with low back pain most likely to respond to manipulation:
1. Duration of current episode less than 16 days
2. Extremity symptoms not distal to the knee
3. Low fear avoidance
4. Palpation of one or more hypomobile lumbar segments
5. One or both hips with internal rotation range of motion greater than 35 degrees

---

Clinical practice guidelines recommend that spinal manipulation be offered according to patients' preference or when patients have failed to improve with a short course of advice and self-care. In addition, the clinical prediction rule is a useful decision support mechanism for identifying patients who are likely to benefit from spinal manipulation.

Nonthrust Manual Therapies

Nonthrust manual therapies encompass various techniques directed at the joints and soft tissues. These techniques include mobilization, muscle energy techniques, myofascial release, strain and counterstrain (see Chapter 106, Strain/Counterstrain), and craniosacral therapy. These procedures use both active and passive movements and are distinct from spinal manipulation in that high-velocity, low-amplitude forces are not used. Nonthrust manual therapies are primarily performed by osteopaths, but they are also commonly delivered by physical therapists and chiropractors.

A meta-analysis by Licciardone et al[66] looked at six randomized controlled trials in populations with subacute LBP and CLBP. These trials used a combination of nonthrust manual therapies described under the umbrella of osteopathic manipulative therapy.[66] In some of the trials, high-velocity, low-amplitude spinal manipulation was also used. The investigators concluded that these combined therapies significantly reduced LBP as compared with active treatment (e.g., massage, chemonucleolysis), sham, and no treatment control. Furthermore, these pain reductions were observed across short-, intermediate-, and long-term end points.

Spinal mobilization provides better pain relief and greater increases in range of motion when compared with no treatment but is not significantly different from sham treatment.[67]

Moderate evidence also shows that spinal mobilization produces benefits in both acute and chronic back pain.[60] Nonthrust manual therapies may be offered according to patients' preferences or when patients have failed to improve with a short course of advice and self-care.

Exercise Therapy

Exercise therapy is the most widely used nonpharmaceutical intervention for LBP[68] (see Chapter 91, Low Back Pain Exercises). *Exercise therapy* refers to a broad range of techniques designed to improve strength, coordination, flexibility, range of motion, endurance, and aerobic capacity. These techniques can vary according to frequency, intensity, and duration. Exercise therapy is principally provided by physical therapists, but it may also be delivered by chiropractors, osteopaths, and physicians.

The benefit of exercise therapy for ALBP remains unclear. However, strong evidence indicates that exercise therapy provides a small but significant benefit in short-term and long-term pain compared with usual care in the population with CLBP.[16,24–27,69] Studies comparing different forms of exercises in the population with CLBP have not found clinically meaningful differences.[68] Individually designed, supervised, high-intensity programs are recommended because they have been found to achieve better pain reduction and functional improvements than standardized group or home programs.[69] Adverse events associated with back exercise programs are rare.[68] If home programs are used, frequent patient follow-up to encourage compliance is needed because adherence is typically poor.[68,69]

Some subgroups of patients with LBP may respond differently to various types of exercise therapy.[68] Although important differences exist between the TBC and the MTD methods of classification, one common component is the identification of patients whose symptoms "centralize" in response to specific postures or movements. The centralization phenomenon occurs when movement in a specific direction, such as lumbar flexion or extension, causes the patient's pain to decrease or move rapidly from a more peripheral location (e.g., leg) to a more central location.[70] Similarly, movement in the opposite direction "peripheralizes" the pain or reverses the effect. Indications in the patient's history that these movement patterns should be explored include constant pain that varies in intensity, pain often in seated positions, and movement restrictions that are usually asymmetric.[71]

The TBC also uses a clinical prediction rule developed by Hicks et al[21] to identify patients likely to benefit from lumbopelvic or core stabilization exercises targeting the transversus abdominis, erector spinae or multifidus, quadratus lumborum, and oblique abdominal musculature. To be placed in this category, a patient must have three or more of the following criteria: age younger than 40 years, average passive straight leg raise range of motion greater than 90 degrees, an aberrant movement pattern during trunk flexion (e.g., the Gower sign, reverse lumbopelvic rhythm), and a positive prone instability test result.[21]

As with manipulation, the major clinical practice guidelines recommend that exercise therapy be offered according to patients' preferences, especially for CLBP. In addition, insights from the TBC and MTD may be helpful in identifying patients who are likely to benefit from specific forms of exercise.

Massage

Massage refers to various techniques in which the therapist presses, rubs, and otherwise manipulates the body's soft tissues and muscles, usually with the hands and fingers. Evidence regarding the benefits of massage for both acute and chronic back pain is conflicting. In patients with CLBP, evidence suggests that massage produces similar improvement in pain and function when compared with exercise therapy, and it provides better short-term outcomes compared with mobilization, relaxation therapy, physical therapy, acupuncture, and self-care education.[25,72] In addition to short-term benefits, one clinical trial found that massage provided long-term beneficial effects when compared with acupuncture and self-care in patients with CLBP.[72] Evidence shows that acupressure massage (gently pressing specific points) produces better results than Swedish massage (effleurage, pétrissage, and tapotement), and that Swedish and Thai massage are equivalent.[72] Minor pain or discomfort is experienced in a small percentage (less than 15%) of patients during or shortly after receiving massage.[73] Working with an experienced or licensed massage therapist is important.[72] For patients with acute and subacute back pain, evidence indicates that massage provides significant short-term reductions in pain and disability when compared with no treatment or sham.[67] For acute and chronic back pain, massage may be offered in accordance with patients' preferences as a short-term measure to improve function and activity tolerance.

Physical Modalities

Physical modalities include agents such as interferential current, low-level laser, shortwave diathermy, superficial heat, cryotherapy, traction, ultrasound, lumbar supports, and transcutaneous electrical nerve stimulation. Some evidence supports the use of superficial heat for ALBP. All international guidelines uniformly recommend against the use of all other physical agents in patients with ALBP and CLBP because of insufficient or conflicting evidence of benefit.[16,24–27]

> Do not recommend physical modalities with no or little evidence of benefit, such as traction, ultrasound, lumbar supports, and transcutaneous electrical nerve stimulation.

Bioenergetic Interventions

Acupuncture

Acupuncture may achieve its effects by three proposed mechanisms: (1) release of endorphins and other neurotransmitters as a result of nervous system stimulation, (2) the gate control theory of pain, and (3) stimulation of vascular and immunomodulatory mediators of inflammation.[74,75]

Acupuncture is more effective than no treatment and conservative management for short-term pain relief and improved function for CLBP.[76] However, the beneficial effects of acupuncture for LBP are generally short lasting.[67] Evidence indicates that pain and function are improved when acupuncture is combined with other treatments such as spinal manipulation or exercise therapy.[76] However, evidence of the benefit of acupuncture as a stand-alone modality compared with other common interventions for CLBP is insufficient.[46] One study found that acupuncture was no more effective than sham acupuncture.[75] Investigators have theorized that patients' expectations may explain this phenomenon; however, results of this line of investigation have been equivocal.[77] Serious complications of acupuncture are rare, although one systematic review did report needle pain and bleeding to be common side effects.[62] Acupuncture is a treatment option for CLBP and may be offered in accordance with patients' preferences. Acupuncture for ALBP is not recommended.[16,24,26,27,35]

Injection Therapies

The use of epidural steroid and facet joint injections for the treatment of LBP has increased significantly since the 1990s, even though evidence for their effectiveness is mixed.[78-80] During this period, numerous systematic reviews and clinical practice guidelines have been published addressing the indications for the use of these two procedures.[25,35,46,81-85] Based on these works, epidural steroid injections appear to provide potential short-term pain relief in patients with subacute or chronic leg-dominant radicular syndromes resulting from disk herniation or spinal stenosis.[25,35,46,81-87] Epidural steroid injections do not appear to confer long-term pain or functional benefits, nor do they mitigate the progression to surgery in these subpopulations with LBP.[81,83,86,87] Epidural steroid injections are not recommended for nonspecific ALBP or CLBP.[24,25,35,46,81-87]

Spinal facet joints have been shown to be pain-generating structures. However, randomized trials evaluating the use of therapeutic facet injections for CLBP have not shown a clear benefit over sham interventions.[24,25,81,85] In addition, no high-quality evidence supports the use of facet joint injections in patients with ALBP.[35,81] Therefore, facet joint injections are not recommended for use in ALBP or CLBP.[24,25,35,46,81,85]

Surgery

According to James Weinstein, spine surgeon and Director of the Dartmouth Institute for Health Policy and Clinical Practice, "the United States has the highest rates of spine surgery in the world, despite incidence and prevalence rates of spine disorders that are similar to those found in other countries. There remains little or no medical, clinical, or surgical evidence to support such variability."[88] Except for a limited number of specific conditions (e.g., cauda equina, infection, tumor) lumbar surgery should not be considered until a comprehensive trial of conservative care has been exhausted.[16,24,25,35,81,83,89]

In patients suffering from significant, nonradicular CLBP with concomitant degenerative changes in whom a 1-year trial of conservative care has failed, surgical fusion is a treatment option.[16,24,25,81,89] Evidence from higher-quality studies shows that fusion is equivalent to multidisciplinary function restoration programs and is moderately superior to nonspecific conservative treatment.[25,81,89] When clinicians consider surgical referral in this population, several factors should be taken into account. First, the benefits of fusion have been shown only in patients with moderate to severe pain or functional limitations who have not responded to at least 1 year of conservative management and who do not have significant psychiatric or medical comorbidities.[81] Second, more than 50% of patients undergoing surgery do not report "excellent" or "good" outcomes, defined as sporadic pain, slight functional limitations, and occasional analgesic use.[81]

> One year of conservative therapy is often recommended before surgery is considered.

Standard diskectomy and microdiskectomy are treatment options in patients suffering from significant radiculopathy resulting from disk herniation following a trial of nonsurgical treatment.[81,83,89] Most patients in this subgroup tend to improve without surgery. However, approximately 10% will have sufficient pain and functional limitations after 6 to 8 weeks to warrant surgical referral.[81,83] Both standard diskectomy and microdiskectomy are associated with moderate short-term benefits (6 to 12 weeks) when compared with nonsurgical management, but these benefits diminish over the longer term (1 to 2 years).[81]

When significant radiculopathy resulting from spinal stenosis persists in spite of an adequate trial of conservative care, laminectomy is a treatment option.[81,89] Patients appear to have moderate benefits as a result of surgery versus nonsurgical treatment, but the average improvement in the stenotic patient is less than that seen in patients with radiculopathy resulting from disk herniation.[81] In addition, the differences in outcomes in patients with radiculopathy related to spinal stenosis who are treated surgically versus nonsurgically diminish over the longer term (1 to 2 years).[81]

PREVENTION PRESCRIPTION

- Educate: Nonspecific low back pain is not progressive and will not disable you unless you let it.
- Maintain normal physical activity as much as possible.
- Lift properly: Bend your knees and keep your back straight.
- Take regular 5-minute breaks to stand and stretch when sitting for long periods.
- Strengthen trunk muscles and walk regularly.
- Have a regular stretching or yoga routine.
- Keep a healthy body weight.

THERAPEUTIC REVIEW

When deciding among the following therapeutic options for low back pain (LBP), augment the biomedical model of evaluation and management with a biopsychosocial approach.

Evaluation

- Rule out potentially serious disease (red flags) and significant neurologic involvement. If present, refer for imaging and specialty care as appropriate.

- Identify risk factors for chronicity (yellow flags).

- Do not routinely use imaging in patients with nonspecific LBP and no red flags.

- For nonspecific back pain, consider patients' preferences and clinical classifications in treatment planning.

Education and Self-Care

- Reassure patients about the benign nature and favorable prognosis of nonspecific back pain.

- Advise patients to stay active and carry on as normally as possible.

- Dispel inappropriate beliefs.

Pharmaceuticals

- Acetaminophen: 500 mg, one to two tablets three to four times daily

- Nonsteroidal antiinflammatory drugs (take with food)
  - Ibuprofen: 400 to 800 mg three times daily
  - Naproxen: 375 to 500 mg twice daily

Botanicals and Supplements

- Willow bark containing 240 mg of salicin: taken once daily

- Devil's claw: 400 mg, two capsules three times daily (standardized to 2% harpagosides and 3% total iridoid glycosides)

Mind-Body Therapy

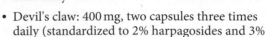

- Consider cognitive-behavioral, operant, and respondent therapies, such as progressive muscle relaxation, as treatment options for patients with chronic LBP.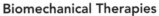

- Recommend yoga as a treatment option for patients with chronic LBP.

- Refer for multidisciplinary functional restoration in patients with chronic LBP in whom conservative options have failed and who exhibit high levels of physical and psychological disability.

Biomechanical Therapies

- Recommend 4 to 8 visits of spinal manipulation as a treatment option for patients with acute and chronic LBP.

- Recommend 8 to 12 visits of therapeutic exercise in patients with chronic back pain.

- Consider a short course of 4 to 8 visits of massage as a treatment option for patients with acute and chronic LBP.

Bioenergetic Therapies

- Acupuncture: Consider a short course of 4 to 8 visits of acupuncture as a treatment option for patients with chronic LBP.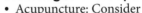

KEY WEB RESOURCES

Fear Avoidance Beliefs Questionnaire: http://www.udel.edu/PT/PT%20Clinical%20Services/journalclub/caserounds/05_06/mar06/FABQ1.pdf

Survey form and scoring methodology used to identify patients with maladaptive coping behaviors

Revised Oswestry Disability Index: http://thepainsource.com/2010/12/revised-oswestry-disability-index/

Survey form, scoring methodology, and interpretation rubric for one of the most commonly used outcomes instruments for low back conditions

Spine-Health information on the McKenzie Method: http://www.spine-health.com/wellness/exercise/mckenzie-therapy-mechanical-low-back-pain

Good overview of the McKenzie Method of Mechanical Treatment and Diagnosis

Yoga Journal yoga poses: http://www.yogajournal.com/poses/finder/therapeutic_focus/t_back_pain

Comprehensive index of yoga poses appropriate for patients with low back pain

Spine-Health information on how to select the best chiropractor: http://www.spine-health.com/treatment/chiropractic/how-select-best-chiropractor

Article offering useful tips to help physicians and patients identify competent chiropractic practitioners

---

References

References are available online at expertconsult.com.

Neck Pain

J. Adam Rindfleisch, MD, MPhil, and Brian Earley, DO

In many Eastern traditions, the neck is held to be our center of communication, self-expression, and creativity. The neck houses our voices, our capacity to swallow, and the major blood vessels that are the lifelines between the heart and head. Metaphors related to the neck tell us something about its association with vulnerability. Something frustrating is "a pain in the neck," and something depressing gives one a "lump in my throat." We "stick our necks out for others" when we are being brave, and we "go for the throat" when we are being aggressive.

The neck has 37 separate joints and moves an average of 600 times per hour. It has evolved to be simultaneously rigid and flexible, and it houses separate flexor and extensor muscles for the head and cervical spine. It contains our cervical spinal cord, multiple nerve roots and joint facets, and the atlantoaxial joint. The neck is indeed a vulnerable part of the body. At any given time, 10% to 15% of people are experiencing neck pain,[1] and two thirds of people have neck pain sometime during their lives.[2] Not surprisingly, neck pain is one of the most common complaints primary care providers encounter.[3] Even with a full biomedical course of treatment, neck pain often recurs.[4] An individualized, relationship-centered, and holistic integrative approach can markedly improve outcomes.

Pathophysiology

Pinpointing the exact anatomic source of neck pain is often difficult. Most neck pain is the result of cervical paraspinal muscle spasm or other musculoskeletal factors, but clinicians must rule out various other causes, as noted in Box 64-1.[1,3]

Musculoskeletal neck pain can be traumatic or nontraumatic in origin.[1] Traumatic neck pain is most commonly associated with hyperextension syndrome (whiplash). As many as 40% of whiplash injuries are estimated to result in long-term symptoms.[5] In countries where litigation for whiplash is uncommon, long-term sequelae of whiplash are almost unheard of, a situation that leads one to wonder about the role of mind-body and economic influences on pain outcomes.[6]

Nontraumatic neck pain, which is more common, can be related to a structural or degenerative disorder, but more commonly it is caused by soft tissue disorders. Twin studies revealed a link between genetics and a predisposition to development of nontraumatic neck pain.[7] Common causes of soft tissue pain include poor posture, repetitive activity, and sports injuries. A strong connection exists between soft tissue neck pain and emotional or mental states, such as anxiety and depression.[8] Myofascial trigger points—clusters of muscle fibers locked in a contractile state—are commonly present in soft tissue pain.

The pathophysiologic basis of neck pain is complex, and our knowledge of the multitude of chemical and structural processes involved is far from complete. Pain begins with tissue irritation, which may be caused by infection, joint deterioration, sustained use (or sustained immobility), psychological stress, or trauma. Irritation activates nociception. Muscle spasms often occur as the neck is voluntarily or involuntarily repositioned to avoid pain. Inflammation follows, and a vicious positive-feedback circle arises as inflammation leads to even more pain. As edema, structural changes, and harmful metabolites accumulate, they can cause ischemia of the tissues. If these alterations are not interrupted or reversed in time, long-term changes in neck structure may arise, and disability can result.

Integrative Therapy

The goals of an integrative approach to neck pain are threefold[9]:
1. Understand the pain in a broader context. Move beyond an exclusively physiologic perspective to explore how emotions, work, social issues, relationships and other factors contribute. What burdens is a person "carrying" on his or her shoulders? Asking people their views on why they have pain can offer interesting insights. Ideally, preventive measures would be instituted before pain ever manifests.

BOX 64-1. Key Points to Remember in the Evaluation of Neck Pain

- Consider a tumor in a patient who has pain at night or whose pain does not improve when the body is supine.
- Neck pain with associated neurologic symptoms (e.g., dizziness, paresthesias, and weakness) merits diagnostic imaging studies, most commonly computed tomography or magnetic resonance imaging of the neck.
- Severe neck pain associated with fever is meningitis until proven otherwise.
- If neck pain is associated with joint pain in other areas, rule out a systemic rheumatic disorder, such as osteoarthritis, rheumatoid arthritis, ankylosing spondylitis, or gout.
- Neck pain can be referred from a source in the head or arms. Consider dental disorders, temporomandibular joint disorders, and rotator cuff injuries. Cervical spine disorders may lead to patient descriptions of the eyes being "pulled" or "pushed" if the sympathetic nerve plexuses that surround the arteries of the neck and innervate the eyes are irritated.
- Referred neck pain can arise from nearly any organ system. Myocardial ischemia, gallbladder disease, gastrointestinal ulcers, hiatal hernias, and pancreatic inflammation are all in the differential diagnosis. Referred diaphragmatic pain and tumors of the apical lung must also be considered.
- Keep in mind that uncommon local sources of neck pain can include the carotid arteries, vertebral arteries, lymph nodes, and the thyroid.

Data from references 1 to 3.

2. Explore where the cycle of pathophysiology described earlier may be interrupted and how that could best be done. Identify the initial insult or insults causing the pain. Supplements or diet may help to lessen inflammation. A mind-body approach may alter the tendency to fear or avoid the pain. Manual therapy, acupuncture, or exercise may help patients diminish the pain by learning to carry themselves differently. The key is to collaborate on a plan of action, with care taken not to overwhelm people with too many options. Trust your intuition as a provider.
3. Remain mindful of therapeutic complications and what is likely to cause pain recurrences. Pain can often be a powerful teacher. Why is this signal arising, and what changes are needed so that the signal will no longer be necessary? It is easy for a pattern to arise where the pain is masked, rather than truly treated. Some therapies (e.g., long-term narcotics) can lead to long-term problems and should be used cautiously.

Lifestyle

Box 64-2 lists some of the risk factors for neck pain.[2,9,10] Smoking, obesity, work activities, and substance abuse should all be given attention in an integrative visit.

BOX 64-2. Risk Factors for Neck Pain

- Depression
- Drug abuse
- Increasing age
- Heavy physical work, manual labor
- High job demands
- History of headaches
- Lack of control over work situation
- Low job satisfaction
- Work with exposure to repetitive vibration or unusual postures
- Obesity
- Smoking (and frequent coughing)

Data from Devereaux MW. Neck pain. *Med Clin North Am.* 2009;93: 273–284; and Teats RY, Dahmer S, Scott E. Integrative medicine approach to chronic pain. *Prim Care.* 2010;37:407–421.

Exercise and Movement

Patients with chronic neck pain demonstrate altered muscle activation patterns during the performance of tasks that may influence how rapidly their muscles become fatigued.[11] Medical research is limited regarding the potential benefits of the Alexander technique, Feldenkrais, and Pilates for neck pain, but these therapies are increasingly popular with patients with chronic pain, are effective for other musculoskeletal complaints, and tend to be safe.[12,13] Qi gong (which also may be classified as a bioenergetic therapy) also holds promise, although more studies are needed[14] (see Chapter 90, Prescribing Movement Therapies).

To assume that exercise for musculoskeletal neck pain would be beneficial seems logical. A Cochrane Review concluded that limited evidence of benefit exists for strengthening, stretching, or eye fixation exercises for neck pain with headache and for active range-of-motion exercises or a home exercise program for acute problems such as whiplash. The benefit of stretching and strengthening for chronic mechanical neck disorder was deemed "unclear."[15] Another review found that exercise, at least when combined with cognitive-behavioral therapy, reduced the number of days of work lost because of neck pain.[16]

Cervical Support

Early mobilization was found to be superior to cervical collar use in the treatment of neck pain.[17] One small randomized, controlled trial from Sweden did find that cervical pillows could be useful for both neck pain and poor sleep.[18] Proper neck positioning during sleep is important. Prolonged flexion of the neck should be avoided; maintenance of the neck's natural lordotic curve is preferable. Cervical spine pillows may be useful. Evidence on whether traction is beneficial is insufficient.[19]

Repetitive Strain

Certain movements and activities can put the musculoskeletal structures of the neck under chronic stress and tension. Examples are holding a phone between the shoulder and the ear (administrative work), carrying a heavy purse or backpack on one shoulder, staring at a computer monitor for long periods of time, and looking over the shoulder (farming). Bifocals may lead to awkward flexion of the neck as well. The effects of such postures should be brought to patients' attention. Many people "carry their stress" in their neck and shoulder muscles. Chronic stress can result in a constant readiness to duck or to dodge danger, and many people chronically tense the muscles used for these actions without realizing it.

Nutrition

Essential Fatty Acids

Increasing intake of omega-3 fatty acids and reducing consumption of omega-6 fatty acids lower the levels of prostaglandins and leukotrienes that cause inflammation[20,21] (see Chapter 86, The Antiinflammatory Diet). Several months may pass before patients derive a benefit from using the antiinflammatory diet, and the diet is most likely to be beneficial when neck pain has been chronic.

Saturated Fats

Eating saturated fats, which come primarily from animal products such as red meat and dairy foods, can also contribute to inflammation and pain.[22] A transition to a vegetarian diet, or at least toward a significant reduction in saturated fat consumption, is worth recommending. Some patients may benefit from a trial of an elimination diet, particularly for dairy and meat products (see Chapter 84, Food Intolerance and Elimination Diet).

Antioxidants

Elevations of free radicals can result from poor nutrition, excessive stress, and toxic environmental exposure. Foods rich in antioxidants, such as fruits and vegetables, seem to play a role in reducing pain by removing free radicals.[23] High doses of supplemental antioxidants, such as vitamin E, have been the subject of some controversy and may be inadvisable in patients with heart disease or other chronic conditions.[24] Eating a combination of green, yellow, red, purple, and orange produce will guarantee that numerous beneficial antioxidants are consumed.

> Take care not to underestimate the impact of mental health on the course of neck pain. Encourage the use of at least one of the many mind-body therapies that may offer benefit.

Mind-Body Therapy

Pain perception does not necessarily correlate with the severity of an injury. Some people with structural neck abnormalities develop chronic pain, whereas others do not. In a landmark study in the *New England Journal of Medicine*, magnetic resonance imaging (MRI) examinations of 98 *asymptomatic* individuals indicated that 52% had one or more bulging disks.[25] Similarly, nearly everyone who is older than 70 years has some degree of cervical spondylosis, but not everyone that age has neck pain.[2] Pain is often centrally mediated, with abnormal intensification of sensation noted in the portions of the brain that govern a chronically painful part of the body.[9] Fortunately, the brain's plasticity allows for the possibility for "rewiring" the brain; sensory processing may be changed to someone's advantage. The key is to discern how to help someone with pain make that happen, and this is where mind-body approaches can come into play.[26]

Emotions and Neck Pain

Emotional well-being plays an important role in whether pain arises.[27] A Stanford University study that evaluated both symptomatic and asymptomatic patients with abnormal MRI findings concluded that the severity of the MRI lesions did not predict the presence of pain; rather, pain severity correlated with whether patients had underlying psychological issues.[28] Pain is more likely to become chronic in people who tend to catastrophize[29] or somaticize.[30] Stress also plays a role. A British study of 12,907 people concluded that the association between perceived neck pain and mental stress was much stronger than the association between neck pain and repetitive occupational activities.[31]

In his book, *The Mindbody Prescription: Healing the Body, Healing the Pain*, John E. Sarno, MD, suggested that unexpressed emotions are responsible for neck, back, and limb pain in most patients.[32] Sarno held that unexpressed anger, accumulated as a result of internal and external pressures, is of particular significance. He proposed that, after physical concerns have been appropriately ruled out, the following elements can be used to help people markedly decrease pain:

- *Learn about pain.* Patients attend a series of lectures describing the relationship between pain and emotions.

- *Focus on emotions when pain strikes.* When patients become aware of the pain, they must consciously shift their focus toward the psychological, as opposed to physical, causes of their discomfort.

- *Maintain physical activity.* Patients must overcome fears that physical activity will worsen the underlying condition. This step is implemented after the pain has been decreased through exploration of emotional issues.

- *Discontinue physical or physiologic treatments.* Sarno contended that focusing on physical causes of pain distracts the mind from the unexpressed emotions that are the pain's true cause. Medications are used sparingly for episodes of severe pain only.

- *Consider counseling.* If needed, patients are encouraged to seek help from a counselor in moving through the various emotional issues they encounter during the program.

Although outcomes research on the efficacy of Sarno's program is limited, the program has proved helpful for many people with chronic neck pain. Once potentially dangerous causes of pain have been ruled out, the risk of harm from participating in such a program is minimal. Many health care institutions offer pain management and coping groups, which may be similarly helpful (see Chapter 100, Emotional Awareness for Pain).

Journaling

By writing about stressful events, patients may be able to reduce pain and inflammation. One study found that symptoms of asthma and rheumatoid arthritis improved significantly in people who wrote about stressful life events in a journal for just 20 minutes for 3 consecutive days.[33] To assume that other disorders may also respond to this approach is reasonable (see Chapter 96, Journaling for Health).

Hypnosis

Hypnosis has been found to be useful in helping patients manage chronic pain.[34,35] In one study, 25 patients with head and neck pain were treated with acupuncture. After a washout period, they were treated with hypnosis. Both interventions were found to be helpful, but hypnosis scored slightly better, with an average reduction of 4.8 points on a 10-point symptom scale, compared with 4.2 points for acupuncture. Acupuncture was more appropriate for acute pain, whereas hypnosis appeared to work better for psychogenic pain. Subjects who also received healing suggestions by audiotape had less pain than those who did not[36] (see Chapter 92, Self-Hypnosis Techniques).

Interactive Guided Imagery

Interactive guided imagery is based on the philosophy that insight and knowledge gained from the creation of internal images can be used to improve symptoms. One interactive guided imagery technique is to have a patient visualize an image representing a particular symptom. The patient is asked to have a dialogue with the image that arises and to explore why it is present and what it would "need" for healing to occur. The image can serve as a means by which the conscious mind can access the subcounscious[37] (see Chapter 95, Guided Imagery).

Relaxation Exercises

Relaxation exercises, such as breathing techniques and progressive muscle relaxation, can reduce sympathetic stimulation, a potential contributor to muscle tension and pain. One study comparing relaxation, exercise, and ordinary activity for neck pain treatment did not find a benefit from either intervention in comparison with placebo.[38] Nevertheless, perhaps these techniques can serve as a safe and potentially useful way to empower patients to decrease their neck pain (see Chapter 93, Relaxation Techniques).

Biofeedback

Biofeedback uses technology or instrumentation to help people gain awareness of and control over various body processes.[39] Functional MRI studies indicated that biofeedback training can allow people with pain to alter pain perception by controlling activation of the rostral anterior cingulate cortex and other brain locations.[40,41] Severe chronic pain can be decreased. Sensors placed over the trapezius muscle can be used to train a patient to relax more efficiently. A small study of older patients with trapezius pain showed a 70% reduction in pain with biofeedback-assisted relaxation.[34] Biofeedback is worth considering in patients with neck pain.[42]

Bioenergetic Therapies

Acupuncture

The principle that energy flows through or over the surface of the body is common to several healing systems worldwide. Acupuncture, a 3000-year-old therapy based on the idea that

the body contains multiple energy channels, or meridians, maps out more than 350 major points. Needles are inserted at those points to improve the flow of energy (known in China as qi). Many of these points are located within or in close proximity to the neck.[43,44]

Evaluations of acupuncture as a treatment for chronic neck pain show promise. A 2006 Cochrane Review concluded that "moderate evidence" indicated that acupuncture is effective for chronic neck pain.[45]

- Acupuncture led to pain relief immediately after treatment and in the short term compared with sham treatment or being on a waiting list.

- Acupuncture led to at least short-term benefit for patients with radicular symptoms when compared with patients who were placed on a waiting list.

- Acupuncture was more effective than massage at short-term follow-up.

A 2008 review by the Task Force on Neck Pain and Associated Disorders also noted that acupuncture was superior to sham treatment, no treatment, and many other modalities for chronic neck pain.[46] Less evidence is available at this time to indicate whether acupuncture is useful for acute neck problems.[47]

 Box 64-1e, which lists contraindications to acupuncture, can be found online at expertconsult.com.

Acupuncture has been found to be extremely safe when it is offered by a well-trained provider.[48]

Good evidence supports the use of acupuncture for chronic neck pain.

Other Energy Medicine Modalities

Many Eastern traditions hold that the neck houses the throat chakra, a wheel of energy that extends anterior and posterior to the body at the level of the thyroid. Although therapies that purport to balance the human energy field, such as therapeutic touch and Reiki, require further study, some interesting findings are beginning to emerge,[49,50] especially with regard to emotional responses to illness. Harm is minimal, provided that patients do not defer potentially lifesaving biomedical therapies to focus on receiving energy medicine treatments.

Manual Therapies

Manual medicine is another common approach to neck pain. Manual techniques are done by various health professionals, including medical doctors (especially doctors of osteopathy, or DOs), physical therapists, massage therapists, manual therapists, and chiropractors.[51] Spinal manipulation performed by chiropractors, in fact, is the most common complementary and alternative therapy provided in the United States.[52] In the early 2000s, approximately 70,000 chiropractors were licensed in the United States, 10,000 in Japan, 6000 in Canada, 2500 in Australia and 16,000 in the United Kingdom.[53]

Nomenclature

The nomenclature of biomechanical therapies can be confusing. Chiropractic and physical therapy manual techniques are typically broken into two groups. Manipulation refers to a technique that uses a high-velocity, low-amplitude (HVLA) thrust.[54-56] Mobilization refers to techniques that incorporate lower-velocity, passive movements to the joints.[54] Osteopaths use the term manipulation to describe more than 100 different techniques including but not limited to HVLA.[56] Osteopathic manipulation is categorized into various groups of techniques, listed in Table 64-1.[57,58] In this chapter, manipulation refers to the term as defined by chiropractors and physical therapists, and osteopathic manipulative treatment (OMT) refers to manipulation as defined by the osteopathic profession.

Safety

The safety of manipulation of the cervical spine has been questioned. Most of these potential risks occur because of the rapid thrust. Therefore, the safety of high-velocity manipulation techniques has been studied much more than mobilization or non-HVLA OMT techniques. As noted in Box 64-3,[59-62] however, few contraindications exist, and manipulation seems to be significantly safer than other modalities (including antiinflammatory medications) commonly used for musculoskeletal conditions.[63,64] A study by Rubinstein et al[65] showed that the "benefits of chiropractic care for neck pain seem to outweigh the potential risks."

Common transient effects of cervical manipulation include local pain, headache, tiredness (fatigue), and radiating pain.[66,67] Transient effects occur in 30% to 61% of patients, begin within 4 hours after spinal manipulation, and usually resolve within 24 hours.[66,67]

Substantive reversible risks of manipulation are much less common. Worsening disk disease can occur with manipulation, but it occurs in fewer than 1 in 3.7 million patients.[66] This adverse effect is more common with manipulation of the low back than in cervical manipulation. Because of this risk, manipulation is relatively contraindicated in patients

---

BOX 64-3. Contraindications to Manipulation (High-Velocity Osteopathic Manipulative Treatment) of the Neck

- Aneurysm
- Bone tumor
- Carotid or vertebrobasilar disease
- History of pathologic fractures
- Vertebral infection
- Acute vertebral fracture
- Ligament rupture and instability
- Metastatic carcinoma
- Osteopenia or osteoporosis
- Anticoagulation therapy
- Previous surgery involving neck joints
- Rheumatoid arthritis of the cervical spine
- Unstable odontoid peg

Data from references 59 to 62.

TABLE 64-1. Examples of Various Osteopathic Manipulative Techniques

High-Velocity Low-Amplitude (HVLA) Techniques	The physician uses an HVLA thrust to push through a joint restructure to restore the range of motion of that joint.
Springing Techniques	The physician repetitively, gently rocks or pulses against the restriction of a joint to restore the range of motion of that joint.
Muscle Energy Techniques	The physician asks the patient to pull against the physician's resistance to rebalance the muscles around a dysfunctional joint.
Soft Tissue Techniques	The physician kneads, stretches, or applies inhibitory pressure to relax the soft tissues.[57]
Functional Techniques	The physician monitors the soft tissues while small motions are applied to the joint to decrease resistance. These techniques often use the patient's breathing to cause the restriction in the joint to "release."
Strain-Counterstrain Techniques	These techniques involve palpating tender points and putting the joint in a position to take away the palpatory pain of these points. This position is held until the restriction releases (approximately 90 seconds).[58]
Facilitated Positional Release	In these techniques, the joint or tissue is taken to the position of most comfort. Traction or compression is applied to facilitate an immediate release of the tissue tension.
Still Technique	This technique, thought to be developed by Dr. Still, is set up like facilitated positional release, but after traction or compression is applied, the joint is taken into the joint's restriction and is then returned to neutral.
Cranial Osteopathy	This gentle, manual technique emphasizes balancing the tensions of the dura.
Lymphatic Techniques	Various techniques that generally involve gentle techniques aimed at promoting the movement of the lymphatic fluid are used to promote healing of several conditions.

Data from Ward RC, Hruby RJ. *Foundations for Osteopathic Medicine.* 2nd ed. Philadelphia: Lippincott Williams & Wilkins; 2003, except where otherwise referenced.

with signs or symptoms of disk herniation until this disorder has been ruled out radiographically.[68]

The most concerning risks of cervical manipulation are those that are nonreversible. The most common of these is iatrogenic stroke, although vertebral dissection can also occur. These complications are quite rare, and in a review of injuries caused by manipulative therapy between 1925 and 1993, only 185 cases of serious injury were reported.[69]

Research in Manual Therapies for Neck Pain

Chiropractors and physical therapists have performed more manual therapy studies than other health professionals, and this is true when it comes to studies of neck pain as well.[70] Whether study findings are generalizable from one type of therapy to another is difficult to know because of the differences in categorization of the various types of manual therapies (see earlier), the difficulties in creating sham manipulation, and the use of osteopathic manual manipulation (in the United States) as adjuvant therapy.[71] Therefore, in this chapter, research done on manual medicine for the neck is divided into studies done by chiropractors or physical therapists and studies done by osteopaths.

■ Chiropractic and Physical Therapy Studies

Approximately 40% of episodes of care for back pain are managed by chiropractors.[72] For these visits, neck pain is the second most common reason (behind low back problems) for a patient to visit a chiropractor. Approximately 24% of visits to a chiropractor are for neck pain.[73] Chronic neck pain has been studied by chiropractors more than acute neck pain, and Gross et al summarized the findings in multiple Cochrane Review meta-analyses. In these reviews, Gross et al assessed whether manipulation or mobilization improved pain, function or disability, patient satisfaction, quality of life, and perceived effect in patients with neck pain (with or without headache or radicular symptoms). The 2004 meta-analysis of 33 trials showed that combined mobilization, manipulation, and exercise achieved clinically important improvements in pain, global perceived effect, and patient satisfaction in subacute and chronic neck disorders with or without headache.[74] A more recent review of 27 trials found immediate- or short-term pain relief with a course of cervical manipulation or mobilization alone, but the effects were not maintained over the long term.[75]

Less literature is available on the use of manipulation and mobilization for acute neck pain.[56,76] A small pilot study of 36 patients showed less pain intensity ($P < .05$) and a greater range of motion ($P < .05$) immediately following a single manipulation to patients with acute neck pain.[77]

■ Manual/Physical Therapy

Newer research showed that manipulation of the thoracic spine results in immediate improvement in neck pain.[54] A follow-up study showed that using thrust manipulation techniques in the thoracic spine resulted in greater short-term reductions in pain and disability than nonthrust mobilization in patients with neck pain. No additional side effects were noted in the thrust-treated group.[78] Previous studies had also shown significant improvements in patients with whiplash-associated disorders after thoracic mobilization was used.[79] Investigators proposed that techniques performed in the thoracic back may be an even safer option in patients with neck pain. However, further research must be done to assess long-term effects and to determine whether thoracic manipulation is most beneficial in isolation or in combination with some form of neck manipulation for the treatment of neck pain.[54]

■ Osteopathy

Only 2 small studies are available in the osteopathic literature to assess the effects of OMT on patients with chronic neck pain. In the first study, 17 patients with chronic neck pain lasting a mean of 168.8 weeks (4 to 1040 weeks) were recruited. These patients were treated with OMT for a total of 4 weeks (twice weekly for 2 weeks and once weekly for the final 2 weeks). They were analyzed before treatment, at 2 weeks, and at 4 weeks for changes in pain and disability. Significant improvements were found in pain ($P = .001$) and disability ($P = .001$) over the treatment course in the group receiving OMT. Improvements in pain and disability were found to be significant in patients with chronic pain and in those with subchronic pain. Further follow-up was not done in the study.[80]

In a second, slightly larger, study, 41 patients with nonspecific neck pain were divided into 2 groups. One group of 17 patients received ultrasound therapy only (every week for an average of 10 weeks), whereas a second group received ultrasound (every week for an average of 10 weeks) and OMT (every other week for an average of 10 weeks). Pain was measured at each of the treatments, 1 week after the treatments, and 3 months after the last treatment. The OMT used a combination of various techniques. Pain intensity decreased in both groups, with more improvement noted in the group receiving OMT ($P = .02$). No long-term follow-up was done.[81]

One study looked at OMT in patients with acute neck pain. In this study, 58 patients were randomized to receive either OMT or 30 mg intramuscular ketorolac (a known effective NSAID for musculoskeletal pain). The OMT provided included a combination of HVLA thrust, muscle energy, and soft tissue techniques. Both groups showed a significant reduction in pain intensity ($P < .01$ for both groups), but patients receiving OMT reported a significantly greater decrease in pain intensity ($P = .02$).[56]

> Manipulation, mobilization, and osteopathic manipulative treatment, especially in combination with exercise, have been shown to be safe and effective in the treatment of chronic neck pain. These options also appear to be appropriate in acute neck pain, although substantially less research is available to support this approach.

In summary, the available literature indicates that manual therapies hold promise and are worth considering in the management of neck pain.

Strain-Counterstrain and the Cranial Base Release

Two techniques that the primary care provider can incorporate into his or her practice for the manual therapy of neck pain are strain-counterstrain and the cranial base release (Fig. 64-1 and Box 64-4). Strain-counterstrain is helpful for relieving trigger points and muscle spasms (see Chapter 106, Strain/Counterstrain). The cranial base release is beneficial for patients with suboccipital neuralgia and tension headaches. For challenging cases, appropriate referral is indicated.

Surgery

Considering surgery, such as disk fusion, is reasonable when patients have symptoms of radiculopathy, progressive myelopathy, neurologic deficits not improved with other forms of treatment, or imaging-confirmed operable conditions.[82] Evidence supporting the use of surgery for chronic neck pain resulting from degeneration radiculopathy is not conclusive, however, according to a 2010 Cochrane Review.[83] The review found no benefit at 1 year postoperatively for patients with mild symptoms preoperatively, and the reviewers noted that additional research is needed to confirm when surgery is most appropriate.

Pharmaceuticals

Western medical therapy goes to great lengths to suppress inflammation and nociception. Steroids, cyclooxygenase-2 inhibitors, NSAIDs, and other medications are effective largely because they interfere with the inflammatory cascade. Muscle relaxants, opioids, and antidepressants are used to alter nervous system signaling at various levels.

Table 64-2 lists medications commonly used in the treatment of neck pain, along with recommended doses and precautions regarding their use.[84–86] A 2007 Cochrane Review concluded that, for mechanical neck disorders, "Muscle relaxants, analgesics, and NSAIDs had limited evidence and unclear benefits."[87] The review also noted that although studies are limited, corticosteroid injections within 8 hours of injury for whiplash, steroids plus lidocaine injections for chronic pain, and lidocaine injections for trigger points seem to have some benefit. Injection of botulinum toxin was not found to be helpful.

Between 1997 and 2004, the use of opioids for treating spinal disorders increased by 108%, but pain, poor quality of life, and percentages of disability claims have not shown improvement.[86] Long-term narcotic administration down-regulates endorphin receptors, which are partially responsible for the pain relief conferred by mind-body therapies such as hypnosis and guided imagery. In other words, long-term narcotic use can impede the symptomatic relief that comes from these therapies.

FIGURE 64-1
Hand positions for cranial base release. See Box 64-4 for explanation of technique. (From Chaitow L. *Cranial Manipulation Theory and Practice: Osseous and Soft Tissue Approaches.* New York: Churchill Livingstone; 1999:119.)

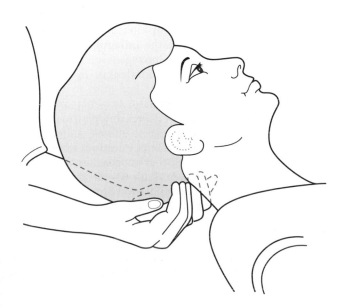

BOX 64-4. Cranial Base Release

The cranial base release (also known as the suboccipital release) is a manual cranial technique that can be incorporated into your daily practice. It is most useful for patients with cervical myofascial tension that has led to suboccipital neuralgia and headache. If you find it helpful, consider referring the patient to a cranial osteopathic practitioner.

The cranial base release loosens soft tissues that attach to the base of the cranium. If hypertrophic and inflamed, these tissues can restrict occipital motion and cause pain.

- See Figure 64-1. The patient is supine on the table. Seat yourself at the head of the table with your arms resting on and supported by it.
- Rest the backs of your hands on the table. The fingertips, which are bent toward the patient's posterior neck, are positioned at the base of the occiput in the suboccipital sulcus.
- Your fingertips serve as a fulcrum for the patient's occiput. The back of the skull should rest comfortably in your palms. The patient should allow the full weight of the head to rest in your hands. The resultant pressure will induce tissue release at your fingertips.
- As relaxation proceeds and your fingers sink deeper into the soft tissues, apply gentle cephalic traction with your fingertips for a few minutes. This movement allows the arch of the atlas to disengage from the occiput. Cephalic traction should be started only after you are a few minutes into the technique, to allow for initial relaxation.

This "release" of deep structures of the upper neck reduces tension, improves drainage and circulation to the head, and helps reduce intracranial congestion.

Data from Chaitow L. *Cranial Manipulation Therapy and Practice: Osseous and Soft Tissue Approaches.* New York: Churchill Livingstone; 1999:113–114.

TABLE 64-2. Pharmaceuticals Commonly Used to Treat Neck Pain

MEDICATION	EXAMPLE(S) AND DOSAGE	COMMENTS/PRECAUTIONS
Tricyclic Antidepressants (TCAs)	Amitriptyline: 10, 25, 75, 100, or 150 mg at bedtime, up to 300 mg/day Nortriptyline: 10–25 mg, titrated up by 25 mg every 3–4 days to maximum of 75–150 mg/day Taper dose when stopping therapy	Modulation of ascending and descending pathways Can give for 2–4 wk for pain reduction Decrease dose if excess sedation or anticholinergic effects Sedating Consider checking serum levels if high doses used for long periods
Muscle Relaxants	Cyclobenzaprine: 10 mg at bedtime or three times/day	Anticholinergic side effects May cause anxiety and restlessness Do not give with TCAs More effective than placebo in back and neck pain[84]
Nonsteroidal Antiinflammatory Drugs (NSAIDs)	Ibuprofen: 200–800 mg with food up to every 6 hr to a maximum dose of 3200 mg Naproxen: 250–500 mg/day with food	Can cause gastrointestinal bleeding, anticoagulation No one NSAID known to be better than others[85]
Acetaminophen	325–650 mg every 4–6 hr as needed to a maximum of 3000 mg/day	Use caution in liver disease Comparable to NSAIDs for arthritis pain
Opioids	Hydrocodone/acetaminophen: 5/500 or 5/325 mg (other doses also available); one to two tablets every 4–6 hr as needed Tylenol with codeine: 30/300 mg; one to two tablets every 4–6 hr as needed	Best to use short-term only Significant addictive potential Constipation common Use caution with alcohol or sedatives No clear benefits long term for quality of life, pain level, or disability[86]

Pharmaceuticals should be used only as a stopgap measure, if at all possible, to allow for symptom management while safer and more "in-depth" therapeutic options are being instituted for the long term.

> Pharmaceuticals should be considered only as stopgap approaches, to be used on a short-term basis as the root causes of pain are being sought. Research on long-term opioid use is becoming less supportive of chronic pain medication use.

Supplements

Omega-3 Fatty Acids
Ideally, as with any nutrients, essential fatty acids should be obtained through a healthy and varied diet, but this often proves difficult. Not many foods contain omega-3 fats in large amounts. Fish oil supplements decrease inflammation for many conditions, and although studies of its use specifically for neck pain are few, a reasonable approach is to give these supplements a try (see Chapter 86, The Antiinflammatory Diet).

■ **Dosage**
The dose is 3 to 8 g fish oil daily.

■ **Precautions**
Doses of more than 3 g of fish oil a day may have an anticoagulant effect and should be used with caution in patients who are prone to bleeding disorders or who are taking anticoagulant or antiplatelet medications.[88]

Phytoantiinflammatory Agents
Few studies have focused specifically on the role of herbal remedies in treating musculoskeletal neck pain. However, several trials have evaluated the overall antiinflammatory properties of herbal remedies and the use of these remedies for pain in general,[9,47,89] as well as for conditions such as osteoarthritis,[90,91] rheumatoid arthritis,[90] and low back pain.[91] Overall, these supplements are quite safe and well tolerated. Most of them work by altering levels of one or more compounds involved in the inflammatory cascade, including cyclooxygenase-2, lipoxygenase, nitric oxide, tumor necrosis factor-alpha, interleukin-1 and interleukin-6, and prostaglandin E_2.[88] For mild to moderate chronic pain, phytoantiinflammatory agents are worth considering, with the intent of decreasing pharmaceutical use and reducing the risk of adverse effects. As with conventional medications, these agents would ideally be used only in the short term while other approaches are used to reveal the root of the neck pain. Table 64-3 lists some of the most commonly used phytoantiinflammatory agents, their dosage, evidence of their efficacy, and precautions related to their use.[47,88–108]

TABLE 64-3. Herbal Antiinflammatory Agents*

BOTANICAL AND DOSE	EFFICACY EVIDENCE	PRECAUTIONS
Avocado (*Persea americana*)/Soy Unsaponifiables[47,89] 300–600 mg/day	Decreased NSAID intake in people with knee and hip OA Stimulated collagen growth	Seems to take 2 mo to reach full effect, and effects linger for 2 mo after patients stop taking them Do not use in people with banana or chestnut allergies
Boswellia[88,90,93,94] (*Boswellia serrata*, Indian Frankincense) Extract: 300 or 333 mg three times/day	Preliminary evidence of benefit for knee OA; effect persisted 1 mo after stopping treatment Conflicting research regarding efficacy for RA	No evidence of harm from any preparation Rare GI effects
Cat's Claw[88,95-98] (*Uncaria guianensis* or *Uncaria tomentosa*) *U. tomentosa* most common in United States (dosing varies with species) Capsules: 350–500 mg once or twice/day Tincture: 1–2 mL, two or three times/day Freeze-dried aqueous extract: 100 mg/day Oxindole alkaloid-free extract: 20 mg three times/day	Freeze-dried extract decreased knee pain with activity in OA Modest improvement with some forms in RA Decreased need for drugs in OA May also have antioxidant and immune-stimulating properties	Studies have not shown harmful effects May lower blood pressure May inhibit CYP 3A4 May interfere with immunosuppressants May work better if oxindole alkaloids removed May increase bleeding risk Avoid in pregnancy Not for children younger than 3 yr old
Devil's Claw[88,89,95,97,99-101] (*Harpagophytum procumbens*) Dried root: 1800–2400 mg in aqueous solution three times/day Tincture: 0.2–1.0 ml (1:5) in 25% alcohol three times/day	Rated by Natural Standard, a producer of good-quality, evidence-based monographs, as having "good" (level B) scientific evidence for therapeutic use Effective for back pain	Rated as safer than analgesic medications; side effects rare May alter GI tract acid levels; avoid in duodenal ulcer disease May lower blood glucose and increase bleeding risk
Ginger[88,93,97,102,103] (*Zingiber officinale*) Powdered root: 500 mg to 1 g twice or three times/day Tincture (1 g:5 mL): 1.25–5 mL, three times/day	Evidence limited; moderate effect on OA of the knee in 247 patients, but mixed results in another, smaller study	Occasional mild GI effects Whole root consumption may increase stomach acid Theoretical increase in anticoagulation (no evidence in humans)
Phytodolor[89,97,104] Mixture of aspen (*Populus tremula*), common ash (*Fraxinus excelsior*), and goldenrod (*Solidago virgarea*) Tincture: 20–40 drops tincture three times/day in a beverage, taken for 2–4 wk to reach full therapeutic benefit	Rich in salicylates Studies of more than 300 subjects showed reduced drug dosing in rheumatologic disease Improved grip in OA Comparable to diclofenac in one OA study	No adverse effects noted in trials Theoretical side effects similar to aspirin; avoid in patients with salicylate allergy No drug interactions known Should be avoided in pregnancy
Rose Hips (from *Rosa canina* subspecies)[88,89] Rosehip powder or seeds: 5 g/day	Improved pain scores and decreased pain medication consumption in OA	No contraindications
Turmeric[88,95,96,105-107] (*Curcuma longa*) Root: 1.5–3 g/day, divided into several doses (can be made into tea; 1 heaping teaspoon is 4 g)	Many mechanisms of action, including alteration of arachidonic acid metabolism Improved swelling, stiffness and walking time in RA Improved OA pain and disability but not other clinical parameters May lower LDL and raise HDL	Generally recognized as safe in doses of 8 g/day or more Can be taken in place of an NSAID Seems to protect stomach against NSAIDs
Willow Bark[88,95,108] (*Salicis* cortex) Powdered bark: 1–3 g three to five times/day	Studies indicated benefit for mild pain Best evidence was for dose-dependent effect in 191 patients with back pain Antiinflammatory effect was largely related to salicylate content	Theoretically, may have similar side effects to aspirin, but this has not been found Occasional nausea, rash, and wheezing Caution with use in asthmatic patients

CYP, cytochrome; GI, gastrointestinal; HDL, high-density lipoprotein; HIV, human immunodeficiency virus; LDL, low-density lipoprotein; NSAIDs, nonsteroidal antiinflammatory drugs; OA, osteoarthritis; RA, rheumatoid arthritis.
*Efficacy data are based primarily on studies of symptom control in RA, OA, or back pain. No studies focusing specifically on the treatment of neck pain were found.
Evidence regarding the use supplements containing gamma-linolenic acid (GLA), such as evening primrose oil, black currant seed oil, and borage seed oil, for pain has been less convincing. Of the three, borage oil has the highest GLA content and should be tried first at a dose of 500 to 1000 mg twice/day.[88] Other promising supplements include stinging nettle, green-lipped mussel extract, *Geranium robertianum*, *Tripterygium wilfordii* (Hook F), and green tea.[88,89]

PREVENTION PRESCRIPTION

■ Avoid tobacco and other substance use.
■ Maintain a healthy body weight.
■ Exercise regularly, and include exercises that strengthen the neck muscles.
■ Ensure that the normal curve of the neck is maintained when sleeping.
■ Take measures at work to minimize the risk of pain:
  • Avoid heavy lifting, or be sure to do it safely.
  • Try to cultivate a sense of control in the work environment.
  • Neck pain is less likely when someone has higher job satisfaction.
■ Pay close attention to posture:
  • Frequent backpack use can increase neck pain.
  • Make sure that posture is good when reading or using a computer.
  • Use a headset rather than holding a phone between the ear and shoulder.
■ Eat a diet that will prevent or reduce inflammation:
  • Increase dietary intake of omega-3 fatty acids or supplement with fish oil or flaxseed oil.
  • Increase fruit and vegetable intake to 8 to 10 servings a day.
  • Avoid foods high in saturated fats.
■ Maintain a healthy social support network.
■ Decrease stress levels. Use stress-reduction techniques regularly, such as meditation, progressive muscle relaxation, journaling, and any others that prove helpful.
■ Treat anxiety or depression, if they are present.

THERAPEUTIC REVIEW

■ Lifestyle Modifications Including Exercise

• Exercise should be encouraged to prevent and treat soft tissue neck pain.

• Postural therapies, such as Alexander technique, Feldenkrais, and Pilates therapy, can provide cervical muscle support.

• Preserve the normal lordotic curve of the neck during sleep; cervical spine pillows may help.

• Avoid repetitive strain (holding telephone on the shoulder, leaning over a desk, carrying heavy over-the-shoulder bags, looking over the shoulder).

■ Nutrition

• Increase intake of foods high in omega-3 fatty acids (cold-water fish, flaxseed products, nuts, green leafy vegetables).

• Decrease intake of foods rich in omega-6 and trans-fatty acids (hydrogenated vegetable oils, margarine, processed foods).

• Decrease saturated fat intake.

• Eat foods rich in antioxidants, including a variety of colors of fruits and vegetables.

■ Mind-Body Therapy

• Address underlying emotional issues that may be causing or exacerbating pain and spasm.

• Journaling, self-hypnosis, biofeedback, and guided imagery are worth exploring.

• Reduce chronic stress and watch for indications of psychological causes of neck pain, such as depression and anxiety.

■ Bioenergetic Therapies

• Acupuncture is a well-studied, potentially beneficial, and safe adjunctive treatment if performed by a trained professional.

• Therapeutic touch and other "hands-on" healing techniques are of potential benefit and quite safe.

■ Biomechanical Therapies

• Consider manipulative therapies:

  • Be cautious with high-velocity, low-amplitude manipulation because it may have some sequelae.

  • Soft tissue manipulation and massage are other possibilities.

• Cranial base release and strain-counterstrain are useful techniques that can be easily performed in the office environment.

• Surgery should be used with caution and only in patients with a known nerve root or spinal cord disorder.

■ Supplements

• Taking 1 to 4 g/day of omega-3–rich oil capsules can help reduce inflammation.

■ Pharmaceuticals

- For chronic pain, if other approaches not effective, consider a tricyclic antidepressant (TCA), such as amitriptyline, 10 to 25 mg at night, or a serotonin-specific reuptake inhibitor, such as fluoxetine, 10 to 20 mg in the morning. Doses of these agents may be gradually increased as needed.

- Consider prescribing a muscle relaxant for 2 to 3 weeks. Cyclobenzaprine, 10 mg at bedtime, is a reasonable choice if the patient is not already taking a TCA.

- Provide a nonsteroidal antiinflammatory drug, such as ibuprofen, 400 to 600 mg every 6 hours with food.

- Consider the use of narcotics for severe pain on a short-term basis only: hydrocodone/acetaminophen, 5/500-mg tablets, one to two every 4 to 6 hours as needed.

■ Botanicals

- Consider a phytoantiinflammatory agent to complement or replace pharmaceutical therapy (see Table 64-3).

KEY WEB RESOURCES

University of Wisconsin School of Medicine suboccipital release technique: http://www.fammed.wisc.edu/our-department/media/618/sub-occipital-release	Video showing how to perform a suboccipital release or cranial base release for neck pain and suboccipital neuralgia and tension headaches
American Osteopathic Association: http://www.osteopathic.org/osteopathic-health/Pages/default.aspx	Information on osteopathy and how to find a DO in your area
Back and Body Care neck pain information: http://www.backandbodycare.com/home/neck/neck.htm	Patient-created site with information for patients on neck pain
Everyday Health alternative treatments for neck pain: http://www.everydayhealth.com/pain-management/neck-pain/alternative-and-complementary-therapies.aspx	Patient-oriented site with numerous neck pain–specific articles on an array of approaches to neck pain
Continuum Center for Health and Healing: New approaches to chronic pain: http://www.healingchronicdisease.org/en/chronic_pain/index.html	Patient-oriented site designed to teach various approaches for dealing with chronic pain
Mayo Clinic neck pain information: http://www.mayoclinic.com/health/neck-pain/DS00542/DSECTION=alternative-medicine; http://www.painexercises.net/	Patient information on complementary medicine and neck pain; searchable site for exercises for various types of pain
Dr. Howard Schubiner's Mind Body Program: www.unlearnyourpain.com/	Site focusing on the mind-body factor as it relates to chronic pain

---

References

References are available online at expertconsult.com.

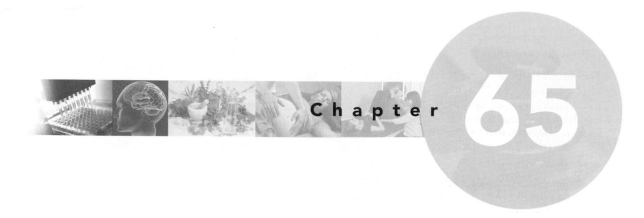

Gout

Fasih A. Hameed, MD

Pathophysiology

Gout is a painful deposition of uric acid crystals in the synovial tissues of the body. Acute attacks usually manifest as a painful monarticular inflammatory arthritis, classically of the first metatarsophalangeal joint, although other joints as well as the kidneys may be affected. A polyarticular presentation is more common with increasing age and length of disease (Fig. 65-1).

Purines are ubiquitous in the body and in nature. As adenine and guanine, they form part of the building blocks of DNA and RNA. Uric acid is the product of purine metabolism by the enzyme xanthine oxidase. Uric acid is excreted primarily by the kidneys, but also by the small bowel. The buildup of uric acid crystals can result from overproduction (10% of cases) or underexcretion (90%) or a combination of the two. A 24-hour urine assay with a finding of more than 800 mg of uric acid supports the diagnosis of overproduction, whereas a finding of less than 600 mg suggests underexcretion.[1]

Because of the numerous diseases with a similar presentation, the diagnosis should be confirmed by aspiration of synovial fluid, examination of which reveals needle-shaped monosodium urate crystals with negative birefringence. Care should be taken not to miss potentially devastating mimics, most notably septic arthritis.

Gout has been recognized since ancient times, with mentions by the Egyptians as early as 2640 BC. In the fifth century BC, Hippocrates referred to gout as "the unwalkable disease." Gout has also been called "the disease of kings" because of the association with the intake of heavy foods and alcohol, apparently common in members of the ruling class. The name "gout" is derived from the Latin *gutta* ["drop"], a reference to a drop of one of the four medieval humors once believed to rule our health or lack thereof.[2]

New Clinical Significance

Although gout is often considered solely in terms of its presentation as an acute inflammatory arthritis, it is truly a systemic disease with significant associated metabolic comorbidities. Gout is linked to obesity, hypertension, dyslipidemia, insulin resistance, hyperglycemia, and coronary artery disease.[3] Data from the third National Health and Nutrition Examination Survey (NHANES III) demonstrated that metabolic syndrome was present in 62.8% of persons with gout but in only 25.4% of those without gout.[4] The Framingham Study demonstrated an *independent* 60% increased risk of coronary artery disease in men with gout after controlling for other factors.[5] The 12-year prospective Health Professionals Follow-up Study of 51,529 men showed that those with gout had a 55% increased risk of fatal myocardial infarction, a 28% increased risk of *all-cause mortality*, and a 38% increased risk of death from cardiovascular disease.[6] These strong associations were independent of age, body mass index, smoking, family history, diabetes, hyperlipidemia, and hypertension. The implications of these data cannot be overstated. Gout is an independent risk factor for death from *all* causes.

> Hyperuricemia can *cause* hypertension.

One proposed mechanism of this relationship may involve a renally mediated increase in blood pressure caused by hyperuricemia. In a rat model of gout, elevated uric acid caused increased blood pressure through activation of the renin-angiotensin system and inhibition of neuronal nitric oxide synthase. Blood pressure normalized with appropriate pharmacologic management and reductions of uric acid. This causal relationship may warrant early administration of urate-lowering therapies in patients with gout and hypertension.[7]

The association of gout with numerous metabolic diseases warrants aggressive lifestyle counseling and screening to prevent long-term morbidity (Fig. 65-2). All persons with gout should thus receive extensive education regarding the health implications of this disease. Comorbidities, once identified, should be promptly managed, and patients should

on the associated increased risk of cardiovascular and all-cause mortality in persons with gout.[6]

Nutrition

Decrease consumption of red meat and most seafood. Persons consuming higher amounts of beef, pork, and lamb have a 41% increased risk of gout. Persons consuming higher amounts of seafood have a 51% increased risk of gout.[9] Given the potential cardiovascular benefits of omega-3 fatty acids found in oily fish, patients can be counseled and may consider moderate intake of small, sustainably caught, cold-water fish (i.e., sardines).

Increase intake of omega-3 fatty acids. Patients wishing to avoid absolutely the purines associated with fish should be encouraged to increase dietary intake of plant sources of omega-3 fatty acids such as flaxseed, purslane, walnuts, and leafy greens. Supplementation (see the later section on omega-3 fatty acids) may also be encouraged.

Increase intake of vegetables, legumes, nuts, and vegetable proteins. Purine-rich vegetables, which were once thought to contribute to gout, are now understood to have no impact on the incidence of the disease.[9] Furthermore, increased intake of vegetable protein was actually associated with up to 27% lower incidence of gout in one report.[9] Additionally, numerous cardiovascular and metabolic benefits are associated with the aforementioned foods, and this association is particularly relevant given the negative impact of gout on cardiovascular and metabolic conditions.

> In response to newer evidence, experts are no longer advocating the avoidance of purine-rich vegetables or an overall purine-restricted diet. Avoidance of animal meat seems to have a larger impact than does reduced purine intake.

Decrease intake of sugar-containing beverages and fructose. Sugar intake was independently associated with elevated uric acid levels in men.[10] Additionally, a direct relationship exists between intake of fructose-containing soft drinks and hyperuricemia, as well as gout.[11,12] Diet soft drinks do not appear to affect uric acid levels, but their use should be discouraged because of an association with metabolic syndrome.[13] Sweet fruits may increase uric acid levels, but the health benefits of these foods far outweigh the associated risks, which can easily be countered through numerous other dietary modifications (e.g., lower consumption of meat, alcohol, and refined sugars).

Limit alcohol to no more than one to two drinks per day, and drink wine rather than beer or liquor. Alcohol intake has been positively correlated with gout. Beer has the strongest association. Each 12-oz beer consumed increases the risk of gout by 50% compared with nonbeer drinkers. Distilled spirits have a smaller but still significant association, whereas wine does not appear to be strongly associated with an increased risk of gout.[14] Numerous studies have demonstrated the health benefits of moderate alcohol consumption.[15] Nonetheless, recommending intake of alcohol to those currently abstinent is probably not advisable. Persons wishing to imbibe should consider wine the healthiest option.

Increase intake of low-fat dairy, up to two servings per day. Low-fat dairy intake, specifically milk and yogurt, appears

FIGURE 65-1
Radiographic forefoot abnormalities in tophaceous gout. Extensive bone destruction is seen at the great toe metatarsophalangeal joint with overhanging edges *(arrowhead)* and soft tissue swelling. Smaller erosions are present involving the first tarsometatarsal and second metatarsophalangeal joints *(arrows).* (From Firestein G: *Kelley's Textbook of Rheumatology.* 8th ed. Philadelphia: Saunders; 2008.)

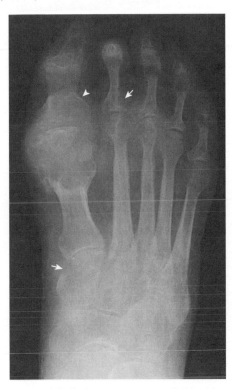

be made aware of the interconnectedness of their various diseases. These preventable diseases of lifestyle may result in significant health consequences even with prompt identification and treatment. Therefore, patients must be encouraged, through appropriate use of behavioral change models such as appreciative inquiry or motivational interviewing, and empowered to make positive changes in their lives (see Chapter 99, Motivational Interviewing Techniques).

> Gout is a metabolic disease that independently increases the risk of all-cause and cardiovascular mortality. Like other metabolic diseases (e.g., diabetes), gout warrants aggressive lifestyle counseling and modification.

Integrative Therapy

Weight Loss

Encourage weight loss and maintenance of a healthy body mass index. Adiposity is associated with hyperuricemia, whereas weight loss leads to reductions in gout incidence.[8] Weight loss also has the greatest benefit on mediating the numerous comorbidities associated with gout. All patients with gout should be encouraged to control weight through exercise and diet modification. Emphasis should be placed

FIGURE 65-2
Gout pyramid. (From Choi HK. A prescription for lifestyle change in patients with hyperuricemia and gout. *Curr Opin Rheumatol.* 2010;22:165–172.)

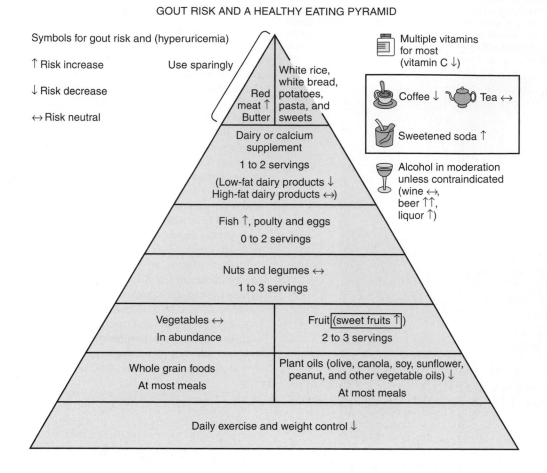

GOUT RISK AND A HEALTHY EATING PYRAMID

Supplements

Vitamin C and Bioflavonoids

Vitamin C supplementation was once thought to exacerbate gout. More recent data, however, reversed that belief. Vitamin C most likely decreases serum uric acid levels through competitive binding of proximal tubule uric acid reuptake channels and may also increase uric acid clearance through a modest improvement in global glomerular filtration.[21] Studies showed an inverse relationship between vitamin C intake and uric acid levels.[22] A double-blind randomized controlled trial showed that supplementation with 500 mg per day of vitamin C significantly lowered uric acid levels compared with placebo.[23] A 20-year, large prospective study published in the *Annals of Internal Medicine* confirmed an inverse relationship between vitamin C intake and the incidence of gout, with as much as a 45% lower incidence in study participants ingesting more than 1500 mg of vitamin C per day.[24]

Although we now know that vitamin C can prevent and aid in the treatment of gout by reducing uric acid levels, an additional benefit may be conferred by increasing intake of citrus foods and by taking supplements with the citrus bioflavonoid hesperidin. Hesperidin is found in citrus foods, as well as in plants of the family Lamiaceae (mint family), such

to have a protective effect on the incidence of gout.[9] A randomized control trial of milk confirmed its urate-lowering effect.[16] The mechanism is likely related to the milk proteins casein and lactalbumin.[17] Low-fat dairy also has the advantage of protecting against metabolic syndrome.[13] Full-fat dairy, which is high in proinflammatory fats, should be avoided.

Drink water. Although no studies have quantified or confirmed the effect, adequate hydration is often considered a mainstay of treatment and prevention. The rationale is that a dehydrated state concentrates uric acid and leads to precipitation. Patients should be advised to drink a minimum of 48 oz of water per day.[18]

Consider coffee. Coffee appears to reduce uric acid levels by a mechanism *not linked to caffeine content.*[19] Modest intake of coffee may be considered part of a therapeutic prevention program. Abrupt increases in coffee consumption may trigger an acute gouty attack and should therefore be discouraged.

Alkalinize urine. A study of an acidic versus alkaline diet found a direct correlation between urine pH and uric acid excretion. This occurred despite the lower purine content of the acidic diet.[20] Patients may therefore be encouraged to follow an alkalinizing diet, low in animal protein and rich in vegetables.

as the common herb rosemary. An extract of rosemary demonstrated antinociceptive effects in an animal model of gout, and hesperidin was identified as a *chief contributor to this effect.*[25]

Dosage
All patients should increase their intake of citrus foods. Patients may also consider increasing their intake of herbs from the family Lamiaceae, especially rosemary. Interested patients should also take 500 to 1500 mg of high-quality vitamin C with citrus bioflavonoids including hesperidin.

> Newer research shows that vitamin C is protective against gout.

Eicosapentaenoic Acid and Gamma-Linolenic Acid
Although purine-rich seafood has been shown to increase uric acid levels and gout,[9] eicosapentaenoic acid (EPA), found in certain fatty fish, and gamma-linolenic acid (GLA) have been shown to suppress inflammation in monosodium urate–induced arthropathy (i.e., gout).[26] EPA and GLA appear to work through complementary mechanisms. Besides decreasing the inflammation of acute gouty arthropathy, omega-3 fatty acids also have demonstrated cardiovascular benefits.[27] This finding is significant, given the association of gout with cardiovascular mortality. In patients wishing to avoid the purine intake associated with fish, supplementation with EPA or GLA may be encouraged. GLA is an omega-6 fatty acid found in evening primrose oil, borage oil, and black currant seed oil.

Dosage
Although ideal dosing has not been determined, consider supplementing with 500 mg of EPA or 3000 mg of evening primrose oil.

Cherry
Consumption of cherries and cherry juice should be encouraged. Studies indicated that intake of 280 g (two servings) of Bing sweet cherries lowered plasma urate levels and increased urine urate levels in healthy volunteers.[28] There is also a trend toward decreased C-reactive protein and nitric oxide with cherry intake, a finding suggesting that cherries may help inhibit inflammation. Indeed, a double-blind placebo-controlled trial of cherry juice in long-distance runners showed that runners who ingested cherry juice 7 days before running reported less postrun pain than those who ingested placebo juice.[29]

Dosage
The recommended dose is approximately half a pound of cherries (approximately 2 cups) or an equivalent amount of cherry juice consumed daily.

Quercetin
In addition to displaying antiinflammatory properties, the flavonoid quercetin inhibits xanthine oxidase.[30] Quercetin can also play a role in the treatment and prevention of cardiovascular diseases by reducing blood pressure and oxidized low-density lipoprotein.[31] Quercetin may thus be of some clinical use in patients with gout, but no clinical trials have been performed to date.

Dosage
Food sources of quercetin include onions, apples, berries, grapes, green and black tea, citrus fruits, capers, tomatoes, broccoli, and leafy greens. Encourage adequate intake of these foods. Consider supplementation with up to 500 mg twice daily.

Bromelain
Use of a proprietary bromelain-containing product was clinically equivalent to diclofenac in a double-blind randomized controlled trial of patients with acute pain from osteoarthritis of the hip.[32] Similar benefits may be conferred to persons with gout, although no studies have yet been performed.

Dosage
Encourage daily consumption of pineapple, which is the source of bromelain. Alternatively, supplementation with 500 mg once or twice daily may be considered.

Botanicals

Hibiscus (Hibiscus sabdariffa)
Mounting evidence demonstrates that hibiscus calyx has blood pressure–lowering qualities, which are believed to result from an effect similar to that of angiotensin-converting enzyme (ACE) inhibitors.[33] Hibiscus tea increased uric acid excretion and clearance in healthy volunteers, but it did not affect serum uric acid levels.[34]

Dosage
Patients with gout and borderline hypertension may wish to try hibiscus, 1.5 g calyx as tea taken twice to three times daily. This can be purchased in the bulk herb section of most progressive grocery stores. Hibiscus tea is also readily available in Mexican grocery stores, where it is known as Jamaica.

Physical Medicine

Acupuncture
Acupuncture alone appears to be an effective treatment for acute gouty attacks. A trial of acupuncture compared with Western treatment with allopurinol and indomethacin found acupuncture to be superior (93% effective versus 80%; $P < .01$). The acupuncture-treated group also had greater reductions in serum uric acid and fewer adverse effects.[35] This trial was limited by its small size ($N = 60$) and the use of allopurinol during acute attacks, a practice that is generally not employed by Western physicians, but is not necessarily contraindicated. Nonetheless, the outcomes were impressive, and given the lack of significant side effects, acupuncture can be recommended as a viable option for the management of acute gouty attacks.[36] Referral to a licensed practitioner of traditional Chinese medicine may also be considered.

Ice
In contrast to most arthritides, application of ice to inflamed gouty joints causes significant pain relief. Although most arthritic conditions benefit from heat application, patients with gout prefer ice.[37] Frequent use of topical ice during

painful attacks should be encouraged. This difference may also help distinguish gout from other inflammatory mimics (e.g., rheumatoid arthritis) and thus help aid in diagnosis.

> An observed response to the therapeutic application of ice may help distinguish gout from other inflammatory arthritides.

Rest
Patients inevitably resist movement of a painful joint, and this rest should be allowed within reason until symptoms are resolving.

Traditional Chinese Medicine

Numerous trials of traditional Chinese medicine have demonstrated its clinical effectiveness. A small trial ($N = 67$) of blood-letting cupping in addition to Chinese herbs compared with a control group receiving diclofenac found both treatments to be effective in improving acute gouty arthropathy.[38]

The traditional Chinese herbal formulation Simiao pill or Si Miao, which is a combination of herbs commonly used in the treatment of gout, was clinically superior to a Western medicine control in a randomized trial of three distinct formulations.[39] Simiao pill traditionally consists of a specific blend of the following individual herbs: *Phellodendron chinense, Atractylodes lancea, Achyranthes bidentata,* and *Coix lacryma-jobi.* This formulation of Simiao pill was also found to have in vivo uricosuric and nephroprotective effects in hyperuricemic rats.[40]

■ Dosage
Based on the specific formulation, generally between three and seven tablets are taken three times daily.

Pharmaceuticals: Acute Treatment of Gouty Arthritis

Nonsteroidal Antiinflammatory Drugs
Despite the relative lack of high-quality large randomized controlled trials, nonsteroidal antiinflammatory drugs (NSAIDs) are considered first-line agents for an acute gouty episode. Indomethacin has historically been favored, but given the lack of data or rationale for its use, any high-dose regimen should suffice.[41]

■ Dosage
Indomethacin, 50 mg three times daily, or naproxen, 500 mg twice daily, or ibuprofen, 600 mg three times daily, is taken as needed for 5 to 10 days.

■ Precautions
Standard NSAID precautions should be reviewed, and therapy should be tapered as soon as clinical improvement is noted. Aspirin should be avoided because of the potential uric acid–raising effect of salicylates.

Colchicine
Alexander of Tralles, a sixth-century Byzantine physician, was the first to use *Colchicum autumnale* for the treatment of gout. Although this plant, autumn crocus, is no longer recommended because of significant toxicity, its active derivative colchicine is still widely used for acute gout attacks, despite the absence of head-to-head studies to show that it offers benefit over any other acute method of treatment. The older methods of hourly high-dose treatments and intravenous colchicine are no longer recommended because of the risk of toxicity and unnecessary side effects, as well as a lack of significant benefit over oral dosing.

■ Dosage
Oral colchicine, 1.2 mg followed by 0.6 mg 1 hour later (total dose, 1.8 mg), is initiated as soon as possible in gouty flare.[42] Some patients may wish to use daily colchicine, 0.6 mg, for suppression, although use of the other preventive methods should be preferentially encouraged because colchicine has no effect on uric acid.

■ Precautions
Do not use in cases of end-stage renal disease. Potentially severe drug-drug interactions do exist. Check specific interactions before prescribing.

Glucocorticoids
Oral, intravenous, or intra-articular steroids may be useful when NSAIDs or colchicine are contraindicated.

■ Dosage
Oral prednisolone, 35 mg, was equivalent to twice-daily naproxen, 500 mg, in a double-blind randomized controlled trial.[43] This dose can be tapered over 7 to 10 days as clinical improvement ensues. In monarticular cases, intra-articular injection of 10 to 40 mg triamcinolone can be effective, although data are limited.[44] Intravenous glucocorticoids can be used in patients unable to take oral prednisone or in polyarticular crisis.

■ Precautions
Standard steroid precautions should be observed. Take oral steroids with food as early in the day as possible. If split doses are used, advise taking a second dose with lunch rather than dinner to avoid insomnia.

Pharmaceuticals: Prevention

Angiotensin-Converting Enzyme Inhibitors Versus Diuretics
Although diuretics have been blamed for precipitating many a gouty crisis, their negative effect is actually less than that of hypertension itself.[45] At low doses, thiazide diuretics have a relatively small effect on serum uric acid levels, and the addition of an ACE inhibitor or angiotensin receptor blocker can offset this increase. That said, the uric acid–lowering effects of an ACE inhibitor should be considered for first-line treatment of hypertension in patients with gout.

Probenecid
Probenecid is a uricosuric drug and therefore helpful in cases of underexcretion. It is the gold standard in older patients who are taking thiazide diuretics.[1] Uricosuric agents should be avoided in persons susceptible to nephrolithiasis such as those with tophaceous disease or urate overproduction.

Dosage

The starting dose is 250 mg twice daily, titrated up to the effective dose, usually 500 to 1000 mg twice daily.

Precautions

Probenecid is less effective at glomerular filtration rates lower than 60 mL/minute. Avoid use of this drug in persons prone to nephrolithiasis and in those with cystinuria.

Allopurinol

Allopurinol inhibits xanthine oxidase activity. Unlike probenecid, allopurinol is useful in all causes of hyperuricemia. Because of theoretical risk, allopurinol is generally not started during an acute attack. Patients taking allopurinol should not, however, stop the medication if an acute attack does occur.

Dosage

Allopurinol can be started at 100 to 300 mg daily and titrated up until normal uric acid levels are achieved. Most patients can be adequately treated with 300 mg daily, although the maximum daily dose is 900 mg. To reduce the risk of precipitating a gouty attack, low-dose colchicine may be started simultaneously.[46]

Precautions

Up to 5% of patients will experience side effects, including rash, leukopenia, thrombocytopenia, diarrhea, or drug fever. The allopurinol hypersensitivity syndrome is a rare (less than 0.1% of patients) but potentially fatal adverse reaction consisting of erythematous rash, fever, hepatitis, eosinophilia, and acute renal failure.

Therapies to Consider

Botanicals

Numerous ethnobotanical studies are being conducted on traditional antigout agents, many of which are yielding promising results and confirming the wisdom of indigenous healing systems.

In mice, in vivo trials of the Ayurvedic gout treatments *Coccinia grandis* (ivy gourd) and *Vitex negundo* (five-leaved chaste tree) demonstrated significant decreases in serum uric acid levels. Impressively, *Coccinia grandis* in particular showed urate reductions nearly equivalent to those of allopurinol (3.90 ± 0.07 mg/dL versus 3.89 ± 0.07 mg/dL).[47]

Polynesians have used noni *(Morinda citrifolia)* juice for treatment of various ailments, including gout. Noni was found to have in vitro inhibition of xanthine oxidase,[48] but no clinical trials have been performed to date.

Populus nigra (black poplar) and *Betula pendula* (silver birch) were found to have the highest level of xanthine oxidase inhibition in a study of traditional Czech herbal folk remedies for gout.[49]

In a similar study of 120 traditional Chinese antigout treatments, the following herbs demonstrated the most pronounced xanthine oxidase inhibition: *Cinnamomum cassia* (Chinese cinnamon), *Chrysanthemum indicum*, leaves of *Lycopus europaeus* (bugleweed, gypsy wort), and the rhizome of *Polygonum cuspidatum* (Japanese knotweed).[50]

Supplements

In vitro studies showed that folic acid is a weak inhibitor of xanthine oxidase.[51] More potent effects on inhibition were traced to the activity of a common folate contaminant, pterin aldehyde.[52] Nonetheless, few in vivo trials have been conducted. Daily doses of folate of 1000 mcg failed to lower serum uric acid concentrations in five hyperuricemic subjects.[53] I therefore do not recommend that folate be prescribed for gout unless stronger evidence emerges to support its usefulness.

Niacin has a small uric acid–raising effect, which is doubtful to be of negative clinical significance.[54]

PREVENTION PRESCRIPTION

- Encourage weight loss and maintenance of a healthy body mass index.
- Decrease consumption of red meat and most seafood.
- Increase intake of vegetables, legumes, nuts, and vegetable proteins.
- Decrease intake of sugar-containing beverages and fructose.
- Limit alcohol to no more than one to two drinks per day, and drink wine rather than beer or liquor.
- Increase intake of low-fat dairy, up to two servings per day.
- Maintain adequate hydration.
- Consider moderate coffee consumption.
- Increase food intake of vitamin C and consider supplementing with 500 mg.
- Increase intake of cherries; half a pound per day should be adequate.
- Increase intake of omega-3 fatty acids or take a supplement.

THERAPEUTIC REVIEW

■ Lifestyle Modification

- Encourage weight loss if overweight.
- Maintain hydration.
- Limit intake of beer and liquor.

■ Nutrition

- Decrease consumption of red meat and most seafood.
- Increase intake of vegetables, legumes, nuts, and vegetable proteins.
- Decrease intake of sugar-containing beverages and fructose.
- Increase intake of low-fat dairy, up to two servings per day.
- Consider moderate intake of coffee.

■ Supplements

- Increase intake of vitamin C through foods; consider supplementing with 500 mg daily.
- Eat more cherries: up to half a pound (2 cups) per day.
- Supplement with eicosapentaenoic acid (EPA) and/or gamma-linolenic acid (GLA): EPA, 500 mg daily or evening primrose oil, 3000 mg daily.
- Eat more pineapple or take bromelain supplements, at 500 mg daily.
- Consume more apples, grapes, onions, and tea or take quercetin supplements, at 500 mg twice daily.

■ Botanicals

- Hibiscus tea can be used for borderline high blood pressure and may lower uric acid levels.

■ Physical Medicine

- Acupuncture can help relieve a gouty attack.
- Ice and rest painful joints.

■ Pharmaceuticals

- Acute treatment
  - Use nonsteroidal antiinflammatory drugs (NSAIDs) (e.g., indomethacin, 50 mg three times daily) for first-line treatment unless contraindications exist.
  - Consider colchicine, but use only a low-dose regimen of 1.8 mg divided over 1 hour (1.2 mg and repeat 0.6 mg in 1 hour).
  - Use glucocorticoids in patients unable to take NSAIDs or colchicine.

■ Prevention

- Use probenecid for inadequate uric acid excretion. Start at 250 mg twice daily, and increase to 500 mg twice daily as needed.
- Use allopurinol for all causes of uric acid excess. Start at 100 to 300 mg daily. Increase as needed to reduce serum uric acid to less than 6 mg/dL.

A 24-hour urine assay with the finding of more than 800 mg of uric acid supports the diagnosis of overproduction (10%), whereas a finding of less than 600 mg suggests underexcretion (90%).

References

References are available online at expertconsult.com.

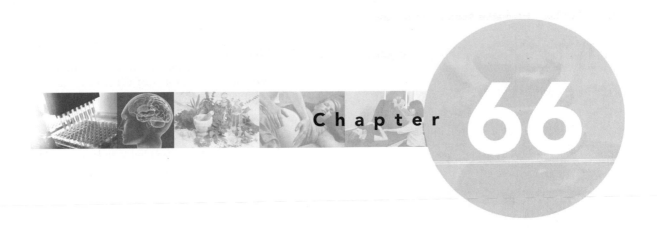

Chapter 66

Carpal Tunnel Syndrome

Gautam J. Desai, DO; Dennis J. Dowling, DO;
Jennifer M. Capra, OMS-IV; and Ankit D. Desai, PharmD

Pathophysiology

Carpal tunnel syndrome (CTS) is a compressive neuropathy of the median nerve that affects women three times as often as men and usually develops after the age 30 of years.[1] Symptoms typically include pain, numbness, tingling, weakness of the thumb and first finger, and involvement of the palm and other fingers except the fifth. Wasting of the thenar eminence may be visible. Activities that may precipitate CTS include repetitive stress activities involving the wrist such as mechanical work, gardening, house painting, meat wrapping, and typing.[2] Trauma, both recent and remote, should be explored, and one of the "keystone" bones of the carpal floor, the lunate, has been implicated in ventral compression of the median nerve against the flexor retinaculum when it is subluxed or displaced.[3] CTS is also commonly seen in persons involved in the occupations listed in Table 66-1.[4]

The carpal tunnel contains nine flexor tendons and the median nerve. The tunnel is created by the three sides of the carpal bones and the flexor retinaculum.[5] Any development that leads to tunnel narrowing or increased pressure within the limited space may cause CTS. These conditions may include edema, bony overgrowth, or inflammation of the tendons. The pressure compresses the median nerve and the small blood vessels that feed the nerve, with resulting ischemia and decreased nerve conduction. Initially, the compression and ischemia result in pain, numbness, and tingling. Chronic compression may result in more prolonged symptoms and signs such as weakness and wasting of the thenar eminence.[6] Some conditions that may be associated with CTS are listed in Table 66-2.[7,8] At times, the origin may be multifactorial, both functional (overuse) and structural (osteoarthritis).

Clinical Manifestations and Diagnosis

Patients typically present with sensory or motor changes along the distribution of the median nerve, which includes the thumb, index finger, middle finger, and radial half of the ring finger.[6] Patients may experience greater pain at night or after sleeping. Some patients find relief of symptoms by shaking their hands, which may temporarily relieve ischemia.[9] Pathognomonic physical findings may be absent early in the course of CTS; as pressure increases within the carpal tunnel, however, patients may demonstrate weakness of the thumb, which causes difficulty with writing or holding objects. Thenar eminence atrophy may be present on physical examination in advanced CTS.[10] Other nerve and vascular compressive syndromes that can cause the same or similar symptoms and signs should also be explored. These disorders can occur separately or concomitantly with CTS in what are known as double-crush and triple-crush syndromes. These syndromes can include cervical root impingement, thoracic outlet syndrome, cubital tunnel syndrome, ulnar neuropathy, pronator syndrome, median nerve neuropathy of the forearm, brachial plexopathy, anterior interosseous nerve syndrome, and Raynaud phenomenom.[11]

The National Institute of Occupational Safety and Health defines CTS as having two or more of the following criteria:

- One or more of the following symptoms affecting at least part of the nerve distribution of the hand: paresthesia, hyperesthesia, pain, and numbness

- One or more of the following symptoms: physical findings of median nerve compression including a positive Hoffman-Tinel sign or a positive Phalen test result, diminished sensation to pinprick in the median nerve distribution, and electrodiagnostic findings indicating median nerve dysfunction across the carpal tunnel[12]

The exact location of nerve entrapment can be diagnosed with electrodiagnostic studies; however, results of nerve conduction studies may be normal in clinically symptomatic patients.[13]

TABLE 66-1. Occupations Associated With Carpal Tunnel Syndrome

- Food processing
- Manufacturing
- Logging
- Construction work
- Poultry work
- Use of vibratory tools

Data from Bernard B, ed. Musculoskeletal Disorders and Workplace Factors: A Critical Review of Epidemiologic Evidence for Work-related Musculoskeletal Disorders of the Neck, Upper Extremity, and Low Back. DHHS (NIOSH) publication no. 97–141. Cincinnati: National Institute for Occupational Safety and Health; 1997; and Scott K, Kothari M. Etiology of Carpal Tunnel Syndrome. <www.UpToDate.com>; 2010 Accessed November 2, 2011.

TABLE 66-2. Causes of Carpal Tunnel Syndrome

Endocrine	Use of corticosteroids or estrogen Myxedema from hypothyroidism Amyloidosis Gout Diabetes mellitus Acromegaly Obesity
Musculoskeletal	Acute trauma Fractures Overuse injury Inflammatory/rheumatoid arthritis
Pulmonary	Tuberculosis
Reproductive	Pregnancy

Data from Solomon D, Katz J, Bahn R, et al. Nonoccupational risk factors for carpal tunnel syndrome. *J Gen Intern Med.* 1999;14:310–314; and Stevens J, Beard C, O'Fallon W, et al. Conditions associated with carpal tunnel syndrome. *Mayo Clin Proc.* 1992;67:541–548.

Integrative Therapy

Lifestyle

Behavior Modification

Elimination of aggravating factors and repetitive motions may help reduce symptoms of CTS, but many patients do not have the opportunity to change occupations. Patients may obtain some relief by using their hands less forcefully, taking frequent breaks, and performing stretching and strengthening exercises. The practitioner should query the patient about hobbies that require repetitive motion as well, because patients may not associate those hobbies with their symptoms. A wrist splint worn during waking hours may provide additional symptom relief, but most patients cannot tolerate daytime splinting. Occasional use of the same splints while sleeping may also bring about some relief during the waking hours.[14] Splints should be individually adjusted (most have a metal stay within a sleeve on the volar surface) to maintain the angle of the wrist to 1 to 5 degrees from neutral into extension. Many braces available off the shelf place the wrist into too high a degree of extension.

Exercise

A 10-month aerobic exercise program demonstrated a reduction in symptoms of CTS, but whether these results were related to the natural course of the disease or to the therapy is unclear.[15] Although performing aerobic activity for cardiovascular health is certainly in the patient's best interests, such exercise has not been proven to be of benefit for CTS treatment, so no evidence supports its use. Stretching of the flexor tendons, the major occupants of the tunnel, may have some benefit in reducing compression of the median nerve (see Fig. 66-2).

Ergonomic Keyboards

Results of studies comparing the use of ergonomic keyboards for amelioration of symptoms of CTS have been mixed.[16] If a patient believes that using such a keyboard will help, it may be worth the higher price to try the device because it has no adverse effects. No evidence exists for its use. The position in which patients place their hands may have more to do with effectiveness than the keyboards themselves. Patients should avoid resting their wrists on the surface while extending their wrists to reach their fingers to the keyboard. Pianists and touch typists classically hover their hands above their respective keyboards.

Pharmaceuticals

Acetaminophen

Acetaminophen has a limited role in CTS owing to a lack of antiinflammatory properties. Acetaminophen appears to display analgesic and antipyretic effects by inhibiting the isoenzymes cyclooxygenase-1 (COX-1) and COX-2 in the central nervous system. This inhibition does not seem to extend into the periphery, thereby eliminating any antiinflammatory properties.[17] Because it has a relatively safe profile, however, acetaminophen remains a good choice for relief of mild to moderate pain in CTS, especially in patients who have concomitant osteoarthritis.

■ Dosage (Adult)

The recommended dose of acetaminophen (Tylenol) is 500 mg every 4 to 6 hours; the maximum dose is 3000 mg/day.[18]

■ Precautions

Use acetaminophen with caution in patients with a history of liver disease and in patients who consume more than three alcoholic beverages daily.[19] In addition, consideration should be given to the appropriate dosage of acetaminophen when patients are taking other concomitant medications that are similarly metabolized by the liver. At recommended dosages, acetaminophen is considered safe in pregnancy.

Nonsteroidal Antiinflammatory Drugs

Median nerve compression caused by inflammation of the flexor tenosynovium can cause patients a great deal of pain.[20] Nonsteroidal antiinflammatory drugs (NSAIDs) exert pain-relieving and antiinflammatory properties through prostaglandin inhibition by inhibition of COX-1 and COX-2 isoenzymes.[19] In general, all NSAIDs have similar efficacy in analgesia and antiinflammatory effects. These effects have yet to be proved adequate in control of symptoms of CTS, however, despite their common use in treatment of this condition. In a study comparing the efficacy of NSAIDs, oral steroids, diuretics, and placebo, only steroids achieved a significant improvement in signs and symptoms of CTS.[21]

■ Dosage
Common NSAIDs and dosages are listed in Table 66-3.

■ Precautions
Use NSAIDs with caution in patients with a history of gastrointestinal bleeding, ulcers or perforation, hypertension or other cardiac disorders aggravated by fluid retention, asthma, renal insufficiency, or coagulation defects, as well as in pregnant patients.[17,19,22]

Diuretics
A rise in tissue pressure in the carpal tunnel is theorized to lead to perineural edema.[23] Diuretic therapy has been employed in efforts to rid the body of excess fluid accumulation and ameliorate CTS. Although case reports exist of the successful use of furosemide to alleviate symptoms of CTS associated with iatrogenic fluid administration, larger comparative studies refute the benefit of diuretic use in CTS.[24] In a study comparing bendrofluazide (a thiazide diuretic not available in the United States) with placebo, no improvements in CTS symptoms were seen.[16] Diuretics should not be used in treatment of CTS.

Corticosteroids
The human body endogenously produces glucocorticoids. At supraphysiologic doses of exogenous corticosteroids, an antiinflammatory response is seen. Modified cellular transcription and protein synthesis lead to local inhibition of leukotriene penetration, suppression of the humoral response, and a reduction in lipocortins, thus diminishing the inflammatory response.[19] In CTS, corticosteroids may be given orally or directly injected into the carpal canal. Short-term oral steroid therapy with conventional treatment, such as splinting, has reduced symptoms in patients with CTS. In a study comparing the use of NSAIDs, diuretics, oral steroids, and placebo, only the group receiving oral prednisolone demonstrated significant relief of CTS symptoms.[21]

Corticosteroid injection, on the radial side of the palmaris longus tendon, has shown short-term efficacy in providing CTS symptom relief.[25,26] In a study comparing surgical decompression with local steroid injection, patients receiving steroid injections had better symptom relief 3 months after treatment than did patients who had undergone surgery.

TABLE 66-3. Common Nonsteroidal Antiinflammatory Drugs Used for Pain Relief

GENERIC NAME	BRAND NAME*	RECOMMENDED ADULT DOSE	ROUTE	MAXIMUM DAILY DOSE
Aspirin	Bayer Aspirin	325–650 mg every 4–6 hr	Oral or rectal	3600 mg
Salsalate	Salflex	500–1000 mg every 8–12 hr	Oral	3000 mg
Ibuprofen	Motrin and Advil	200–400 mg every 4–6 hr	Oral	2400 mg
Diflunisal	Dolobid	500–1000 mg every 12 hr	Oral	1500 mg
Choline magnesium	Tricosal	500–1000 mg every 8–12 hr	Oral	3000 mg salicylate
Naproxen sodium	Aleve and Anaprox	220–550 mg every 8–12 hr	Oral	1500 mg
Naproxen	Naprosyn	250–500 mg every 12 hr	Oral	1500 mg
Ketoprofen	Orudis KT	12.5 mg every 6–8 hr; second dose may be taken after 1 hr if needed	Oral	75 mg
Fenoprofen	Nalfon	300–600 mg every 6–8 hr	Oral	3200 mg
Flurbiprofen	Ansaid	200–300 mg in 2–4 divided doses	Oral	300 mg
Oxaprozin	Daypro	600–1200 mg/day	Oral	1800 mg
Indomethacin	Indocin and Indocin SR	25–50 mg 2–3 times/day	Oral	200 mg
Diclofenac	Voltaren	50 mg every 8 hours; 75 mg every 12 hr	Oral	150 mg
Etodolac	Lodine	200–400 mg every 6–8 hr	Oral	1200 mg
Nabumetone	Relafen	500–1000 mg 1–2 times/day	Oral	2000 mg
Meloxicam	Mobic	7.5 mg/day	Oral	15 mg
Piroxicam	Feldene	10–20 mg/day	Oral	20 mg

Data from references 18, 19, and 22.
*More than one brand may exist for an agent.

At 6 months and 12 months, however, the percentage of patients in whom relief of symptoms was maintained after injection began to decline, whereas the level of relief in the surgically treated group remained constant.[26] Steroid injections are most beneficial to patients with mild to moderate CTS, thus delaying the need for surgery. Injection may be repeated 3 weeks after the initial dose, but the need for a third dose in less than 1 year indicates a need for surgical treatment.[25]

Dosage

A standard dosage for oral steroids in CTS has not been determined. A study comparing two prednisolone regimens—2 weeks of 20 mg/day followed by 2 weeks of 10 mg/day versus 2 weeks of 20 mg/day followed by 2 weeks of placebo—for long-term improvement found no difference in treatment response with respect to duration of steroid therapy.[27] Hence the lower dosage should be used to minimize adverse effects.

Injection therapy consists of methylprednisolone acetate, 20 to 40 mg mixed with 1 mL of 1% lidocaine, or 6 mg of betamethasone combined with 1% lidocaine.[26]

Precautions

Long-term oral steroid use has been associated with immunosuppression, hyperglycemia, hypertension, Cushing syndrome, osteoporosis, and electrolyte disturbances. Injection of steroids must be performed by a skilled practitioner trained in CTS injection to avoid nerve atrophy and necrosis, which may be created by entry of corticosteroid into the median nerve sheath.[19,22,25] The use of corticosteroids in pregnancy is controversial. Although drug monographs indicate corticosteroids to be relatively safe in pregnancy (safety category B), animal studies indicated possible long-term developmental abnormalities. More research using corticosteroids in pregnancy is needed.[28]

Cyclooxygenase-2–Selective Inhibitors

In an effort to protect gastrointestinal mucosa while maintaining pain relief and antiinflammatory properties, medications specific for COX-2 inhibition were developed in the 1990s.[29] COX-2 inhibitors do not inhibit platelet aggregation, but they are not without risk. Although COX-2 inhibition does prevent the production of prostacyclin (prostaglandin I_2 [PGI_2]), it does not inhibit thromboxane A_2, which is responsible for platelet aggregation and vasoconstriction. PGI_2 inhibits platelet aggregation and facilitates vascular smooth muscle contraction. Investigators have theorized that selective inhibition of COX-2 causes a shift toward a prothrombotic state,[22] thus raising the risk of stroke and myocardial infarction. In September 2004, the COX-2 inhibitor rofecoxib (Vioxx) was withdrawn from the market because postmarketing surveillance demonstrated a higher relative risk of stroke and myocardial infarction in patients receiving the drug. In April 2005, valdecoxib (Bextra) was also withdrawn from the market. Celecoxib (Celebrex) is the only COX-2 inhibitor remaining available for prescription.[30] The U.S. Food and Drug Administration (FDA) requires labeling of containers to warn patients and prescribers that celecoxib as well as other NSAIDs may increase the risk for heart attack and stroke. COX-2 inhibitors may be effective in mild to moderate pain relief, but the benefits and risks of therapy

must be weighed before prescribing, especially because these drugs have not been proved to be of benefit in the treatment of CTS.

Dosage

The dose of celecoxib is 100 to 200 mg twice daily; the maximum dose is 800 mg/day.[18,19]

Precautions

COX-2 inhibitors should be used with caution in patients with a history of congestive heart failure, hypertension, asthma, or renal insufficiency. Patients who are pregnant or are allergic to sulfonamides should not take celecoxib.[17,19,22]

Botanicals

Patients using dietary supplements should be advised to choose brands that have been certified for content and purity. Testing for content and purity is not a mandatory requirement for dietary supplements. Trusted organizations that voluntarily test product purity are the United States Pharmacopeia (USP), the Association of Analytical Communities (AOAC), and Consumer Labs (consumerlabs.com). Table 66-4 is a list of sample USP-verified brands.[31]

Ginger (Zingiber officinale)

Ginger, also known as African ginger, black ginger, cochin ginger, and imber, is a mixture of several compounds. Compounds include gingeroles, beta-carotene, capsaicin, caffeine, curcumin, and salicylate.[32] However, these chemical entities seem to vary according to the form of the herb. Ginger is most often used for relief of nausea, vomiting, motion sickness, dyspepsia, flatulence, migraine headache, rheumatoid arthritis, osteoarthritis, and pain. Although the exact mechanism remains unknown, investigators have speculated that some of the constituents in ginger may inhibit COX-1, COX-2, lipoxygenase pathways, tumor necrosis factor-alpha, PGE_2, and thromboxane B_2.[33] Each of these inhibited mechanisms plays a role in inflammation. A randomized placebo-controlled crossover study was conducted comparing the efficacy of ginger, ibuprofen, and placebo in patients with osteoarthritis. Although ibuprofen was found to be the most effective at treating pain, both ibuprofen and ginger both had a significant pain-rating reduction in comparison with placebo.[34] Ginger may be of benefit in

TABLE 66-4. United States Pharmacopeia–Verified Brands

- Berkley & Jensen
- Equaline
- Kirkland Signature
- Nature Made
- Nature's Resource
- Nutri Plus
- Safeway
- Sunmark
- Tru Nature
- Your Life

Data from United States Pharmacopeia. USP-Verified Dietary Supplements. <http://www.usp.org/USPVerified/dietarySupplements/supplements.html/>; Accessed 14.10.11.

patients who have both CTS and osteoarthritis. Patients with nausea and vomiting of pregnancy and CTS may benefit from the antinausea properties of ginger as well.

■ Dosage

In osteoarthritis management, Eurovita Extract 33, a specific ginger extract, is often used. The dosage of this formulation is 170 mg orally three times/day or 255 mg twice daily.[33]

■ Precautions

Because of possible inhibition of platelet aggregation, ginger should be used with caution in patients who are concurrently undergoing anticoagulant therapy or have coagulation disorders. Common adverse reactions with ginger are gastrointestinal discomfort, heartburn, and diarrhea. The use of ginger during pregnancy is relatively safe when it is orally ingested for medicinal purposes. Although some concerns have been expressed about ginger and its involvement in altering fetal sex hormones, and one case report of spontaneous abortion exists, the overall risk of fetal malformation does not appear to be higher than the baseline (1% to 3%).[33]

Willow Bark (Salix alba)

Willow bark, also known as white willow bark, brittle willow, and simply willow, is a dietary supplement from the Salicaceae family. It is most often used by patients to treat headache or pain caused by osteoarthritis, myalgia, gout, and dysmenorrhea. Although components of willow bark include flavonoids and tannins, the pain-relieving properties are attributed to the salicin glycosides present in the compound. After ingestion of willow bark, the salicin glycosides are converted in the intestine to saligenin, which is then metabolized to produce salicylic acid. At this point, elimination becomes the same as for aspirin (acetylsalicylic acid).[33] Like aspirin, willow bark demonstrates analgesic, antipyretic, and antiinflammatory properties. Platelet aggregation may be inhibited by willow bark, but to a lesser extent than by aspirin. Studies comparing willow bark, diclofenac, and placebo in patients with osteoarthritis and rheumatoid arthritis found willow bark to be no better than placebo for pain relief.[35] Although no studies have evaluated willow bark use for CTS, this substance can be regarded as having efficacy similar to that of aspirin and other NSAIDs in pain management.

■ Dosage

Willow bark should be dosed according to the salicin content in the supplement: salicin, 120 to 240 mg orally in two to three divided doses daily.[33]

■ Precautions

Safety concerns about using willow bark are similar to those for salicylate therapy. Willow bark may cause gastric irritation, nausea, vomiting, and bloody stools. It should be used with caution in patients who are also taking antiplatelet medications or other salicylate-containing products. Insufficient evidence exists for using willow bark in pregnancy. Pregnant women are advised to avoid it.

Arnica (Arnica montana)

Also known as arnica flower, leopard's bane, and mountain tobacco, arnica is used to treat inflammation and as an immune system stimulant. The boost in immune response is thought to decrease healing time in bruises, aches, and sprains. The primary active constituents in arnica are sesquiterpene lactones.[33] Although the exact mechanisms are not completely understood, the antiinflammatory effects seen with arnica seem to differ mechanistically from those of NSAIDs. A specific sesquiterpene lactone, helenalin (which is implicated in inflammation), inhibits nuclear transcription factor NF-kappaB.[36] Helenalin has also been shown to inhibit platelet function. In a randomized placebo-controlled study using arnica to control pain and swelling in patients who had undergone surgical repair of CTS, no difference in swelling was seen in patients receiving arnica and in those receiving placebo. However, a significant reduction in pain was seen 2 weeks after surgery in patients receiving arnica.[37] Arnica may be useful in patients who have undergone surgical treatment for CTS, but the potential side effects and toxicity, as well as the difficulty in obtaining standardized doses, may be obstacles to its use.

■ Dosage

Unless diluted, arnica is toxic when taken by mouth. Although no standard or well-studied doses or arnica preparations are available, the usual homeopathic preparations are diluted to 1:10 and 1:100 strengths. Serial dilutions continue until the desired strength is reached. For example, a 1:100 solution that is diluted 30 times is said to be 30 C potency.[37] Caution should be exercised because of the difficulty in obtaining a standardized dose and the possible side effects.

■ Precautions

Arnica in homeopathic doses is generally safe.

> Arnica belongs to the Asteraceae/Compositae family. Patients allergic to other members of this family will also be allergic to arnica. Additional members of the Asteraceae/Compositae family include ragweed, chrysanthemums, marigolds, daisies, and many other herbs.[33]

Supplements

Vitamin B_6 (Pyridoxine)

Vitamin B_6 is required by the body for many functions, including metabolism of amino acids, carbohydrates, and lipids. Vitamin B_6 is also a coenzyme in various metabolic reactions, such as transamination of amino acids, conversion of tryptophan to niacin, synthesis of gamma-aminobutyric acid, metabolism of serotonin, norepinephrine, and dopamine, and the production of heme for hemoglobin. It is also required in myelin sheath formation.[33] Clinically, vitamin B_6 is used to offset neuropathy caused by certain medications, such as isoniazid. Vitamin B_6 was first thought to be an effective treatment in CTS on the basis of low tissue levels seen in deceased patients with CTS. Investigators now know, however, that pyridoxine levels decline in deceased or infarcted tissue.[33] Two studies involving a total of 50 subjects with CTS demonstrated no benefit for vitamin B_6 in comparison with placebo.[38]

Mild deficiencies in vitamin B_6 are relatively common. Sources of this vitamin include potatoes, milk, cheese, eggs, fish, carrots, spinach, and peas. Vitamin B_6 is useful in treating general deficiency and neuritis. Patients with CTS receiving benefit from pyridoxine therapy are thought to have an underlying deficiency or neuropathy. More studies are needed to assess the effectiveness of vitamin B_6 in CTS, but the supplement may be useful in patients with an underlying deficiency.

■ Dosage
For vitamin B_6 deficiency, 2.5 to 25 mg/day orally is taken for 3 weeks, with a maintenance dose of 1.5 to 2.5 mg/day thereafter. For neuritis, the dose is 10 to 50 mg/day orally.[33]

■ Precautions
Adverse reactions associated with vitamin B_6 therapy include abdominal pain, nausea, vomiting, increased serum aspartate aminotransferase values, and decreased serum folic acid concentrations. At doses exceeding 1000 mg, this vitamin has been shown to cause sensory neuropathy. It should be used with caution in patients concurrently taking phenytoin, phenobarbital, or levodopa. Pyridoxine may increase the metabolism of these drugs and thereby reduce the plasma levels of phenytoin, phenobarbital, or levodopa.

The U.S. Recommended Dietary Allowance (RDA) values for vitamin B_6 are as follows:
- *Men:* 19 to 50 years old, 1.3 mg; 51 years old and older, 1.7 mg
- *Women:* 19 to 50 years old, 1.3 mg; 51 years old and older, 1.5 mg. Some researchers think that the RDA for women 19 to 50 years old should be increased to 1.5 to 1.7 mg.
- *Pregnant women:* 1.9 mg; lactating women: 2 mg[33]

Biomechanical Therapy

Massage Therapy
A small study ($N = 16$) showed a short-term benefit of pain reduction and functionality improvement in patients treated with four weekly massages by a therapist (not further defined) as well as daily self-massage.[39] The type of massage described resembled pétrissage and effleurage-type stroking and was focused on the hand and forearm. No group received sham massage, so whether the benefits resulted from direct action of the massage on the carpal tunnel and surrounding tissues to mobilize fluid or from neurotransmitter release in the central nervous system is unclear. Because teaching a patient to massage his or her own hand and forearm has minimal cost, a trial of this modality may be of benefit.

Yoga
In another small study, a group of patients taking part in a highly individualized and methodical yoga program (Iyengar approach) demonstrated significant reduction in pain and significant improvement in grip strength compared with a control group offered a wrist splint in addition to continuation of the current treatment.[40] No significant difference was reported in median nerve motor and sensory conduction time between the two groups. The yoga regimen, for which the group met twice weekly for 8 weeks, was designed to focus on improving strength and balance in each joint in the upper body and also covered a relaxation technique. Although a larger study with long-term follow-up is needed, yoga may be an option for patients who are able to afford such a program, as well as for those who may be unable or unwilling to use other approaches or treatment options for CTS.

Physical Therapy and Occupational Therapy Modalities
■ Wrist Splinting
Nighttime splints that prevent flexion of the wrist are inexpensive options useful in the treatment of CTS and should be a first-line choice for most patients with mild to moderate CTS. Although full-time splint use may produce better results, most patients generally do not tolerate daytime use of the appliance. Splints that keep the wrist in a neutral position may be more beneficial than those placing the wrist in extension. Patients should try a noncustom orthotic first, which is less expensive than the custom-fitted counterpart. Generally, negative effects are not associated with splint use, other than the initial discomfort of wearing a new appliance. Splinting may be used in combination with other therapies. One study demonstrated splinting to be superior to steroid injection of the carpal tunnel in patients with mild and moderate CTS, in terms of both symptomatic relief and improvements in sensory and motor nerve conduction velocities.[41] These results were obtained with near-nightly use of the splint for 1 year, a regularity and duration that may be more difficult to obtain in a nonstudy patient population. Patients whose CTS is unresponsive to this therapy after 3 weeks of use must be reexamined; in addition, patients with thenar wasting on initial presentation may benefit from another treatment modality. Pregnant patients may be especially good candidates for splinting.

■ Ultrasound Therapy
Ultrasound therapy may be of benefit in patients with mild to moderate CTS, although the cost and frequency of treatments may be a barrier. One study demonstrated an improvement in symptoms and motor distal latency in wrists receiving ultrasound treatment that was not seen in wrists receiving sham ultrasound.[42] The investigators postulated that the antiinflammatory and tissue-stimulating effects of ultrasound could be responsible for the results, although more research is needed. Other modalities are less expensive and less time consuming, so ultrasound should be considered after those have been tried and are unsuccessful. Long-term benefits of ultrasound therapy are unknown.

Chiropractic Manipulation
Chiropractic manipulation has not been proved to be of benefit in the treatment of CTS. One randomized clinical trial demonstrated an improvement in symptoms in the group receiving chiropractic manipulation, but this group also underwent ultrasound and received wrist splints, thus making it impossible to determine whether symptom improvement resulted from chiropractic manipulation or from the other modalities.[43] No significant difference was noted between the group treated with chiropractic manipulation and the group treated with medication, who also received splints. Manipulation was defined as high-velocity,

low-amplitude thrust, myofascial massage, and loading procedures to the wrist, elbow, and shoulder, as well as treatment to the cervical and upper thoracic regions. A few published case reports of the efficacy of chiropractic manipulation for treatment of CTS exist, but more studies are needed before this approach can be recommended for this condition.

Osteopathic Manipulative Treatment

Randomized controlled studies of osteopathic manipulative treatment (OMT) for the treatment of CTS are scarce. Palpatory examination was noted to be 92% sensitive but only 75% specific when compared with electrodiagnostic studies for determining CTS.[44] However, cadaver studies demonstrated an elongation of the transverse carpal ligament after treatment with OMT (nonthrust techniques designed to stretch the transverse carpal ligament) directed at the wrist, in conjunction with static loading (weights).[45,46] Whether these results may be applied to living patients remains to be seen, although animal studies showed minimal change in postmortem biomechanical properties of ligaments after freezing,[47,48] so these findings may possibly be relevant. The female cadaver wrists tended to be smaller and had greater elongation of the transverse carpal ligament, especially when OMT was done first, followed by static loading.

Osteopathic physicians practice many specialties, and many serve as primary care physicians and can easily perform OMT in the office, as shown in Figure 66-1, during the first presentation of the complaint. The patient can be instructed in self-stretching exercises (shown in Fig. 66-2), which can be done at home at no cost and often with increasing relief of symptoms. One small study ($N = 16$ wrists) demonstrated a reduction in symptoms with OMT,[49] and another reported magnetic resonance imaging evidence that OMT

and self-stretching enlarged transverse and anteroposterior dimensions of the carpal canal.[50] However, three of the four patients undergoing this treatment had symptoms of CTS after trauma, which may respond differently than CTS of other causes, such as repetitive motion. Large randomized trials including sham OMT are needed before OMT can be clearly stated as being beneficial for CTS. Given the low risk of adverse events with OMT as well as the low cost, however, a patient can be treated by a combination of approaches, including self-stretching and wrist splints. Before more invasive approaches (i.e., injection, surgery) are considered, a trial of OMT may be of benefit. Additionally, the holistic philosophy of osteopathic medicine mandates taking into account the person as a whole, considers other potential aggravating factors, and seeks ways to reduce or remove these factors.

Surgery

The three basic types of surgical procedures for carpal tunnel release, all of which attempt to visualize and cut the transverse carpal ligament, are as follows:

- Traditional open (approximately a 5-cm incision)
- Mini-open (approximately a 2.5-cm incision)
- Endoscopic (one or two portals)

Relief of symptoms is similar with all three types, but patients undergoing endoscopic surgery performed by an experienced surgeon will likely return to work sooner than will patients having traditional open surgery.[6] A 2005 randomized controlled trial demonstrated open surgery to be superior in terms of symptom relief but not grip strength, compared with a single steroid injection for CTS, over a

---

FIGURE 66-1
A, The physician's thumbs apply pressure away from the center of the wrist, while the fingers below simultaneously apply an upward force to create a spreading effect. **B,** Once an initial stretch has been achieved and held, the physician can then gently extend the patient's wrist farther (by pushing patient's fingers with his or her knee) and create more of a spread by moving his or her thumbs farther away from the center of the wrist. The goal is to increase the length of the transverse carpal ligament and widen the carpal canal, thereby reducing the amount of pressure on the median nerve. (Adapted from Sucher BM. Myofascial release of carpal tunnel syndrome. *J Am Osteopath Assoc.* 1993;93:92–101.)

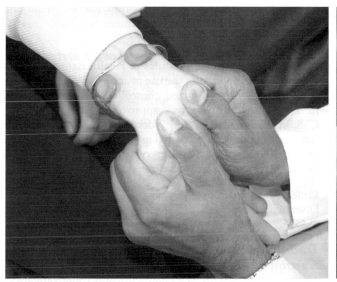

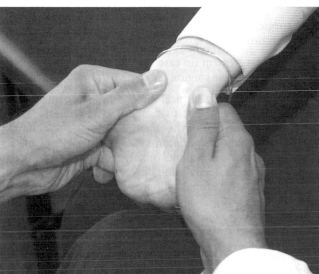

A

B

Steroid Injection

- Injection of methylprednisolone acetate, 20 mg mixed with 1 mL of 1% lidocaine, into the carpal canal by a physician trained in this procedure may offer some relief of symptoms. It may also delay the need for surgery.

- Use of more than three doses in 1 year suggests a need for surgical intervention.

Ultrasound

- Although costly and time consuming, ultrasound may be beneficial in patients with mild to moderate CTS. It can be combined with splint therapy, OMT, or medications.

Traditional Acupuncture

- Acupuncture can be used as a possible alternative to surgery for mild CTS.

- It may be costly and is usually not covered by medical insurance.

Surgery

- Surgery is likely most useful for patients with unrelenting pain or numbness, thenar atrophy, or treatment failure with other modalities.

- The clinician must be certain of the diagnosis and must choose a surgeon who has performed many CTS procedures.

- Referral to a CTS specialist for evaluation is recommended before surgery is suggested to the patient.

- Surgery is not advised for pregnant patients with CTS, which will probably resolve with delivery.

- Indications for surgery are unrelenting pain, thenar eminence atrophy, loss of motor function with diminished finger strength, and failure of other treatments.

KEY WEB RESOURCES

National Institute of Neurological Disorders and Stroke, National Institutes of Health carpal tunnel syndrome (CTS) fact sheet: http://www.ninds.nih.gov/disorders/carpal_tunnel/detail_carpal_tunnel.htm	Fact sheet and information page touching on diagnoses, etiology, and treatments
MedicineNet article on CTS: http://www.medicinenet.com/carpal_tunnel_syndrome/article.htm	A comprehensive and patient-friendly site referencing and explaining CTS
American Society of Surgery for the Hand information on CTS: http://www.assh.org/Public/HandConditions/Pages/CarpalTunnelSyndrome.aspx	Information on surgical treatment of CTS

References

References are available online at expertconsult.com.

Chapter 67

Epicondylitis

David Rabago, MD, and Aleksandra Zgierska, MD, PhD

Pathophysiology

Lateral epicondylosis (LE) and medial epicondylosis (ME) are common, painful, debilitating soft tissue disorders. LE (tennis elbow) affects up to 7 patients per 1000 per year in general medical practices.[1] ME (golfer's elbow) is much less common and is associated with less functional impairment.[2] Both conditions are well known as sport-related injuries, but they have their greatest effect on workers with repetitive stressful hand tasks.[3] The most common causes of LE and ME may be low-load, high-repetition activities such as keyboarding, although formal data are lacking.[4] The cost of time away from work because of these disorders is significant.

Our understanding of the pathophysiology underlying LE and ME has changed. Both LE and ME were traditionally seen as inflammatory conditions. The terms *lateral epicondylitis* and *medial epicondylitis* are often used indiscriminately to refer to chronic overuse elbow injury. However, most overuse tendon injuries, including LE and ME, show no histopathologic evidence of inflammatory cells.[5-7] Rather, they are chronic degenerative conditions. Therefore, *epicondylosis* is the preferred term.[8,9] The current understanding identifies overuse of or trauma to elbow extensor or flexor tendons, microtearing, and failed tendon healing as the key mechanisms of injury. The result is weakened, fibrosed, and, finally, calcified and necrotic tendon insertions at the lateral or medial epicondyle.[10,11] Although inflammation may be present early in the disease process, biopsy studies show an absence of inflammatory mediators and cells, as well as dramatically disorganized collagen (Figs. 67-1 and 67-2). Tendinopathy has been used as a general term for this class of injury.[11,12]

> Lateral epicondylosis and medial epicondylosis are examples of overuse tendinopathies, complete healing of which often requires 3 to 12 months.

Integrative Therapy

The treatment of epicondylosis was assessed in more than 100 randomized controlled trials (RCTs) and critical reviews, most addressing LE. The results of these reviews can be disheartening, given that no therapy was definitively better in the long term than conservative treatment. Existing studies often suffer from small sample size, poor evaluation over longer periods (12 to 24 months), and inconsistency of diagnostic criteria, treatment protocols, and outcome measures. Key issues, such as quality of life, the cost and benefit of various therapies, and return to work parameters are relatively unstudied. Very few studies compare a given intervention with either watchful waiting or physical therapy designed specifically for epicondylosis. However, although better research is sorely needed, recommendations can be made based on both clinical trial data and clinical experience.

Lifestyle

Healing Context

An integrative approach for the treatment of LE and ME focuses on pain relief, preservation of movement, muscle conditioning, and prevention. Most patients respond well to conservative treatment. The clinician should explain the pathophysiology of epicondylosis to the patient and should establish realistic expectations about treatment and expected time to full recovery. Many patients are surprised by both the nature of the condition (noninflammatory) and the extended period often required for complete healing. Most patients recover completely in 3 to 6 months regardless of treatment.[10] Some patients with LE and ME suffer from symptoms that are refractory to initial therapy, however. In a general practice trial of watchful waiting, 20% of patients who had elbow pain for longer than 4 weeks did not experience resolution of the pain and disability within 1 year.[13]

FIGURE 67-1

Histology of a normal tendon. (From Wilson JJ, Best TM. Common overuse tendon problems: a review and recommendations for treatment. *Am Fam Physician.* 2005;72:811–818. Copyright 2005 American Academy of Family Physicians.)

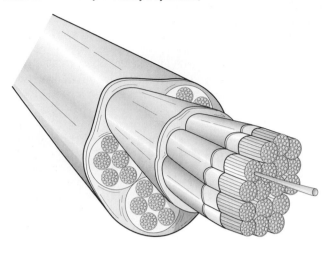

FIGURE 67-2

Histology of a damaged tendon. Note the collagen disorientation and separation. (From Wilson JJ, Best TM. Common overuse tendon problems: a review and recommendations for treatment. *Am Fam Physician.* 2005;72:811–818. Copyright 2005 American Academy of Family Physicians.)

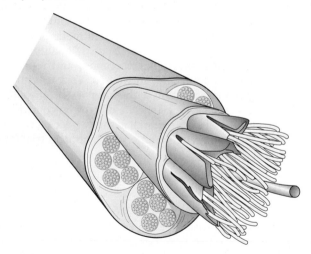

Relative Rest

The pain of LE and ME is likely caused, and is certainly exacerbated, by activities that overuse the extensor and flexor tendons (Fig. 67-3). Pain from LE can be decreased by limiting wrist extension; ME-related pain can be decreased by limiting wrist flexion and pronation.

Patients whose work activity necessarily exacerbates pain should be transferred to more benign tasks or lighter or shorter duty or should be given medical leave. Because relative rest makes good clinical sense but is unstudied, the duration and extent of rest or leave, as well as the effect of short breaks, should be monitored clinically.

FIGURE 67-3

A, Lateral epicondylosis. **B,** Medial epicondylosis.

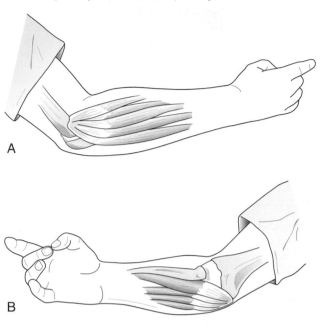

Ice

Because the role of inflammation in tendinopathies is unclear, the importance of icing, a traditional antiinflammatory technique, is also uncertain. However, cryotherapy is probably effective in the acute phase (first 7 days), especially in the setting of trauma. A 2004 systematic review of icing treatment for soft tissue injury found that application of ice through a wet towel for 10 minutes every 4 to 6 hours was effective.[14]

Mind-Body Therapy

Psychosocial Stress

The severity of epicondylosis has been found to be related to the intensity of work environment stress.[3] Patient education about stress relief techniques, and workplace assessment to reduce psychosocial stressors, may affect the level of pain of LE and ME. It may also help prevent further tendinopathy when these measures are combined with other therapy.

> Evidence suggests that acupuncture alleviates lateral epicondylosis pain in the short term.

Bioenergetic Therapy

Acupuncture

Acupuncture is based on the idea that patterns of energy flow (qi) through the body are essential for health. Disruptions of this flow are believed to be responsible for disease.

Acupuncture may work on epicondylar pain through activation of endogenous opioids.[15] Reviews and RCTs reported that needle acupuncture was significantly more effective than sham acupuncture in treating LE,[16] that acupuncture could increase the duration of pain relief and the proportion of people with at least 50% pain reduction after only one treatment,[17] and that acupuncture increased the proportion of subjects who reported a good or excellent result of treatment (22 out of 44 with acupuncture, compared with 8 out of 38 without acupuncture).[18] Acupuncture is a reasonable therapeutic option if pain and disability are refractory to more conservative treatment.

■ Precautions

Acupuncture must be performed by a trained specialist. Only one study reported any harm from needle acupuncture.[19] The investigators noted that one patient withdrew from the study because of needle pain. Given that needle acupuncture has provided pain relief in the short term and has very low risk, it is a reasonable treatment option for patients in whom more conservative management has failed.

Pharmaceuticals

Nonsteroidal Antiinflammatory Drugs

Nonsteroidal antiinflammatory drugs (NSAIDs) target the inflammatory process thought to play a role in the early stage of LE and ME. A systematic review of the use of topical NSAIDs (diclofenac and benzydamine) for lateral elbow pain in adults found that pain was significantly improved after 4 weeks of NSAID use in comparison with placebo.[20] However, no differences in grip strength or range of motion were reported. Another study noted significant improvements in pain and function after iontophoresis and diclofenac.[21] A systematic review of oral NSAIDs found that diclofenac significantly reduced short-term pain compared with placebo, but the studies reviewed did not assess function or long-term pain.[22]

> Nonsteroidal antiinflammatory drugs and corticosteroid injections have been shown to relieve acute epicondylar pain but not to improve outcomes in the long term.

Although beneficial in the short term, use of NSAIDs is controversial because the role of inflammation is not fully understood; inflammation may have an efficacious role in soft tissue healing. In addition, the studies assessed the use of NSAIDs in the acute phase, when spontaneous healing is most likely. Acetaminophen has not been studied, but it may provide relief of mild to moderate pain without gastrointestinal risk.

■ Dosage

Topical diclofenac 3% gel is applied twice daily for 1 to 2 weeks. The regimen for topical diclofenac with iontophoresis is as follows: 3% gel, 150 mg using a 4- to 8-mA intensity for 20 sessions of 25 to 30 minutes each.

The dose of oral diclofenac is 75 mg twice daily for 1 to 2 weeks. The dose of oral ibuprofen is 600 mg each 6 hours for 1 to 2 weeks.

■ Precautions

Topical NSAIDs may cause skin irritation. Oral NSAIDs may cause abdominal pain and diarrhea, and patients have an increased risk of gastrointestinal complaints (relative risk, 3.0 to 5.0).[23]

Corticosteroid Injections

Corticosteroid injections also target inflammation and have been a mainstay of conventional therapy for LE and ME. Clinical trial data support their use on a limited basis for pain and disability from LE and ME, although the effects may be relatively short lived; clinical trial and systematic review data suggested that the effectiveness of these injections is limited to 6 months or less. One review concluded that steroid injections were effective over the short term (2 to 6 weeks) compared with placebo, elbow strapping, physical therapy, and NSAIDs, but not in the long term.[22] The best study compared steroid injections with physical therapy and watchful waiting; at 6 weeks, the injection-treated group was most improved, but at 1 year, the other two groups experienced a higher rate of complete symptom relief.[24] A systematic review and clinical trial both reported that corticosteroid injection use was associated with limited effectiveness at 1 year.[25,26] Corticosteroid injections may have a role in patients whose work or sport activity requires rapid, short-acting relief of pain. Patients can be reinjected at 4 to 6 weeks, to a maximum of three injections.[20]

■ Dosage

The dose is 1 mL of 40 mg/mL methylprednisolone in 2 to 3 mL of 1% lidocaine.

■ Precautions

One systematic review found that 17% to 27% of patients in two RCTs suffered some skin atrophy. A more common adverse event is postinjection pain, experienced by approximately half of patients.[27] The theoretical outcome of tendon rupture was not found in two separate reviews, and this complication seems to be rare.[22]

Other Injection Therapies

Two other injection-based therapies, prolotherapy and platelet-rich plasma (PRP), received attention in small but well-done RCTs. In both cases, patients had approximately 3 mL of solution injected at the insertion of the common extensor tendon with optional injection of surrounding ligamentous tissue. A peppering injection technique is often employed for these injections. Although the precise mechanism of action for both techniques is not well known, both purport to heal damaged, degenerative tendons at the tissue level. As such, both therapies address the contemporary understanding of LE and ME as degenerative conditions.

PRP is a concentrated solution of autologous platelets that can deliver growth factors directly to areas of degeneration and is hypothesized to enhance tissue healing.[28,29] Autologous blood is drawn at the point of care and is centrifuged to separate the portion with the greatest abundance of platelets. Studies reported that PRP for LE could result in improved quality of life, pain, and function, and PRP could modify the disease course at the level of the damaged tendons.[26,30] Promising early clinical trial and anecdotal evidence resulted in increasingly common use of PRP in clinical practice.[28,29] One RCT reported that at 52 weeks, subjects with LE who received PRP injection reported a 66% effect size compared with baseline, whereas study participants who received steroid injections reported only a 17% improvement ($P < .05$) in disease-specific quality of life.[26]

Prolotherapy, an injection-based therapy reported to enlarge and strengthen ligaments, was assessed in systematic and descriptive reviews.[31,32] Prolotherapy is used for various soft tissue conditions including LE and ME. Inflammation is thought to initiate a local physiologic reaction favoring anabolic processes that strengthen tendon and ligament tissue at the bony insertion. Injectants include hypertonic dextrose and morrhuate sodium. In one RCT, subjects with severe refractory LE responded well to three prolotherapy treatments.[33] Compared with participants receiving blinded saline injections, subjects treated with prolotherapy experienced pain reduction (absolute effect size between groups of 68%; $P < .01$) and improved isometric strength ($P < .05$) compared with control saline injections by 16 weeks, and these effects were maintained at 52 weeks.

Both prolotherapy and PRP injection appear safe when performed by an experienced injector and are reasonable treatment options for patients in whom more conservative management has failed. Neither is typically covered by third-party payers. Costs for each vary considerably.

■ Dosage
Formal dosing for both PRP and prolotherapy is not standard. Both therapies use specific injection techniques. Obtaining these services is best done in consultation with physicians who are experienced with these procedures. Both procedures are performed in outpatient settings without significant analgesia, similar to corticosteroid injections. Both solutions are injected at tender points at the insertion of the common extensor tendon and radial collateral ligament.[2,5,7] PRP injection therapy has been performed in a single treatment session, whereas prolotherapy is more typically performed in a minimum of in three treatment sessions separated by approximately 4 weeks.

Biomechanical Medicine

Physical Therapy
Exercise and physical therapy make sense clinically and are well accepted. Eccentric exercises preferentially load tendons and promote the formation of new collagen. These exercises were reported to be beneficial in one small RCT comparing exercise for epicondylar pain at 8 weeks with ultrasound and friction massage,[22] as well as in other tendinopathies.[34,35]

> Exercise and physical therapy are reasonable conservative modalities, although their overall long-term efficacy is unclear.

One review and one well-done RCT reported that exercise, stretch, and mobilization were effective therapies and yielded significant improvement compared with wait-and-see, placebo, and ultrasound approaches.[36,37] Unfortunately, physical therapy protocols vary, and studies do not describe them in detail. Examples of exercises and recommendations for their use are given in Figure 67-4.

Orthoses (Braces)
Orthotic devices (brace, splint, cast, or strap) are thought to decrease the pain of LE or ME by removing damaging load from lateral and medical epicondylar tendon attachments.

A systematic review of five RCTs assessing various orthotic devices was unable to make a general recommendation for their use.[38] However, the notion of reducing stress and strain at the tendon insertion makes sense and is generally accepted; clinically, many patients respond well to a simple and inexpensive elbow strap or wrist splint combined with relative rest. Complete immobilization with any orthotic should be avoided because of the risks of deconditioning and muscular atrophy.

■ Precautions
Local deconditioning should be avoided.

Surgery

A 2005 review found no RCTs assessing surgical intervention for LE or ME.[22] However, case series data suggest efficacy of surgery in patients with symptoms refractory to more conservative therapy. The goal of surgery is to excise abnormal tissue or release the affected portions of the extensor or flexor tendon. One case series reported that of 1300 patients undergoing surgery for refractory epicondylar pain (1000 for LE and 300 for ME), 85% experienced complete pain relief and strength return, 12% had partial improvement, and 3% had no improvement.[11] Surgery is a reasonable option for patients with significant pain for whom more conservative therapy has failed.

■ Precautions
Precautions include postoperative concerns such as infection and nerve damage. In the study cited previously, however, reported complications were rare.[11]

PREVENTION PRESCRIPTION

Lifestyle
- Stop smoking.
- Reduce stress.

Avoid Exacerbating Activities
- Reduce or avoid the lifting of objects with the arm extended.
- Reduce repetitive gripping.
- Decrease overall tension of gripping.
- Avoid extremes of wrist bending and full extension.
- Work or train with the elbow in a partially flexed position.
- Use wrist supports when weight training.
- Enlarge the gripping surface of tools or rackets with gloves or padding, use a hammer with extra padding to reduce tensions and impact, and hold heavy tools with two hands.

Ergonomic Evaluation
- Evaluate repetitive motion activity, duties, equipment, and techniques, especially in work situations.
- More complete information on ergonomic evaluation of computer, laboratory, and industrial settings is available through the Centers for Disease Control and Prevention (see Key Web Resources).

Exercise
- Use stretching and strengthening exercises once daily, along with frequent periods of short rest.

FIGURE 67-4
Physical therapy for lateral epicondylosis.

Lateral Epicondylosis Physical Therapy

Start exercises with set **A** and proceed slowly through the set. Advance to exercises with weights when pain begins to decrease, usually after 7-10 days.

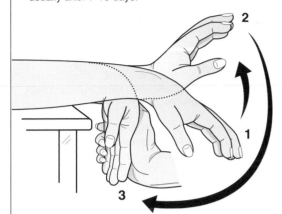

A. Active range of motion and strengthening

1. Place forearm on table with hand off edge of table, palm down.
2. Move hand upward.

Hold position for 15 seconds.
Return to starting position.
Perform 1 repetition every 4 seconds.
Perform 1 set of 12 repetitions twice per day.

After 7-10 days, or as range of motion improves and pain diminishes, advance to step **3**:

3. With other hand, grasp at thumb side of hand and bend wrist downward gently.
Perform 1 set of 4 repetitions twice per day.

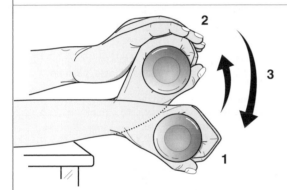

B. Exercise with weight

1. Place forearm on table, palm down, weight in hand.
2. Use other hand to raise wrist fully upward.
3. Release wrist and slowly lower weight.

Start with 1/2-lb weight, advance to 1-lb weight.
Perform 1 repetition every 4 seconds.
Perform 3 sets of 10 repetitions once every other day.
Rest 1 minute between sets.

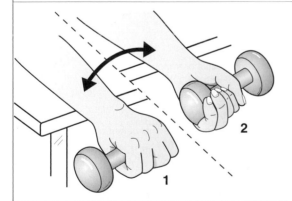

C. Exercise with weight

1. Support forearm on table or armchair, hand palm down holding weight.
2. Rotate hand to thumb up.
Return to starting position.

Start with 1/2-lb weight, advance to 1-lb weight.
Perform 1 repetition every 4 seconds.
Perform 3 sets of 10 repetitions once every other day.
Rest 1 minute between sets.

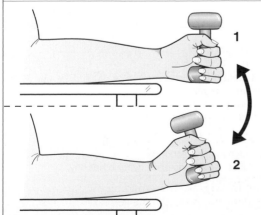

D. Exercise with weight

1. Support forearm on table or knee.
Hold weight in hand, thumb up.
2. Lift weight upward.
Return to starting position and repeat.

Start with 1/2-lb weight, advance to 1-lb weight.
Perform 1 repetition every 4 seconds.
Perform 3 sets of 10 repetitions once every other day.
Rest 1 minute between sets.

Continued

FIGURE 67-4, cont'd

Medial Epicondylosis Physical Therapy

Start exercises with set **A** and proceed slowly through the set. Advance to exercises with weights when pain begins to decrease, usually after 7-10 days.

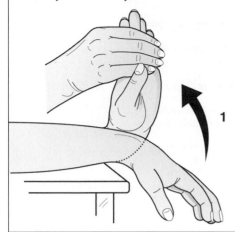

A. Stretch exercise

1. Grasping fingers of one hand with other hand, pull hand back gently. Keep injured elbow straight.

Hold position for 15 seconds.
Perform 1 set of 4 repetitions twice each day.
Rest 30 seconds between repetitions.

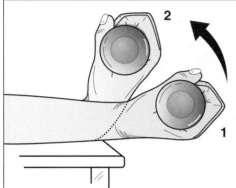

B. Exercise with weight

1. Grasp weight with hand.
Place forearm on table with hand off edge of table, palm up as shown.
2. Move wrist upward.
Return to starting position.

Start with 1/2-lb weight, advance to 1-lb weight.
Perform 1 repetition every 4 seconds.
Perform 3 sets of 10 repetitions once every other day.
Rest 1 minute between sets.

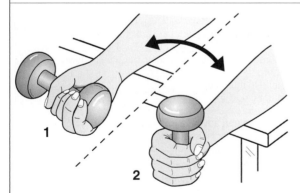

C. Exercise with weight

1. Support forearm on table or armchair.
Position hand palm up with weight in hand as shown.
2. Rotate hand to thumb up.
Return to starting position.

Start with 1/2-lb weight, advance to 1-lb weight.
Perform 1 repetition every 4 seconds.
Perform 3 sets of 10 repetitions once every other day.
Rest 1 minute between sets.

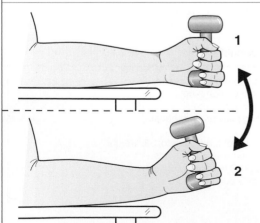

D. Exercise with weight

1. Support forearm on table or knee.
Hold weight in hand, thumb up.
2. Lift weight upward.
Return to starting position and repeat.

Start with 1/2-lb weight, advance to 1-lb weight.
Perform 1 repetition every 4 seconds.
Perform 3 sets of 10 repetitions once every other day.
Rest 1 minute between sets.

THERAPEUTIC REVIEW

Lifestyle

- Prevention: Most of the techniques listed in the Prevention Prescription box also off-load affected tendons and may speed healing.

- Establish a time course of healing; most patients recover in weeks to months, but recovery may take up to 1 year or longer. ⊝ C 1

- Relative rest: Remove or reduce repetitive, heavy activity affecting wrist flexors or extensors. ⊝ C 1

- Use ice in the first 2 to 4 weeks of pain. ⊘ B 1

Mind-Body Therapy

- Stress reduction techniques and workplace evaluation are recommended. ⊝ C 1

Bioenergetic Therapy

- Needle acupuncture may be used. ⊘ B 1

Pharmaceuticals

- Nonsteroidal antiinflammatory drugs and corticosteroid injections have good efficacy for pain control in the early stages of lateral epicondylosis and medial epicondylosis, but they do not change outcomes in the long term. ⊘ B 2

  - Topical diclofenac, 3% gel, may be applied twice daily for 1 to 2 weeks.

- Topical diclofenac may be applied with iontophoresis, using 150 mg at 4 to 8 mA for 20 sessions.

- Oral ibuprofen, 600 mg, may be taken every 6 hours for no more than 2 weeks.

- Injection: Methylprednisone, 40 mg in 1 mL of lidocaine, may be injected weekly for up to 4 treatments.

Physical Therapy and Preventive Exercise

- Various exercises may be performed in sets of repetitions with and without weights from twice daily to every other day (see Fig. 67-4). B 1

Orthotics

- Simple wrist splints and elbow straps may be used in conjunction with relative rest. ⊝ C 1

Prolotherapy

- Prolotherapy appears safe when performed by an experienced injector and is a reasonable treatment option for patients in whom more conservative management has failed. B 2

Platelet-Rich Plasma

- Platelet-rich plasma injection appears safe when performed by an experienced injector and is a reasonable treatment option for patients in whom more conservative management has failed. B 2

Surgery

- Surgery is a reasonable option for patients with severe pain refractory to conservative care. B 2

KEY WEB RESOURCES

Mayo Clinic information on tennis elbow: http://www.mayoclinic.com/health/tennis-elbow/DS00469	This site is a basic but helpful patient-oriented online tool.
Centers for Disease Control and Prevention information on ergonomics: http://www.cdc.gov/niosh/topics/ergonomics/	This site provides information on ergonomic evaluation of computer, laboratory, and industrial settings.
American Association of Orthopaedic Medicine: http://www.aaomed.org	This nonprofit organization provides information and educational programs on comprehensive nonsurgical musculoskeletal treatment including prolotherapy. This searchable site lists members who perform prolotherapy.

References

References are available online at expertconsult.com.

Section XII Dermatology

Chapter 68

Atopic Dermatitis

Amanda J. Kaufman, MD

Atopic dermatitis is a pruritic, hereditary skin disease with a lifetime prevalence of 10% to 20%; most cases begin in infancy.[1] Among affected infants, 20% to 40% will have disease that persists into adulthood. The heavy impact of atopic dermatitis on quality of life and medical care costs has led to great interest in improving outcomes. Although conventional therapies are available, they are not always effective, they only suppress disease, and their lifetime use poses potential risks. Investigators have shown keen interest in and have studied integrative therapies to prevent disease and reduce dependence on these medications.

Pathophysiology and Diagnosis

The diagnosis of atopic dermatitis requires three major and three minor features.[1] Major features are as follows:

- Pruritus

- Typical morphology and distribution

- Flexural lichenification in adults

- Facial and extensor involvement in infants and children

- Chronic or chronically relapsing dermatitis

- Personal or family history of atopy (asthma, allergic rhinitis, atopic dermatitis)

The 22 minor features illustrate the varying degrees, extent, and distress patients endure. Educating patients about these minor features may lead to less emotional distress through an improved understanding of their condition. The minor features are as follows:

- Itch caused by sweating

- Xerosis

- Eczema (perifollicular accentuation)

- Recurrent conjunctivitis

- Wool intolerance

- Keratosis pilaris

- Palmar hyperlinearity

- Pityriasis alba

- White dermatographism

- Susceptibility to cutaneous infection (*Staphylococcus aureus,* herpes simplex virus and other viruses)

- Nipple dermatitis

- Dennie-Morgan lines

- Elevated immunoglobulin E (IgE)

- Immediate (type I) skin test reactivity

- Food intolerance

- Cataracts (anterior-subcapsular)

- Cheilitis

- Facial pallor or erythema

- Hand dermatitis

- Ichthyosis

- Keratoconus

- Orbital darkening

Genetic, immunologic, and environmental risks collide to influence the course of disease and provide opportunities to mediate the clinical course. Healthy skin in patients with atopic dermatitis has increased density of proinflammatory type 2 helper T (Th2) cells.[1] The skin barrier is impaired, with fewer ceramide lipids and skin barrier proteins, thus causing poor water retention and abnormal permeability. This abnormal skin barrier allows penetration of allergens and microbes that trigger an inflammatory cascade as they stimulate Th2 cells excessively. Affected skin has increased concentrations of inflammatory cytokines and greater eosinophil infiltration. Any stimulation or inflammation sets off the central clinical feature, which is intense itching.

Light stimuli and contact irritants such as sweating, wool, and detergents cause itching. Skin damage caused by scratching releases inflammatory cytokines and further stimulates itch. Reduced barrier function allows entry of *S. aureus*, *Malassezia* yeasts, *Candida* organisms, and *Trichophyton* dermatophytes, thereby inducing local inflammation. Food allergies, especially to egg, soy, milk, wheat, fish, shellfish, and peanuts, are implicated in one third to one half of children with atopic dermatitis. Aeroallergens can also increase peripheral eosinophilia and serum IgE levels, which lead to increased release of histamine and vascular mediators. These features induce edema and urticaria and thus cause persistence of the cycle of itch, scratch, and rash.

> Food allergies, especially to egg, soy, milk, wheat, fish, shellfish, and peanuts, are implicated in one third to one half of children with atopic dermatitis.

The relationship between psychological stress and atopic disorders is bidirectional.[2] Psychosocial stressors increase both self-reported and objective measures. The lack of sleep and physical suffering cause irritability and worsen mood disorders. Self-reporting of itch severity is increased when depression scores are elevated, similar to the relationship with pain scores.

Integrative Therapy

Atopic dermatitis is improved through an integrative approach focusing on improving the barrier function and reducing the itch-scratch cycle. Least invasive therapies are presented first, followed by those with a greater potential for harm. As the disease course waxes and wanes, patients should advance and reduce their regimen as appropriate to allow improved control of flares and reduced use of pharmaceuticals.

Lifestyle and Supportive Care

Hydration
Rehydration of the stratum corneum improves barrier function and reduces the effects of irritants and allergens. Soaking in a lukewarm bath for 10 to 20 minutes is ideal, or lukewarm showers may be taken if preferred. Bath oils can be added to the bath after the skin surface is wet. If even plain water is irritating during acute flares, 1 cup of salt added to the water will help.

Mild Soap or Soap Substitutes
Use mild, neutral-pH soap (Dove, Aveeno, Basis) minimally as needed for the face, axillae, and groin. If these soaps are too irritating, hydrophobic lotions or creams such as Cetaphil can be applied without water, rubbed until foaming, and wiped away with a soft cloth.[1]

Bleach Baths
Dilute bleach baths combined with nasal application of mupirocin with a goal to reduce colonization with *S. aureus* caused dramatic improvement in those areas of the body exposed.[3] Thirty-one children age 6 months to 17 years were treated with cephalexin, 50 mg/kg (maximum 2 g daily) divided three times daily for 14 days, and were then randomized to bathing in a dilute bleach solution (approximately ½ cup to a bathtub of water) twice weekly for at least 5 to 10 minutes and applying mupirocin ointment intranasally for the patient and all household members twice daily for the first 5 consecutive days of each month or placebo. The mean Eczema Area and Severity Score (EASI) of 19.7 was reduced by 10.4 points at 1 month and by 15.3 points at 3 months compared with 2.5 and 3.2 points in the placebo group. These reductions were in exposed areas, but not in head and neck lesions, although the head and neck can also be carefully exposed to the bleach solution.

Moisturizers Following Bathing
Follow bathing by lightly patting the skin with a towel and immediately applying an occlusive emollient over the entire skin surface to retain this moisture. Application within 3 minutes improves hydration, whereas beyond 3 minutes, surface evaporation is drying. Commonly recommended emollients include petroleum jelly, vegetable oil, and Aquaphor. Virgin coconut oil additionally reduces colonization with *S. aureus* and thus provides added benefit.[4] Ceramide-containing emollients have been shown to decrease transepidermal water loss and decrease clinical severity scores. One ceramide formulation (EpiCeram) showed improvement nearly equal to that with fluticasone cream after 28 days of use.[5] Another brand is TriCeram cream, which is also highly effective.

> Ceramide, a family of lipid molecules found in cell membranes, can be applied through emollients (e.g., EpiCerem or TriCeram) after bathing, thus decreasing transepidermal water loss while reducing the symptoms of atopic dermatitis.

Urea, alpha-hydroxy acid, and lactic acid products have long been used for their exfoliation and moisturizing properties. A tolerability study of a 5% urea-containing moisturizer compared with the typical 10% formula noted a nearly 20% objective improvement over 42 days of twice-daily use for both groups.[6]

Wet Dressings
Wet dressings are useful for severely affected skin. The constant moisture is therapeutic, the cooling sensation with evaporation reduces itching, and the mechanical barrier prevents scratching. Apply wet cloth with either plain water or Burow solution to recalcitrant lesions, and periodically rewet the compress. Wet dressings increase penetration of corticosteroids. Burow solution can be made 1:40 by dissolving one Domeboro packet or tablet in a pint of lukewarm water. Parents may have success when their children sleep in cotton pajamas dampened in problem areas with another set of pajamas over top.

Avoidance of Allergens
Eliminate known allergens. Eliminate smoke exposure for children with allergies. Dust mite control measures may be helpful in patients with documented sensitivity to dust mites.

In children with animal allergies, consider removing animals from the home. A dog living in the home at the time of birth is associated with a 50% decrease in the incidence of atopic dermatitis at age 3 years.[7] However, parents caring for a dog are less likely to be severely allergic to dog dander.

Loose-Fitting Clothing

Wear loose-fitting clothing made of cotton, silk, or other natural, smooth fibers. Avoid wool. Launder new clothes before wearing to remove formaldehyde and other chemicals. Use liquid detergent, ideally without fabric softeners or optical brighteners, and consider an extra rinse cycle.

Humidity

Controlled humidity and temperature may reduce triggers of cold, heat, and dry air. Humidify in the winter with a goal of 30% to 40% humidity. Air conditioning in the summer decreases sweating as a trigger and prevents the growth of mold.

Nutrition

Prevention Through Breast-Feeding or Hydrolyzed Formula in Infancy

Debate exists on how to counsel atopic families on food exposure in early life. Exclusive breast-feeding for the first 6 months of life was previously thought to reduce atopy, although results of more recent breast-feeding studies have been inconclusive. Debate also exists on the role of food avoidance even in high-risk infants. Some experts point to populations in which very young babies are given tastes of adult food and have a lower incidence of life-threatening allergies. The LEAP (Learning Early about Peanut Allergy) study randomized high risk 4- to 10-month old infants to either exposure or avoidance of peanuts. The study should come to completion in 2013 and give guidance on which approach lowers the incidence of life-threatening peanut allergy. Food allergies are actively being studied to enhance our understanding and to provide a basis for advice to parents. In my practice, mothers with a strong history of atopy who avoid common or known familial triggers in the last month of pregnancy and in the first months of breast-feeding reduce objective measures of disease and increase parental perception of control. Any delay of symptoms or reduction in severity is welcome in these first months of life.

For those infants who cannot breast-feed, hydrolyzed formulas have been found effective for the prevention of atopic dermatitis. A 6-year follow-up to a study of 2252 newborns with familial atopy history who were randomized to various hydrolyzed formulas when breast-feeding was insufficient found a significant risk reduction for allergic disease.[8] Infants were randomized to partially hydrolyzed whey formula, extensively hydrolyzed whey formula, or extensively hydrolyzed casein formula, with regular cow's milk formula as control. The relative risk of development of any allergic manifestation was 0.82, 0.90, and 0.80, and for atopic eczema it was 0.79, 0.92, and 0.71, for the respective study formulas compared with cow's milk formula. A meta-analysis and a more recent study also found that partially hydrolyzed whey formulas appear to be as good at preventing atopic disease as extensively hydrolyzed formulas, and they cost less.[9,10]

Allergy Elimination Diet

Food allergies affect 10% to 40% of children with atopic dermatitis.[1] A study attempting to show a benefit to an allergy elimination diet in a broad sample of children with atopic dermatitis found a benefit only to an egg-free diet in infants with suspected egg allergy positive for specific IgE to eggs.[11] By 5 years old, many of these food allergies resolve. The most common foods causing positive oral challenges are egg, soy, milk, wheat, fish, shellfish, and peanuts. Elimination diets can be stressful on parents. Parents often desire testing to guide them; however, testing is not as reliable as a clinical response. The skin in atopic dermatitis can develop a wheal with a needle prick alone.[1] Serum-specific IgE tests also have significant false-positive rates.[12] The gold standard for diagnosis is a placebo-controlled double-blind oral food challenge because history, prick tests, and specific IgE do not correlate well with clinical reactivity, especially in delayed eczematous skin reactions.[1,11] Diagnostic elimination diets, such as described in this text (see Chapter 84, Food Intolerance and Elimination Diet), should be used before an oral provocation test is considered.[11] Although elimination diets are challenging, parents feel an increased perception of control over the illness when food allergies are found and exposure can be eliminated. A review of the serum radioallergosorbent test (RAST) and enzyme-linked immunosorbent assay (ELISA) and their inherent challenges provides further detailed guidance.[13]

Oolong Tea

With drinking Oolong tea three times a day (made from five teabags daily), 63% of patients had significant objective improvement, and the response persisted at 6 months in 54%.[14] The antiallergenic properties of polyphenols are thought to produce the effect. Drinking 5 to 6 cups of green tea or green tea extract, at 200 to 300 mg three times daily, may provide similar results.

> The main difference among green, oolong, and dark tea (all *Camellia sinensis*) is the length of fermentation of the leaf. Green is the shortest and dark the longest.

Mind-Body Therapy

Psychosocial stressors trigger flares of atopic dermatitis, and this connection prompted studies on the effectiveness of mind-body interventions. A Cochrane Review called into question the effectiveness of these interventions.[15] Mixed results showed that at least some patients may benefit from biofeedback, massage therapy, and hypnosis. Cognitive-behavioral therapy and autogenic training are superior to standard care alone and education in reducing use of topical steroids. A study on the benefits of support groups found improved quality of life scores, especially personal relationships and leisure scores.[16] A study of a structured education program on coping skills in children with atopic dermatitis and their parents showed that the intervention improved psychological scores beyond what would be expected with disease improvement.[17] Dr. Ted Grossbart, a Harvard Medical School (Boston) psychologist, created a mind-body program for skin disorders, and his e-book is available for free (see Key Web Resources). Many therapies with known effectiveness in similar conditions have not been studied. Given the low risk of side effects and the known benefits of mind-body therapies for other measures of well-being, these approaches are worth exploring.

Supplements

Vitamins

Vitamin D and E supplementation may be helpful. In one trial, patients were divided into four groups: those given both vitamin D_3 (1600 units) and vitamin E (600 units synthetic all-rac-alpha-tocopherol), just one, or both compared with placebo for 60 days.[18] Reduction in the symptoms of atopic dermatitis by objective scoring was 64.3% in those taking both vitamin D and vitamin E and 35% in each of the groups taking just one ($P = .004$).

■ Dosage

Many practitioners recommend supplementation with antiinflammatory supplements such as vitamin A, 5000 units daily, and zinc, 50 mg daily. Vitamin B_{12} cream, 0.07% used twice daily, was found effective and well tolerated in adults and children with eczema in small studies.[19]

Essential Fatty Acids

Essential fatty acid supplementation may be useful to counterbalance abnormal essential fatty acid metabolism. Docosahexaenoic acid (DHA), eicosapentaenoic acid (EPA), and gamma-linolenic acid (GLA) also improve atopic dermatitis through their antiinflammatory effects. The primary source of DHA and EPA is salmon and other cold-water fish. Good sources of GLA include borage oil (23% GLA), black currant seed oil (17% GLA), and evening primrose oil (8% to 10% GLA).[20]

Many studies showed insignificant improvement with supplementation, although these studies were often limited by small sample size and short duration. Other studies have been more promising. An 8-week study of 53 adults randomized to DHA (5.4 g daily) or isoenergetic saturated fatty acids found significant improvement in the DHA-treated group.[21] Another small study of evening primrose oil with 2 g of linoleic acid and 250 mg of GLA for 3 months significantly improved inflammation in atopic dermatitis.[22]

A meta-analysis of 12 trials of borage oil concluded that the evidence was limited by the small size of trials and their short duration, although borage oil is well tolerated and may have some benefit.[23] A small study in children found that undershirts coated with borage oil significantly reduced erythema, itch, and transepidermal water loss.[24]

Black currant seed oil was tested in the prevention of atopic dermatitis in neonates by randomizing 313 mothers, 81.7% of whom had a personal history of atopy, to black currant seed oil or olive oil placebo from the beginning of pregnancy until the cessation of breast-feeding, followed by supplementation of infants until 2 years old.[25] Although no difference in the groups was observed at 2 years, the prevalence of atopic dermatitis was lower in the group receiving black currant seed oil at 12 months (33% versus 47.3%; $P = .035$).

■ Dosage

A total of 2000 mg of DHA, EPA, and GLA is likely effective when combined, compared with the doses recommended in single-agent trials. The dose of fish oil (DHA and EPA) is 2 to 4 g daily for an adult. The adult dose of borage oil is 500 mg to 1 g daily, and the adult dose of evening primrose oil is 1 to 2 g daily.

■ Precautions

Adverse effects of supplements are few, and they are primarily gastrointestinal.

Probiotics

The effects of probiotics were mixed in study results, although this area of research is still in its infancy. Large questions remain to be answered, such as which organisms are effective for which conditions, how best to administer them, and for how long. Although probiotics are exceedingly safe, the current evidence base does not provide significant evidence for their use in treatment. A Cochrane Review left open the possibility that further studies could be promising,[26] and they have been. In a randomized double-blind placebo-controlled prospective trial, 90 toddlers aged 1 to 3 years with moderate to severe atopic dermatitis were treated with a mixture of *Lactobacillus acidophilus* DDS-1 and *Bifidobacterium lactis* UABLA-12 with fructo-oligosaccharide with 5 billion colony-forming units (CFUs) twice a day for 8 weeks, and these children showed an improvement of 33.7% versus 19.4% for placebo ($P = .001$).[27] A cream containing a 5% lysate of *Vitreoscilla filiformis* that was used for 30 days significantly improved objective measurements and pruritus compared with the cream alone.[28] Prenatal and postnatal use of *Lactobacillus rhamnosus* GG among atopic mothers reduced the prevalence of atopic dermatitis in their infants by 50%, with a number needed to treat of 4.5.[29,30] Women with a history of atopy should consider supplementation with *L. rhamnosus* when they are pregnant and breast-feeding, to prevent atopic dermatitis. Other women should consider a 2-month trial of probiotic use.

■ Dosage

For adults, the dose is 20 billion CFUs daily of a combination probiotic containing *L. rhamnosus,* such as Jarro-dophilus or PB-8. For infants and children, the dose is 5 billion CFUs daily.

■ Precautions

Patients with extreme immune compromise or those with indwelling catheters should use caution with regard to taking these live organisms.

Botanicals

Much of the long heritage of herbal treatment of atopic dermatitis has not been studied, although several compounds have had small, successful trials, and no safety concerns exist. Ensuring the quality of the compound used is essential to achieve these treatment effects.

Glycyrrhetinic Acid

Derived from licorice root, glycyrrhetinic acid has antiinflammatory actions when it is used topically. Two studies of a 2% glycyrrhetinic acid cream used in a 2-week and 5-week study noted significant improvements in objective disease scores and itch.[31,32] Atopiclair is a hydrophilic cream containing hyaluronic acid, telmesteine, *Vitis vinifera* (grape), and 2% glycyrrhetinic acid. A vehicle-controlled, randomized study of 218 adults with mild to moderate atopic dermatitis found highly significant response rates with more than 50 days of use.[33] A similarly designed trial of 142 children found Atopiclair statistically more effective than vehicle at 22 days of use.[34] Atopiclair cream is available by prescription and over the counter.

Dosage
Atopiclair cream should be applied to the rash or pruritic area two to three times daily as needed. The 100-g tube is available by prescription only.

Precautions
Atopiclair cream contains a nut oil and thus should not be used in patients with a nut allergy.

Other Botanicals
Honey has been used to reduce inflammation and promote healing. A small study of 21 children ages 5 to 16 years used a honey, beeswax, and olive oil preparation on the left side of the body compared with petroleum jelly (Vaseline) on the right three times daily for 2 weeks; children were randomized to use of corticosteroids or not.[35] In the emollient-only group, 8 of 10 children improved on the honey side, and 2 of 10 improved on the petroleum jelly side. Among the corticosteroid users, 5 of 11 found the honey mixture useful in reducing corticosteroid use.

Chamomile is regarded as gentle and safe, and it has antiinflammatory and antibacterial properties. Cold, wet packs with chamomile tea are traditionally used for bacterial superinfections.[36] A half-side comparison study of chamomile cream or hydrocortisone 0.5%, with vehicle as placebo, showed neither better than placebo, but chamomile fared slightly better than the steroid.[37]

Studies demonstrated the effectiveness of an extract of *St. John's wort* (*Hypericum perforatum*). This botanical has antimicrobial activity and may have beneficial immunologic effects. A study of 28 patients found significant clinical improvement when this extract was applied as a cream, compared with its vehicle.[38]

Twenty-one patients with mild atopic dermatitis who were 5 to 28 years old were randomized to 0.3% *rosmarinic acid* emulsion twice daily or vehicle. These patients had significantly reduced erythema and transepidermal water loss.[39]

Oregon grape root (*Mahonia aquifolium*) has antimicrobial properties and inhibits proinflammatory cytokines.[36] A 10% cream used in 42 adult patients three times daily over 12 weeks demonstrated significant clinical improvement.[40]

Herbavate, a topical preparation that contains the oil extracts of *Calotropis gigantea*, *Curcuma longa*, *Pongamia glabra*, *and Solanum xanthocarpum* in a cream base, showed promise in an open-label 4-week pilot study.[41] These extracts have been used in Indian traditional medicine and Ayurveda.

Commercially available, standardized preparations with demonstrated efficacy should be easy for patients to find either online or in health food stores. One example is the Four Elements

Herbals' product Look No X E Ma!, which contains licorice, chamomile, calendula, evening primrose oil, and vitamin E. Compounding pharmacies often can compound several agents into a single product, thus making use less burdensome. Consider compounding glycyrrhetinic acid 2% and St. John's wort (0.3% hypericin or 2% to 5% hyperforin) into a ceramide-containing cream such as CeraVe.

> Familiarize yourself with the products available from your local compounding pharmacist. Use of more than two topical products can be cumbersome for patients, although many products can be compounded together for ease of use. Many commercially available products contain several agents in combination.

Conventional Modalities
Coal Tar
Coal tar preparations have antipruritic and antiinflammatory effects and were used before the development of topical corticosteroids. They are second-line preparations but work well on chronic and lichenified lesions.[1] Tar shampoos can be used for scalp involvement. Adverse effects include contact dermatitis, folliculitis, and photosensitivity. One review found that most studies reported favorable profiles of effectiveness with few side effects (including staining and odor) and also noted that these preparations are cost effective.[42]

Immunotherapy
Allergen immunotherapy is typically indicated for patients with allergic rhinitis or allergic asthma, although trials of subcutaneous or sublingual immunotherapy to house dust mites in persons sensitized with atopic dermatitis showed some promise. Among 28 children 5 to 16 years old who had atopic dermatitis with sensitization to dust mites but without food allergy or asthma compared with 28 children who were given placebo for 18 months, sublingual immunotherapy for dust mites showed improvement in those with mild to moderate disease, but not severe disease.[43] Two children withdrew from the study because of worsening dermatitis.[43] Larger trials are ongoing.

Immunization and Childhood Diseases
Concerns have been raised about the effect of immunizations on atopic dermatitis. Analyses concluded that both natural infection and immunization protect against childhood atopic dermatitis. In a study of 2184 infants with atopic dermatitis and a family history of atopy, exposure to vaccines (diphtheria, tetanus, pertussis, polio, *Haemophilus influenzae* type b, hepatitis B, mumps, measles, rubella, varicella, bacille Calmette-Guérin, meningococci, and pneumococci) was not associated with increased risk of allergic sensitization to food or aeroallergens.[44] On the contrary, immunizations against varicella and pertussis and cumulative numbers of vaccine doses were inversely associated with eczema severity. With varicella, infection has a decreased odds ratio of 0.55 for development of atopic dermatitis.[45] Children who are infected with wild-type varicella zoster infection, as opposed to vaccine, who develop atopic dermatitis have fewer doctor visits for atopic dermatitis (odds ratio, 0.17). One study of measles vaccine (ROUVAX) compared with

placebo that included 12 infants 10 to 14 months old with atopic dermatitis showed improvement in clinical severity in 1 treated child; improvement of some serum markers was also noted.[46] Immunizations have not been found to worsen disease. In fact, exposure has been found to decrease the risk and severity of atopic dermatitis.

Ultraviolet Light

Ultraviolet (UV) light may be helpful for some patients, although this technique is less popular because of acceleration of photoaging and increased risk of skin cancer. A study of narrow-band UVB showed a statistically significant advantage when light therapy was accompanied by synchronous bathing in a 10% Dead Sea salt solution.[47] In one study, narrow-band UVB and medium-dose UVA1 dosed three times a week were equally effective.[48]

Pharmaceuticals

Antimicrobials

Use of antibiotics has not been found effective as treatment for atopic dermatitis.[49] However, bleach baths and mupirocin ointment, as discussed earlier, are tremendously helpful. A study of the effectiveness of pimecrolimus cream measured colonization of *S. aureus,* which correlated with more severe disease, in a cohort of patients whose disease did not respond to corticosteroids.[50] Antibiotics are useful for superinfection and when lesions are not responsive to corticosteroids because subclinical superinfection may be the cause. *Staphylococcus* species and group A beta-hemolytic streptococci are the most common organisms cultured.

■ Dosage for Superinfection

For superinfection of atopic dermatitis, consider the following: mupirocin or bacitracin ointment twice daily for 7 to 10 days; cephalexin, 250 mg four times daily for 7 days; or dicloxacillin, 250 mg four times daily for 7 days.

Consider herpesvirus superinfection in recalcitrant lesions. Smear or culture swab provides the diagnosis. For herpesvirus superinfection, consider the following: for herpes zoster, acyclovir, 800 mg orally five times daily for 7 to 10 days; for varicella-zoster, acyclovir, 800 mg orally four times daily for 5 days.

■ Dosage for Fungal Infection

Dermatophyte infections can contribute to head and neck lesions. In patients infected with *Candida albicans* or *Malassezia furfur,* ketoconazole, used topically or taken orally 200 mg twice daily for 10 days, may be helpful.[51]

Antihistamines

Antihistamines may be useful to reduce scratching. Oral antihistamines may be mostly useful for their sedative properties.[1] Doxepin cream can cause sedation if it is used over large areas of the body.

■ Dosage

Doses are as follows: doxepin cream 5%, a thin layer applied up to four times daily; diphenhydramine, 12.5 to 50 mg orally every 6 hours; hydroxyzine, 10 to 50 mg orally every 6 hours; or loratadine, 10 mg orally daily.

Topical Corticosteroids

The standard medical treatment of atopic dermatitis consists of topical corticosteroids. These drugs are typically used twice daily for up to 2 weeks during an acute flare and then once to twice daily on weekends to maintain remission. Because this disease is more common in young children, concerns arise that long-term use may suppress the hypothalamic-pituitary-adrenal (HPA) axis, cause growth retardation, and have other side effects. Despite these concerns, no other medication is as effective during an acute flare, and use during these times only does not appear to pose a risk.

For quick control of flares, consider using a higher-potency product and then reducing the strength for maintenance or switching down to an herbal preparation. Use only class IV and V corticosteroids on the face, axilla, groin, and intertriginous areas.[1] For children, use class III agents when a more potent agent is desired and titrate downward. For the eyelids, use a class V or VI agent for 5 to 7 days. Apply a thin layer directly after bathing, followed by emollient use. Ointments are generally recommended, although not in warm, humid climates, in which their occlusiveness can cause sweat retention dermatitis. Gels can be used for weeping lesions and on the scalp and bearded skin. A full list of potencies of topical steroids is available in Chapter 69, Psoriasis.

■ Dosage

Class I (superpotent): clobetasol ointment 0.05% twice daily (also available as a gel)

Class III (upper midstrength): triamcinolone 0.1% ointment twice daily

Class IV (midstrength): hydrocortisone valerate 0.2% ointment twice daily

Class V (lower midstrength): desonide 0.05% ointment twice daily

Class VI (mild): hydrocortisone 1% ointment twice daily

■ Precautions

Prolonged use of steroid creams can cause skin atrophy or acne, and prolonged use of potent steroids carries a risk of growth retardation in children.

> If systemic steroids are warranted, use in conjunction with an aggressive topical regimen and give as a 14-day taper to avoid a rebound flare.

Topical Immunomodulators

Tacrolimus ointment and pimecrolimus cream, inhibitors of calcineurin, are additional nonsteroid options for treatment of atopic dermatitis. These agents decrease T-cell activation and cytokine release while inhibiting mast cell and basophil degranulation. They have been studied largely as steroid-sparing agents for use after control of an acute flare to maintain remission. Investigators and clinicians were hopeful to find an agent to provide control without the risks of skin thinning and effects on the HPA axis.

After case reports of skin cancer and lymphoma with use of these agents appeared, the U.S. Food and Drug Administration issued a black box warning noting that although a causal relationship had not been established, these agents should be used with caution. Continued study has not demonstrated an increased risk of malignancy, although longer-term safety studies are ongoing.[52] Patients with atopic dermatitis have an increased risk of lymphoma, and this risk increases with severity of disease. One study found a higher risk in patients treated with topical corticosteroids, and this risk rose with increasing potency and longer duration of use.[53] Avoid the use of topical immunomodulators in immunocompromised patients or in those with known neoplasm. In atypical atopic dermatitis, such as new onset in an adult, skin biopsy can rule out cutaneous T-cell lymphoma or other causes. Encourage sun protection to reduce photocarcinogenesis.

A meta-analysis of tacrolimus use in children found it safe and effective, with no statistical difference between tacrolimus 0.03% and 0.1% preparations and a good response compared with vehicle, 1% hydrocortisone acetate, and 1% pimecrolimus (odds ratio, 4.56, 3.92, and 1.58, respectively).[54] A Cochrane Review found pimecrolimus less effective than moderate and potent corticosteroids and 0.1% tacrolimus.[55] Pimecrolimus studied for prevention had a relapse rate of 9.9% in twice-daily use and 14.7% in daily use.[56]

Use creams as infrequently as possible to maintain remission. Typical use is twice daily for short-term use, no longer than 6 weeks, or intermittently. Tacrolimus used three times weekly is effective in children to maintain remission.[57] Use only on lesional skin and not with occlusive dressings. Use only in children who are older than 2 years old. Adverse effects include burning on application and photosensitivity.

▪ Dosage
Tacrolimus 0.03% ointment is applied twice daily in patients older than 2 years, including adults with mild disease. For adults, tacrolimus 0.1% ointment is applied twice daily, or pimecrolimus 1% cream is applied twice daily.

Other Immunomodulators
Cyclosporine is helpful in patients with severe disease refractory to steroid use. However, cyclosporine should be used only by a provider experienced in its use.

Leukotriene inhibitors (e.g., montelukast) have not been shown to be particularly efficacious as monotherapy for atopic dermatitis, but they may reduce itching.

Therapies to Consider

Traditional Chinese Medicine
Several trials of traditional Chinese medicine herbal blends for atopic dermatitis showed promise. A Cochrane Review concluded that although the studies were small, they showed some evidence of effectiveness.[58] A five-herb concoction was studied in children with moderate to severe disease for 12 weeks, and although no significant difference was noted in clinical severity scores, the treatment group used one-third less corticosteroid and had significantly improved quality of life index scores at the end of treatment and 4 weeks later.[59]

Traditional Japanese Medicine (Kampo)
A case report on treatment with Kampo, traditional Japanese medicine, had color pictures showing resolution of flexural lichenification and is an excellent review of the likely immunomodulatory effects of this therapy.[60] A trial of Shiunko, an herbal mixture commonly used in Kampo for atopic dermatitis, lowered bacterial counts in the areas treated in 4 of 7 people.[61] A trial involving 95 patients using Kampo showed promise, with a moderate to marked effect in more than half and no effect in just 4 patients.[62]

Homeopathy
Homeopathic studies have largely not shown an effect of this therapy in atopic dermatitis, though one small study in children was promising. An open-label trial of 27 children using a homeopathic cream of Oregon grape root (*M. aquifolium*), pansy (*Viola tricolor hortensis*), and gotu kola (*Centella asiatica*) found complete resolution in 6 children and marked improvement in 16.[63]

PREVENTION PRESCRIPTION

- ▪ Moisturize the skin.
  - • Bathe in tepid or lukewarm water up to every day, followed by liberal application of emollients (petroleum jelly, virgin coconut oil, extra virgin olive oil, creams containing ceramide, or other greasy product) to lock in moisture.
  - • Limit soap to use only as needed; use a mild, pH-balanced soap such as Dove, Aveeno, or Basis.
- ▪ Consider bathing in dilute bleach water (½ cup per tubful) twice weekly for 5 to 10 minutes to reduce staphylococcal colonization.
- ▪ Do not scratch! Pat, firmly press, or grasp the skin.
- ▪ Avoid triggers.
  - • Humidify air in the winter.
  - • Reduce exposure to dust mites if sensitive; avoid rugs in bedrooms, wet mop floors, use mattress covers, and launder bedclothes weekly in hot water.
  - • Wear smooth, natural fibers that do not rub the skin.
  - • Avoid fabric softeners and other chemicals in laundry detergent, use liquid detergent, and consider an extra rinse cycle.
- ▪ Discover ways to control emotional stress. Seek low-stress work environments. Mindfulness meditation, massage, or learning self-hypnosis may be helpful. Consider reading *Skin Deep* on www.grossbart.com.
- ▪ Pursue an antiinflammatory diet with frequent sources of omega-3 fatty acids such as cold-water fish, walnuts, and flaxseed. Drink green or Oolong tea.
- ▪ Consider essential fatty acid supplementation, adding docosahexaenoic acid and eicosapentaenoic acid 2 g daily if your fish intake is inadequate and gamma-linolenic acid in the form of borage oil, 500 mg daily, or evening primrose oil, 1 to 2 g daily.
- ▪ Pregnant women with strong history of atopy should consider taking *Lactobacillus rhamnosus* GG prenatally and while breast-feeding. Continue giving it to the infant until age 2 years. If you cannot breast-feed, consider hydrolyzed formulas for atopy prevention for at least the first 4 months of life.
- ▪ Consider the benefit from childhood immunizations and natural chickenpox (varicella) infection.
- ▪ Moderate amounts of sunshine may be useful and allow you to obtain vitamin D.

THERAPEUTIC REVIEW

Avoidance of Triggers

- Reduce exposure to known allergens.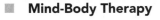
- Wear smooth, comfortable, breathable clothing.

Improvement in Barrier Function

- Ceramide-containing creams, such as *EpiCeram* or *TriCeram,* have added benefit over other emollients.
- Virgin coconut oil reduces *Staphylococcus aureus* colonization.

Nutrition

- Avoid known food allergies. (The most common foods triggers of atopic dermatitis are egg, soy, milk, wheat, fish, shellfish, and peanut.)
- Infants at high risk who cannot exclusively breast-feed should use hydrolyzed formula (broken down proteins) in the first 4 months of life. Examples of hydrolyzed formulas include Nutramigen LIPIL, Pregestimil, and Alimentum Advance.
- Drink 3 cups of strong oolong tea daily.

Mind-Body Therapy

- Support groups
- Coping skill educational program
- Psychotherapy

Supplements

- Vitamin D$_3$: 1600 units daily
- Vitamin E: 600 units daily
- Docosahexaenoic acid/eicosapentaenoic acid: 2 to 4 g daily
- Gamma-linolenic acid: 500 mg daily
- *Lactobacillus rhamnosus:* 20 billion CFUs daily for an atopic mother prenatally and postnatally for prevention of atopic dermatitis in the infant

Botanicals

- 2% Glycyrrhetinic acid (Atopiclair or others) applied three times daily

- Topical formulations of *Hypericum perforatum* (St. John's wort), chamomile, rosmarinic acid, or Oregon grape root applied twice daily

Other Creams

- Vitamin B$_{12}$ 0.07% cream used twice daily
- Coal tar preparations applied twice daily to chronic or lichenified lesions

Pharmaceuticals

- Antihistamines
  - Doxepin cream: twice daily to affected areas
  - Diphenhydramine: 12.5 to 50 mg orally every 6 hours
  - Hydroxyzine: 10 to 50 mg orally every 6 hours
  - Loratadine: 10 mg orally daily
- Antimicrobials
  - Dilute bleach baths (½ cup per full bathtub) are recommended twice weekly for 5 to 10 minutes combined with mupirocin 2% intranasally 5 consecutive days each month to reduce *S. aureus* colonization.
  - Consider ketoconazole, 200 mg twice daily for 10 days, for head or neck involvement.
  - Consider skin culture for bacteria and herpes or empirical treatment for recalcitrant lesions.
- Corticosteroids
  - Triamcinolone 0.1% ointment: twice daily for up to 2 weeks for flares, then up to twice daily on weekends to maintain remission
  - Hydrocortisone 1% ointment: used on thin skin at higher risk for adverse events (face, neck, axilla)
- Topical immunomodulators
  - Tacrolimus 0.03% ointment: twice-daily short-term use for patients older than 2 years old
  - Tacrolimus 0.03% ointment: three times weekly to maintain remission in patients older than 2 years old
  - Tacrolimus 0.1% ointment: twice-daily short-term use for patients older than 15 years old
  - Pimecrolimus 1% cream: twice-daily short-term use

KEY WEB RESOURCES

Eczema and Sensitive-Skin Education: www.easeeczema.org	Patient education and support
KidsHealth: Kidshealth.org; search: eczema	Patient information on eczema for children
Eczema Awareness, Support, and Education (EASE) program: www.eczemacanada.ca	Clear information and downloadable brochures in multiple languages including, "But It Itches So Much!" (for children) and "Eczema: It's Time to Take Control"
Skin Deep: www.grossbart.com	Home of Skin Deep, Dr. Ted Grossbart's mind-body program for healthy skin that is available by free e-book
iHerb.com: www.iherb.com	Online source for difficult to find over-the-counter products at prices often lower than suggested retail price

References

References are available online at expertconsult.com.

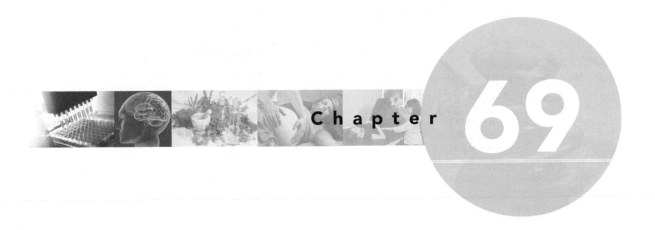

Chapter **69**

Psoriasis

Apple A. Bodemer, MD

Pathophysiology and Clinical Background

Psoriasis is a chronic inflammatory skin disease characterized by abnormal differentiation and hyperproliferation of the epidermis. Clinically, it manifests as redness and scaling (Figs. 69-1 and 69-2). Psoriasis is fairly common, affecting approximately 2% of the general population. It is more common in white persons and has a bimodal age distribution, with peak onsets between 20 and 30 years and between 50 and 60 years.[1] The cause of psoriasis is multifactorial, with both genetic and environmental components. A family history can usually (but not always) be elicited. If one parent has psoriasis, the risk of a child's having the disorder is approximately 14%. This figure jumps to 41% if both parents have the disorder.[1] Several human leukocyte antigens (HLAs [histocompatibility antigens]) have been associated with psoriasis, including HLA-B13, HLA-B17, HLA-B27, HLA-Cw6, and HLA-DR7. The strongest connection lies with HLA-Cw6, which is associated with earlier-onset disease that is more difficult to treat. Finally, several genetic loci have been linked to the development of psoriasis. Currently, *PSORS1* is considered the major gene associated with psoriasis.[1]

Environmental factors implicated in triggering psoriasis or psoriatic flares are physical trauma (the isomorphic or Koebner phenomenon), infections (e.g., streptococcal pharyngitis), hypocalcemia, stress, and medications such as lithium, beta blockers, antimalarials, interferon (IFN), and rapid tapers of systemic corticosteroids. The effect of pregnancy on psoriasis is not consistent; half of women with psoriasis experience worsening during pregnancy, and half note improvement. Patients infected with human immunodeficiency virus (HIV) tend to have more severe disease, but the incidence of psoriasis is not higher in this population. Finally, rapid weight changes, alcohol consumption, and tobacco use have been associated with psoriasis, but these features have not clearly been shown to be risk factors.

> The Koebner phenomenon is when skin trauma or irritation triggers a skin reaction such as a psoriatic plaque. Treatment of itching is important because scratching can trigger flares.

Clinically, psoriasis may manifest in several ways (Table 69-1). In addition to skin findings, nail abnormalities are often present. These include pits, oil slicks, subungual hyperkeratosis, and onycholysis. Nail psoriasis is thought to occur in up to 55% of patients with the disorder. In patients who also have psoriatic arthritis, however, the incidence of nail disease is 86%.[2]

Psoriatic arthritis affects approximately 10% of patients with psoriasis. Generally, skin lesions precede the joint disease by as long as 10 to 20 years; in approximately 10% to 15% of patients, however, the joint disease manifests first.[3] The five classifications of psoriatic arthritis are summarized in Table 69-2. Psoriatic arthritis can be extremely disabling and warrants more aggressive systemic treatment, such as methotrexate or the newer biologic immune response modifiers (see later discussion of systemic pharmaceuticals).

Although psoriasis was initially thought to be caused by abnormalities of keratinocytes, current research indicates that it is an autoimmune-mediated process driven by abnormally activated helper T cells. Activation of these T cells can occur through specific interactions with antigen-presenting cells (APCs) or through nonspecific superantigen interactions (i.e., guttate psoriasis triggered by streptococcal antigens). APC activation requires costimulatory signals. Table 69-3 summarizes the specific costimulatory interactions that are clinically relevant for treatment. Once activated, psoriatic T cells produce a type 1 helper T cell (Th1)–dominant cytokine profile that includes interleukin-2 (IL-2), tumor necrosis factor-alpha (TNF-alpha), IFN-gamma, and IL-8. These cytokines act to attract and activate neutrophils, which are responsible for much of the inflammation seen in psoriasis. Other factors leading to neutrophil recruitment and activation are complement split products (C5a) and leukotrienes (arachidonic acid metabolites from the 5-lipoxygenase pathway).[4]

FIGURE 69-1
Auspitz sign. Pinpoint bleeding areas where scale was lifted from psoriatic plaque. (From Weston WL, Lane AT, Morelli JG. *Color Textbook of Pediatric Dermatology.* 4th ed. Philadelphia: Mosby; 2007.)

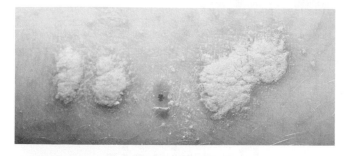

FIGURE 69-2
Psoriatic plaque. Note the sharp demarcation and silvery scale. (From van de Kerkhof PCM, Schalkwijk J. Psoriasis. In: Bolognia JL, Jorizzo JL, Rapini RP, eds. *Dermatology.* 2nd ed. Philadelphia: Mosby; 2008.)

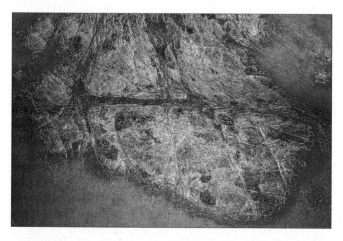

Integrative Therapy

Skin Care

Gentle skin care can help minimize pruritus and skin trauma and can thus prevent the Koebner phenomenon in psoriatic lesions. A helpful measure is bathing in cool to tepid water with gentle cleansers (e.g., Cetaphil soapless cleanser, Aquanil). Additionally, frequent and regular application of emollients, especially while the skin is still damp, will help keep psoriatic skin soft and more manageable. Natural oils such as avocado oil, almond oil, or olive oil can be very helpful and soothing. Colloidal oatmeal in the form of an emollient or bath (e.g., Aveeno) may also help soothe itching and irritation associated with psoriasis.

> Oatmeal baths can be made by placing whole oats in a blender and grinding to a fine powder. Water is added to a half cup of the oat flour to make a lose slurry that can be added to a bath. A thicker paste can be made and patted onto psoriatic lesions as a poultice.

Phototherapy

Psoriasis typically improves over summer months, when exposure to ultraviolet radiation (UVR) is greater. People have been taking advantage of this response to UVR for many years. The advent of better-controlled exposure has allowed for more predictable clinical results.

Ultraviolet B

Ultraviolet B (UVB) consists of radiation with wavelengths between 290 and 320 nanometers (nm). UVB is known to decrease DNA synthesis and has immunosuppressive effects. Langerhans cells (the main APCs in the epidermis) are extremely sensitive to UVB, and exposure limits antigen presentation to T lymphocytes. UVB also stimulates keratinocytes to secrete various cytokines, which can further alter the immune response, as well as limit inflammation.[5,6] In 1980, narrow-band UVB (nb-UVB), with a wavelength between 308 and 313 nm, was found to be much more effective than full-spectrum UVB in the treatment of psoriasis.[7,8]

■ **Dosage**

Treatment protocols are based on determining a minimal erythema dose (MED), that is, the dose of UVB that elicits barely perceptible erythema. Once an MED is defined, treatments are started at approximately 70% to 75% of the MED and are given three times a week with the goal of maintaining minimally perceptible erythema. Clearance may require up to 30 treatments with broad-band UVB, but it can occur with only one treatment with nb-UVB.[9] Once the skin is clear, some practitioners simply stop phototherapy, but others recommend tapering UVB to a maintenance dose. No clearly defined guidelines exist for accomplishing the tapering.

■ **Precautions**

Potential short-term side effects of UVB include erythema, xerosis, pruritus, and higher frequency of herpes simplex outbreaks. Longer-term side effects consist of photoaging and, possibly, increased risk of skin cancers. The carcinogenetic risk of UVB appears to be much less than that associated with ultraviolet A (UVA) combined with psoralen (PUVA; see next section). One multicenter trial examining the risk of carcinogenesis with phototherapy could not find a direct relationship between UVB and nonmelanoma skin cancers.[10] Additionally, a newer study specifically examining the correlation between nb-UVB and skin cancer found no significant association.[11] This therapy is relatively young, however, and further studies will help define the potential long-term risks more definitively.

Ultraviolet A and Psoralen

UVA radiation alone is not effective for the treatment of psoriasis. However, when it is combined with a topical or systemic photosensitizing agent (e.g., psoralen), PUVA becomes a powerful tool for the treatment of psoriasis. Psoralens are furocoumarins found in a wide variety of plants, including lime, parsley, fig, and celery. Synthetic furocoumarins consist primarily of 8-methoxypsoralen (8-MOP) and 5-MOP (available in Europe). Psoralens can be taken orally or used topically. Once absorbed, these compounds incorporate into DNA strands and absorb photons in the

TABLE 69-1. Subtypes of Psoriasis

SUBTYPE	CHARACTERISTICS	ASSOCIATIONS
Chronic Plaque	Erythematous plaques with silvery scale Typically involving scalp, knees, elbows, low back, umbilicus, and gluteal cleft Pruritus variable Nail findings common	Most common; accounting for approximately 90% of all cases of psoriasis
Guttate	Diffuse salmon to red "droplike" papules and plaques with fine scale Typically involving trunk and extremities	Second most common type (2%) Most common in children and young adults Affecting children and young adults Associated with group A *Streptococcus* infections Tends to resolve with eradication of infection Possibly persistent in "strep" carriers Best prognosis for remission
Inverse	Affecting predominantly axillae, groin, and submammary area Less scale than in other types	Prone to secondary bacterial or yeast infections
Erythrodermic	Erythema with scaling over more than 80% of body surface area	Potential complications including high-output cardiac failure, renal failure, and sepsis
Pustular	Confluent pustules on an erythematous base von Zumbusch type: generalized with acute fever, chills, nausea, headache, and joint problems Annular type: subacute or chronic; systemic symptoms possible Acrodermatitis continua of Hallopeau: distal fingers; fingernails possibly floating away on lakes of pus, and permanent nail destruction common	Life-threatening Potential complications including high-output cardiac failure, sepsis, and hypercalcemia Systemic symptoms less common with Hallopeau type
Palmoplantar Pustulosis	Pustules of the palms and soles with yellow-brown macules	Commonly associated with sterile inflammatory bone lesions

TABLE 69-2. Classification of Psoriatic Arthritis

TYPE	CHARACTERISTICS	ASSOCIATIONS
Asymmetric Oligoarticular	Digits of the hands and feet affected first Inflammation of the flexor tendon and synovium occurring simultaneously Usually affecting fewer than five digits	"Sausage digit" (involvement of both DIP and PIP of one digit)
Symmetric Polyarthritis	Clinically identical to rheumatoid arthritis Possibly affecting hands, wrists, ankles, and feet Involvement of DIP Rheumatoid factor negative	Erosive changes seen on radiographs
DIP Arthropathy	Unique to psoriasis Affecting only 5%–10% More prominent in men	Nail involvement with chronic paronychia
Arthritis Mutilans	Osteolysis leading to telescoping of finger with "opera-glass" hand More common in early-onset disease More common in men	Osteolysis (dissolution of the joint) "Pencil-in-cup" deformity on radiographs
Spondylitis with or without Sacroiliitis	Occurring in 5% of patients with psoriatic arthritis More common in male patients Asymmetric involvement of vertebrae	Morning stiffness of lower back the most characteristic symptom

Data from Hammadi AA, Gorevic PD. *Psoriatic Arthritis.* www.emedicine.com/med/topic1954.htm. Accessed 28.08.06.
DIP, distal interphalangeal joint; PIP, proximal interphalangeal joint.

TABLE 69-3. Important Antigen-Presenting Cell–T-Cell Costimulatory Interactions

MOLECULES PRESENT ON APC	MOLECULES PRESENT ON T CELL
Leukocyte function–association antigen-3	Interleukin-2
B7-1 (CD80) B7-2 (CD86)	CD28
Leukocyte function–associated antigen-1	Intercellular adhesion molecule-1

APC, antigen-presenting cell.

UVA range, (320 to 400 nm), thus causing DNA cross-linkage and, ultimately, cell cycle arrest. Additionally, psoralens can interact with reactive oxygen species to cause cell membrane damage.[12]

■ Dosage

The systemic dose is 0.6 to 0.8 mg/kg 1 to 3 hours before UVA treatment. The initial dose of UVA is commonly based on skin type but ideally should be determined by a patient's specific minimal phototoxicity dose (MPD). For a bath, the regimen is as follows: 15 to 20 minutes of immersion in 0.5 to 5.0 mg 8-MOP per liter of water followed by immediate UVA exposure. The topical dose is 0.01% to 0.1% 8-MOP as a cream, lotion, or ointment before UVA exposure.

Treatments are given two to four times a week, with no more than twice a week during dose changes to allow for appropriate evaluation of overdose. The dose may be increased by 30% if no erythema is noted at the next treatment. Doses should be held stable if minimal erythema is present. If evidence of burn is noted, therapy should be stopped until symptoms resolve.[12]

■ Precautions

Because psoralens persist for approximately 24 hours, patients must wear protective eyewear and practice sun avoidance with strict photoprotection. Oral psoralens can cause nausea and vomiting, sunburn, and persistent pruritus. These agents should be used extremely carefully or not at all in patients with liver or renal disease, because slower metabolism and excretion can lead to extremely prolonged photosensitivity.

The dose-related risk of skin cancer with PUVA therapy is well known. The risk particularly applies to squamous cell carcinoma and is greatest in fair-skinned people. Subsequent immunosuppressive therapy may lead to a further rise in the risk of squamous cell carcinoma.[13] The risk for development of basal cell carcinomas of the trunk or extremities is moderately higher. An association between PUVA and melanoma has also been identified. One study that examined melanoma diagnosed in patients 15 years after their first PUVA treatment found a higher than expected rate. Patients who received 250 or more treatments appeared to be at the highest risk.[14] More long-term studies are needed to clarify this issue.

Patients with severe psoriasis may use phototherapy along with other systemic therapies. One group found an increased risk of lymphoma in patients concomitantly treated with PUVA and methotrexate for at least 36 months. This risk was higher for those taking higher methotrexate maintenance doses.[10]

Climatotherapy and Balneophototherapy

Climatotherapy means to relocate, either permanently or temporarily, to a climate more favorable to treatment of a disease. *Balneophototherapy* is treatment with water and sun, usually in a spa setting. Dead Sea climatotherapy has long been touted as beneficial for patients with psoriasis. Patients visit resorts at the Dead Sea for 2 to 4 weeks and expose themselves to both the water and sun. One study of 740 German patients treated at the Dead Sea found a 70% complete clearance of symptoms after 4 weeks at one of the clinics.[15] Another study of 100 Danish patients found that symptoms of 75% were clear after 4 weeks, and 68% of those patients remained in remission 4 months later.[16] One proposed explanation for the success of this approach is that the elevation of 400 m below sea level and the thick haze present in the area increase the thickness of the atmosphere. This could attenuate shorter UVB wavelengths and allow a larger proportion of longer-wave UVB to reach the patients. Additionally, the water has a high mineral content. In vitro studies indicated that Dead Sea water has an antiproliferative effect on exposed cells.[17] In addition to the sun and water, these clinics and solariums offer patients an extended retreat from stressful lives; the relaxation likely plays a role in the outcomes as well.

Studies looking at the safety of this type of therapy have found increased actinic damage but not an increase in skin cancers when compared with Israeli patients with psoriasis who were treated by other means.[18,19] Nevertheless, recommending protection of exposed noninvolved skin is prudent.

Nutrition

Antiinflammatory Diet

Although no studies specifically evaluating the benefits of an antiinflammatory diet for psoriasis could be found, one group compared the effects of a low–arachidonic acid diet in patients with rheumatoid arthritis with those of a typical Western diet in a well-matched control group. The average arachidonic acid intake was 49 mg/day in the diet group and 171 mg/day in the control group. A significant positive correlation between arachidonic acid intake and disease activity was found.[20] Although major differences exist between rheumatoid arthritis and psoriasis, this study suggests that minimizing the consumption of proinflammatory substances may help improve inflammatory disease processes (see Chapter 86, The Antiinflammatory Diet).

Fish Oil

Rates of psoriasis and other inflammatory conditions are low in populations consuming high levels of fish oils rich in omega-3 fatty acids such as eicosapentaenoic acid (EPA) and docosahexaenoic acid (DHA). This observation led to laboratory investigations looking for potential mechanisms of action, as well as clinical studies of efficacy.[21] In vitro evidence supports the theory that omega-3 fatty acids should improve psoriasis by inhibition of the inflammatory cytokines IL-6 and TNF-alpha, as well as by decreasing levels of leukotrienes. Collier et al[22] looked at the effect of consumption of oily fish compared with white fish on chronic plaque psoriasis. These investigators found that the people eating oily fish (6 oz/day for 6 weeks) had significant improvement in their Psoriasis Area and Severity Index score.[22]

Bittiner et al[23] conducted a double-blind placebo-controlled study of patients supplemented with 10 fish oil capsules (1.5 g EPA each) compared with 10 olive oil capsules for 12 weeks and found significantly less itching, scale, and erythema in the group treated with fish oil.

One randomized double-blind placebo-controlled study looked at 20 patients hospitalized for guttate psoriasis who had at least 10% body surface area involvement.[24] These patients were given intravenous infusions of either omega-6 solution or omega-3 solution (2.1 g EPA, 21 g DHA) for 10 days. Improvement from baseline was moderate for the omega-6 group (16% to 25% decrease in severity) and significant for the omega-3 group (45% to 76% decrease in severity).[24] Similar results were also found in another randomized double-blind placebo-controlled study also looking at intravenous infusion of a fish oil–based lipid emulsion in patients with chronic plaque psoriasis.[25] Other randomized and double-blind investigations did not find significant benefits.[26,27]

Some evidence indicates that fish oils can minimize side effects of other systemic therapies. Fish oils may help decrease triglyceride levels and improve cholesterol profiles in patients treated with retinoids.[28] Additionally, fish oils may help reduce the risk of nephrotoxicity associated with cyclosporine.[21]

■ Dosage

Doses vary depending on the source. Flaxseed, walnuts, and cold-water fish such as mackerel, lake trout, herring, sardines, albacore tuna, and salmon are all rich natural sources of omega-3 fatty acids.

■ Precautions

Some types of fish may contain high levels of mercury, polychlorinated biphenyls (PCBs), dioxins, and other environmental contaminants. Fish listed by the American Heart Association as having the highest mercury levels are shark, swordfish, tilefish, and king mackerel. PCBs are found in high concentrations in farmed salmon. Choosing wild-caught salmon, trimming fat before cooking, and avoiding overgrilling can help decrease exposure to PCBs. Dioxins can be found in various foods, and dioxin levels are much higher in freshwater fish than in ocean fish.

At doses greater than 3 g/day, fish oils can inhibit coagulation and potentially increase the risk of bleeding. Fish oils should be used carefully in patients taking other blood-thinning agents. Additionally, fish oils may decrease blood pressure and should be used carefully in patients already taking antihypertensives.[29]

Supplements

Zinc

Zinc has been considered a potential therapeutic option for patients with psoriasis. Some investigators have suggested that patients with psoriasis have decreased epidermal zinc levels.[30] McMillan and Rowe[31] compared plasma levels of zinc in 35 patients with psoriasis and in age- and sex-matched controls. These investigators did not find significant differences, but they did note a trend toward lower plasma zinc levels, independent of serum albumin and alkaline phosphatase levels, in patients with more extensive psoriasis.[31] Subsequent studies did not reproduce this finding, and no benefit has been found in clinical studies evaluating zinc supplementation.[32] Nevertheless, some clinicians who have used zinc supplementation for patients with psoriasis feel strongly that it can be beneficial for some patients.

■ Dosage

The recommended dietary allowance (RDA) is 15 mg/day of elemental zinc.

■ Precautions

Minor side effects include nausea, vomiting, and a metallic taste in the mouth. Taking more than 40 to 50 mg/day may raise the risk of copper deficiency. At even higher doses, zinc toxicity can manifest as watery diarrhea, irritation and erosion of the gastrointestinal tract, acute renal tubular necrosis, interstitial nephritis, and a flulike syndrome.

Inositol

Lithium is known to worsen psoriasis. Depletion of inositol is known to occur in people taking lithium. The role of inositol as a mechanism of action in bipolar disease is not completely clear, but supplementation of inositol for people taking lithium has been shown to reduce some of the side effects of lithium without diminishing its clinical usefulness. In 2004, Allan et al[33] conducted a randomized placebo-controlled cross-over study and found that Psoriasis Area and Severity Index scores were improved when patients taking lithium (300 to 1200 g/day) also took inositol (6 g/day) for 10 weeks. These investigators did not see a worsening of bipolar disorder, but this outcome was not formally evaluated in this study.[33]

■ Dosage

The dose is 6 g/day.

■ Precautions

Inositol appears to be safe. However, patients who have bipolar disorder should undergo close monitoring of their psychiatric state during inositol supplementation.

Topical Botanicals

Capsaicin

Itching is a common complaint in psoriasis. The neuropeptide substance P has been shown to be elevated in psoriatic skin.[34] This compound up-regulates the expression of adhesion molecules important in the activation and recruitment of leukocytes.[35] Additionally, substance P is known to elicit itching when it is applied to normal skin.[36] Capsaicin is an extract of chili peppers that acts by depleting substance P locally. A double-blind placebo-controlled study looking at the potential use of capsaicin four times daily for 6 weeks found that the treatment group trended to have better global improvement, greater pruritus relief, and a reduction in psoriasis severity scores. None of the differences in parameters, however, reached statistical significance.[37]

Dosage

The dose is 0.025% or 0.075% capsaicin cream, applied three or four times/day.

Precautions

Patients typically experience burning during initial applications. The burning disappears with consistent use. Patients must be careful to wash hands after application and to avoid rubbing capsaicin into their eyes.

Aloe Vera

Topical aloe extract seems to reduce the desquamation, erythema, and infiltration associated with psoriatic plaques. Results from controlled studies have been variable. One small study of patients with mild psoriasis compared the application of a 0.5% extract in hydrophilic cream three times a day for 4 weeks with a placebo and found improvement of psoriatic plaques in the treatment group.[38] Another double-blind placebo-controlled study with right-left comparison in 40 patients found a slightly better response in the placebo group.[39] Although aloe is very safe, topical sensitization can occur.

Glycyrrhetinic Acid (Licorice)

In the skin, cortisol is inactivated by the enzyme, 11beta-hydroxysteroid dehydrogenase. This enzyme is dramatically inhibited by glycyrrhetinic acid, a compound found in licorice. Through this mechanism, topical glycyrrhetinic acid has been shown to potentiate the action of hydrocortisone.[40] Glycyrrhetinic acid is available in 1% and 2% formulations and appears to be safe when it is used topically. No studies have specifically investigated the use of this compound in psoriasis.

Systemic Botanicals

Curcumin

The active component of turmeric, curcumin, is known to inhibit proinflammatory pathways critical to psoriasis.[41] One study looked at patients who were given 500-mg capsules of a curcuminoid complex that contained 95% curcuminoids.[42] These patients were instructed to take three capsules three times a day for 12 weeks, followed by 4 weeks of observation. Only eight people completed the study. Although two had an excellent response, the very small sample size and the complicated nature of some of these patients' cases make the results difficult to interpret. Larger and better-controlled studies are needed.

Milk Thistle (Silybum marianum)

Although milk thistle has not been suggested to play a role in psoriasis treatment, this botanical has been purported to protect against the hepatotoxicity seen with methotrexate. Milk thistle has been shown to act as an antioxidant by scavenging free radicals and inhibiting lipid peroxidation. Investigators have also suggested that it may protect against DNA injury and increase hepatocyte protein synthesis.[43]

Dosage

The dose is 140 mg (70% silymarin) two or three times/day.

Precautions

Diabetic patients taking silymarin require careful monitoring of blood glucose because this botanical may cause hypoglycemia secondary to increased insulin sensitivity.[42]

> Milk thistle can be protective against hepatotoxicity in patients using methotrexate to control psoriasis.

Topical Pharmaceuticals

Keratolytics

Keratolytics such as salicylic acid (2% to 10%), urea (up to 40%) and alpha-hydroxy acids (glycolic and lactic acids) are useful for decreasing the thickness of psoriatic plaques. Along with providing added comfort, thinner plaques allow for enhanced penetration of other topical agents.

Precautions

Salicylic acid should not be applied extensively on the body, especially in children. Systemic absorption can lead to salicylism, which is characterized by tinnitus, nausea, and vomiting.

Tar

Coal tar is created from the gasses produced during the distillation of coal. These are condensed and undergo ammonia extraction, resulting in a thick dark liquid. Coal tar contains 10,000 different chemical compounds, including polycyclic aromatic hydrocarbons, phenols, and nitrogen bases. Similar products that contain fewer carcinogenic compounds can be created from wood. Because of the large number of compounds available, determining a precise mechanism of action for tar is difficult. It does appear to have antiproliferative and antiinflammatory activities.[44,45]

Dosage

Patients should use 5% to 20% preparations.

Precautions

Use of tar in patients who are also treated with UV radiation has been shown to lead to a higher incidence of skin cancer. Other side effects are phototoxicity, contact allergy, irritant dermatitis, and acneiform eruptions.

Anthralin

Anthralin is a synthetic derivative of chrysarobin, which is found in Goa powder from the bark of the araroba tree of South America.[46] The mechanism of action is not well understood, but it has been shown to inhibit cell growth and promote cell differentiation.

Dosage

A 0.5% to 1% preparation is applied for 10 to 30 minutes, and is then washed off, once to twice daily.

Precautions

Irritation to normal skin can be minimized by protection with petrolatum or zinc oxide paste around psoriatic plaques. Anthralin is messy and can stain hair, skin, nails, clothing, and bedding a brownish to purplish color. The hair discoloration can be minimized by using neutral henna powder to coat the hair.

Calcipotriene (Dovonex)

Vitamin D receptors are present on many different cells, including keratinocytes and Langerhans cells. The bioactive form (1,25-dihydroxycholecalciferol) has been shown to inhibit keratinocyte proliferation and promote keratinocyte differentiation.[47] Calcipotriene is a synthetic analogue of the natural active form of Vitamin D. It is locally metabolized very rapidly, thus leading to less interference with calcium metabolism.

Dosage
A 0.005% cream, ointment, or lotion is applied twice daily.

Precautions
Self-limited irritant dermatitis is the most common complaint. Photosensitivity can develop in patients who receive UVB after calcipotriene is applied. Hypercalcemia is the most significant potential risk, but this is not a problem as long as the dose is kept at less than the recommended 100 g/wk.[48]

> The benefits of phototherapy and topical vitamin D analogues in the treatment of psoriasis also warrant 25-hydroxyvitamin D serum screening to make sure adequate oral supplementation is provided to maintain levels between 40 and 60 ng/mL.

Tazarotene Gel
Tazarotene is a topical retinoid (vitamin A derivative) that can be applied once daily. It acts to increase differentiation of keratinocytes.

Dosage
A 0.05% or 0.1% gel may be used with a topical steroid.

Precautions
Local skin irritation and pruritus are common side effects. Tazarotene may be teratogenic, so it should be used extremely carefully by women of childbearing age.

Topical Steroids
Corticosteroids have antiinflammatory, immunosuppressive, and antiproliferative properties. These activities are mediated by alterations in gene transcription. The efficacy of an individual topical corticosteroid is related to its potency and its ability to be absorbed into the skin.

Dosage
See Table 69-4 for information on potencies of different topical steroids.

Precautions
Topical corticosteroids are associated with tachyphylaxis, which is decreased efficacy with continued use. Combining topical steroids with other topical medicaments minimizes this problem. Local side effects are more common with higher potency; they include skin atrophy, acne, and localized hypertrichosis. Systemic absorption can occur with frequent or long-term use over large areas and can cause side effects similar to those of oral steroids (e.g., hyperglycemia, adrenal suppression).

Systemic Pharmaceuticals

Methotrexate
Methotrexate is a folic acid antagonist. It blocks the formation of the building blocks needed for DNA synthesis and leads to cell cycle arrest. It also has immunosuppressive effects. Finally, methotrexate acts as a potent antiinflammatory by raising tissue adenosine levels.[49] Methotrexate is particularly useful in patients with psoriatic arthritis.

Dosage
Methotrexate comes as a 2.5-mg pill or as solutions of 2.5 or 25.0 mg/mL. Typically, a 5- to 10-mg test dose is given, and complete blood count and liver function values are measured 7 days later. A dose of 10 to 15 mg/wk is usually enough to control psoriasis. Methotrexate is given weekly either as a single dose or divided into three doses given 12 hours apart.[49]

Precautions
Multiple side effects are associated with methotrexate. The most common is gastrointestinal upset, and the most dangerous is pancytopenia. Both can be decreased by adding 1 mg of folic acid daily. Other significant concerns are hepatotoxicity, pulmonary fibrosis, induction of malignancy, and teratogenicity. The concern for induction of malignancy is much greater when methotrexate is combined with PUVA; the risk of skin cancer and lymphoma appears to be increased (see the earlier section on PUVA). These potential complications require frequent monitoring with complete blood count, as well as renal and liver function tests. Liver biopsy to evaluate for fibrosis is indicated after a cumulative dose of 1.5 to 2.0 g. Additionally, the dose needs to be adjusted if the creatinine clearance value is less than 50 mL/minute.

Cyclosporine
Cyclosporine was initially isolated from the soil fungus *Tolypocladium inflatum*. It inhibits IL-2 gene transcription and leads to decreased T-cell proliferation and activation. Cyclosporine also inhibits the transcription of various proinflammatory cytokines.[50,51] It is useful in all types of psoriasis, but because of its rapid effect, cyclosporine is particularly useful in widespread pustular or erythrodermic psoriasis.

Dosage
Treatment should start at 5.0 mg/kg/day and slowly taper by 0.5 mg/kg/day until the minimum dose required to prevent recurrences is reached.

Precautions
Potential side effects include renal dysfunction, hypertension, hypertrichosis, gingival hyperplasia, gastrointestinal upset, neurologic effects (headache, tremor, paresthesias), electrolyte imbalances, sleep disturbances, acneiform eruptions, hypertriglyceridemia, decreased seizure threshold, and bone marrow suppression. Monitoring consists of measurements of blood pressure, renal function parameters including urinalysis, complete blood count, liver function tests, and blood chemistry analysis including magnesium, potassium, and uric acid.

Because cyclosporine is metabolized by the cytochrome P-450 CYP3A4 enzyme system, it has many potential drug interactions. The clinician should review a complete medication and herbal list with each patient before cyclosporine therapy is initiated.

TABLE 69-4. Potencies of Topical Steroids

CLASS	BRAND NAME	GENERIC NAME
1: Superpotent	Clobex Lotion, 0.05% Cormax Cream/Solution, 0.05% Diprolene Gel/Ointment, 0.05% Olux Foam, 0.05% Psorcon Ointment, 0.05% Temovate Cream/Ointment/Solution, 0.05% Ultravate Cream/Ointment, 0.05%	Clobetasol propionate Clobetasol propionate Betamethasone dipropionate Clobetasol propionate Diflorasone diacetate Clobetasol propionate Halobetasol propionate
2: Potent	Cyclocort Ointment, 0.1% Diprolene Cream AF, 0.05% Diprosone Ointment, 0.05% Elocon Ointment, 0.1% Florone Ointment, 0.05% Halog Ointment/Cream, 0.1% Lidex Cream/Gel/Ointment, 0.05% Maxiflor Ointment, 0.05% Maxivate Ointment, 0.05% Psorcon Cream, 0.05% Topicort Cream/Ointment, 0.25% Topicort Gel, 0.05%	Amcinonide Betamethasone dipropionate Betamethasone dipropionate Mometasone furoate Diflorasone diacetate Halcinonide Fluocinonide Diflorasone diacetate Betamethasone dipropionate Diflorasone diacetate Desoximetasone Desoximetasone
3: Upper Midstrength	Aristocort A Ointment, 0.1% Cutivate Ointment, 0.005% Cyclocort Cream/Lotion, 0.1% Diprosone Cream, 0.05% Florone Cream, 0.05% Lidex-E Cream, 0.05% Luxiq Foam, 0.12% Maxiflor Cream, 0.05% Maxivate Cream/Lotion, 0.05% Topicort Cream, 0.05% Valisone Ointment, 0.1%	Triamcinolone acetonide Fluticasone propionate Amcinonide Betamethasone dipropionate Diflorasone diacetate Fluocinonide Betamethasone valerate Diflorasone diacetate Betamethasone dipropionate Desoximetasone Betamethasone valerate
4: Midstrength	Aristocort Cream, 0.1% Cordran Ointment, 0.05% Derma-Smoothe/FS Oil, 0.01% Elocon Cream, 0.1% Kenalog Cream/Ointment/Spray, 0.1% Synalar Ointment, 0.025% Uticort Gel, 0.025% Westcort Ointment, 0.2%	Triamcinolone acetonide Flurandrenolide Fluocinolone acetonide Mometasone furoate Triamcinolone acetonide Fluocinolone acetonide Betamethasone benzoate Hydrocortisone valerate
5: Lower Midstrength	Cordran Cream/Lotion/Tape, 0.05% Cutivate Cream, 0.05% Dermatop Cream, 0.1% DesOwen Ointment, 0.05% Diprosone Lotion, 0.05% Kenalog Lotion, 0.1% Locoid Cream, 0.1% Pandel Cream, 0.1% Synalar Cream, 0.025% Uticort Cream/Lotion, 0.025% Valisone Cream/Ointment, 0.1% Westcort Cream, 0.2%	Flurandrenolide Fluticasone propionate Prednicarbate Desonide Betamethasone dipropionate Triamcinolone acetonide Hydrocortisone Hydrocortisone Fluocinolone acetonide Betamethasone benzoate Betamethasone valerate Hydrocortisone valerate
6: Mild	Aclovate Cream/Ointment, 0.05% DesOwen Cream, 0.05% Synalar Cream/Solution, 0.01% Tridesilon Cream, 0.05% Valisone Lotion, 0.1%	Alclometasone dipropionate Desonide Fluocinolone acetonide Desonide Betamethasone valerate
7: Lowest Potency	Hydrocortisone Dexamethasone Methylprednisolone Prednisolone	

From The National Psoriasis Foundation: Potencies of topical steroids. www.psoriasis.org/treatment/psoriasis/steriods/potency.php. Copyright 2006 National Psoriasis Foundation/USA.

Acitretin

Acitretin is an oral retinoid with antiproliferative and anti-inflammatory effects. It can reduce lymphocyte proliferation and decrease arachidonic acid metabolism, thus leading to decreased neutrophil chemotaxis. Acitretin has been especially useful for rapid control of pustular psoriasis.

■ Dosage

The dose is 10, 25, or 50 mg/day. Acitretin should be taken with food.

■ Precautions

Acitretin, like all retinoids, is highly teratogenic. It can cause drying of skin and mucous membranes, which some investigators have suggested may be improved by adding 800 units of vitamin E daily.[52] Decreased night vision may occur, as well as pseudotumor cerebri, especially if acitretin is given with tetracycline antibiotics. Arthralgias, myalgias, bony changes (hyperostosis), poor wound healing, and gastrointestinal symptoms are all potential side effects. Serum cholesterol and triglyceride values may be elevated in 25% to 50% of patients, who must be monitored throughout therapy. Liver transaminase values may be elevated in up to 33% of patients, but toxic hepatitis is very rare.[53,54]

Monitoring should include pregnancy tests, lipid measurements, liver function tests, complete blood count with platelets, renal function tests, and creatine phosphokinase concentrations.

Biologic Immune Response Modifiers

Biologic immune response modifiers are directed specifically at neutralizing cytokines and blocking costimulatory messages important for the activation of T cells (see Table 69-3).

Alefacept (Amevive) is a fusion protein that blocks the costimulatory signal between leukocyte function–associated antigen 3 (LFA-3) and CD2 needed for antigen-mediated T-cell activation. This agent is given as an intramuscular injection of 15 mg once weekly for 12 weeks. The injection schedule may be repeated after 12 weeks of observation. Alefacept is contraindicated in patients who have active infections or malignant diseases.

Etanercept (Enbrel) is a humanized chimeric monoclonal antibody to TNF-alpha. It is given subcutaneously as 50 mg once or twice weekly. It should not be given to patients who have an active infection or a personal or family history of multiple sclerosis.

Efalizumab (Raptiva) is a monoclonal antibody directed against CD11a (a component of LFA-1). It blocks the costimulatory interaction between LFA-1 and intercellular adhesion molecule-1 (ICAM-1), thus preventing T-cell activation. This medication can be self-administered as a subcutaneous injection of 1 to 4 mg/kg each week, with the weekly dose not to exceed 200 mg. Mild to moderate flulike symptoms may occur initially, but they tend to resolve after the first few treatments.

Infliximab (Remicade) is a monoclonal antibody that neutralizes TNF-alpha by binding to both soluble and transmembrane TNF-alpha. It induces apoptosis of TNF-alpha–expressing cells and inhibits other proinflammatory cytokines, thus leading to a decrease in keratinocyte proliferation. It is given intravenously at a dose of 5 mg/kg over 2 to 3 hours at weeks 0, 2, and 6 and then every 8 weeks. The development of antibodies is of concern and can result in infusion reactions. Infliximab should not be used in people with heart failure. In addition to regular careful monitoring (see later), patients taking infliximab must undergo additional screening for liver function.

Ustekinumab (Stelara) is a human monoclonal antibody that blocks both IL-12 and IL-23, which cause naive CD4$^+$ T cells to differentiate into types 1 and 17 helper T cells, key mediators in psoriasis. This agent is given as a subcutaneous injection at either 45 or 90 mg at weeks 0 and 4 and followed by one dose every 12 weeks. It appears to have efficacy and safety profiles similar to those of other biologics.[55] It is a very new medication, and we will learn more about its optimal use and safety as more studies are done.

All the biologic immune response modifiers require thorough baseline evaluation. This includes a history and physical examination (with special attention to liver, neurologic or cardiac disease, infection, and malignancy), complete blood count, chemistry screen with liver function tests, viral hepatitis screening, and screening for latent tuberculosis. Patients all require screening for tuberculosis annually and blood chemistry with liver function testing every 2 to 6 months. The exception is Alefacept, which requires this testing only at the beginning of each course and in patients with signs of liver damage. Alefacept also requires monitoring of CD4$^+$ T cell count at baseline and every 2 weeks. Efalizumab requires monitoring of complete blood count monthly for the first 3 to 6 months and then every 3 months thereafter. Both etanercept and infliximab require blood counts every 2 to 6 months. Patients are generally advised to have any necessary vaccinations before they begin treatment with the biologic immune response modifiers.[56]

Mind-Body Therapy

That patients with psoriasis experience greater stress as a consequence of their disease is well known. A large survey study including members of the National Psoriasis Foundation documented that psoriasis has profound emotional, social, and physical effects on quality of life.[57] Additionally, emotional factors—particularly stress—have been shown to have a strong correlation with onset and exacerbation of psoriasis.[58,59]

The mechanism of action for the effect of stress on psoriasis is beginning to be understood more clearly. Garg et al[60] found that the epidermal barrier is impaired by psychological stress. These investigators showed that injury to the epidermis promotes higher levels of keratinocyte growth stimulators, such as substance P and vasoactive intestinal peptide. Additionally, epidermal injury increases neural proliferation that, in turn, may stimulate Langerhans cell activity. These researchers suggested that psychological stress may change the level of tolerance for physical insult or may prolong epidermal recovery time. This effect could lower the threshold for disease initiation or interfere with treatment.[60]

Stress levels have also been found to affect treatment outcomes. Fortune et al[61] examined 112 patients with psoriasis before they started PUVA phototherapy and compared stress level with time to clearance of symptoms. These investigators found that high-level worry was the only significant predictor of time taken for PUVA to clear psoriasis. Patients in the high-level worry group cleared 19 days later (1.8 times slower) than did patients in the low-level worry group. Severity of disease, rates of positive family history, and levels of alcohol intake at the onset of the study were not significantly different between the two groups.[61] This information suggests that improving stress levels may enhance results from more conservative or traditional therapies. Other studies looking at various psychogenic interventions supported this suggestion as well.[62,63]

> Improving stress levels may enhance results from more conservative or traditional therapies.

Meditation

A small study found that patients who listened to a mindfulness meditation–based stress-reduction tape during PUVA or UVB therapy for psoriasis demonstrated significantly faster improvement than did patients who had no access to the tape. Clearance occurred 1 month earlier for the patients receiving UVB and the relaxation tape compared with the UVB-only group and 6 weeks earlier in the PUVA and relaxation tape group than in the PUVA-only group.[64] Another small study looked at symptoms of psoriasis as rated by dermatologists after treatment with 12 weeks of meditation ($n = 5$) or meditation plus imagery ($n = 4$) compared with controls ($n = 9$). A significant difference was noted between the treatment groups and the control group, but imagery did not yield more improvement than meditation alone.[65] The study was very small and had flaws; nevertheless, the results suggested that some patients may be able to decrease symptoms of psoriasis with meditation.

Hypnosis

A 3-month randomized blind controlled trial looked at the efficacy of active (suggestion of disease improvement) versus neutral (no mention of disease) hypnosis for the treatment of psoriasis in patients classified as highly or moderately hypnotizable. Although the groups were very small, highly hypnotizable patients showed significantly greater improvement regardless of their assigned treatment group. This observation suggests that patients who are highly hypnotizable may benefit from adding hypnosis to their treatment plan.[66]

Therapies to Consider

Traditional Chinese Medicine

According to traditional Chinese medicine (TCM), the main cause of papulosquamous disorders is an inadequate supply of nutrients to the skin. The inadequacies include external pathogenic wind-heat and wind-cold, accumulation of blood-heat resulting from dietary or emotional influences, qi stagnation and blood stasis from retention of pathogenic wind, damp, and heat, and yin deficiency of the liver and kidneys.[67]

■ Topical Preparations

Xu Yihou[67] discussed topical therapies only briefly in his text. He recommended combinations that emphasize gentle, nonirritating ointments used to decrease the scale and thickness of psoriatic plaques. An abundance of combination topical TCM preparations is available. Many actually contain corticosteroids, which would explain their efficacy.[68] Additionally, reports exist of contamination with heavy metals, toxins, and other pharmaceuticals. Such contamination can have significant adverse effects, as exemplified by the report of salicylate toxicity after the use of an herbal preparation containing oil of wintergreen over a large body area with occlusion.[69]

■ Systemic Herbs

A full description of all the Chinese herbs and combinations that can be useful for patients with psoriasis is beyond the scope of this chapter. Tse[70] reviewed clinical trials in both the English and Chinese literature that pertained to the use of Chinese herbal medicines for psoriasis from 1966 to 2001. He found only 7 poorly performed controlled trials but was also able to gain information from the 20 noncontrolled trials he identified. Of the 174 different herbs used in these trials, Tse specified 10 herbs that were commonly encountered and discussed their potential mechanisms of action. They were *Rehmannia glutinosa* (dried root), *Angelica sinensis* (root), *Salvia miltiorrhiza* (root), *Dictamnus dasycarpus* (root cortex), *Smilax glabra* (underground stem), *Oldenlandia diffusa* (whole plant), *Lithospermum erythrorhizon* (root), *Paeonia lactiflora* (root), *Carthamus tinctorius* (flower), and *Glycyrrhiza uralensis* (root).

■ Precautions

Many herbal preparations are not well regulated, and the risk of hepatotoxicity can be significant, either from the herbal components themselves or from contaminants.[71]

Acupuncture

As with the prescription of herbs, the acupuncture points used depend on the pattern of psoriasis. The main points discussed by Xi Yihou[67] focused on correcting blood-heat (BL18, BL23, BL12, and BL15) and wind-dryness from blood deficiency (BL17, BL19, BL12, BL13, and BL20). He also provided guidance on selecting points on the basis of location of the disease: LI4, LI11, TB6, and GB20 are useful for the scalp and arms; SP6, SP10, and GB34 treat the trunk, buttocks, or genital area; SP6, SP10, and ST36 treat lower limbs; and GV14, LI11, SP6, and SP10 are good for generalized lesions.

In a case series, 61 patients with psoriasis not responsive to more conventional therapies were treated with acupuncture.[72] After an average of 9 sessions (range, 1 to 15), 30 patients experienced complete or almost complete clearance of the skin lesions, 14 had two-thirds clearance, 8 experienced one-third clearance, and 9 had minimal or no improvement.[72]

One controlled clinical trial compared electrostimulated acupuncture with a sham procedure (described as "minimal acupuncture") in 56 patients with psoriasis.[73] No difference in response between the two groups was found.[73] Acupuncture without electrostimulation is used extensively in TCM, and this study was not designed to evaluate the potential benefit of plain needle acupuncture. Acupuncture is very difficult to study, and perhaps a more appropriate control would be to compare acupuncture performed on nontreatment points with acupuncture performed on points that are considered therapeutic.

Precautions

Acupuncture is quite safe, but because the needles are inserted into the skin, the Koebner phenomenon could potentially occur.[74] Clearly, more work is needed in this area if we are to gain a better understanding of its usefulness in the treatment of psoriasis.

> Assessment of traditional Chinese medicine (TCM) as a system is very difficult within a Western framework. The classification of disease in TCM is based on a different point of view, and because each patient is evaluated and treated individually with various combinations of herbs and acupuncture, creating standardized protocols to measure treatment outcomes is difficult.

Homeopathy

Like TCM, the system of homeopathy looks at psoriasis as the local expression of a systemic disturbance. Each patient is evaluated individually, and treatments are given on the basis of a constitutional approach. Because each patient is viewed as having a unique imbalance, the specific remedy chosen depends greatly on the patient. The practitioner must be well trained and have a deep understanding of homeopathy. Certification is not uniformly required, so one should look for practitioners who are accredited by one of the following organizations: Council for Homeopathic Certification (CHC), American Board of Homeotherapeutics (ABHt),

Homeopathic Academy of Naturopathic Physicians (HANP), and North American Society of Homeopaths (NASH).

Precautions

With homeopathic treatments, patients may experience an exacerbation of symptoms before resolution. This exacerbation is known as a healing crisis.

PREVENTION PRESCRIPTION

■ We currently do not have a way to prevent psoriasis. Although some situations are known to exacerbate psoriasis, flares are often unpredictable. Some things patients with psoriasis can do include the following:
- Maintain a balanced lifestyle.
- Minimize stress.
- Maintain a stable weight.
- Avoid alcohol overuse.
- Avoid tobacco.
- Eat a well-balanced diet.
- Treat skin infections early.
- Avoid medications known to exacerbate psoriasis (i.e., lithium, beta blockers, antimalarials, interferon, and rapid tapering of systemic corticosteroid dosage).

THERAPEUTIC REVIEW

General Measures
- Gentle skin care: Avoid hot water for bathing and use gentle cleansers and emollients and colloidal oatmeal.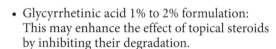

Phototherapy
- Narrow-band ultraviolet B or ultraviolet B
- Ultraviolet A alone or with psoralen (PUVA)
- Climatotherapy and balneophototherapy

Nutrition and Supplements
- Antiinflammatory diet: See Chapter 86, The Antiinflammatory Diet.
- Fish oil or oily fish: This is also useful as an adjuvant to decrease side effects of systemic retinoids and cyclosporine. Consider 2 to 3 g/day.
- Zinc: No good evidence has indicated a benefit in psoriasis; however, some clinicians do report a benefit. The dose is 15 to 30 mg/day.
- Inositol: This may be useful in patients with lithium-induced psoriasis. The dose is 6 g/day, with monitoring of psychiatric disease in patients with bipolar disorder.

Topical Botanicals
- Capsaicin for itching: A 0.025% or 0.075% cream is applied three or four times/day. Patients may experience stinging or burning during initial applications.
- Aloe vera: This may help decrease scaling and redness.
- Glycyrrhetinic acid 1% to 2% formulation: This may enhance the effect of topical steroids by inhibiting their degradation.

Systemic Botanicals
- Curcumin: The effective dose is unclear. One study looked at 150 mg three times a day.
- Milk thistle: The dose is 140 mg (70% silymarin) two to three times/day. It is best used as a hepatoprotective agent in patients taking hepatotoxic medications.

Topical Pharmaceuticals
- Keratolytics, to decrease scale and plaque thickness:
  - Salicylic acid (2% to 10%) twice daily
  - Urea (up to 40%) twice daily
  - Alpha-hydroxy acids (glycolic and lactic acids) twice daily
- Tar: 2% to 20% preparations

Continued

- Anthralin: 0.5% to 1% preparation applied for 10 to 30 minutes once or twice daily, to protect normal skin from irritation

- Calcipotriene (Dovonex): 0.005% cream, lotion, or ointment twice daily, limited to no more than 100 g/week

- Tazarotene gel (Tazorac): 0.05% to 1% gel applied at bedtime

- Topical steroids: See Table 69-4. Clinician should pay attention to the location treated and watch for side effects.

▣ Systemic Pharmaceuticals

- Methotrexate: 10 to 15 mg/week; single weekly dose or divided into three doses given 12 hours apart

- Cyclosporine: started at 5.0 mg/kg/day, with dosage tapered by 0.5 mg/kg/day to the lowest required dose

- Acitretin (Soriatane): 10, 25, or 50 mg daily

- Biologic immune response modifiers:
  - Alefacept (Amevive): 15 mg/week intramuscularly for 12 weeks

- Etanercept (Enbrel): 50 mg once or twice a week subcutaneously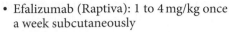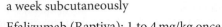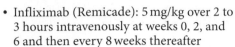

- Efalizumab (Raptiva): 1 to 4 mg/kg once a week subcutaneously

- Infliximab (Remicade): 5 mg/kg over 2 to 3 hours intravenously at weeks 0, 2, and 6 and then every 8 weeks thereafter

- Ustekinumab (Stelara): 45 or 90 mg as a subcutaneous injection at weeks 0 and 4 and then every 12 weeks thereafter

▣ Mind-Body Therapy

- Meditation: Great for stress reduction or minimization

- Hypnosis: Most potential benefit for hypnotizable patients

▣ Therapies to Consider

- Traditional Chinese medicine: Please see the text *Dermatology in Traditional Chinese Medicine*, by Xu Yihou,[67] for more detailed and complete information on and understanding of traditional Chinese medicine.

- Homeopathy

KEY WEB RESOURCES

Information About Traditional Chinese Medicine Practitioners
National Certification Commission for Acupuncture and Oriental Medicine: www.nccaom.org
American Academy of Medical Acupuncture: www.medicalacupuncture.org

Information About Homeopathic Practitioners
Council for Homeopathic Certification (CHC): www.homeopathic-directory.com
American Board of Homeotherapeutics (ABHt): http://homeopathy.org/specialty-board.html

Homeopathic Academy of Naturopathic Physicians (HANP): www.hanp.net
North American Society of Homeopaths (NASH): www.homeopathy.org

General Web Sites for Psoriasis
National Psoriasis Foundation: www.psoriasis.org
Mayo Clinic: www.mayoclinic.com/health/psoriasis/DS00193
American Academy of Dermatology: http://www.aad.org/education-and-quality-care/medical-student-core-curriculum/psoriasis/

References

References are available online at expertconsult.com.

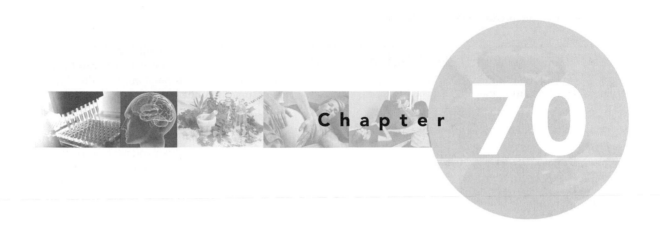

Chapter 70

Urticaria

Apple A. Bodemer, MD

Pathophysiology

Urticaria, also known as hives, is a common problem affecting approximately 20% of the general population at some point in their lives. It is characterized by wheals—discrete areas of swelling, erythema, and pruritus that are often surrounded by a pale halo. Individual lesions typically come and go over the course of 24 hours, but recurrent crops can appear for weeks. *Acute urticaria* refers to outbreaks of wheals occurring on at least 2 days a week for up to 6 consecutive weeks. When the process lasts for 6 weeks or longer, it is considered *chronic urticaria*. Patients who have less frequent outbreaks are classified as having recurrent urticaria.[1] The skin findings and symptoms of urticaria are the result of increases in inflammatory and vasoactive mediators such as histamine, prostaglandins, leukotrienes, proteases, and cytokines. These mediators are primarily found in mast cells and basophils. Although the main physiologic event is mast cell degranulation, any mechanism that elevates these mediators can result in urticaria.

Mast cell degranulation can occur through both immunologic and nonimmunologic pathways. Immunologic mechanisms include allergic mast cell degranulation, which is a type I hypersensitivity process elicited by antigen-mediated cross-linking of immunoglobulin E (IgE) receptors. Additionally, autoantibodies either to IgE or to the high-affinity IgE receptor (FcεRI) can bind to mast cells and result in degranulation.

Nonimmunologic processes cause degranulation without interacting with the IgE receptor. This category involves agents that can directly bind to mast cells to elicit degranulation (e.g., opiates, radiocontrast media), as well as other compounds that can induce the production of factors that bind to other receptors on the mast cell to cause degranulation. C1 esterase inhibitor deficiency can lead to higher levels of mediators important in urticaria. This defect causes uninhibited activation of the complement system that leads to an increase in bradykinin, which is a vasoactive inflammatory mediator.[2] Some compounds, such as aspirin, can alter the balance of prostaglandin and leukotriene synthesis, and others, including nettle plants, can directly implant vasoactive mediators into the skin.[3]

Determining the causative factor in a case of urticaria is often very frustrating. No specific origin is ever determined in 50% to 80% of patients. The most commonly implicated causes of acute urticaria are infections (especially viral infections of the upper respiratory tract), drugs (such as penicillins, sulfonamides, salicylates, nonsteroidal antiinflammatory drugs, and opiates), and foods (particularly shellfish, fish, eggs, cheese, chocolate, nuts, berries, and tomatoes). Chronic urticaria can be caused by these same agents but is more likely to be secondary to physical stimuli (e.g., dermatographism, pressure, vibration, heat, cold, exercise, sun, water), stress, autoimmune diseases (most commonly thyroid disorders), and other chronic medical diseases, such as connective tissue disease, cryoglobulinemia or cryofibrinogenemia, rheumatoid arthritis, amyloidosis, and cancer (Table 70-1).[1]

The most important factor in a good evaluation is the history. Thorough questioning may help patients recognize associations between stimuli and symptoms. Detailed diaries of a patient's activities, exposures, and ingestants can be invaluable in helping identify an association with urticarial outbreaks. Random screening laboratory tests have proved to be of little value.[4] In selected patients, however, laboratory investigations directed by the history and physical findings may be considered. The tests may include stool examination for ova and parasites, antinuclear antibody titer, screening for hepatitis B and C, thyroid function and thyroid antibody measurements, complete blood count with differential, and, possibly, an age-directed screen for malignant disease.[5]

Understanding the difference between urticaria and urticarial vasculitis is important. Urticarial vasculitis looks identical to other forms of urticaria, but individual lesions typically last for more than 24 hours and may be purpuric. Patients

TABLE 70-1. Histamine-Rich and Histamine-Releasing Foods

Histamine-Rich Foods	Avocados
	Fermented drinks
	Cheese
	Emmenthal
	Harzer
	Gouda
	Roquefort
	Tilsiter
	Camembert
	Cheddar
	Fish
	Anchovies
	Mackerel
	Herring
	Sardines
	Tuna
	Processed meat
	Ham
	Salami
	Sausage
	Jams and preserves
	Sauerkraut
	Sour cream
	Spinach
	Tomatoes
	Vinegar
	Yeast extract
	Yogurt
Histamine-Releasing Foods	Alcohol
	Bananas
	Chocolate
	Eggs
	Milk
	Some nuts
	Papaya
	Shellfish
	Strawberries
	Tomatoes

Data from Wantke F, Gotz M, Jarisch R. Histamine-free diet: treatment of choice for histamine-induced food intolerance and supporting treatment for chronic headaches. *Clin Exp Allergy.* 1993;23:982–985.

often complain more of burning than of itching.[6] Additionally, systemic symptoms such as arthralgia, gastrointestinal pain or a digestive disturbance, pulmonary obstructive disease, or renal disease may be present.[7] Urticarial vasculitis has been associated with connective tissue diseases (most commonly systemic lupus erythematosus), infections (viral hepatitis), and, rarely, with medications or hematologic disorders. The evaluation and treatment of urticarial vasculitis are beyond the scope of this chapter.

Integrative Therapy

General Principles

When a cause of urticaria is recognized, treatment can be as simple as avoiding the causative agent. In many cases of urticaria, however, the trigger is never identified. Even if the trigger is known, some patients may be unable to avoid the reaction. In these situations, many options are available for the management of urticaria.

The patient must be informed that a causative agent may never be found and that urticaria can be a chronic disease. He or she should understand that the skin reaction itself is not dangerous but is often very frustrating and difficult to live with. Chronic idiopathic urticaria can be a very unsatisfying disorder to manage, and the health care practitioner may become easily frustrated with the patient. Practitioners must not let this happen and must be open and supportive of the patient, with the recognition that urticaria is most frustrating for those who live with it.

General conservative measures can increase comfort during an exacerbation. They include staying in a cool, calm environment, wearing loose, comfortable clothing, and taking lukewarm to cool baths with added baking soda, cornstarch, or colloidal oatmeal (Aveeno). Many topical preparations can help calm the itching associated with urticaria, including menthol-containing products, aloe, and topical steroids.

Nutrition

Dietary Limitations

In the setting of acute urticaria without an inciting agent after ingestant and activity diaries have been analyzed, trying an elimination diet may be useful (see Chapter 84, Food Intolerance and Elimination Diet). Although food is a rare cause of chronic urticaria (approximately 1% of cases), it may still be helpful to try eliminating histamine-rich and otherwise antigenic foods from the affected patient's diet (see Table 70-1).[8] An Italian research group evaluated patients with chronic idiopathic urticaria before and after a 3-week, low-histamine, hypoallergenic diet. Although their sample size was small, these investigators did find significant decreases in both symptoms and plasma histamine levels after the low-histamine diet ($P = .05$).[9]

Antiinflammatory Diet

Research into the role of an antiinflammatory diet in patients with urticaria is lacking. Intuitively, it seems that if general inflammation can be minimized, urticaria—which is driven by inflammatory mediators—should improve. However, many antiinflammatory diets focus on foods rich in omega-3 fatty acid, including fish and nuts, which are known to cause or exacerbate urticaria in some patients. This type of diet should be tried only in patients who have already determined that their urticaria is not exacerbated by the recommended foods (see Chapter 86, The Antiinflammatory Diet).

Botanicals

Many different botanicals have been reported to be useful in the treatment of urticaria. They vary with sources, including canthaxanthin, field scabious, Japanese mint, kudzu, peppermint, alfalfa, bilberry extract, cat's claw, chamomile, echinacea, ginseng, licorice, nettle, yellow dock, and sarsaparilla. Many of these remedies have no evidence of efficacy from controlled studies. This section focuses only on the botanicals for which at least some in vitro evidence supports potential mechanisms of action to explain their possible benefit for patients with urticaria.[10]

Quercetin

The bioflavonoid quercetin can be found in many foods, including red wine, black tea, green tea, onions, apples, berries, citrus fruit, and brassica vegetables. Its antiinflammatory effects are thought to be mediated by inhibition of leukotriene and prostaglandin synthesis, as well as by inhibition of histamine release from mast cells and basophils.[10,11] Although theoretically quercetin should help ameliorate symptoms of urticaria, no studies looking specifically at its use in urticaria could be found.

Dosage
The dose is 400 mg by mouth twice daily before meals.

Precautions
None are known.

> Quercetin works by stabilizing mast cells, and butterbur inhibits histamine and leukotrienes. These botanicals may work synergistically on the allergic type of reaction seen in urticaria.

Butterbur (Petasites hybridus)

Butterbur lowers serum levels of histamine and leukotrienes.[12] It also decreases priming of mast cells in response to contact with allergens.[13] One study found butterbur to be as effective as cetirizine (Zyrtec) for allergic rhinitis, without sedation.[14] No studies have been conducted specifically on the use of butterbur in urticaria. Because of its positive mechanism of action on the mediators of this condition, however, butterbur should be considered in those patients who are intolerant of the sedating side effects of antihistamines.

Dosage
The dose is 50 to 100 mg of extract twice daily with meals (extract should be standardized to contain a minimum of 7.5 mg of petasin and isopetasin).

Precautions
The major concern with butterbur is its hepatotoxic pyrrolizidine alkaloid content. This herb should not be used in patients with liver disease, and liver function parameters should be monitored in any patient who uses it over a long period.

Sarsaparilla

The sarsaparilla root contains quercetin. Please see the earlier section on quercetin for more details.

Dosage
The dose of dried root is 1 to 4 g or 1 cup of tea three times/day. The dose of liquid extract (1:1 in 20% alcohol or 10% glycerol) is 8 to 15 mL three times/day.

Precautions
Gastrointestinal irritation or temporary kidney impairment may occur when sarsaparilla is used in excessive doses.

> To prepare sarsaparilla tea, simmer 1 to 4 g of dried sarsaparilla in 8 to 12 oz of water for 5 to 10 minutes.

Stinging Nettle (Urtica dioica)

The leaves of the stinging nettle contain flavonoids, including quercetin, rutin, and kaempferol. Please see the earlier section on quercetin for more details.

Dosage
The dose is 300 mg three times/day (up to seven times/day).

Precautions
Possible side effects include gastrointestinal complaints, sweating, diarrhea, and rash. Stinging nettle may worsen glucose control in patients with diabetes, lower blood pressure, and act as a diuretic.[15]

Peppermint

Luteolin-7-orutinoside from the peppermint leaf may inhibit histamine.[16] Additionally, menthol volatile oil found in peppermint is useful as a soothing topical preparation for itchy skin.

Dosage
The dose of peppermint oil is 0.2 to 0.4 mL three times/day between meals. Enteric-coated tablets are available.

Precautions
Topical use of peppermint oil can cause contact dermatitis and hives. Oral peppermint can relax the gastroesophageal sphincter and possibly worsen symptoms of gastroesophageal reflux disease. Some people have peppermint sensitivity leading to burning mouth syndrome or pruritus ani. Other side effects of peppermint that may be seen at very high doses are cramping, diarrhea, drowsiness, tremor, muscle pain, slow heart rate, and coma. Additionally, peppermint oil appears to inhibit several cytochrome P-450 enzymes, thus resulting in several potential drug interactions. Pure menthol is toxic and should never be taken internally.

> **Menthol-Containing Products for Topical Use**
> - Aveeno Skin Relief Moisturizing Lotion: menthol and colloidal oatmeal
> - Sarna Anti-Itch Lotion: 0.5% menthol and 0.5% calamine
> - Gold Bond Medicated Body Lotion: 0.15% menthol (Extra Strength has 0.5% menthol)
> - PrameGel: 0.5% menthol and 1% pramoxine
> - Watkins Menthol Camphor Ointment: 2.8% menthol and 5.3% camphor
> - Eucerin Itch-Relief Spray: 0.15% menthol

Ginkgo biloba

Ginkgo biloba contains ginkgolides, which are strong inhibitors of platelet-activating factor. Some early evidence indicates that platelet-activating factor may be implicated in some cases of cold-induced urticaria.[17] No studies have looked at the use of *Ginkgo biloba* in urticaria, but this botanical may be useful in some patients with cold-induced urticaria.

Dosage
The dose is 120 mg/day of standardized extract.

■ Precautions

Because of its antiplatelet activity, *Ginkgo biloba* may potentiate other anticoagulants, and concomitant use requires extreme care. Other side effects may include gastrointestinal upset and dizziness.

Valerian Root

Valerian has long been used as an anxiolytic and may be useful in patients whose urticaria is induced by high levels of emotional stress. No studies have specifically looked at this use of valerian.

■ Dose

The dose is 200 to 300 mg/day for generalized anxiety.

■ Precautions

No known contraindications exist. Possible side effects may include upset stomach, headache, and itching.

Pharmaceuticals

Antihistamines

The four known histamine receptor subtypes are H_1, H_2, H_3, and H_4. H_1 receptors are found throughout the body and are involved in evoking pain and pruritus, vascular dilatation, vascular permeability, bronchoconstriction, and stimulation of cough receptors. H_2 receptors are widely distributed as well and have functions similar to those of the H_1 receptors, with increased activity in the gastrointestinal system leading to higher secretion of gastric acid and mucus. In allergic processes, H_2 receptors act indirectly by altering the cytokine milieu. H_3 and H_4 receptors have been described, and their expression appears to be limited to neural and hematopoietic tissues, respectively.[18]

Antihistamines are the mainstays of treatment for patients with urticaria. Pharmacologic control is typically initiated with H_1-receptor antagonists. These agents can be broken down into the first-generation, more sedating drugs (chlorpheniramine, diphenhydramine, hydroxyzine, and promethazine) and the newer, less sedating medications (fexofenadine, cetirizine, loratadine). Because additional factors are involved in the development of urticaria, antihistamines may not completely control symptoms, but they can be expected to improve symptoms in most patients. Antihistamines should be used on a regular basis, rather than as needed, to reduce inflammation and prevent symptom development.[19]

Many studies of the various antihistamine medications showed that efficacy is equivalent for the sedating and nonsedating classes.[20,21] No specific drug works consistently better, but some patients may have a better response to one than to another. If one agent does not adequately control symptoms, switching medications or adding a second antihistamine is appropriate. In fact, combining two nonsedating agents is not an uncommon practice and can be very useful.[22] Additionally, some patients may have good response to a combination of H_1 and H_2 antagonists.[23,24]

The tricyclic antidepressant doxepin has potent antihistamine properties that make it useful for patients with chronic urticaria.[25] Doxepin is very sedating and therefore is best used either in patients who have symptoms primarily at night or in combination with nonsedating antihistamines during the day.[26]

■ Dosage of First-Generation H_1-Receptor Antagonists

The dose of hydroxyzine is 50 mg at bedtime or up to four times/day. The dose of diphenhydramine is 25 to 50 mg every 6 to 8 hours. For chlorpheniramine, the dose is 4 to 8 mg twice daily. The dose of promethazine is 12.5 to 25 mg every 6 to 8 hours.

■ Dosage of Second-Generation H_1-Receptor Antagonists

The dose of loratadine (Claritin) is 10 mg daily or twice daily. The dose of fexofenadine (Allegra) is 60 to 180 mg daily or twice daily. For cetirizine (Zyrtec), the dose is 10 mg daily or twice daily.

■ Dosage of H_2-Receptor Antagonists

The dose of ranitidine (Zantac) is 150 to 300 mg twice daily. For famotidine (Pepcid), the dose is 20 to 40 mg one or twice daily. The dose of cimetidine (Tagamet) is 200 to 400 mg once or twice daily.

■ Dosage of Doxepin

The dose of doxepin is 10 to 75 mg, taken at bedtime.

■ Precautions

The possible side effects of first-generation H_1-receptor antagonists include central nervous system depression, cardiac arrhythmias, electrolyte imbalance, dry mouth, constipation, blurred vision, dysuria, and drug interactions.

Second-generation H_1-receptor antagonists have no significant adverse effects. Loratadine may interact with some antidepressant medications.

The side effects of H_2-receptor antagonists are generally mild and reversible. Common side effects include constipation, diarrhea, fatigue, headache, insomnia, muscle pain, nausea, and vomiting. Cimetidine has some antiandrogenic activity, and high doses may rarely lead to breast enlargement in men or impotence. Cimetidine is an H_2 blocker that is typically used to block stomach acid, but it can be tried in recalcitrant urticaria. Its use in urticaria is considered off-label.

Doxepin is extremely sedating and has a potential for significant drug interactions. Other possible side effects are cardiac conduction disturbances (QT prolongation), orthostatic hypotension, and anticholinergic effects (dry mouth, blurry vision, constipation, urinary retention).

> The tricyclic antidepressant doxepin has potent antihistamine properties that make it useful for patients with chronic urticaria.

Leukotriene Inhibitors

Leukotrienes are secondary inflammatory mediators in the pathogenesis of urticaria. Inhibitors of these compounds include zafirlukast, montelukast, and zileuton. These agents are used successfully in asthma and, theoretically, should work for chronic urticaria as well. Case reports have shown somewhat mixed results.[27,28] These agents are most useful when they are combined with traditional histamine receptor antagonists.[26]

Dosage
The dose of zafirlukast (Accolate) is 20 mg twice daily. For montelukast (Singulair), it is 10 mg daily. The dose of zileuton (Zyflo) is 600 mg up to four times/day.

Precautions
Use these agents cautiously in patients with liver disease, and consider potential drug interactions.

Corticosteroids
Corticosteroids are very effective for rapid resolution of urticarial symptoms. Because side effects can be significant, the use of these drugs should be limited to occasional short, tapering dosages for severe exacerbations. These agents should be used cautiously and sparingly, with reliance on other therapies for maintenance control. Short, rapidly tapered dosages of corticosteroids are generally safe and well tolerated, but repetitive tapered dosages or long-term use can lead to significant side effects and complications.

Dosage
The dose of prednisone is 60 mg/day for 2 to 3 days, then tapered over 1 to 2 weeks.

Precautions
Common side effects include euphoria or depression, gastrointestinal distress, hypertension, sodium and fluid retention, impaired wound healing, higher risk of infection, osteoporosis, and skin atrophy. Growth retardation may occur in children. More serious side effects are adrenocortical insufficiency, cataracts, glaucoma, Cushing syndrome, hyperglycemia, and tuberculosis reactivation. Additionally, many potential drug interactions are associated with corticosteroids.

Cyclosporine
Cyclosporine is a strong immune suppressant that can be useful for patients with severe debilitating urticaria that has been recalcitrant to other therapies. It blocks the transcription of interleukin-2, which is required for T-cell activation. Among other effects, cyclosporine blocks the release of histamine from mast cells. Side effects are severe and significant, so appropriate monitoring is essential. Long-term treatment is not ideal, although some patients may require long-term low-dose therapy. Fortunately, many patients experience a period of improvement or even remission after 4 to 12 weeks of treatment.[29]

Dosage
Many dosage regimens have been described. All use cyclosporine at does at or less than 5 mg/kg/day for various durations. One regimen described specifically for chronic and debilitating urticaria is as follows: 3 mg/day divided into two doses for 6 weeks, followed by 2 mg/kg/day divided into two doses for 3 weeks, followed by 1 mg/kg/day divided into two doses for 3 weeks.[30]

Precautions
Cyclosporine is contraindicated in patients with uncontrolled hypertension, severe renal disease, serious infections, or a current or prior history of malignant disease.

Potential side effects include renal dysfunction, hypertension, hypertrichosis, gingival hyperplasia, gastrointestinal upset, neurologic effects (headache, tremor, paresthesias), electrolyte imbalances, acneiform eruptions, hypertriglyceridemia, bone marrow suppression, and sleep disturbances. Monitoring includes urinalysis, complete blood count, liver function tests, and blood chemistry analysis including magnesium, potassium, and uric acid.

Because cyclosporine is metabolized by the cytochrome P-450 CYP3A4 enzyme system, it has many potential drug interactions. The clinician should review a complete medication and herb list with each patient before cyclosporine therapy is initiated.[31]

Mind-Body Techniques
Background
Several studies showed that psychological stress can trigger or exacerbate flares of urticaria.[32,33] Although the mechanism is not well understood, the release of neuropeptides is thought ultimately to lead to elevations of histamine or greater sensitivity to histamine.[34] Human skin mast cells have been shown to release histamine in response to stimulation from various neuropeptides, including substance P, vasoactive intestinal polypeptide, and somatostatin.[35] Much more work needs to be done before we have a clear understanding of the relationship between the neural impact of stress on inflammation and urticaria.

Hypnosis
Most information on the effectiveness of hypnosis is in the form of case reports. The flare reaction to histamine prick testing has been shown to be significantly decreased with hypnosis.[36,37] One investigation looking at the use of relaxation techniques in patients who were classified as hypnotizable and those classified as unhypnotizable found that both groups experienced improvement in symptoms; however, only patients classified as hypnotizable had fewer clinical lesions.[38] In spite of the limited evidence, hypnotherapy may be a beneficial alternative—either alone or in combination with other therapies—for some patients with urticaria.

> Hypnosis is a therapy that should be encouraged for chronic urticaria. The evidence is promising, and potential for side effects is minimal.

Traditional Chinese Medicine
Within the framework of traditional Chinese medicine (TCM), urticaria is thought to be caused primarily by wind-heat, which obstructs energy channels and networks and causes red inflammation on the skin. When excess wind is present in the body, it can wander through the skin and cause itching. Wind-heat can arise through several different mechanisms. Invasion of pathogenic wind is often combined with pathogenic cold or heat. Emotional disturbances and irritability cause heat accumulation in the heart and blood that makes one more susceptible to invasive wind. Damage to the spleen and stomach (resulting from a diet that is unhygienic or heavy in fish, seafood, or spicy foods) impairs the function of these organs and leads to increased dampness. When dampness accumulates internally, it can be transformed into wind-heat.

Each situation leading to the accumulation of wind-heat can be specifically treated with various herbal concoctions that are beyond the scope of this chapter. Acupuncture can also be used alone or in combination with herbal remedies. The main general acupuncture points used for urticaria vary according to the source but include PC6 Neiguan, GB20 Fengchi, and ST36 Zusanli[39] or LI11 Quchi, SP10 Xuehai, SP6 Sanyinjiao, and S36 Zusanli.[40] Because TCM treatments are highly individualized for each patient and specific symptom variations, these very general acupuncture points may differ significantly from patient to patient. The assistance of a well-trained TCM physician should be sought, especially if one is interested in pursuing TCM herbal therapies.

Wide variation exists from state to state regarding certification, so when choosing an Oriental Medical Doctor (OMD), one should ask whether the person has passed the National Certification Commission for Acupuncture and Oriental Medicine herbal examination. If someone is interested in acupuncture alone, the American Academy of Medical Acupuncture is a good additional source of well-trained practitioners.

Homeopathy

Like TCM, homeopathy looks at urticaria as the local expression of a systemic disturbance. Each patient is evaluated individually, and treatments are given on the basis of the constitutional approach. Because each patient is viewed as having a unique imbalance, the specific remedy chosen depends greatly on the patient. Two patients with urticaria may be successfully treated with vastly different therapies. Approximately 20 remedies are commonly employed to help patients with urticaria, including Natrum Muriaticum (a derivative of sodium chloride), Apis Mellifica (derived from the honey bee), Urtica Urens (derived from the stinging nettle plant), silica, and Kali Carbonicum (derived from potassium carbonate).

To give a patient an appropriate cure, a practitioner must be well trained and have a deep understanding of homeopathy. Certification is not uniformly required, so one should look for practitioners who are accredited by one of the following organizations: the Council for Homeopathic Certification (CHC), the American Board of Homeotherapeutics (ABHt), the Homeopathic Academy of Naturopathic Physicians (HANP), and the North American Society of Homeopaths (NASH).

■ Precautions

With homeopathic treatments, patients may experience an exacerbation of symptoms before resolution; this exacerbation is known as a healing crisis.

PREVENTION PRESCRIPTION

■ If a cause is identified in a particular patient, recurrences can be limited by having the patient
  • Avoid exposure to known triggers.
  • Limit stress.
  • Eat a healthy, balanced diet with a low histamine content.

THERAPEUTIC REVIEW

This is a summary of therapeutic options for urticaria. Laboratory investigation should be directed by the history and physical findings. Particular attention to associations with systemic disease is warranted in patients with chronic urticaria.

■ General Measures

• Identify and avoid any precipitating factors, if possible. Activity and ingestant diaries may be particularly useful in this endeavor.

• Use topical measures, including a cool, calm environment, loosely fitting, comfortable clothes, baths with cornstarch, colloidal oatmeal (Aveeno), or baking powder.

■ Nutrition

• Avoid allergenic foods and foods high in histamine (see Table 70-1).

• Consider an elimination diet (see Chapter 84, Food Intolerance and Elimination Diet).

■ Botanicals and Supplements

• Quercetin: 400 mg orally twice daily before meals

• Butterbur (Petadolex): 75 mg orally twice daily

• Sarsaparilla: 1 to 4 g as dried root or tea three times daily; liquid extract (1:1 in 20% alcohol or 10% glycerol): 8 to 15 mL three times daily

• Stinging nettle: 300 mg three times daily

• Peppermint: 0.2 to 0.4 mL oil three times daily between meals or equivalent in enteric-coated tablets

• Ginkgo biloba for cold-induced urticaria: 120 mg/day standardized extract

• Valerian root for stress-related urticaria: 200 to 300 mg/day

■ Pharmaceuticals

• Antihistamines: H₁-receptor blockers alone or in combination with H₂-receptor blockers

• First-generation

  • Hydroxyzine: 50 mg one to four times daily

- Diphenhydramine: 25 to 50 mg every 6 to 8 hours

- Chlorpheniramine: 4 to 8 mg twice daily.

- Promethazine: 12.5 to 25 mg every 6 to 8 hours

- Second-generation

  - Loratadine (Claritin): 10 mg once or twice daily

  - Fexofenadine (Allegra): 60 to 180 mg once or twice daily

  - Cetirizine (Zyrtec): 10 mg once or twice daily

- H_2-receptor antagonists

  - Ranitidine (Zantac): 150 to 300 mg twice daily

  - Famotidine (Pepcid): 20 to 40 mg one to twice daily

  - Cimetidine (Tagamet): 200 to 400 mg one to four times daily

- Doxepin: 10 to 75 mg before bed

- Leukotriene inhibitors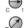

  - Zafirlukast (Accolate): 20 mg twice daily

- Montelukast (Singulair): 10 mg daily

- Zileuton (Zyflo): 600 mg up to four times daily

- Corticosteroids: 60 mg/day for 2 to 3 days, then tapered over 1 to 2 weeks

- Cyclosporine: 3 mg/kg/day for 6 weeks, 2 mg/kg/day for 3 weeks, and 1 mg/kg/day for 3 weeks. Appropriate monitoring is essential.

Mind-Body Therapy

- Relaxation: Good for everyone!

- Hypnosis, especially for people classified as hypnotizable

Traditional Chinese Medicine

- Please see the text *Dermatology in Traditional Chinese Medicine*, by Xu Yihou,[35] for more detailed and complete information on and understanding of TCM.

- Please also see Key Web Resources for Web sites listing traditional Chinese medicine practitioners.

KEY WEB RESOURCES

General Overview of Disease and Treatment
American Academy of Dermatology: http://www.aad.org/public/publications/pamphlets/skin_urticaria.html
Mayo Clinic: http://www.mayoclinic.com/health/chronic-hives/DS00980

Web Sites for Information about Traditional Chinese Medicine Practitioners
National Certification Commission for Acupuncture and Oriental Medicine: www.nccaom.org
American Academy of Medical Acupuncture: www.medicalacupuncture.org

---

References

References are available online at expertconsult.com.

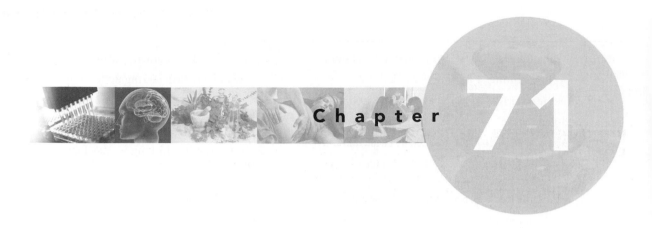

Recurrent Aphthous Ulceration

David Rakel, MD

Recurrent aphthous ulcers (RAUs), also called aphthous stomatitis and canker sores, are the most common oral mucosal lesions, affecting 20% of the population in North America. They appear as recurrent ulcers with circumscribed margins with erythematous halos and gray or yellowish floors (Fig. 71-1).

RAUs affect the nonkeratinized or poorly keratinized mucosa of the mouth and oropharynx. No specific test is available for RAUs, and diagnosis is made from the patient's history and clinical findings.

Pathophysiology

RAUs appear to be multifactorial in origin, with a strong component of immune mediation. Histologically, there is an increase in immunoglobulin (Ig)E–bearing lymphocytes along with an increase in mast cells and tumor necrosis factor-alpha (TNF-alpha) in the prodromal stages.[1] Cytotoxic action of lymphocytes and monocytes seem to cause the ulceration, but the exact trigger is not clear.

The three main clinical variations are as follows:

Minor aphthous ulcers: Commonly less than 5 mm in diameter, these are the most common form (80%). Typically one to five ulcers may be present at any one time, and they usually heal without scarring in 7 to 14 days.

Major aphthous ulcers: These ulcers, which are less common, are larger and deeper than minor aphthous ulcers, tend to have irregular edges, and are more painful. They affect the lips, soft palate, and oropharynx and can take up to 6 weeks to heal, often leaving a considerable scar. Major and minor RAUs can be associated with Behçet's syndrome and human immunodeficiency virus (HIV) infection.

Herpetiform RAUs: From 1 to 3 mm in diameter, herpetiform RAUs often occur in groups of 10 to 100 that commonly coalesce to form large, irregular areas of ulceration. These are not as deep as major aphthous ulcers. They heal without scarring in 7 to 14 days and, in spite of their name, are not associated with herpesvirus or other viral origin.

Minor and major RAUs usually begin in childhood or early adolescence and have a tendency to resolve naturally later in life. Herpetiform RAUs appear later than minor and major RAUs, usually in the third decade (Box 71-1).

Integrative Therapy

Nutrition

Several nutritional deficiencies have been associated with RAUs. Nutrients vitamin B_{12}, iron, and folic acid have been the most studied and are commonly deficient in patients with RAUs.[2] Laboratory evaluation for red cell folate, serum vitamin B_{12}, and ferritin levels should be included in any evaluation of RAUs.

Vitamins B_1,[3] B_2, B_6, and B_{12} have also been found to be deficient in some patients with RAUs.[4]

> Laboratory evaluation for red cell folate, serum vitamin B_{12}, and ferritin levels, as well as complete blood count, should be ordered in the evaluation of recurrent aphthous ulceration. HIV infection should be considered if the patient is at risk for this infection.

Diet

A few patients with RAUs have gluten-sensitive enteropathy and improve considerably with a gluten-free diet.[5] The diagnosis is usually made by jejunal biopsy or by assay of tissue transglutaminase IgA with a positive antiendomysial antibody. Although no evidence in the literature shows that gluten-free diets help patients with RAUs who do not

FIGURE 71-1

Recurrent aphthous ulcers. The ulceration seen on the labial mucosa is surrounded by a characteristic erythematous halo. (From Zitelli BJ, Davis HW. *Atlas of Pediatric Physical Diagnosis.* 5th ed. St. Louis: Mosby; 2007.)

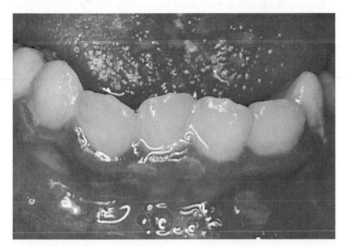

BOX 71-1. Etiology of Recurrent Aphthous Ulceration

The origin of recurrent aphthous ulceration seems to be multifactorial and can include one or several of the following factors:

- Familial and genetic basis
- Nutritional deficiencies: vitamins B_1, B_2, B_6, and B_{12}, folic acid, iron
- Stress
- Stopping smoking
- Menstruation
- Food allergies (cow's milk and gluten most common)
- Sensitivities to toothpastes (sodium lauryl sulfate)
- Medications
  - Antineoplastic (methotrexate, daunorubicin, doxorubicin, hydroxyurea)
  - Angiotensin-converting enzyme inhibitors (captopril most common)
  - Antimicrobials
  - Barbiturates
  - Griseofulvin
  - Nonsteroidal antiinflammatory drugs (NSAIDs)
  - Sulfonamides
  - Quinidine
  - Penicillamine
- Physical trauma
- Systemic conditions
  - Celiac disease
  - Crohn's disease
  - Human immunodeficiency virus infection
  - Neutropenia and other immune deficiencies
  - Neumann bipolar aphthosis
  - Behçet's syndrome
  - MAGIC (mouth and genital ulcers with inflamed cartilage)

---

have gluten sensitivity,[6] anecdotal observations indicate that some patients without gluten sensitivity may benefit from a gluten-free diet.[7] For the patient with recurring ulcers, a 2- to 4-week therapeutic trial of gluten avoidance is a reasonable option to assess effect.

The role of food allergies in the pathogenesis of RAUs is controversial. Several foods—milk, chocolate, coffee, nuts, strawberries, pineapple, citrus fruits, tomatoes, azo dyes—and food additives—monosodium glutamate (MSG), benzoic acid, tartrazine (yellow dye no. 5), and cinnamaldehyde—have all been suggested as a cause of RAUs[8,9] (see Chapter 84, Food Intolerance and Elimination Diet).

Honey

Honey has been found to be helpful in healing stasis ulcers of the legs as well as preventing mouth ulcers in patients receiving radiation therapy. In 40 patients with head and neck cancer who were receiving radiation, those who took 20 mL of honey 15 minutes before therapy and at 15-minute intervals at the time of therapy, and then again 6 hours after therapy, had significantly fewer mouth ulcers than the saline-treated control group.[10]

Supplements

Glutamine

Glutamine, the most abundant amino acid in the body, is essential for maintaining intestinal function, immune response, and amino acid homeostasis during times of severe stress. Glutamine supplementation has been found to improve nutritional and immunologic status and reduce complications in critically ill patients.[11] Not everyone benefits from supplementation, however. Those who are most nutritionally deficient are thought to have the best clinical response.[12] Supplementation with glutamine is beneficial during times of skeletal muscle wasting because most of glutamine is produced in skeletal muscle, and glutamine depletion raises the incidence of oral and gastrointestinal ulcerations. This amino acid has been found to reduce the duration and severity of oral stomatitis in patients undergoing chemotherapy.[13]

■ Dosage

Glutamine can be purchased in powdered form. The patient should mix 4 g in water, swish in the mouth, and swallow four times daily. If glutamine is used with chemotherapy, it should be taken on the day of chemotherapy and then used for 4 days after completion of each treatment.

■ Precautions

Grittiness of the oral solution may be unpleasant. Glutamine is otherwise well tolerated. It may cause mania in patients with bipolar disease.

Vitamin B_{12}

A randomized double-blind trial using 1000 mcg of sublingual vitamin B_{12} taken daily before sleep for 6 months in 58 patients with RAU showed that those in the treatment arm of the trial had significant reduction in ulcer formation, and 74% (compared with 32% in the placebo group) reported "no aphthous ulcer status" after 6 months. The response was not predicted by baseline serum vitamin B_{12} levels, and study subjects with normal levels still responded to therapy.[14]

■ Dosage
The dose of vitamin B_{12} is 1000 mcg sublingually daily for ulcer prevention.

■ Precautions
Vitamin B_{12} therapy is safe. The body excretes any excess into the urine, with the resulting classic bright yellow coloration seen with B-vitamin supplementation.

Botanicals

German Chamomile (Matricaria recutita)
Chamomile is used for its antiinflammatory properties in the treatment of dyspepsia, leg ulcers, and oral mucositis. When used as a mouthwash, it has been found to prevent oral mucositis associated with radiation therapy and chemotherapy.[15]

■ Dosage
Make an oral rinse with 10 to 15 drops of German chamomile liquid extract in 100 mL warm water, and use three times daily.

■ Precautions
The plant has allergic potential but is otherwise safe.

Licorice (Glycyrrhiza)
Licorice, which has antiinflammatory action, has been used as a mouthwash and is available in oral disks.[16] A randomized double-blind study using a *Glycyrrhiza* oral patch compared with placebo patch showed significantly faster resolution of ulcers in the *Glycyrrhiza*-treated group at 8 days.[17]

■ Dosage
To use licorice as a mouthwash, mix ½ teaspoon licorice extract with ¼ cup water, swish, gargle, and expel the mouthwash four times daily for symptomatic aphthous ulcers.

A product called CankerMelt contains 30 mg *Glycyrrhiza* extract. The disk is applied to the ulcer and allowed to dissolve over time; then a new disk is applied every 6 hours.

■ Precautions
If the mouthwash is not swallowed, side effects are rare. Licorice can cause sodium retention and hypokalemia if it is swallowed. Care should be taken with the use of licorice in patients with hypertension, because licorice ingestion can worsen the condition.

> Although research is limited, many patients find pain relief from the tannins found in tea leaves (*Camellia sinensis*). A brewed black or green tea bag can be applied to the ulcer as needed.

Homeopathy

Several homeopathic remedies have been used historically to treat RAUs. Unfortunately, all the evidence for their use is anecdotal. A classical homeopath would look for a constitutional remedy that fits the whole patient. Symptomatic remedies that may help are as follows:

Mercurius solubilis is indicated if the RAUs are associated with foul breath and increased salivation.

Borax is indicated if the RAUs are brought on by citrus or acidic foods. The mouth usually feels dry even though some saliva may be present.

Arsenicum album is indicated in patients with RAUs that are brought on by stress and eased with hot drinks.

■ Dosage
All the preceding remedies are best given initially at a potency of 6X or 6C four times daily (the X and C refer to the potency, which is the extent of dilution of the remedy). They should be discontinued when the RAUs begin to improve (see Chapter 111, Therapeutic Homeopathy).

Mind-Body Therapy

Stress, both emotional and physical, triggers RAUs. Emotional and environmental stress may precede 60% of first-time aphthous ulcer cases and be involved in 21% of recurrent episodes.[7] The pathogenesis may involve the known alteration of the immune response from stress or the depletion of B vitamins, or the cause may be unknown.

Meditation and stress reduction techniques, such as guided imagery and hypnosis, have been shown to be useful in the management of RAUs.[18,19]

Lifestyle

Toothpaste
Sodium lauryl sulfate is a common detergent used in toothpastes that has been shown to precipitate RAUs.[20] Other ingredients may also affect RAUs, so a good question to ask patients with newly developed RAUs is whether they have recently changed toothpaste. *CloSYS, Tom's of Maine, The Natural Dentist, Burt's Bees,* and *Squigle* are examples of brands of toothpaste that do not contain sodium lauryl sulfate.

Pharmaceuticals: Antiinflammatory Agents

Amlexanox
The only prescription medication approved by the U.S. Food and Drug Administration (FDA) for treatment of aphthous stomatitis is amlexanox (Aphthasol) 5% paste. It accelerates healing through an unknown mechanism that inhibits inflammatory mediators (histamine, leukotrienes) from mast cells, neutrophils, and mononuclear cells. This agent has no direct analgesic properties.

■ Dosage
Apply 0.5 cm to the sore with fingertip four times daily after meals and at bedtime. Start at the onset of symptoms, and stop with resolution. If no resolution has occurred in 7 days, reevaluation is warranted. Amlexanox is dispensed in a 5-g tube.

■ Precautions
This agent may cause minimal burning on application. Rash, diarrhea, nausea, and worsening stomatitis have been reported in less than 1% of cases.

Triamcinolone and Dexamethasone

Steroids such as triamcinolone and dexamethasone reduce inflammatory mediators but do not decrease the frequency of RAU occurrence.

■ Dosage

For triamcinolone acetonide 0.1% in carboxymethyl cellulose paste (Kenalog in Orabase), apply 0.5 cm to the sore two or three times daily. Start at the onset of symptoms and stop with resolution. If no resolution has occurred in 7 days, reevaluation is warranted. This agent is dispensed in a 5-g tube.

For dexamethasone (Decadron) oral solution 0.5 mg/5 mL, rinse the mouth with 1 teaspoon (5 mL) for 2 minutes and spit out, three times daily after meals and once at bedtime.

■ Precautions

Thrush may occur.

Pharmaceuticals: Analgesic Agents

A helpful approach is to avoid spicy, salty, and vinegar-containing foods that may irritate and increase pain of the ulcers. The following analgesic agents may also be useful.

Viscous Lidocaine (Xylocaine 2% solution)

This agent provides anesthetic properties that diminish pain while eating.

■ Dosage

To use viscous lidocaine (Xylocaine 2% solution), swish 15 mL and expel, every 3 hours or before meals as needed for pain relief. Do not use more than eight doses daily. This agent is dispensed in 50-, 100-, and 450-mL bottles.

■ Precautions

Care should be taken not to ingest large amounts of viscous lidocaine internally because of its potential cardiotoxicity. Benzocaine gel (10% to 20%) is a safer alternative, particularly for use in children.

Pharmaceuticals: Mouthwashes

Chlorhexidine Gluconate

Chlorhexidine gluconate 0.12% oral solution (Peridex or Periogard oral rinse) is a mouthwash that has been shown to reduce the incidence, duration, and discomfort of RAUs.[21] It does not, however, appear to be as effective as the other pharmaceutical topical agents.[22]

■ Dosage

Swish 15 mL for 30 seconds and expel, twice daily. Chewing sugarless gum after using this mouthwash can help reduce tooth discoloration.

■ Precautions

This agent can cause stinging when it is first used, reversible discoloration of the teeth and tongue after 1 week of use, transient disturbances of taste, and burning sensation of the tongue.

Tetracycline–Fluocinolone Acetonide–Diphenhydramine Mouthwash

For more severe cases, a formula containing tetracycline, fluocinolone acetonide, and diphenhydramine can be used. Tetracycline is thought to work through antimicrobial as well as antiinflammatory mechanisms. Fluocinolone and diphenhydramine work through antiinflammatory and anesthetic mechanisms. I have found this mixture to be very helpful in severe cases of RAUs resulting from immunosuppressant therapy.

■ Dosage

This formula requires the help of a pharmacist for mixing. Most pharmacies are able to comply with these directions. The following should be mixed together to make a total of 150 mL:

Tetracycline: At a concentration of 500 mg/5mL (which pharmacist makes by dissolving a 500-mg capsule in 5 mL of water) for a total of 60 mL

Diphenhydramine syrup (Benadryl): 12.5 mg/5 mL for a total of 60 mL

Fluocinolone acetonide 0.01% solution (Synalar): A total of 30 mL

Swish 10 mL and expel four times daily until the ulcers resolve. Do not use for more than 7 days at a time.

■ Precautions

Tetracycline should not be given to children younger than 9 years old because it stains the teeth. Fluocinolone, like most steroids, can cause thrush if it is used for extended periods.

> For severe cases, a trial of tetracycline–fluocinolone acetonide–diphenhydramine mouthwash is indicated before using systemic therapy.

Systemic Pharmaceuticals

For cases resistant to topical therapy, consider the following systemic pharmaceuticals, in descending order as discussed here.

Colchicine

Colchicine has been used for stomatitis associated with Behçet's disease.[23] It has also been found to be beneficial for RAUs in patients without this disorder and is even more effective when combined with systemic steroids.[24]

■ Dosage

The dose is 0.6 mg orally twice daily. It may be increased to three times daily as tolerated with regard to gastrointestinal side effects.

■ Precautions

The most common side effects are gastrointestinal, consisting of diarrhea, nausea, and cramping. Colchicine can also cause thrombocytopenia and aplastic anemia.

Systemic Steroids

No good studies have been conducted on the use of systemic steroids for RAUs. These agents should be used cautiously in immunocompromised hosts.

■ Dosage

The dose of prednisone is up to 40 to 60 mg/day for 5 days. If longer use is needed, taper the dosage over 10 to 14 days.

■ Precautions

In patients with HIV infection, adverse reactions include cushingoid facies, thrush, reactivation of herpes simplex virus, and accelerated progression of Kaposi sarcoma.[25]

Thalidomide

Thalidomide has pronounced efficacy in healing oral aphthae. In two trials involving difficult cases, thalidomide completely healed 48% to 55% of ulcers, compared with 7% to 9% in patients receiving placebo. This effect was temporary, however; many of the patients treated had recurring symptoms.[26]

■ Dosage

The dose is 200 mg/day orally.

■ Precautions

Because of the potential for teratotoxicity and irreversible peripheral neuropathy, this treatment should be used only for the most serious, intractable cases.

> Because of the elevation of tumor necrosis factor-alpha (TNF-alpha) in recurrent aphthous ulceration, some people with resistant cases related to autoimmune conditions may benefit from a TNF inhibitor drug such as infliximab, etanercept, or adalimumab. These medications also have significant risk resulting from inhibition of immune function.[27]

Cautery With Silver Nitrate

The use of silver nitrate sticks to provide chemical cautery was found to reduce pain significantly compared with placebo, but it did not reduce healing time. The study involved only one application. Clinicians contemplating this therapy should consider pretreating the ulcer with 2% viscous lidocaine and then painting the ulcer with the silver nitrate stick until it turns completely white.[28]

Therapies to Consider

Traditional Chinese Medicine

Chinese medicine views RAU as a condition caused by heat in the stomach; it can also be caused by yin deficiency or toxic heat. Treatment is with Topical Watermelon Frost or internally with formulas that cool stomach heat and clear toxic heat, such as Dao Chi Pian or Niu Huang Jie Du Pian. Although no reliable studies on the use of traditional Chinese medicine in the treatment of RAUs have been conducted, referral to a Chinese medicine practitioner is a valid approach if other treatments are not indicated or are unsuccessful.

PREVENTION PRESCRIPTION

■ Have patients:
  • Avoid oral trauma from biting, dental procedures, brushing, and eating of rough foods.
  • Avoid toothpaste that contains sodium lauryl sulfate.
  • Ensure adequate nutrition by consuming seven to nine servings of fruits and vegetables daily.
  • Avoid trigger foods; cow's milk and wheat (gluten) are most common.
■ Consider a B-100 complex vitamin daily for recurring cases.
■ Help patients learn how to change their interpretation of stressful information and events to reduce physical consequences (see Chapter 93, Relaxation Techniques, and Chapter 98, Recommending Meditation).
■ Avoid the use of medications associated with recurrent aphthous ulcers (see Box 71-1).

THERAPEUTIC REVIEW

The most important issue in dealing with recurrent aphthous ulcers (RAUs) is to exclude systemic conditions, particularly Behçet's syndrome (mouth, genital, and eye ulcers). Because the origin of RAUs is multifactorial, a simple list of treatments is not applicable; a good history helps focus on the triggers and can lead to a specific treatment plan. The following is a guide to the most common causes and treatments of RAU.

■ Laboratory Evaluation

• Identification of nutritional deficiencies should be the first step in treating RAUs.

• Order measurements of serum ferritin, red cell folate, and serum vitamin B_{12}. Replace these nutrients if the patient is deficient.

• Giving 250 mg of vitamin C with the iron is often helpful to assist in iron absorption.

■ Nutrition

• If you suspect celiac disease, assess the patient for tissue transglutaminase immunoglobulin A and antiendomysial antibodies.

• Identify any foods that trigger the RAUs and consider elimination (see Chapter 84, Food Intolerance and Elimination Diet).

• Consider using honey, 20 mL before, during, and after radiation therapy of the head and neck to reduce the severity of mouth ulcerations.

Supplements

- B vitamins (vitamins B₁, B₂, B₆, B₁₂)
  - Because the cost and potential harm of B vitamins are low, a 3-month trial of one B-50 complex vitamin pill daily can be used to see whether the frequency of RAUs is reduced. A B-50 complex vitamin contains approximately 50 mcg or mg of each B vitamin.
  - Vitamin B₁₂, 1000 mcg sublingually daily for 6 months, has been found to reduce the incidence of ulcers.
- Glutamine
  - Mix 4 g of powder in water, swish, and swallow four times/day.
  - This is best for RAUs resulting from severe disease or injury or in patients undergoing chemotherapy.

Botanicals

- Licorice *(Glycyrrhiza)* mouthwash: Mix ½ teaspoon of licorice extract in ¼ cup of water; swish and expel four times/day.
- CankerMelt disks contain 30 mg *Glycyrrhiza* extract. The disk is applied to the ulcer and allowed to dissolve over time; then a new disk is applied every 6 hours.

Homeopathy

- Mercurius solubilis is indicated if the RAUs are associated with foul breath and increased salivation. Use 6X or 6C potency four times/day until healing begins.
- Borax is indicated if the RAUs are brought on with citrus or acidic foods. The mouth usually feels dry even though some saliva may be present. Use 6X or 6C potency four times/day until healing begins.
- Arsenicum album is indicated in patients whose RAUs are brought on by stress and eased with hot drinks. Use 6X or 6C potency four times/day until healing begins.

Mind-Body Therapy

- Because stress is often a component of RAUs, stress reduction techniques, such as meditation and guided imagery, are usually advisable to include in management (see Chapter 93, Relaxation Techniques).

Pharmaceuticals

- Topical therapy
  - Amlexanox (Aphthasol) 5% paste: 0.5 cm applied to sore four times daily
  - Triamcinolone acetonide 0.1% in carboxymethyl cellulose paste (Kenalog in Orabase): 0.5 cm applied to sore three to four times daily
  - Viscous lidocaine (Xylocaine 2% solution): 15 mL swished every 3 hours as needed for pain
  - Chlorhexidine gluconate 0.12% oral solution (Peridex or Periogard oral rinse): 15 mL rinsed and expelled twice daily
  - Tetracycline 500 mg/5 mL to make 60 mL, fluocinolone acetonide solution (Synalar) 30 mL, and diphenhydramine syrup (Benadryl) 60 mL, mixed together to make 150 mL: 10 mL swished and expelled four times daily
- Systemic therapy
  - Colchicine: 0.6 mg twice daily, increased to three times daily as tolerated in terms of gastrointestinal side effects
  - Prednisone: 40 to 60 mg/day for 5 days
  - Thalidomide: 200 mg/day; used only for most severe cases

Cautery

- Premedicate with 2% viscous lidocaine and paint the ulcer once with silver nitrate stick until it turns white.
- This technique helps reduce pain but not ulcer duration.

KEY WEB RESOURCES

Dentist.net: http://www.dentist.net/sls-free-toothpaste.asp	This consumer site sells sodium lauryl sulfate–free toothpastes.
OraHealth: http://www.orahealth.com/	This company developed oral adhering disks that allow the medicinal application of specific treatments for recurrent aphthous ulcers. Information on obtaining CankerMelts can be found here.

References

References are available online at www.expertconsult.com.

Seborrheic Dermatitis

Alan M. Dattner, MD

Pathophysiology

Seborrheic dermatitis (SD) involves a predisposition toward a specific inflammatory desquamative reaction pattern in typically oily areas rich in *Malassezia*. An overabundance of or an inappropriate immune reaction to the common skin and follicular microflora species known as *Malassezia* (formerly *Pityrosporum*) has been both demonstrated and disputed in the literature.[1] Since the identification of seven major strains of *Malassezia* in 1996, studies have begun to demonstrate which species are most predominant in SD in different populations. *Malassezia globosa* and *Malassezia restricta* predominate, according to some reports,[2,3] and various other strains are reported to be associated with SD as well. Evidence both for and against an association with increased or altered sebum production has been presented, but increased sebum production leading to greater growth of *Malassezia* seems to be a contributor.

Seborrhea is aggravated by Parkinson disease and by drugs that induce parkinsonism; clinical improvement is obtained with levodopa treatment of Parkinson disease. Aggravation by emotional stress and changes associated with cases of partial denervation suggest a neurohumoral influence as well. Some drugs have been implicated in inducing SD. Infantile SD, or Leiner disease, has been reported to respond to biotin and essential fatty acids (EFAs). The observation of an increase in both frequency and severity of SD among patients with acquired immunodeficiency syndrome (AIDS) has renewed interest in this otherwise benign disorder. These findings suggest that immune alterations may play some role in SD. *Malassezia* metabolites including free fatty acids released from triglycerides of sebaceous origin are also thought to induce the inflammation seen in SD.[4]

> *Malassezia* is a genus of fungi found to cause seborrhea and skin depigmentation commonly associated with tinea versicolor. It requires fat to grow and thus is common in sebaceous glands.

Because *Malassezia* species are present in most people, one should ask why SD develops in some people and not others. Besides the specific species, sebum production, and particular circumstances just mentioned, reactions initiated by both the keratinocytes and immune system can account for this difference. Some of the response in SD may be related to direct interactions between *Malassezia* organisms and keratinocytes that generate cytokines such as interleukin-8 (IL-8).[5] Activation of innate immunity through Toll-like receptors (TLRs) also seems to play a role. Keratinocytes infected with *Malassezia furfur* up-regulate TLR-2, as shown by RNA analysis.[6]

Another possible explanation of the mechanism of SD may come from the observation that symptomatic *Candida* vulvovaginitis does not develop unless an aggressive response by polymorphonuclear leukocytes occurs.[7] A similar excessive neutrophilic hypersensitivity may play a role in SD because a neutrophilic infiltrate is a characteristic histopathologic finding in SD.

My own interpretation of the pathophysiology is that the trigger involves cytokines and TLRs, as already described, as well as a specific hyperactive cross-reactive immune response to some antigenic component of *Malassezia* that contributes greatly to the inflammation. The cross-reactive stimulation is a hyperactive response to the *Malassezia* organisms resulting from primary stimulation of the lymphocytes by *Candida* and other gut fungal microflora products. Patients with scalp psoriasis and seborrhea have been shown to have elevations of *Candida* organisms in the feces and on the tongue, a finding suggesting higher gut levels.[8] Elevations of *Candida* in the stool and *Candida* phospholipase A, as well as the improvement of seborrhea with oral nystatin (which tends to remain in the gut), further argue for a role for *Candida* cross-stimulation in SD.[9] This phenomenon of primary stimulation and secondary response has been demonstrated in vitro[10] and in the clinical setting.[11]

I believe that the immune response to the organism is biphasic, leading to both a tolerance to some components (epitopes) of yeast and a hyperactive response to others.

Cross-reactivity among *Malassezia, Candida,* and other yeasts relative to immunoglobulins has been well demonstrated.[12,13] Such a biphasic response would explain the mixed results in the literature showing both hyporeactivity and hyperreactivity to *Malassezia* antigens in patients with SD. The first component allows some overgrowth of *Malassezia* and related organisms (i.e., yeasts in gut and on skin). The hyperactive response precipitates a cascade of immune-mediated activity leading to the erythema and desquamation characteristic of the disease. Resident microflora (especially *Candida*) and ingested antigens from related microflora (i.e., yeasts and molds and their byproducts) provide the cross-reactive stimulus leading to both the tolerance and the hyperreactivity. Consideration of this etiologic hypothesis changes the way one treats chronic SD, described later.

The proinflammatory response disposition comes in part from a metabolic shift toward the production of proinflammatory prostanoids, caused by the common dietary oils rich in arachidonic acid. Antiinflammatory precursors, such as the omega-3 EFAs eicosapentaenoic acid (EPA) and docosahexaenoic acid (DHA), are insufficient. A study of psoriasis, a related skin disease, demonstrated a higher ratio of arachidonic acid to omega-3 EFAs in patients receiving fish oils than in a control group. Supplementing with fish oil reduced arachidonic acid and malondialdehyde (another inflammatory molecule that is a marker of oxidative stress) and was associated with clinical improvement.[14] Arachidonic acid is a precursor to the proinflammatory leukotriene B_4 (LTB_4), which has been well documented to play a role in the pathogenesis of the psoriatic lesion.

The mixed nature of those findings may result in part from a lack of control of other critical factors influencing both lipid metabolism (e.g., oxidant status of the patient and relative intake of proinflammatory lipid precursors) and biochemical influences on the delta-5 and delta-6 desaturases, which are key in the metabolic pathway toward proinflammatory or antiinflammatory prostanoids. An additional key factor is that carbohydrate excess leads to excess insulin release. The excess insulin both inhibits the delta-6 desaturase and causes long-term release of proinflammatory cytokines,[15] thus favoring the inflammatory disease process despite the antiinflammatory effects of ingested EFAs. Most published studies do not address this important variable, which is best managed by encouraging a diet low in simple carbohydrates. In my experience, such a diet leads to positive results in a significant proportion of patients with SD as well as in patients with other inflammatory disorders of the skin (see Chapter 86, The Antiinflammatory Diet).

Integrative Therapy

Changing to antiinflammatory oils, controlling yeast on the skin and in the bowel, and calming the nervous system are mainstays in controlling seborrheic dermatitis.

Nutrition

Omega-3 Essential Fatty Acids
Omega-3 unsaturated fatty acids should be substituted for other dietary fats. Saturated, heat-altered, and partially hydrogenated fats should be eliminated from the diet because they lead to production of proinflammatory prostaglandin E_2 (PGE_2) prostanoids. In addition, they block the delta-6 desaturase that catalyzes the formation of antiinflammatory leukotriene precursors. Extra fats contribute to the unfavorable ratio of proinflammatory lipids in the cell membrane and contribute to weight gain because of their caloric content. Other indicators of a need for omega-3 oils are dry skin in winter, dryness around the nailfold area, a lack of dietary intake of such oils, depression, and a high ratio of arachidonic acid to omega-3 EFAs in the plasma or red blood cell membrane. EPA appears to be the primary antiinflammatory component of omega-3 unsaturated fatty acids.

An excellent source of omega-3 unsaturated EFAs is EFA-enriched fish oil capsules or liquid. Krill oil, cod liver oil and other cold-water fish oils are also good sources. Eating four to five portions weekly of oily cold-water fish is also recommended. Flaxseed oil, which contains alpha-linolenic acid, is also a potential source, but it must undergo chain elongation involving an extra step requiring the delta-6 desaturase, and some people cannot use this oil effectively. Canola oil and walnut oil are lesser sources of omega-3 unsaturated EFAs.

Oils can be either taken as supplements or worked into the diet as foods. For example, flaxseed oil can be used in making smoothies or salad dressing. These oils should not be heated because the unsaturated bonds that make them useful are unstable on heating. Because of their unsaturated nature, they should be accompanied by vitamin E in the diet. Similarly, other factors contributing to high oxidative stress in the individual patient should be corrected, or counterbalanced with additional antioxidants, to maximize the effectiveness of these oils. Omega-3 fish oil can induce glucose intolerance in diabetic patients. To counter this effect and to reduce the proinflammatory mediators from carbohydrate-stimulated insulin elevation, a proper balance of carbohydrate intake with protein intake and exercise should be achieved.

■ Dosage
The dosage is based on the severity of presentation, a history of inadequate dietary intake of omega-3 EFAs, and a low red blood cell membrane ratio of EPA to arachidonate. Whereas daily intake of five capsules (approximately 1 teaspoon) of flaxseed oil or EPA-DHA fish oils may be helpful, some patients may need as much as 15 mL (3 teaspoons) daily for a short time, mixed into a shake to make it palatable. Vitamin E, 400 to 800 units/day, should be taken to protect these unsaturated oils from oxidation. At least 1000 mg of EPA should be in the product used.

■ Precautions
Fish oils have been known to prolong bleeding time through the anticoagulant effect of PGE_3 for which they are precursors. Use of large doses in pregnant women has also been associated with elevated birth weight of their infants.

Yeast Elimination
For patients who require additional measures to control their seborrhea, a yeast and mold elimination diet should be instituted. The basis of this diet is the elimination of bread, cheese, wine and beer, excessive carbohydrates (especially sugar and simple starches), and other foods containing or produced by yeast or fungus. This diet has been touted as

highly effective in the popular literature, and the success of different variations is probably related both to yeast reduction and to relief of different food allergies in patients with yeast sensitivities. Probiotics such as *Lactobacillus acidophilus* and *Bifidobacterium bifidus* should be taken before or during meals to help repopulate the normal flora of the gut. Patients who cannot give up bread should be counseled to eat true sourdough bread, the leavening agent for which is derived from limited cultures of different yeasts captured from the air.

Supplements

Vitamins

Oils, which can be used as either foods or supplements, have already been discussed. Vitamin E, at 400 units/day, should be added as an antioxidant to protect the oils. Adequate levels of magnesium, zinc, vitamin C, and vitamin B6 should be maintained by supplementation if intake of any of these nutrients is insufficient in the diet, to enhance the function of the delta-6 desaturase. Vitamin B6 cream, 50 mg/g, compounded in a water-based cream by a compounding pharmacy, has been used for treatment of SD of the scalp.[16,17]

Biotin is especially useful in infantile SD,[18] and it may have a role in the treatment of adult seborrhea as well. Besides contributing to the generation of antiinflammatory prostanoids through activation of the delta-6 desaturase (as do other vitamins mentioned here), biotin is reputed to retard the formation of the mycelial form of *Candida*. Other B vitamins shown to be helpful in seborrhea are vitamin B6, folate,[19] and vitamin B12.[20]

■ Dosage

One or two tablets/day of a high-potency multivitamin with mineral (even for those with a three- to six-tablet/day recommendation on the bottle label) can be used for B-vitamin supplementation in most patients. If clinical improvement is not seen, extra biotin up to 7.5 mg/day, and vitamin B6 or pyridoxal 5-phosphate 20 to 50 mg/day can be added; zinc picolinate 25 to 50 mg/day and vitamin C 500 mg one to three times daily are also useful.

Probiotics

To address the yeast overgrowth, adding probiotic bacteria such as *Lactobacillus acidophilus* and *Bifidobacterium,* or the yeast *Saccharomyces boulardii* to the diet is nearly as important as proper diet in restoring normal gut flora and reducing the yeast population. Caprylic acid can be added to inhibit attachment of the yeast to the intestinal wall.

■ Dosage

GI Flora (Allergy Research Group, Alameda, Calif) is an economical, effective source of multiple probiotic strains; the dose is one or two capsules with meals. Ultra Flora DF and Ultra Flora IB, one capsule per day (Metagenics, San Clemente, Calif), are other useful sources. Doses for caprylic acid are begun at one capsule three times daily before meals and are gradually increased to two capsules/meal.

If the patient has known overgrowth of yeast in the gastrointestinal tract, consider Caprystatin (Ecological Formulas, Concord, Calif; telephone 800-888-4585), which contains caprylic acid, a short-chain fatty acid that inhibits *Candida*

growth and prevents attachment of yeast to the intestinal wall. Start with one capsule three times per day before meals, and increase the dose as necessary. Some patients, especially those who have associated fatigue or hypersensitivities, may have a die-off reaction and have some symptoms worsen before they improve. Follow these patients closely to be sure that they are not reacting to something in the treatment regimen. Resume the program at a slower rate if symptoms occur.

■ Precautions

A source of fiber is important to add, to ensure that bowel movements are occurring at least one or more times per day during yeast reduction therapy, so that allergenic moieties are not absorbed from the dying organisms. Fiber also promotes healthy mucosa along the gastrointestinal tract in which bacteria live.

Probiotics should not be given to a patient with a compromised immune system because of the slight risk of infection.

Many companies that produce probiotics claim to offer the absolute best species, combinations, or strains of bacteria. Clinicians are advised to start with an affordable *Lactobacillus acidophilus* or *Bifidobacterium bifidus* preparation and then add others to their personal pharmacopoeia as evaluation of a specific product is found to be convincing and its effects are confirmed to be beneficial. Different patients do better with different probiotic bacteria. *Bifidobacterium bifidus* is thought to be more beneficial initially.

Botanicals

For topical treatment, any application that reduces yeast on the skin may be helpful. Various essential oils may be useful for their incorporation in scalp sebaceous lipids and antimicrobial action against *Malassezia*. Tea tree oil, honey, and cinnamic acid have been shown to reduce *Malassezia* and SD.[21] Tea tree oil and cinnamic acid, as well as other essential oils, however, can cause contact dermatitis, especially in inflamed skin, and honey is messy to use on the scalp. *Monarda fistulosa*, a distinctive-smelling herb from the mint family, has also been reported to yield an essential oil that is effective against seborrhea.[22]

Many different antifungal herbs and combination products with probiotics are available on the market today, and a comprehensive evaluation of these products is beyond the scope of this chapter. A few are mentioned here, but most that are effective in significantly reducing the yeast population in the gut will work. The use of fiber products such as psyllium and of other vegetable fiber is essential to maintain rapid passage of treated organisms through the bowel.

Grapefruit seed extract and *Artemisia annua* can also be added to reduce the yeast population. Some newer herbal preparations constituted for this purpose are available. Pau d'arco tea is another product with reported antiyeast activity. Application of aloe has been shown to be useful in seborrhea.[23]

Dosages

Tea tree oil may be used in adults on an occasional basis, applied sparingly to the areas of intense scaling after wetting the scalp. Because it is a potent allergen, I do not recommend it for regular, ongoing use. Aloe vera *(Aloe barbadensis)* gel may be applied directly from the cut leaf of the plant. Avocado may contain oils and sugars[24] that are helpful in controlling SD.

Mind-Body Therapy

SD is more prevalent in patients with depression.[25] Perhaps the improvement seen in the summer is the result either of reduced depression or of the effects of increased sunlight on melatonin release.[26] Addressing depression or seasonal affective disorder with light therapy, visits to a sunnier climate, psychotherapy, Bach Flower Remedies, supplements, or medications may be considered in a patient with SD in whom the disease severity varies with his or her affective state.

Pharmaceuticals

Shampoos

The two mainstays of topical treatment of SD are tar shampoos and antiyeast shampoos. Antiyeast shampoos consist, in order of potency, of zinc pyrithione, selenium sulfide 1% (over-the-counter shampoos), selenium sulfide 2.5% (prescription), and ketoconazole shampoos (available over the counter in some countries). Tar shampoos have antiinflammatory and antiyeast activity.

Dosage

A more recent treatment for fungal infections is ciclopirox 1% shampoo (Loprox), which is also approved for use in SD. Side effects include pruritus (itching), burning, erythema (redness), seborrhea, and rash. This product comes in a gel and a shampoo. Use the shampoo twice a week for 4 weeks or apply the gel twice daily for 4 weeks.

Tar shampoo (Tegrin, T/Gel) is used three times per week initially and then once per week.

Keratolytic Treatments

Oils are applied to the scalp to loosen scale. Olive oil is particularly useful in this regard, especially in infants with thin hair. Wetting the scalp and applying a warm oil turban for an hour, with 6% salicylic acid mixed into the olive oil, may remove more adherent scale. Patients must remove the oil with dishwashing liquid detergent before they apply a therapeutic shampoo.

Other salicylic acid preparations may also be used for the same purpose when thick, adherent scale is difficult to remove. Urea preparations may be used for the same purpose. These preparations also need time to act and generally require shampoo for removal. After thick scale is removed, a therapeutic agent can be applied to penetrate the scalp more deeply. Keratolytics such as salicylic acid have antifungal properties as well.

Dosage

Consider the following treatment to help reduce scaling. Olive oil is compounded with 6% salicylic acid. The oil is applied under a towel turban for 1 hour, and then scales are removed with a soft brush.

Topical Corticosteroids

Topical corticosteroids are another mainstay of conventional treatment of SD. Even 1% hydrocortisone cream brings temporary improvement in SD of the face and nasolabial folds in a previously untreated patient. Liquids, gels, and even a foam vehicle are available, with a more potent fluorinated corticosteroid used to avoid the hair and reach the scalp.

Dosage

Patients should apply 1% to 2.5% hydrocortisone cream sparingly once or twice daily for 1 to 2 weeks.

Precautions

Frequent or repeated application of corticosteroids results in tachyphylaxis (a progressively diminished response), requiring more potent steroids to obtain the same response. In addition, some patients behave as though they are addicted to the topical steroids. The problem becomes worse, and the corticosteroid is needed more and more often in higher strengths to control the redness and scaling. Repeated use on the face, especially of stronger corticosteroids, and even the use of hydrocortisone on the thin tissues of the eyelids, can result in atrophy of the skin with permanent show-through of the underlying capillaries or the development of problematic steroid acne.

Other Creams

Ketoconazole (Nizoral) cream applied sparingly twice daily is extremely helpful for management of SD of the face and hairline. It inhibits the *Malassezia*, gives dramatic clinical improvement, and does not cause the atrophy resulting from prolonged corticosteroid use. Other antifungal creams, including ciclopirox (Loprox) and nystatin cream, are also useful.

Dosage

Ketoconazole cream 2% is applied twice daily to affected areas, sparingly.

Lithium Succinate

Lithium succinate 8% ointment has been reported to be helpful in SD. An antiyeast effect has been confirmed in vitro,[27] as well as in patients.[28] The ointment is applied twice daily. The relationship between lithium as a drug for depression, which has been implicated as a cause of seborrhea, and direct application of lithium as a treatment for seborrhea is interesting to contemplate. A common mediator pathway for both disorders may exist.

Oral Antifungals

Oral antifungals should be used only when the seborrhea is serious enough to warrant the risk of taking the drug or when the underlying condition of overgrowth has not responded to diet and herbal treatment alone.

Nystatin

Oral nystatin is useful to reduce the *Candida* population in the gut. It has the benefit of being poorly absorbed and therefore remaining in the gut. It works by causing defective yeast cell wall formation, resulting in release of intracellular contents, which has in turn been blamed for the aggravation of symptoms constituting a Herxheimer-type reaction (flulike feeling from die-off effect of yeast) in some patients after a large dose.

■ Ketoconazole and Fluconazole

Ketoconazole (Nizoral) is well absorbed, exerts an antiyeast effect in the gut and skin, and is excreted in high concentrations in the sweat. Other oral antifungal agents, such as fluconazole (Diflucan), have also been used for severe cases of seborrhea. An antiyeast regimen should be instituted gradually, starting with diet, *Lactobacillus acidophilus,* and supplements and botanicals before oral pharmaceuticals are used. The first reason is to avoid rapid kill-off of a large number of organisms, which may result in a die-off effect, or Herxheimer-type reaction. The second reason is to reduce the intestinal yeast population less drastically. If the gut ecology is altered to favor a more gradual reduction in yeast population, a rebound growth of yeast resistant to the most powerful agents available will be less likely to occur. Although these agents may be effective in the short term, I question whether it is responsible practice to use these agents without initially or simultaneously altering the ecologic conditions that favor yeast overgrowth.

■ Dosage

The dose of nystatin is increased slowly from 500,000 units once daily to 2 million units three times daily; this dose is then maintained until the patient's condition is improved and stable and appropriate dietary changes have been effected. Dosing should begin with one capsule (500,000 units) per day of the powder, with addition of an extra capsule every 2 or 3 days until a total dose of four capsules three times daily (6 million units/day total) is achieved. Doses for the pure powder should begin with ⅛ teaspoon/day increased to 1 teaspoon/day (6 million units/day total) in the same gradual manner. This dose should be continued for 1 to 3 months or tapered for 1 to 2 weeks after symptoms clear.

For fluconazole (Diflucan), the dose is 100 to 200 mg/day for 10 to 14 days. (Many drug interactions and cautions are cited in the package insert.) Seborrhea is not a listed indication and should only be used in cases with severe underlying yeast issues.

The dose of ketoconazole (Nizoral) is 100 to 200 mg/day. Ketoconazole should be used only if other indications exist and liver enzyme values are monitored. In general, this drug should be avoided, or the liver can be protected with silymarin (milk thistle). Seborrhea is not a listed indication and should only be used in cases with severe underlying yeast issues.

■ Precautions

Adverse effects include elevation in liver enzymes, hepatic failure (uncommon with oral ketoconazole and less likely with fluconazole), a Herxheimer-type die-off phenomenon (especially with nystatin), and overgrowth of resistant organisms.

Before an oral antifungal is considered, intestinal yeast growth should be reduced with dietary measures. This will help prevent the growth of resistant strains of yeast and lead to improved response from the oral antifungal.

Therapies to Consider

Homeopathy

A homeopathic dilution of tobacco was reported to clear SD in a patient with tobacco sensitivity. I mention this not to recommend this specific remedy but rather to emphasize the potential benefits of choosing an appropriate homeopathic or other remedy that addresses prominent underlying imbalances in the patient. Other homeopathics, including Natrum Muriaticum, Arsenicum Album, and Bryonia, may be considered, but homeopathics should be prescribed according to other characteristics of the patient besides local presentation.

Food Allergy

As in patients with atopic dermatitis, addressing food allergy by removing the offending foods from the diet may benefit some patients with recalcitrant SD (see Chapter 84, Food Intolerance and Elimination Diet).

Energy-Based Treatments

When addressing a variety of apparent causal factors is not sufficient, the clinician must address ways in which the seborrhea may be an expression of some deeper autonomic or psychological pattern. Psychotherapy may be useful if it is powerful and targeted. Classical homeopathy addressing mental and emotional symptoms may touch this level. Newer forms of treatment that use acupressure meridian activation or tapping to release patterns of sensitivity in the autonomic nervous system, including Lang desensitization and Neuromuscular Therapy (NMT), may be considered by the practitioner skilled in these techniques.

PREVENTION PRESCRIPTION

- Use a Mediterranean-type diet based on olive oil and fresh vegetables.
- Supplement with omega-3 essential fatty acids from fish oil, northern fish, and flaxseed.
- Reduce the intake of bread, cheese, wine, beer, and yeast.
- Reduce the intake of sugar, refined carbohydrates, and heated oils.
- Shampoo the scalp at least twice a week, with an antidandruff shampoo when necessary.

THERAPEUTIC REVIEW

The following is an outline of therapeutic options for the treatment of seborrheic dermatitis. Determining which factors lead to the disease presentation in a given patient may improve the chances of success of a given therapy. For more severe or resistant cases, a progressive, sequential approach with multiple therapeutic avenues is recommended, with either intensification of treatments or addition of systemic pharmacologic agents, as indicated by the clinical response.

■ Antidandruff Shampoos

- Zinc pyrithione, selenium sulfide (Selsun), tar, or ketoconazole (Nizoral) shampoo is used for 5 minutes two or three times/week.
- If the patient has used one type with no clinical improvement, another can be tried.

■ Antiyeast Creams

- Ketoconazole cream 2% (Nizoral) or another pharmacologic or herbal substitute works well on the face and nonscalp areas.

■ Supplements

- Eicosapentaenoic acid and docosahexaenoic acid (fish oils) can be added at 1 to 2 g/day and titrated to clinical improvement.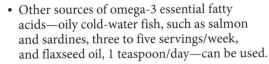
- Other sources of omega-3 essential fatty acids—oily cold-water fish, such as salmon and sardines, three to five servings/week, and flaxseed oil, 1 teaspoon/day—can be used.
- Vitamin E 400 units/day should be given with these oils to prevent oxidation.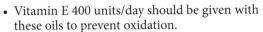
- Vitamin B complex, vitamin B_6 500 mg, and biotin up to 8 mg/day may be beneficial in patients with resistant cases.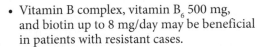
- Caprylic acid is taken at 100 to 200 mg two to three times/day.

■ Nutrition

- A diet low in yeast and simple carbohydrates, especially one that eliminates bread, cheese, wine, beer, fermented foods, and starches, is helpful in patients with persistent cases.

- Some improvement may result from removal of other food allergens.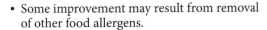
- Adding probiotic bacteria such as *Lactobacillus acidophilus,* one capsule/meal, or live-culture yogurt may also help.

■ Botanicals

- The antiyeast botanicals grapefruit seed extract and *Artemisia annua* may be used at two to six capsules/day.
- Undecenoic acid, derived from the castor bean, is another antiyeast product (Formula SF 722 [Thorne Research, Sandpoint, Idaho]), used at two to six capsules/day.

■ Pharmaceuticals

- Nystatin is used in slowly increasing doses from 0.5 to 6 million units/day.
- Fluconazole (Diflucan) is taken at 100 to 200 mg/day for 2 weeks, for resistant cases. This agent is best used after dietary, herbal, and supplement methods have been employed to reduce the yeast flora and to attenuate the ecologic factors favoring yeast growth.
- Triamcinolone solution or betamethasone valerate foam (Luxiq) once or twice daily can be used to relieve pruritus and inflammation.

KEY WEB RESOURCES

Holistic Dermatology: www.holisticdermatology.com	Information on alternative treatments for numerous skin conditions, including seborrheic dermatitis
Medscape: http://emedicine.medscape.com/article/1108312-treatment	Conventional medications for seborrhea
American Academy of Dermatology EczemaNet: http://www.aad.org/public/publications/pamphlets/common_seb_dermatitis.html	Photographs and a description of conventional treatments for seborrheic dermatitis
Wikipedia: http://en.wikipedia.org/wiki/Seborrhoeic_dermatitis	Overview of seborrheic dermatitis, including treatment

References

References are available online at expertconsult.com.

Acne Vulgaris and Acne Rosacea

Sean H. Zager, MD

Pathophysiology and Clinical Presentation

Acne vulgaris, known by most as acne, represents the most common disease of the skin as it affects approximately 45 million individuals in the United States and as many as 80% to 90% of adolescents.[1,2] Worldwide spending on prescription and over-the-counter acne treatments is estimated to be tens of billions of dollars each year, making it one of the fasting growing markets in the dermatologic industry to date.[3] Although the majority of cases are seen through the teenage years and in young adulthood, acne may be manifested at any time during the life span. Whereas it is not typically associated with significant physical comorbidity, acne may have severe social and psychological sequelae, necessitating a multidimensional approach to care.[4]

Acne rosacea, commonly referred to as rosacea, is a skin disorder that primarily affects individuals older than 30 years.[5] It is a condition that affects approximately 10% of fair-skinned people and tends to run in families. It has a higher prevalence in women and among individuals of northern European descent.[6,7] Although rosacea may sometimes appear similar to acne vulgaris and have comparable psychoemotional consequences, the two conditions represent distinct pathophysiologic processes.

Acne Vulgaris

Acne vulgaris is a disease of the pilosebaceous unit of the skin, where the hair follicle meets the sebaceous gland in the dermis. The sebaceous gland functions to facilitate desquamation and lubrication of the skin. In the development of acne vulgaris, a cascade of five main factors contributes to a dysregulation of the pilosebaceous unit:

1. Increased levels of androgens are produced not only by the adrenal glands and gonads but also by the sebaceous glands in the skin. Elevated androgenicity is a physiologic consequence of puberty and a pathophysiologic consequence of conditions such as polycystic ovary syndrome, congenital adrenal hyperplasia, Cushing syndrome, and androgen-secreting tumors.[8]
2. Proliferation and impaired desquamation of keratinocytes lining the orifice of the follicle pore follow and lead to the development of a hyperkeratotic plug. This occurs within the follicular canal and causes the formation of a microcomedo.
3. Increased sebum is produced within the sebaceous gland, also because of increased androgen production. This results in the evolution of a closed comedo (a whitehead) and, if the orifice of the pore dilates, an open comedo (a blackhead).
4. The gram-positive anaerobic bacterium *Propionibacterium acnes* propagates in its sebum-rich growth medium. Although *P. acnes* is typically a normal component of skin flora, it thrives in an anaerobic environment abundant with lipids as a nutrient source.
5. A local inflammatory process develops as neutrophils and other host immune cells accumulate. Papules form, and with the rupture of the pilosebaceous follicle into the surrounding dermis, more severe pustular, nodular, and cystic acne lesions may appear (Fig. 73-1).

There is a wide spectrum of susceptibility to the proliferation of *P. acnes* and the factors that facilitate it. Inheritance studies, such as those comparing dizygotic and monozygotic twins,[9,10] demonstrate a significant role of genetics in the pathogenesis of acne. Suggested mechanisms include an increased tendency of 5-alpha-reductase to convert testosterone to the tissue-active metabolite dihydrotestosterone and a possible hypersensitivity of androgen receptors within sebaceous glands.[11,12] Whether through genetic predispositions (e.g., polycystic ovary syndrome, Cushing syndrome) or environmental exposure, increased levels of hormones

FIGURE 73-1
The pathogenesis of acne vulgaris. (From Habif TP. Acne, rosacea, and related disorders. In: Habif TP, ed. *Clinical Dermatology.* 5th ed. Philadelphia: Saunders; 2009.)

PATHOGENESIS OF ACNE

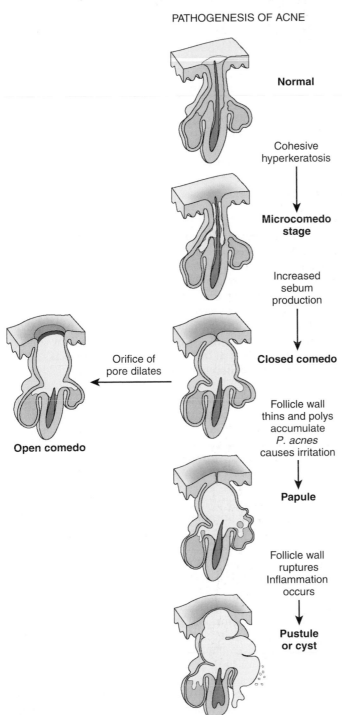

Normal

Cohesive hyperkeratosis

Microcomedo stage

Increased sebum production

Closed comedo

Orifice of pore dilates

Follicle wall thins and polys accumulate *P. acnes* causes irritation

Open comedo

Papule

Follicle wall ruptures Inflammation occurs

Pustule or cyst

such as insulin and cortisol are also shown to promote acne development.[8]

Acne Rosacea

Like advanced cases of acne vulgaris, acne rosacea should be viewed as a chronic condition with cycles of exacerbation and remission. The pathophysiologic mechanism of rosacea is not yet well elucidated, and the therapeutic aims should emphasize control rather than cure. With regard to etiology, the following theories have been proposed:

1. Dysbiosis or invasion of foreign organisms triggering immune hyperreactivity
   a. *Demodex folliculorum* is a skin mite that feeds on sebum. It has been found in higher density in the facial skin of those affected by rosacea compared with unaffected subjects.[13] Further, it has been postulated that this mite may have symbiotic relationships with bacteria that spur inflammation and are susceptible to antibiotics used in the management of rosacea.[14]
   b. Data are conflicting about the relationship between the bacterium *Helicobacter pylori* and the pathogenesis of rosacea. With treatment of *H. pylori* infection, there is evidence of concomitant improvement of rosacea symptoms; as well, studies show no notable change.[15,16]
   c. Small bowel bacterial overgrowth has also been put forth as a trigger of rosacea. One study found that bacterial overgrowth in the small intestine was more common in those with rosacea and that eradication of the overgrowth decreased rosacea symptoms.[17]
2. Structural or functional dysregulation
   a. Reduced levels of hydrochloric acid in gastric secretions have been linked to rosacea.[18] Hypochlorhydria, secondary to genetic defect or environmental cues such as proton pump inhibitors, is evidenced to cause small bowel overgrowth.[19] Rosacea may represent one consequence of this aberrant condition.
   b. Vascular instability including accelerated angiogenesis and capillary dysfunction, mast cell prevalence, and connective tissue hypertrophy may also contribute to the inflammatory process of rosacea.[20,21]

The four major subtypes of acne rosacea and the common clinical features of each are as follows:

1. Erythematotelangiectatic rosacea (vascular rosacea): flushing, telangiectasias, and persistent erythema of the central face
2. Papulopustular rosacea: inflammatory papules and pustules; erythema of the central face
3. Ocular rosacea: burning, itching, and dryness of the eyes; conjunctival injection, blepharitis, periorbital edema, and photosensitivity
4. Phymatous rosacea: connective tissue hypertrophy or nodularity most notable at the distal nose (known as rhinophyma) but also seen on the chin, forehead, cheeks, and ears (Fig. 73-2)

These subtypes often overlap. Typical environmental triggers for rosacea include extremes of temperature, stress, and particular foods and beverages; some of these are touched on in later sections of the chapter.[22]

Integrative Therapy

Hygiene

In approaching the patient with acne vulgaris or rosacea, it is reasonable to begin with a focus on simple behavioral considerations for prevention—whether it is primary, secondary, or tertiary. It is essential to engage in a dialogue about proper skin care. Ensure that patients are rinsing twice daily with lukewarm water and a non–soap-based cleanser. To avoid

FIGURE 73-2
Rhinophyma in phymatous rosacea. (From Habif TP. Acne, rosacea, and related disorders. In: Habif TP, ed. *Clinical Dermatology.* 5th ed. Philadelphia: Saunders; 2009.)

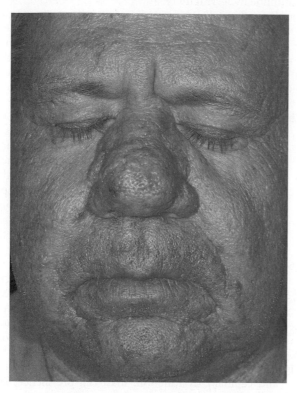

microabrasion of the skin, instruct patients to rinse with their hands instead of washcloths or other rough materials and to do so gently without scrubbing. Water-based, noncomedogenic lotions, cosmetics, and hair products are preferable to those that are oil based, and picking at acne lesions should be discouraged. The mechanical trauma of picking at lesions may lead to follicular wall rupture, releasing inflammatory cells into the surrounding dermis and increasing the likelihood of scarring.

Finally, particularly in patients with rosacea, environmental conditions must be considered. Sun and wind exposure and extremes of temperature have been noted to aggravate rosacea symptoms.[23] In one study, bacteria were isolated from the facial skin of affected subjects. At higher temperatures, these bacteria were noted to secrete greater amounts of a specific lipase that may be implicated in the inflammatory process of rosacea.[24]

Stress Management

Psychoemotional stress is an important contributor to and effect of acne vulgaris and rosacea. In a survey of 1066 rosacea patients, 79% identified emotional stress as an exacerbating factor and 64% ranked it within their top three triggers.[24] In a study of high-school students, a significant difference was noted in severity of acne vulgaris during periods of high stress (midterm exams) and low stress (summer break).[25]

It has also been shown that many patients with acne vulgaris or rosacea experience considerable levels of ensuing stress in association with depression, anxiety, anger, and low self-esteem.[4,26,27] Treatment strategies must therefore include attention to patients' social, psychological, and emotional well-being in addition to physical manifestations.

In response to these clinical needs, the field of psychodermatology has emerged. One mind-body technique, biofeedback-assisted guided relaxation imagery, was evidenced to improve acne vulgaris.[28] Cognitive-behavioral and biofeedback therapies have also been used to help patients decrease their frequency of picking at acne lesions.[29] Given the close reciprocal relationship between psychoemotional stress and both acne vulgaris and rosacea, other relaxation practices, such as breathing exercises, meditation, and massage therapy, may be recommended as part of a treatment plan (see Chapter 89, Breathing Exercises; Chapter 93, Relaxation Techniques; and Chapter 98, Recommending Meditation).

Diet

Nutritional factors play an important role in the pathogenesis of acne. A diet with a low glycemic load, favoring protein over carbohydrates and fats, has been shown to significantly decrease (inflammatory and noninflammatory) lesion counts in acne vulgaris.[30] A low glycemic–load diet has also been associated with a reduction in calorie intake, body mass index, and insulin resistance. Improved insulin sensitivity leads to a decrease in androgen production and a concordant improvement in the symptoms of acne vulgaris[30-34] (see Chapter 85, The Glycemic Index/Load).

Large population studies have furthermore demonstrated a worsening of acne symptoms with greater consumption of dairy products.[35,36] This may be a consequence of an increased carbohydrate-to-protein ratio, exposure to exogenous androgenic hormones, or triggering of proinflammatory processes by dairy allergy or lactose intolerance. Hence, in addition to adhering to a diet favoring protein over carbohydrates and fats, patients with acne should limit consumption of animal products treated with exogenous androgenic hormones. Instead, they should seek U.S. Department of Agriculture (USDA)–certified organic meats and dairy products. It may also prove beneficial to review the details of an antiinflammatory diet (see Chapter 86, The Antiinflammatory Diet) and to consider a trial of an elimination diet (see Chapter 84, Food Intolerance and Elimination Diet) that excludes dairy products.

A diet rich in omega-3 fatty acids—found in high quantities in salmon, mackerel, sardines, and flaxseed oil—has been linked to improvement in acne symptoms. Probably through the reduction of both proinflammatory compounds (such as leukotrienes and prostaglandins) and androgen production, omega-3 fatty acids discourage the opportunity for and sequelae of *P. acnes* proliferation.[37-40] Indeed, epidemiologic investigation reveals that communities consuming higher levels of omega-3 fatty acids have less prevalence of acne.[38,41] Although it is best to consume them in food in which they naturally occur, omega-3 fatty acids may be supplemented in the diet. Typical daily doses are 1 tablespoon of flaxseed oil per 100 pounds of body weight or 1 to 2 g of fish oil in capsule form. One small study did show marked improvement in acne symptoms and mental outlook after 2 months of omega-3 fatty acid supplementation.[42]

In addition, decreased serum levels of vitamin A have been associated with worsening acne severity.[43] Hence, patients with acne may be counseled to eat more vegetables rich in vitamin A, such as carrots, sweet potatoes, spinach, kale, and winter squash.

With regard to acne rosacea, affected patients should be screened for potential food allergies or intolerances that may contribute to exacerbations. Dietary triggers typically include alcohol, spicy foods, hot beverages, marinated meats, dairy products, and certain fruits and vegetables.[22] A careful elimination diet should be performed as part of tailoring a treatment plan specific to the needs of each individual patient.

Supplements

Brewer's Yeast (Saccharomyces cerevisiae)

Brewer's yeast is a medicinal yeast often used in brewing and baking. It is commonly used as a remedy for acne vulgaris in Western Europe. Brewer's yeast is known to contain chromium and is thereby thought to decrease insulin resistance.[44,45] One strain of brewer's yeast, known as Hansen CBS 5926, has been recognized as an inhibitor of bacterial growth.[46] In one study of 139 subjects with acne, more than 80% saw significant improvement in symptoms with brewer's yeast supplementation.[47]

▇ Dosage

The recommended intake of dried brewer's yeast is 2 g three times daily. The recommended dose of isolated Hansen CBS 5926 strain of brewer's yeast, freeze-dried, is 750 mg daily.[46]

▇ Precautions

Brewer's yeast may cause migraine headaches or flatulence in sensitive individuals. It can lead to hypertension if it is used in conjunction with monoamine oxidase inhibitors and will have decreased efficacy if it is used with antifungal medications.[44,47]

Zinc

Zinc is a metallic chemical element that serves as an essential cofactor in many biochemical reactions involved in the maintenance of skin health and general immune function, local hormone activation, and production of retinol-binding protein. Zinc has been noted to be bacteriostatic against *P. acnes* and to inhibit the production of inflammatory cytokines. Although sample sizes have been small, most studies show that zinc supplementation does have a therapeutic effect on acne symptoms.[3,18,48–52]

▇ Dosage

The recommended dose of zinc gluconate is 30 mg/day.

▇ Precautions

Oral zinc supplementation can result in gastrointestinal symptoms including nausea, vomiting, and diarrhea.[53] These adverse effects may be mitigated by taking zinc just after meals. Prolonged zinc supplementation can also lead to copper deficiency with resultant sideroblastic anemia and neutropenia.[54] Thus, as a rule of thumb, clinicians should supplement 2 mg of copper for every 30 mg of zinc.

Vitamin A

Vitamin A is a retinol and fat-soluble vitamin that has been studied in the treatment of acne, given its capacity for immune modulation and reduction of follicular hyperkeratinization. In one study of patients supplemented with 100,000 units of vitamin A daily, there was no significant improvement in acne severity, and a number of subjects complained of symptoms compatible with hypervitaminosis A.[55] In another trial using higher doses of vitamin A (between 300,000 and 500,000 units daily), therapeutic effects were noted. In this study, however, the majority of patients experienced cheilitis and xerosis; a number suffered from headache (causing two patients to quit the study), fatigue, and nausea—all symptoms associated with hypervitaminosis A.[56]

▇ Dosage

Tolerable upper intake level (the maximum dose that is unlikely to carry a risk of adverse side effects) is 10,000 units daily and less for children.[57] As mentioned earlier, significantly higher doses have been used in the treatment of acne vulgaris.

Precautions

Given its questionable therapeutic effect and demonstrated potential for toxicity, oral supplementation with vitamin A is *not recommended*. High doses appear to be required for symptomatic control, and hypervitaminosis A has short- and long-term health risks. These risks include headaches, myalgias, fatigue, nausea and vomiting, dry skin and mucous membranes, hair loss, hepatitis, reduced bone mineral density, and teratogenicity.

Botanicals

Tea Tree Oil (Melaleuca alternifolia)

An essential oil from the leaves of the native Australian tea tree, tea tree oil is commonly used as a topical antimicrobial. In two blinded, randomized controlled trials, application of 5% tea tree oil was shown to significantly improve acne severity compared with placebo and was comparable to 5% benzoyl peroxide. Although tea tree oil had a slower onset of action than that of benzoyl peroxide, it was better tolerated with less skin irritation.[58,59]

▇ Dosage

Tea tree oil, 5% to 15% solution or gel, is applied topically once daily.

▇ Precautions

Topical tea tree oil is generally well tolerated, but it has been noted to cause local skin irritation and allergic contact dermatitis in some patients.[60]

Pharmaceuticals: Topical Preparations

Azelaic Acid

A naturally occurring dicarboxylic acid produced by the yeast *Malassezia furfur*, azelaic acid is found in wheat, rye, and barley. It is antibacterial as well as anticomedonal through its capacity for keratolysis.[61] In two blinded, randomized controlled trials, the therapeutic effect of azelaic acid on acne severity was demonstrated to be significant and on par with that of topical benzoyl peroxide and clindamycin .[62] In addition, azelaic acid is helpful in treating the hyperpigmentation that results from acne-associated inflammation.[61,63] For patients with acne rosacea, azelaic acid has been shown to be comparable to topical metronidazole in the reduction of inflammatory lesions and erythema.[64]

■ Dosage
Azelaic acid, 20% cream or 15% gel, is applied topically twice daily.[61–64]

■ Precautions
Azelaic acid may cause local skin irritation and changes in pigmentation. Of note, it has been shown that whereas azelaic acid decreases the postinflammatory hyperpigmentation seen with acne, it does not alter skin tanning or hyperpigmentation that occurs with exposure to ultraviolet light.[61,65]

Salicylic Acid
Salicylic acid occurs naturally as a phenolic phytohormone; its name comes from the Latin word *salix,* which means willow tree. It is chemically similar to the active component of aspirin and has a comedolytic effect by disrupting the pilosebaceous unit and causing desquamation. Salicylic acid is found in many over-the-counter products, including lotions, creams, and pads. It is generally considered to be less potent but better tolerated than topical retinoids in the treatment of acne vulgaris. As a 2% preparation, salicylic acid has been demonstrated to be more effective than 10% benzoyl peroxide for acne control, although this may be due to better patient compliance given the superior side effect profile of salicylic acid.[3,66–68]

■ Dosage
Salicylic acid, applied topically one or two times daily, is commonly used as an over-the-counter preparation in concentrations up to 2%. It may also be obtained by prescription in concentrations between 2% and 10%.

■ Precautions
The most frequent adverse effect of salicylic acid is local skin irritation and peeling, which are likely when concentrations of 2% or higher are used. Risk of hyperpigmentation is less common, and salicylate toxicity is rare, noted with application over large body surface areas for prolonged periods.[3,69]

Retinoids
In the conventional care of acne vulgaris, topical retinoids are included in the initial management of most patients. As vitamin A derivatives, they are useful for treatment of both comedonal and inflammatory acne lesions because they oppose hyperkeratinization and obstruction of the follicular pore as well as the release of proinflammatory compounds.[70,71] In addition, they are helpful in reducing acne-associated postinflammatory hyperpigmentation.[72] Of the topical retinoids currently available, no significant difference in efficacy has been established, and each should lead to visible improvement of acne vulgaris after 8 to 12 weeks of treatment. In the approach to patients with acne rosacea, studies highlight notable risks and benefits of topical retinoid application.[73–75]

■ Dosage
Tretinoin, 0.01% to 0.1%, is applied once nightly or every other night if it is not well tolerated. Adapalene, 0.1%, is applied once nightly or every other night if it is not well tolerated. Tazarotene, 0.05% to 0.1%, is applied once nightly or every other night if it is not well tolerated.

■ Precautions
Topical retinoids may lead to local irritation and drying of the skin. They may also increase sun sensitivity and should therefore be applied at night. Whereas no topical retinoids are recommended in pregnancy, tazarotene must be avoided as it is classified as pregnancy category X. Finally, topical retinoids should *not* be used to treat acne rosacea given their potentially harmful effects, including the promotion of epithelial thickening, neovascularization, and telangiectasia formation.[74,75]

Antibiotics
The use of topical antibiotics is generally indicated for the treatment of mild to moderate inflammatory (papular or pustular) lesions of acne vulgaris and rosacea. Particularly in those cases recalcitrant to other measures of care, topical antibiotics are prescribed in combination with topical retinoids and in combination with one another.

> The topical antimicrobial benzoyl peroxide is unique in that it serves to reduce rather than to increase the antibiotic resistance of *P. acnes.* When it is prescribed in combination with other topical antimicrobials, such as erythromycin and clindamycin, benzoyl peroxide is noted to elevate treatment efficacy significantly and to decrease antibiotic resistance. In turn, given the rising antibiotic resistance of *P. acnes,* patients with acne vulgaris should not be prescribed antibiotics as monotherapy. Instead, the use of topical or oral antibiotics should be accompanied by topical benzoyl peroxide, a topical retinoid, and a continuing dialogue on lifestyle modifications and adjuvant therapies as outlined earlier.[76–81]

Of note, benzoyl peroxide should not be applied at the same time as tretinoin because it may cause tretinoin to oxidize and become less effective. Basic descriptions of topical antibiotics commonly used in the treatment of acne vulgaris and rosacea are included in Table 73-1.

Pharmaceuticals: Systemic Preparations

When considering systemic pharmaceuticals in association with acne, the astute clinician should be aware of the range of oral medications that may induce or worsen acne vulgaris. Many of these are listed in Table 73-2.

Antibiotics
Oral antibiotics are reserved for the treatment of moderate to severe inflammatory acne lesions, specifically for refractory pustular, cystic, and nodular lesions of acne vulgaris and for rosacea with nodular lesions or ocular involvement.[82,83] Because they directly inhibit bacterial growth, oral antibiotics demonstrate relatively rapid clinical benefit, usually visible within 6 to 8 weeks. This, however, is at the cost of

TABLE 73-1. Topical Antibiotics Commonly Used for Acne Vulgaris or Acne Rosacea

PREPARATION AND DOSAGE	INDICATION	SIDE EFFECTS
Benzoyl peroxide 2.5% to 10%, applied topically once or twice daily	Acne vulgaris and glandular or phymatous subtypes of acne rosacea	Significant itching, redness, or drying of skin Contact dermatitis May bleach clothing
Clindamycin 1%, applied topically once or twice daily	Acne vulgaris and acne rosacea	Local irritation and drying of skin Very rare incidence of pseudomembranous colitis Will stain clothing
Erythromycin 1.5% to 2%, applied topically once or twice daily	Acne vulgaris and acne rosacea	Local irritation and drying of skin Will stain clothing
Sulfacetamide 5% or 10% lotion, with or without sulfur, applied topically twice daily	Acne vulgaris and acne rosacea	Local irritation, itching, redness Rare occurrence of hypersensitivity reactions Contraindicated in individuals allergic to sulfa
Metronidazole 0.75% or 1.0% cream, applied once or twice daily	Acne rosacea	Significant skin irritation and dryness

From Hull SK. Acne vulgaris and acne rosacea. In: Rakel D, ed. *Integrative Medicine*. 2nd ed. Philadelphia: Saunders; 2007.

TABLE 73-2. Oral Medications That Induce or Exacerbate Acne Vulgaris

Androgens (e.g., testosterone, danazol)	Isoniazid
Glucocorticoids (e.g., prednisone)	Cyclosporin
Corticotropin	Azathioprine
Lithium	Disulfuram
Phenytoin	Iodides, bromides
Phenobarbital	Epidermal growth factor receptor inhibitors

greater side effects, including increasing antibiotic resistance and risk of inflammatory bowel disease.[84] The following oral preparations are those most commonly used in the treatment of both acne vulgaris and rosacea.

Dosage
Erythromycin and tetracycline are administered at 250 to 500 mg twice daily. Doxycycline and minocycline are administered at 50 to 100 mg twice daily.

Precautions
As is typical with the use of systemic antibiotics, these medications may lead to vaginal candidiasis, reduced effectiveness of oral contraceptives, and gastrointestinal distress. Tetracycline should be taken on an empty stomach; along with doxycycline and minocycline, it may cause photosensitivity. Like tetracycline itself, these tetracycline derivatives are contraindicated in pregnancy and in children younger than 9 years, given their potential to reduce bone growth and to discolor developing teeth. Antibiotic resistance may be minimized by continually assessing for clinical response and discontinuing systemic antibiotics when inflammation resolves. Topical benzoyl peroxide and retinoid application

should carry on, and if the clinical need again arises, the same oral antibiotic should be used as long as it is effective.

Retinoids
Systemic retinoids are extremely effective in the treatment of severe refractory nodular acne that is often to the point of scarring. This therapeutic option is unique in that it can permanently alter acne pathogenesis, yet its side effect profile has raised concern.

Dosage
Isotretinoin, 0.5 to 1 mg/kg/day, is administered once or in two divided doses daily. Duration of treatment is usually 20 weeks or for a cumulative dose of 120 mg/kg.[85]

Precautions
Oral retinoids are highly teratogenic. In turn, the Food and Drug Administration has implemented the iPLEDGE program (www.ipledgeprogram.com), which requires registration by licensed providers, participating pharmacies, and patients who agree to specified responsibilities before they may prescribe, distribute, or use the medication. For example, female patients of childbearing age must use two separate forms of birth control from 1 month before until 1 month after treatment.[86] In addition, oral retinoids may cause hepatotoxicity, mucocutaneous irritation, myalgias, hypertriglyceridemia, and pseudotumor cerebri. Depression and suicidality have been questioned but not conclusively evidenced as further adverse effects.[85,87]

Oral Contraceptives
Combined oral contraceptive pills (OCPs) decrease serum androgen levels and sebum production. They are a reasonable addition to a treatment regimen for female patients with moderate to severe acne vulgaris whether or not they have comorbid hyperandrogenism. All of the typical adverse effects of OCPs (e.g., nausea, weight gain, thromboembolic events) should be considered. There is some evidence that OCPs containing the progestin drospirenone are among the most efficacious and best tolerated as a part of acne management.[88-91]

Dosage

Some combinations that contain drospirenone include drospirenone–ethinyl estradiol (Yasmin, Gianvi, Ocella, Yaz). Oral contraceptive pills are taken as 1 tablet daily.

Phototherapy, Laser Therapy, and Surgery

In the treatment of acne vulgaris, limited evidence supports the efficacy of various light and laser therapies. It has been demonstrated that red-blue light therapy may be more effective than 5% benzoyl peroxide in the short term (4 to 12 weeks) and that pulsed dye laser therapy after 5-aminolevulinic acid application may transiently reduce inflammatory acne lesions.[81,92,93] Better quality, long-term studies are clearly needed. With respect to acne rosacea, laser therapy has shown promise in the reduction of associated telangiectasias and erythema.[94,95] Surgical techniques used in the reshaping of significant rhinophyma include heated scalpel, electrocautery, dermabrasion, and radiofrequency electrosurgery.[75]

Therapies to Consider

Other therapeutic options for which limited data are available include topical alpha-hydroxy acids, such as glycolic acid, and retinaldehyde for improved control of acne symptoms and associated postinflammatory hyperpigmentation.[96-98] One study demonstrated the efficacy of topical green tea for reducing acne severity.[99] Botanical preparations in Ayurvedic medicine, such as *Sunder vati*, and Japanese kampo remedies, such as *Mahonia aquifolium*, may also be useful adjunctive treatments of acne vulgaris.[100-105] The pharmaceutical spironolactone has been used to treat acne, but a systematic review of the literature found no evidence that it is effective.[106] For acne rosacea, topical application of permethrin,[107] the herbal extract *Chrysanthellum indicum*,[108] and the bioflavonoid silymarin with methylsulfonylmethane (MSM)[109] may lead to symptomatic improvement. Finally, as a topical or oral therapy, niacinamide has been noted to be of benefit in both acne vulgaris and rosacea.[52,110]

PREVENTION PRESCRIPTION

- Maintain proper skin care: rinse gently, twice daily with warm water and a non–soap-based cleanser. Avoid scrubbing with abrasive materials, oil-based lotions and cosmetics, and picking at acne lesions.
- Reduce psychoemotional stress by getting adequate amounts of sleep and engaging in regular relaxation practices, such as meditation, guided imagery, breathing exercises, and massage therapy.
- For acne vulgaris, maintain a diet with a low glycemic load, rich in protein and omega-3 fatty acids and low in carbohydrates and saturated fats.
- Also for acne vulgaris, eat USDA-certified organic meats and dairy to limit consumption of animal products treated with exogenous androgenic hormones.
- Limit exposure to pharmaceutical medications that may cause eruption of acne vulgaris (see Table 73-2)
- Particularly in acne rosacea, avoid potential environmental triggers such as extremes in temperature as well as dietary triggers that may best be identified by way of a dedicated elimination diet.

THERAPEUTIC REVIEW

Mind-Body Medicine (for acne vulgaris and rosacea)

- Practice stress management and relaxation techniques   B 1

Nutrition (for acne vulgaris)

- Maintain a diet low in glycemic load   B 1
- Limit or eliminate dairy consumption   B 1
- Maintain a diet high in omega-3 fatty acids with the option of flaxseed or fish oil supplementation   C 1

Supplements (for acne vulgaris)

- Brewer's yeast: 2 g three times daily   B 2
- Zinc gluconate: 30 mg daily   B 2

Botanicals (for acne vulgaris)

- Tea tree oil: 5% to 15% solution or gel, applied topically once daily   B 2

Pharmaceutical Preparations (for acne vulgaris and rosacea)

- Azelaic acid: 20% cream or 15% gel, applied topically twice daily for acne vulgaris or rosacea   B 2
- Salicylic acid: applied topically one or two times daily for acne vulgaris   B 2
- Retinoids: applied topically once nightly for acne vulgaris   A 2
- Topical antibiotics (benzoyl peroxide, clindamycin, erythromycin, sulfacetamide, metronidazole) for acne vulgaris and rosacea (see Table 73-1)   A 2
- Oral antibiotics (erythromycin, tetracycline, doxycycline, minocycline) for acne vulgaris and rosacea   A 2
- Isotretinoin: 0.5 to 1 mg/kg/day, taken orally once or in two divided doses daily for acne vulgaris   A 3

Surgical Therapy (for acne rosacea)

- Laser therapy for associated erythema and telangiectasias   B 2
- Various surgical techniques for rhinophyma, a consequence of phymatous rosacea   C 3

KEY WEB RESOURCES

www.rosacea.org	Run by the National Rosacea Society, this is a Web site that includes links to information for patients, physicians, and researchers as well as to the Rosacea Review Newsletter, a glossary of terms, and a weblog.
www.glycemicindex.com	Maintained by the University of Sydney, this Web site provides descriptions of glycemic index and load, a food measurement database, literary resources, newsletters, press releases, and research efforts.
www.ipledgeprogram.com	This online resource provides information about the iPLEDGE program as well as the use and risk of isotretinoin. It is geared toward prescribing providers and patients and allows a search of participating pharmacies.

References

References are available online at expertconsult.com.

Human Papillomavirus and Warts

Yue Man Onna Lo, MD

Pathophysiology

Warts are benign growths found on the epithelium of the skin and mucous membranes that appear as thick, hyperkeratotic lesions. They are caused by infections from a family of double-stranded DNA viruses known as human papillomavirus (HPV).[1] More than 100 types of HPV have been identified within this family.[2] Infections by HPV (Figs. 74-1 to 74-3) are manifested mostly as cutaneous, nongenital disease (common warts, flat warts, plantar warts) and genital disease (genital warts, cervical dysplasia, cervical cancer). HPV infection is also uncommonly found in the oral and respiratory mucosa (Table 74-1). The clinical manifestation of the infection depends on the HPV type, the size of the inoculum, the immune status of the host, and the anatomic site. Individuals with impaired cell-mediated immunity are particularly more susceptible to HPV infection.[3]

The virus is transmitted by direct and indirect contact, and predisposing factors include disruptions to the normal epithelial barrier. The risk factors for cutaneous warts are community showers, occupational handling of meat, and immunosuppression[4]; the risk factors for genital HPV infection are sexual activity and lifetime number of sexual partners.[5,6]

Cutaneous warts and genital warts are usually asymptomatic. Most do not have malignant potential. However, some types in the genital region, such as HPV types 16 and 18, have been associated with cervical dysplasia and cervical cancer in women and squamous intraepithelial neoplasia in men.[7,8]

Cutaneous warts affect around 3.5% of the general population and occur in 10% of children and adolescents.[9,10] Warts resolve spontaneously in 40% of children, and two thirds of the warts resolve spontaneously within 2 years.[11]

Genital warts affect around 1% of sexually active adults in the general population.[12] Approximately 500,000 cases of genital warts occur each year in the United States[13]; associated annual medical costs are estimated at $200 million.[14] HPV is associated with more than 99% of cervical cancers and 84% of anal cancers, primarily due to HPV types 16 and 18.[8,15] Each year, more than 10,000 cases of cervical cancer are diagnosed, and 3700 women die of the disease[16] (see Fig. 74-1).

Integrative Therapies

The primary goals of treatment are to remove symptomatic warts, to decrease social stigma, and to decrease infectivity from one person to another. Otherwise, observation is a reasonable first approach.

> Observation is a reasonable first approach.

HPV infection and wart development are closely linked to the immunologic state of the individual. Warts occur more frequently, last longer, and appear in greater numbers in patients with acquired immunodeficiency syndrome (AIDS) or lymphomas and in those taking immunosuppressive drugs.[1,3] Therefore, therapies that promote a healthy immune system are crucial for treatment of warts.

Nutrition and Lifestyle

Diet

A healthy combination of whole food with fruits and vegetables, particularly dark green and yellow ones such as papaya, pumpkin, oranges, broccoli, and spinach, has been reported to protect against the effects of HPV and to support a healthy immune system.[17-20] These foods are usually rich in antioxidants like vitamin C, carotenoids, tocopherols, and folic acids. Avoidance of high intake of sugar may also improve the immune system.[21]

FIGURE 74-1
Human papillomavirus (HPV) infections. **A,** Large, cauliflower-like wart of the vagina. **B,** Dome-shaped HPV-induced lesions of the soft palate and retromolar trigone. (**A** from Habif TP, Campbell JI Jr, Chapman MS, et al. *Skin Disease: Diagnosis and Treatment.* 2nd ed. St. Louis: Mosby; 2005; **B** from Little JW, Falace DA, Miller CS, Rhodus NL. *Dental Management of the Medically Compromised Patient.* 7th ed. St. Louis: Mosby; 2008.)

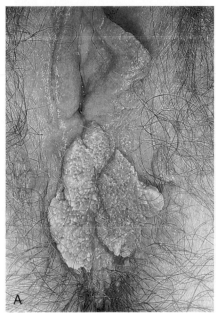

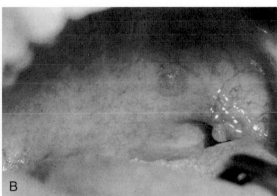

FIGURE 74-3
Verrucae planae or flat warts. The warts, skin colored to pink, are smooth-surfaced, flat papules (HPV 10 was detected). (From Bolognia JL, Jorizzo JL, Rapini RP. *Dermatology.* 2nd ed. St. Louis: Mosby; 2008.)

FIGURE 74-2
Plantar wart. A hyperkeratotic, verrucous papule or plaque beneath a pressure point on the sole of the foot is characteristic. HPV types 1 (myrmecia), 2 (mosaic), and 4 are most common. Because plantar warts are driven into the skin by the pressure of walking or standing, they are usually the most treatment resistant. (From Douglas JM. Papillomavirus. In: Goldman L, Ausiello D, eds. *Cecil Medicine.* 23rd ed. Philadelphia: Saunders; 2008.)

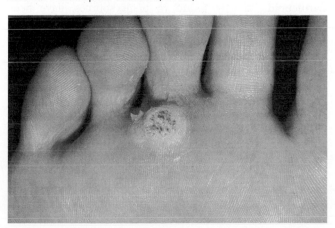

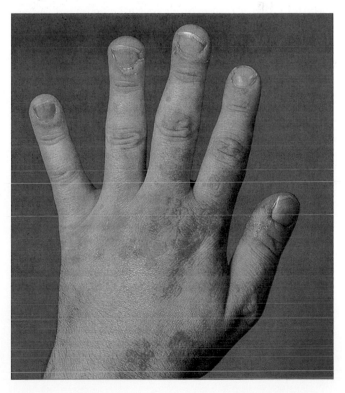

TABLE 74-1.   Warts and Some of Their Frequently Associated Locations and HPV Types

CLINICAL MANIFESTATIONS	LOCATIONS	SOME ASSOCIATED HPV TYPES
Cutaneous warts		
Common warts (verruca vulgaris)	Hands, knees, fingers, toes, nails	2, 4
Common warts: butcher's warts, found on meat, fish, and poultry handlers	Hands, fingers	7, 2
Plantar warts (verruca plantaris)	Foot	1
Flat warts (verruca plana)	Face	3, 10, 28
Epidermodysplasia verruciformis	Face, neck, trunk, extremities	5
Anogenital warts		
Genital warts (condylomata acuminata)	Anogenital area	6, 11
Anogenital malignant neoplasms	Anogenital area	16, 18
Other manifestations		
Recurrent respiratory papillomatosis	Larynx, trachea, lungs	6, 11

HPV, human papillomavirus

A healthy combination of whole food with fruits and vegetables, particularly dark green and yellow ones such as papaya, pumpkin, oranges, broccoli, and spinach, has been reported to protect against the effects of HPV and to support a healthy immune system.

Sexual Contact

Genital contact is a major risk factor for genital HPV infections. Behaviors such as limiting the number of sex partners, delaying age at first intercourse, and consistently using condoms may reduce infection risk.[22]

Alcohol

Connections have been made between alcohol consumption and HPV infections in epidemiologic studies, but confounding factors, such as risky sexual behaviors and poor hygiene, pose a challenge to clarification of these relationships. However, animal and in vitro studies support the effect of alcohol on cellular immunity and lymphocytic activities.[23]

Smoking

Tobacco cessation is recommended because tobacco use is associated with increased risk of persistent HPV infections and with the development of warts and HPV-related malignant neoplasms.[24,25]

Tobacco use is associated with increased risk of persistent HPV infections as well as with the development of warts and HPV-related malignant neoplasms.

Supplements

Most of the epidemiologic studies that have evaluated nutritional factors and their relationship with the treatment of warts have been based on targeted nutrient intakes or serum levels of specific nutrients rather than on specific supplement use. These studies support healthy food choices without identification of a specific dietary supplement to be more protective against warts.[26] So far, studies on the use of carotenoids, vitamin C, vitamin E, and folic acid have been inconclusive regarding the prevention and treatment of HPV infections in women.[26-30] These nutrients, however, have many immunostimulatory and protective functions. The supplements described here are chosen on the basis of their positive effects on the immune system and the inverse relationships with the risk for HPV infection or disease.[26-28,31]

Carotenoids

Carotenoids, mostly found in plant sources, have been shown to have antioxidant effects and to enhance lymphocytic responses. Studies have not shown vitamin A, a fat-soluble vitamin obtained from animal sources, to be related to cervical cancer risk or progression. In contrast, studies have shown that low intake of carotenoids in food and low serum levels are linked to increased risk for cervical cancer or persistent HPV infection.[26,31] However, because of the potential toxicity of high-dose vitamin A supplementation and lack of consistent evidence, a diet high in carotenoids is recommended over supplementation.[26]

A diet high in carotenoids is recommended over supplementation.

Vitamin C

Vitamin C has been well studied for its antioxidant effects that protect DNA against oxygen species and has been suggested to inhibit oncogenic transformation and to reduce virus production. It also increases immune system modulators and improves folate uptake and function.[26,27,32] In most epidemiologic studies, vitamin C has been found to be inversely related to the risk of cervical cancer.

■ Dosage

The recommended dosage of vitamin C is 1000 mg twice daily.

■ Precautions

High doses often cause diarrhea.

Vitamin E

Vitamin E has been shown to enhance cell-mediated immune response and phagocyte-derived functions. A study has shown that women with persistent HPV infection had a lower concentration of serum tocopherols than did those with transient or no HPV infection.[26,31]

■ Dosage

The recommended dosage of vitamin E is 400 units/day of mixed tocopherols and tocotrienols.

■ Precautions

Prolonged use of high doses (400 units or more) has been associated with an increase in cardiovascular risk.

Folic Acid

Folic acid is essential for DNA synthesis, protein synthesis, and gene expression.[26,27] Low levels have been suggested to increase incorporation of HPV DNA in cervical tissue at early infection stages.[27,33]

■ Dosage

The recommended dosage of folic acid is 400 mcg/day.

Mind-Body Therapies

Hypnotherapy

Hypnotherapy is the induction of a trance state for the purpose of treatment and healing. During hypnosis, a person is induced into a hypnotic state consisting of narrowed awareness, restricted attentiveness, selective wakefulness, and heightened suggestibility through specific techniques.[34] Suggestions for imaginative experiences will then be presented to the patient by the hypnotherapist for alterations in perception, sensation, emotion, thought, or behavior.[35] Many case reports and studies have data supporting the use of hypnotherapy in the treatment of warts.[36–39] In a study that compared hypnosis, topical salicylic acid, and placebo, hypnosis produced significantly more wart regression than the salicylic acid or placebo treatment did at a 6-week follow-up.[37] Hypnosis is generally safe and does not have side effects. Self-hypnosis is also easy to learn, even for children (see Chapter 92, Self-Hypnosis Techniques).

> In a study that compared hypnosis, topical salicylic acid, and placebo, hypnosis produced significantly more wart regression than the salicylic acid or placebo treatment did at a 6-week follow-up.

Botanicals

Since ancient times, there have been many traditional cures for warts. This section discusses some herbal treatments for which there are at least some prospective randomized controlled trials (RCTs) that support the potential efficacy of wart treatments.

Green Tea Extract

Green tea polyphenols or catechins (major components of green tea leaves) have immunostimulatory, antiproliferative, and antioxidant activities. The ointment Veregen (sinecatechins), which contains polyphenols, has shown positive effects against genital warts. In a few double-blinded RCTs, the clearance rate for genital warts is statistically significant compared with placebo.[40–42] Veregen was approved by the Food and Drug Administration (FDA) in 2006.

■ Dosage

Veregen ointment, 15%, is applied three times daily.

■ Precautions

The ointment can cause local pain, itching, burning, and inflammation. It is expensive.

Fig Tree Latex

Fig tree (Ficus carica) latex, or ficin, a milky excretion of leaves and fruits of the common fig tree, has been documented for treatment of warts since ancient Persia. A small prospective study showed similar outcomes compared with cryotherapy.[43]

■ Dosage

One drop per wart is applied three times daily for a minimum of 4 days.

Propolis

Propolis is a natural flavonoid-rich resin created by bees, used in the construction of hives. It is a mixture of the buds of conifer and poplar trees and bee secretions. It has antiviral and antibacterial properties that increase natural host resistance to infections. In a randomized study, 73% and 75% of patients with common warts and flat warts were cured compared with echinacea and placebo.[44]

■ Dosage

Propolis is administered orally, 500 mg/day, for 3 months.

Populus euphratica

The Populus euphratica tree is found in the Middle East, central and southern Asia, and northern Africa. It is part of the Salicaceae family that contains salicin, a precursor of salicylic acid, a common treatment of warts. In a randomized study, the smoke of the tree's burnt leaves was found to be as effective as cryotherapy when the affected area was exposed for 10 minutes for up to 10 weeks.[45]

Other Therapies

Duct Tape (silver type)

In a prospective RCT comparing duct tape use with cryotherapy in children, the clearance rate was 85% compared with 60%, respectively. Duct tape was placed on the patient's warts for 6 days and removed on the seventh day; the area was then soaked and débrided. This cycle was repeated for up to 2 months.[46] Other studies did not show significant results, but those used a different transparent tape.[47,48]

Pharmaceutical Therapies

Therapies usually include local destruction of wart tissue directly by chemical agents, ablative therapies, and immunomodulating therapies that enhance the patient's immune response against HPV.[1,49,50] For cutaneous warts, the first-line treatments are typically salicylic acid and cryotherapy; for genital warts, they are cryotherapy, trichloroacetic acid, and podophyllin. Other treatments are reserved for extensive or recalcitrant disease.

> Therapies usually include local destruction of wart tissue directly by chemical agents, ablative therapies, and immunomodulating therapies that enhance the patient's immune response against HPV.

Chemical Agents (for cutaneous warts)

Salicylic Acid

Salicylic acid is a safe and effective first-line treatment of cutaneous warts.[51-53] It is a keratolytic agent that chemically débrides the surface of the wart, resulting in a host immune response that may help clear the infection.[51,54] The wart surface should first be pared away with pumice stone, emery board, or surgical blade and then soaked in warm water for softening. Salicylic acid is then applied to the softened keratin on the wart and allowed to dry. This cycle should be repeated daily for up to 12 weeks.[51] The pooled data from six RCTs demonstrated a clearance rate of 75% in the salicylic acid treatment group compared with 48% in the control group.[53]

■ **Dosage**

Salicylic acid, 15% to 20% preparation, is applied daily at home.

Bleomycin (Blenoxane)

Bleomycin (Blenoxane) is a cytotoxic agent that directly interferes with DNA synthesis. The solution may be injected into a wart or applied to the wart and then pricked through with a lancet, allowing the solution to enter the tissue.[51,52,54] Data for efficacy are inconsistent, and use is supported only for recalcitrant warts.[53,54]

■ **Dosage**

Bleomycin 0.3 mL (0.15 unit) is administered in each treatment; the injection may be repeated every 3 to 4 weeks.

■ **Precautions**

Common adverse effects include pain, swelling, scarring, pigment change, and nail damage.[51]

Chemical Agents (for genital warts)

Trichloroacetic Acid

Trichloroacetic acid destroys the wart tissue by causing chemical coagulation of tissue proteins. It is inexpensive and has an efficacy of 80%. It can be used on the cervix and vagina, and it is safe during pregnancy.

■ **Dosage**

Trichloroacetic acid (Tri-Chlor), 80% to 90% solution, is administered weekly for 4 to 6 weeks by the physician.[55, 56]

■ **Precautions**

A common side effect is irritation.[49]

Podophyllin

Podophyllin from the mayapple plant, *Podophyllum peltatum*, acts as an antimitotic and cytotoxic agent that disrupts viral activities and the microcirculation of the wart.[6,9] The preparations are not standardized; therefore, efficacy may be variable.

■ **Dosage**

Podophyllin, 25% solution for small warts and 10% solution for areas near the mucosal surfaces or larger warts, is washed off within 6 hours after application. It is applied by the physician one or two times per week.

■ **Precautions**

Because podophyllin is highly absorbable, treatment of large areas may increase the potential for systemic effects, such as bone marrow suppression and neurotoxicity. Side effects include burning, redness, and swelling.

Podophyllotoxin (Podofilox)

Podophyllotoxin (podofilox) is a standardized formulation of the active compound from podophyllin, a preparation safe for self-administration. Studies show that podophyllotoxin is more effective than podophyllin. It has an estimated efficacy of 60%.[55]

■ **Dosage**

Podofilox, 0.5% gel or solution, is applied twice daily for 3 days, followed by 4 days of no treatment, repeated for up to four cycles. The treatment surface area should not exceed $10\,cm^2$, and the volume of medication should not exceed 0.5 mL per use.[6,57,58] It is applied by the patient.

■ **Precautions**

Do not apply podophyllin to the cervix or vagina because of the risk of chemical burns. Do not use in pregnancy.

5-Fluorouracil

5-Fluorouracil (5-FU) inhibits cell growth by interfering with DNA and RNA synthesis. It is used intralesionally and is awaiting FDA approval.[49] It is highly teratogenic.

Immunomodulating Agents (for cutaneous warts and genital warts)

Imiquimod

Imiquimod (Aldara) induces local production of cytokines and enhances T-cell–mediated cytolytic activity against viral targets. Although RCT data are lacking, a study showed a clearance rate of 56% for cutaneous warts.[59] Use for recalcitrant warts.

▪ Dosage

Imiquimod, 5% cream, is applied three times a week at bedtime for up to 16 weeks.[56]

▪ Precautions

Adverse reactions included erythema, burning, itching, and erosion.

Immunomodulating Agents (for cutaneous warts)

Candida Antigen and Mumps Antigen

Most people have been exposed to the yeast *Candida albicans* or to the mumps virus and will mount a delayed hypersensitivity response when they are injected with one of these antigens. As a result, immunity against HPV is enhanced.[60]

Immunomodulating Agents (for genital warts)

Interferons

Interferons are immunologic proteins that inhibit viral replication. Topical interferon may be effective against recalcitrant and recurrent warts.[61]

▪ Dosage

Interferon alfa, 1 million international units, is injected two or three times per week for up to 8 weeks. Limit to five warts per session.[49,54]

Vaccinations

Human Papillomavirus Vaccine

Two vaccines (Gardasil and Cervarix) are available to protect females against HPV infections that cause most cervical cancers. The quadrivalent HPV vaccine (Gardasil) targeting HPV types 6, 11, 16, and 18 is effective for primary prevention against genital warts in males and females. It is licensed for use between the ages of 9 and 26 years. It is most beneficial to complete three doses during a 6-month period before beginning of sexual activity.[62]

> The quadrivalent HPV vaccine (Gardasil) is effective for primary prevention against genital warts in males and females.

Ablative Methods (for cutaneous and genital warts)

Cryotherapy

Liquid nitrogen is the most commonly used cryogen. It causes irreversible cytolysis by thermal damage, and local inflammation produces a cell-mediated immunologic response.[9,51,54] First, débride the wart with a surgical blade, then use a cotton-tipped applicator or cryospray to treat the wart until a halo of frozen tissue appears around the wart and time for 5 to 30 seconds. Alternate the freezing with an intervening period that allows the wart to thaw. This freeze-thaw-freeze technique may increase the chance for complete eradication of the wart.[9] Repeat treatment at 1- to 3-week intervals. Side effects may include pain and blistering. Efficacy studies have shown variable results. Pooled data showed that aggressive cryotherapy has a clearance rate of 52%.[53]

Pulsed Dye Laser

Pulsed dye laser is a vascular lesion laser that selectively heats hemoglobin contained in the wart blood vessels. This cauterization of the blood vessels leads to necrosis.[58] Its efficacy is between 48% and 93% for different warts and highest against periungual warts.[52] Use when other therapies have failed.

Carbon Dioxide Laser

The carbon dioxide laser uses focused infrared light energy to vaporize the wart. It is indicated for extensive vaginal and intraurethral warts. Physicians are advised to wear masks during treatment to prevent inhalation of the smoke plume, which contains HPV viral particles.[49,56]

Surgical Excision

Surgical treatment of warts involves removal at the dermal-epidermal junction. Surgical methods include scissor excision, shave excision, curettage, electrocautery, loop electrosurgical excision procedure (LEEP), and large loop excision of the transformation zone (LLETZ). The efficacy is 35% to 70%.[56] Side effects include pain, scarring, and bleeding. Local, regional, or general anesthesia is required, depending on the location and size of the lesion. LEEP and LLETZ are effective ways for removal of cervical condylomas.[9,49,50,63]

Therapies to Consider

Garlic has been used for warts in China, and a few studies have demonstrated that garlic is effective when it is used as an extract or cut off and rubbed onto the lesion.[64,65] Acupuncture points have also been suggested for wart treatments.[66]

A limited number of studies have been done in distant healing,[67] Reiki,[68] and homeopathy,[69] but no strong supporting data have been found.

PREVENTION PRESCRIPTION

- Maintain a healthy diet that consists of dark green and yellow vegetables and fruits.
- Avoid moderate to high consumption of alcohol and cigarette smoking.
- Workers handling meat, fish, and poultry should wear appropriate protective gear.
- Wear shoes when using communal showers or locker rooms.
- If either partner has genital warts, use condoms consistently during sexual intercourse.
- Maintain regular screening for cervical HPV infection with Papanicolaou smear.
- Vaccinate against HPV types that lead to cervical cancer and genital warts (quadrivalent HPV vaccine [Gardasil], 0.5 mL intramuscularly three times at 0, 2, and 6 months).

THERAPEUTIC REVIEW

Diet and Lifestyle

- Balanced, whole-food diet that consists of vitamin C, vitamin E, carotenoids, and folic acid. Also include lots of dark green and yellow vegetables and fruits.   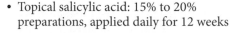B/1

Integrative Therapies

- Hypnotherapy   B/1
- Duct tape   B/1
- Topical green tea extract ointment (Veregen)   B/1

Supplements

- Vitamin C: 1000 mg two times daily   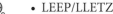B/2

- Vitamin E: 400 units/day   B/2
- Folic acid: 400 mcg/day   B/1

Pharmaceutical Therapies

- Topical salicylic acid: 15% to 20% preparations, applied daily for 12 weeks   A/2
- Topical podophyllotoxin (podofilox): 0.5% gel or solution, applied twice daily for 3 days, followed by 4 days of no treatment, then repeated up to four cycles   B/2
- Topical trichloroacetic acid: 80% to 90% preparations, applied weekly by physician for 4 to 6 weeks   B/2

Surgical Therapies

- Cryotherapy   B/2
- LEEP/LLETZ   A/2

References

References are available online at expertconsult.com.

Section XIII Cancer

Chapter 75

Breast Cancer

Lucille R. Marchand, MD, BSN

Cancer encompasses a wide variety of diseases that have uncontrolled growth of abnormal cells in common. Each cancer has a unique set of genetic and environmental factors that encourage this abnormal response in the body. Genetic vulnerability is coupled with environmental factors (epigenetics) that give rise to conditions favorable to cancer growth. Breast cancer involves this interplay of genes with environmental factors (such as food choices, exercise, lifestyle, and estrogen exposures) and environmental toxins (such as radiation and pesticides). Integrative medicine emphasizes personal empowerment to make lifestyle choices that can help prevent cancer from occurring and slow its growth once it has occurred or prevent recurrence. Many factors may not be in our control, but many lifestyle choices are. These same healthy choices also limit the development of other chronic illnesses, such as heart disease, diabetes, obesity, and hyperlipidemia.[1]

Breast cancer is currently the most common cancer in women in the United States (incidence of 28% of all new cancers in women), with a lifetime risk of one in eight women. It is the second most common cancer in women causing cancer-related mortality—15% of all cancers (highest mortality rates in women are from lung cancer—26%).[2] Five-year survival rates are high in women with early-stage cancers: stage 0, 100%; stages 1 and 2, 98% for local invasion, 83.6% for regional invasion; stage 3, 57%; and in women with metastatic breast cancer, 23.4%.[3] One percent of breast cancers occur in men.[4]

Pathophysiology

Breast cancer is generally a hormone-driven cancer; higher lifetime risk is associated with higher estrogen exposure. Seventy percent of breast cancers express hormone receptors for progesterone or estrogen.[5] Exogenous estrogens, such as hormone replacement therapy (HRT), pesticides that have an estrogenic effect in our bodies, and hormones from animal and dairy sources, are most concerning, although obesity is an intrinsic factor that increases risk as well. Soy foods (rather than supplements), which are weak plant estrogens, may have

a protective effect. Some genetic mutations have a higher likelihood of cancer development, such as *BRCA1* and *BRCA2* mutations, which are associated with a 60% to 80% lifetime risk for breast cancer. These genetic markers are related to mutations that inactivate cancer suppressor genes.[6,7]

 Table 75-1e, which lists risk factors for breast cancer, can be found online at expertconsult.com.

Risk Factors

Factors that increase the risk of breast cancer include alcohol consumption of more than one serving per day, taking estrogen-containing products such as HRT and birth control pills, increased estrogen lifetime exposure including early menarche and late menopause, low intake of fruits and vegetables, obesity, exposure to radiation, and sedentary lifestyle (Table 75-1e, available online at expertconsult.com). Aging is a risk factor in that 80% of women with a breast cancer diagnosis are older than 50 years. Family history of breast cancer and certain mutations, such as *BRCA1, BRCA2,* and *p53*, increase the risk for breast cancer. These gene mutations increase lifetime risk for development of breast cancer by 40% to 85%. Women with a mother, sister, or daughter with breast cancer are twice as likely to develop cancer as is a woman with no family history of breast cancer in female relatives. Both paternal and maternal relatives are important in determining breast cancer risk.[1]

 More information on this topic can be found online at expertconsult.com.

A study in Sri Lanka identified prolonged breast-feeding (24 months in a lifetime) in significantly reducing risk of breast cancer. The mechanism may be reduction in lifetime estrogen exposure.[10] Another study in Tunisia showed similar protective effect of prolonged breast-feeding.[11]

Short telomere length is associated with increased risk of cancer occurrence and cancer mortality. Telomeres are nucleoproteins that serve to protect chromosomal integrity. In a population-based study, telomere length was not shown to have the same association in breast or colorectal cancer.[12]

Obesity is a significant risk factor for breast cancer occurrence, recurrence, and mortality. Limiting the intake of high-density foods, such as fat and sugars, and increasing plant-based lower density foods, such as fruits, vegetables, and whole grains, can help maintain healthy weight in combination with regular exercise for energy expenditure and glycemic control.[13,14] Limiting of portion size is an important weight control strategy.[13]

Night shift work and subsequent disruption of the natural circadian rhythm can put women at risk for increased breast cancer. Melatonin levels are suppressed with these disruptions, and low melatonin levels raise estradiol levels and increase risk of breast cancer.[15-17]

2-Hydroxyestrone/16-Hydroxyestrone Ratio

In estrogen receptor–positive (ER⁺) tumors, estrogen metabolism can contribute to risk. Both strong and weak estrogen metabolites are produced from oxidative processes in the body. 2-Hydroxyestrones are weakly estrogenic and may be protective (similar perhaps in action to weak plant estrogens such as soy foods), and 16-hydroxyestrones are more strongly estrogenic. The 16-hydroxyestrones can stimulate estrogen receptors in vulnerable tissue, leading to ER⁺ tumors, and can disrupt DNA, which produces oncogenes and tumor suppressor genes (Fig. 75-1). The ratio of these urinary estrogen metabolites can be measured by specialized testing to monitor and guide interventions and to assess risk.[18-20] Dietary measures (decreased alcohol intake, increased oleic acid such as in olive oil), physical activity, phytoestrogens such as flaxseed meal, and cruciferous vegetables can help favor weaker estrogen metabolites.[19,21,22]

FIGURE 75-1
Pathways of estrogen synthesis and catabolism. 2-MeO-E₁, 2-methoxyestrone; 2-MeO-E₂, 2-methoxyestradiol; 2-OH-3-MeO-E₁, 2-hydroxyestrone 3-methyl ether; 2-OH-3-MeO-E₂, 2-hydroxyestradiol 3-methyl ether; 2-OH-E₁, 2-hydroxyestrone; 2-OH-E₂, 2-hydroxyestradiol; 3β-HSD, 3β-hydroxysteroid dehydrogenase; 4-OH-3-MEO-E₁, 4-hydroxyestrone 3-methyl ether; 4-OH-3-MeO-E₂, 4-hydroxyestradiol 3-methyl ether; 4-OH-E₁, 4-hydroxyestrone; 4-OH-E₂, 4-hydroxyestradiol; 16α-OH-E₁, 16α-hydroxyestrone; 16α-OH-E₂, 16α-hydroxyestradiol; 17β-HSD, 17β-hydroxysteroid dehydrogenase; COMT, catechol O-methyltransferase; CYP11, 11β-hydroxylase; CYP1A1, cytochrome P-450 1A1; CYP1B1, cytochrome P-450 1B1; CYP17, 17β-dehydroxylase; CYP19, P-450 aromatase; CYP21, 21-hydroxylase; DHEA, dehydroepiandrosterone; E₁, estrone; E₂, estradiol; P-450, cytochrome P-450; scc, side-chain cleavage enzyme. (From Clemons M, Goss P. Estrogen and the risk of breast cancer. *N Engl J Med.* 2001;344:276–285.)

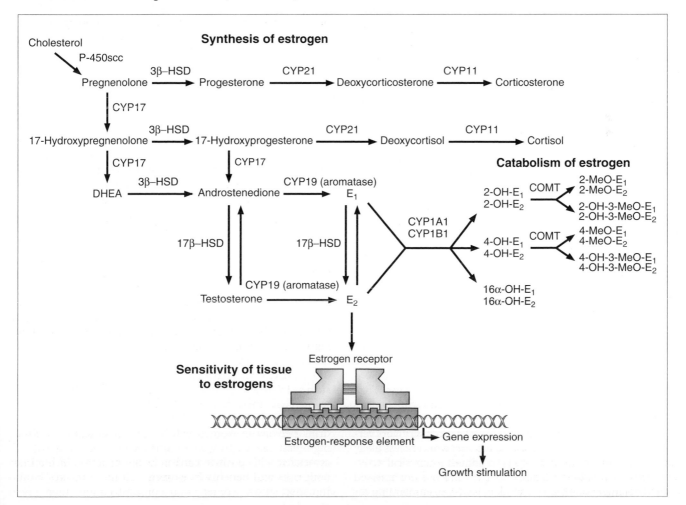

> Exercise, weight loss, cruciferous vegetables, and lignan-rich flaxseed can improve the 2-hydroxyestrone/16-hydroxyestrone ratio, reducing the stimulatory effect on breast tissue.

In women receiving postmenopausal HRT, breast cancer risk for hormone receptor–positive cancers and HER2/neu-positive tumors increases. In women taking estrogen and progestin replacement for more than 15 years, the risk of breast cancer increased by 83% compared with estrogen-only HRT, which increased risk by 19%. Risks associated with HRT were found only in women with body mass index (BMI) below 29.9 kg/m² but not in women with a BMI above 30.[23]

Screening

 Information on this topic can be found online at expertconsult.com.

Integrative Therapies

Lifestyle

The European Prospective Investigation into Cancer and Nutrition found that four lifestyle measures were critical in reducing risk of cancer as well as chronic illnesses such as heart disease and diabetes. These measures included not smoking; BMI below 30; 3.5 hours a week of exercise or more; and eating a healthy diet of fruit, vegetables, and whole grains, with little meat consumption. Having all four lifestyle factors reduced the risk of cancer by 36%.[30] Block et al[31] found that at their integrative cancer center with attention to nutrition, nutraceuticals, exercise, and psychological interventions, metastatic breast cancer patients had a survival rate twice that of comparison groups in the literature. Median survival in their center was 38 months, compared with 12 to 24 months reported in similar populations. For patients to make informed decisions about nutritional changes, consultation with a person trained in integrative nutrition must be made available.[32]

Exercise

Exercise has a role in cancer prevention through weight control, muscle strength, and improved immunity and mood control. During and after cancer treatment, exercise can benefit mood, strength, weight control, energy levels, immunity, overall health and well-being, survival, prevention of recurrence, and quality of life. It allows patients to go through their cancer treatments with increased strength, less fatigue and muscle weakness, better balance, and fewer falls.[33] It also has a beneficial effect on the vasomotor instability of menopause. Yoga and higher intensity, frequent exercise have significant beneficial effects on depression with less marked positive effects on anxiety.[34] One study that looked at breast cancer survivors versus controls showed that breast cancer survivors are less likely than non–breast cancer controls to adhere to physical activity recommendations.[35] Unfortunately, what was not assessed was what their health care providers were recommending for

exercise and whether they advised continuing exercise during and after treatment. The American College of Sports Medicine reviewed the literature on exercise and cancer treatment and concluded that exercise is safe in patients undergoing cancer treatment and that exercise improves physical functioning, quality of life, and fatigue.[36] In a population-based study of breast cancer patients, consistent and long-term, higher activity (more than 3 hours/week) exercisers had lower risk of cancer mortality than did women with low activity levels.[37] In another study of breast cancer survivors, women who had 2 to 3 hours of walking per week after diagnosis reduced their mortality risk by 45% compared with sedentary women. Women who decreased their activity after diagnosis increased their mortality risk fourfold.[38] In another study, a simple walking intervention reduced pain and maintained cardiorespiratory fitness in patients with breast cancer undergoing radiation therapy and chemotherapy.[39] (See Chapter 88, Writing an Exercise Prescription.)

Nutrition

Mediterranean Diet

Diets high in fruits and vegetables, fish, fresh foods, and olive oil and low in animal fat (the Mediterranean diet) reduce the risk of breast cancer and many other cancers.[40] In one large French study of 2381 women with invasive postmenopausal breast cancer, a Western/alcohol-dominant diet was associated with higher risk of breast cancer incidence compared with a healthy Mediterranean diet. The Western diet included meat products, French fries, alcohol, pizza, high-fat foods, and processed foods. The Mediterranean diet included fruits and vegetables, fish, olive and sunflower oils, and nonprocessed fresh foods. This difference was especially significant in women with estrogen-positive, progesterone-negative (ER$^+$/PR$^-$) tumors.[40]

Fiber

Food intake high in fiber, in the National Institutes of Health–AARP Diet and Health Study, can reduce the risk of breast cancer, especially for ER$^-$/PR$^-$ tumors.[41] In the Malmö Diet and Cancer cohort, intake of high-fiber bread reduced the risk of breast cancer.[42] High-fiber foods are preferable to fiber supplements because of the beneficial nutrients intrinsic to food sources such as fruits, vegetables, beans, nuts and seeds, whole grains, and legumes.[13]

Alcohol

Controversy exists about the role of alcohol and risk in breast cancer. In primary prevention, alcohol intake and lower folate levels are associated with increased risk.[43] In one study of secondary prevention, low to moderate alcohol intake was not associated with increased risk of recurrence or increased mortality.[44] Alcohol (in women, more than one alcohol drink per day) increases circulation of androgens and estrogens, and use of alcohol is associated with lower levels of important nutrients such as folate and B vitamins, with a protective effect noted in women with increased folate intake who drink alcohol.[6] Many studies have linked alcohol intake of more than one alcoholic drink per day in women with a number of cancers, including breast cancer. In women, one alcoholic drink per day is associated with positive cardiac health benefits. Alcohol has both risks and benefits in women.[13] In the Women's Health Initiative study, women who consumed more than seven alcoholic drinks per week doubled their risk of hormone receptor–positive invasive lobular carcinoma. This effect was not seen in ER⁻ women or women with ductal breast cancer. Alcohol has a differing effect on breast cancer risk, depending on the subtype of the breast cancer.[45] Deandrea et al[46] found increased risk for alcohol and ER⁺ tumors.

Sugar

High sugar intake increases calories in the diet (sometimes excluding more nutritious food), contributes to weight gain, and increases insulin levels, which can have other deleterious metabolic effects that contribute to cancer cell growth.[13,47] High sugar intake in the form of products with high-fructose corn syrup, sugar, honey, and molasses is not recommended.[13]

Polyunsaturated Fatty Acids

Polyunsaturated fatty acids include omega-3 and omega-6 fatty acids. In large quantities and especially if hydrogenated for extended shelf life, sunflower, safflower, soy, sesame, and corn oils can be proinflammatory in the body. Omega-3 fatty acids (eicosapentaenoic acid [EPA] and docosahexaenoic acid [DHA]) are antiinflammatory and are contained in fish oil, flaxseed oil, and the oil in walnuts. Omega-3 fatty acids are present in fatty fish (such as salmon, sardines, and mackerel), walnuts, green leafy vegetables, and flaxseed meal. The VITamins And Lifestyle (VITAL) study demonstrated that fish oil reduced the risk of ductal but not lobular breast cancers.[48] In a case-controlled study of patients with breast cancer with case controls with no malignant disease, fish omega-3 intake was found to reduce risk of breast cancer in premenopausal and postmenopausal women, with the greatest reduction in postmenopausal women.[49] Cottet et al[40] demonstrated in a large cohort study of postmenopausal women that there was a lower risk of invasive breast cancer with a Mediterranean diet (high in fish, fruits, and vegetables) but a higher risk on a Western/alcohol-type diet (high in saturated meat fat and processed foods). These omega-3 fatty acids may also enhance the effects of chemotherapy.[50]

■ Dosing

Approximately 1000 mg of combined DHA and EPA daily in less than 3 g of total high-potency fish oil is recommended. Flaxseed oil can be substituted on a vegan diet. If any fishy aftertaste occurs, remember not to take with hot food or drinks and to take before eating; if these measures do not work, freeze fish oil capsules.

■ Precautions

If any bleeding occurs, stop fish oil immediately because its action on decreasing adhesiveness of platelets in clotting can increase bleeding. Stop 1 week before surgery or any invasive procedure. Fish oil is contraindicated with platelet counts of less than 20,000. A more conservative approach is to discontinue fish oil if the platelet count is less than 50,000. Use with caution if the patient is taking any other anticoagulants. If the international normalized ratio becomes too high with anticoagulants, stop fish oil to avoid bleeding.

Monounsaturated Fatty Acids

Oleic acid (omega-9 fatty acid) is found in olive oil, avocados, hazelnuts, and cashew nuts. It can help with suppression of HER2/neu tumor cell growth and can help enhance the

action of trastuzumab.[51] Eating these nuts and using olive oil in cooking and as a salad dressing are recommended.

Green Tea

Green tea is a polyphenol that is a natural aromatase inhibitor. Green tea consumption of more than three cups per day reduced the risk of breast cancer recurrence by 27%, but no consistent effect could be found on cancer incidence.[52] In a Chinese population, green tea and dietary mushrooms decreased the risk for development of breast cancer.[53]

■ Dosing

Three cups a day is a recommended intake.

Soy

In the recent past, a scarcity of research on soy made this food controversial with estrogen-sensitive tumors because soy is a phytoestrogen and theoretically could stimulate estrogen receptors. Studies in mice using the isoflavone genistein in isolation raised concerns about soy. In mice, genistein stimulated ER⁺ tumors; but in clinical studies of soy consumption, opposite effects are found.[54] Because they are weak estrogens, however, they might also block receptors from being stimulated by stronger exogenous and intrinsic sources of estrogen. The Shanghai Breast Cancer Survival Study, which included 5042 breast cancer survivors, showed that soy food intake is inversely associated with breast cancer mortality and recurrence. The benefits existed for ER⁺ and ER⁻ tumors and for both users and nonusers of tamoxifen.[55] In another study of soy food intake, high soy intake reduced the risk of breast cancer recurrence in patients with ER⁺/PR⁺ tumors receiving the aromatase inhibitor anastrozole.[56] In another study of soy intake and breast cancer risk, an inverse association was found for high intake to lower risk of breast cancer.[57] In Korean women, soy intake was associated with lower breast cancer risk in postmenopausal women, and the inverse association was marked in women with ER⁺/PR⁺ tumors.[58]

> Soy isoflavones in supplements may be avoided, given concerns in mice; but soy foods do not appear to be contraindicated and indeed seem to be valuable in reducing risk of breast cancer, recurrence, and mortality.

■ Dosing

One to three servings a day, in a balanced diet with other foods, are recommended unless an individual has sensitivity to soy.

Other phytoestrogens, plant lignans, can help reduce risk of breast cancer, especially in postmenopausal women.[59]

Flax

Flax, usually consumed as flaxseed meal or oil, is a rich source of phytoestrogens containing alpha-linolenic acid. It has protective effects by decreasing inflammation in the body as an omega-3 fatty acid, inhibits aromatase activity, binds weakly to estrogen receptors, and increases the weaker 2-hydroxyestrones. It reduces the risk of breast cancer and decreases breast cancer cell growth.[18,19,60]

■ Dosing

One to 2 tablespoons a day of the meal can be added to food. Flaxseed meal and oil can become rancid easily and should be kept in an airtight container, refrigerated, and used promptly.

Antioxidants

Diets high in fruits and vegetables are high in antioxidants and can lower risk of breast cancer.[40] Carotenoids in fruits and vegetables that were consumed in large amounts reduced the risk of invasive breast cancer in premenopausal women.[61] Antioxidants in foods are safer and preferable to high-dose supplement forms, given their bioavailability, synergistic effects, and better absorption. Given scant evidence for benefit of antioxidant supplements during cancer treatment and potential risks of interfering with treatment, antioxidant supplements are not recommended during cancer treatment.[62]

▨ Dosing

Five to nine servings of fruits and vegetables daily are recommended.

Edible (Medicinal) Mushrooms

Medicinal mushrooms that have an antiinflammatory and immune-enhancing effect include maitake *(Grifola frondosa),* shiitake *(Lentinus edodes),* reishi *(Ganoderma lucidum),* and turkey tail *(Trametes versicolor).*[62] Mushrooms also have a number of other properties, including antifungal, antibacterial, antiviral, and tumor attenuating. Each mushroom has different characteristics. Maitake mushrooms in particular have high antitumor and antiinflammatory activity.[63] In one phase I/II trial of maitake extract, a statistically significant association was found with positive immune response. There was no dose-limiting toxicity.[64] In a review of *T. versicolor* research in Japan and China, Standish et al[65] discuss data suggesting that this mushroom improves disease-free intervals and overall survival in breast cancer patients by immune modulation. More research is warranted.

▨ Dosing

Mushrooms can be eaten in the diet or taken as a dried supplement.

Whey Protein

Whey protein, which is a byproduct of cheese making, is of the highest protein quality and high in glutamine, which helps prevent mouth sores (stomatitis) in patients receiving chemotherapy and may be useful in preventing the peripheral neuropathy of certain chemotherapy agents, such as taxanes (Taxol). Glutamine is abundant in whey, and this is the preferred manner of ingesting this nutrient.

▨ Dosing

Whey protein powder, 20 to 30 g twice daily in smoothies, will provide adequate glutamine to prevent these complications of chemotherapy. If whey is not tolerated because of allergy or sensitivity, glutamine can be taken as a supplement, 3 to 5 g one to three times daily.[66]

Brassica (Cruciferous) Vegetables

Cruciferous vegetables include kale, broccoli, cauliflower, Brussels sprouts, and cabbage. Indole-3-carbinol is an important constituent of these vegetables that helps decrease cancer cell proliferation, increase apoptosis, and alter the ratio of weak to strong estrogens (2-hydroxyestrone/16-hydroxyestrone) favorably. Breast cancer risk can be reduced by 20% to 40% with one or two servings of cruciferous vegetables daily.[22,67-69] Indole-3-carbinol can interfere with tamoxifen and is safer to eat in vegetable form than in supplement form.[1]

▨ Dosing

One or two servings per day is the recommended intake. In supplement form, 400 mg/day is recommended.[19,70,71]

> One head of cabbage contains approximately 1200 mg of indole-3-carbinol. Eating of one third of a head of cabbage daily would equal the common supplemental dose of 400 mg daily and offer the other synergistic properties of the whole plant.

Supplements

Botanicals and supplements can be useful in promoting health; some have an anticancer effect or immunity-enhancing effect, and some are useful in attenuating the side effects of conventional cancer therapies. It is important to consider the interactions of some botanicals and supplements with chemotherapy and radiation therapy that might decrease the effectiveness of these modalities and in some cases increase toxicity. Antioxidants taken in high-dose supplement form can theoretically interfere with radiation therapy and chemotherapy by neutralizing free radical formation key to the effectiveness of these agents. Controversy remains, but most practitioners agree that foods high in antioxidants are safe, given the variety of antioxidants naturally occurring in many foods that act synergistically, are better absorbed, and do not reduce the effectiveness of radiation therapy and chemotherapy because they are in concentrations lower than in supplement forms.

 More information on this topic can be found online at expertconsult.com.

Vitamin D

Vitamin D deficiency is common, especially in patients chronically or acutely ill and in northern climates (above 35 to 40 degrees north or south of the equator). Those individuals with darker skin, who are obese, who have little unprotected sun exposure, who are older than 65 years, and who are taking particular medications such as glucocorticoids or anticonvulsants are also at risk for deficiency. It can express itself as diffuse body aches and can contribute to osteopenia and osteoporosis. It can also be manifested as low back pain, proximal muscle weakness, and bone pain, especially over the sternum or tibia.[74,75] Vitamin D is also important in immunity and has an anticancer effect. Vitamin D is ingested as vitamin D_2 (ergocalciferol) or vitamin D_3 (cholecalciferol), which is converted in the liver to 25-hydroxyvitamin D (calcidiol), the circulating form of vitamin D. Vitamin D_3 is also formed in the skin when 7-dehydrocholesterol, the skin precursor, is exposed to ultraviolet B light. Calcidiol is converted in the kidney to 1,25-dihydroxyvitamin D (calcitriol), the active metabolite. Calcitriol significantly inhibits cancer cell growth, especially in breast, colon, prostate, and ovarian tissue.[74] In testing for vitamin D deficiency, the 25-hydroxyvitamin D level is most accurate.

Strong evidence exists that vitamin D and calcium intake can help reduce the risk of breast cancer.[76] In a meta-analysis of 36 studies, 45% lowered risk was found in those women whose 25-hydroxyvitamin D levels were in the highest quartile versus the lowest quartile. Decreased cancer risk was also found in those with the highest quartile of calcium intake.[77] Blackmore et al[78] found reduced risk of ER$^+$/PR$^+$ breast cancer in women with the highest intake of vitamin D. Nonsignificant positive trends were also seen in women with ER$^+$/PR$^-$ and ER$^-$/PR$^-$ tumors. Dark-skinned individuals such as African Americans convert less vitamin D in their skin and are more likely to be vitamin D deficient without supplementation. This increases cancer risk, which may help explain why this population group is more at risk for cancer with higher mortality.[79]

Aromatase inhibitors can contribute to myalgias, arthralgias, and loss of bone mass. In combination with other therapies that cause significant side effects and may further prevent meaningful sun exposure, vitamin D deficiency can contribute to these adverse effects of conventional therapy. Medications such as anticonvulsants and glucocorticoids increase metabolism and reduce vitamin D levels.[75]

Vitamin D–fortified foods contain vitamin D in small and inconsistent amounts. Reliable and potent food sources of vitamin D are oily fish, including salmon, mackerel, and sardines.[74,75] Supplements are usually needed to obtain adequate amounts of vitamin D. Amounts generally obtained in multivitamins (400 units of vitamin D) are too low to prevent deficiency in most individuals.[74] According to research, the body metabolizes about 4000 units of vitamin D daily.[80] Current recommendations of 800 units of vitamin D daily are extremely conservative.

Optimal serum levels of vitamin D are controversial. In general, a 25-hydroxyvitamin D level of less than 20 ng/mL (50 nmol/L) is deficiency range, and 20 to 30 ng/mL (50 to 75 nmol/L) is in the insufficiency range. Treatment of vitamin D deficiency includes oral vitamin D_2 (ergocalciferol) at 50,000 units per week for 8 weeks. After vitamin D levels are normalized, current recommendations are conservative at 800 to 1000 units daily.[75] Vitamin D is relatively contraindicated in patients with hypercalcemia, which can occur in metastatic breast cancer with bone involvement, granulomatous disease such as tuberculosis and sarcoidosis, and Williams syndrome.[75] In an epidemiologic projection of optimal serum 25-hydroxyvitamin D levels, Garland et al[81] estimated prevention of 58,000 cases of breast cancer per year with year-round levels of 40 to 60 ng/mL (100 to 150 nmol/L). Abbas et al[82] found that vitamin D lowered the risk of premenopausal breast cancer. Other studies in Norway and England have found that patients with cancers diagnosed in summer or fall, when vitamin D levels are highest, had longer survival and a milder clinical course than did patients diagnosed in the winter or spring, when vitamin D levels are lowest.[83]

■ Dosing

The recommended dose of vitamin D_3 is 1000 to 2000 units daily.[84-86] In the summer months at latitudes higher than 35 to 40 degrees away from the equator or daily at latitudes closer to the equator, moderate exposure to sun, at least 20 minutes midday without sunscreen in patients who are not at risk for sunburn or skin cancer, will maintain normal vitamin D levels.[87] Serum levels of 25-hydroxyvitamin D can be used to determine optimal dosing of vitamin D, which can vary from person to person and by time of year, latitude, and degree of sun exposure.

■ Precautions

Signs of vitamin D toxicity include nausea and vomiting, pancreatitis, nephrocalcinosis or vascular calcinosis, metallic taste, and headache.[75]

Melatonin

Melatonin has antioxidant, immune-enhancing, cytotoxic, and estrogen-regulating properties. It is also useful in the treatment of insomnia. Melatonin comes in an immediate preparation for individuals having difficulty in falling asleep and a sustained-release preparation for those having difficulty staying asleep.[88,89]

■ Dosing

Doses range from 1 to 20 mg before bed; a starting dose is 3 mg before bed. Titration occurs to effect, without causing a hangover the next day.

■ Precautions

Melatonin is contraindicated in bipolar illness, and it can worsen depression in some vulnerable individuals. Monitoring for optimal effect with minimal side effects is recommended. Caution must be exercised in use with other sedative medication.

Botanicals

Botanicals can be helpful in the treatment of cancer but must be used carefully during chemotherapy because many botanicals can interfere with the metabolism of the chemotherapy agent by increasing or decreasing its metabolism in the body. Refer to the text *The Definitive Guide to Cancer: An Integrative Approach to Prevention, Treatment, and Healing* by Alschuler and Gazella for specific information on botanical and supplement interactions with chemotherapy drugs. For example, certain botanicals can interfere with the metabolism of taxanes, platinum-based drugs, cyclophosphamide, doxorubicin, etoposide, and irinotecan.[1] In general, botanicals do not interfere with radiation therapy. Botanicals such as St. John's wort can interact with a number of other drugs the patient may be taking through the cytochrome P-450 metabolic pathway.

Spiritual and Emotional Care

Patients who have social support, empowerment, and meaning often have more positive lifestyle behaviors and coping strategies. Those patients with lack of meaning and purpose often have more symptoms from treatment and more difficulty in coping, leading to more negative choices.[90] Small-group psychological interventions for breast cancer patients led by a psychologist and concentrating on stress management and strategies to optimize conventional treatment and to improve mood helped decrease recurrence and mortality.[91] Emerging evidence on life review and Internet-based social networking shows improvement in quality of life measures; it is another intervention that is simple yet powerful in cultivating meaning through the challenges of cancer.[92,93] Spiritual and emotional assessment and recommendations for interventions such as support groups, journaling, life review, and psychotherapy with oncology health professionals are reviewed in other chapters (see Chapter 80, End-of-Life Care, and Chapter 110, Taking a Spiritual History).

Conventional Treatment

Breast cancer treatment and prognosis depend on staging and pathologic examination of tumor tissue. Lymph node and vascular spread of tumor, histologic staging of degree of invasion and type of tissue, hormone receptor expression, and epidermal growth factor receptor 2 (ERBB2, formerly HER2 or HER2/neu) overexpression are all included in describing breast cancer. Stage 0 describes lobular or ductal carcinoma in situ without spread of tumor. Lobular carcinoma in situ does not progress to breast cancer, but its presence increases the risk of breast cancer by 7% over 10 years. Ductal carcinoma in situ can progress to invasive breast cancer.[3]

Surgery

Because ductal carcinoma in situ can progress to invasive breast cancer, local breast-conserving surgical therapy with radiation therapy afterward is generally the treatment offered. Mastectomy may be needed for more extensive or multifocal involvement. Use of tamoxifen in stage 0 breast cancer is controversial, and benefits of treatment may not outweigh risks.[3]

For stage 1 and stage 2 invasive cancer, lumpectomy (breast-conserving surgery) with sentinel node biopsy is favored when it is followed by radiation therapy. The addition of radiation therapy improves long-term survival on par with mastectomy. Full axillary lymph node dissection is favored in patients with palpable lymph nodes or a positive sentinel node. Sentinel node biopsy has a sensitivity of 95%.[94-98] This procedure reduces the occurrence of lymphedema in the affected arm and breast. Lymphedema can cause arm and breast swelling and pain, numbness, and decreased mobility in the affected arm.[3]

Other therapies to reduce estrogen stimulation in select women include oophorectomy and ovarian ablation.[3]

Radiation Therapy

Radiation therapy to the entire involved breast is recommended after breast-conserving surgical therapy and should occur within 7 months after surgery for optimal benefit. Radiation therapy reduces risk of local recurrence within 5 years from 7% to 26% (number needed to treat [NNT] = 5). Reduction in 15-year mortality is 30.5% to 35.9% (NNT = 18).[99] Brachytherapy and shorter radiation therapy regimens are currently being evaluated.[3]

Pharmacologic Agents

Chemotherapy, endocrine therapies, and targeted molecular therapies are used in conjunction with surgical and radiation therapies for prevention of recurrence and for cure or control of disease. Tumors larger than 1 cm and positive lymph nodes are generally treated with chemotherapy. Hormone receptor–negative tumors have improved outcomes with chemotherapy compared with hormone receptor–positive tumors.[100] Regimens including anthracyclines and taxanes have improved disease-free intervals and improved survival in both premenopausal and postmenopausal women and may have small increased benefit in patients with ERBB2.[101-103] Herbs can interfere with both anthracyclines and taxanes by preventing drug conversion to its active form in the liver.[1]

Endocrine therapies are effective only in hormone receptor–positive women. These agents (including selective estrogen receptor modulators such as tamoxifen; aromatase inhibitors such as anastrozole, exemestane, and letrozole; and gonadotropin-releasing hormone agonists such as goserelin)

either block or prevent estrogen production to reduce stimulation of estrogen-sensitive tumor cells. Tamoxifen reduces 15-year mortality by 9.2% (NNT = 11).[3,104]

> Tamoxifen is used in premenopausal women; aromatase inhibitors (anastrozole) are more effective in postmenopausal women. Use of tamoxifen in stage 0 breast cancer is controversial, and benefits of treatment may not outweigh risks.[3]

Overexpression of ERBB2 occurs in 20% to 30% of early-stage breast cancers. This characteristic of certain breast cancers has a worse prognosis. Trastuzumab is a humanized anti-ERBB2 monoclonal antibody that improves effectiveness of treatment with anthracyclines and taxanes but carries a 2% to 3% risk of cardiac toxicity during a 2-year period.[105,106]

In stage III locally advanced breast cancers, chemotherapy often precedes surgery, radiation therapy, or both. In this stage, tumors are often larger. There may be extensive lymph node involvement, invasion into the chest wall, or inflammatory breast cancer. These tumors do not have distant metastases. Outcomes are similar to those of early breast cancer treatment if a favorable response is achieved with induction chemotherapy. Tumor decrease can allow breast-conserving surgery, usually with axillary lymph node dissection. If chemotherapy is not successful, mastectomy is often the surgical treatment option. Endocrine therapy is generally not used in the induction phase unless advanced age or the patient's preference makes chemotherapy a less desirable option. Trastuzumab is generally not used in the induction phase, but it is used postoperatively for 12 months. Radiation therapy is generally advised after induction chemotherapy (even if complete remission occurs) and surgery to help prevent local recurrence.[3]

 More information on this topic can be found online at expertconsult.com.

New Biomarkers and Treatments

New biomarkers are being identified that will help indicate which patients with breast cancer are at low risk for recurrence and may not benefit from adjuvant chemotherapy. The Oncotype DX assay helps identify patients with node-negative disease who have low risk of recurrence by identifying the expression of 21 genes. These markers will help individualize approaches to treatment of patients with conventional therapies that have the highest benefit with least harm.[3] These markers might also help identify those patients most likely to benefit from alternative and complementary therapies as well.

Integrative Management of Side Effects From Breast Cancer Treatment

Block[107,108] has described chronomodulation of chemotherapy to help reduce toxicities of chemotherapy. Chronomodulation involves not only the optimal timing of chemotherapy but also strengthening of circadian rhythms. Interventions to strengthen these rhythms include lifestyle modifications (diet, exercise) and mind-body therapies, all of which increase melatonin levels in the brain at night, producing a more restful and restorative and healing sleep. Inflammatory and stress hormones that disrupt the circadian rhythm can be addressed with herbs, diet, supplements, and mind-body therapies (meditation and meditative movement), which optimize the internal biochemical milieu.

Cannabinoids are used in symptom management of nausea and vomiting, anorexia, and pain, including neuropathic pain (see Chapter 80, End-of-Life Care, for description of use in symptom management). Cannabinoids may also have a role as anticancer agents.[109]

Fatigue

Exercise throughout treatment for cancer and beyond is essential to help prevent fatigue and weakness from muscle mass loss. Rest, if it is not balanced with gentle exercise, can increase fatigue rather than alleviate it. Initial weight loss with cancer treatment is often associated with muscle mass loss. In general, cancer treatment causes weight gain, and this can be alleviated with regular exercise within an individual's limitations.[33,110]

An 8-week acupuncture course in one study reduced fatigue and other symptoms that can contribute to fatigue, such as depression, anxiety, and pain.[111] In a small study, Takahashi[112] found that acupuncture could help relieve fatigue, dyspnea, and constipation in terminal cancer patients.

Vasomotor Instability

In a systematic review of nonhormonal interventions for hot flashes in women with a history of breast cancer, relaxation was the only nonpharmaceutical intervention that reduced hot flashes significantly. Black cohosh and other botanicals were not evaluated. Only one study of acupuncture and a few other complementary and alternative medicine therapies was included; the interventions of vitamin E, acupuncture, and magnetic devices did not show evidence of benefit. Clonidine, selective serotonin reuptake inhibitors, selective norepinephrine reuptake inhibitors, and gabapentin showed mild to modest benefits in reducing the number and intensity of hot flashes.[113] Evening primrose oil is a botanical occasionally used in treatment of menopausal symptoms such as hot flashes that can occur with cancer treatment. There is insufficient evidence to recommend it for this indication.[114]

Twelve weeks of acupuncture versus venlafaxine was found to be equivalent in effectiveness to control hot flashes in hormone receptor–positive breast cancer patients in a randomized controlled trial. Both groups experienced decrease in hot flashes and improvement in depressed mood and quality of life. The drug group had numerous side effects, whereas the acupuncture group experienced improved libido, energy, thinking, and well-being.[115] Acupuncture reduced hot flashes and night sweats in a study of breast cancer patients receiving tamoxifen. Emotional and physical well-being were also improved without significant side effects.[116] In another randomized controlled trial, 10 weeks of acupuncture versus sham acupuncture significantly decreased day and night hot flashes in breast cancer patients receiving tamoxifen.[117]

In one large study, phytoestrogen botanicals and black cohosh, used to treat vasomotor symptoms, were found to lower risk of invasive breast cancer in postmenopausal women.[118] In a large study, black cohosh was not effective in decreasing hot flashes, but another smaller study did show a positive effect.[62] Of note, black cohosh is not estrogenic.[119] Black cohosh may cause liver toxicity and needs to be used with caution. It is not recommended during chemotherapy, and evidence for its benefits is inconclusive.

Atrophic Vaginitis

See Chapter 56, Vaginal Dryness, for recommendations on nonhormonal lubricants.

Osteopenia and Osteoporosis

Strength training and weight-bearing exercise are known to help prevent bone loss in postmenopausal women. Yoga is a form of meditative exercise that can also help maintain bone mineral density. Other strategies to help maintain bone health are vitamin D and calcium. One clinical trial of weight training in postmenopausal breast cancer survivors showed that a 24-month weight training program with adherence greater than 50% improved bone mineral density. Both groups took bisphosphonates, vitamin D, and calcium but were randomized to the program or no exercise.[120]

Nausea and Vomiting

Moxibustion, which stimulates acupuncture points with heat generated from burning herbal preparations, was evaluated in several clinical trials; some evidence showed that this therapy could significantly reduce nausea and vomiting in patients undergoing chemotherapy.[121] The National Institutes of Health endorsed acupuncture for chemotherapy-associated nausea.[122] The Society of Integrative Oncology, on review of the evidence, also strongly endorsed acupuncture for this indication.[32] Acupressure of acupuncture point 6 at the wrist, sometimes stimulated with specialized wrist bands, can alleviate chemotherapy-related nausea[32,123] (see Chapter 108, Acupuncture for Nausea and Vomiting).

Lee et al[124] found that nausea intensity was less in breast cancer patients receiving adjuvant chemotherapy or radiation therapy who engaged in moderate exercise as opposed to no exercise.

Ginger (Zingiber officinale)
Ginger can help alleviate nausea. It has been found efficacious for nausea associated with chemotherapy but not for postoperative nausea. Its mechanism of action is unknown, but ginger appears to have a prokinetic effect.[125]

▪ Dosage
Take 500 to 1000 mg of ginger root extract every 4 to 6 hours as needed, or eat 1 tsp or 5 g of crystallized ginger every 2 to 3 hours as needed.

▪ Precautions
Ginger candy or tea is less potent than the root and may yield antinausea effects that do not interfere with certain chemotherapy agents.[1]

Side effects are rare. Excessive doses can cause heartburn.

Anxiety, Stress, and Depression

One 8-week acupuncture course significantly improved anxiety and depression in patients with advanced cancer. It also helped improve psychological distress and life satisfaction.[111]

An 8-week mindfulness-based stress reduction (MBSR) program improved depression and medical symptoms, mindfulness, coping with illness and stress, and sense of coherence after completion of the primary cancer treatment.[126] In another study on MBSR in cancer patients, similar results were found.[127] In a study of MBSR by Kieviet-Stijnen et al,[128] positive effects on mood and vitality strengthened 1 year after completion of the program. A study of an 8-week program using imagery found positive results on anxiety, stress, and depression.[129]

Art therapy can be helpful in improving general quality of life measures, including physical and psychological functioning, in breast cancer patients undergoing radiation therapy.[130]

Anxiety can be managed effectively with exercise. Yoga in particular can help with anxiety, depression, mood, and quality of life with its meditative and restorative movement.[131,132]

Massage can help relieve anxiety and stress during chemotherapy.[133] The Society of Integrative Oncology also strongly endorsed massage for anxiety during cancer treatment.[32] Art therapy, dance, journaling, and aromatherapy all have positive effects on anxiety, depression, and quality of life.[62]

Support groups can be helpful with improvements in mood, less anxiety and depression, better coping, and decrease in pain, but the survival benefits reported by Spiegel et al[134] in 1989 have not been duplicated in subsequent studies.[135-138] In a review of psychosocial interventions, Zimmerman et al[139] found that psychoeducation had the strongest effect size for breast cancer patients. Other psychological interventions led by a psychologist were conducted individually. In a meta-analysis of 116 mind-body therapies, guided imagery, biofeedback, cognitive-behavioral therapy, meditation, relaxation, and hypnosis were effective in improving mood states, coping, anxiety, and depression.[140]

Insomnia and Other Sleep Disturbances

Good sleep hygiene can help induce sleep at night when production of melatonin is optimal. Minimizing sleep during the day, exercising regularly, sleeping in a quiet dark room, and going to sleep at a similar time each night promote sleep. Relaxation, meditation, and yoga can have positive effects on melatonin and sleep states.[141] Cognitive-behavioral therapy has also shown positive effects on sleep.[142]

Regular exercise can help reinforce normal circadian rhythm and maximum endogenous melatonin production by increasing awakeness during the day and sleep at night.[33] Melatonin in supplemental form can also be helpful.

Breast cancer survivors tend to have 10% more sleep disturbances even long term compared with age-matched women without breast cancer. These sleep disturbances in both groups are associated with hot flashes, depression, more distress, and worse physical conditioning.[143] Breast cancer survivors tended to do less physical activity and had more hot flashes than did women without breast cancer[144] (see Chapter 8, Insomnia).

Pain and Peripheral Neuropathy

Pain and other uncomfortable neurologic sensations can occur in posttreatment breast cancer survivors. In 1543 patients studied, Gartner et al[145] found that 47% of women reported pain, and 13% of this group had severe pain. Pain was associated with young age (younger than 40 years) and adjuvant radiation therapy; axillary lymph node dissection was associated with increased likelihood of pain compared with sentinel lymph node dissection; and pain complaints from other parts of the body were associated with increased risk of pain in the surgical area. Pain was not associated with chemotherapy. Women undergoing mastectomy versus breast-conserving surgery did not significantly differ in frequency of reporting pain, but pain was generally more severe in patients reporting pain after mastectomy. Thus, type of surgical technique and radiation therapy do affect chronic pain incidence during and after treatment of breast cancer.

Acupuncture can help with pain relief. One study showed improved pain scores and psychological functioning with an 8-week course of acupuncture.[111] The Society for Integrative Oncology, on review of the literature, strongly endorsed acupuncture for this indication.[32] Massage can also be helpful in relieving pain.[32]

Exercise (a walking intervention) during radiation therapy and chemotherapy can attenuate the negative side effects on physical functioning, increase cardiorespiratory fitness, and reduce pain in breast cancer patients, especially in those who are younger.[39]

Cannabinoids can help with neuropathic pain associated with the neuropathy that can be caused by some chemotherapeutic agents, such as taxanes and platinum-derived drugs.[109]

Lymphedema and Musculoskeletal Issues

Concerns are expressed by clinicians that exercise involving the upper extremities might increase lymphedema. In a review of exercise programs in the recovery of breast cancer patients, early exercise with the upper extremities improved shoulder function and range of motion but did not increase lymphedema. Early exercise interventions were superior to delayed exercise interventions.[146] In a randomized controlled trial of progressive weightlifting twice weekly in patients with breast cancer, this program did not exacerbate lymphedema but instead reduced lymphedema and its symptoms and increased strength.[147]

Moderate exercise can help relieve limited range of motion of the shoulder, pain, and fatigue during radiation therapy in breast cancer patients.[148]

Aromatase inhibitors can cause arthralgias and joint stiffness. In a randomized controlled trial of acupuncture, these symptoms were significantly relieved.[149] Acupuncture also increased shoulder range of motion and decreased lymphedema and its symptoms of heaviness and tightening in a small study by Alem and Gurgel.[150]

Massage can help with pain and edema control. Massage is recommended only with a trained health professional in this area of treatment. Deep massage into vulnerable tissue is not recommended.[32]

Dermatitis From Radiation Therapy

Calendula cream applied multiple times daily to the skin being irradiated can reduce the severity of dermatitis from therapy.[151]

PREVENTION PRESCRIPTION

- Eat primarily a plant-based diet rich in cruciferous vegetables (broccoli, cauliflower, Brussels sprouts, cabbage, and kale). Eat one or two servings of cruciferous vegetables daily.
- Follow an antiinflammatory and Mediterranean diet. This diet avoids saturated fat in dairy and meats; it has no trans-fats and includes increased amounts of omega-3 fatty acids (ocean fish, walnuts, soybeans, greens, flaxseed meal). See Chapter 86, The Antiinflammatory Diet.
- Avoid processed foods.
- Organic foods are not contaminated with pesticides and herbicides. Many organic meats, poultry, and produce can be purchased from local farms or farmers' markets.
- Fatty fish such as herring, mackerel, tuna, salmon, and sardines have high levels of omega-3 fatty acids. Minimize your eating of albacore tuna, shark, swordfish, king mackerel, and tile fish because they can have higher levels of contamination with mercury. You may want to take omega-3 supplements that are detoxified. Fish, however, is an excellent protein source. Eat fish often (three times per week or less) or take fish oil supplements daily. (If you eat fish high in omega-3 content, do not take your fish oil supplements that day.)
- Do not skip meals. If breakfast is a problem, try protein-fortified smoothies in the morning. Whey protein powder is best, and if you are lactose intolerant, buy whey protein powder without lactose.
- Drink lots of water, filtered if possible. Bring it with you everywhere (reuse water bottles). Flavor it with lime or lemon (or cucumber, orange, or any other natural flavor you like).
- Drink green tea, two or three cups a day.
- Moderate alcohol intake if you drink alcohol (no more than one serving per day for women). Do not drink it at all if it makes you feel not well.
- Mushrooms contribute to a healthy diet, especially adding medicinal mushrooms (i.e., maitake, shiitake, reishi, turkey tail) as food or supplement.
- Eat one to three servings of soy food daily. Avoid soy (isoflavone) supplements.
- Eat one or two tablespoons of flaxseed meal daily.
- Vitamin D can be obtained from adequate sun exposure or a supplement. For most people, 2000 units/day will maintain adequate levels. I recommend determination of a 25-hydroxyvitamin D level in winter to asses for adequate intake.
- Maintain healthy weight with a BMI of less than 30 and ideally 25 (not overweight).
- Avoid smoking and passive tobacco exposure.
- Exercise for 30 to 60 minutes at least 5 days a week (more than 3 hours per week is recommended). Combine aerobic activity such as walking with a resistance or strength training program two or three times a week. Nordic walking sticks can increase the overall conditioning of walking while improving posture, balance, and core strengthening. Yoga, tai chi, and qi gong are meditative movement with the benefit of relaxation and exercise. Do exercise that is enjoyable to you.
- Optimize sleep at night. Melatonin can be added if sleeping difficulties are occurring, starting at 3 mg before bed. Sleep in a darkened room at regular hours to improve sleep quality. Do not sleep with a television on in the bedroom.
- Maintain spiritual practices that give meaning and relaxation to your life.
- Maintain a strong support network with family and friends.
- Consider testing for a 2-hydroxyestrone/16-hydroxyestrone ratio, and consider interventions to improve the ratio in favor of weak estrogens. (See the Appendix for laboratories that offer this testing.)
- Minimize use of estrogen replacement medication. For menopausal symptoms, consider nonhormonal measures first.
- Attend to self-care every day. Make healthy lifestyle choices a part of your routine.

THERAPEUTIC REVIEW

Nutrition

- The Mediterranean diet can lower the risk of breast cancer and other chronic health conditions, such as heart disease, diabetes, and obesity. This diet is high in omega-3 and omega-9 fatty acids; add five to nine servings of fruit and vegetables per day.

- Cruciferous vegetables are beneficial in a healthy diet to decrease cancer risk.

- In general, antioxidants are preferably obtained in food rather than in supplements.

- Three cups of green tea per day can decrease breast cancer risk.

- Soy foods in moderation are safe and protective for breast cancer. One to three servings of soy foods daily are recommended. Avoid isolated isoflavone supplements.

- Flaxseed meal can lower breast cancer risk.

- Avoid excessive alcohol intake. Drink no more than one alcoholic beverage daily.

Continued

- Weight control and gradual weight loss if the patient is obese or very overweight can reduce risk of breast cancer. Weight loss can be achieved with regular exercise, portion control, and eating more fruits and vegetables and fewer calorie-dense foods. [A ↑ 1]

- Vitamin D in supplement form when adequate sun exposure is not available is important for bone health, anticancer effect, immunity, and muscle health. Higher levels of vitamin D are associated with decreased risk of breast cancer. Monitor levels of 25-hydroxyvitamin D in the winter to ensure adequate intake of vitamin D_3. [A ↑ 1]

- Medicinal mushrooms have many potential beneficial effects during cancer treatment and can be part of a healthy diet. [C → 1]

Medication

- Avoid prolonged HRT of both estrogen and progesterone. [A ↑ 1]

- Nonhormonal therapies for postmenopausal symptoms of hot flashes can be effective. These include regular exercise, medications, and acupuncture. [A ↑ 1]

- Tamoxifen is commonly used for ER^+ tumors for 5 years after treatment to prevent recurrence. The dose is 20 mg daily. [A ↗ 2]

- Aromatase inhibitors (anastrozole, exemestane, letrozole) are used in postmenopausal treatment of breast cancer to prevent recurrence. [A ↗ 2]

Exercise

- Exercising more than 3 hours per week can decrease cancer risk. [A ↑ 1]

Lifestyle

- Sleep is important in decreasing cancer risk. Melatonin is implicated in this mechanism of reduced cancer cell proliferation when melatonin levels are high. Supplemental melatonin can help improve circadian rhythms and quality of sleep. The dose is 1 to 3 mg at bedtime. Up to 20 mg has been used. [B → 2]

- Psychological interventions can be helpful in cancer care. Those most helpful are psychoeducation and psychotherapy conducted by a psychotherapist individually. [A ↑ 1]

- Mindfulness-based stress reduction programs can enhance well-being and coping and decrease anxiety during and after treatment. See Table 75-1. [A ↑ 1]

TABLE 75-1. Integrative Medicine and Breast Cancer Treatment Symptoms

SYMPTOM	TREATMENT	EVIDENCE VS. HARM RATING
Fatigue	Exercise	A ↑ 1
	Acupuncture	B ↗ 1
Postmenopausal symptoms of hot flashes	Medications such as selective serotonin reuptake inhibitors, selective norepinephrine reuptake inhibitors, and gabapentin	A ↗ 2
	Acupuncture	A ↑ 1
	Exercise	A ↑ 1
Nausea and vomiting due to chemotherapy	Acupuncture	A ↑ 1
	Ginger	B ↗ 1
	Cannabis	B → 2
Anxiety, stress, and depression	Acupuncture	B ↗ 1
	Mindfulness-based stress reduction	A ↑ 1
	Art therapy	B ↗ 1
	Exercise	A ↑ 1
	Yoga	B ↗ 1
	Massage	A ↑ 1
	Support groups	A ↑ 1
Insomnia	Exercise	A ↑ 1
	Melatonin	A ↗ 2
	Relaxation techniques	B ↗ 1
	Sleep hygiene	A ↑ 1
Pain and peripheral neuropathy	Acupuncture	A ↑ 1
	Exercise	A ↑ 1
	Cannabinoids	A ↗ 2
	Massage	A ↑ 1
	Mind-body therapies	A ↑ 1
Lymphedema	Acupuncture	B ↗ 1
	Exercise	A ↑ 1
Radiation dermatitis	Calendula cream	B ↗ 1

Modified from Deng G, Cassileth BR, Yeung KS. Complementary therapies for cancer-related symptoms. *J Support Oncol.* 2004;2:419–426.

KEY WEB RESOURCES

www.bmj.com/cgi/content-nw/full/337/jul11_2/a540/FIG3 (login to *British Medical Journal* required to view)	Adjuvant therapy predictor for breast cancer Predicts what chemotherapy and endocrine or targeted therapies might be helpful, given tumor markers and staging
http://www.cancer.gov/bcrisktool/Default.aspx	National Cancer Institute Breast Cancer Risk Assessment Tool
InspireHealth Integrated Cancer Care *Research Updates* To subscribe to newsletters, email: mwiebe@inspirehealth.ca; hard copy or electronic copy Phone: 604-734-7125 #200-1330 West 8th Avenue, Vancouver, BC V6H 4A6	Summary of important research studies that inform integrative cancer care International studies are reviewed.
American Cancer Society: http://www.cancer.org/Cancer/BreastCancer/index?ssSourceSiteId=null	Monographs cited in references on the research of exercise and nutrition in the prevention of cancer and during and after cancer treatment
Susan G. Komen Breast Cancer Foundation: ww5.komen.org	Dedicated to education and research about causes, treatment, and search for a cure
Society for Integrative Oncology: www.integrativeonc.org Deng GE, Frenkel M, Cohen L, et al. Evidence-based clinical practice guidelines for integrative oncology: complementary therapies and botanicals. *J Soc Integr Oncol.* 2009;7:85-120.	International organization of clinicians, researchers, and others interested in evidence-based integrative oncology A monograph is available for integrative oncology practice guidelines.
Breast Cancer Recovery: www.bcrecovery.org	Breast Cancer Recovery's mission is to help women heal mind, body, and spirit after breast cancer. All programs are designed and conducted by survivors for survivors.
National Institutes of Health National Cancer Institute (NCI): http://www.cancer.gov/cancertopics/cam/ Office of Cancer Complementary and Alternative Medicine (OCCAM): http://www.cancer.gov/cam/	Evidence-based information on complementary and alternative medicine and its applications in oncology
National Institutes of Health, Office of Dietary Supplements: http://ods.od.nih.gov/research/pubmed_dietary_supplement_subset.aspx	Provides information on dietary supplements. The PubMed Dietary Supplement Subset succeeds the International Bibliographic Information on Dietary Supplements (IBIDS) database active from 1999-2010.
Memorial Sloan-Kettering Cancer Center: http://www.mskcc.org/cancer-care/integrative-medicine/about-herbs-botanicals-other-products	A searchable database provides evidence-based information on herbs, botanicals, vitamins, and other supplements. It includes evaluations of alternative or unproven cancer therapies.
The University of Texas MD Anderson Cancer Center Complementary and Integrative Medicine Educational Resources: www.mdanderson.org/CIMER	Evidence-based review of complementary and alternative medicine and integrative medicine therapies

 Also see Table 75-2e online at expertconsult.com for further reading on integrative oncology.

References

References are available online at expertconsult.com.

Acknowledgments

Thank you to Amye Tevaarwerk, MD, for reviewing this manuscript and to Mary Stone and Char Luchterhand for technical assistance.

Chapter 76

Lung Cancer

Wadie I. Najm, MD, MSEd

Lung cancer is the second most common type of cancer in the United States and the leading cause of cancer death in both men (accounting for 29% of deaths due to cancer) and women (accounting for 26%). The annual percentage change based on incidence of new cases in men decreased by 1.8% between 1991 and 2006. For women, the annual percentage change based on incidence increased by 0.4% between 1991 and 2006. Mortality began leveling off in 1995 after increasing for several decades. Deaths from lung cancer decreased in men but remained stable in women from 2003 to 2006. The lifetime probability for development of lung cancer is 1 in 13 in men and 1 in 16 in women. The 5-year survival rate is poor (16%), often owing to the late diagnosis.[1]

Pathophysiology

There are two major types of lung cancer: small cell lung cancer (SCLC), which accounts for 10% to 15%; and non–small cell lung cancer (NSCLC), which encompasses squamous cell carcinoma, large cell carcinoma, and adenocarcinoma (the most common form). Lung cancer that has features of both types is identified as mixed small cell/large cell cancer.

Tobacco Use

It is well documented that cigarette smokers have a higher risk of morbidity from cardiovascular disease, pulmonary disease, and various cancers. Approximately 85% to 90% of lung cancers are believed to be due to tobacco smoking. Squamous cell carcinoma and small cell carcinoma are most commonly associated with smoking. Actually, it is uncommon for someone who has never smoked to have SCLC. The risk for lung cancer increases with earlier age of smoking, number of cigarettes, number of years smoked, extent of inhalation, and higher tar content of cigarettes. Smoking of low-tar cigarettes, pipes, or cigars does not reduce the risk of acquiring lung cancer. The risk declines gradually after a person quits smoking, reaching the risk level of nonsmokers after 20 to 25 years.

Passive smoking has been the subject of intense discussion as an additional cause of lung cancer. In 2000, the National Institutes of Health declared passive smoking a known human carcinogen.[2] Passive smoking is responsible for approximately 3000 lung cancer deaths each year in nonsmoking adults.

Exposure to the gas phase and the aqueous tar extracts of tobacco induces mitochondrial DNA damage and lowers levels of plasma antioxidants. Because mitochondria play a central role in apoptosis, tobacco-induced mitochondrial DNA damage would cause cells to forgo apoptosis.

Other Environmental Carcinogens

Other environmental carcinogens are capable of generating reactive oxygen species, which in turn can lead to DNA damage. Asbestos, arsenic, chromium, nickel, tar, mineral oils, mustard gas, radon, silica, diesel exhaust, ionizing radiation, and bis(chloromethyl)ether have been implicated in lung cancer.

Screening

Chest Radiography

The sensitivity of chest radiography for lung cancer detection depends on the location and size of the lesion and the skill of the interpreting physician. Use of chest radiography has a limited potential in screening for lung cancer, particularly in comparison with newer technologies with higher resolution. A review concluded that the evidence does not support the use of chest radiography (with or without sputum cytology) as a screening test for lung cancer.[3]

Spiral (Helical) Computed Tomography

Spiral (helical) computed tomography (CT) is a low–radiation dose radiologic modality in which multiple thin-slice (5-mm) images are obtained and then assembled into a three-dimensional model of the anatomic structures examined. Evidence obtained from an ongoing clinical trial, the

Early Lung Cancer Action Project (ELCAP), suggests that the cure rate of screen-diagnosed lung cancer, using the trial's regimen of CT screening, may exceed 70%, compared with 10% for usual care and 20% for chest radiography.[4] Current observational and prevalence studies on the role of spiral CT screening have failed to establish whether it has an impact on improved disease-free survival, despite consistently higher early detection rates of lung cancer.[5]

The National Cancer Institute reported that annual CT scans of current and former smokers may detect early cancers and reduce the risk of death by 20%. The U.S. Preventive Services Task Force makes no recommendations for the use of CT in an asymptomatic person.[6]

Sputum Cytology

Sputum cytology was evaluated in a large multicenter lung cancer screening trial, but this modality did not positively predict lung cancer development. Results of the National Cancer Institute cooperative trials showed no added benefit over chest radiography.[7]

Positron Emission Tomography

Positron emission tomography is increasingly being used for cancer staging. The absence of glucose uptake is a reliable criterion to exclude malignant change; however, false-positive findings can occur in inflammatory conditions (e.g., pneumonia, granulomatous diseases).

Laser Bronchoscopy

In laser technology, light of a special wavelength can be used to stimulate different intracellular components (fluorophores, which include flavins, riboflavins, nucleic acids, and proteins) to emit a spectral pattern specific to the particular tissue. By use of this principle, laser bronchoscopy can differentiate dysplastic from neoplastic tissue, which contains altered levels of fluorophores. The usefulness of this technique for lung cancer screening remains uncertain.[8]

Genetic and Other Biomarkers

Mutations of the *p53* gene have been found in approximately 50% of persons with NSCLC and in bronchial dysplasia. However, use of *p53* mutation as a biomarker is limited by technical difficulty and variability of its detection.

Another biomarker being investigated as a screening tool is the K-*ras* gene. However, owing to the gene's low prevalence in NSCLC (30% of the cases), K-*ras* gene assay is not an effective screening method.

In up to 80% of smokers, evidence of loss of heterozygosity (loss of one chromosomal allele) or genomic instability (loss or gain of genetic material within a chromosomal region) in bronchial tissue can be demonstrated. Use of these markers as intermediate end points in lung cancer prevention studies is under investigation.

Another potentially useful biomarker is the retinoic acid receptor-beta, levels of which are reduced in bronchial metaplasia, dysplasia, and NSCLC.

A rise in the level of the epidermal growth factor receptor (EGFR) has been noted in bronchial metaplasia, and proliferating cell nuclear antigen (PCNA) levels are increased in dividing cells and in NSCLC. Both EGFR and PCNA assays may therefore prove useful in lung cancer screening.

Integrative Therapy

In addition to the measures discussed here, Table 76-1 lists resources that clinicians may find valuable in treatment of patients with lung cancer.

Lifestyle

Smoking Cessation

There is abundant evidence that smoking cessation is the single most important factor in reducing the incidence of lung cancer. Patients should be counseled to abstain from smoking. Various products and programs, such as acupuncture, hypnosis, bupropion (Zyban), and nicotine analogues (gum, patch), are available to assist in smoking cessation, and the costs of these interventions are covered by some insurance providers (see Table 76-1).

> Smoking cessation is the single most important factor in lung cancer prevention.

TABLE 76-1. Resources for Treatment of Patients With Lung Cancer

Cancer Trials A great resource for up-to-date information on ongoing trials and preliminary results of ongoing studies	Web site: http://cancertrials.nci.nih.gov Telephone: 1-800-4-CANCER
National Center for Complementary and Alternative Medicine (NCCAM) An excellent resource for different complementary and alternative medicine information, research centers, and database; also a connection to other relevant agencies in the National Institutes of Health	Web site: http://nccam.nih.gov
American Cancer Society A rich source of information on prevention and treatment options for professionals and consumers; a great site for national and local resources and for general information on some dietary supplements	Web site: http://www.cancer.org/ Telephone: 1-800-227-2345
Helpful Smoking Cessation Resources Centers for Disease Control and Prevention: "How to Quit" for support in quitting, including coaching, a free quit plan, educational materials, and referrals to local resources	Web site: http://www.cdc.gov/tobacco/quit_smoking/ Telephone: 1-800-QUIT-NOW (1-800-784-8669)
Quit Smoking Today!	Web site: http://www.smokefree.gov/
Office of the Surgeon General	Web site: http://www.surgeongeneral.gov/tobacco/

Exercise

The evidence, albeit limited, suggests that exercise may limit the development of lung cancer. The exact mechanism for this action remains unclear.

Nutrition

Major limitations of the assessment of nutritional approaches to the prevention of lung cancer are the low accuracy of dietary questionnaires and the poor specificity of instruments used to collect the information. Case-control studies of subjects with lung cancer found that high sugar and saturated fat intake increased the risk of lung cancer.[9,10] The joint effect of pack-years, total fat intake, and sucrose intake was associated with an increased risk of 28.3 (95% confidence interval [CI], 13.4-59.7) of the three variables. A large case-cohort study conducted during 13.3 years in The Netherlands found an inverse association between acrylamide intake (fried French fries, potato crisps) and lung cancer (adenocarcinoma) in women, but no association was found in men.[11]

> Acrylamide is a potential carcinogen that is produced when starchy foods (French fries, potato chips) are heated with frying or baking, but not boiling. Cigarette smoking and coffee are significant sources of acrylamide.

Other evidence points to a potential beneficial effect of some nutrients. Consumption of green leafy vegetables and carrots has been strongly correlated with a reduction in the risk of lung cancer. The protective effect persisted after tobacco use was removed as a possible confounder of results. Consumption of cruciferous vegetables (broccoli, Brussels sprouts, cauliflower, mustard greens, turnips, and rutabagas) has been suggested to have a protective effect against cancer of the aerodigestive tract owing to their high content of glucosinolates. Prospective cohort studies and case-control studies have yielded mixed results. However, consumption of *Brassica* vegetables, particularly cabbage, appears to have an inverse association with cancer risk. A large European study found that consumption of a variety of vegetables is inversely associated with lung cancer risk among current smokers.[12] Risk of squamous cell carcinomas was reduced with increasing variety in fruit and vegetable consumption.

Other types of food—meat, fish, eggs, and legumes— have not been shown to have a protective effect. A cohort study conducted in The Netherlands found no relation between the consumption of onions, leeks, or garlic and a reduction in risk of lung cancer.[13] An observational study on the consumption of black tea did not show a protective effect against lung cancer.[13,14]

Botanicals

Green Tea

Animal studies point to a possible protective effect of the polyphenolic fraction and water extract of green tea. Green tea has been shown to inhibit the formation of DNA strand and lipid peroxidation in cultured human lung cells,[15] and its consumption with meals may inhibit the formation of nitrosamines. In animal studies, green tea reduced lung oncogene expression by induction of phase II enzymes, inhibition of tumor necrosis factor-alpha expression and release, inhibition of cell proliferation, and induction of apoptosis,[16,17] and it was very effective in inhibiting lung carcinogenesis induced by asbestos and benzo[a] pyrene.[18,19] Results of human studies on the role of green tea in lung cancer prevention remain limited and inconclusive.[20] Few studies indicate a small beneficial association, particularly among never-smokers.[21] Better-designed studies are needed to evaluate the effect of green tea for cancer prevention. Although green tea is considered safe, precautions should be taken to limit its intake in pregnant and lactating women because of its significant caffeine content. Decaffeinated forms are available.

Ginseng

Results of animal studies of ginseng in cancer suggest variable outcomes based on the type and age of ginseng used. The majority of studies have indicated a tendency for Panax ginseng to decrease the incidence of lung cancer. In laboratory studies, an acidic polysaccharide, ginsan, was found to be safe and effective in lowering the incidence of lung cancer[22]; a purified ginseng saponin also resulted in G_1 phase arrest with progression to apoptosis[23]; and the oral administration of lipid-soluble red ginseng extract to mice bearing lung cancer cells showed a potent anticancer activity.[24] Human studies showed a dose-response inhibitory effect. Smokers who used ginseng had a lower odds ratio (OR) for development of lung cancer than nonusers did; these results were substantiated by a cohort study (relative risk [RR], 0.3; 95% CI, 0.1-0.7). The available evidence points to a significant preventive effect against cancer for Panax ginseng.[25,26]

Chinese Herbs

Studies of Chinese herbs have focused mainly on their use in the treatment of persons with cancer. In laboratory studies, herbal extracts used routinely in Chinese medicine inhibited the growth of several tumor cells. The possible role of Chinese herbs in the prevention of lung cancer remains to be investigated. A review of clinical and experimental evidence of commonly used compounded Chinese medicines in the treatment of lung cancer was conducted by Tian et al.[27]

Maitake Mushroom

Maitake mushroom has been used in tonics, soups, teas, and herbal formulas by Asian therapists to promote health. Laboratory studies indicate that it has an immune-enhancing effect and inhibits the spread of different tumors.[28,29] These findings remain to be verified by human studies.

Kombucha Tea

Kombucha tea is promoted to enhance and boost the immune system and to fight cancer in the early stages. There is no scientific evidence to support its use. A 2003 systematic review concluded that the undetermined benefits do not outweigh the documented risks.[30] The U.S. Food and Drug Administration has issued a warning to consumers to exercise caution with use of this botanical after two reports of Kombucha-related acidosis.[31]

Supplements

Cancer risk is associated with elevated oxidative stress, accounting for interest in the use of antioxidants such as vitamin C and vitamin E in lowering the risk of lung cancer.

Findings from the VITamins And Lifestyle (VITAL) study (N = 77,125) suggest that some herbals and supplements may be associated with lower risk of lung cancer.[32] A significantly lower risk of lung cancer was associated with use during the previous 10 years of glucosamine (OR, 0.74; 95% CI, 0.58-0.94) and chondroitin (OR, 0.72; 95% CI, 0.54 -0.96). These associations persisted after adjustment for other risk factors. No other herbal or specialty supplement was associated with decreased risk of lung cancer.

Selenium

Selenium is not an antioxidant; however, it is essential for the production of two enzymes that affect the antioxidant network. It is not produced in the body and must be obtained through food. The amount of selenium in foods varies according to the soil in which the food is grown. Foods rich in selenium are garlic, onions, broccoli, egg yolks, and wheat germ.

The exact mechanism by which selenium may prevent cancer is unclear. Proposed mechanisms are through apoptosis, antiandrogen activity, growth inhibitory effects by producing superoxide that activates p53 antioxidant function, and DNA damage.

Several cohort studies have evaluated the effect of selenium serum level on the development of lung cancer.[33,34] Results are controversial; a few studies show an inverse relationship, and others show a direct relationship with lung cancer. Three randomized studies looked at the effect of selenium supplementation on lung cancer prevention.[35-37] A 2004 meta-analysis found some protective effect against lung cancer (RR, 0.74; 95% CI, 0.57-0.97), mainly in populations in which the average selenium level is low.[38] A 10-year phase III clinical trial conducted at the University of Texas M.D. Anderson Cancer Center found that selenium offered no protection against recurrence or onset of a new cancer or second primary cancer. The study was halted because those taking a placebo appeared to be living longer.

Vitamin A, Beta-Carotene, and Retinoids

The term *vitamin A* is popularly used to indicate two different families of dietary factors: retinyl esters, retinol, and retinal (preformed vitamin A); and beta-carotene and other carotenoids (pro–vitamin A) that serve as precursors to vitamin A.[39] The seven predominant carotenoids in human beings are beta-carotene, lycopene, lutein, alpha-carotene, alpha-cryptoxanthin, beta-cryptoxanthin, and zeaxanthin. Different carotenoids are concentrated in different organs. The circulating level of beta-carotene is influenced by retinol intake, or retinol suppresses its conversion to vitamin A.

Several theories have been advanced to explain the role of vitamin A in fighting cancer. Specifically, vitamin A activity may

- have antioxidant properties in conditions of low oxygen tension
- inhibit proliferation and induce differentiation of epithelial cells
- modulate cytochrome P-450

- inhibit arachidonic acid metabolism
- modulate immune function
- induce gap junction communication
- inhibit chromosome instability and damage
- influence apoptosis.[40]

Several studies evaluated the effect of beta-carotene on lung cancer. Diet, serum level, and supplement use were examined. Interest in vitamin A and beta-carotene for the prevention of lung cancer is based on initial animal and epidemiologic data, which suggested a protective effect in lung cancer.[41] Even in early-stage cancer, questions are raised about whether smoking status, type of food, and food ingredient (other than carotenoids) may influence the outcome.

Some of the early epidemiologic studies tried to determine whether the effect of vitamin A or carotenoids differs between genders. Two studies found similar results in both men and women, whereas other studies found a protective effect in men and an adverse effect in women.[42]

Lung cancer risk was reduced in case-control studies[33] with consumption of large quantities of vegetable and fruits; however, this effect was found to be stronger for vegetable and fruit intake than for beta-carotene intake. Prospective and pooled analysis studies looking at the effect of dietary beta-carotene intake on decreasing the risk of lung cancer found a nonsignificant association for alpha-carotene, lutein/zeaxanthin, and lycopene.[42-44] In contrast, beta-cryptoxanthin intake has been found to be inversely associated with lung cancer risk (RR, 0.76; 95% CI, 0.67-0.86).[45] Thus, the inverse relationship found with vegetable and fruit intake was not maintained in beta-carotene studies except for beta-cryptoxanthin.

Plasma or serum beta-carotene levels were found to be lower in several studies exploring the prediagnostic level of beta-carotene in persons in whom lung cancer developed.[46,47] However, interpretation of these studies was based on one measurement taken several years before the onset of cancer.

> Smokers (particularly those who smoke more than 20 cigarettes per day) should avoid vitamin A and beta-carotene supplements.

Studies looking at the association of other carotenoids found an inverse association of lung cancer with dietary intake of lutein and alpha-carotene. Prospective studies, however, failed to establish such an association for lutein, alpha-carotene, or lycopene.[48]

Several multicenter double-blind, controlled trials explored a possible role for beta-carotene supplements in the primary prevention of lung cancer. Two studies, the Alpha-Tocopherol and Beta-Carotene Cancer Prevention (ATBC) study and the Beta-Carotene and Retinol Efficacy Trial (CARET), indicated a higher incidence of lung cancer among the group receiving beta-carotene supplementation. Follow-up data from subjects previously enrolled in the active arm of the CARET indicate persistence of all-cause mortality (RR, 1.12; 95% CI, 0.99-1.17) 6 years after the intervention.[49] In contrast, the Physicians' Health Study (PHS) reported no effect of beta-carotene supplementation on the incidence of lung cancer. The low number of smokers (11%) in the PHS study group may explain the discrepancy. The VITAL study found that longer duration of use of individual retinol was associated with significantly high risk of NSCLC and total lung cancer.[50] Long-term use of individual beta-carotene supplements was associated with elevated SCLC risk, and use of individual lutein supplements was associated with elevated NSCLC. In ATBC and CARET, a higher incidence of lung cancer was noted among smokers, whereas the VITAL study did note a difference between genders or smoking status. Above-average alcohol consumption was also noted to be a predisposing factor.

Vitamin B

In 2001, a case-nested study found significantly lower risk of lung cancer among men who had higher serum vitamin B_6 levels.[51] Those with the highest vitamin B_6 concentration had about half the risk of lung cancer (OR, 0.51; 95% CI, 0.23-0.93). More recently, the European Prospective Investigation into Cancer and Nutrition (EPIC), which investigated the role of vitamin B in lung cancer, observed 519,978 subjects from 10 countries during 12 years.[52] Higher levels of vitamin B_6 (OR, 0.44; 95% CI, 0.33-0.60) and methionine (OR, 0.52; 95% CI, 0.30-0.69) were strongly associated with a reduced risk of lung cancer in people who never smoked, those who quit, and current smokers. Folate, combined with above-average levels of vitamin B_6 and methionine, was associated with a two-thirds reduction in lung cancer risk.

> Vitamin B_6 in high concentrations in the blood has been associated with a lower risk of lung cancer. Foods rich in B_6 include cereal grains, legumes, vegetables, meat, fish, and eggs. B_6 has also been found to be beneficial in the prevention of colon cancer.

Vitamin E

The association between dietary intake of alpha-tocopherol and lung cancer was explored in a few studies, with variable results. In the ATBC study, a protective effect for lung cancer was not demonstrated in a cohort of persons receiving alpha-tocopherol (dose, 50 mg/day). Most cohort studies of serum concentrations of alpha-tocopherol showed no association, except for one study, which showed an inverse relationship. Evidence from a pooled analysis[53] and prospective cohort study[54] confirmed that supplementation with vitamin E is not associated with decreased risk. In fact, the VITAL study reported that prolonged supplementation with high-dose vitamin E is associated with a small increased risk.

Vitamin C

Several prospective studies examined the effect of dietary vitamin C on the risk of lung cancer. The effect of vitamin C and a mixture (vitamins C and E and alpha-lipoic acid) on lipid peroxidation biomarkers was not found to decrease the oxidative stress in passive smokers.[55] In another double-blind study, smokers were randomly allocated to receive antioxidants (500 mg of vitamin C and 400 units of vitamin E per day) or placebo. No effect of antioxidants on benzo[a]pyrene-DNA adducts were seen in male smokers, but a 31% decrease was noted among female participants.[56] Overall, the results do not support a role of vitamin C, although additional studies are needed to evaluate its role.

Vitamin D

In the past few years, interest in vitamin D and its anticancer activities increased significantly. Vitamin D receptor (VDR) gene polymorphisms are reported to influence the cancer risk by their antiproliferative, antiangiogenic, antimetastatic, and apoptotic effects. A small study reported that genetic variation at the VDR locus may influence lung cancer risk, and the association may be modified by age, gender, and smoking.[57] A prospective cohort study that observed 6937 subjects during 24 years found no association between vitamin D and lung cancer (RR, 0.72; 95% CI, 0.43-1.19).[58] However, women and young subjects, with higher levels of vitamin D, were observed to have a lower risk of lung cancer. Evidence is mounting that improved vitamin D status would have a protective effect against the development of cancer, although no agreement has been reached in regard to optimal dose or level. Unfortunately, the lack of high-quality scientific evidence and standardization in testing was reflected in a recent Institute of Medicine report, which concluded that "we could not find solid evidence that consuming more of either nutrient [i.e., vitamin D and calcium] would protect the public from chronic diseases ranging from cancer to diabetes to improved immune function."[59]

Melatonin

Melatonin is popular as an antidote to jet lag and as a sleep aid. It also has antioxidant properties and acts to stimulate the main antioxidant of the brain, glutathione peroxidase. In vitro studies have reported a possible anticancer role. The proposed mechanism is an antiestrogenic activity and augmentation of the anticancer effect of interleukin-2. Melatonin (in a dose of 10 mg/day) has been studied in patients with metastatic NSCLC; results included a higher 1-year survival rate and disease stabilization.[60] The melatonin/cortisol mean nocturnal level ratio was also found to decrease in cancer patients.[61] A reduction in risk of death and low adverse effects were reported by several randomized controlled trials of melatonin treatment in cancer patients. In a 5-year follow-up study, melatonin plus chemotherapy was seen to enhance the quality of life and to prolong survival.[62] The role of melatonin in the prevention of lung cancer is still to be determined.

Pharmaceuticals

Etretinate, a synthetic retinoid, was found in a nonrandomized study to decrease bronchial metaplasia in smokers. However, a randomized study did not substantiate this benefit.[63]

Therapies to Consider

Hypnosis and acupuncture can be helpful as adjuvant or stand-alone therapies in smoking cessation.

PREVENTION PRESCRIPTION

- Patients should be assisted to stop smoking and to avoid smoke-filled areas.
- Appropriate precautions should be taken to prevent possible environmental exposure to known carcinogens and dusts.
- Consumption of *Brassica* vegetables, particularly cabbage, is recommended.
- A low–saturated fat and simple carbohydrate diet should be encouraged.
- Use of green tea (two or three cups a day; three cups = ~300 mg of polyphenols) and ginseng (Panax ginseng, 100 mg daily) in moderate doses may have a preventive effect.
- Intake of vitamin A and beta-carotene should be increased through dietary means by eating yellow, orange, and red fruits and vegetables.
- Use of folate (1 mg) combined with above-average levels of vitamin B_6 (50 mg) may be protective.

THERAPEUTIC REVIEW

■ Remove Exacerbating Factors

- Stop smoking and exposure to passive smoke or chemicals. Consider use of masks and other filters to minimize the exposure to harmful chemicals. A①₁

■ Nutrition

- Encourage the regular consumption of green leafy vegetables and *Brassica* vegetables. B⊘₁
- Avoid foods rich in simple carbohydrates and saturated fats. B⊘₁
- Avoid foods rich in acrylamide, including heated starches such as fried or baked potato products (French fries, potato chips) and coffee. B⊘₁

■ Supplements

- Advise smokers to avoid high and prolonged intake of beta-carotene and vitamin E supplements. A①₁
- Folate (1 mg), combined with above-average levels of vitamin B_6 (50 mg), may have a protective effect. B⊘₁

- Consider recommending a cryptoxanthin-rich smoothie consisting of the following:

  mango, peeled and cubed (can also use peaches, oranges, or watermelon)

  1½ cups plain yogurt (beta-cryptoxanthin is a fat-soluble vitamin and is better absorbed if it is taken with fat)

  ¼ cup frozen tangerine juice concentrate (thawed)

  2 tsp maple syrup

  ½ tsp vanilla extract

- Melatonin, 10 mg at bedtime, may benefit 1-year survival rates in those with metastatic NSCLC.
- Supplement vitamin D to keep serum levels near 50 ng/dL (approximately 1000 units of vitamin D_3 will raise serum levels 8 to 10 points).

■ Botanicals

- Panax ginseng (100 to 200 mg/day) may decrease the incidence of lung cancer among smokers. B→₂
- Glucosamine and chondroitin use may offer a protective effect. B→₂

KEY WEB RESOURCES

http://cancertrials.nci.nih.gov	Up-to-date information on ongoing trials and cancer-related studies sponsored by the National Institutes of Health
http://www.cancer.org/	A rich source of information on prevention and treatment options for professionals and consumers A great site for national and local resources and for general information on some dietary supplements
http://www.cdc.gov/tobacco/quit_smoking/; http://www.smokefree.gov/	Helpful Web sites for smoking cessation
http://acor.org/	Online community support and resources for patients with cancer

References

References are available online at expertconsult.com.

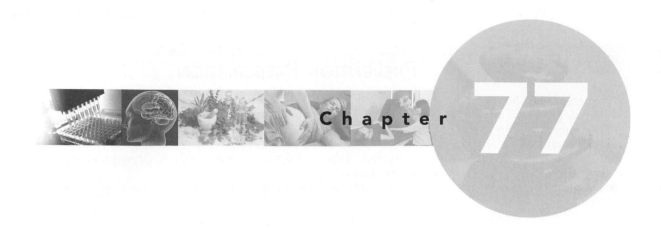

Chapter 77

Prostate Cancer

Mark W. McClure, MD

Etiology

Prostate cancer is the leading cause of cancer and the second leading cause of cancer-related death in men in the United States.[1] Nevertheless, only 3% of men ultimately die as a result of prostate cancer, even though the majority of men will harbor prostate cancer cells (usually undetected) if they live long enough. Among other things, this dichotomy reflects the marked variability in prostate cancer growth rates.

Tumor doubling times can vary from every 2 weeks to 5 years or longer. Faster growing tumors, especially those with dividing times of less than 12 months, are more likely to cause signs and symptoms and premature death if they are left untreated.

At the other end of the spectrum, slower growing tumors, particularly in men older than 65 years, usually remain indolent and are rarely life-threatening. Unfortunately, it is not possible to predict exactly when a prostate cancer becomes life-threatening. Nevertheless, it is possible to modify prostate cancer's behavior.

Prevention

A substantial body of in vitro laboratory and animal data and evolving epidemiologic and human in vivo data suggest that complementary therapies such as dietary and lifestyle interventions, botanical and nutritional supplements, and selected vitamins can complement conventional therapies to modulate the initiation, promotion, and progression of prostate cancer, to improve quality of life, and to prolong survival.[2-8] Encouraged by these findings, researchers are actively pursuing primary and secondary prevention strategies for prostate cancer.[9]

Primary Prevention

The goal of primary prevention is to prevent persons without evidence of clinical prostate cancer from development of invasive, life-threatening disease.[10] Carcinogenesis is a complex multistep process that is characterized by genetic and epigenetic alterations that disrupt immune function and regulation of cellular proliferation, apoptosis, and differentiation. The transformation from a normal to a malignant prostate cell can span decades. Therefore, it may be possible to prevent or even to reverse the neoplastic process, even in patients with a genetic risk for prostate cancer.[11] According to the results of a seminal study that examined cancer incidence among a cohort of 44,788 twins from Sweden, Denmark, and Finland, environmental influences were more important than genetic predisposition as a determinant of prostate cancer risk.[12]

Secondary Prevention

The goals of secondary prevention are to detect and treat men with prostate cancer at a curable stage and to prevent the spread or recurrence of disease. Researchers have identified certain risk factors for the development of prostate cancer, most notably age, family history of prostate cancer, and ethnicity.[12,13]

According to autopsy data, a small percentage of teenagers harbor latent prostate cancer cells, and the incidence of occult prostate cancer in men rises with each decade.[14,15] Among ethnic groups, African American men have one of the highest incidences of prostate cancer. They are 1.6 times more likely than white men and 2.8 times more likely than Asian/Pacific Islander men to develop prostate cancer.[16] A family history of prostate cancer is also relevant. The risk for development of prostate cancer increases 2.2-fold if a single relative is affected and 3.9-fold or greater if two or more relatives have a history of prostate cancer, especially if they are first-degree relatives or diagnosed with prostate cancer before the age of 55 years.[17]

Although data are inconclusive and contradictory, other risk factors for development of prostate cancer include obesity, smoking, high-fat diet, and occupational exposure (Box 77-1).[13] Obesity also significantly increases the risk for fatal prostate cancer and recurrent prostate cancer after radical prostatectomy.[18]

BOX 77-1. Risk Factors for Prostate Cancer

- Age
- Family history
- African American race
- Obesity
- Smoking
- High-fat diet
- Occupational exposure (e.g., farming, lawn care, exterminator)
- Initial PSA level > 2 ng/mL, abnormal percentage free PSA, elevated PSA velocity

Men who have been treated with curative intent for localized prostate cancer deserve special attention. According to various reports, between 15% and 40% of these men will ultimately have recurrent disease that is heralded by a steadily increasing prostate-specific antigen (PSA) level.[19,20]

Early recurrence of prostate cancer is usually a manifestation of preexisting occult metastatic disease. Researchers postulate that the same situation may account for delayed prostate cancer recurrence. The results of two research studies using refined histologic techniques to evaluate pelvic lymph node tissue and specialized antibody testing of bone marrow aspirates suggest that the majority of men with clinically localized prostate cancer harbor disseminated prostate cancer cells in their bone marrow and up to 30% of men with presumed localized disease have micrometastatic prostate cancer cells in their pelvic nodes.[21-23] Even so, the presence of micrometastatic disease does not necessarily equate with biochemical recurrence or overt metastatic disease. Only a tiny subset of cells are capable of surviving over time, and even a smaller percentage of cells are capable of producing a metastatic tumor.[24] Moreover, alterations in the microenvironment can prevent metastatic tumor cells from successfully colonizing elsewhere in the body.[25] Therefore, secondary prevention therapies should be considered for every man diagnosed with prostate cancer.

Prostate Cancer Screening

Prostate cancer screening (PCS) is an important component of secondary prostate cancer prevention. PCS consists of a yearly digital rectal examination, PSA blood test (controversial), and validated questionnaire of urinary symptoms. The American Cancer Society (ACS) and the American Urological Association (AUA) currently recommend PCS for informed men who wish to be tested and who have a life expectancy of at least 10 years.

The ACS recommends starting at the age of 50 years for the general male population, 45 years for men with increased risk factors, and 40 years for men with a risk for hereditary prostate cancer (several first-degree relatives diagnosed before the age of 65 years). In the 2009 ACS guidelines, there are some notable differences from earlier recommendations: digital rectal examination is optional; men with a PSA level of more than 2.5 ng/mL should be screened annually; men with a PSA level of less than 2.5 ng/mL can be screened every 2 years; and an individualized risk assessment should be part of the referral decision for patients with a PSA level between 2.5 and 4.0 ng/mL.[26]

The 2009 AUA guidelines for PCS also contain several new recommendations from earlier guidelines: a baseline PSA level should be obtained at the age of 40 years, and there is no single, threshold PSA value that should prompt a prostate biopsy—other factors that influence risk for prostate cancer should be considered.[27]

Although PCS can detect prostate cancer at an early stage, professional medical organizations are divided on the value of routine PCS. Opponents claim that routine PCS often detects insignificant cancers, fails to have an impact on overall survival, and may adversely affect quality of life. Instead of routine PCS, opponents recommend informed decision-making for the individual patient.

In contrast, proponents of routine PCS claim that the majority of PSA-detected prostate cancers are clinically significant, that is, life-threatening if left untreated, and evolving data suggest that routine screening improves disease-specific survival.[27]

Two large randomized controlled trials were conducted to determine whether evidence-based data support PCS. The trials reached different conclusions. At 7 years or 10 years, the Prostate, Lung, Colorectal, and Ovarian (PLCO) cancer screening trial failed to show a reduction in prostate cancer–related mortality in men who underwent PCS compared with the control arm.[28] Conversely, the European Randomized Study for Prostate Cancer (ERSPC) showed 20% fewer deaths in the screening arm than in the control arm after a mean of 8.8 years.[29] To prevent one prostate cancer death, though, 1410 men (or 1068 men who were actually participated in PCS) would have to be screened (NNS), and an additional 48 men would have to be treated (NNT). A further decrease in prostate cancer–specific mortality was seen for men who had been in the trial for 12 years (36% lower mortality; NNS = 500). In addition, the incidence of T3 and T4 tumors was 22% lower and the incidence of M1 lesions was 41% lower in the screening arm of the ERSPC trial than in the control arm. Fundamental differences between the two studies may account for the divergent conclusions.

The ERSPC trial studied 162,000 men from seven European countries, whereas the PLCO trial studied 76,693 men from a single country. The majority of men (85%) with indications for biopsy in the ERSPC trial accepted a prostate biopsy. In contrast, only 30% of men in the screening arm in the PLCO study with an abnormal PSA level had a prostate biopsy. Moreover, in the PLCO trial, 52% of the men in the control arm had PSA screening during the study, which may explain why the incidence of and death rate from prostate cancer were not significantly different between the screening and control arms.

Other data from the United States are consistent with the findings of the ERSPC trial. Age-adjusted data from the prostate cancer Surveillance, Epidemiology, and End Results (SEER data) show that the incidence of metastatic disease has dropped more than threefold since the advent of PCS in 1990. Furthermore, data from the ACS show that the death rate from prostate cancer has dropped by almost 50% during the past two decades.

Certain other caveats must also be considered. Normal PSA values may vary with prostate volume, age, and race (Table 77-1), and refinements of PSA testing, such as percentage free PSA and PSA velocity, can help identify men with the greatest risk of harboring prostate cancer.[27]

TABLE 77-1. "Normal" PSA (ng/mL) Thresholds Based on Age and Race

AGE RANGE (yr)	ASIAN MEN	BLACK MEN	WHITE MEN
40–49	0–2	0–2	0–2.5
50–59	0–3	0–4	0–3.5
60–69	0–4	0–4.5	0–4.5
70–79	0–5	0–5.5	0–5.5

Percentage free PSA measures the ratio between total PSA (bound and unbound) and unbound or "free" PSA. This test is most useful for PSA values between 4 and 10 ng/mL. The lower the percentage, the higher the risk of prostate cancer.[30] For example, in men aged 50 to 64 years, if the percentage free fraction is more than 25%, there is only a 5% risk of prostate cancer; however, if it is less than 10%, the risk of prostate cancer jumps to 56%.

PSA velocity (PSAV) is determined by measuring three PSA values at least 6 months apart. A PSAV of more than 0.75 ng/mL per year in men with PSA values between 4 and 10 ng/mL is associated with an increased risk of prostate cancer.[27] PSAV is also relevant for men with PSA values below 4 ng/mL. A PSAV of more than 0.4 ng/mL per year may be associated with adverse pathologic features and a twofold increase in significant prostate cancer.[31]

PSAV is calculated as the running average of change in three consecutive visits according to the following formula[32]:

$$0.5\{[(PSA_2 - PSA_1)/\text{elapsed time in years}]$$
$$+ [(PSA_3 - PSA_2)/(\text{elapsed time in years})]\}$$

Unlike the total PSA value, the percentage free PSA is affected by manipulation of the prostate gland. Therefore, the clinician should not order a percentage free PSA test on the same day as a rectal examination or within 24 hours of intercourse.[1]

Integrative Therapies

Integrative therapies for primary and secondary prostate cancer prevention should be considered for all men for many reasons. According to some estimates, the pool of men with prostate cancer in the Unites States exceeds 20 million. "Localized" prostate cancer is often disseminated in the peripheral bloodstream and bone marrow, yet only 0.3% of these men will ultimately have metastatic disease.[33] Therefore, fatal metastatic disease is an uncommon event that may be modified with integrative therapies.

Prostate cancer is a disease of aging; 75% of new prostate cancers are diagnosed in men older than 65 years. The median doubling time of prostate cancer is 2 to 4 years. Any treatment that can delay tumor growth rates by 75% or more

in older men will increase the likelihood that some event other than prostate cancer will cause death.[33] A provocative pilot study demonstrated that a plant-based diet in the context of mindfulness-based stress reduction delayed PSA doubling time by 272%, from 6.5 months to 17.7 months.[34] Another group of researchers reported that a similar program doubled survival time for a cohort of men with metastatic prostate cancer.[35]

Finally, integrative therapies for prostate cancer prevention improve overall health and decrease the risk of premature morbidity and mortality from diseases associated with a Western lifestyle.[36,37]

Lifestyle

Exercise

Although data are inconclusive, physical activity may reduce prostate cancer risk by lowering body fat and serum testosterone concentration and by improving use of insulin-like growth factor 1 (IGF-1).[13] IGF-1 has mitogenic and anti-apoptotic effects on normal and malignant prostate cells. In one study, men with the highest quartile of IGF-1 levels had a 4.3-fold greater risk of prostate cancer compared with men in the lowest quartile.[38]

Exercise can also lessen the risk for development of aggressive or advanced prostate cancer. Data from the Health Professionals Follow-up Study show that men older than 65 years who exercise vigorously at least 3 hours per week in activities such as running, biking, and swimming have a 70% lower risk of being diagnosed with high-grade, advanced, or metastatic prostate cancer.[39] Similarly, a British study of 45,887 men aged 45 to 79 years showed that men with the highest lifetime physical activity had a 16% overall lower incidence of prostate cancer as well as a lower risk of advanced prostate cancer compared with men with the lowest activity. Each 30-minute increment of activity reduced the risk of prostate cancer by 7%.[40]

Men should exercise (e.g., walking, jogging, swimming) 30 minutes or longer at least three times weekly.

Every 30-minute incremental increase in aerobic exercise per week has been associated with lowering of the risk of prostate cancer by 7%.

Xenobiotic Exposure

A xenobiotic is any chemical or toxin that is foreign to the body. Findings vary, but herbicides and pesticide exposure may increase prostate cancer risk by causing DNA damage and altering hormone metabolism.[13] In the most mature study to date, Vietnam War veterans who had been exposed to the xenobiotic Agent Orange (dioxin) had twice the risk for development of prostate cancer, were diagnosed at a younger age, had twice the risk of Gleason 8 to 10 disease, and were at least three times more likely to have metastatic disease. Mean time from exposure to diagnosis was 407 months.[41]

Endocrine disrupters, substances that mimic natural hormones, increase prostate cancer risk by disrupting hormone metabolism. Common examples of endocrine disrupters are polychlorinated biphenyls (PCBs, used to make plastic, ink, and electrical and electronic equipment) and plasticizers (substances used to make plastic food wrap more pliable).[42]

Finally, in addition to being high in fat, dairy and beef products are occasionally contaminated with toxic pesticide and hormone residues.[13]

Reduce prostate cancer risk by washing all produce, peeling nonorganic produce (when applicable), and buying organic fruits and vegetables whenever possible. Preserve and cook food in glass containers instead of plastic ones. Limit or eliminate meat and dairy consumption.

Hormone-Altering Medications and Supplements

Injudicious use of dehydroepiandrosterone (DHEA), androstenedione, and human growth hormone may increase the risk for development of prostate cancer or promote the growth of existing prostate cancer by increasing IGF-1 levels.[43,44] Although testosterone has not been proved to cause prostate cancer, testosterone is a potent promoter of benign and malignant prostate cell growth.

Therefore, men should avoid taking these supplements or androgen replacement therapy unless it is medically indicated, especially men at increased risk for prostate cancer.

■ Chondroitin Sulfate

This popular supplement is used to treat osteoarthritis. Researchers have shown that there may be a link between chondroitin sulfate and the spread of prostate cancer.[45] Although the results are inconclusive, men with prostate cancer (or a strong family history of prostate cancer) should avoid chondroitin sulfate pending further studies.

Alcohol

Alcohol yields 9 calories per gram, the same as fat. Therefore, excessive alcohol consumption increases energy intake and promotes obesity. Nevertheless, only a few studies have found a direct association between alcohol consumption and prostate cancer risk. According to one study, excessive drinking of alcohol—more than 96 oz of alcohol weekly (about 10 drinks)—tripled the risk for development of prostate cancer.[46] On the other hand, moderate consumption of red wine may confer protection against prostate cancer. Red wine is a rich source of resveratrol, a polyphenol that induces apoptosis and modulates androgen receptor function in prostate cancer cell lines.[47] Researchers reported that men who drank 4 oz of red wine four times weekly experienced a 50% reduction in prostate cancer and a 60% reduction in the diagnosis of Gleason 8 disease.[48]

Avoid indiscriminant alcohol consumption.

Smoking

Among other carcinogens, tobacco contains cadmium, a heavy metal that may increase prostate cancer risk.[13] Although data for smoking and an increased risk of prostate cancer are conflicting, smoking increases the risk of lung, bladder, and other epithelial cancers, and it may induce a more aggressive form of prostate cancer. According to a meta-analysis of 24 prospective cohort studies, the heaviest smokers had a 24% to 30% greater risk of death from prostate cancer compared with nonsmokers.[49]

The message is clear: do not smoke.

Nutrition
Animal Fat

The incidence of prostate cancer discovered at autopsy is similar worldwide. However, the incidence of clinical prostate cancer, particularly advanced prostate cancer, is greatest in countries with the highest calorie and saturated fat consumption.

Among other things, excessive calories and saturated fat, especially from dairy products and red meat, promote obesity and prostate cell growth by increasing the production of IGF-1 and inflammatory arachidonic acid (AA) byproducts.[4,5,8] Men in the highest quartile for red meat consumption have a significantly higher risk of being diagnosed with prostate cancer and a 30% increased chance for development of advanced disease. Processing of meat and barbecuing and grilling of meat also increased the risk of total and advanced prostate cancer.[50]

AA is converted to inflammatory prostaglandin E_2 (PGE_2) molecules and series 4 leukotrienes. These messenger molecules enable prostate cancer cells to evade the immune system, inactivate natural killer cells and cytotoxic T cells, promote angiogenesis, and prevent apoptosis.[8] Research has shown that prostate cancer cells produce 10 times as much PGE_2 as surrounding benign cells do.[51] Meat-based diets and most cooking oils (with the exception of canola and olive oils) increase AA formation. In contrast, a vegan vegetarian diet can lower AA production by 30%.[33]

Although the relationship is complex and data are conflicting, animal data have shown that excess dietary omega-6 polyunsaturated acids generally stimulate tumor growth, whereas omega-3 polyunsaturated fatty acids, especially from fish, and monounsaturated omega-9 fatty acids from olive oil have the opposite effect.[52-54]

Finally, regardless of the food source, excessive calorie intake promotes obesity, which increases premature mortality and overall cancer-related death rates, including prostate cancer.[7,55]

Decrease prostate cancer risk by limiting or eliminating food items that increase AA production (e.g., animal fat, hydrogenated oils, and dairy products) and by avoiding excessive calorie intake.

Soy Protein

Even though the age-adjusted incidence of latent prostate cancer in native Japanese and American men is roughly the same, clinical prostate cancer is 10 times higher in American men. Researchers attribute this glaring discrepancy to dietary differences. A typical American diet is high in saturated animal fat but low in fruits, vegetables, fish, and soy protein, whereas a typical Japanese diet is the reverse. Japanese men consume substantially more soy protein and fish but less saturated fat from dairy and red meat than American men do.[56] According to one report, Japanese men have isoflavone concentrations 30 times higher in the urine and more than 100 times higher in the blood than Western men do.[57]

Soy protein isoflavones, most notably genistein, inhibit prostate cancer cell growth in vitro and in vivo by promoting apoptosis; by blocking beta-estrogen receptor activity in the prostate; by inhibiting angiogenesis and endothelial cell proliferation; and by blocking 5-alpha-reductase, aromatase, and tyrosine-specific protein kinase activity.[9,56,58]

Soy protein yields up to 3 mg of isoflavones per gram and provides five times as much protein as wheat and 25 times as much protein as beef. Soy protein is available in a variety of food items, including tofu, tempeh, soy milk, soy cheese, textured soy foods, and soy flour.

For prostate cancer prevention, consume enough soy protein to yield at least 80 mg of genistein daily (approximately 4 oz). Drinking of soy milk is also beneficial. A 16-year-long prospective health study showed that men who drank several glasses of soy milk daily lowered their risk of prostate cancer by 70%.[59]

For men with prostate cancer, higher doses of daily soy consumption may provide additional protection. Researchers found that men taking 100 mg of soy isoflavones twice daily slowed the growth of an aggressive form of prostate cancer called androgen-insensitive prostate cancer by 35% and slowed overall cancer growth by 84%.[60,61] Commercially available soy protein bars and sweetened or unsweetened soy powder can supplement dietary soy intake to provide at least 200 mg of isoflavones daily. Physicians Laboratories (www.revivalsoy.com) offer non–genetically modified organisms (GMO) soy products that can help patients meet these requirements. Each Rival soy bar or soy shake provides 160 mg of soy isoflavones.

■ Dosage
Drink soy milk and consume at least 4 oz of soy protein daily for prevention. Men with prostate cancer should consume at least 200 mg of isoflavones daily.

> Nonfermented soy products (tofu, soy milk, and edamame) appear to be more protective than fermented ones (miso, tempeh, natto, soy sauce).

Lycopene
Lycopene is a cancer-fighting antioxidant vitamin that gives tomatoes, strawberries, and watermelon their rosy color. Other natural sources of lycopene are apricots, pink grapefruit, and guava juice. Although not all studies have found that lycopene confers a protective effect against prostate cancer,[62] data from a variety of case-control and large prospective studies focusing on dietary assessment show a beneficial effect, especially against advanced prostate cancer.[18,63,64] According to one report, men who consumed tomato products four times weekly reduced their prostate cancer risk by 20%, and those who ate 10 or more helpings weekly reduced their risk by 45%.[65] Cooking tomatoes and adding a little olive oil improves lycopene absorption.

■ Dosage
For prevention, eat at least four helpings of tomato products weekly or take one 10-mg lycopene capsule twice daily. Men with prostate cancer should eat at least 10 helpings of tomato products weekly or take one 10-mg lycopene capsule three times daily.

Fruits and Vegetables
Packed with cancer-fighting vitamins, minerals, and fiber, fruits and vegetables, especially cruciferous vegetables, may decrease prostate cancer risk.[66] Data suggest that a plant-based diet can slow PSA doubling time in men with recurrent prostate cancer.[24]

Follow National Cancer Institute guidelines and eat at least five to nine servings of fruits and vegetables daily.

Pomegranate
Pomegranate juice contains polyphenolic compounds, especially ellagic acid, that exert antiproliferative and antimetastatic effects on prostate cancer cells. According to a phase II study of 46 men with recurrent prostate cancer after surgery or radiation therapy, consumption of 8 oz of pomegranate juice daily significantly slowed PSA doubling time from 15.6 months to 54.7 months.[67] Pomegranate extract also inhibits prostate cancer cell growth.[9] Long-term follow-up data (mean of 30 months) showed that the beneficial effect of consuming pomegranate juice remained durable or increased.[68]

■ Dosage
Consume 8 oz of pomegranate juice or an equivalent amount of pomegranate extract daily.

Supplements

Vitamin E (Mixed Tocopherols) and Selenium
Secondary end points from several key epidemiologic and prospective cohort studies suggested that vitamin E and selenium supplementation could decrease prostate cancer incidence and mortality, especially among smokers.[69,70] Accordingly, the Southwest Oncology Group in collaboration with others sponsored a phase III randomized, placebo-controlled trial of 35,553 men to determine whether taking selenium (200 mcg/day from L-selenomethionine) and vitamin E (400 units/day of all-*rac*-tocopheryl acetate), either alone or in combination, could provide protective benefit against prostate cancer.[71] The Selenium and Vitamin E Cancer Prevention Trial (SELECT) was terminated prematurely after 4 years because of concern about a small but significant increased incidence of prostate cancer in the vitamin E–alone arm and a small but insignificant increase in prostate cancer in the combined vitamin E and selenium arm and the selenium-alone arm. Compared with placebo, the hazard ratios for prostate cancer were 1.13 in the vitamin E–alone cohort, 1.05 in the selenium and vitamin E cohort, and 1.04 in the selenium-alone cohort. There was also a nonsignificant increase in the risk for development of diabetes (RR, 1.07) in the selenium-alone arm. On the basis of these data, supplementation with vitamin E and selenium for the prevention of prostate cancer is not recommended.

Vitamin D
Vitamin D is a steroid hormone that can be acquired from the diet and dietary supplements, or it can be synthesized in the skin from 7-dehydrocholesterol in response to ultraviolet radiation. Ultraviolet irradiation of ergosterol from yeast yields vitamin D_2. Ultraviolet irradiation of 7-dehydrocholesterol from lanolin yields vitamin D_3. Vitamin D_2 is approximately 30% as effective as vitamin D_3 in maintaining serum 25-hydroxyvitamin D levels.

Although there is no consensus on the optimal blood level of vitamin D, deficiency is defined as a 25-hydroxyvitamin D level of less than 30 ng/mL. According to several studies,

40% to 100% of men and women still living in the community are deficient in vitamin D. Both prospective and retrospective epidemiologic studies have shown that vitamin D deficiency is associated with an increased risk for development of prostate cancer. Prostate cancer cells have a vitamin D receptor. Vitamin D is involved in the regulation of more than 200 genes, including genes that are responsible for cellular proliferation, differentiation, apoptosis, and angiogenesis. Vitamin D decreases cellular proliferation of normal and cancer cells and promotes their terminal differentiation. It also inhibits prostate cancer invasion and metastasis.[9,72]

■ Dosage

Supplement the diet with sufficient vitamin D_3 to maintain a vitamin D level of at least 30 ng/mL for prevention of prostate cancer and a level between 50 and 100 ng/mL for men with prostate cancer or an increased risk for development of prostate cancer.

■ Precautions

Vitamin D intoxication is extremely rare, but it can occur with excessive consumption of vitamin D. Oral supplementation with vitamin D should be monitored with periodic laboratory testing for 25-hydroxyvitamin D levels.

Multivitamins

Researchers examined a cohort of 1,063,023 adult Americans between the years of 1982 and 1989 and compared the mortality of vitamin nonusers with that of users of multivitamins alone; vitamin A, C, or E alone; and vitamin A, C, or E in combination. Surprisingly, the risk of dying of prostate cancer significantly increased with more than 5 years of multivitamin use (RR, 1.31). Furthermore, male smokers who used vitamins A, E, or C alone or in combination with multivitamins had a greater risk of fatal cancer (RR, 1.44 and RR, 1.58) than that of vitamin nonusers.[73] Data from the National Institutes of Health–AARP Diet and Health Study showed that men who consumed multivitamins more than seven times per week had a significantly increased risk of advanced or fatal prostate cancer (RR, 1.32 and RR, 1.98).[74] Therefore, multivitamin consumption is not recommended for the prevention or treatment of prostate cancer.

> Taking a multivitamin containing vitamins A, E, and C more than seven times a week may increase the risk of dying of prostate cancer.

Botanicals

Green Tea (Camellia sinensis)

Green tea contains a variety of antioxidants called catechins that have antitumor activity against prostate cancer cells. In vitro and in vivo studies have shown that green tea can inhibit prostate cancer cell growth by inducing apoptosis, activating tumor suppressor genes, and mitigating the activity of stimulatory messenger molecules. According to preliminary data, the beneficial effect of green tea may be dose related, and it may be more effective against early-stage prostate cancer as opposed to end-stage disease.[9]

In 60 men with high-grade prostate intraepithelial neoplasia who took 200 mg three times a day of mixed green tea catechins, only 1 of 30 (3.3%) progressed to cancer compared with 9 of 30 (30%) in the placebo group. Taking the green tea catechins did not influence the PSA level.[75]

■ Dosage

Drink three to five cups of decaffeinated green tea daily or take 500 mg of a standardized green tea extract composed of mixed catechins once daily for prevention or twice daily if prostate cancer is present.

■ Precautions

No precautions are necessary.

Pharmaceuticals

Finasteride

The Prostate Cancer Prevention Trial (PCPT) randomized 18,882 men to a 7-year course of placebo or 5 mg of the 5-alpha-reductase type 2 enzyme inhibitor finasteride daily.[76] The results showed a 24.4% prevalence rate of prostate cancer in the placebo arm (1147/4692) versus an 18.4% prevalence in the finasteride arm (803/4368). Although there were a higher number of high-grade tumors in the finasteride group, researchers attribute this difference to an artifact of trial design.

Dutasteride

The Reduction by Dutasteride of Prostate Cancer Events (REDUCE) trial data showed that dutasteride reduced the risk of prostate cancer during 4 years by 23% compared with placebo.[77] The REDUCE trial was a randomized, double-blind, placebo-controlled phase III trial of 8000 men from 42 different countries between the ages of 50 and 75 years with a PSA level of 2.5 to 10 ng/mL and normal findings on prestudy prostate biopsy. In contrast to finasteride, dutasteride inhibits both type 1 and type 2 5-alpha-reductase enzymes. Type 1 5-alpha-reductase enzyme predominates in prostate cancer, whereas type 2 enzyme predominates in normal and hyperplastic prostate tissue.

Nonsteroidal Antiinflammatory Drugs

Cancer initiation, promotion, progression, angiogenesis, and metastasis are modulated in part by the inflammatory cascade of eicosanoids, cyclooxygenases, and lipoxygenases.[8] Aspirin reduces inflammation by inhibiting cyclooxygenase-1 (COX-1) and cyclooxygenase-2 (COX-2) enzymes. According to a systematic review of the literature and meta-analysis, long-term consumption of aspirin (5 years or more) was inversely associated with the risk for development of prostate cancer. The risk reduction was more pronounced for advanced prostate cancer (OR = 0.7) than for total prostate cancer (OR = 0.9).[78] A cohort study of 70,144 men reported similar findings; regular use of nonsteroidal antiinflammatory drugs (NSAIDs) decreased the risk of prostate cancer by 18% and the risk of advanced prostate cancer by 33%.[79] Taking one 81-mg baby aspirin daily may be sufficient to reduce prostate cancer risk.

Suppression of COX-2 activity with COX-2–selective inhibitors may also reduce prostate cancer risk.[80-82] Although rofecoxib was withdrawn because of adverse cardiovascular side effects, high doses of the COX-2 inhibitor celecoxib markedly slowed PSA doubling times in men whose PSA level started to rise after local curative therapy without causing any serious adverse cardiovascular effects.[83]

■ Dosage

If there are no medical contraindications, take one baby aspirin daily. Men with an increased risk for development of prostate cancer may wish to consider taking dutasteride (Avodart), 0.5 mg daily, especially if they have symptomatic prostate enlargement.

■ Precautions

Patients taking anticoagulation or antiplatelet medication and patients with a history of heart, renal, or gastrointestinal disease should check with their health care provider before taking aspirin or NSAIDs. Finasteride and dutasteride can decrease libido and semen volume and cause gynecomastia.

Mind-Body Medicine

Psychosocial interventions can improve the quality of life for cancer patients and significantly prolong survival. According to one study, men who were taught new coping skills (mental relaxation and imagery techniques, stress management, ways to develop self-esteem and spirituality, receptive imagery/ intuition and problem solving, and how to create a personal health plan/goal) lived twice as long as men in the control group.[84] Similarly, mindfulness-based stress reduction coupled with a plant-based diet can slow PSA doubling time in men with biochemical recurrence after radical prostatectomy and prolong survival in men with metastatic prostate cancer.[34,35]

Men with prostate cancer should practice stress reduction and relaxation techniques daily.

PREVENTION PRESCRIPTION

- ■ For men at normal risk, discuss the pros and cons of PSA screening and provide information on prostate cancer prevention. For men at high risk, perform a digital rectal examination and PSA test yearly after the age of 40 years.
- ■ Encourage exercise for 30 minutes or longer at least three times weekly.
- ■ Avoid hormone-altering medications such as DHEA, androstenedione, human growth hormone, and testosterone, unless medically indicated.
- ■ Instruct patients to buy organic produce whenever possible. They should also wash all produce and peel it when applicable, drink filtered water, and cook and store food in glass containers.
- ■ Advise patients to reduce or to eliminate dairy and meat consumption.
- ■ Instruct patients to use olive or canola oil instead of other vegetable oils.
- ■ Emphasize that patients should avoid tobacco products and excessive alcohol consumption.
- ■ Teach patients to drink soy milk and eat at least 4 oz of soy protein daily.
- ■ Encourage intake of five to nine servings of fruits and vegetables daily.
- ■ Instruct patients to drink three to five cups of decaffeinated green tea or to take 500 mg of a standardized green tea extract once daily.
- ■ If there are no medical contraindications, advise taking one 81-mg baby aspirin daily.
- ■ Suggest that patients practice stress reduction and relaxation techniques daily.

THERAPEUTIC REVIEW

Men with a normal risk for development of prostate cancer should follow the recommendations listed here. Men with a high risk for development of prostate cancer should consider adopting the suggestions for high-risk patients. High-risk factors include any of the following: prior history of prostate cancer; recurrent prostate cancer; family history of prostate cancer; African American race; initial PSA value above 2 ng/mL; PSAV of more than 0.4 ng/mL per year for men with a PSA level of less than 4 ng/mL; and PSAV of more than 0.75 ng/mL for men with a PSA level between 4 and 10 ng/mL.

■ Remove Exacerbating Factors

- Avoid smoking and excessive alcohol consumption. Patients with high risk may consider drinking 4 oz of red wine or 8 oz of Concord grape juice four times weekly.

■ Lifestyle

- Exercise for 30 minutes or longer at least three times weekly.

■ Nutrition

- Reduce or eliminate dairy and meat consumption and eat at least five to nine servings of fruits and vegetables daily and at least 4 oz of soy products daily. Patients with high risk should consume at least 200 mg of soy isoflavones daily and consider adopting a plant-based diet. Refer receptive patients to a qualified dietitian.

■ Supplements

- Take 10 mg of lycopene twice daily (three times daily for high-risk patients). Men with high risk should avoid taking DHEA, human growth hormone, androstenedione, chondroitin sulfate, and supplemental androgens.

▇ Botanicals

- Take 500 mg of green tea extract daily (twice daily for high-risk patients).

▇ Mind-Body

- Discuss mindfulness-based stress reduction techniques, especially for men with high risk, and refer receptive patients to a qualified professional.

▇ Pharmaceuticals

- Take one 81-mg baby aspirin daily (consider taking 5 mg of dutasteride daily for high-risk patients).

KEY WEB RESOURCES

www.prostate-cancer.org	A comprehensive prostate cancer resource, sponsored by the Prostate Cancer Research Institute
http://www.cancer.gov/cancertopics/types/prostate	Prostate cancer home page of the National Cancer Institute
http://acor.org/	An online resource of cancer information for the patient with cancer
http://deb.uthscsa.edu/URORiskCalc/Pages/calcs.jsp	Risk calculator of biopsy-detectable prostate cancer for men older than 55 years

References

References are available online at expertconsult.com.

Chapter 78

Colorectal Cancer

Matt P. Mumber, MD

Incidence and Prevalence

Colorectal cancer is an important public health problem; nearly one million cases are diagnosed worldwide each year, with about half a million deaths.[1] The geographic distribution of colorectal cancer varies widely between westernized and developing countries. The highest rates are in North America, Australia, and Europe. Rates in Africa and Asia are low but are increasing in countries adopting Western-style dietary habits.[2] Colorectal cancer is the third most common malignant neoplasm in the United States. Men and women have a generally equal risk for development of the disease—a risk of about 1 in 20.[3] Survival rates have improved with multiple possible explanations: implementation of more consistent screening leading to earlier stage at presentation, improved diet and lifestyle patterns, and improvements in surgical and adjuvant therapies.[4] Patients with localized disease have a 90% 5-year survival rate. Epidemiologic factors and outcomes are different for disease originating above the peritoneal reflection (colon origin) and disease originating below the peritoneal reflection (rectal origin).[5]

Risk Factors

Box 78-1 lists factors that place individuals at increased risk for colorectal cancer.[5] Several genetic factors can help define risk of patients for colorectal cancer. Hereditary syndromes such as Lynch syndrome (hereditary nonpolyposis colorectal cancer) and personal or family history of polyposis syndromes place an individual at high risk. African American race, diabetes mellitus, and history of *BRCA*-positive breast cancer are linked to higher incidence. Lifestyle and behavioral factors such as tobacco and alcohol use, sedentary lifestyle, obesity, Western-type dietary pattern, low fiber consumption, inflammatory bowel disease, and psychosocial distress are known potential modifiable risk factors for the development and progression of colorectal neoplasia.

Natural History

The majority of colorectal cancer begins as benign polypoid changes in the colorectal mucosa, and progression to malignant features can take many years. The relatively slow and consistent progression from benign to malignant disease is the reason that screening and early detection can have a positive impact. The disease generally progresses locally to extend through the bowel wall, and after having done so, it can progress with either lymphatic or hematogenous spread. Metastatic disease that is limited to one or two lesions in organs such as the lung or liver is termed oligometastatic disease. Patients with oligometastatic disease that is surgically resectable can still experience long-term disease-free survival.[6]

Screening

Screening has been proved to have an impact on stage at diagnosis and also to eliminate benign polypoid disease before malignant transformation. The initiation and frequency of screening should be driven by individual risk assessment based on family and personal history of colorectal cancer, inflammatory bowel disease, and other risk factors. Normal-risk individuals should have a screening colonoscopy at the age of 50 years. Despite strong recommendations for screening, rates are still relatively low; approximately 60% of the recommended population receives appropriate screening procedures. This level has increased from 52% in 2002 to 63% in 2008.[4,7-9]

> Screening intervals should be adjusted for the individual patient's risk level, and any type of screening (endoscopy or fecal testing) is better than none at all.

BOX 78-1. Factors Associated With Increased Risk for Colorectal Cancer

- Age older than 50 years
- African American race
- Personal history of colorectal cancer or polyps
- Inflammatory bowel disease
- Inherited syndromes: familial polyposis and Lynch syndrome
- Family history of colorectal cancer and polyps
- Low-fiber, high-fat diet (Western-type diet)
- Sedentary lifestyle
- Diabetes
- Tobacco and alcohol use
- Previous radiation therapy to abdomen or pelvis
- Psychosocial distress

BOX 78-2. Modifiable Risk Factors That Lower Incidence of Colorectal Cancer

- Avoidance of red meats, processed meat, and refined carbohydrates
- Maintenance of recommended physical activity levels
- Maintenance of healthy body weight (body mass index less than obese)
- Avoidance of alcohol and tobacco
- Avoidance of hyperinsulinemia (metabolic syndrome)

Up to 70% of colorectal cancer can be prevented through diet and lifestyle changes.

Colonoscopy, the most complete screening procedure, has a demonstrated 50% risk reduction on colorectal cancer incidence. Flexible sigmoidoscopy lowers incidence by 33%. Computed tomographic colonography, also known as virtual colonoscopy, is noninvasive and does not require sedation. It is still being studied in large trials but may prove to be an effective screening measure in the future. Fecal-based screening tests detect signs of cancer in stool samples by measuring the presence of either human blood products or cancer DNA signatures. Fecal occult blood testing has a 16% relative risk reduction for colorectal cancer death in large study populations. Different types of fecal testing are available, and all must be coordinated by physicians to increase sensitivity of detection. A single in-office guaiac test is not optimal. Any type of screening is better than no screening at all.[7] Different strategies are being investigated to increase the compliance of patients with screening recommendations, including patient navigation (see later).[10]

Individuals with high risk, such as those with Lynch syndrome, familial polyposis syndromes, and positive family or personal history of colorectal cancer, should have increased screening diligence (colonoscopy instead of fecal testing) and shorter intervals between screening procedures. Intervention with colonic resection as a risk reduction strategy is advisable in certain populations of patients, such as those with familial polyposis, who have a nearly 100% chance for development of cancer in their lifetime.[6]

Primary and Secondary Prevention

Genetic risks are difficult to modify; these are mainly focused around family history of colorectal cancer. Modifiable risk factors, such as those in Box 78-2, have the advantage of relatively simple recommendations to lower risk. However, the actual initiation and maintenance of comprehensive diet and lifestyle changes is not an easy formula (simple, but not easy). It is important for the clinician to use the tools of motivational interviewing (see Chapter 99, Motivational Interviewing Techniques) and to have a full understanding of the stages of change for the best chance of guiding sustainable health practices.[11,12] It is estimated that at least 70% of colon cancers may be preventable through moderate changes in diet and lifestyle.[13,14]

Lifestyle

There are ample data that physical activity, a whole-food plant-based diet, and stress reduction can decrease the incidence of colorectal cancer. Because of the nature of these interventions and the difficulty in studying primary prevention, overwhelming randomized trial evidence is lacking, but multiple systematic reviews are available that at least support safety and hint at efficacy of these interventions.[13-16] There is also a plausible mechanism of action related to insulin sensitivity and production of insulin-like growth factor 1 (Fig. 78-1).

Physical activity should consist of 30 minutes of aerobic activity daily as well as resistance exercise several times weekly.

Nutrition should focus on a whole-food plant-based diet. Two questions can help define what to eat and what to avoid.
1. Is the food from an animal or a plant source? If it is from an animal source, either avoid the food or significantly limit use of it.
2. If the food is from a plant source, is it a whole part of the plant (root, stem, leaf, seed) or is it composed of a part of the plant that has been processed and then had extra ingredients added (such as sugar, salt, or oil)? Eat whole parts of plants and either avoid or limit processed foods.

A stress reduction practice can include a variety of modalities, such as mindfulness-based meditation, other forms of meditation, yoga, sitting in silence, listening to music, creative arts, massage, and guided imagery.

In my practice, I use the three-legged stool of health as an educational tool (Fig. 78-2). I also discuss the stages of change, advancing from pre-contemplation to contemplation to preparation, action, and then maintenance.[17] We discuss the fact that the practice of awareness is foundational to creation of sustainable change. It is more beneficial to apply different types of tools to different stages of change. Tools are generally divided into two categories. Transformational tools are defined by letting go of the old and seeing things with new eyes; they mainly involve a new way of being. Translational tools are characterized as interventions or practices that can be easily defined and have specific rules for implementation; they mainly include embracing new habits or ways of doing.[18] The foundational practice of

FIGURE 78-1
Proposed inflammatory mechanisms relating diet, lifestyle, and medication use to colorectal cancer. IGF-1, insulin-like growth factor 1. (From Chan AT, Giovannucci EL. Primary prevention of colorectal cancer. *Gastroenterology.* 2010;138:2029–2043.e10.)

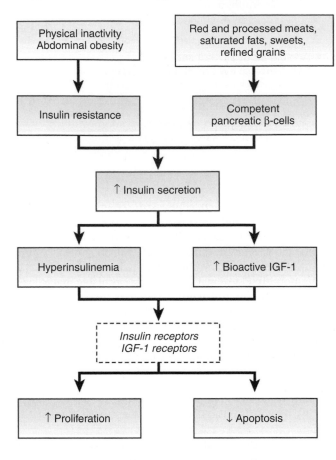

FIGURE 78-2
Three-legged stool of health.

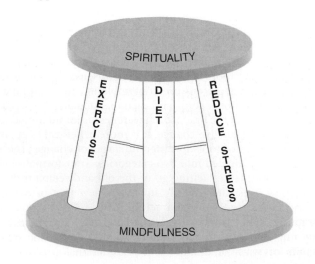

awareness is transformational and has its main functionality in pre-contemplation, contemplation, and maintenance stages of change, whereas discrete translational tools such as physical activity, improved diet, and stress reduction practices have their main impact on the preparation and action stages.

Insulin Resistance and Metabolic Syndrome

Many mechanisms of action are proposed for the cancer preventive effect associated with healthy lifestyle and dietary changes; chief among them is optimal energy balance. Suboptimal energy balance can result in obesity, and this can result in the metabolic syndrome. Metabolic syndrome is characterized by excess abdominal obesity, atherogenic dyslipidemia, hypertension, insulin resistance, prothrombotic state, and proinflammatory state. All these factors have in vitro evidence of stimulation of carcinogenesis and cancer proliferation. There are well-documented in vitro effects on immune function, cell proliferation, cancer cell migration and invasion, loss of apoptosis, and increased angiogenesis (Fig. 78-3; see also Fig. 78-1).

Supplements

Significant research effort has gone into looking for a prescribed agent that can lower risk; this also is a potentially simple solution that would not require as much effort on the part of the patient. Daily aspirin intake, supplementation, and increasing dietary intake of foods containing folate, vitamin B$_6$, vitamin D$_3$, calcium, and omega-3 fats have been proposed to play a role in colorectal cancer risk reduction; however, supportive data are generally from small cohort studies, and meta-analyses generally show marginal or no clear effect on prevention.[19–25] A Cochrane meta-analysis found no convincing evidence that antioxidant supplements decrease colorectal adenoma formation.[26] A meta-analysis revealed that vitamin B$_6$ intake and blood levels of pyridoxal 5′-phosphate (PLP, the bioactive form of vitamin B$_6$) were inversely associated with the risk of colorectal cancer.[27] This study showed that whereas the correlation with vitamin B$_6$ supplementation was moderate, it was dramatic with higher PLP levels, which decreased risk of colon cancer by nearly half. This points to the probable importance of obtaining this nutrient from food sources as opposed to supplements.

> Food sources of vitamin B$_6$ include garlic, tuna, cauliflower, mustard greens, banana, celery, cabbage, crimini mushrooms, asparagus, broccoli, kale, collard greens, Brussels sprouts, cod, and chard.

Aspirin has been the most well studied and may be especially beneficial in patients with previous history of adenomas (secondary prevention).[21] A retrospective review of several randomized trials originally designed to prevent vascular events showed that daily aspirin intake was associated with significantly lower death rates from several cancer types, including colorectal cancer.[28] These data must be interpreted with caution because of their retrospective nature.

FIGURE 78-3
Proposed insulin-related mechanisms that relate diet, obesity, and physical activity to colorectal cancer. (From Chan AT, Giovannucci EL. Primary prevention of colorectal cancer. *Gastroenterology.* 2010;138:2029–2043.e10.)

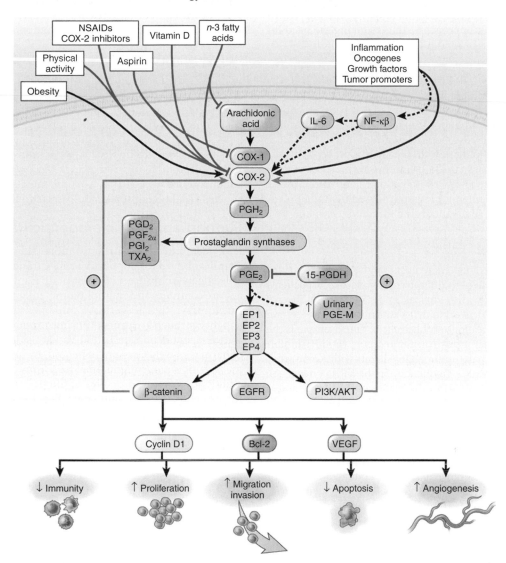

The risks and benefits of supplementation with any of these compounds must be weighed carefully for every individual, especially in light of the fact that a whole-food plant-based diet should provide adequate amounts of each of the nutrients mentioned. The hypothesis that oral supplementation or preventive treatment (nonsteroidal antiinflammatory drugs) can overcome poor dietary and lifestyle practices has not been well tested in a prospective fashion.

Secondary prevention for high-risk individuals, such as those with familial adenomatous polyposis, may also include the use of selective cyclooxygenase-2 (COX-2) inhibitors, such as celecoxib, although some significant cardiac morbidity is possible with this agent at preventive doses used in clinical trials.[29] Natural agents that have anti inflammatory mechanisms of action, including ginseng, curcumin, quercetin, omega-3 fatty acids, and green tea, also affect the COX-2 pathway and have been proposed as possible preventive agents. Further research is indicated.[30,31]

Treatment

Conventional therapy has arguably progressed more for colorectal cancer than for any other malignant neoplasm. Diagnostic efforts usually include endoscopy and biopsy. Endoscopic ultrasonography for rectal cancer has dramatically improved clinical staging by helping to define the extent of the primary disease invasion through the bowel wall as well as by an improved ability to detect perirectal and regional lymph nodes. Improved clinical staging has led to the ability to better define the most appropriate initial intervention, either initial surgery or preoperative chemotherapy and radiation therapy.

Surgery

Surgical intervention can now include laparoscopic approaches for colon cancers (supported by multiple systematic reviews[32,33]), and the ability to provide low coloanal anastomosis has lowered colostomy rates in low-lying rectal cancer. Resection of oligometastatic disease can be performed through partial liver resection, taking advantage of the fact that liver regenerates after such procedures. Wedge excision of solitary metastatic disease to the lung may include video-assisted laparoscopic approaches, thus reducing the need for thoracotomy and associated postoperative morbidity.[6]

Chemotherapy and Radiation Therapy

Preoperative chemotherapy and radiation therapy are the standard of care for tumor that has invaded through the muscle wall of the bowel; this approach results in lower colostomy rates compared with postoperative adjuvant therapy as well as improved survival. Radiation therapy has improved with the use of techniques that spare dose-limiting normal tissue structures, such as the small bowel. Radiation therapy can now be delivered with computed tomography–based treatment planning and improved setup and immobilization techniques.[6]

Chemotherapy

Systemic therapy has added new agents, both cytotoxic and biologic, that have improved the long-term survival of most patients currently diagnosed with colorectal cancer. The biologic agents can be targeted for delivery only to patients who have certain genetic features indicating responsiveness. One example is the use of the epidermal growth factor receptor (EGFR) inhibitors cetuximab and panitumumab in patients with *KRAS* wild-type tumors (those without a mutation in the *KRAS* oncogene). The K-*ras* oncogene is part of the *ras* oncogene family and is the most common mutation in colorectal cancer; about 40% to 50% of colorectal cancers have mutated *KRAS* genes. *KRAS* wild-type tumors respond to EGFR inhibitors, whereas those tumors with a mutation in *KRAS* do not respond to these relatively well tolerated, targeted biologic agents. A clinical trial showed improvements in overall survival and quality of life for a population of colorectal cancer patients with wild-type *KRAS* treated with cetuximab (Erbitux) alone versus best supportive care when all other therapies had failed.[34,35]

Systemic therapy by use of chemotherapy has significant potential toxicity, and there is a debate, especially in early-stage colon cancer, as to whether the risks outweigh the benefits. The entire field of oncology has shifted toward a more "personalized," individualized, and targeted approach to therapy. The field of gene expression profiling is a potential solution by which only patients with high-risk disease that would benefit from therapy are treated. The Oncotype DX assay, a 12-gene expression profile for colon cancer, is currently undergoing validation in clinical trials. It is possible that this assay, which has shown successful implementation with a similar process in breast cancer patients, could help define which patients will benefit from chemotherapy and which will not.[36]

Chronotherapy

Various investigators have also looked at the idea of chronotherapy, the administration of antineoplastic therapy based on circadian rhythms. Several trials and approaches to therapy have been reported, including a meta-analysis of the limited published trials that showed significant benefit in patients with advanced disease.[37-40] One such publication[37] described patients who adopted comprehensive diet

and lifestyle changes as well as various supplements, including individually tailored nutraceuticals and botanicals in oral and intravenous forms, along with chronomodulated chemotherapy. This study documented significant response in patients with otherwise refractory disease. This type of intervention deserves future research attention.

Supplements for Treatment

Preliminary data support improved tolerance and efficacy of conventional therapies when multiple supplements, nutraceuticals, and botanicals are taken concurrently during chemotherapy or radiation therapy. These include omega-3 fats, astragalus, milk thistle (silymarin), green tea, melatonin, L-glutamine, alpha-lipoic acid, vitamins C and E, soy isoflavones, Siberian ginseng, and a variety of Chinese herbal combinations.[41] Data for these supplements are generally not conclusive, although further research should be conducted.

Support and the Therapeutic Ratio

Despite improvements in conventional therapies, there is still significant need for supportive care throughout the process. Side effects from surgery, radiation therapy, and chemotherapy are common, and multiple complementary interventions can improve the side effect profile. With help to support patients through treatment, an improvement may occur in the therapeutic ratio, basically a ratio that defines the amount of harm versus the amount of benefit. By improvement of the therapeutic ratio, patients may have improved cure rates in addition to improved quality of life because of better treatment tolerance and compliance. See Table 78-1 for symptoms and supportive care interventions.[18,41] Physical activity, nutrition, and stress reduction are recommended activities throughout the entire cancer continuum, with an excellent risk/benefit ratio.

> Physical activity, nutrition, and stress reduction are recommended activities throughout the entire cancer continuum, with an excellent risk/benefit ratio.

TABLE 78-1. Symptoms Associated With Colorectal Cancer Treatment and Potential Complementary Therapies

Nausea	Acupuncture, ginger capsules, frequent small meals, astragalus, mind-body therapies
Anxiety and distress	Massage therapy, creative arts therapy, mindfulness-based stress reduction, physical activity
Fatigue	Increased physical activity, botanicals, supplements, mind-body therapies
Pain	Massage therapy, acupuncture, Reiki (energy medicine), mind-body therapies
Insomnia	Yoga, meditation, physical activity, selected botanicals (chamomile, valerian, melatonin)
Depression	Physical activity, dietary changes, yoga, Reiki, massage therapy, meditation, omega-3 fats

Survivorship and Tertiary Prevention

As a result of the significant advances in early detection and treatment, the number of deaths due to colorectal cancer has been steadily decreasing. There are now more than 1 million survivors of colorectal cancer in the United States. Tertiary prevention should mainly focus on the modifiable risk factors discussed as a part of primary prevention. There are good data that adopting a whole-food plant-based diet and increasing physical activity can help reduce recurrence rates and preserve overall health and function. [42-45] An emphasis should be placed on compliance with follow-up screening procedures because a previous personal history for colorectal cancer places an individual in a high-risk category for development of new colorectal cancers.

End-of-Life Care

Despite appropriate therapy, approximately 500,000 deaths due to colorectal cancer occur yearly. End-of-life care can be enhanced by a variety of complementary therapies, including massage therapy, acupuncture, spiritual interventions, a variety of mind-body therapies, appropriate nutrition and supplementation, and targeted physical activity. [46-48]

Implementation of an Integrative Model

Integrative oncology must include an assessment of the intention of therapy—curative versus palliative—as well as of the outcome data for specific stages of disease and the performance status of patients. These factors will have a heavy impact on the decision to recommend interventions that have higher and lower levels of evidence. [18] For example, it might be reasonable to recommend an intervention that is rated B2 to a specific patient with a poor performance status being treated palliatively with therapy who has a low response rate to conventional therapy more than to a healthy patient being treated curatively in a situation in which the chance of cure is high.

Ideally, an integrative model will address all participants in the process at all levels of their being and experience. Many of the tools that have proven impact—modifiable lifestyle and diet risk factors—are simple to describe to patients but are not easy for patients to implement and to maintain. Physician self-care is vital for oncology care providers to prevent burnout. [49] Physicians who practice self-care are more effective at guiding patients to adopt healthy lifestyle and diet changes. [50]

Patient navigation is a new and expanding field that may provide a part of the solution to improving compliance of patients with screening and comprehensive diet and lifestyle changes. [51] Patient navigation basically consists of an individual in the health care system whose sole responsibility is to act as a patient advocate, providing access to all available resources throughout the cancer care continuum. [52] Patient navigation has been shown to improve access to care; the data are especially strong for improvement of screening and early detection, and some trials have improved colorectal cancer screening in disparate populations. [53] Patient navigators can include trained lay volunteers of similar cultural background, social workers, community health workers, and nurses. [54,55] The National Cancer Institute is currently sponsoring several trials to document optimal methods of patient navigation throughout the cancer care continuum. [56]

PREVENTION PRESCRIPTION

Screening and early detection should focus first on identification of high-risk populations, such as those with familial polyposis syndromes and family history of colorectal cancer. Screening studies are then matched to risk level and should follow ACS recommendations. Individuals with a normal risk should have screening colonoscopy at the age of 50 years.

Primary, secondary, and tertiary prevention of colorectal cancer should include the following foundation:
- Physical activity of at least 30 minutes of brisk walking daily or its equivalent
- Maintenance of a body mass index between 19 and 25
- A whole-food plant-based diet with avoidance of processed and sugary foods; avoidance or limitation of animal-based food products, especially charred red meat
- Avoidance of tobacco and alcohol consumption
- Appropriate, individualized supplementation with a low-potency multivitamin, omega-3 fat, vitamin D_3, and calcium citrate; vitamin D_3 levels should be maintained between 30 and 50 ng/mL
- Practice of a stress management tool for a minimum of 10 to 15 minutes/day

This whole-system approach should be consistently reevaluated for adherence, patient satisfaction, and efficacy and to determine if new tools in each category are indicated.

Secondary Prevention
- COX-2 inhibitors: either selective (such as celecoxib; most trials have used 400 mg twice daily; optimal dosing is still under investigation) or nonselective (aspirin; a single baby aspirin, 81 mg daily, appears to be sufficient, although optimal dosing is still not known).

THERAPEUTIC REVIEW

■ Primary Prevention

- Risk reduction in at-risk population

■ Screening and Early Detection

- Identify high-risk populations for increased screening and early intervention.

- Follow ACS recommendations for screening in normal-risk populations with colonoscopy starting at the age of 50 years.

■ Exercise

- 30 minutes of physical activity daily, the equivalent of brisk walking (see Chapter 88, Writing an Exercise Prescription)

■ Nutrition

- Whole-food plant-based diet (see Chapter 86, The Antiinflammatory [Omega-3] Diet)

■ Mind-Body

- Mind-body stress reduction techniques (see Chapter 93, Relaxation Techniques)

■ Supplements

- Folate: 400 mcg daily. Evidence is mixed for benefit. Some studies with 1000 mcg daily show an increased risk with supplementation. It is best to obtain folate through eating of foliage, such as green leafy vegetables.

- Vitamin B_6: Doses of these B vitamins in the range commonly found in a simple multivitamin are reasonable or 50 mg daily.

- Vitamin D_3: Maintain blood level between 30 and 50 ng/mL with baseline supplementation of 1000 units/day of D_3 once normal range is achieved.

- Calcium: Dose used in positive trials was 1200 mg calcium citrate per day. Calcium should be taken with vitamin D.

- Omega-3 fatty acids: 1000 mg/day of eicosapentaenoic acid (EPA) and docosahexaenoic acid (DHA). No definitive evidence favors an optimal ratio of EPA to DHA.

■ Patient Outreach

- Implement a patient outreach program, such as lay navigation, to address disparities in access to care. This can result in improved adherence to screening guidelines and migration to a lower disease stage at presentation.

■ Treatment

Symptom control during chemotherapy and radiation therapy can be enhanced through the use of a variety of complementary tools.

- Acupressure and acupuncture relieve chemotherapy-associated nausea and vomiting.

- Ginger tablets (2000 mg/day), 2 days before, during, and after chemotherapy, relieve chemotherapy-related nausea.

- Physical activity during conventional therapy improves fatigue levels and treatment adherence.

- Mind-body stress reduction techniques—yoga, mindfulness-based stress reduction, meditation, and hypnosis—improve tolerance of therapy, adherence to therapy, and quality of life during therapy.

- Individualized nutritional programs can increase the patient's tolerance of and compliance with conventional therapy.

Some botanicals may improve the tolerance and efficacy of conventional therapy.

- Astragalus: Some data show improved tolerance and efficacy when it is given during platinum (cisplatin)-based chemotherapy. Doses and schedules are not clearly defined. Most data come from clinical trials in China.

- Milk thistle: Some preclinical data show improved tolerance and efficacy during platinum-based chemotherapy.

Some nutritional supplements may improve tolerance of, adherence to, and efficacy of conventional therapy.

- L-Glutamine (5000 mg/day) improves radiation therapy–associated mucositis and decreases chemotherapy-related neuropathy.

- Acetyl-L-carnitine improves chemotherapy-related neuropathy and increases efficacy. Doses used in randomized trials were in the range of 1000 mg two or three times daily.

- Mushroom extract (PSK, *Cordyceps*): Significant preclinical data show increased immunity, and some clinical randomized data in gastrointestinal tract cancers show improved efficacy and tolerance when it is given with chemotherapy. However, no definitive dose or schedule is available currently.

- Alpha-lipoic acid improves neuropathy. Doses used for treatment of diabetic neuropathy are in the range of 200 to 400 mg/day.

  Individualized and highly rigorous, costly programs including "targeted" nutritional and intravenous supplements, physical activity, and mind-body stress reduction can have an antineoplastic effect.

KEY WEB RESOURCES

www.cancer.net	Official patient site of the American Society of Clinical Oncology; includes significant patient resource and educational materials
www.cancer.org	American Cancer Society Web site with specific information on colon cancer, including early detection, genetic markers, treatment, and prevention
www.trialcheck.org	Search for clinical trials for specific cancer types and stages
http://www.cdc.gov/cancer/colorectal/pdf/SFL_brochure.pdf	Free brochure on colon cancer from the Centers for Disease Control and Prevention (CDC)
http://www.cancer.gov/colorectalcancerrisk/#	Colorectal risk calculator from the National Cancer Institute

References

References are available online at expertconsult.com.

Chapter 79

Skin Cancer

Wadie I. Najm, MD, MSEd

Skin cancer, the most common of all cancer types, can be divided into two major groups, melanoma and non-melanoma skin cancer (NMSC). Melanoma is a tumor derived from melanocytes in the basal layer of the epidermis. Melanoma (Fig. 79-1) is the fifth leading cause of cancer in men (5%) and the sixth leading cause of cancer in women (4%).[1] Lifetime probability for development of invasive melanoma increases with age and is 1 in 37 for men and 1 in 56 for women. Whites have a higher (10-fold) incidence than that of nonwhites. NMSC encompasses different types of cancer, the two most common types being basal and squamous cell carcinomas. Basal cell carcinoma (BCC), the most common type of skin cancer (75%), arises from basal cells found in the outer layer of the epidermis and adnexal structures (hair follicles, sweat ducts; Fig. 79-2). Squamous cell carcinoma (SCC), the second most common type of skin cancer (20%), originates from scaly cells on the surface of the skin (Fig. 79-3). It is estimated that the incidence of NMSC is approximately equal to the combined incidence of all cancers.

Pathophysiology

Skin cancer can occur in any individual. The main risk factor for BCC is the inability to tan, whereas the risk factors for SCC include light skin, outdoor occupations, sunburns, and exposure to sunlight during childhood. Evidence for a role of the immune system in the pathogenesis of skin cancer is also noted. The increased frequency of SCC, especially in transplant recipients, is probably due to long-term immunosuppressive therapy. Exposure to ultraviolet (UV) light and sunburn increases the incidence of all skin cancers. Approximately 90% of NMSCs can be attributed to UV exposure.[2] UVB radiation can induce both direct and indirect adverse biologic effects, including induction of oxidative stress, DNA damage and its repair, premature aging of the skin, and multiple effects on the immune system. UVA can also lead to development of melanoma and SCC, mainly by production of reactive oxygen species through interaction with endogenous and exogenous photosensitizers. Several factors have been identified to increase the risk for melanoma (Box 79-1).

Screening

Early detection remains the gold standard. The American Cancer Society screening guidelines recommend regular skin self-examination for all adults. A review of the literature on screening for skin cancer identified several limitations. The direct evidence to support the benefits of a screening examination by a physician or patient in reducing morbidity and mortality is limited.[3] Pamphlets for self-examination of the skin are available from the American Cancer Society, the American Academy of Dermatology, and the Skin Cancer Foundation.

Clinical examination of the skin should be performed annually, particularly for individuals at high risk for skin cancer. People considered at high risk are those with a family history of skin cancer or melanoma; those with a personal history of skin cancer or precancer; and those with a high number of melanocytic nevi, xeroderma pigmentosum, and basal cell nevus syndrome.

Recognize early melanoma by the ABCD screening guideline, as follows:

Asymmetry
Border irregularity
Color variation
Diameter more than 6 mm

Imaging systems have been introduced to assist in detection of early lesions. Dermoscopy, with a hand-held lighted magnifier using cross-polarizing light filters, provides a 10-fold magnification of the skin. Several checklists can be used to assist in the decision.[4] A review of current studies reported a sensitivity of 82.6% to 85.7% and a specificity of 70% to 83.4%, dependent mainly on the experience of the examiner.[5] In multispectral digital dermoscopy, a sequence of images are obtained with use of particular bands of wavelengths; it offers the advantage of identifying characteristics

FIGURE 79-1
Melanoma. This melanoma has all of the melanoma-specific criteria from the algorithm and should be easy to diagnose. There are areas with an atypical pigment network, irregular streaks asymmetrically located in the lesion, irregular dots and globules, irregular blotches, and blue-white structures. Clinically, this lesion was in the gray zone of suspicion, but this dermoscopic picture leaves no doubt that this is a melanoma. (From Johr RH. *Dermoscopy*. St. Louis: Mosby; 2004.)

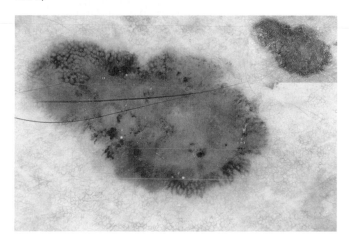

FIGURE 79-2
Basal cell carcinoma. (From Schuchter L, Ming M. Melanoma and nonmelanoma skin cancers. In: Goldman L. *Cecil Medicine*. 23rd ed. Philadelphia: Saunders; 2007.)

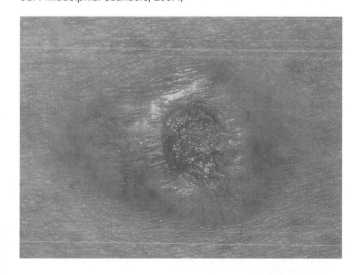

FIGURE 79-3
Squamous cell carcinoma of the skin. (From Schuchter L, Ming M. Melanoma and nonmelanoma skin cancers. In: Goldman L. *Cecil Medicine*. 23rd ed. Philadelphia: Saunders; 2007.)

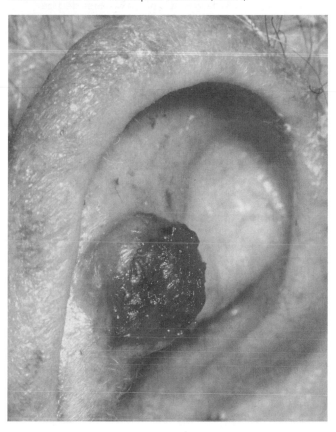

of the lesion not obvious to the naked eye. This automated version can enhance the sensitivity to 91.3% to 100% and the specificity to 70% to 85%.[6,7]

Confocal scanning laser microscopy uses a hand-held near-infrared laser of low power to provide real-time in vivo imaging of skin lesions at variable depths. It has a sensitivity of 97.3% and a specificity of 83%.[8,9]

Other technology (bioimpedance, ultrasonography) is available, but additional evaluation is required to define its role. Despite all the advances, clinical acumen remains the essential skill to identify skin lesions.[10]

Integrative Therapy

Lifestyle

The depletion of the ozone layer has increased the exposure of people to UV light. To protect themselves, people should wear protective clothing, avoid acute exposure to sunlight (particularly at midday, between 11 AM and 3 PM), and apply a broad-spectrum, high–sun protection factor (SPF) sunscreen. These precautions are not limited to sunny days; the sun's rays can penetrate light clouds and mist, and they are reflected by snow (85%) and water (5%). Multiple-day exposure to sunlight significantly increases sensitivity of the skin to sun damage on the second day, particularly in susceptible individuals. When such exposure occurs, application of high-SPF (30+) sunscreen is recommended. A major portion of UV exposure is received during childhood and adolescence; therefore, application of sunscreen during this time considerably reduces the incidence of NMSC. It should be cautioned that application of sunscreen may cause subjects to feel protected; hence, they may spend a longer time exposed to the sun and develop a higher risk of skin cancer.[11] Sunscreen should be reapplied every 2 hours if subjects decide to prolong their sun exposure.

Almost any opaque substance can be used to reduce the amount of UV radiation reaching the skin. The more opaque the material, the better the protection it provides.

Nutrition

Dietary Fat

Preliminary studies in the early 1980s reported a possible association of fat intake with incidence of melanoma. Although this initial work was based mainly on a dietary questionnaire, a follow-up study indicated a higher content of polyunsaturated fat in the adipose tissue of subjects with melanoma compared with controls.[12,13] Studies of the effect of fat intake on nonmelanoma skin cancer reported a similar association between fat intake and the incidence of new cancer. Reduction of fat intake (but not total calories) led to a lower incidence of new actinic keratosis (premalignant lesions) in study subjects than that found in the control group.[14,15]

Case-control and epidemiologic studies identify a trend toward lower risk of melanoma and SCC with high dietary intake of omega-3 polyunsaturated fatty acids and high omega-3/omega-6 polyunsaturated fatty acid ratio. In a review of Mediterranean diet and fatty acid intake,[16,17] observational studies show that adherence to a Mediterranean diet reduces the incidence of melanoma, even among populations that adopt the traditional diet.[18,19]

Garlic and Onion

Garlic and onion oils were found to lower the number of skin tumors in an animal study. Diallyl sulfide, a component of garlic, applied topically 1 hour before or after exposure to carcinogens, delays the onset of tumors and confers significant protection from skin carcinogenesis.[20] Animal studies proposed several potential mechanisms for skin cancer prevention: suppression of development of tumors that harbor *ras* mutations by inhibiting the membrane association of oncogenic p21/ras protein[21]; antimutagenic properties on 7,12-dimethylbenz[*a*]anthracene (DMBA [a carcinogenic polycyclic aromatic hydrocarbon])—induced DNA strand breaks[22]; and up-regulation of p53wt and p21/Waf1, while p53mut expression was down-regulated.[23] Translation of these results into human prevention studies is lacking.

Fish and Fish Oil

Fish intake was noted to have a protective effect in case-control studies, suggesting a possible role for fish oil in the prevention of melanoma.[24] Studies reported that linolenic acid (18:2 omega-6) and alpha-linolenic acid (18:3 omega-3), the precursors to omega-3 and omega-6 fatty acids, have shown promise as a safe adjunctive treatment of several skin conditions, including NMSC and melanoma.[25] Several mechanisms were proposed, including maintenance of the stratum corneum, inhibition of proinflammatory eicosanoids and cytokines, elevation of sunburn threshold, and promotion of apoptosis in malignant cells. However, case-control studies found no appreciable association of lower melanoma risk with fish, meat, vegetables, fruit, dairy products, whole-meal bread, alcohol, or coffee and tea drinking.[26] A systematic review confirmed these conclusions; the review did not find evidence to suggest a significant association between omega-3 fatty acids and cancer incidence.[27] In fact, subanalysis of skin cancer found an increased risk (RR, 1.13; 95% CI, 1.01-1.27). However, a closer look at the study identifies several limitations that render the conclusions uncertain. Additional studies are still needed to evaluate the role of omega-3 fatty acids in cancer prevention.

Botanicals

Green Tea

Green tea contains powerful polyphenol antioxidants (epigallocatechin gallate). Their protective effect is thought to be due to inhibition of free radicals, inhibition of lipid peroxidation, inhibition of UV light–induced and chemical-induced tumor growth, reduction of the inflammation associated with UV exposure, DNA repair, and inhibition of oncogenic expression.[28,29] Several animal and human studies investigating the oral and topical application of green tea to prevent skin cancer have suggested that green tea may reduce the risk of skin cancer induction in humans by UV radiation.[30,31] Reports suggest that green tea polyphenols have the potential, in conjunction with the use of traditional sunscreens, to further protect the skin against the damaging effects of UV radiation.[32] In addition, animal study suggests that the antitumor activity of green tea on melanoma can be enhanced when it is combined with vitamin A.[33]

Panax Ginseng

Animal and laboratory[34] studies suggest a dose-dependent inhibitory effect of Panax ginseng on skin cancer, prolonging the latency period and reducing the tumor numbers. Laboratory studies of ginsenoside Rp1 (G-Rp1), a novel ginseng saponin, strongly inhibited the metastatic lung transfer of melanoma cells, suggesting that G-Rp1 may act as an anticancer agent by strongly inhibiting cell viability and metastatic processes.[35]

Thuja Standishii

Labdane diterpenoid, derived from the stem bark of *Thuja standishii* (Japanese name: kurobe) and from marine sources, has been found to demonstrate different levels of bioactivity, such as antiinflammatory, antibacterial, antifungal, antileishmanial, cardiotonic, and cytotoxic activities. A two-stage mouse skin carcinogenesis study reported an inhibitory effect on tumor promotion induced by TPA (12-O-tetradecanoylphorbol-13-acetate).[36, 37] A potential role in the prevention or treatment of human skin cancer is yet to be established.

Turmeric (Curcumin)

In a study on three different melanoma cell lines at M.D. Anderson Cancer Center, the yellow Indian spice turmeric (curcumin) inhibited growth of all three. Curcumin also stimulated cell apoptosis (programmed cell death) by suppressing a protein called nuclear factor kappaB that normally protects these cancer cells from death. The effects were dose dependent; the higher the dose, the more cancer cell death.[38] More recently, attention has been directed at curcumin in the attempt to repair photodamaged skin as a means of preventing degeneration into solar-induced skin cancers. Curcumin has been shown to protect from injury by attenuating oxidative stress and suppressing inflammation.[39]

The combined treatment at lower doses of curcumin with tamoxifen provides a nontoxic option for chemotherapy with great potential for future use.[40] The combination was noted to produce significant induction of autophagy along with apoptosis of cancerous cells; noncancerous cells are unaffected by this combination. In addition, once they are exposed to low doses of this cotreatment, melanoma cells still retained signals to commit suicide even after removal of the drugs.

Curcumin shows promise as it has been found to reduce inflammation in the skin, to provide protection against damage, and to enhance the benefits of treatment for melanoma.

Supplements

Selenium

Selenium is a trace element that plays an important part in antioxidant enzymes (selenoproteins). The content of selenium in plant food depends on the soil content of the mineral. Some nuts and particularly Brazil nuts contain a high amount of selenium (each nut contains about 80 to 120 mcg). Selenium can also be found in some meats (beef, turkey, chicken breast) and seafood (cod, tuna). Despite early indications of a possible role of selenium in the prevention of skin cancers, randomized studies on the use of selenium for the prevention of melanoma and NMSC do not show a protective effect; in fact, later evidence found it to raise the risk of recurrence among high-risk individuals.[41,42]

Probiotics

Probiotics are defined as living microorganisms that confer a health benefit to the host when they are consumed in adequate amounts. Several trials suggested a beneficial role of probiotics in the management of atopic dermatitis. A small randomized trial reported that *Lactobacillus johnsonii* NCC 533 could modulate the cutaneous immune homeostasis altered by UV exposure.[43] Clinical data suggest that certain probiotic strains may confer a benefit at the skin level, leading to the preservation of skin homeostasis. However, additional studies are needed to better define a potential role for probiotics in skin cancer prevention.

Beta-Carotene

Beta-carotene is a member of the carotenoids, a group of red, orange, and yellow pigments. Beta-carotene can be found in green plants, carrots, sweet potatoes, green peppers, fruits, apricots, and whole grains. Alpha-, beta-, and gamma-carotenes are considered provitamins because they can be converted to vitamin A. UV radiation disrupts skin homeostasis, in part by causing a loss of retinoid receptors. Retinoid receptors participate in epidermal growth and differentiation. Animal studies point to an inhibitory role of beta-carotene in UV-induced skin cancer. In addition, an inverse relationship between the level of serum beta-carotene and the incidence of skin cancer was noted.[44] In a large clinical trial, the protective effect of beta-carotene (50 mg/day) against NMSC during 5 years was not supported.[45,46] These findings were confirmed by a large Australian study using 30 mg/day for 4.5 years.[47] High levels of retinol and carotenoids have been found to have a weak or no protective effect against melanoma.[24,48]

Vitamin D

Vitamin D is a fat-soluble vitamin made in the body when the skin is exposed to the sun. Food sources are fatty fish (salmon, tuna, or mackerel), beef liver, cheese, and egg yolks. Several foods (e.g., cereals, milk) are fortified with vitamin D. Several studies suggest a potential influence of vitamin D on site-specific aggressiveness of melanomas. A meta-analysis of 10 studies (N = 6805) found an overall protective association with melanoma and NMSC for 2 vitamin D polymorphisms (FokI and BsmI).[49] However, additional studies are needed to define the role of vitamin D in skin cancer primary or secondary prevention.

Vitamin E

Vitamin E can be found in nuts, whole grains, spinach, egg yolk, vegetable oils, and asparagus, among others. Animal studies show a possible protective effect of vitamin E. The effect was noted to be greater in vivo than in vitro. Vitamin E has been found to protect against lipid peroxidation and DNA miscoding, and it had a strong inhibitory effect on tumor promotion in a two-stage protocol after application of dimethylbenzanthracene (DMBA).[50] Vitamin E has also been found to have a synergistic effect with the other carotenoids by protecting them from photo-oxidation and hence enhancing their tumor suppression effect.[51] Additional studies are needed to evaluate the exact role of vitamin E in skin cancer prevention. Earlier human studies did not show a protective effect for vitamin E supplementation against melanoma or NMSC; however, a consistently higher risk was noted in subjects with low vitamin E intake. A 2005 review found that topical vitamin E reduced erythema, sunburn cells, chronic UVB-induced skin damage, and photocarcinogenesis, whereas only high doses of oral vitamin E may affect the response to UVB in humans.[52]

Vitamin C

Vitamin C can be found in most plants, such as broccoli, bell peppers, kale, tomatoes, strawberries, blueberries, citrus, kiwi, pineapples, and cantaloupes. Studies report that vitamin C lowers the incidence of skin cancer in UV light–treated mice and has a photoprotective effect in human epithelial cells.[53] A small study using 10% topical vitamin C 5 days before UVB irradiation showed a reduced erythematous response. Lower concentrations did not confer any protection. Oral use of vitamin C has not been demonstrated to confer photoprotection.

Pharmaceuticals

Sunscreen

No randomized controlled trials have assessed the effect of sunscreens on the incidence of or mortality from malignant melanoma. One randomized controlled trial found that sunscreens reduced the incidence of solar keratosis. A review of existing studies demonstrated a major role of UVA in the induction of skin photodamage and emphasized the need for a broad protection covering the entire solar UV spectrum.[54] It is increasingly accepted that sunscreens should protect against UV radiation–induced immunosuppression, with an index of protection that can be compared with the SPF. The SPF number indicates protection against UVB rays only. The American Academy of Dermatology recommends products with SPF of 30 or higher. Despite the lack of prospective studies, use of broad-spectrum sunscreens for the prevention of melanoma and NMSC seems sensible and is highly recommended. For best results, recommend application of a thick layer of sunscreen to exposed areas. Recommend reapplication of sunscreens at least every 2 hours and even more often with swimming or sweating. Sunscreens labeled waterproof can provide

protection for 80 minutes even when subjects become wet; products labeled water resistant may protect for only 40 minutes.

Studies have shown that a class of natural agents known as oligosaccharins, complex carbohydrates found in plants, protects the cutaneous immune system from UVB- and UVA-induced immunomodulation.[55,56] This immune protective effect occurs independently from erythema and DNA damage protection, and these agents, particularly tamarind xyloglucan, may become important adjunctive ingredients to sunscreens.

Concerns were raised by the Environmental Working Group report, which stated: "Recently available data from an FDA study indicate that a form of vitamin A, retinyl palmitate, when applied to the skin in the presence of sunlight, may speed the development of skin tumors and lesions (NTP 2009). This evidence is troubling because the sunscreen industry adds vitamin A to 41 percent of all sunscreens." However, on closer review, there is no convincing evidence to support this conclusion.[57]

Vaccine Therapy

A number of trials are evaluating vaccine therapies in melanoma patients. Recent trials reported that high-dose interferon improves relapse-free survival in melanoma patients at high risk for recurrence. Promising trials are under way to evaluate the efficacy of vaccines (CD34+ derived and an oncolytic special strain of herpes simplex type 1 virus reprogrammed to infect only cancer cells) for treatment of patients with high-risk or completely resected metastatic melanoma. Additional trials are evaluating the efficacy of different regimens of melanoma vaccine: mutated gp100 melanoma vaccine in HLA-A*0201 patients; peptides or tumor lysates using dendritic cells for antigen delivery; and anti–gastrin-releasing peptide DNA.

PREVENTION PRESCRIPTION

- Avoid sunburn, midday sunlight, artificial ultraviolet sources (tanning booths, sunlamps), and prolonged sun exposure starting in childhood.
- Wear protective clothing and a wide-brimmed hat when exposed to sunlight.
- Apply a generous layer of broad-spectrum high-SPF sunscreen of 30 or greater. Reapply every 2 hours and as needed if the skin gets wet. Use of sunscreen does not mean that one can prolong exposure time.
- Perform yearly skin examinations and educate patients to do self-examination using the ABCD warning signs.
- A low-fat diet may have a beneficial effect in the prevention of melanoma and nonmelanoma skin cancers.

THERAPEUTIC REVIEW

Avoid Sunburn

- Avoid prolonged sun exposure, particularly between 11 AM and 3 PM.

- Use a broad-spectrum sunblock with an SPF of 30 or higher to provide 1 to 2 hours of protection. An important and efficient barrier is clothing. A hat can protect the face and scalp.

Nutrition

- Consider a reduction in total fat intake and encourage foods rich in fish oil.

Botanicals

- Consider green tea; drinking of three cups a day or using it in topical form may provide some protection from UV radiation.

- Consider adding curcumin to the diet. At a dosage of 500 to 1000 mg three times a day, it has an antiinflammatory effect.

Supplements

- A combination of antioxidants (beta-carotene with vitamin C; vitamin A with green tea) may have a better protective effect against UV radiation than either alone.

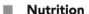

KEY WEB RESOURCES

American Cancer Society: http://www.cancer.org

1-800-ACS-2345 (1-800-227-2345)

Melanoma Research Foundation: http://www.melanoma.org/

Information, database, chat room, and a patient network with case profiles are provided for people interested in melanoma. Information is also provided about ongoing trials and results from relevant trials.

Melanoma Education Foundation: http://www.skincheck.com

This Web site of the Melanoma Education Foundation (1-978-535-3080) is a good resource for patients and health care workers, with pictures and useful link sites.

Guide to Internet Resources for Cancer

The Skin Cancer Resources Directory: http://www.cancerindex.org/clinks2s.htm

A wealth of information, resources, links, and database about skin cancer are provided for both professionals and patients.

American Academy of Dermatology: www.aad.org

1-888-462-DERM (1-888-462-3376)

Skin Cancer Foundation: www.skincancer.org

1-800-SKIN-490 (1-800-754-6490)

References

References are available online at expertconsult.com.

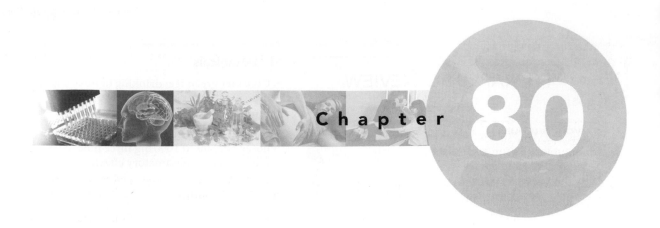

Chapter **80**

End-of-Life Care

Lucille R. Marchand, MD, BSN

Integrative end-of-life care, integrative palliative care delivered at the end of a person's life, is usually referred to as hospice care (Fig. 80-1). It encompasses whole-person, relationship-centered care using conventional and alternative approaches with an emphasis on health and healing.[1] Goals of care for the dying person include optimization of well-being and quality of life, relief of distressing symptoms, empowered decision-making, support of caregivers, and effective life closure for peaceful and meaningful dying and death. Bereavement services for family and friends of the person dying are an essential element of care. Grief and loss begin with the diagnosis of disease. Hospice care incorporates the use of a multidisciplinary team of health professionals working together to best meet the needs of the patient and family. The team includes the patient's physician, the hospice physician, nurses, certified nurses' aides, chaplains, bereavement counselors, social workers, housekeepers, dietitians, volunteers, occupational and physical therapists, and other integrative practitioners who work in the hospice, are affiliated with the hospice, or have been sought out by the patient and family for care and support.[2] Integrative palliative care calls on us to be creative and innovative in the care of dying patients, expanding options to enhance healing, to maintain hope, and to improve well-being in a unique way for each person.

In a survey of complementary therapy services provided by hospices, 60% of responding organizations offered such therapies. The most common services were massage therapy (83%), music therapy (50%), therapeutic touch (49%), pet therapy (48%), guided imagery (45%), Reiki (36%), aromatherapy (30%), harp music (23%), reflexology (20%), art therapy (20%), hypnotherapy (4%), yoga (3%), acupuncture (1%), and humor therapy (1%). Constraints to providing complementary services were lack of funding, lack of staff time, lack of qualified complementary therapists, inadequate knowledge about these services, and patient and staff resistance to complementary therapies. Even in hospices that offered these services, less than 25% of the patients received them.[3] In a 2008 survey of 27 Nevada and Montana hospices

using the survey instrument of Demmer, 70.4% of hospices offered complementary and alternative medicine (CAM) services, but less than 25% of hospice patients received them. The most used CAM therapies included massage and music therapy; 61.1% of hospices had a salaried CAM provider, and 88.3% had CAM volunteers. None of the hospices had an assessment tool to determine which patients might benefit from CAM services. Barriers to use were the same as those cited for constraints to providing complementary services.[4] Preliminary research outcome data on the program have been favorable.[5] Demmer and Sauer[6] found that patients who received complementary therapies were more satisfied with their hospice services. Sirios[7] compared consumers seeking consultation with CAM practitioners in 1997 and 2005. Consumer motivation changed in that period from use of CAM due to negative attitudes toward conventional medicine to use of CAM modalities for their positive effects and a whole-person, empowered approach to health care.

For patients dying with uncontrolled symptoms, such as pain, the symptoms are often more frightening than death itself. Patients desire pain and symptom control; the ability to prepare for their dying and to have their choices honored; life completion; mental clarity; being touched; being at peace with their god; having clinicians one can trust, who listen, and are comfortable talking about dying; and being in the presence of loved ones without being a burden.[8] Ira Byock[9] describes the essential elements of meaningful living as the expression of forgiveness, appreciation, and love. The phrases "Please forgive me," "I forgive you," "Thank you," and "I love you" embody these elements; they can improve relationships at any time in life but particularly at life's closure.[9]

Pathophysiology

General criteria in patients with advanced chronic illness who are dying are as follows: unintentional weight loss of more than 10% body weight, serum albumin value lower than

FIGURE 80-1
Model of integrative palliative medicine.

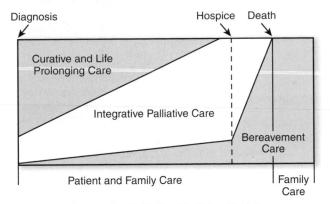

Integrative Palliative Medicine Model

Common Issues in End-of-life Care

Common symptoms managed in end-of-life care are pain; nausea, vomiting, and constipation; dyspnea; depression and anxiety; and delirium. Unrelieved physical, emotional, or spiritual discomfort must be treated as a palliative care emergency, and careful assessment and intensive palliative resources must be applied to prevent unnecessary suffering.[16] Uncontrolled symptoms can lead to the patient's desire for a hastened death.[17] On occasion, physical and psychological symptoms cannot be controlled with conventional and alternative therapies, and palliative sedation must be used to control symptoms such as intractable and intense pain, seizures, and existential psychological suffering. The intention of this therapy is to treat intractable suffering, not to hasten death. Careful guidelines have been developed for its use.[18-22]

It is beyond the scope of this chapter to discuss conventional symptom management in detail. There are many valuable palliative care resources for this information.[2,23-27]

2.5 g/dL, spending more than 50% of time in bed (Karnofsky score), inability to perform most activities of daily living, progression of disease, and uncontrolled symptoms despite aggressive treatment of the underlying illness.[10] Physicians tend to be overly optimistic about prognosis, an error that leads to delayed hospice referrals, less time for patient and family to prepare for death, delay or absence of end-of-life care discussions with informed decision making, lack of preparatory bereavement services, and inappropriate life-prolonging interventions. An important question for clinicians to ask themselves is, Would I be surprised if this patient died in the next year or in the next 6 months? If the answer is no, the patient has reached the end of life; communication about treatment preferences becomes more important and referral to hospice appropriate.[11]

Communication lies at the heart of integrative end-of-life care. "Hoping for the best" needs to be balanced with "preparing for the worst."[12] Conversations must be sensitive in eliciting how much the patient wants to know.[13] Goals of care are explored in a patient-centered way and then serve as guides for further decision-making. Armed with knowledge about patient preferences for care, clinicians can avoid unwarranted treatment. Hope is then in keeping with what the patient wants to accomplish in his or her remaining life. Goals and hope will change as the process unfolds. Hope can be viewed as an inner power that moves a person forward in life. Questions that can be helpful in palliative medicine conversations with patients in uncovering what will move them forward and inspire hope include the following: How can I be most helpful to you? What worries you most now and for the future? What is important or meaningful to you right now? When the clinician listens to the answers intently without interruption, empowerment and a sense of hopefulness can arise in the patient. It allows the patient to heal and to live well in the face of dying. Hope becomes a fluid process of living fully rather than fixed dependence on a particular outcome.[14]

Communicating "bad" or challenging news constitutes an essential skill that is well described by Buckman.[15] It requires deep listening, empathy, presence, and emotional awareness on the part of the clinician (see Chapter 3, The Healing Encounter).

Pain Management

Opioids are the foundation of end-of-life pain management. Pain, however, is a complex phenomenon involving physical, emotional, social, and spiritual aspects that must be addressed for total pain management, as described by Cicely Saunders,[28,29] the founder of the modern hospice movement. The World Health Organization (WHO) ladder of pain management recommends various levels of pain treatment, depending on pain severity.[23] Physical pain is often a combination of nociceptive and neuropathic pain, and opioids alone are usually not effective in treating the neuropathic component of pain without adjunctive medications, such as antidepressants and anticonvulsant medication.[29]

Methadone is a unique opioid that can effectively treat both components but must be dosed carefully, given that it has a large volume of distribution and its kinetics differ from those of other opioids. The switch from another opioid to methadone must be made carefully and may require consultation with a pain or palliative medicine consultant.[30-32] There is no ceiling dose for opioids, and careful but aggressive and rapid titration of the dose to relieve pain is recommended (see box). Pain that is unrelieved by opioids can be treated with agents such as ketamine, parenteral lidocaine, nerve blocks, and, in some cases, palliative sedation.[29,33-36]

Depression, anxiety, and spiritual distress can all increase the perception of pain intensity, and addressing these components of pain can reduce the need for pain medication.[37,38] A multicontinental WHO study in primary care revealed that persistent pain is associated with greater psychological illness.[39] Lin et al,[40] in a large randomized controlled trial, found that amelioration of depressive symptoms decreased pain and improved both functional status and quality of life.[40] Because most antidepressants, including St. John's wort, take 2 to 6 weeks to have effect, treatment at end of life depends on length of life expected. Psychostimulants such as methylphenidate have immediate effects in alleviating depression.[41] Other modalities, such as psychotherapy, energetic medicine, and mind-body modalities, can also have a beneficial effect.

Many integrative modalities for the pain management of chronic conditions are covered in other chapters in this volume and can be applied at end-of-life care. Relatively few studies have focused solely on alternative and complementary treatments of pain at end of life.

Never order opioids without also scheduling a stool softener and/or laxative such as senna to prevent constipation that can lead to bowel obstruction. A common one is docusate sodium, 100 mg at bedtime. A laxative is usually needed in conjunction with a stool softener to have a bowel movement at least every other day as a usual goal.

Supplements for Pain

Glucosamine Sulfate
Glucosamine is used for arthritis pain. Arthritis pain can be worsened with decreased mobility at the end of life. Glucosamine has fewer side effects than nonsteroidal antiinflammatory analgesics do, but it can be as efficacious for arthritis pain.

PAIN MANAGEMENT FOR HOSPICE PATIENTS

Remember!
- There is no maximum dose of morphine if the patient remains in pain.
- Dose the medicines around the clock to prevent pain; "prn" dosing for cancer pain is poor pain control.

What You Will Need
- Morphine extended-release (MS Contin) 30 mg #60 to start (also comes as 15, 60, 100, and 200 mg)
- You can use suppositories for immediate-release dosing every 2 to 4 hours if the patient is unable to swallow (available as 5, 10, 20, and 30 mg).
- Paper and pencil, or calculator and pencil if math is "not your thing."

Dosing for the First 48 Hours
Dosages for maintenance and long-acting pain medications may be calculated as follows:

Start with an immediate-release morphine sulfate liquid formulation that will be given every 4 hours.	Example: Roxanol 20 mg/mL concentrate
Give a loading dose of the liquid. This is done in part to demonstrate to the patient that the pain can be controlled, and it should relieve pain within 30 minutes.	Roxanol 30 mg (1½ mL)
Follow that with a maintenance dose, which is then given around-the-clock.	Roxanol 10-20 mg every 4 hours
To control breakthrough pain, the patient is allowed to take half the maintenance dose every hour as needed for pain.	Roxanol 5-10 mg every hour as needed
The patient is given a dose of long-acting morphine sulfate at bedtime to allow him or her to sleep through the night.	Morphine extended-release (MS Contin) 30 mg at bedtime

Subsequent Dosing of Long-Acting Morphine Sulfate for Maintenance and Immediate-Release Liquid for Breakthrough Pain
Subsequent dosages of pain medications for maintenance and breakthrough pain are calculated as follows:

To figure the maintenance dose, add up the total amount of long-acting morphine sulfate given in a 24-hour period (immediate-release liquid plus long-acting pills used each day). Divide the total by 2; the result is the maintenance dose. The dosage can be rounded up or down to make things easier.	The total 24-hour dose is 120 mg. 120/2 = 60. The maintenance dose for long-acting morphine sulfate is started at 60 mg every 12 hours: MS Contin 30 mg, 2 tablets twice daily
To calculate the amount of immediate-release liquid to use for breakthrough pain, divide the total 24-hour dose by 6.	120/6 = 20 The patient may have 20 mg (1 mL) of Roxanol every 2 to 4 hours as needed for breakthrough pain.

If More Pain Control Is Needed Over Time

Recalculate dosages for more pain control as follows:

Have the family keep track of how much morphine sulfate is needed for breakthrough pain in a day.	The patient needs three doses of 20 mg of the immediate-release liquid (Roxanol) in a day; the total requirement is 60 mg.
Recalculate the amount of long-acting morphine sulfate that is given for maintenance as follows: Add the total daily breakthrough dose to the 24-hour maintenance dose to obtain the new maintenance dose.	Total daily breakthrough dose = 60 mg. 24-hour maintenance dose = 120 mg. New maintenance dose is 180 mg.
Divide this total by 2 to obtain the new twice-daily dose for the long-acting morphine sulfate.	180/2 = 90 Extended-release morphine (MS Contin) 90 mg twice daily
The same new maintenance dose number is then divided by 6 to obtain the new breakthrough dose for the immediate-release morphine sulfate that can be given every 2 to 4 hours as needed.	180/6 = 30 Roxanol 30 mg (1½ mL) every 2 to 4 hours as needed

Modified method of Michael Frederich, MD, Regional Medical Director, TrinityCare Hospice, Torrance, California; used with permission.

Dosage

Start with 3000 mg/day; once pain is relieved, decrease to 1500 mg daily. Tablets can be crushed. It can be taken for 1 to 3 months to achieve pain relief.

Side Effects

The side effects of glucosamine are minimal, but it can cause gastrointestinal distress.[42]

Botanicals for Pain

Cannabis

Cannabis can help alleviate neuropathic pain. Dronabinol (Marinol) is the oral synthetic form of cannabis. Cannabinoid receptors are located in the central and peripheral nervous system (CB1) and the immune system (CB2). Investigation of these receptors is becoming more prominent.[43] One small randomized controlled trial found that cannabinoid CT-3 is significantly more effective than placebo in controlling neuropathic pain 3 hours after dosing, with less response after 8 hours. In a study of patients with human immunodeficiency virus (HIV) infection, cannabis improved muscle pain and nerve pain significantly.[44-46]

Dosage

The dose of dronabinol is 10 mg, four times a day.

Side Effects

Side effects include dry mouth, tiredness, and poor memory.

Other Modalities for Treatment of Pain: Acupuncture, Massage, and Music

A Cochrane review of 16 trials of acupuncture for osteoarthritis pain of the knee or hip showed statistically significant short-term improvements in pain.[47] A Cochrane review of massage and low back pain in 13 trials demonstrated short- and long-term significant relief of low back pain, outperforming acupuncture, relaxation techniques, and other CAM modalities.[48] Music therapy was also found to relieve pain and to help decrease opioid dose needed.[49]

Nausea, Vomiting, and Constipation

Whenever nausea, vomiting, and constipation symptoms occur, it is important to establish the cause for an antiemetic targeted at the responsible mechanism to be used. Common causes are dysmotility, obstruction, side effects of medication such as opioids, metastases in the brain, and vestibular apparatus irritation (sometimes caused by dehydration). Constipation is a common cause of nausea and vomiting. Corticosteroids (such as prednisone and dexamethasone) can reduce the nausea and vomiting caused by the cerebral edema that occurs from brain metastases. Laxatives, stool softeners, and enemas can prevent and relieve constipation and bowel obstruction from severe constipation. The goal is to achieve a bowel movement at least every other day[50,51] (see Chapter 45, Constipation). Bulking agents should be avoided in patients who are not taking in sufficient fluids. Metoclopramide (Reglan) can relieve nausea from dysmotility but can have extrapyramidal side effects, especially in older persons. For dysmotility, promethazine (Phenergan) is a potent anticholinergic drug that should not be used for nausea in this situation because it will cause further slowing of gut motility.[52]

Antiemetics represent a variety of drugs with antihistamine, antidopaminergic, antiserotonergic ($5\text{-}HT_3$ receptor antagonists), and anticholinergic effects. They are not interchangeable. Promethazine is an antihistamine with potent anticholinergic effects and very weak antidopaminergic effects, making it a poor choice for treatment of the nausea of opioids as well. Prochlorperazine (Compazine) is the drug of choice for opioid-induced nausea, together with stool softeners to prevent constipation, metoclopramide to improve motility, and long-acting opioids to prevent drug level peaks that can cause nausea. 5-Hydroxytryptamine type 3 ($5\text{-}HT_3$) antagonists such as ondansetron (Zofran) are expensive second-line agents that are preferred for treatment of the nausea from chemotherapy or when other agents have failed or are contraindicated, such as in Parkinson's disease.[52] There is evidence that acupuncture as well as other mind-body and energetic therapies can also help relieve nausea.

Botanicals for Nausea

Ginger (Zingiber officinale)

Ginger can help alleviate nausea. It has been found efficacious for nausea of pregnancy, motion sickness, and nausea associated with chemotherapy but not for postoperative nausea.[53] Its mechanism of action is unknown, but ginger appears to have a prokinetic effect.

■ Dosage

Take 500 to 1000 mg of ginger root extract every 4 to 6 hours as needed, or eat 1 tsp or 5 g of crystallized ginger every 2 to 3 hours as needed.

■ Precautions

Side effects are rare. Excessive doses can cause heartburn.

Cannabis

Cannabis can help alleviate nausea and improve appetite. In a study of HIV-positive patients, cannabis improved nausea and appetite significantly.[45]

■ Dosage

Dronabinol, 10 mg, is given four times a day.

■ Side Effects

Side effects include dry mouth, tiredness, and poor memory.

Dyspnea

Opioids and oxygen are important palliative treatments of dyspnea. Opioids relieve the sensation of breathlessness and can improve the patient's functional capacity. Diuretics can help relieve dyspnea from fluid overload. Optimal treatment of the underlying condition is essential, but some interventions may no longer reverse the condition in end-stage disease. Nonpharmacologic strategies to help relieve dyspnea include the use of fans for a well-ventilated environment and cool ambient temperature. Complementary therapies include mind-body and energetic modalities.

Scopolamine, glycopyrrolate, and hyoscyamine dry oral secretions and decrease the "death rattle."[54,55] Dying is marked usually by progressive dehydration that keeps the patient comfortable by eliminating excessive secretions. Thirst is relieved with small sips of fluids and by keeping the mouth moist with frequent swabbing. Artificial feeding through a gastric tube and artificial intravenous fluids can cause respiratory congestion, pain, nausea, and vomiting. Families and health care professionals who equate caring with feeding can be encouraged to provide caring by other means, such as touch, life review, listening, and expressing love and appreciation to the dying person.[56,57]

Dyspnea is often accompanied by anxiety and is effectively treated with anxiolytics. If carefully titrated, opioids and anxiolytics do not hasten death or cause respiratory depression but make the patient comfortable. Care must be taken in the opioid naive patient, and initial dosing is low.[54,56]

In a Cochrane review of nonpharmacologic interventions most effective in relieving malignant and nonmalignant dyspnea, there existed strong evidence for the positive role of neuroelectrical muscle stimulation and chest wall vibration and moderate evidence for breathing training and walking aids. There was weak evidence for the role of acupuncture and no evidence for benefit of music therapy. There was insufficient evidence for other modalities, such as relaxation breathing and psychological interventions. Most studies reviewed were of patients with chronic obstructive pulmonary disease.[58]

Anxiety and Depression

 Information on this topic can be found online at expertconsult.com

Delirium

The patient's inability to focus, fluctuating level of consciousness, poor memory, agitation, hallucinations, hyperactivity and restlessness or hypoactivity and somnolence, tangential thinking, insomnia, anxiety, and significant distress characterize delirium. Careful assessment of the delirious patient is essential, and the condition should not be reflexively treated with anxiolytics, which can potentially make delirium worse.[60] Benzodiazepines, however, are first-line treatment of the delirium associated with alcohol withdrawal or seizures.[64] Medications commonly cause delirium, especially those with anticholinergic side effects, such as tricyclic antidepressants and antihistamines. Opioids can also cause delirium, and decreasing the dose or substituting another opioid with no active metabolites, such as hydromorphone (Dilaudid), can help. Steroids can cause delirium as well as hepatic encephalopathy, hypoxia, and hypoglycemia. Haloperidol (Haldol) continues to be the most effective medication for acute delirium. The treatment goal, however, is to treat the underlying cause.[65-67]

Near-death awareness encompasses a dying person's experience and possibly control over the dying process. When a patient experiences the presence of a deceased relative, clinicians can interpret this event as delirium with hallucinations and can inappropriately medicate the person with an antipsychotic or anxiolytic agent. The patient, however, may not demonstrate other criteria for delirium. Patients can feel annoyed, frustrated, and isolated in their profound end-of-life experiences. This is a time for clinicians to listen. Patients will attempt to describe these experiences or request something to ensure a peaceful death. They may know when they will die. They may use symbolic language to describe their experiences, which can be difficult to interpret. By being curious and appreciative of the experience, clinicians can validate and support the patient, help family members understand the experience, and perhaps learn themselves about the dying process.[68-70]

Do not treat agitation reflexively with anxiolytics. Careful assessment is needed to determine the cause of agitation, especially in patients with decreased cognitive function such as dementia. Causes can include delirium, near-death awareness, spiritual distress, depression and anxiety, unrelieved pain, and other uncontrolled physical symptoms.

Spiritual Care

End of life brings questions about life's meaning and purpose. Spiritual and religious concerns often affect end-of-life decision making.[71] In one study questioning ambulatory outpatients, 66% of respondents said they would want their physician to ask about their spirituality and beliefs if they became gravely ill, and 16% said they would not.[72] Careful spiritual assessment can help the patient who desires supportive spiritual resources to obtain them to aid in life closure. Expressive therapies such as music, art, collage, movement, and writing can facilitate the exploration of spiritual issues.[73] Life review or reminiscence therapy can encourage the discovery of meaning. Chibnall and associates[74] reported that higher levels of death distress in patients correlated with higher levels of physical and psychological symptoms, living alone, lower spiritual well-being, and less physician communication as perceived by the patient. In a study of patients with cancer, Meraviglia[75] found that higher levels of finding meaning in life and greater use of prayer correlated with higher psychological well-being and less physical distress. Use of a spiritual assessment tool can facilitate communication about life's meaning, life closure, and treatment goals and help assess a patient's strengths. It can also be used as a therapeutic tool to increase self-efficacy and well-being.[76–80] Puchalski's model for spiritual assessment with the acronym of FICA includes questions related to faith and belief, importance of that faith and beliefs, spiritual or social community, and how to address these beliefs in end-of-life care (Table 80-1).[77] The clinician can learn how the patient copes with illness, what support systems are in place, and what beliefs the patient may have that could affect decision making.[81] Supporting the dignity of the patient and his or her "person-ness" is essential in effective spiritual care. Miller et al[82] demonstrated better spiritual and psychological well-being in patients with life-threatening illness who were given supportive-affective group experiences with a spiritual inquiry tool.

The clinician should pray only with the explicit permission of the patient. Requests from the patient for prayer with the clinician should not compromise the clinician's religious beliefs. A clinician may choose to be with the patient in silence as the patient prays.[79,83] Often, the patient can identify a spiritual mentor, such as a priest, minister, or rabbi, who can guide him or her through the spiritual territory of the dying process. If not, involving the hospice chaplain, after obtaining the patient's permission, can provide the needed spiritual support. Spiritual support, however, can come from the entire end-of-life health care team, family, and friends[84] (see Chapter 110, Integrating Spiritual Assessment and Care.)

TABLE 80-1. FICA: Taking a Spiritual History*

Faith and belief	Do you consider yourself spiritual or religious? *or* Do you have spiritual beliefs that help you cope with stress? If the patient responds no, the physician might ask: What gives your life meaning? Sometimes patients respond with answers such as family, career, or nature.
Importance	What importance does your faith or belief have in your life? Have your beliefs influenced how you take care of yourself in this illness? What role do your beliefs play in regaining your health?
Community	Are you part of a spiritual or religious community? Is this of support to you? How? Is there a group of people you really love or who are important to you? Communities such as churches, temples, mosques, or a group of like-minded friends can serve as strong support systems for some patients.
Address in care	How would you like me, your health care provider, to address these issues in your health care?

© Christina M. Puchalski, MD, 1996. Modified with permission from Puchalski CM, Romer AL. Taking a spiritual history allows clinicians to understand patients more fully. *J Palliat Med.* 2003;3:129–137.
*The acronym FICA can help structure questions for health care professionals taking a spiritual history.

Bereavement

The loss of the healthy self begins at the time of diagnosis of illness. Delivery of "bad" or "important" news requires skill in managing the grief of the patient and family for this loss.[15] Grief is the experience of the loss, and bereavement is the process of journeying through grief. Mourning is the public expression of grieving. Grief work or bereavement targets the restoration of wholeness and a new identity as the desired outcome. Each person journeys through the grief process uniquely, but certain tasks of grieving are universal; they are to accept the reality of the loss, to experience the pain of the loss, to adjust to a new reality where the deceased is not, and to reinvest energy into new relationships.[85] The grief that the dying patient experiences is called preparatory grief.[86]

In hospice care, bereavement services are offered to the patient and family before death (anticipatory grief occurs for the family before the death) and to the family up to 13 months after the patient's death. Supportive interventions for preparatory grief of the patient and for the anticipatory grief of the family help prevent depression in the patient and complicated grief in family and significant others left behind by the death. Periyakoil and Hallenbeck[87] suggest psychosocial-spiritual interventions with the acronym RELIEVER: reflect with the patient on emotions, empathize, lead with questions to facilitate grieving, improvise interventions to the unique individual, educate about the grief process and what to expect, validate the experience, and recall the life story and accomplishments of the patient. All health care professionals and bereavement counselors can facilitate this process. As in spiritual exploration, the use of the humanities such as art, music, writing, and collage can help individuals express their grief and work through it one-on-one or in bereavement groups.

Encouragement of healthy grieving can prevent complicated grief, such as delayed grief, absent grief, distorted grief, and chronic grief. When complicated grief occurs, refer to a bereavement counselor, psychiatric consultant, or spiritual counselor. Grief can also be complicated by major depression, anxiety disorder, posttraumatic stress disorder, and, in children, adjustment disorder. Those at risk for complicated grief include mothers after the death of a child, widowers, family members who feel guilt or anger or "unfinished business" with the deceased, survivors of a sudden violent death of a loved one, children and teenagers who have lost a parent, persons with a history of psychiatric illness or substance abuse, and refugees. Patients presenting with somatic or psychiatric symptoms may be experiencing complicated grief, and this should be explored. In the patient interview, the clinician starts the therapeutic intervention by acknowledging the loss and then supports the patient in the grief process.[88] In one study, those who had strong spiritual beliefs were more resilient in the face of grief and had lower incidence of complicated grief.[89]

Depression must be differentiated from preparatory grief in the dying patient because depression requires different interventions for successful treatment. Depression is characterized by flat affect, anhedonia, hopelessness, worthlessness, guilt, and social withdrawal. One must remember that pain can also cause a flat affect, anhedonia, and withdrawal. In grief, sadness fluctuates and responds to social support, some activities can be enjoyed, and sadness improves with time. Symptoms such as insomnia and loss of appetite cannot be used to differentiate depression and grief in the dying process. Patients can at times sense whether they are depressed or grieving, and asking patients if they are feeling depressed can simply differentiate between the two states.[90]

Integrative Therapies

Nutrition

Appetite naturally decreases at end of life, and progressive dehydration is the rule. Food and fluids optimally are flavorful and of an appropriate consistency to facilitate swallowing. Food is often equated with caring, but forcing the patient to eat and drink is to be avoided. Offering small quantities of food and foods desired by the patient is optimal. Avoid dietary restrictions unless certain foods cause uncomfortable symptoms. In conditions such as congestive heart failure and pneumonia, fluid overload is to be avoided. Cool foods are often better tolerated than warm or hot foods, unless the patient prefers the latter. Fruit-flavored juices, ices, or smoothies can relieve dry mouth and are usually well tolerated. Cancer in particular can change taste sensation, and foods that taste good to the patient should be maximized.[91,92]

Supplements

Polypharmacy with nutritional supplements is to be avoided, just as polypharmacy with medications at end of life can increase burden on the patient without significant benefit. Only those nutritional supplements essential to the patient's well-being should be continued. In most cases of patients imminently dying, almost all nutritional supplements can be discontinued except for those giving specific symptom relief. Patients and families must be a part of this decision-making process because they may hold strong beliefs about what supplements are essential for their well-being. These supplements can be continued unless the patient is having difficulty swallowing them, they are contributing to distressing symptoms, or they are contraindicated (e.g., fish oil in a patient with the potential for bleeding or actively bleeding).

Mind-Body Therapies

Mind-body therapies are efficacious for chronic pain, anxiety, depression, and insomnia. In a telephone survey of 2055 Americans, 18.9% had used one mind-body therapy in the past year.[93]

Mindfulness-Based Stress Reduction

In a meta-analytic review of mindfulness-based stress reduction (MBSR), an 8-week program of teaching moment-to-moment awareness of mind-body interactions was significantly correlated with reductions in the anxiety, chronic pain, stress, and depression often found in patients at end of life.[94,95] Practices that can be used in end-of-life care include walking, sitting, or lying meditation, depending on the condition of the patient; body scan meditation; gentle Hatha yoga; and breath awareness.[96] MBSR has also been combined with art therapy in cancer patients, achieving higher quality-of-life measures than in controls as well as diminished psychological distress.[97]

Life Review and Reminiscence Therapy

Life review and reminiscence therapy are techniques used in end-of-life care as therapeutic interventions. Reminiscing is often done in a group setting, focuses on happy memories, is superficial in nature, and aims to improve socialization and communication skills.[98] It is especially effective with patients who have dementia.[99] Life review, in contrast, is performed individually by a health professional who guides the patient in specific recollections in an effort to reframe, reexplore, and redefine life events and explore them for meaning. Using Milton Erickson's life stage approach,[100] life review is a critical developmental task enabling older persons and the dying to achieve ego integrity rather than despair. With the achievement of ego integrity, a person finds meaning in his or her life and dying experience and, it is hoped, fears death less.[101] Chochinov[80] has developed a life review tool to guide patients in looking over their lives for meaning and purpose and to help them maintain their person-ness and dignity in the dying process. The dignity-conserving perspectives fostered by this style of life review include continuity of self, role preservation, maintenance of pride, hopefulness, autonomy and control, generativity and legacy, acceptance, resilience, and fighting spirit. Three personal approaches that enhance dignity are living in the moment, maintaining normalcy, and finding spiritual comfort.[80] More research is needed to document the effects of life review, although many working in end-of-life care acknowledged that this tool has significant effects in relieving the existential suffering of dying patients.[101-103]

Hypnosis and Guided Imagery

In small trials, hypnosis and guided imagery have been shown to reduce anxiety, pain, and stress and to promote relaxation. Hypnosis creates a state of "focused awareness and attention," which can facilitate improvements in coping, well-being, and acceptance of death.[98] Guided imagery can be facilitated with music to evoke deeper connection.[96,104,105] Hypnosis was found to be efficacious in attenuating the nausea and vomiting associated with cancer chemotherapy as well as pain.[106] Hypnosis and guided imagery may be helpful in decreasing pain and increasing relaxation in patients at end of life, although more research is needed in this area.[107,108] Guided imagery can also be used before death to imagine a person's optimal dying process: who would be with the person, what environment he or she would be in, what he or she would like to hear or say, and so on. Once this process is defined through imagery, family can do their best to re-create it (see Chapter 92, Self-Hypnosis Techniques, and Chapter 95, Guided Imagery and Interactive Guided Imagery).

Music Therapy

Simple music that is relaxing can be provided by anyone, but only a certified music therapist provides music therapy. In active approaches to music therapy, the patient creates music with voice or instruments as a way of relating or expressing deep feelings. In receptive music therapy, the patient is receptively engaged but listening to music rather than creating it. Some forms of receptive music therapy involve the playing of music while the patient reminisces, paints, relaxes, meditates, or moves gently. Goals of therapy include relief of pain or other discomfort, relaxation, increased energy, better sleep, and relief of depressive symptoms. Music therapy has a clear theoretical framework for its effects. Although a number of studies have examined the use of music therapy for depression, the variety of modalities of music therapy makes it difficult to create a systematic review with strong recommendations.[109]

Music can raise endorphin levels in the brain and lower adrenaline levels.[110,111] The noise level in an intensive care unit (ICU) can exceed 60 dB, engendering anxiety and pain in the patients being treated there. Music can help modulate this noisy environment when it is played through earphones, but music therapy should not be continuous, and optimal treatment periods are 25 to 90 minutes.[112-114] Studies by Chlan[111] and Wong et al[115] have shown that 30 minutes of music therapy for relaxation is more effective than uninterrupted rest of ICU patients undergoing mechanical ventilation, and Zimbardo and Gerrig[116] found that 30 minutes of classical music therapy in an ICU setting equaled the relaxation effects of 10 mg of diazepam. In a 2010 Cochrane review, because of high risk of bias and limited number of studies, insufficient evidence was found for beneficial effects of music in end-of-life care to improve quality of life.[117] Music therapy can improve mood in depression.[118] This modality reduced the intensity of pain by up to 70% in one study and can decrease opioid requirements.[49]

Music thanatology combines music therapy as medicine and spirituality. Its goals are to relieve suffering and pain and to promote a peaceful and conscious death. The therapy depends on the assessment of the musician and the needs of the patient and is therefore described as prescriptive music. A bedside vigil lasts 45 to 60 minutes, and caregivers are encouraged to be present. A portable harp produces polyphonic sound that is described by Therese Schroeder-Sheker,[119] founder of the Chalice of Repose Project in End of Life Care in Oregon and North Carolina, as dissolving, which is well suited to the various environments in which the vigils are held. The tempo of the music is synchronized to the heart and respiratory rate of the patient to produce entrainment to a more relaxed or sleep state.[120] In one study of harp therapy, 77% of patients and families found the therapy of great benefit, and 23% found it to be of some benefit. Anxiety was relieved in 84% of patients, fear in 70%, dyspnea in 71%, nausea in 92%, and pain in 63%.[5]

Massage

Massage encompasses many different styles, but in dying patients, gentler forms such as Swedish massage may be better tolerated. Massage is beneficial in the treatment of depression and pain, and it can help alleviate anxiety and promote more restful sleep.[121-130] In one study of 1290 patients with cancer, massage reduced moderate to severe symptoms of pain, fatigue, anxiety, and nausea by about 50%.[131] A Cochrane review found evidence that massage, especially paired with stress reduction techniques, improved quality of life in HIV/AIDS patients.[132] Hand massage may be helpful for patients with dementia who are agitated. This modality can promote relaxation.[133] This modality is also combined with aromatherapy at times for a synergistic effect.

Aromatherapy

Aromatherapy is often used together with massage. One randomized controlled trial showed that massage therapy with or without lavender oil helped promote sleep; massage therapy appeared to be the essential intervention.[134] Lavender oil aromatherapy alone was found to relieve anxiety in two small studies.[135,136] Use of rosemary oil increased alertness and decreased anxiety.[135] In a small study of 20 terminally ill patients with cancer, a regimen of lavender oil aromatherapy, followed by a foot soak with oil and warm water, followed by application of reflexology significantly relieved fatigue.[137] In another small experimental study of 17 hospice patients, inhaled lavender aromatherapy helped relieve anxiety and pain.[138] In a systematic review, aromatherapy massage showed benefit for psychological well-being and anxiety. Limited evidence exists for benefits in nausea, pain, and depression.[139] The species of plant used for the oil and the quality of the essential oil can have an impact on therapeutic effect.[140] Many essential oil blends exist for specific indications, and the reader is encouraged to read a definitive text on this modality or to seek out the services of a certified aromatherapist.

Energy Medicine

Subtle energies involved in some complementary therapies work on a level of physics that is new to a purely mechanical, materialistic, and chemical view of life, and new discoveries have been slowly accepted in the understanding of biologic systems. DNA has been found to have electronic as well as acoustical resonances, in which quantum fluctuations switch DNA expression on and off. Music thanatology, described previously, may very well affect acoustical resonances on a DNA level as well as on a universal healing plane.[141] The emerging understanding that exists today makes the randomized clinical trial perhaps too primitive a research tool with which to study these energetic modalities, especially at end of life, when a person's vibrational energies merge with the energies beyond the human form (see Chapter 112, Human Energetic Therapies).

Healing or Therapeutic Touch and Reiki Therapy

In small, nonrandomized, not controlled trials, therapeutic touch has been found to reduce anxiety and pain and to improve relaxation. Therapeutic touch is the focused intention to heal on the part of the practitioner; it involves the transfer of energy from the environment through the practitioner to the patient.[142] In one large descriptive study, a hospital evaluated its inpatient therapeutic touch program. The investigators found that it decreased anxiety and pain and increased relaxation.[143] It is challenging to research therapeutic touch with randomized controlled trials because it is difficult to have a control group, and the effects cannot be differentiated from a placebo response.[144] Four trials of therapeutic touch for wound healing were variable in effect.[145] A Cochrane review on touch therapies found modest effects on decreasing pain, and positive results seemed to be in part related to the experience of the practitioner.[146]

Reiki therapy balances the bioenergy fields on a deep vibrational level. Its therapeutic goals are to restore balance and resiliency and to promote nonspecific healing. Light touch is used on specific areas of the head and torso. If the patient has lesions, the practitioner's hands can hover a few inches above the patient. Reiki therapy may reduce anxiety and pain.[147] Miles and True[148] reviewed randomized controlled trials of the use of Reiki therapy and found inconclusive results.

Acupuncture and Traditional Chinese Medicine

Traditional Chinese medicine has been practiced for thousands of years as a system of healing modalities, including herbs, acupuncture, and qi gong, designed to balance the life energy called *qi*. Acupuncture is an effective modality for breathlessness, nausea and vomiting, and pain.[149-151] One randomized controlled trial showed a significant decrease in neuropathic pain with acupuncture compared with sham acupuncture.[152] Acupuncture is effective for pain in a number of musculoskeletal pain syndromes, such as headache, chronic neck and back pain, and osteoarthritis. Adverse reactions are rare.[153-157]

Therapies to Consider

Art therapy is useful in bereavement groups, especially with children and teens, as a means of expressing feelings, communications about the death, and their resulting grief. Pet therapy is also increasingly more popular in end-of-life care. Anyone dying who has a pet should be allowed to have the pet present at end of life if at all possible. The comfort provided can reduce anxiety.[158] Other modalities to consider in end-of-life care are homeopathy, chiropractic care, osteopathic manipulation, and humor therapy. See Key Web Resources for a list of resources for patients and clinicians.

PREVENTION PRESCRIPTION

- Prevention is focused on maximizing comfort, well-being, healing, and life closure rather than on prevention of death.
- Carefully apply and titrate therapeutic interventions to minimize side effects and to maximize well-being.
- Avoid skin breakdown with frequent turning and gentle massage.
- Prevent anxiety and spiritual discomfort with supportive and trusting therapeutic relationships, effective symptom management, empowered decision making by the patient, and bereavement and spiritual care.
- Prevent complicated grief with effective bereavement services during terminal illness and after death.
- Advocate the use of advance directives, educate the patient and family on options in end-of-life care, elicit and honor patient treatment preferences, and deliver palliative care on the basis of the patient's treatment goals. Doing so will reduce unnecessary and unwanted interventions at the end of life.

THERAPEUTIC REVIEW

A number of therapeutic interventions can be used synergistically to maximize therapeutic effect, in some cases reducing the dose of medication needed for effect and minimizing side effects. In addition to controlling symptoms, many integrative modalities can improve well-being by enhancing psychological and spiritual health as well as by providing physical comfort. In end-of-life care, unnecessary therapies are discontinued, and less invasive modalities can be increased in keeping with the needs and goals of the patient, the resources available, and the patient's response to them. Attentive listening and keen observation are essential in guiding therapeutic choices.

■ Pain Management

Pharmaceuticals

- Treat pain as an emergency. Addiction at end of life is a nonissue. Believe the patient's report of pain. Treat pain aggressively. Use a lower starting dose in patients who are opioid naive and in older persons, but increase dosage rapidly and carefully for an adequate response. There is no ceiling dose for opioids.[29]

- For unrelieved severe pain, increase the immediate-acting opioid dose by 50% to 100% every 24 hours; for moderate pain, increase the dose by 25% to 50%. The dose of short-acting opioids for breakthrough pain should be 5% to 10% of the total 24-hour dose of sustained-release medication and should be given every 1 to 2 hours. Consider increasing bedtime dose by 50% to avoid administration during the night. Opioid-induced sedation caused by initiation of or increase in the dose of an opioid analgesic usually clears within a few days.[29,159,160]

- Use scheduled dosing of a long-acting pain medication for chronic pain to prevent oversedation and troughs of pain relief. Adjust dose every 2 to 4 days after a steady state is achieved. Increase the dose of immediate-acting opioids for uncontrolled pain. Administer by mouth whenever possible. Avoid intramuscular injections.[29]

- The lowest dose of the fentanyl transdermal patch is 12 mcg/hr and replaced generally every 3 days. The 25-mcg/hr patch is equivalent to approximately 50 mg of oral morphine daily. The patch should be avoided in opioid-naive patients, for whom the starting dose may be too strong. Most patients can take oral medication, which also costs less. The transdermal patch takes 8 to 24 hours to achieve analgesic effect and therefore should not be used alone to treat acute pain. Also, once the patch is removed, the analgesic effect continues for 17 to 24 hours. Dosage may be usually titrated every 6 days. Absorption increases with fever. Subcutaneous fat is needed as a reservoir for the drug.[29,159]

- Decrease dose and intervals of analgesics in patients with reduced hepatic and renal clearance and in patients who are dehydrated and oliguric.[29]

- Extended-release tablets cannot be crushed or chewed. Extended-release granules can, however, be mixed with food or fluids or given by gastric tube.[29]

- Avoid use of meperidine (Demerol) because of its problematic metabolites when it is used for chronic pain.[159]

- For severe chronic pain, start with extended-release morphine, 15-mg tablet twice daily, with immediate-acting morphine, 10 mg every 4 hours, as needed. Kadian, a long-acting morphine preparation, consists of a capsule containing sprinkles that can be given by gastric tube or mixed with food; the starting dose is 20 mg every 24 hours.[29]

- Hydromorphone does not have toxic metabolites and is preferred in patients with severe renal insufficiency. Morphine and oxycodone are excreted renally and should be used carefully or avoided in patients with severe renal insufficiency.[29]

- In patients with liver impairment, morphine is preferred. Avoid acetaminophen and tricyclic antidepressants in patients with liver impairment.[29]

- Methadone is useful in the treatment of nociceptive and neuropathic pain; it is inexpensive and can control pain that is not responsive to other opioids.[30] Initiation and titration of methadone therapy is unique, and appropriate resources must be carefully used; alternatively, the clinician can consult with a palliative medicine or pain consultant.[30,32] Conversion to methadone from another opioid is also unique, and guidelines for optimal, safe conversions are available.[29-33]

- Always use a stool softener when treating a patient with opioids, for example, docusate (Colace), 100 mg twice daily. Use laxatives liberally; senna (Senokot), at a starting dose of 2 tablets at bedtime as needed, works well. The goal is for the patient to have a bowel movement every other day. A stool softener alone is often not effective, and use with a laxative is needed.

- Neuropathic pain often requires the addition of adjuvant medications, such as anticonvulsants (e.g., gabapentin [Neurontin] starting at 100 mg three times a day) or antidepressants (e.g., the tricyclic antidepressant nortriptyline [Pamelor] starting at 10 mg/day or amitriptyline starting at 25 mg at bedtime), for adequate relief. Opioids alone, except methadone, are usually not adequate to treat neuropathic pain.[29] Use caution with renal or hepatic impairment.

Botanicals and Supplements

- For arthritis pain, glucosamine sulfate: start with 3000 mg/day; once pain is relieved, decrease to 1500 mg/day. Tablets can be crushed. The patient needs to use it for at least a few months to assess the effect.

- For pain, especially neuropathic pain, cannabis (oral synthetic cannabinoid): dronabinol, 10 mg four times a day. Medical marijuana is only available legally in specific states in the United States and countries worldwide. Check local laws and clinical resources.

Other Modalities

- Consider acupuncture for neuropathic and nociceptive pain, often in conjunction with medication.

- Massage can help relieve pain.

Nausea and Vomiting

Lifestyle

- Target the mechanism of cause and either discontinue the offending medication or treat the underlying cause.

Pharmaceuticals

- Stimulation of chemoreceptor trigger zone (CTZ) in the fourth ventricle of the brain by medications including opioids, hypercalcemia, or uremia commonly causes nausea and vomiting. The CTZ has dopamine

Continued

and serotonin (5-HT$_3$) receptors. Antidopaminergics such as prochlorperazine and haloperidol and 5-HT$_3$ antagonists such as ondansetron most effectively treat this cause of nausea and vomiting.[52]

Prochlorperazine: start at 5 mg every 6 hours as needed orally or 25 mg twice daily as needed by the rectal route

Haloperidol: start at 1.5 mg orally three times daily as needed; may also be given subcutaneously

- Nausea caused by constipation is relieved with laxatives.[52]

- Nausea caused by infection and inflammation responds well to anticholinergic and antihistamine antiemetics, such as promethazine, starting at 25 mg orally or rectally every 4 to 6 hours as needed; this agent can also be given intramuscularly or intravenously starting at 50 mg every 4 to 6 hours as needed.[52]

- Nausea caused by dysmotility of the gut, such as in the use of opioids, is relieved best with prokinetic agents such as metoclopramide, starting at 5 mg orally, intramuscularly, or intravenously every 6 to 8 hours as needed. Anticholinergic drugs make this kind of nausea worse. Avoid this drug in patients with Parkinson's disease and renal failure.[52]

- Vestibular causes of nausea respond best to antihistamine, anticholinergic drugs such as promethazine, and scopolamine, one patch every 72 hours as needed.[52]

Botanicals

- Ginger: 500 to 1000 mg of ginger root extract as needed (boiled to make a tea), or eat 1 tsp or 5 g of crystallized ginger as needed for nausea.

- Cannabinoid: dronabinol CT-3, 10 mg four times a day for nausea and to improve appetite.

Dyspnea

Pharmaceuticals

- Oxygen therapy can help relieve dyspnea caused by low oxygen saturation.

- Morphine and other opioids can help relieve the sensation of breathlessness.[54] Start with a low dose of sustained-release morphine (e.g., 15 mg twice daily). A 10-mg dose of immediate-release morphine is sometimes given to the patient to assess the response, especially in a patient who has never taken morphine. Also, in elderly and opioid naive patients, consider initially using very low doses of morphine solution in doses of 2 to 4 mg every 3 hours either scheduled or as needed. Immediate-release morphine can also be given if the patient must exert himself or herself above baseline activities, if a more strenuous activity causes more dyspnea.

The dose is given 30 minutes before the more strenuous activity.

- In patients already receiving opioids for pain, the dose of opioid to control breathlessness may need to be 1.5 to 2.5 times the analgesic dose.[29]

- Drying secretions with a scopolamine patch every 72 hours can help with the sensation of dyspnea. Avoidance of overhydration is also important.

- Anxiolytics such as lorazepam (Ativan), 0.5 to 2 mg every 6 to 8 hours as needed, can help with the anxiety associated with breathlessness.

Energy Medicine

- Acupuncture can help relieve dyspnea.

Delirium

- Assess for delirium carefully because the patient can be in a hyperactive/agitated or hypoactive/somnolent delirium state. Do not treat states of agitation reflexively with anxiolytics, which have a high potential to make delirium worse. Medications (especially with anticholinergic side effects), steroids, benzodiazepines, and opioids are often the culprit, and offending medications must be discontinued or changed, the dose decreased, or the route of administration changed. Treatment is aimed at the underlying cause.[60,65,66]

- Delirium must be differentiated from near-death awareness.[70]

Pharmaceuticals

- Haloperidol is the drug of choice for treatment of acute delirium; dosing starts at 0.5 to 2 mg orally two or three times a day or 0.5 to 2 mg intravenously or intramuscularly every 1 to 4 hours as needed. The dose can be titrated down by 25% daily. It is less sedating and has fewer side effects than other neuroleptics. Side effects are extrapyramidal, consisting of restlessness, tremor, and so on.[60,65] Use caution if the QTc interval is prolonged.

- Benzodiazepines are indicated for delirium caused by seizures and alcohol or sedative withdrawal and in cases not responding to haloperidol.[64,65]

Spiritual Care

- Indigenous cultural and spiritual practices are important in facilitating healing as well as peaceful, meaningful dying and death. Ritual and ceremony are important in supporting the patient and relieving emotional and spiritual distress, which can have an ameliorating effect on physical symptoms.

- Spiritual inquiry using a spiritual assessment tool, meditation, and prayer can improve spiritual and psychological well-being in the dying process and also relieve physical symptoms.

Bereavement

- Preparatory grief work for the patient can help relieve existential distress, and anticipatory grief work for family, friends, and health care staff can diminish complicated grief after the death.

Nutrition

- Reducing food and fluid intake is normal in the dying process, and patient discomfort can occur if food or fluids are forced. Substitute the nurturing aspects of feeding with touch and other ways to show love and caring to the patient. Offer foods in small quantities that the patient enjoys and finds palatable. Swab the mouth frequently to prevent feeling of thirst.

Mind-Body Therapies

- Mindfulness-based stress reduction can decrease anxiety, chronic pain, stress, and depression.

- Music therapy encompasses many modalities. Harp therapy can decrease pain, existential and physical suffering, anxiety, and nausea and can improve sleep.

- Massage therapy also includes many different styles of treatment; it can ameliorate pain, fatigue, anxiety, depression, and nausea as well as promote better sleep.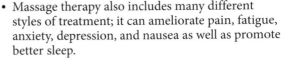

- Reminiscence therapy can improve cognition in patients with dementia.

- Life review therapy improves depression and spiritual distress, improves quality of life, and alleviates pain.

- Hypnosis and guided imagery can reduce anxiety, pain, and stress and promote relaxation.

Energy Therapies

- Aromatherapy massage has been shown to be of benefit for psychological well-being and anxiety. Limited evidence exists for its benefits in nausea, pain, and depression.

- Therapeutic touch may reduce anxiety and pain and promote relaxation. Other benefits are also possible, but this modality is challenging to research.

- Acupuncture is an effective modality for nausea and vomiting and pain.

KEY WEB RESOURCES

Advance Care Planning
- Aging with Dignity Five Wishes: www.agingwithdignity.org
- Respecting Choices: http://respectingchoices.org/
- Partnership for Caring: America's Voices for the Dying: www.partnershipforcaring.org
- Complementary and alternative medicine integrative pain management: www.stoppain.org
- Integrative pain assessment and treatment: www.HealingChronicPain.org

Palliative Medicine and Hospice
- Education in Palliative and End-of-Life Care (EPEC): www.epec.net
- End-of-Life Nursing Education Consortium (ELNEC): www.aacn.nche.edu/elnec
- Dying Well: www.dyingwell.org

- National Hospice and Palliative Care Organization: www.nhpco.org
- Last Acts: www.lastacts.org
- End of Life/Palliative Educational Resource Center—Fast Facts: www.eperc.mcw.edu
- Americans for Better Care of the Dying (ABCD): www.abcd-caring.com
- Death, dying, and grief resources: www.katsden.com/webster/index.html
- American Academy of Hospice and Palliative Medicine: www.AAHPM.org
- Society for Integrative Oncology: www.integrativeonc.org
- Module on grief with patient resources including handouts on coping with grief and tools to help with the grief experience: http://www.fammed.wisc.edu/integrative/modules/grief

---

References

References are available online at expertconsult.com.

Section XIV Substance Abuse

Chapter 81

Alcoholism and Substance Abuse

Donald Warne, MD, MPH

Alcoholism, or alcohol dependence, is a disease characterized by four key components[1]:

- Craving: a strong urge to drink alcohol

- Loss of control: being unable to stop drinking once one has started

- Physical dependence: symptoms such as sweating, shaking, and anxiety after one stops drinking

- Tolerance: the need for greater quantities of alcohol to feel intoxicated

In addition to alcohol, there are numerous drugs of abuse, including opiates, marijuana, cocaine, methamphetamines, and tobacco.[2] See Box 81-1 for a simple three-question screening tool for alcohol disorders (AUDIT-C).

Alcoholism and substance abuse have a negative impact on other chronic diseases managed in the primary care setting by the direct effects of the substances abused and issues related to compliance and self-care. Acute injury and illness resulting from alcohol and substance abuse are analogous to exacerbations of chronic conditions and therefore constitute issues of extreme importance in the arena of primary care. Unfortunately, many physicians do not routinely address these issues, and few conventional allopathic interventions are easily accessible and efficacious. This chapter examines the treatment options available to the primary care physician and also provides a source of information for appropriate referrals. A multitude of both illicit and prescribed substances are abused; the focus of this chapter is primarily on alcohol, tobacco, opiates, cocaine, and marijuana.

Addiction to drugs and alcohol should be treated as a chronic illness not unlike diabetes mellitus or hypertension.[3] Like these disorders, addiction has behavioral components as well as underlying biochemical mechanisms. Within chronic addiction and recovery, there are also exacerbations

of abuse as well as chronic multiorgan system complications. Successful treatment of all chronic diseases requires good rapport between patients and providers and the use of a nonjudgmental approach. Box 81-2 provides simple guidelines to assess the severity of alcohol risk.

Pathophysiology

Alcoholism and substance abuse have many dimensions, each with unique implications and standards of treatment. The processes of alcoholism and substance abuse may be divided into broad categories or stages: craving, active abuse, intoxication, withdrawal, detoxification, recovery, and relapse prevention.

A proposed mechanism of addiction for all substances of abuse involves the sudden release of dopamine in the "reward pathway" connecting the midbrain to the prefrontal cortex. This rush of dopamine is believed to cause a sense of euphoria and pleasure that is at the root of drug abuse. With extended drug use, there is a profound alteration in brain chemistry. This neurophysiologic change in the central nervous system eventually causes a "switch" in the affected person from a state of drug abuse to one of addiction with uncontrollable cravings and dependence. The exact mechanisms of this process are as yet unknown.[4]

The process of addiction is, of course, not limited to brain chemistry. The effect of environmental, social, cultural, genetic, and behavioral factors is significant in the development of alcoholism and substance abuse. These factors assume varying levels of importance in the development of addiction for each person. Addiction is therefore most accurately viewed as a complex illness with varying degrees of environmental and biochemical features.[5]

BOX 81-1. AUDIT-C Screening for Alcohol Use Disorders

Instructions: For each question, please check the answer that is correct for you.

1. How often do you have a drink containing alcohol?
   - ☐ Never (0)
   - ☐ Monthly or less (1)
   - ☐ Two to four times a month (2)
   - ☐ Two to three times per week (3)
   - ☐ Four or more times a week (4)
2. How many drinks containing alcohol do you have on a typical day when you are drinking?
   - ☐ 1 or 2 (0)
   - ☐ 3 or 4 (1)
   - ☐ 5 or 6 (2)
   - ☐ 7 to 9 (3)
   - ☐ 10 or more (4)
3. How often do you have six or more drinks on one occasion?
   - ☐ Never (0)
   - ☐ Less than monthly (1)
   - ☐ Monthly (2)
   - ☐ Two or three times a week (3)
   - ☐ Four or more times a week (4)

Add the numerical value of each answer selected to get your total score.

TOTAL SCORE: _____
The maximum score is 12. A score of ≥4 identifies 86% of men who report drinking above recommended levels or who meet criteria for alcohol use disorders.

A score of >2 identifies 84% of women who report hazardous drinking or alcohol use disorders.

From National Council for Community Behavioural Healthcare. http://www.thenationalcouncil.org/galleries/business-practice%20files/tool_auditc.pdf.; Accessed 7.5.11.

Integrative Therapy

Pharmaceuticals

Until recently, few effective pharmacologic options have been available to the primary care physician to treat alcoholism and substance abuse. Some of the most effective pharmaceutical agents are available only through licensed intensive outpatient and inpatient programs specializing in the treatment of addictions. However, with the U.S. Food and Drug Administration (FDA) approval of acamprosate (Campral) and buprenorphine (Subutex), primary care physicians have the opportunity to take a more active role in the treatment of addiction to alcohol and opiates. For physicians interested in using these medications for their patients with addictions, it is important to remember that these agents are most effective when they are used as part of a comprehensive management program that involves psychosocial support such as counseling and support groups. Table 81-1 provides an overview of

BOX 81-2. Alcohol Risk Terms: Abstinence, Moderate, and Risky or Hazardous

Abstinence
No alcohol use

Moderate
Men: no more than 2 standard drinks per drinking day
Women and older persons (older than 65 years): no more than 1 standard drink per drinking day

Risky or Hazardous
Men
   More than 4 standard drinks per drinking day
   More than 14 standard drinks per week
Women and older persons (older than 65 years)
   More than 3 standard drinks per drinking day
   More than 7 standard drinks per drinking week

TABLE 81-1. Pharmaceutical Agents Used for Treatment of Alcoholism and Substance Abuse

SUBSTANCE OF ABUSE	AGENTS USED FOR DETOXIFICATION/WITHDRAWAL	AGENTS USED FOR CRAVING/RELAPSE PREVENTION	AGENTS USED FOR OTHER PURPOSES
Alcohol	Benzodiazepines Phenobarbital	Naltrexone Acamprosate Topiramate	Disulfiram
Tobacco	Nicotine Bupropion	Nicotine Varenicline	Bupropion
Opiates	Methadone Clonidine Buprenorphine	Methadone L-Alpha-acetylmethadol	Naloxone
Cocaine	Selective serotonin reuptake inhibitors Monoamine oxidase inhibitors Amantadine	Tricyclic antidepressants	
Marijuana	N/A	N/A	

N/A, not applicable.

pharmaceutical treatments of alcohol and substance abuse. As noted, these treatments may be divided into the broad categories of detoxification/withdrawal and craving/relapse prevention.

Management of Alcohol Withdrawal and Recovery

The most common treatment of acute alcohol withdrawal is administration of diazepam or another benzodiazepine. The benefit of benzodiazepine treatment is relief of the anxiety and sleep disturbances experienced during the withdrawal phase. A disadvantage of benzodiazepine therapy is the potential for dependence if the drug is not prescribed appropriately. Benzodiazepine for detoxification should be prescribed only for a short time in a supervised setting. Phenobarbital or carbamazepine (Tegretol) is occasionally used in managing withdrawal seizures. There is evidence that opioid receptors play a role in the physiologic response to alcohol. Naltrexone (ReVia), an opioid antagonist, has been shown to be effective in preventing alcoholic relapse. Disulfiram (Antabuse) inhibits aldehyde dehydrogenase and produces unpleasant effects, such as nausea, vomiting, and dizziness, when alcohol is consumed.

Acamprosate, an amino acid derivative that modulates activity of gamma–aminobutyric acid (GABA) neurotransmission in the brain, appears to be effective in reducing alcohol cravings. As opposed to limiting the "high" sensation of alcohol (as naltrexone does) or producing unpleasant side effects (as disulfiram does), acamprosate can assist in preventing alcohol relapse by reducing the anxiety and sleep disturbances associated with alcohol craving, although its exact mechanism of action is unknown.[6] Pharmacologic treatments of alcohol withdrawal generally work well and can potentially be used for outpatient withdrawal management if the primary physician is able to monitor the patient closely. Treatments for relapse prevention generally are not efficacious in the absence of comprehensive follow-up care.[7]

For patients who have not abstained from alcohol, topiramate (Topamax) has been found to reduce heavy drinking and days of any drinking over a 12-week period. It is also cleared through the kidney and thus does not exacerbate toxicity to the liver. It is generally used for 6 to 12 months as part of a comprehensive treatment program.[8] Research also suggests that topiramate at a mean dose of 200 mg daily may work better to maintain abstinence with reduced cravings than naltrexone at a mean dose of 50 mg/day.[9]

■ Dosage

Naltrexone, 50 mg/day orally, reduces the high sensation associated with alcohol.

For the reduction of the craving of alcohol, acamprosate, 333 to 666 mg three times a day, or topiramate, titrated from 25 to 300 mg weekly over 8 weeks (Table 81-2), is prescribed.

Disulfiram, 250 to 500 mg/day, creates unpleasant side effects when it is used with alcohol.

For help with tapering and withdrawal from alcohol, the dosage of benzodiazepine is titrated to achieve a calming effect. High doses may be needed initially. An example is clonazepam (Klonopin), 1 mg three times a day, with a gradual taper over 10 to 14 days.

TABLE 81-2. Titration of Topiramate for Treatment of Alcohol Dependence

WEEK	MORNING DOSE (mg)	AFTERNOON DOSE (mg)	TOTAL DAILY DOSE (mg)
1	0	25	25
2	0	50	50
3	25	50	75
4	50	50	100
5	50	100	150
6	100	100	200
7	100	150	250
8	150	150	300

Management of Nicotine Withdrawal: Smoking Cessation

Effective outpatient treatment regimens are available for smoking cessation. Tapered nicotine replacement therapy is effective in the management of nicotine withdrawal and cravings. Bupropion (Zyban) has been shown to be effective in managing symptoms of anxiety associated with nicotine withdrawal and craving. Varenicline (Chantix), a partial nicotine receptor agonist, has been found to help increase smoking cessation more than placebo and as well as bupropion.[10] These medications can be used successfully in the outpatient primary care setting.[11]

■ Dosage

Bupropion, 150 mg, is administered twice daily for 6 weeks, with a target quit date of 2 weeks after the start of therapy. Varenicline is started 1 week before smoking cessation: 0.5 mg orally for 3 days, 0.5 mg twice daily for 4 days, and then 1 mg twice daily for 11 weeks; the general course of therapy is 12 weeks.

■ Precautions

Varenicline has a black box warning for neuropsychiatric side effects including behavior change, hostility, agitation, depression, and suicidality. This can be exacerbated when it is used with nicotine long term.

Management of Opiate Withdrawal and Recovery

Acute opiate withdrawal is treated commonly with methadone, an opioid receptor agonist that can block withdrawal symptoms without producing the euphoria caused by heroin and other opiates. Owing to this effect, methadone is also commonly used in long-term maintenance programs to reduce cravings and relapse. Clonidine has been shown to be effective in lessening opiate withdrawal symptoms and does not foster physiologic dependence. L-Alpha-acetylmethadol (LAAM) is derived from methadone and acts in a fashion similar to that noted for methadone. The advantage of LAAM in maintenance therapy is that its effect lasts 72 hours, allowing dosing every other day or three times per week. Naloxone is an opiate antagonist used for treatment of acute opiate overdose.[12]

Perhaps the most significant pharmaceutical development in the management of opioid addiction is the approval of the use of buprenorphine in the United States. An opiate receptor partial agonist, buprenorphine has shown benefit in managing opioid addiction and preventing relapse. Opioid partial agonists bind to the opioid receptor but only partially activate the receptor and generate significantly less euphoric sensation than opiate agonists like heroin do.[13] Potential for abuse of buprenorphine is much lower than that of other opiates, and buprenorphine has been shown to be as effective as methadone in weaning clients off this class of drugs.[14]

Buprenorphine requires specific training for prescribing, and referral to the appropriate qualified physician is required. More information is available at the U.S. Department of Health and Human Services Substance Abuse and Mental Health Services Administration (SAMHSA) Web site (http://buprenorphine.samhsa.gov).

Management of Cocaine Dependence

Cocaine withdrawal is associated with minimal symptoms. Several classes of pharmaceutical agents have been studied for their efficacy in treating cocaine dependence and relapse prevention, although none of these is approved by the FDA for this purpose. Extensive abuse of cocaine can cause depression by depletion of baseline levels of dopamine. Several antidepressants have been studied for their role in treating cocaine addiction, including tricyclic antidepressants, selective serotonin reuptake inhibitors, and monoamine oxidase inhibitors; however, results are mixed and inconclusive. Amantadine, a dopamine agonist, has been studied for its role in cocaine dependence. In theory, dopamine agonist therapy should cause dopamine restoration and reduce the need for cocaine, but findings of studies have not been convincing.[15] In addition, the results of studies examining the role of buprenorphine in the management of cocaine addiction have been mixed.[16]

Botanicals

Various herbs and combinations of herbs are reported to be effective in reducing cravings, but in general, no studies have been conducted to prove their effectiveness.

Kudzu

Kudzu, a traditional Chinese herb, has been used as an "anti-inebriation" treatment for hundreds of years, although its mechanism of action is not yet known.[17,18]

A small study showed that in heavy drinkers of alcohol, kudzu did result in a reduction of the number of beers consumed after 7 days of treatment.[19] It has not been found to enhance sobriety in chronic alcoholics.[20]

◼ Dosage

The recommended dose is 1.2 g twice daily.

◼ Precautions

Kudzu is considered safe with few side effects other than the potential for an allergic reaction to the plant.

Herbal Antidepressants and Anxiolytics

Because people who struggle with alcoholism and substance abuse commonly have coexisting depression and anxiety,[21,22] it is possible that herbal remedies used for these conditions

may have a role in recovery and abstinence. Poorly managed anxiety may lead to higher alcohol intake.[23] Herbs that are effective in treating anxiety and insomnia, such as valerian and kava kava, might be helpful in managing anxiety associated with detoxification and cravings. These herbs have been shown to enhance the levels and action of GABA and therefore might also have a role in control of alcohol cravings and prevention of relapse. Caution should be taken with the use of kava in alcoholic patients because it has been associated with liver toxicity. These are potential uses that warrant further investigation. St. John's wort has a mechanism of action similar to that of the selective serotonin reuptake inhibitors and has been shown to be effective in treating depression.[24] Its role in managing depression associated with alcoholism and substance abuse is yet to be determined.

Other Herbal Remedies

Lobelia is described as a respiratory stimulant and has been used in homeopathic preparations as an aid to stop smoking.[25] Milk thistle, which has been studied for its hepatoprotective effects, appears to be a promising treatment of alcoholic cirrhosis.[26]

Acupuncture

Acupuncture is perhaps the most extensively studied and most promising integrative treatment of addictions. The practice of acupuncture is documented in Chinese literature as early as the Han dynasty in the second century BC in the *Huang Di Nei Jing (Yellow Emperor's Classic of Medicine)*. In acupuncture terms, the body is seen as having several energy channels, or meridians, that allow the free flow of *qi* (pronounced "chee"), or energy. In a healthy or balanced state, *qi* flows smoothly throughout the body and provides for homeostasis. With disease, injury, or a state of imbalance, the normal movement of *qi* is obstructed or impaired. Acupuncture treatments are designed to unblock obstructions of meridians and to promote the healthy flow of energy.[27]

In 1973, Wen and Cheung[28] reported that opiate-addicted patients who were using electroacupuncture for treatment of postoperative pain described relief from symptoms of withdrawal. Omura brought the treatment protocol to Lincoln Hospital in New York in 1974, and Smith and Kahn[29] developed a five-point auricular acupuncture treatment protocol for addictions that is currently being taught and advocated by the National Acupuncture Detoxification Association (NADA).

In acupuncture terms, substance abuse can be seen as an attempt by the patient to self-treat an imbalance in the flow of *qi*. The "drug of choice" provides a temporary relief from energy imbalance, but unfortunately, it also commonly causes further underlying imbalance. As a result, the baseline imbalance slowly worsens, and the need for more drugs slowly increases. The acupuncture treatment therefore provides energy balancing without the need for alcohol or drugs as well as relaxation and relief from cravings.[30]

> Acupuncture treatments influence the flow of *qi* to achieve energy balancing, relaxation, and reduced cravings for alcohol, tobacco, and illicit drugs.

Another proposed mechanism of action is that the acupuncture needles stimulate peripheral nerves to cause release of endorphins in the brain, thereby resulting in relaxation and a sense of well-being; acupuncture thus can provide direct biochemical treatment of opiate and ethanol craving and withdrawal.[31] The NADA treatment protocol and certification course emphasize the multifaceted nature of this modality and describe treatment benefits in the biochemical, psychological, and social realms as well as in the traditional Chinese paradigm.

The specific points used in the NADA protocol are shen men (spirit gate), sympathetic, kidney, liver, and lung (Fig. 81-1). These points have roles in balancing energy and calming as well as in regulating sympathetic nervous system function and specific organ function from the modern and traditional Chinese perspectives of physiology. The kidney, liver, and lung each have specific roles in the generation, regulation, and flow of *qi*. These organ-specific functions are described in acupuncture texts[32] and are beyond the scope of this chapter.

Auricular acupuncture has been studied in the treatment of addiction to various drugs, including alcohol, cocaine, opiates, and marijuana. In 1989, Bullock et al[33] reported that auricular acupuncture is effective in the treatment of relapsing alcoholics. In this study, 80 relapsing alcoholics who were enrolled in a treatment facility were randomly assigned to receive either the appropriate acupuncture treatment protocol (treatment group) or sham acupuncture points at sites close to the appropriate points (control group). The outcomes measured included completion of the treatment program and self-reported abstinence at 1, 3, and 6 months after the end of the program. Of the 40 subjects in the treatment group, 21 finished the program, whereas only 1 of 40 in the control group completed treatment ($P < .001$). Information about self-reported drinking episodes was collected from all available subjects, including those who did not complete treatment. Fewer treatment group subjects than control group subjects reported drinking episodes at 1-, 3-, and 6-month follow-up evaluations.[33]

In 1998, Shwartz et al[34] compared residential detoxification programs that used acupuncture with programs that did not. In this retrospective study, 6907 patients completed non-acupuncture programs, and 1104 patients completed programs that used acupuncture as an adjunctive therapy. The study subjects were dependent on alcohol, cocaine, crack, heroin, marijuana, or a combination of these drugs. The primary outcome measured was readmission to a detoxification program in the 6 months after discharge. After control for baseline differences of patients in the study, those who completed programs offering acupuncture were readmitted to detoxification less frequently than were those from conventional programs ($P < .02$).[34] A randomized controlled trial of auricular acupuncture for cocaine dependence published in 2000 studied 82 patients who were randomly allocated to receive appropriate acupuncture treatment, sham acupuncture, or relaxation therapy. Thrice-weekly urine screening for cocaine was conducted during an 8-week period. The patients who received the appropriate acupuncture protocol were less likely to test positive for cocaine on urine screening than were the patients in the sham acupuncture control group ($P = .05$) or the relaxation control group ($P = .01$).[35]

Auricular acupuncture has been shown by these studies to be a useful adjunct in treating alcoholism and substance abuse. Other investigations have found mixed results or little benefit from acupuncture in treating addiction.[36,37] Further investigation in this area is warranted.

Mind-Body Therapies

As more is learned about the connection between thoughts and physiology, the field of mind-body medicine continues to grow and to gain acceptance. Commonly used therapies classified as mind-body interventions are meditation, biofeedback, hypnosis, guided imagery, yoga, and prayer. Research in this field appears promising for mind-body medicine as an adjunctive intervention for alcoholism and substance abuse.

Meditation

Meditation can be divided into three broad categories: concentrative, mindfulness, and transcendental. Concentrative meditation focuses attention on breathing, imagery, or sounds; mindfulness meditation involves focused awareness on the passage of thoughts and images as they spontaneously appear. Transcendental meditation (TM) is a technique brought to the United States by Maharishi Mahesh Yogi in the 1960s. TM was developed from the ancient East Indian Vedic belief system and helps practitioners of this technique balance the physical, mental, emotional, and spiritual components of health.[38] Within this belief system, prolonged or excessive stress leads to holistic imbalance, which causes illness, including alcoholism and substance abuse. The sense of balancing offered by TM allows optimal function and decreases the need for drugs and alcohol.[39] Several studies and review articles have shown TM to be effective in the treatment of alcoholism and substance abuse; however, most of these studies had flaws in design and methods without randomization, blinding, and appropriate control groups.[40]

FIGURE 81-1
Acupuncture points for the National Acupuncture Detoxification Association (NADA) treatment protocol. (Reprinted with permission from Joseph Helms, MD, and Medical Acupuncture Publishers, Berkeley, CA)

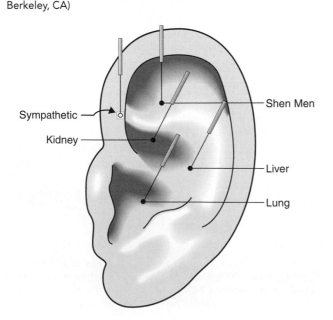

Sympathetic

Kidney

Shen Men

Liver

Lung

A randomized controlled trial indicated improvement in number of days of alcohol abstinence with the use of TM or biofeedback compared with electronic neurotherapy and the Alcoholics Anonymous program or counseling.[41] TM has been shown to significantly raise serotonin levels and to decrease cortisol levels in as little as 4 months of practice.[42] This is a possible mechanism for improving sense of balance and well-being and for reducing the effects of stress. In a group of polysubstance abusers, when goal management training was combined with mindfulness-based meditation, there was significant improvement with emotional risks associated with substance use[43] (see Chapter 98, Recommending Meditation).

> Mind-body therapies, including meditation, biofeedback, hypnosis, guided imagery, yoga, and prayer, use the power of the mind to influence the body. Relaxation and reduced physiologic responses to stress are helpful in the recovery process.

Biofeedback

Biofeedback is a technique that uses electronic monitors, including electroencephalography, electromyography, and electrocardiography, as well as cutaneous thermometers and pulse oximeters to teach the patient how to consciously control physiologic functions such as respiratory rate, heart rate, skin temperature, and blood pressure. Conscious regulation of these functions is achieved through concentration, meditation, and the use of relaxation techniques. Biofeedback has been shown to be useful in managing stress-related disorders such as hypertension, irritable bowel syndrome, pain, and substance abuse. Electromyographic biofeedback, which focuses on relieving muscle tension, has been shown to be an effective tool in treating alcoholism.[44] Unfortunately, there are only limited studies on the use of this intervention in treating addictions. The mechanism of action and efficacy of biofeedback in managing alcoholism and substance abuse have not yet been determined.

Hypnosis

The German physician Franz Anton Mesmer introduced modern hypnotherapy in the eighteenth century as mesmerism. The American Medical Association recognized hypnosis as a legitimate medical therapy in 1958, and it has been applied by various health care practitioners in the treatment of numerous disorders, including alcoholism and substance abuse. Hypnotherapy involves concentration, mental focusing exercises, relaxation techniques, guided imagery, and suggestion. Studies have shown that hypnosis improves memory and cognitive function[45] and can affect physiologic function by reducing sympathetic nervous system activity, heart rate, blood pressure, and oxygen consumption.[46] Many techniques are used in hypnotherapy, making standardization difficult for research purposes; however, there are case reports of positive results of its use in substance abuse treatment and relapse prevention.[47] Controlled trials have not shown long-term benefits in the management of addictions. Some techniques used in hypnosis may be useful as adjunctive modalities in comprehensive recovery programs. One study used self-hypnosis tapes in a residential treatment

program for drug and alcohol abuse. Those who listened to the tapes three to five times a week showed the highest levels of self-esteem and serenity and the least amount of anger or impulsivity compared with less frequent users[48] (see Chapter 92, Self-Hypnosis Techniques).

Guided Imagery

Guided imagery uses the power of the mind to directly affect physiologic function. Practitioners of this technique report improved insight into emotional and physical health. Imagery can modulate heart rate, blood pressure, oxygen consumption, and various other physiologic measures. Deeper insight into emotions, behaviors, and thoughts can help patients deal with the anxiety and depression associated with the recovery process[49] (see Chapter 95, Guided Imagery and Interactive Guided Imagery).

Yoga

A traditional East Indian healing system, yoga combines specific postures, breathing control, and meditation to reduce stress and to promote balance and a sense of well-being. Yoga, meaning "union," attempts to help its practitioners address and equilibrate the physical, mental, and spiritual forces that coalesce in the process of disease or disharmony. Yoga has been shown to have a beneficial effect on stress-related conditions, including chronic pain, hypertension, and recovery from addiction.[50] There are, however, no randomized controlled trials specifically assessing the efficacy of yoga for management of addictions. The use of this technique has been shown to be beneficial as part of a comprehensive treatment program[51] (see Chapter 90, Prescribing Movement Therapies).

Spirituality

The role of spirituality in medicine and recovery has been steadily gaining acceptance from mainstream health care practitioners. Numerous studies on the role of spirituality in the recovery from addiction have been conducted. Defining spirituality and religion and identifying interventions that exist within these realms are difficult. Spirituality is a subjective concept that can be considered to represent a person's connection with and relationship to a transcendent or higher power.[52] Religion can be defined in terms of a structured value and belief system with its own hierarchy, rituals, and practices.[53]

Commonly described practices in spirituality are prayer and meditation. The field of mind-body medicine often includes prayer with meditation as a synergistic tool to promote wellness and healing. Spirituality is addressed separately here because it transcends mind-body interventions and is not easily defined by objective markers. The role of spirituality—and, to some extent, religion—in the recovery process cannot be ignored. The regular practice of prayer and meditation is strongly correlated with recovery and abstinence from drugs of abuse.[54] Active participation in spiritual practices such as prayer appears to be more important in the recovery process than being prayed for by others.[55]

"Negative spirituality" may be at the root of addictions, and a "spiritual awakening" may be required before an individual can genuinely recover from addiction.[56] Regular church attendance has been associated with negative perceptions of addiction and lower rates of alcoholism, substance abuse,[57] and tobacco use.[58] The extent of family religious practice also has an effect on youth perspectives on substance abuse.[59] Obviously, spirituality cannot be prescribed in the primary care setting, but it is important for the clinician to be aware of the client's spiritual beliefs and value systems when identifying appropriate recovery programs for referral (see Chapter 110, Integrating Spiritual Assessment and Care).

Twelve-Step Programs

Alcoholics Anonymous (AA) has helped millions of people in their approach to recovery from alcoholism worldwide since it began in 1935. The AA program of recovery is spiritually based, with frequent meetings, mentoring, and social support. The basic spiritual framework is described in the Twelve Steps of AA, presented in Box 81-3.

AA is rooted in spirituality, not religion. The AA preamble, commonly recited at the start of meetings, states that "AA is not allied with any sect, denomination, politics, organization or institution." The belief in a "higher power" is seen as a point of connection for all AA members, no matter what each calls this higher power. This generalized belief allows a group/mutual connection to a transcendent power that can help in the healing and recovery process without the need for all members to share a common belief system or religion.

BOX 81-3. The Twelve Steps of Alcoholics Anonymous

We:
1. Admitted we were powerless over alcohol; that our lives had become unmanageable.
2. Came to believe that a Power greater than ourselves could restore us to sanity.
3. Made a decision to turn our will and our lives over to the care of God as we understood Him.
4. Made a searching and fearless moral inventory of ourselves.
5. Admitted to God, to ourselves and to another human being the exact nature of our wrongs.
6. Were entirely ready to have God remove all these defects of character.
7. Humbly asked Him to remove our shortcomings.
8. Made a list of all persons we had harmed, and became willing to make amends to them all.
9. Made direct amends to such people wherever possible, except when to do so would injure them or others.
10. Continued to take personal inventory and, when we were wrong, promptly admitted it.
11. Sought through prayer and meditation to improve our conscious contact with God as we understood Him, praying only for knowledge of His will for us and the power to carry that out.
12. Having had a spiritual experience (awakening) as the result of these steps, we tried to carry this message to alcoholics, and to practice these principles in all our affairs.

Reprinted with permission of Alcoholics Anonymous World Service, Inc. Permission to reprint this material does not mean that AA has reviewed or approved the contents of this publication or that AA agrees with the views expressed herein.

Meetings generally begin with reading of the AA preamble and end with reading of the serenity prayer. Meetings may be open, which anyone may attend, or closed, which only alcoholics may attend. AA groups serve specific populations, such as racial or ethnic groups, gays, and lesbians, as well as specific professions, such as doctors, nurses, and other health care providers. Approximately 100,000 AA groups in nearly 150 countries now serve millions of members.

Several concepts used in AA add to the success of the program, including sponsorship, anniversaries, and social support. A new member of AA is mentored by another member, a sponsor, who is usually of the same gender and has been active in AA for a minimum of 1 year. New members are encouraged to contact their sponsors when they are considering drinking or are having difficulties with sobriety. This system of social support and mentoring has been shown to be beneficial both to the new member and to the sponsor. Cross et al[59] showed that 91% of sponsors maintained their abstinence from alcohol after 10 years.

Anniversaries of sobriety are emphasized in the AA model. Special events or parties are scheduled to coincide with the individual's anniversary of sobriety. The arrangement encourages members to meet goals of prolonged abstinence and provides another avenue of social support. The social nature of these events also allows members to have fun and to make strong connections with others in the group without consuming alcohol. Primary care physicians should be aware of the AA groups in their geographic area and also should know their patients' sobriety anniversaries to be supportive and to acknowledge their accomplishments in the recovery process.

Several other 12-step programs use models similar to that of AA, including Narcotics Anonymous, Cocaine Anonymous, and Al-Anon. Family support groups like Al-Anon are available to family members and friends of alcoholics and substance abusers for the support of people close to the addicted person who are also deeply affected by substance abuse–related behaviors.

Traditional Native American Interventions

Native American Indians have the highest alcohol-related death rates and the highest prevalence of illicit drug use reported among any racial or ethnic group in the United States. According to Indian Health Service data, the total age-adjusted alcohol-related death rate among Native Americans is 627% greater than that of the U.S. all-races population.[60] SAMHSA reports that 10.6% of Native Americans are illicit drug users. Although alcoholism and substance abuse are common in many Native American communities, there are significant differences between tribes from different regions, and not all tribes are significantly affected by addiction.

Native American people have experienced an immense history of injustice in the past several hundred years. The theft of land, language, culture, and spirituality has created a sense of despair that continues today in many Native American communities. A detailed account of historical events is beyond the scope of this chapter, but it is important to recognize the relatively recent dramatic cultural changes that have occurred. I was fortunate to grow up in a family with many traditional healers and spiritual leaders from the

Lakota tribe, and I incorporate this traditional philosophy into my medical practice.

The effect on people of Native American heritage of the loss of their land and culture is recognized by many current traditional leaders. This sense of loss and mourning is at the root of the high rates of depression, alcoholism, substance abuse, and other chronic diseases experienced by Native Americans. As Ed McGaa, Eagle Man, states, "Native American Indians learned how to live with the earth on a deeply spiritual plane."[61] The loss of land resulted in a loss of spiritual tradition. According to *Wounded Warriors,* a book delineating the loss faced by many Native Americans, "We need to understand that the primary reason our people are so afflicted with addiction, poverty, abuse and strife, is that our way of life was taken from us. Everything was taken. And nothing was replaced."[62] From a traditional perspective, not unlike that previously described for acupuncture and mind-body medicine, the use of alcohol and illicit drugs by some Native Americans fills the void created by the loss of spirituality.

The medicine wheel is a symbol that has been used by numerous tribes to represent wholeness and balance. To be healthy, each person must achieve a sense of balance among spiritual, mental, physical, and emotional forces (Fig. 81-2). This image provides a visual format for depicting the connection between spirituality and mental, physical, and emotional health. Another interpretation of the medicine wheel shows values, decisions, actions, and reactions as representing the spiritual, mental, physical, and emotional realms, respectively. From a spiritual perspective, in this interpretation, personal values (spiritual) are interpreted into decisions (mental). These decisions are then implemented into actions (physical), and the actions produce reactions (emotional). The emotions then provide feedback to the value system (spiritual). In this way, all decisions, actions, and emotions are rooted in the spiritual realm (Fig. 81-3).[61] When the spiritual realm is weakened or broken, negative emotions such as depression, anger, and low self-esteem have no spiritual basis or value system in which to be processed. As a result, these negative emotions affect decision-making and actions. For many Native American people, the sense of a "broken spirit"

and emotional despair lead to high rates of alcoholism and substance abuse (Fig. 81-4).

Within this model, health care practitioners can see the importance of addressing the concept of spiritual healing and promoting balance in treating addictions. Clearly, simple allopathic pharmacologic interventions are not enough to address addiction in this setting. Comprehensive programs that incorporate traditional cultural perspectives and philosophy with AA and other treatment methods are the most successful in treating substance abuse in Native Americans.

Healing ceremonies such as the sweat lodge and talking circle are commonly used in Native American treatment programs (see Chapter 114, Creating Ceremony and Ritual in the Medical Encounter). The sweat lodge is a traditional gathering for prayer, meditation, and purification. The talking circle is analogous to a support group, in which individuals share thoughts, emotions, and prayers in a culturally relevant and sacred manner. Anecdotally, most of my patients who participate in these healing rituals in the treatment of any chronic condition, including alcoholism and substance abuse, find the traditional interventions to promote a sense of balance

FIGURE 81-3
Medicine wheel showing spiritual values in decision-making.

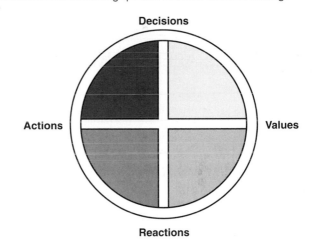

FIGURE 81-2
Traditional Lakota Indian medicine wheel.

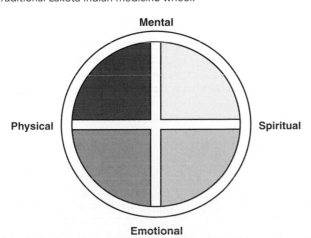

FIGURE 81-4
The "broken spirit" factor in alcoholism and substance abuse.

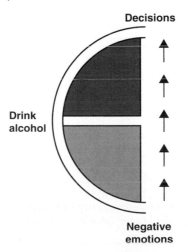

and wellness more effectively than anything offered by modern allopathic medicine.

Therapies to Consider

Nutrition

There may be a connection between nutritional deficiencies and addiction. Alcoholism is known to cause nutritional deficiencies, but it is not clear whether nutritional disorders lead to addiction. Preliminary studies of nutritional supplements appear promising in maintaining sobriety, reducing depression, and minimizing cravings. Amino acid supplementation may be an effective adjunct in the treatment of alcohol and cocaine addiction.

Homeopathy

Homeopathic remedies have been reported to be helpful in managing addictions, anxiety, and depression. The nature of homeopathy is such that the treatment regimen is formulated to address the patient's specific characteristics and complaints. Therefore, there is no specific "anti-addiction" homeopathic remedy. A skilled homeopath may be able to prescribe remedies for specific patients that can aid in the recovery process.

PREVENTION PRESCRIPTION

- Encourage patients to make a connection with something that gives life deeper meaning and purpose.
- Treat depression and anxiety. Work with a spiritual care provider or other health care providers before symptoms result in self-medication with alcohol or other substances.
- Encourage patients to avoid the use of illicit drugs.
- Be aware of a patient's alcohol intake. If he or she displays any of the following traits, begin an integrative approach for treatment of the addiction:
  - Craving: a strong urge to drink alcohol
  - Loss of control: being unable to stop drinking once your patient has started
  - Physical dependence: symptoms such as sweating, shaking, and anxiety after your patient stops drinking
  - Tolerance: the need for greater quantities of alcohol to feel intoxicated

---

THERAPEUTIC REVIEW

The following is a summary of options for treatment of alcoholism and substance abuse. If a patient presents with a history and symptoms consistent with alcohol or substance abuse withdrawal, immediate referral to a detoxification center is warranted.

■ Laboratory

Laboratory testing is not helpful in screening, but liver assessment can help in monitoring of the toxic effects of heavy drinking and be a tool in motivating behavior change.

- Alanine aminotransferase, gamma-glutamyltransferase, and carbohydrate-deficient transferrin (CDT): CDT is least affected by nonalcoholic liver disease and thus is a specific indicator for heavy ethanol use. It can be elevated if four or five drinks have been consumed at one time in the previous 2 weeks.

- Consider complete blood count and determination of levels of B_{12}, folate, electrolytes, magnesium, uric acid, lipase, and prealbumin in chronic alcohol users.

■ Pharmaceutical Agents

■ Alcohol

Benzodiazepines are commonly used for detoxification and withdrawal symptoms:
- Consider clonazepam, 1 mg three times daily, with a gradual taper during 10 to 14 days.

To reduce the high sensation associated with alcohol:
- Naltrexone (ReVia): 50 mg/day orally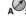

To reduce the craving of alcohol:
- Acamprosate (Campral): 333 to 666 mg three times a day
- Topiramate (Topamax): titrate 25 to 300 mg weekly during 8 weeks (see Table 81-2)

To create unpleasant side effects with use of alcohol:
  Disulfiram (Antabuse): 250 to 500 mg/day

■ Tobacco

- Tapered nicotine replacement: oral, patch, or inhaled over 3 to 4 weeks

- Bupropion (Zyban): 150 mg twice a day × 6 weeks. The patient should set a quit date after taking the medication for 2 weeks. It is effective in managing symptoms of withdrawal and cravings.

- Varenicline (Chantix) is started 7 days before the quit date: days 1 to 3: 0.5 mg daily; days 4 to 7: 0.5 mg twice daily; subsequent 11 weeks: 1 mg twice daily. It can be used for up to 24 weeks if needed to prevent relapse.

■ Opiates

- Methadone, 15 to 20 mg/day orally for opiate addiction, is the most commonly used pharmaceutical agent in relapse prevention and management of cravings.

- Buprenorphine (Subutex) is an opioid partial agonist that reduces cravings and helps prevent relapses. It also has a lower potential than methadone for dependence. Extra training is required to prescribe it.

Cocaine

- Antidepressant medications (selective serotonin reuptake inhibitors and tricyclic antidepressants)

- Amantadine, 100 mg orally twice daily, has been used to decrease cravings and to prevent relapse, with varying success.

Botanicals

For anxiety, insomnia, and depression associated with substance abuse, consider the following:

- Valerian: for anxiety, 300 to 450 mg three times daily or 400 to 900 mg 2 hours before sleep. It must be used for 2 to 3 weeks before an effect can be seen.

- Kava kava extract standardized to 70% kava-lactones: 100 mg three times a day for anxiety. Avoid in patients with liver disease because of the potential for hepatic toxicity.

- St. John's wort, 300 mg three times daily or 450 to 600 mg twice daily, is used for depression, but its role in alcohol and substance abuse recovery is yet to be determined.

- Kudzu is a traditional Chinese herb that has been used in alcohol recovery. The recommended dose is 1.2 g twice daily.

Acupuncture

Acupuncture is effective in producing relaxation and minimizing cravings for most substances of abuse.

Treatment protocols typically involve five needles placed in each ear several times a week and are most effective as part of a comprehensive treatment program.

Not all treatment facilities offer acupuncture, and referring practitioners should be aware of the treatment options available in their geographic area.

Mind-Body Therapies

Meditation, biofeedback, hypnosis, guided imagery, yoga, and prayer have been shown to be effective adjunctive therapies in treatment programs, but most of the studies conducted to assess them have not been well controlled.

Spirituality

Numerous studies have shown a benefit in the recovery process in persons who have a strong spiritual connection or actively participate in various religious practices. There is no correlation between a specific religion or belief system and recovery; the important factor appears to be the presence of a spiritual connection or practice.

Twelve-Step Programs

Alcoholics Anonymous has proved to be successful in the alcoholism recovery process. The Twelve Steps are rooted in spirituality and social support.

Other programs, such as Narcotics Anonymous, Cocaine Anonymous, and Al-Anon, use similar principles and focus on other substances of abuse and their effects on the abuser's family.

Primary care physicians should be aware of the programs available in their geographic area.

Culturally Specific Interventions

Various cultural and ethnic groups have been affected by alcoholism and substance abuse to different degrees. In many cultures, including Native American cultures, culture-specific interventions and practices can aid in the recovery process.

Physicians should be aware of the patient's cultural background and belief system when making referrals to treatment facilities.

KEY WEB RESOURCES

National Institute of Alcohol Abuse and Alcoholism: http://www.niaaa.nih.gov	Patient education, resources, and helpful links
http://rethinkingdrinking.niaaa.nih.gov/ToolsResources/CalculatorsMain.asp	Clinical calculators for alcohol, including those used to determine alcohol content of cocktails, calories in alcohol, financial costs, and blood alcohol concentrations
National Acupuncture Detoxification Association (NADA): http://www.acudetox.com/	
Alcoholics Anonymous (AA): www.aa.org	
http://www.aa.org/lang/en/meeting_finder.cfm?origpage=29	To find AA meetings and times
National Institute on Drug Abuse (NIDA): www.nida.nih.gov	Information on drugs of abuse for clinicians, patients, teachers, and students
www.PCSSmentor.org	NIDA also has a free "warmline" (warm because contact is made within 24 hours) that offers primary care clinicians mentors who can provide clinical assistance and resources, or call 877-630-8812

References

References are available online at expertconsult.com.

Section XV Ophthalmology

Cataracts

Robert Abel, Jr., MD

Etiology

The lens is one of the body's most solid tissues, being approximately 36% solid. It is composed of mostly proteins (crystalline fibers and enzymes) and some carbohydrate and polyunsaturated fatty acids. The lens curvature and the alignment of the fibers are designed for the bending of light rays in the visual spectrum and the absorption of radiation above and below that spectrum. A cataract is any opacification of the normally clear crystalline lens of the eye. Oxidation of lens fibers, catalyzed by short, phototoxic ultraviolet (UV) wavelengths of light, destroys the sulfhydryl protein bonds. Breaking of these bonds leads to a denaturation and clumping of the protein, with consequent loss of lens clarity.

The eye is a remote outpost that relies on good nutrition, liver function, circulation, and breathing. The lens, in particular, has no direct vascular or neurologic innervations and therefore must rely on the circulation of the small amount of aqueous humor, going from the ciliary body out through the trabecular meshwork, for delivery of nutrition and removal of toxins.

The aqueous humor has very high levels of water-soluble compounds, such as ascorbic acid, glutathione, and its key amino acid, cysteine, the major diet-derived antioxidants that protect lens clarity.

However, the eye is not an isolated organ; it is connected to the brain and cardiovascular and digestive systems. It requires protection from bright illumination, which is provided by the lids, lashes, watery tear film, cornea, and iris. Cataract formation is often symptomatic of deeper abnormalities and systemic imbalances. In a common clinical scenario, the ophthalmologist tells the patient that he or she has a cataract, followed by reassurance of its nonacute nature, "Don't worry, I'll see you in 6 months." Six months later the patient is told, "It's time to operate!" Earlier interventions directed at the disturbances underlying cataract formation can halt or significantly retard this inevitable progression.

There has been evidence to suggest the role of diabetes in the development of cataracts. From a biochemical perspective, the sugar within the bloodstream diffuses into the aqueous humor and, in combination with light, performs photo-oxidation of the lens proteins.[1] Therefore, it is not unusual for diabetic patients to present with eye complaints related to cataract earlier than one would expect. In fact, Iranian researchers compared patients with type 2 diabetes and a control group to show that the diabetic patients demonstrated visually debilitating cataracts 5 years earlier than the control group.[2]

Cataracts are the leading cause of vision impairment in both developed and developing countries and are the major cause of blindness worldwide.

Vision provides up to 80% of our sensory input and is to be preserved at any cost. This chapter reviews the current evidence correlating antioxidant deficiency with the prevalence of cataract formation as well as the administration of specific antioxidants to reduce the incidence of lens opacification.

Screening

Changes in Vision

Subtle cataract development leads to unrecognized loss of color interpretation and fine detail and to difficulty with contrast and distance vision. In younger patients, fluctuating vision is often related to refractive error, computer use, diminishing accommodation, and even medications. As reported by mature adults, the following visual symptoms may indicate early cataract formation and can serve as the basis for questioning of the patient during a general medical history and physical examination:

- Blurred vision

- Difficulty with reading road signs and distance vision

- Trouble reading
- Loss of depth perception
- Difficulty following a golf ball
- Difficulty with night driving
- Glare, especially at night
- Double vision
- Reduced vision

> Patients may not volunteer information about decreasing vision because they do not notice the gradual decrement, may fear losing a driver's license, or are anxious about having their eyes examined.

Primary Care Diagnosis

The small-pupil Welch Allyn ophthalmoscope enables primary care physicians to look at the fundus of the eye to detect diabetic and other changes. The device is focused by a simple rotary movement of the thumb. With this instrument, it is possible to assess lens transparency as well as to observe the fundus.[3] Patient complaints are the first symptom. Distance vision problems and glare far exceed near-vision disturbances in patients with cataracts; the reverse is true in patients with macular degeneration.

Ophthalmologic Referral

The definitive diagnosis of cataract is made by ophthalmologic referral and slit-lamp examination. Distance visual acuity, near vision, and depth perception as well as contrast sensitivity and peripheral vision can be evaluated. Glare testing may also approximate real-world conditions and may corroborate functional impairment.

Documentation of Progression

Because cataracts are slowly progressive and phacoemulsification removal with intraocular lens implantation is an elective procedure, most ophthalmologists choose to wait for patients to volunteer information about level of inconvenience or significant loss of function. The mere appearance of early cataract changes alone rarely warrants surgical intervention. Additional difficulty is posed with lens grading because it requires multiple observers.

> Every year in the United States, cataract surgery is performed in more than 3 million people, engendering more than $2 billion in Medicare costs. Delay of cataracts for 10 years would lead to tremendous cost savings.

Epidemiology

Cataracts are by far the leading cause of blindness worldwide. In fact, cataracts are a major cause of reversible blindness in the United States and Western Europe. The frequency increases with age; modern dogma is that everyone will get cataracts, but the truth is that most will.[4]

> ### BOX 82-1. Major Stressors to the Eye and Lens
>
> Ultraviolet and blue light (sunlight)
> Inadequate nutrition
> Lifestyle habits
> Stress
> Chronic disease

Risk Factors

The incidence of cataract formation varies with a number of risk factors (Box 82-1). Cataract formation is not inevitable with age. It is not unusual to find men and women in their 80s and 90s with relatively clear lenses who have had healthy lifestyle habits. The following risk factors for cataract formation have been identified:

- Age
- Sunlight exposure
- Stress
- Medications
- Smoking
- Alcohol excess
- Obesity and high body mass index
- Chronic disease
- Malnutrition
- Saturated-fat diet
- Heredity and genetics
- Trauma
- Congenital disorders
- Inborn errors of metabolism
- Dehydration
- Diabetes
- Vitamin deficiencies
- Low estrogen
- Glass blowing
- Lead exposure
- Long-term aspirin use
- African-American race

Integrative Therapy

Lifestyle Interventions

Ultraviolet Light–Blocking Sunglasses

Increased solar exposure and high altitudes have long been known to raise the frequency of cataracts in all decades of life. UV light, especially in the presence of oxygen, contributes strongly to the denaturation of lens protein, which results in cataract formation; this phenomenon was known to occur even before the deterioration of the ozone layer.

There currently are anecdotal veterinary reports of a higher incidence of cataract in rabbits in Patagonia and in dogs in Australia, both due to thinning of the ozone layer. Beachgoers and sunlamp users must be counseled to always wear adequate eye protection. Parents should encourage their children, including infants, to wear sunglasses and other forms of eye protection. Airline pilots have also been found to have a higher incidence of nuclear cataracts, as have astronauts, who may go into space only once in their lifetimes. Part of this risk may be attributable to cosmic radiation and blue light as well as to UV light.

Nevertheless, appropriate protective lenses should also be used in occupations such as welding and ironwork, in which workers experience prolonged exposure to hazardous radiation, even above and below the visual spectrum (400 to 700 nm). Use of hats and visors has been the recommendation of several long-term epidemiologic and longitudinal studies. UVA (also called near-UV) light and UVB (far-UV) light constitute toxic radiation, and their long-term effects are cumulative. Near-UV light penetrates the cornea and is generally absorbed by the lens, whereas far-UV light is more damaging but is usually absorbed by the cornea, although not entirely. For this reason, astronauts had been known to take large amounts of N-acetylcysteine (3000 mg/day), a glutathione booster, while on space missions.

Stress Management

Stress depresses immune function, alters sleep patterns, impairs gastrointestinal absorption, and reduces available antioxidants. Stress also stimulates the sympathetic nervous system, causing vasoconstriction, increasing muscle tension, and, during long periods, decreasing microcirculation through the ophthalmic artery and its tributaries. A direct correlation between stress and cataract formation remains to be proved in humans, but there is ample evidence that stress, smoking, nutritional deficiency, radiation, and corticosteroids increased cataract formation in animal models.

Pharmaceuticals

More than 300 common medications are known to be photosensitizing agents. Many antibiotics, diuretics, antihypertensives, botanicals (St. John's wort), psoralens, and other agents increase the sensitivity of lens protein to UV damage. Therefore, it is important to advise all people taking medicine to wear sunglasses and to ask their pharmacists about whether their medications are photosensitizers. Many medications also require hepatic excretion and may interfere with normal nutritional biochemistry in the liver. For instance, many cholesterol-lowering agents decrease the production of coenzyme Q10 and glutathione in the liver. Glutathione, a sulfur-containing tripeptide, is a major free radical scavenger in the human lens.

Corticosteroids

Corticosteroids by any route of administration (topical, oral, intranasal, inhaled, or intravenous) are known to raise the incidence of both cataracts and glaucoma in susceptible persons. This adverse effect is most common with topical corticosteroids used in treatment of ocular inflammation and allergies. Therefore, it is advisable for patients who are prescribed ocular steroids for allergies not to have refills without appropriate ophthalmologic supervision. There are other ways to treat ocular allergy, such as with topical antihistamines, mast cell stabilizers, and the administration of oral vitamin C (1000 mg/day) and the eucalyptus bioflavonoid preparation quercetin (1000 mg/day).

Often, the patient who sees many physicians develops a polypharmacy, which is perpetuated. Chinese and Ayurvedic healers tend to use a mixture of herbal remedies for a limited time; they then reevaluate the patient within 2 weeks and readjust the formula. This approach is a good one to incorporate into contemporary Western medicine.

Smoking

Smoking not only reduces available ascorbic acid and alpha-tocopherol but also has a direct toxic effect on the lens of the eye. The longitudinal Physicians' Health Study and Nurses' Health Study have shown a significant rise in cataract formation in smokers, with twice the incidence in the male physicians' study and two thirds more cataract operations in the women who smoked.[5,6] In many pack-a-day smokers, a yellow-brown cast to the nucleus develops during 20 years of smoking.

Alcohol

Excess intake of alcohol is known to raise the incidence of cataract formation, probably by loss of some of the B and fat-soluble vitamins and through the possible alteration of liver function.

Lack of Exercise

Exercise stimulates breathing and parasympathetic activity. This effect is especially desirable in persons with chronic glaucoma conditions and macular degeneration. A group of University of Oregon investigators[7] found that 30 to 40 minutes of walking, four times weekly, lowered intraocular pressure and also reduced stress. Improved aqueous flow is important to the health of the crystalline lens of the eye as well.

Overweight

Obesity or an unfavorable waist-to-hip ratio has been associated with a higher incidence of cataract formation.[8] Chinese researchers noted that there is a higher rate of so-called age-related cataracts in individuals who are deemed overweight and obese by body mass index.[9] This association is yet another reason that it is important to encourage maintenance of ideal body weight and moderation of calorie intake.

Management of General Medical Conditions

Patients with diabetes have three to five times the risk of cataract formation noted in the general population.[10] Effective management of diabetes is important for avoidance of both the highs and the lows of serum glucose levels. An elevation in blood glucose concentration causes an influx of fluid into the lens of the eye, significantly changing the refractive error. This change in permeability ultimately enhances protein decomposition and cataract formation through the sorbitol pathway (Fig. 82-1). Quercetin, a preparation of naturally occurring eucalyptus bioflavonoids, inhibits the

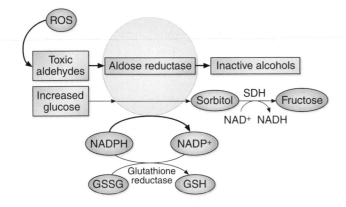

aldose reductase pathway. Several studies also indicate that hypothyroidism is more common in persons with cataracts. Hypertension and Cushing syndrome are also associated with cataract formation.

Female Gender
Some studies have indicated a higher incidence of cataracts in women that cannot be accounted for solely by the slight preponderance of women in the general population older than 65 years. Replacement estrogen therapy is correlated with a protective effect; therefore, the use of natural or synthetic estrogens may be appropriate in patients without contraindications to it.

Aging and Longevity
Because the incidence of cataract rises every decade after the age of 45 years, it is important to screen people older than 45 years for general health and driving ability. Several studies in the orthopedic literature have indicated that visual disability is one of the risk factors for hip fracture. The loss of depth perception makes people particularly vulnerable to falls because they assume that they can see well with one eye yet may be likely to miscalculate steps and distances. Cataract development is seemingly related to overall health and other medical conditions. Several articles point to an inverse relationship between cataract development and life span. In fact, Age-Related Eye Disease Study (AREDS) participants with age-related macular degeneration and cataracts had a shorter life expectancy than those without both diseases.[11]

Lack of Sleep
Patients should be advised to get plenty of sleep. Darkness is a time when the eyes, especially the retina, have a chance to rest, recover, and replenish. The lens and intraocular structures are bombarded by light, with the formation of free radicals, all day; sleep provides an opportunity for the liver and circulation to replenish the necessary antioxidants and minerals to the lens and other ocular tissues.

Nutrition
Fruits and Vegetables
Ascorbic acid, carotenoids, tocopherol, and glutathione are present in the lens epithelium and lens fibers. Proteolytic enzymes that act to remove damaged protein are also present in the lens and are spared by glutathione and other free radical scavengers. In general, the colored bioflavonoids and carotenoids are nature's protectors and should be part of a balanced diet. Multiple studies have identified green leafy vegetables as being preventive of cataract as well as of age-related macular degeneration.[12] The Australian Blue Mountains Eye Study, which involved 3654 persons, found that subjects with a diet high in protein, fiber, vitamin A, niacin, thiamine, and riboflavin had a lower incidence of nuclear cataracts. Persons whose diet had higher levels of polyunsaturated fatty acids had a significantly lower rate of cortical cataract formation.[13] Low serum levels of alpha-tocopherol may not reflect the actual concentration within the lens; interestingly, this may be true for many other nutrients as well.[14] Increased dietary fructose induces cataracts in diabetics and nondiabetics.[15]

Vitamin C
Citrus fruits and many other fruits and vegetables contain high levels of ascorbic acid, which is a major antioxidant in the lens of the eye. The lens and aqueous humor concentrate ascorbic acid in amounts more than 10 times those found in human plasma. Ascorbate is richer in the cortical fibers than in the older, nuclear fibers. As expected, patients with senile cataracts have a lower serum ascorbate level than that of controls.[16] Higher blood levels of the vitamin seem to confer some protection against cataract. Persons with higher than average vitamin C intake appear to have a lower risk of nuclear cataract, and those younger than 60 years have a lower risk of cortical opacities, with intake range of 150 to 300 mg/day.[17]

Lutein-Containing Foods
Spinach, kale, collard greens, guava, and even corn and eggs contain lutein, which has been found to be protective against cataract formation. People who consume high levels of green leafy vegetables and whose serum lutein levels are in the highest quintile have a 20% reduced risk of cataract formation.[18,19] In both the Physicians' Health Study and the Nurses' Health Study, cataract surgery was associated with lower intake of foods such as spinach, which are rich in lutein and zeaxanthin carotenoids rather than beta-carotene.

Avoidance of Saturated Animal Fat
By reducing saturated fats, the patient will find it easier to reach and to maintain an ideal body weight. The change from saturated fat and *trans*-fat acids to polyunsaturated fatty acids is protective to the lens and is currently being evaluated in AREDS 2.[20] As an added benefit, the change also helps the patient improve his or her serum lipid profile.

Hydration
The patient should be encouraged to drink plenty of water. The lens of the eye is a dehydrated tissue much like a fingernail, another avascular ectodermal structure. Drinking six to eight glasses of filtered water a day is an excellent way to increase aqueous humor circulation, which supports lens health. Tips for prevention of dry eyes are presented in Box 82-2.

BOX 82-2. Tips for Prevention of Dry Eyes

- Adequate hydration can be promoted by drinking six to eight glasses of water daily.
- It is important to remember to blink, especially during work with computers and other tasks requiring visual concentration.
- The beneficial fats in the tear film can be reinforced with supplementation of docosahexaenoic acid (DHA) and fat-soluble nutrients such as vitamin A and lutein. DHA produces significant improvement in comfort within a week. Recommend 800 to 1000 mg/day (or 2 g/day of fish oil).
- Use of eye drops and ointments as moisturizers is recommended. For example, Tears Again (Cynacon/OCuSOFT, Inc., Rosenberg, Tex), a liposomal vitamin A and E spray, can be applied externally on the lid and appears to penetrate the eye quickly, providing relief.
- Mechanical problems with the lower lids should be ruled out, especially in patients who may be sleeping with their eyes open. When observing the patient, the clinician should check to see whether the lower lid moves during routine blinking.
- A humidifier should be kept in the bedroom.
- Periodic evaluation of the patient's medication profile is recommended.

Sulfur-Containing Foods

Glutathione, a major antioxidant in the lens, is found in such foods as onions, garlic, avocados, cruciferous vegetables, asparagus, and watermelon. Glutathione and its boosters are thiol compounds, which scavenge free radicals. These glutathione boosters include L-cysteine, lipoic acid, and methanylsulfonylmethane. Glutathione also spares proteolytic enzymes in the cortical lens fibers. In studies from the late 1960s, extracted mature cataracts were demonstrated to contain very low levels of glutathione and ascorbic acid; this finding was considered to represent a secondary aspect of cataract formation. In retrospect, this deficiency appears to be a preliminary event and one that can be managed nutritionally.

Algae-Eating Fish

Single-cell algae are at the bottom of the food chain. When the early hominids began eating fish, their brains developed further, approaching human dimensions. The traditional Japanese diet appears to protect against cataract formation because of the inclusion of cold-water fish and algae, both of which are rich in docosahexaenoic acid (DHA). (Examples of such fish are tuna, mackerel, salmon, sardines, and cod.) Currently, fish such as salmon are being farm raised. Because farm-raised fish are fed grain instead of algae, they contain less DHA and provide less benefit to the eyes and body.

Supplements

For a more complete listing of supplements that promote eye health, see Chapter 83, Age-Related Macular Degeneration.

Lutein and Zeaxanthin

Results of the Physicians' Health Study and Nurses' Health Study have indicated an approximately 20% protection against cataract formation among persons with serum lutein values in the highest quintile.[18,19] Lutein and its isomer, zeaxanthin, are present in high levels in ocular tissues, including the lens. Their importance may lie in the fact that they absorb and reflect the phototoxic blue and UV wavelengths. The carotenoids present in the lens turn out to be lutein and zeaxanthin more than beta-carotene. A daily dose of 2.4 mg of lutein has been shown to double the serum level. Olmedilla et al[21] showed that lutein had a slowing effect on cataract progression during their 2-year study. In fact, they concluded that visual function improved in patients who received lutein supplementation, suggesting that higher intakes of lutein may enhance vision in spite of cataractous lens changes. Christen et al[22] found that supplementing with C, E, lutein, and zeaxanthin significantly lowered the risk of cataracts.

■ Dosage

Patients with early cataracts should take 10 mg/day for the first month then 6 mg/day as part of their daily regimen.

Vitamin C

Numerous studies have shown that increased vitamin C consumption (60 to 600 mg/day) during many years protects against cataracts. In one study, the 5-year risk for the development of any cataract was 60% lower among 3634 participants, aged 43 to 86 years, who had been taking a multivitamin that included vitamin C for 10 years than in participants who had not.[23] Another study showed a 45% protection rate against cataract surgery in women who had consumed vitamin C supplements for 10 years.[24] Jacques et al[25] found that women with a mean vitamin C intake of 359 mg/day for 10 years had a 77% lower prevalence of earlier lens opacities.

■ Dosage

The investigators of the study on vitamin C supplementation recommend approximately 300 mg/day of vitamin C, although I recommend 1000 mg/day.

■ Precautions

Vitamin C supplementation can cause gastrointestinal disturbance, including cramping and diarrhea.

Vitamin A

Hankinson et al[24] found a 39% lower incidence of cataract formation in more than 50,000 nurses who had an adequate intake of vitamin A during an 8-year period than in nurses in the study who did not. This association has been reported in other studies as well. However, this finding must be balanced with a study[26] that has described an association of hip fractures with vitamin A supplementation at more than 17,000 units/day in women. This association may be due to competition of vitamin A with vitamin D absorption in some way.

■ Dosage

Most good multivitamins contain 5000 units of vitamin A or beta-carotene. Additional supplementation is usually not warranted.

Multivitamins

Multivitamin intake has been observed to reduce the risk for cataracts by approximately 20% to 60%, depending on the content of ascorbic acid. Vitamin E (*d*-alpha-tocopherol) is also protective, as found by numerous studies. Robertson et al[27] found that vitamin C (300 to 600 mg/day) and vitamin E (400 units/day) had a 50% protective effect.

The 10-year randomized AREDS was concluded early. It supported the use of a multivitamin with A, C, E, and zinc in macular degeneration but did not find a reduction in cataract development. There is not enough scientific evidence to support the notion that a high dose of a single nutrient provides a greater benefit in reducing cataract risk than a daily multivitamin or a healthy diet.[28] One randomized clinical trial showed that one multivitamin preparation prevented the development of cataract but did not stop the progression once it was fully developed.[29] Others found that ascorbate, lutein, and retinol inversely affected the rate of cataract development.[30]

■ Dosage

Taking a multivitamin is a convenient way to obtain a daily amount of beta-carotene or vitamin A, trace minerals, lutein, and other essential nutrients in two to four capsules, depending on the brand.

Vitamin E

The Lens Opacities Case-Control Study confirmed that alpha-tocopherol is protective against lens opacity.[31] Another study from Linxian, China, also found vitamin E to be protective against cataract formation in persons older than 45 years.[32] Results of other studies suggest that vitamin E has no protective effect against cataract formation,[33] but the question remains whether natural (*d*-alpha) or synthetic (*dl*-alpha) vitamin E was administered in these studies.

B Vitamins

The B vitamins, especially riboflavin (3 mg), thiamine (10 mg), and niacin (40 mg), were found to be protective against cataracts in both the Blue Mountains Eye Study in Australia and another study from Linxian, China.[13,32]

Docosahexaenoic Acid

DHA, the end product of omega-3 fatty acid metabolism, is known to protect cell membranes and thiol groups. An important constituent of retina and brain, DHA has also been found in the lens of the eye. With its presence in all cell membranes and its six double bonds, replenishment of this compound is important. Reduction of DHA stores in women who have experienced pregnancy may be a reason for the gender discrepancy in cataract development. The DHA available in breast milk has been documented to reduce learning disabilities in children and to improve head size and growth in the first year of life. The Mediterranean diet has a 1:1 ratio of omega-3 to omega-6 fatty acids, whereas in the average American diet, the ratio ranges from 1:6 to 1:20.

■ Dosage

A supplemental regimen of 800 to 1000 mg/day of DHA is helpful for almost all adults. Amounts up to 6 g/day have not shown any toxicity in volunteers. This supplement, like all fat-soluble vitamins and supplements, should be taken with a meal for enhanced bioavailability.

Carnosine

N-Acetyl-ʟ-carnosine eye drops are appearing everywhere on vitamin store shelves. Toh et al[34] reviewed the modern treatment of cataracts and stated that the clinical trials with carnosine eye drops are encouraging. It is commonly found in antiaging products because of its inhibition of advanced glycosylation end products. Limited human data are available.

Botanicals

Numerous herbs are known to improve blood flow to the eye and to strengthen liver function. Bioflavonoids in certain berries have been proved to enhance capillary formation; however, their effect on night vision is inconclusive. Astragalus, milk thistle (silymarin), oleander, turmeric root, garlic bulb in oil, and wheat sprouts are botanicals that strengthen liver function.[35] Some supplements are used to improve and support liver function, such as *S*-adenosyl-ʟ-methionine (SAMe) and silymarin.

Turmeric

Curcumin, a constituent of turmeric *(Curcuma longa),* is a spice found in Indian curry dishes. This compound is an effective antioxidant known to induce the glutathione-linked detoxification pathways in rats. It significantly reduces the rate of cataract formation in laboratory rats, but human studies have not been done in the West.[36]

Cineraria

Cineraria maritima, or *Senecio cineraria* (silver ragwort), has been used for centuries as an eye drop preparation for the treatment of conjunctivitis and early cataract. Homeopathic preparations have also been employed, but they have not been subjected to controlled studies.

Bioflavonoids

The eucalyptus bioflavonoid preparation quercetin has been found in multiple laboratory studies to inhibit the formation of cataracts induced by steroids, diabetes, and radiation.

Surgery

Cataract surgery is the most common surgery performed in the United States today; more than 3 million procedures are performed annually. The subsequent laser treatment of an opacified capsule ranks among the 10 most common surgical procedures. With appropriate history and physical examinations and regular eye examination, early cataract formation can be detected long before functional visual loss develops.

Cataract surgery is performed under sterile conditions with local anesthesia. The procedure involves removal of the cataract by phacoemulsification and insertion of an implant within the lens capsule. The synthetic implant may be silicone, polymer, or acrylic. The complications of cataract surgery include infection, lens dislocation, retinal hemorrhage, and retinal detachment. With modern technology, however, this is one of the safest surgical procedures today. In fact, most patients who undergo cataract surgery in one eye can immediately notice the difference and are satisfied with the results.[37,38]

PREVENTION PRESCRIPTION

- Recommended eye examination annually for people older than 50 years and for people at risk. Use of preventive measures is appropriate even in patients with early cataracts.
- Advise use of sunglasses, with side shields as necessary, as well as hats or visors and sunblock in persons whose occupation or interests dictate spending time outdoors.
- Recommend a balanced diet with five or six servings of fruits and vegetables as well as grains, nuts, berries, and organic eggs for amino acids, with consumption of cold-water fish two or more times per week.
- Recommend lutein-rich foods, such as spinach, three times a week; these foods are especially important for ocular protection.
- Promote adequate hydration with intake of six to eight glasses of filtered water daily, with reduction in intake of soft drinks and artificial sweeteners.
- Recommend a daily multivitamin including taurine, zinc, lutein, an additional 1000 to 2000 mg of vitamin C, 400 units of vitamin E, and 5000 units of vitamin A palmitate.
- Advise the patient to maintain an appropriate body weight and to avoid animal fat in the diet.
- Encourage the healthful lifestyle habits of stretching, exercise, moderate alcohol intake, and a regular sleep pattern, with cessation of smoking.
- Advise the patient to maintain a positive attitude and optimism.
- Periodically review prescription and other medications for ophthalmologic effects.
- Encourage regular physical examination and vision testing.

THERAPEUTIC REVIEW

Abundant evidence suggests that we can develop new strategies to maintain our health now instead of waiting for cataracts to form.

Here is a summary of therapeutic and preventive options for cataracts. If a patient presents with severe symptoms, such as profound visual obstruction, it would be to his or her benefit for the clinician to immediately begin a more aggressive therapy, such as referral for elective surgery. For the patient who has mild to moderate symptoms, however, this ladder approach is appropriate.

■ Remove Exacerbating Factors

The patient should be encouraged to

- Stop taking steroid-containing and photosensitizing medications for prolonged use.
- Stop smoking; have moderate alcohol intake; try to lose weight, if needed, through diet and exercise; and substitute good fats in place of bad fats in the diet.
- Wear sunglasses while outside and a hat or visor with at least a 3-inch brim.

■ Nutrition

- Encourage a low-fat, low-cholesterol diet.

- Encourage foods rich in omega-3 fatty acids (wild salmon, nuts, flaxseed) or supplementation with DHA 800 to 1000 mg/day.

■ Supplements

- Multivitamins: daily multivitamin including taurine, zinc, lutein, an additional 1000 to 2000 mg of vitamin C, 400 units of vitamin E, and 5000 IU of vitamin A palmitate

- Docosahexaenoic acid (DHA): 500-800 mg/day

- Lutein: 6 mg/day for 1 month, then 2 mg/day

■ Botanicals

- Turmeric is a major antiinflammatory agent used throughout Asia; there are many data in the Chinese literature of its effectiveness in reducing the risk of cataracts.

■ Surgical Therapy

If the patient's symptoms persist or worsen despite the preceding measures, referral for ophthalmic evaluation and treatment is warranted:

- Cataract extraction by phacoemulsification with intraocular lens insertion (one-step)

KEY WEB RESOURCES

http://eyeadvisory.com/	This Web site is devoted to providing the latest options in both traditional and complementary therapies for 21st-century eye care.
http://www.ageingeye.net/	Current options in cataract care are explored in laymen's language.

References

References are available online at expertconsult.com.

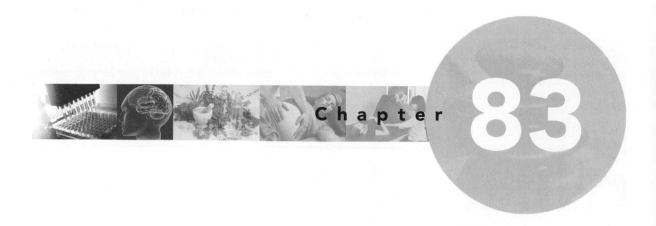

Chapter 83

Age-Related Macular Degeneration

Robert Abel, Jr., MD

> Nowhere has there been so much scientific documentation about nutritional prevention as in the case of macular degeneration. The irony lies in the fact that this information is often virtually ignored by the very specialists who manage patients with the disease.

Etiology

Age-related macular degeneration (AMD) is the scourge of the "golden years." People 65 years and older constitute the fastest-growing segment of the population in developed countries; the risk for AMD and its impact will only become greater in the future. There is a tremendous need to develop preventive strategies to counter AMD and to arrest early cases before the loss of useful vision.

Retinal photoreceptors are subjected to oxidative stress from the combined exposure to light and oxygen on a daily basis. The body's ability to resupply the photoreceptors and underlying pigment epithelium with essential nutrients is the basis for maintenance of good vision throughout life. Diseases of the retina are the leading cause of blindness throughout the developed countries of the world. Among these diseases, macular degeneration is the most common, and its incidence is rising as the population ages. Population-based studies indicate that approximately 10% of people 65 to 74 years and 30% of those 75 years and older demonstrate early signs of the disease, and 7% already have late signs of disease.[1]

Free radicals are thought to attack the rod and cone cell membranes; the retinal pigment epithelium (RPE), a monolayer beneath the retina, fails to keep up with the removal of lipid debris, which accumulates as drusen (yellow spots of different sizes). The melanin pigment protects the retina from radiation, but the amount of this pigment diminishes with age, smoking, and low serum lutein levels. When the RPE cells drop out, pigmentary defects can be noted by ophthalmoscopic examination and on retinal photography. Drusen and progressive RPE atrophy characterize the dry form of macular degeneration, which accounts for 90% of cases of AMD (Figs. 83-1 and 83-2).

The other 10% of cases are attributable to the exudative or vascular type of AMD. A hyaline membrane (i.e., Bruch's membrane) separates the choroidal blood supply from the RPE and overlying retina. Degeneration of Bruch's membrane, retinal anoxia, and impairment of choroidal circulation are believed to be factors that induce the vascular ingrowth characteristic of this form of the disease. These fragile new vessels grow rapidly and may bleed spontaneously.

Most ophthalmologists agree that oxidative stress combined with failure to fortify the retinal photoreceptors is a major pathophysiologic mechanism in this disease, which currently affects 20 million older Americans. Many of these physicians also consider vision loss from macular degeneration to be inevitable, believing that nothing can be done for the dry form and that perhaps only recent interventional therapies are useful for treatment of the wet form of macular degeneration, if it is detected in time. Nowak et al[2] demonstrated significantly higher concentrations of lipid peroxidation products in AMD patients. This finding adds credence to the considerable evidence that nutritional approaches play a major part in prevention and management of this age-related disease. Cumulative photo-oxidative stress, other systemic diseases, and nutritional deficiencies contribute to the onset and progression of AMD. With aging, the protective cell-derived enzymes—catalase, superoxide dismutase, and glutathione peroxidase—decrease, as does the ability to absorb the diet-derived antioxidants.

Screening

Owing to the swelling ranks of the elderly, the number of persons with macular degeneration is growing. Routine dilated-eye examinations are fundamental to early detection

FIGURE 83-1
Atrophic (dry) age-related macular degeneration. Geographic atrophy of the retinal pigment epithelium causes loss of central vision. (From Fillit H. *Brocklehurst's Textbook of Geriatric Medicine and Gerontology.* 7th ed. Philadelphia: Saunders; 2010.)

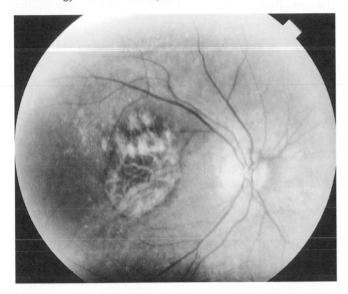

FIGURE 83-2
Exudative (wet) age-related macular degeneration. Leakage and scarring from a subretinal neovascular membrane destroy central retinal function. (From Fillit H. *Brocklehurst's Textbook of Geriatric Medicine and Gerontology.* 7th ed. Philadelphia: Saunders; 2010.)

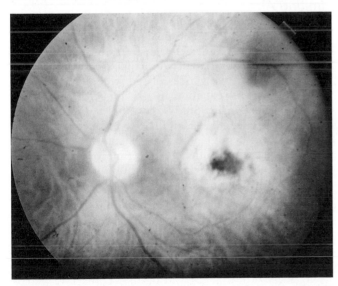

FIGURE 83-3
Amsler grid. This checkerboard-patterned square has parallel vertical and horizontal lines. The patient looks at the central dot with one eye covered and notes the pattern of the lines. If any line in any direction is missing or wavy, the patient marks it in with a pencil or makes a note. The Amsler grid can be used to determine whether there is a disorder of the optic nerve or macula; in particular, use of the grid is an excellent way to monitor macular degeneration to determine whether it is stable or progressing.

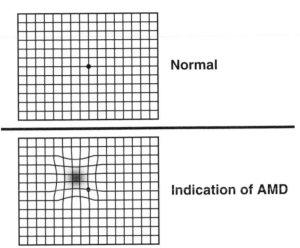

Normal

Indication of AMD

diseases are at greatest risk. Early detection offers greater flexibility in the use of complementary therapies.

Referral to an ophthalmologist is indicated for dilated funduscopic examination and retinal imaging (photograph, laser tomography, and fluorescein angiography), which can clearly document stages of AMD. On occasion, retinal specialists are needed for advanced management.

Primary care physicians should help patients coordinate the various medicines used in the management of underlying and concurrent diseases. Periodic review of medications is important because polypharmacy may contribute to the risk for AMD.

Risk Factors

The following risk factors for AMD have been identified:

- Age
- Sunlight exposure
- Previous cataract surgery
- Light-colored irises, fair complexion
- Obesity
- Female gender, parity
- Postmenopausal status
- Inflammation
- Smoking
- Physical inactivity
- Elevated serum cholesterol values
- Hypertension
- Nocturnal hypotension

and management of AMD. The onset is often so gradual as to go unnoticed.

Use of an Amsler grid, a 4 × 4-inch checkerboard square with a central dot for fixation, is an excellent way to diagnose AMD and allows home monitoring of the condition. This approach to management is especially useful in patients with the slowly progressive, dry form of the disease (Fig. 83-3).

Primary care physicians should know the AMD risk profiles to alert patients about preventive steps and the need for periodic eye examinations. Patients with multiple systemic

- Poor digestion, use of antacids
- Hypothyroidism, use of thyroid hormones
- Family history
- Low dietary intake of carotenoids, low serum carotenoid levels
- Low macular pigment density
- Low serum zinc levels
- Hyperopia

The National Health and Nutrition Examination Survey demonstrated that for 65- to 70-year-old respondents, the chance for development of AMD was nearly five times that for 45- to 54-year-old respondents.[3]

Sunlight

Reducing exposure to sunlight through the use of hats and sunglasses has been stressed in numerous studies.[4] A University of Wisconsin study of 3684 persons between the ages of 43 and 84 years found a positive correlation between daily sun exposure and the development of AMD. Persons who spent more than 5 hours a day in the sun were twice as likely to have AMD as those with less than 2 hours a day of sun exposure.[5]

Gender

The incidence of AMD is at least three times greater in postmenopausal women than in men of similar age. Two studies have indicated that hormone replacement therapy (HRT) significantly reduces this risk, although a third study did not find any correlation. Apparently, women require more lutein than men do because it is preferentially deposited in fatty tissue rather than in the retina.[6] Obstetricians and gynecologists should inform their patients about early prevention and participate in decisions about biocompatible HRT when appropriate.

Inflammation

Clemons et al[7] showed that early or moderate AMD advances with smoking, increasing body mass index, and, probably, use of antacid and antiinflammatory medications. Seddon et al[8] demonstrated that C-reactive protein levels were higher in individuals with advanced AMD.

Smoking and Other Factors

Numerous investigators have determined that current smokers, especially those who smoke one pack a day or more, have a significantly higher risk for development of AMD than do nonsmokers and persons who have given up smoking 10 years previously. The Nurses' Health Study indicated that women who smoked 25 or more cigarettes a day were more than twice as likely as nonsmokers to have AMD.[9] The Physicians' Health Study also showed a greater than two-fold incidence in men who smoked 20 or more cigarettes daily.[10] One study indicated an association between smoking, low serum selenium levels, and the development of AMD. Smoking has been shown to contribute to reduced levels of circulating antioxidants as well as of the lutein pigment in the macular area.

The Age-Related Eye Disease Study (AREDS) found that smoking is associated with three of its five stages of macular degeneration.[11] This multicenter, randomized controlled trial also found that hypertension, obesity, hyperopic refractive error, white race, and increased use of thyroid hormones and antacids were indicators for the most severe stages of the disease.

Integrative Therapy

Lifestyle Interventions

Sunglasses, Hats, and Visors
Everyone's need to wear sunglasses with light protection, hats, and visors should be emphasized as early as childhood. People with dilated pupils, outdoor workers, and people who frequent tanning beds may be at a higher risk for development of macular degeneration. Microscope light during cataract surgery is another source of phototoxicity. Sun exposure is a known causative factor in the progression of the hereditary disorder retinitis pigmentosa.

Stress Management
Hormonal imbalance and lack of sleep contribute to debilitation of retinal health. Depression contributes to food habituation, overeating, and abnormal sleep patterns. Ocular health remains in a sensitive balance between oxidative stress and antioxidant support of cell membranes. Therefore, smoking and inadequate nutrition both tip the scale toward increased or imbalanced free radical activity.

Limiting Alcohol Intake
Alcohol excess has been associated with cardiovascular and liver disorders. The Beaver Dam Eye Study documented an association between beer consumption and risk of RPE degeneration. Two further studies have indicated that one or two glasses of red wine daily can confer a 40% to 50% reduction in risk for AMD. However, the Physicians' Health Study and Nurses' Health Study, conducted between 1980 and 1994, could not confirm any significant benefit. Red wine has a protective effect on cardiovascular health and may improve retinal and choroidal blood flow. Apparently, white wine, which lacks the high levels of grape skin bioflavonoids, does not confer as much ocular protection.

Recognition of Medication Effects
Numerous medications, including phenothiazines, hydroxychloroquine, and ethambutol, may negatively affect the RPE. Other agents may alter digestion or liver function. The liver not only filters out all of the nutrients and toxins from the gastrointestinal tract but also stores fat-soluble vitamins, activates the B vitamins, and manufactures glutathione. Chinese and Ayurvedic physicians have known for millennia that the liver is essential to good vision.

> Antacid use has been positively correlated with the development of AMD. The lack of gastric acidity reduces the stimulus for secretion of pancreatic and biliary enzymes into the duodenum.

Hydration

Drinking six or more glasses of good water a day hydrates the body, flushes the liver and kidneys, and decreases appetite. Patients should be counseled against excessive consumption of caffeinated soft drinks.

Exercise

Exercise plays a role in cardiovascular health and in stimulating the parasympathetic nervous system. Physical activity also plays a part in relaxation of the mind, decreasing intraocular pressure and improving ocular blood flow.

Breathing

Deep breathing relaxes the mind, strengthens the diaphragm, and improves blood flow to the eye. Conscious attention to breathing is the foundation of meditation and stress reduction practices.

Whole Body Health

Management of concurrent medical conditions is essential. Regulating blood pressure and serum cholesterol level, controlling diabetes, supporting necessary weight reduction, and managing cardiovascular health are important to the long-term maintenance of good vision. It is wise to remember that the eye is intimately connected to the rest of the body.

Estrogen

Women are more likely than men to have AMD. Several studies have demonstrated that postmenopausal women who are taking HRT exhibit a lower incidence of macular degeneration, especially the wet form of the disease.[12] However, one study was unable to determine any significant effect of estrogen replacement therapy. Nonetheless, clinicians find that more postmenopausal women have AMD than men do.

Sleep

Sleep is crucial to restoration of photoreceptor and ocular health. The eye requires darkness to restore photoreceptor integrity and to replenish nutrients consumed during the daylight hours, when ultraviolet wavelengths and bright light are constantly bombarding the eye.

Attitude

Adopting a positive attitude is the first step in lifestyle modification. The placebo effect is another demonstration of the "power of positive thinking." In one study, 68% of persons who took a multivitamin for 6 months showed an improvement in macular appearance on electroretinograms; however, 32% of the placebo group also showed improvement. Similarly, in an initial study of photodynamic therapy to control retinal bleeding, approximately 50% of subjects receiving the therapy demonstrated some benefit compared with 28% of the placebo group. This nearly 30% placebo effect, which contributed to the cessation of retinal bleeding, is a demonstration of the power of positive thinking.

Nutrition

Box 83-1 lists the foods recommended for preservation of sight.

BOX 83-1. Top 10 Foods for Sight Preservation

- *Cold-water fish (sardines, cod, mackerel, and tuna):* an excellent source of DHA, which provides structural support to cell membranes and is recommended for dry eyes, treatment of macular degeneration, and sight preservation (see Chapter 86, The Antiinflammatory Diet).
- *Spinach, kale, and green leafy vegetables:* rich in carotenoids, especially lutein and zeaxanthin; lutein, a yellow pigment, protects the macula from sun damage and from blue light.
- *Eggs:* rich in cysteine, sulfur, lecithin, amino acids, and lutein; sulfur-containing compounds protect the lens of the eye from cataract formation.
- *Garlic, onions, shallots, and capers:* rich in sulfur, which is necessary for the production of glutathione, an important antioxidant for the lens of the eye and for the whole body.
- *Soy:* low in fat, rich in protein; has become a staple in vegetarian diets; contains essential fatty acids, phytoestrogens, vitamin E, and natural antiinflammatory agents.
- *Fruits and vegetables:* contain vitamins A, C, and E and beta-carotene; the yellow vegetables, such as carrots and squash, are important for daytime vision.
- *Blueberries and grapes:* contain anthocyanins, which improve night vision; a cupful of blueberries or huckleberry jam or a 100-mg bilberry supplement may improve dark adaptation within 30 minutes.
- *Wine:* known to exert a cardioprotective effect; has many important nutrients that protect vision, heart, and blood flow (as with any alcohol, moderation is always important).
- *Nuts and berries:* nature's most concentrated food sources; grains such as flaxseed are high in the beneficial omega-3 fatty acids, which help lower serum cholesterol and stabilize cell membranes.
- *Extra-virgin olive oil:* a monounsaturated oil and a healthy alternative to butter and margarine.

Fruits and Vegetables

Fruits and vegetables contain vitamins A, C, and E and beta-carotene and lutein. The yellow-orange vegetables, such as carrots and sweet potatoes, are important for daytime vision. Cho et al[13] found strong evidence of a protective role of fruit against the risk for neovascular AMD or age-related maculopathy.

Lutein-Containing Foods

Spinach, collard greens, kale, guava, and many other green and yellow fruits and vegetables contain lutein and its isomer, zeaxanthin. These two carotenoids are concentrated in the macular pigment; their accumulation depends directly on dietary intake and serum level.

The complete name of the visually sensitive center of the retina is macula lutea because of its yellow color (Latin *luteus*, "yellow"). Lutein and zeaxanthin are known to be responsible for the yellow color. The normal retina is capable of concentrating these carotenoids to a level several orders of magnitude greater than the serum level. Evidence suggests that the lutein in macular pigment is entirely of dietary origin and is highly protective against AMD.[14]

In one study, persons consuming lutein-rich foods five times a week were eight times less likely to have AMD than those consuming such foods once a month.[15] In addition, persons with serum lutein values in the highest quintile had a 43% lower risk for AMD. Another study demonstrated that consumption of 4 to 8 oz/day of spinach for 4 months resulted in greater macular pigment density. The vitamin K content in spinach may interfere with blood-thinning agents such as warfarin sodium. Preliminary data have demonstrated improvement in visual function in patients with the dry form of AMD whose diet was modified to provide an abundance of dark green vegetables.[16]

> There is 44 mg of lutein per cup of cooked kale, 26 mg per cup of cooked spinach, and 3 mg per cup of broccoli.

Avoidance of Saturated Fats
Patients should be advised to decrease their intake of saturated fats. Diets high in saturated fats contribute to the risk of AMD, whereas those high in unsaturated fats reduce that risk.[17]

Cold-Water Fish
Docosahexaenoic acid (DHA), found in cold-water, deep-dwelling fish, is an essential nutrient for good brain and retinal function. The flesh of algae-eating fish is high in DHA, which is important in building and protecting photoreceptor membranes. In one study, persons consuming cold-water fish more than once a week were half as likely to experience macular degeneration as those consuming fish less than once a month.[18] The same study found a 2.7-fold greater incidence of AMD in persons consuming high levels of dietary cholesterol. Eating oily fish at least once weekly compared with less than once weekly halved the incidence of neovascular AMD.[19]

Wine in Moderation
Most researchers agree that consumption of moderate amounts of red wine reduces the risk of macular degeneration. In addition, many studies report that moderate wine consumption is associated with lengthened life span.

Glutathione
An important study found that glutathione and related precursor amino acids are protective against damage to human RPE cells, which underlie the macula. Foods that contain the tripeptide glutathione are onions, garlic, avocados, asparagus, watermelon, and cruciferous vegetables.

Supplements

Multivitamins
Many studies indicate the protective effect of antioxidants on retinal photoreceptors and the RPE. Some studies have demonstrated an association between vitamin or mineral deficiencies (e.g., of zinc, tocopherol, carotenoids, taurine) and a higher risk of AMD. Ascorbate as well as lipoic acid helps recycle tocopherol in retinal tissue. Patients with AMD in general were found in one study to have a lower intake of tocopherol, magnesium, zinc, pyridoxine, and folic acid. In an important Veterans Affairs study, patients with AMD who were taking an antioxidant capsule (containing 19 ingredients) twice daily maintained better vision than the placebo control group.[20] One review found positive evidence for vitamins A, C, and E and beta-carotene, lutein and zeaxanthin, selenium, and zinc, with the best evidence for vitamins C and E, lutein, and zeaxanthin.[21]

The 10-year randomized, controlled AREDS was concluded 3 years early because of the significant difference in the vitamin groups versus placebo. It demonstrated that the combination of vitamins C and E, beta-carotene, and zinc significantly reduced the progression of macular degeneration.[22] Ophthalmologists regard this as a landmark study acknowledging the effect of supplementation on macular degeneration. This proof of specific benefits of a balanced diet and broader nutrient supplementation has exciting implications.

The National Eye Institute is instituting AREDS II. It will reduce the amounts of zinc and beta-carotene in the study combination and add lutein and DHA.[23] In a 1-year Italian study, a combination of vitamin C, vitamin E, zinc, copper, lutein, and zeaxanthin improved established AMD.[24] The 6-month TOZAL study found similar results with a multivitamin including C, E, zinc, beta-carotene, and lutein and recommended prolonged administration.[25]

Lutein
Carotenoids are powerful antioxidants. Lutein and zeaxanthin have been precisely identified at high levels in the retina, particularly in the macular area. They have also been identified at significant concentrations in the iris, choroid, and lens (where they are needed to quench singlet oxygen and to filter out blue light). Greater lutein consumption is directly associated with elevated serum values and an increased macular pigment density. Investigators studying 23 pairs of donor eyes found that the eyes with lower lutein and zeaxanthin levels were the ones with histopathologic signs of AMD.[26] Another study evaluated lutein and zeaxanthin levels in 56 donor eyes affected by AMD and 56 donor eyes known to be without the disease. Donor eyes with the highest amounts of lutein and zeaxanthin were 82% less likely to exhibit the signs of macular degeneration.[27]

As little as 2.4 mg/day of lutein can double the serum level. A dose of 6 mg/day produced a 43% lower prevalence of AMD.[15] The Veterans Lutein Antioxidant Supplementation Trial (LAST) documented improvement in visual function with lutein alone or in combination with other nutrients.[28] With the addition of DHA, lutein buildup in the macular pigment density is even more effective.[29]

▪ Dosage
Healthy persons should select a multivitamin containing 6 mg of lutein, and patients already diagnosed with AMD should take 10 or more mg/day for several months to build up plasma and macular levels of this nutrient.

Beta-Carotene, Vitamin A, and Other Carotenoids
Investigators have confirmed in both laboratory and clinical studies that carotenoids such as vitamin A protect retinal cell membranes from light damage. Vitamin A is required to provide adequate levels of rhodopsin for optimal rod function. Severe vitamin A deficiency causes keratomalacia, xerophthalmia, and visual impairment. Administration of

vitamin A has been helpful in patients suffering from retinitis pigmentosa. An early study documented an association between low vitamin A levels and macular degeneration and encouraged the inclusion of yellow fruits and vegetables in the diet.[3] The value of beta-carotene in the management of AMD remains inconclusive .[30,31] Only one study indicated a specific beneficial effect of the carotenoid lycopene on the macula.

Tocopherols

Tocopherols protect against lipid peroxidation in cell membranes. Multiple studies have shown a powerful protective effect of *d*-alpha-tocopherol against macular degeneration. Some of these studies indicate a similar protective effect of plasma ascorbic acid and beta-carotene as well. High serum levels of *d*-alpha-tocopherol have been associated with decreased prevalence of drusen and late macular degeneration. French researchers examining 2500 patients found that those with the highest serum levels of vitamin E had an 82% lower prevalence of AMD.[32] Gamma-tocopherol and tocotrienol may prove superior to *d*-alpha-tocopherol.

Vitamin C

Ascorbic acid reduces the loss of rhodopsin and photoreceptor cell nuclei that occurs on exposure to light. Vitamin C also rejuvenates vitamin E– and cell membrane–related enzymes. In several of the major studies that showed a protective effect of multivitamins against AMD, the multivitamin included at least 60 mg of vitamin C. Ocular tissues, especially the lens, contain high levels of vitamin C and glutathione.

Alpha-Lipoic Acid

Alpha-lipoic acid is an important nerve stabilizer that reduces insulin resistance in diabetic patients. It may protect the remaining ganglion cells and nerve fibers in patients with glaucoma. In addition, alpha-lipoic acid helps regenerate the reduced form of ascorbic acid.

B Vitamins

Pyridoxine deficiency has been identified in two observational studies in AMD populations. Folate deficiency has been identified in one of the studies. The B vitamins in general are important for nerve conduction, and the methylators (B_4, B_6, and B_{12}) reduce homocysteine levels. Christen et al[33] reported a reduction in AMD development in 5205 women observed for 7.3 years with supplementation of folate, pyridoxine, and cyanocobalamin. Niacin, a B vitamin used to treat lipid abnormalities, has been shown to increase choroidal blood volume within 30 minutes of administration; the perfusion is at a slower rate, however, so niacin has not been shown to increase total flow to the choroid.[34]

Glutathione

Glutathione has been reported to be protective against damage to human RPE cells. Glutathione is manufactured in the liver after ingestion of the appropriate amino acids and sulfur-containing foods. This underappreciated water-soluble compound serves as an antioxidant and regenerator of vitamin E and carotenoids as well as an intracellular enzyme. Because glutathione is hydrolyzed in the stomach, supplementation with glutathione boosters is recommended. The following have been found to increase glutathione: *N*-acetylcysteine, 600 mg twice a day; methylsulfonylmethane, 1000 mg once

daily; *S*-adenosylmethionine (SAMe), 200 mg twice a day; and alpha-lipoic acid, 250 mg twice daily.

Bioflavonoids

Studies show that quercetin, a preparation of eucalyptus and citrus bioflavonoids, facilitates vitamin E protection of bovine and rat retina from induced lipid peroxidation. It also exerts an antihistaminic effect that may be beneficial for patients with chronic allergies.

Amino Acids

Taurine, the only nonbound circulating amino acid, is a stabilizer of biologic membranes that protects rod outer segments, supports cardiovascular function, and modulates nerve transmission. Isolated taurine deficiency has been documented to cause retinal degeneration, and taurine administration has been shown in several studies to stabilize retinal changes.[35]

Arginine is one of the most important regulators of ocular perfusion. Intravenous administration of arginine has been shown to increase retinal (and choroidal) blood flow in healthy volunteers. This discovery merits further investigation in the AMD population.[36]

Minerals
■ Zinc and Copper

Zinc is found in high concentrations in the retina, RPE, and choroid. This trace mineral serves as a cofactor with many important retinal enzymes, including superoxide dismutase, catalase, carbonic anhydrase, retinol dehydrogenase, and protein phosphorylase; it also releases vitamin A from the liver. A 2-year study demonstrated that 100 mg/day of zinc sulfate significantly slowed the progression of AMD compared with the course of the disease in controls.[37] A study using a dietary intake questionnaire found a significant inverse association between zinc consumption and number of drusen.[30] Copper is adversely affected by prolonged elevation of zinc levels (30 mg or more orally) and needs to be supplemented as well. A good multivitamin for long-term use includes 15 to 30 mg of zinc and 2 mg of copper. Both copper and zinc are needed to synthesize superoxide dismutase, and both act with other retinal enzymes to scavenge free radicals.

■ Magnesium

Magnesium has a significant role in nerve conduction and also dilates blood vessels. This mineral is important for maintenance of blood flow to the eye and brain in older persons with macular degeneration or diabetes whenever blood pressure is decreased because they are lying down. The dose is 400 to 500 mg at bedtime.

■ Selenium

Selenium (maximum dose, 200 mcg/day) is a cofactor for vitamin E and glutathione enzymes. Low serum selenium levels and smoking have been associated with AMD.

Docosahexaenoic Acid

The primary source of DHA is algae and the cold-water, deep-dwelling fish that eat them. DHA not only supports retinal health in general but also improves hand-to-eye coordination, sharpens night-driving ability, and stabilizes cell membranes throughout the body. With its six unsaturated double bonds, it composes 30% to 50% of the "good" fat in the outer segments of the retinal photoreceptors. Because people are undersupplied with DHA from infancy, it is important to incorporate DHA capsules in the diet. The suggested supplementation amount is 500 to 1000 mg/day. One study found that lutein supplementation at 12 mg/day increased macular pigment ocular density (MPOD) in the peripheral macula, whereas the addition of DHA (800 mg/day) increased peripheral and central MPOD.[38] This evidence strengthens the support for supplementing polyunsaturated fatty acids in the diet to raise their concentration in macular photoreceptors. Feher et al[39] reported that the combination of omega-3 fatty acids, acetyl-L-carnitine, and coenzyme Q10 showed significant stabilization and improvement in vision in a 106-patient study. These three compounds along with vitamin E favorably affect mitochondrial lipid metabolism. A 12-year study confirmed the reduction in neovascular AMD with high intake of omega-3 fatty acids.[40]

> Alpha-linolenic acid (present in flaxseed oil, among others) is the parent omega-3 fatty acid. It takes 20 to 30 of the 18-carbon alpha-linoleic acid molecules to make one 22-carbon DHA molecule, which is a building block for every cell membrane in the body.

Botanicals

Ginkgo

The ginkgo tree is the sole survivor of a family of trees that flourished before the Ice Age. *Ginkgo biloba*, which increases cerebral blood flow, has been demonstrated to improve retinal blood flow by 23%[41] and is prescribed regularly by certain glaucoma specialists. For vasodilation, I recommend either 15 to 60 drops of a ginkgo solution (24% ginkgosides) in water or a 30-mg tablet twice daily. Be sure to check the patient's other medications first for possible blood-thinning influences because ginkgo can exacerbate this effect.

Sage

Sage (*Salvia officinalis*) also improves circulation, but unlike ginkgo, which has an excitatory effect, it has a calming effect.[42] A controlled study from Hunan Medical College in China indicated that *Salvia miltiorrhiza* as part of a four-herb formula improved visual field in a third of a glaucoma population receiving the formula for more than 19 months. Herbalists recommend 1 g orally twice daily. More studies are necessary, however.

Bilberry

Bilberry (*Vaccinium myrtillus*) has been said to improve night vision; with the exception of one preliminary French study, however, it has not proved effective in stabilizing AMD. Bilberry only improves the effectiveness of rhodopsin, which is necessary for night vision.

Milk Thistle

Silymarin, from the herb milk thistle (*Silybum marianum*), is a major supporter of liver function. The liver is the key organ for maintenance of eye health because the fat-soluble vitamins and glutathione are stored and the B vitamins are activated there. The usual dose of milk thistle is 150 mg two or three times a day. SAMe in a dose of 200 mg twice daily is an alternative.

> The eye is subjected to bright light throughout the day, and the important ingredients for molecular repair are stored in the liver. When the liver is overburdened, eyesight is compromised.

Chinese Herbs

Experienced herbalists report that tien chi root, dang gui root, triphala, lycium fruit, ginseng root, cooked and raw rehmannia, shilajatu, wild asparagus root, and elderberry have been used in ancient formulas to treat vascular disease inside the eye.[42] None of these remedies has been used in controlled studies, although there is ample anecdotal evidence in the Chinese literature of success as measured by nonprogression of disease during 3 years.

Pharmaceuticals

Ranibizumab (Lucentis) and bevacizumab (Avastin) are two new vascular endothelial growth factor (VEGF) inhibitors that can remarkably reverse leakage into the retina in wet AMD. Ranibizumab has been approved by the U.S. Food and Drug Administration (FDA); bevacizumab, an intravenous therapy for colon cancer, is used off label. Intraocular injections of steroids, pegaptanib sodium (Macugen, an intraocular anti-VEGF), and verteporfin (Visudyne, an intravenous dye that highlights leaky retinal vessels) are relegated to ancillary roles. Dosages are to be determined by the retinal specialist.

Other Therapy

The FDA may soon approve implantable silicone devices that will serve as replacement for damaged retina. Implantable devices and telescopic lenses are also in phase II FDA testing.

Low-vision experts have many optical devices to support those people with failing vision.

PREVENTION PRESCRIPTION

- Adoption of a positive attitude and awareness of risk factors and potential medication effects
- Use of sunglasses and other sun protection
- Increased consumption of green leafy vegetables
- Diet rich in polyunsaturated fatty acids and low in saturated fats
- Multivitamins with zinc, taurine, and lutein
- Use of supplements, with attention to overall good dietary nutrition
- Avoidance of long-term use of antacids or gastric acid suppression
- Regular exercise
- Performance of deep-breathing exercises on a regular basis
- Periodic eye examinations with use of the Amsler grid
- Use of low-vision aids for vision loss

Early intervention after recognition of macular degeneration is crucial. The performance of an Amsler grid examination is recommended in all patients (see Fig. 83-3). It is important to remember that the retina can be rebuilt.

THERAPEUTIC REVIEW

If a patient presents with severe symptoms, such as profound visual loss, it would be to his or her benefit for the clinician to immediately begin a more aggressive therapy. For the patient who has mild to moderate symptoms, however, the following nutritional and lifestyle approach is appropriate.

◼ Remove Exacerbating Factors

- Encourage smoking cessation, moderate alcohol intake, weight management, and exercise.

◼ Nutrition

- Encourage foods rich in omega-3 fatty acids (wild salmon, nuts, or flaxseed).
- Increase foods rich in carotenoids, such as lutein and zeaxanthin (dark green leafy vegetables).

◼ Supplements

- Multivitamins have been the focus of many epidemiologic studies over the years. It is known that the combination of low-dose antioxidants is supportive of macular function; this fact became evident in the landmark AREDS. The multivitamin should include vitamin C, vitamin E, beta-carotene, zinc, selenium, taurine, lutein, and zeaxanthin.

- Incorporate lutein, 6 to 10 mg/day (6 mg for prevention, 10 mg for treatment).
- DHA supplementation: 500 to 800 mg daily
- Vitamin C, 1000 mg/day, has been shown useful in some observational studies to act as an antioxidant and therefore to protect the retinal pigment epithelium from oxidative stressors.

◼ Botanicals

- *Ginkgo biloba* has been shown to improve ocular blood flow by 23%; 30 mg twice daily.
- Milk thistle is the primary source of the bioflavonoid silymarin, a major supporter of hepatocyte function, which in turn supports eye health;150 mg two or three times a day

◼ Chinese Herbs

- Although clinical data are lacking, there is an abundance of historical data on the benefits of the use of Chinese herbs for AMD.

◼ Pharmaceutical Injection

Anti–vascular endothelial growth factor (VEGF) therapy

- Intraocular injections of ranibizumab (Lucentis) and bevacizumab (Avastin) have become the best treatment of more advanced disease.

KEY WEB RESOURCES

References

References are available online at expertconsult.com.

Part Three Tools for Your Practice
Section I Lifestyle

Food Intolerance and Elimination Diet

J. Adam Rindfleisch, MD, MPhil

Detecting and eliminating specific antagonistic foods, and designing a nutritionally sound diet to ensure the optimum health of the food-sensitive person, is the ultimate aim in food sensitivity management. This process is often tedious and time consuming, and requires tremendous knowledge, skill, commitment, and dedication. . . . However, when a person who has been chronically sick suddenly feels well for the first time in many years, as so often happens, the rewards for both practitioner and client more than justify the time and effort of the endeavor.

J. V. Joneja[1]

Indian Ayurvedic healing for centuries has emphasized the elimination of certain foods and the use of others.[2] Foods, like drugs, can have both helpful and adverse effects. Pesticide contamination, the use of growth hormones and antibiotics in meat production, genetic engineering of food sources, and the health risks associated with fast and processed foods are topics of concern that can arise in an integrative medicine visit.

For many disorders, identification of adverse food reactions and recommendation of elimination diets can be of potential benefit. This chapter describes various classes of adverse food reactions. An overview of the state of the research on the elimination diet as a clinical tool is provided. Tips for prescribing elimination diets, pitfalls to avoid in their use, and resources for further information are also provided. A Patient Handout on elimination diets appears at the end of the chapter.

Adverse Food Reactions: What Are They?

Adverse reactions to foods may be classified on a pathophysiologic basis.[3,4] Often, a distinction is made between food allergy and food intolerance. A food allergy involves an immune-mediated reaction, usually to a glycoprotein found in a given food. Food intolerance, in contrast, is defined more generally as any adverse physiologic response to a food product.

An intolerance may be classed as immune or nonimmune, structural, or functional. Nonimmune reactions are estimated to have a prevalence of 15% to 20%.[3] Table 84-1 lists key clinical entities on the food intolerance spectrum and offers clinical pointers regarding their etiology, differential diagnosis, and treatment.

> There are many types of adverse food reaction. Keep in mind diagnoses such as eosinophilic esophagogastroenteritis, histaminergic food reactions, and reactions associated with psychological or structural disorders. Keep lactose intolerance and celiac disease in mind as two of the most commonly encountered disorders.

Pathophysiology

The epithelial cells of the gastrointestinal tract have been found to function as nonprofessional antigen-presenting cells.[5] The gut is constantly sampling various potential antigens, ultimately allowing only 2% of them to move into the bloodstream. The epithelial cells, gut dendritic cells, and at least five different T-cell types help regulate intestinal immunity. One of the T cells' main functions is to allow tolerance to develop; that is, the body must be able to minimize allergic reactions to the foreign antigens commonly consumed in foods. In some individuals, this process seems to break down, and certain foods begin to elicit symptoms.[6]

Greater intestinal permeability, or "leaky gut," has been proposed as one means by which antigens that are typically

TABLE 84-1. Differential Diagnosis of Adverse Food Reactions

INTOLERANCE CATEGORY	DESCRIPTION	COMMENTS AND CLINICAL TIPS
Food allergy[4,32,33]	Immune mediated, mainly by IgE, to a food glycoprotein Symptoms arise in minutes to hours Manifested the same way with every exposure, usually with rash, angioedema, anaphylaxis; GI symptoms may also arise with histamine release	Prevalence increasing (4%-8% in children, 1%-4% in adults) One fourth of the population claims to have a food allergy One third of infants with frequent spitting up respond to oral challenge testing; 10% who react to cow's milk also react to soy; 45% retain a milk allergy past 1 year of age
Celiac disease[34,35]	Gliadin, a portion of the grain protein gluten, triggers chronic inflammation through reactive $CD4^+T$ cells in people with the alleles for HLA DQ2 or DQ8 Affects all age groups Two to three times more common in females than in males May affect multiple organ systems 10%-23% may develop neurologic symptoms, such as idiopathic ataxia and paresthesias Grains that can contribute are wheat, rye, barley, spelt, kamut, semolina, triticale, and malt. Oats do not have gluten but are often contaminated with it, so many providers encourage avoidance.	Prevalence 1% and increasing as more testing is being done 50% of adults with disease present with diarrhea Increased risk with Down syndrome, Turner syndrome, type 1 diabetes 2%-5% do not respond to gluten-free diet and are at risk for T-cell lymphoma Laboratory results may show decreased calcium and protein, increased levels on liver function tests People with celiac disease have higher risks of iron deficiency and osteoporosis Best tests are transglutaminase IgA, antiendomysial antibodies, and tissue transglutaminase (an enzyme that reacts with gliadin). These are 90% sensitive, and titers indicate degree of damage.
Cross-allergy[3,4]	Arises when foods with similarities to environmental allergens trigger a response Often characterized by oral tingling (oral allergy syndrome)	Examples: Birch, alder, and hazelnut can cross-react with apples, pears, cherries, hazelnuts, walnuts, and pistachios. Grass and cereal pollens can be linked to allergy to wheat, rye, and oat flour as well as to tomato, kiwi, and celery. In people with latex allergies, pineapple, kiwi, avocado, potato, banana, and nuts can cause reactions. Feather allergies can mean allergies to hen's eggs, poultry meat, and giblets. House dust mite allergy can be associated with shellfish allergy.
Pseudoallergies[3,4]	Foods trigger mast cell degranulation without involving IgE antibodies	Examples: Strawberries, chocolate, tomatoes Salicylates (cause cyclooxygenase-1 inhibition, leading to abnormal prostaglandin levels), used as food preservatives Benzoates (preservatives used in fruit drinks, pickled foods, and alcoholic beverages) Tartrazine (yellow #5)
Eosinophilic esophagogastroenteritis[34,36]	Eosinophils accumulate in any or all layers of the digestive tract wall One half to two thirds will have elevated serum eosinophil counts with no other explanation	Affects all ages Diagnosed by endoscopy, colonoscopy; may be related to chronic acid suppression Responds to elimination diets, medication Worth considering in unexplained diarrhea, especially if serum eosinophil counts are inexplicably high
IgG-related intolerance[8,23]	Intolerances slowly develop hours to days after an exposure as IgG is created by the immune system IgG may be the pathogen itself, causing increased small intestinal permeability. IgG half-life is 22 to 96 days, which makes false-positive results possible on testing.	Isolated IgG testing in patients with irritable bowel syndrome is controversial, and no one test is likely to identify all problem foods. Foods that test positive often do not cause symptoms. Tests are not typically covered by insurance. See Table 84-2.

Continued

TABLE 84-1. Differential Diagnosis of Adverse Food Reactions—cont'd

INTOLERANCE CATEGORY	DESCRIPTION	COMMENTS AND CLINICAL TIPS
Physiologic reactions[4]	Foods lead to gas production or cause dyspepsia by relaxing the lower esophageal sphincter	Examples of gas-generating foods include legumes, cabbage, bran, and other vegetables and grains. Heartburn and dyspepsia can result from fatty foods, alcohol, mint, chocolate, and citrus.
Pharmacologic reactions[3,4]	Some foods have drug-like effects. A common example is histaminergic foods, which influence the histamine pathways in the stomach and other GI tract organs. Sulfites, monosodium glutamate (Chinese restaurant syndrome), and biogenic amines may also cause symptoms through drug-like actions.	Histamine intolerance: Is present in 1% of Europeans Is more common in middle-aged women Can be associated with other histamine-caused symptoms, such as nasal congestion, dyspnea, skin reactions, and headache; dysmenorrhea may also occur Leads to opposite effects for histamine-blocking drugs, such as ranitidine
Toxin mediated[3,4]	A specific toxin is present in a food.	Examples include food poisoning, mycotoxins, perhaps herbicides and pesticides.
Enzymatic[37-39]	Deficiency of an enzyme, such as lactase, leads to poor digestion. GI symptoms result. Lactose intolerance arises as cells lose their ability to make lactase. Symptoms occur 30-120 minutes after lactose is consumed. Other sugar intolerances, such as to fructose, sorbitol, mannitol, and xylitol, are less common.	Lactose intolerance: Has lowest prevalence in northern Europeans, highest in Asians, Native Americans, African Americans Is usually not triggered by less than 12 g of lactose (the amount in a cup of milk) Is usually not affected as much by yogurt, especially as it ages Can be triggered by medications; 20% of prescription drugs and 6% of over-the-counter drugs use lactose as a base
Structural[3]	An underlying pathologic process leads to intolerance of different foods	Examples include achalasia, strictures, pancreatitis, inflammatory bowel disease, abdominal angina
Infectious[3]	Chronic infections predispose to adverse food reactions	Examples include lambliasis (*Giardia*), bacterial overgrowth (especially in immunosuppression, diabetes, or the use of proton pump inhibitors), chronic salmonellosis, *Blastocystis* infection, and parasites
Psychogenic[3]	Somatoform disorders, eating disorders, or the discouragement tied to food intolerance itself may lead to food reactions. Note that high norepinephrine levels can trigger histamine release, so stress can cause intolerances through some of the mechanisms listed above as well.	It is not uncommon in integrative practice to see individuals who become obsessed with their diets. This "orthorexia" can become a pathologic process unto itself. Treatment involves working closely with a nutritionist, adding mental health and mind-body approaches to care, and helping them slowly regain their ability to enjoy eating.
Other causes[3]	Mastocytosis, carcinoid and other neuroendocrine tumors, and GI neoplasms may also lead to symptoms.	As always, a careful history and differential diagnosis are mandatory.

GI, gastrointestinal; Ig, immunoglobulin.

unable to cross through the intestinal tract into the bloodstream become capable of doing so. Molecules that would normally be too large to pass from the gut into the bloodstream are suddenly able to move in, eliciting any number of negative physiologic effects.[7,8] Permeability seems to be increased by a number of factors, including inflammation, exposure to medications (e.g., nonsteroidal antiinflammatory drugs), shifts in intestinal microflora, and the presence of various disease states, such as celiac disease and ulcerative colitis.[9] Leaky gut is known to be increased with radiation therapy,[10] in patients with intermittent claudication,[11] and in people with multiple sclerosis.[12] Its presence has been correlated with higher risk of cirrhosis in people with chronic alcoholism.[13] Studies have shown that children with autism have increased urinary peptides, indicating that their intestines may be more permeable to amino acids that may cross the blood-brain barrier and have harmful effects.[14]

It has been proposed that many cases of food intolerance may be tied to the overall process of toxicant-induced loss

TABLE 84-2. Laboratories Offering Testing for Delayed Hypersensitivity Reactions

Memory Antibodies ELISA testing is used to determine presence of immunoglobulins, usually IgG and IgE	Alletess Medical Laboratories, Rockland, MA: www.foodallergy.com Genova Diagnostics, Asheville, NC: www.genovadiagnostics.com Great Plains Laboratories, Lexana, KS: www.greatplainslaboratory.com Immuno Laboratories, Fort Lauderdale, FL: www.immunolabs.com Metametrix Clinical Laboratory, Duluth, GA: www.metametrix.com Meridian Valley Laboratories, Renton, WA: www.meridianvalleylab.com US Biotek Laboratories, Seattle, WA: www.usbiotek.com
Automated Cytotoxic Assay Measures difference between normal white cell sizes and changes in overall cell size in response to exposure to various food antigens Has been criticized as not differentiating between "protective" and "activating" (pathologic) responses	ALCAT (Antigen Leukocyte Cellular Antibody Test) Cell Science Systems, Deerfield Beach, FL: www.alcat.com NuTron/NOVO testing, Immogenics, London, UK: www.immogenics.com MRT/LEAP Testing (Mediator Release Testing/Lifestyle Eating and Performance), Forrest Health, Riviera Beach, FL: www.forresthealth.com/leap-mrt-food-allergy-test.html
Lymphocyte Cell Culture Claims to use functional assays to determine if immunoglobulins are present and if they trigger reactivity through the complement cascade and other means Evaluates for presence of immunoglobulins as well as type II (immune complex) and type IV (cell activation) immune responses	Elisa-Act Biotechnologies, Sterling, VA: www.elisaact.com
Complement Activation Includes assays for both IgG and circulating immune complexes (type III immune responses)	Complement testing, Sage Medical Lab, Ormond Beach, FL: www.sagemedlab.com

Note that the utility of these tests in clinical management of food intolerance remains controversial.
Based on a table available in Mullin GE, Swift KM, Lipski L. Testing for food reactions: the good, the bad, and the ugly. *Nutr Clin Pract.* 2010;25:192–198.

of tolerance, which is thought to be precipitated not only by foods but by inhalants, chemical exposures, and electrical stimuli.[15] As such, any steps that may reduce overall sensitivity may be helpful with food intolerances. Examples include exercise, minimizing body inflammation, desensitization, and detoxification regimens. It may be helpful to explore whether an individual with food intolerances is also "reactive" in other ways, physically and emotionally, to his or her environment.

Diagnosis of Adverse Food Reactions

For food allergies, a number of tests can be considered, although they may not be easily performed in a primary care setting. Testing can begin with skin prick testing and checking for specific serum immunoglobulin (Ig) E panels.[16] Double-blind, placebo-controlled food challenges, which are considered the "gold standard" for food allergy diagnosis, may be obtained.[17,18] However, this challenge may require intravenous access, and the food products and placebos can be difficult to prepare or mask. Only 30% of positive open food challenge results correlate with positive blinded challenge results, suggesting that adverse food reactions are strongly influenced by mind-body interactions.[19] Radioallergosorbent testing is thought by some to be helpful to assess for the presence of food allergies.[20] Interestingly, one trial found that diet history and skin prick testing seemed to correlate well in predicting food allergies,

but skin prick testing, antibody measurements, and double-blind placebo-controlled food challenges did not correlate well with one another.[21]

Laboratory testing for nonallergy forms of food intolerance is more controversial. IgG testing has demonstrated some utility in the management of irritable bowel syndrome. In one study, tailoring of the diet to IgG-based testing led to a 26% overall decrease in symptoms in the treatment group.[22] Table 84-2 lists a number of private laboratories that offer various forms of testing. Note that how best to apply test results in clinical practice remains controversial, and further research is needed. Other unproven forms of food intolerance testing are listed in Table 84-3. For a detailed, evidence-based review of approaches to food intolerance testing, see Mullin et al.[23]

> Aside from certain tests for IgE-mediated food allergies, most tests for adverse food reactions remain controversial. Remember that an elimination diet can serve, in and of itself, as a useful diagnostic tool.

The Elimination Diet for Treatment of Various Disorders

A number of disorders are known to be influenced by food. Examples include celiac disease, lactose intolerance, gastroesophageal reflux disease (see Chapter 41), cholelithiasis

TABLE 84-3. Unproven Diagnostic Approaches for Investigating Food Intolerance[16,40]

TEST	DESCRIPTION
Hair analysis	Levels of various compounds are measured in a hair sample. There is no evidence that hair levels accurately reflect body toxin levels
Iridology	Holds that there are correlations between iris patterns and pathologic changes throughout the body
Cytotoxic testing	Seeks alterations or death of white cells in vitro when an allergen is introduced to a blood sample
Applied kinesiology/DRIA	The subject holds an allergen in a container in one hand while an investigator gauges its relative effect on the strength of a given muscle group. In the DRIA test, the substance is put under the tongue rather than held.
Electrodermal testing	A galvanometer is used to measure skin conduction as a person holds two electrodes. Introduction of a poorly tolerated food extract into the circuit is said to cause a drop in conductivity of the skin.
Provocation/ neutralization	A small quantity of food extract is placed under the tongue, watching for symptoms thereafter. If symptoms arise, a more dilute solution is placed under the tongue, with the expectation that symptoms will disappear.

TABLE 84-4. Conditions for Which Elimination Diets Might Be Used[1]

Cardiovascular	Palpitations Tachycardia
Dermatologic	Angioedema* Atopic dermatitis* Contact dermatitis Dermatitis herpetiformis Pruritus* Seborrheic dermatitis Urticaria*,[41]
Gastrointestinal	Bloating, belching Celiac disease*,[34] Cholecystitis, cholelithiasis*,[42] Chronic diarrhea*,[43] Colic[44] Constipation, including laxative resistant in children[45] Cyclic vomiting syndrome*,[46] Encopresis[47] Eosinophilic esophagitis*,[5] Eosinophilic gastroenteritis*,[48] Gastroesophageal reflux*,[49] Irritable bowel syndrome* Inflammatory bowel disease*,[50-53] Nausea, vomiting Pruritus ani[54] Recurrent abdominal pain in children with confirmed allergy*,[55]
Genitourinary	Enuresis*,[31,56] Frequency Interstitial cystitis Vulvodynia
Neurologic/ psychological	Attention deficit hyperactivity disorder* Autistic spectrum disorders* Medication-resistant depression Migraine* Other types of headache Seizures (by ketogenic diets)*,[57]
Respiratory/ otolaryngologic	Aphthous ulcers (recurrent)[58] Asthma*,[59-61] Chronic congestion, rhinitis*,[62] Chronic serous otitis* Conjunctivitis Laryngeal edema, hoarseness
Rheumatologic	Chronic fatigue[63,64] Rheumatoid arthritis* Systemic lupus erythematosus[65] Vasculitis
Miscellaneous	Listlessness, poor concentration Irritability Cold intolerance, low-grade fever Dizziness Excess sweating Pallor

*Indicates that at least level B evidence (SORT criteria) exists for treatment of this condition with an elimination diet.

(see Chapter 43), urolithiasis (see Chapter 58), and gout (see Chapter 65). For other disorders, the relationship between foods eaten and symptoms is less clear. Table 84-4 lists a number of disorders for which treatment by use of elimination diets has been suggested. Table 84-5 summarizes the research findings for some of the most-studied conditions commonly treated by elimination diets and lists foods that are eliminated for each.

Prescribing an Elimination Diet

An elimination diet is, put simply, an eating plan that omits a food or group of foods believed to cause an adverse food reaction. Elimination diets can serve as both diagnostic and treatment strategies in an integrative setting. In general, four principal steps are followed in prescribing any elimination diet.

Step 1: The Planning Phase

Before recommending an elimination diet, the clinician must take a thorough patient history. Ideally, patients should provide a recent dietary log that chronicles what they ate during the course of a few weeks. They should note what symptoms they experience and when they arise relative to mealtimes and time of day. Symptoms might range from gastrointestinal complaints and skin changes to low mood, fatigue, or difficulty with concentration. Table 84-6 lists key issues to address in taking the history of a patient for whom an adverse food reaction is suspected. A sample 1-week dietary log form is included in the Patient Handout.

After a list of potential problem foods is elicited, the next step is to create a list of foods to avoid. The list should be individualized as much as possible for each patient. Table 84-7 lists

TABLE 84-5. Foods to Eliminate for Specific Disorders and Synopsis of Key Research

CONDITION	FOODS TO ELIMINATE*	RESEARCH SUMMARY
Attention deficit hyperactivity disorder (ADHD)[1,66]	Apples, artificial colors, aspartame (NutraSweet), butylated hydroxyanisole, butylated hydroxytoluene (in packaged cereals), benzoates (chewing gum, margarine, pickles, prunes, tea, raspberries, cinnamon, anise, nutmeg), caffeine, corn, dairy products, nitrates and nitrites (preserved meats like bacon, frankfurters, pepperoni), oranges, propyl gallate, sulfites (dried fruits, mushrooms, potatoes, baked good, canned fish, pickles, relishes), peanuts, tomatoes	Began with Feingold diet in 1975 but lost favor when research did not show benefit Food additives such as tartrazine (yellow dye #5), benzoates, and glutamate are known to affect the nervous system, but sugar does not seem to have an effect. A 2010 review concluded that no dietary interventions are helpful with ADHD, except that a small subset of children may benefit from removal of artificial food colors.[67] A 2008 review found moderately good evidence of effect for removal of food additives.[68]
Atopic dermatitis[1,68,69]	*Children:* dairy, eggs, soy, wheat *Adults:* pollen-related foods (fruit, nuts, vegetables) Other considerations would be artificial colors, benzoates, berries, citrus, currants, fish, legumes, sulfites, tomatoes, and occasionally beef, chicken, and pork.	Evidence of an effect of mother's diet when pregnant or breast-feeding is less clear,[70] but breast-feeding itself is preventive.[71] No other dietary interventions were conclusively found to affect atopy in children. A Korean study divided 524 patients into four groups for interferon-gamma treatment, elimination diet, or both. The elimination diet–only group had the most significant decrease in symptom severity.[72] A 1991 study found improvement in 49 of 66 children with eczema, which recurred when cow's milk and tomato were added back.[73] A 1987 study found that 37 of 101 people with eczema reacted to one or more food additives, with 16 reacting to the placebo. Only one third of the subjects had reproducibility on repeated testing.[74]
Autistic spectrum disorders[4,30,75,76]	Gluten and casein (gluten-free, casein-free [GFCF] diet), food additives, and artificial colors	Significant numbers of autistic children have relatively high titers of antibodies (IgA, IgG, and IgE) to gluten and casein.[75,76] A 2008 review noted that GFCF diets are "promising" but that current evidence is not conclusive.[30] A 2008 Cochrane review concluded that the current quality of evidence regarding the effect of the GFCF diet is poor.[77] GFCF diets decrease urine peptides, perhaps indicating improved intestinal permeability (after 1 year)[78]
Irritable bowel syndrome (IBS)[1,8,79]	Dairy, eggs, wheat Some diets become elaborate, focusing on which starches should and should not be consumed. See reference 1 for a comprehensive IBS diet.	>60% of IBS sufferers think that specific foods contribute to their symptoms,[28] and 50% report that their symptoms arise after eating.[80] A 2010 review found that insufficient data exist to make recommendations about elimination diets and IBS.[81] A 2005 review concluded that "dietary manipulation may result in substantial improvement in IBS symptomatology provided it is individualized to the particular patient."[28] Many IBS sufferers have changes in motility even with the sight or smell of food, which complicates diagnosis.[28] A 1998 review[82] showed a 15%-71% response rate when study data were pooled for IBS and elimination diets. Rule out lactose intolerance in IBS patients.[83]
Migraine[1,7,60,84,85]	Aspartame, beef, chocolate, coffee, corn, eggs, histamine (fish, cheese, wine, beer), monosodium glutamate (mushrooms, kelp, scallops, preserved meats, Chinese food), nitrates (processed meats), oranges, sugar, tea, tyramine (aged cheeses, some red wines), yeast See also www.fammed.wisc.edu/integrative/modules/headaches for an online "Headache Elimination Diet" handout	A 2009 review concluded that individualized elimination diets for migraine are a useful therapeutic approach.[86] One study found that 29 of 55 patients had complete symptom resolution with elimination diets, and another 21 experienced improvement[87] A 1979 study found that 85% of a group of 60 became headache free after following a 5-day elimination of an average of 10 different foods. The total number of headaches/month fell from an average of 402 to 6.[88] In a blinded study of aspartame (NutraSweet) compared with placebo, there was a 100% increase in headache frequency during the aspartame consumption phase of the trial.[89] More than 90% of a group of 88 children with severe migraine symptoms had response to a food elimination diet.[90]

Continued

TABLE 84-5. Foods to Eliminate for Specific Disorders and Synopsis of Key Research—cont'd

CONDITION	FOODS TO ELIMINATE*	RESEARCH SUMMARY
Serous otitis media	See the Level 2 diet in the Patient Handout. Consider removal of dairy foods.	70 of 81 children (aged 1 to 9 years) with documented food allergies had improved tympanometry findings after a 16-week individualized elimination diet.[91] A 1997 trial found a 70% to 83% improvement in symptoms of fullness, allergic symptoms, and overall well-being in 151 people with eustachian tube dysfunction and noted to have allergic symptoms.[92] A number of integrative clinicians link dairy and other foods to chronic ear and sinus congestion, and an elimination diet is worth considering in patients with these problems.[93]
Rheumatoid arthritis (RA)	Consider the few foods listed in the Patient Handout. Corn, dairy, and nightshade vegetables (bell peppers, eggplant, potatoes, tomatoes) are worth considering.	Interest arose in 1981 when the media described a woman with RA whose 25 years of symptoms resolved with corn elimination.[94] In the 1960s, the nightshade diet, which eliminates eggplant, bell peppers, potatoes, and tomatoes, became popular. There is limited evidence to support the effect of nightshades on RA. A 2009 Cochrane review concluded, "The effects of dietary manipulation, including vegetarian, Mediterranean, elemental and elimination diets, on rheumatoid arthritis are still uncertain due to the included studies being small, single trials with moderate to high risk of bias."[95] One small study of 70 people with RA observed that 19% were able to stay well without medications for 1 to 5 years after elimination of particular foods.[96]

*Other foods may also be implicated. It is important to tailor therapy to the individual.

TABLE 84-6. Points to Consider Before Prescribing an Elimination Diet

Several key questions may reveal which foods should be removed[77]	What foods do you frequently eat? What foods do you crave? What foods make you feel better? What foods would be difficult to give up or go without?
A history should cover several specific topics[1,97,98]	Family history of food intolerance, irritable bowel, headache, and mouth ulcers Past medical history of respiratory allergies, chronic upper respiratory congestion, asthma, atopic dermatitis, infant colic, gastrointestinal problems (including lactose intolerance or celiac disease), or unusual reactions to medications or foods History of eating disorders (to avoid risk that an elimination diet may exacerbate these conditions) History of food allergies Previous laboratory test findings (e.g., results of skin prick testing) Relation of symptoms to exercise (some intolerances are exacerbated with increased activity) Relation of symptoms to substance use, including smoking, alcohol,* caffeine, and illicit drugs Life stressors

*Some clinicians have noted that the development of food intolerance in some patients is preceded by changes in alcohol tolerance. Patients may first note an intolerance to red wine and beer and later an inability to drink white wine and spirits.[99] Ultimately, intolerance to other food items is noted.

TABLE 84-7. Common Food Culprits for Food Allergy and Food Intolerance[1,5]

Food allergy*	Citrus Dairy products Eggs Fish Peanuts Soy Gluten (barley, oats, rye, wheat) Shellfish Tree nuts (almonds, pecans, walnuts)

Food intolerance	All of the foods listed for food allergy, plus:
	Beef products
	Corn
	Food additives, including
	    Antioxidants (butylated hydroxyanisole, butylated hydroxytoluene)
	    Aspartame (NutraSweet, an artificial sweetener)
	    Flavor enhancers (monosodium glutamate)
	    Food colors (tartrazine and various other Food Dye and Coloring Act [FD&C] dyes, which are derived from coal tar)
	    Nitrates and nitrites (found in preserved meats)
	    Preservatives (sulfites, benzoates, and sorbates)
	    Thickeners/stabilizers (tragacanth, agar-agar)
	Biogenic amines (histamine, tyramine, octopamine, phenylethylamine)
	Disaccharides (lactose)
	Foods high in nickel and salicylates (see reference 1 for a complete listing)
	Refined sugars

*These foods account for roughly 80% of all food hypersensitivity reactions.

the foods most likely to cause adverse food reactions; Table 84-5 lists foods linked to symptoms in various disease states.

> Patients often have a sense of which foods are most likely to contribute to their symptoms. The clinician should be sure to explore this issue with them. Trust their "gut feelings." Remember that comfort foods and foods that are often craved can be important culprits.

Step 2: The Avoidance Phase

Elimination diets vary in terms of intensity.[1,24] The type of diet chosen varies according to the number of suspected food culprits, the likelihood of patient compliance, and the potential effects of the diet on the patient's nutritional status. Patient compliance decreases as diets become more restrictive. The Patient Handout provides examples of three elimination diets of variable intensity.

The lowest intensity elimination diets are referred to as food-specific diets. In these, just one food or group of foods is removed. Which food or foods are to be removed is often determined on the basis of both the patients' suspicions and their responses to the questions listed in Table 84-6. For some patients, particularly those for whom maintaining healthy nutrition may be a challenge, it is most appropriate to pursue several low-intensity elimination diets, one after another, rather than to remove multiple foods or food groups simultaneously. However, some individuals display intolerance to combinations of foods or food groups; for them, a low-intensity elimination diet may not prove as useful as one in which multiple food groups are removed simultaneously.

In a moderate-intensity elimination diet, multiple foods or food groups are eliminated. However, if successfully done, moderate-intensity diets have the potential to serve as useful diagnostic and therapeutic tools. The list of foods eliminated is tailored to the individual patient; disease-specific elimination diets, such as those listed in Table 84-5, are available in the reference materials listed at the end of this chapter. Because moderate-intensity elimination diets are more likely than food-specific elimination diets to lead to symptom resolution, they are popular with many integrative clinicians.

Finally, a high-intensity or "few-foods" diet may be considered. In this diet, only the foods on a specific list may be eaten. Higher levels of supervision are necessary with this type of diet to ensure that nutritional needs are met.[1] The Patient Handout contains an example of this diet as well.

The Patient Handout also provides a table of common "foods in disguise." When a specific group of foods is eliminated, some common ingredients that may cause adverse food reactions must also be eliminated. For example, if a patient is to successfully perform a dairy elimination diet, he or she must also avoid anything containing whey, caramel, casein, and semisweet chocolate.

Patients should follow an elimination diet for at least 10 days; some sources suggest 2 to 4 weeks.[1,16] It is hypothesized that symptoms caused by food intolerance may not arise until a few days after the food has been eaten, so it is important to give the food-related symptoms time to "wear off" before the foods are reintroduced. A study performed in 2000 found that in children with cow's milk allergy, there was a delay of 3

to 13 days between exposure to milk proteins and the onset of clinical reactions, lending support to this "rule of thumb."[25]

> Patients should be warned that with the elimination diet, it is not uncommon for symptoms to worsen before they begin to improve.

Step 3: The Challenge Phase

If symptoms decrease during the avoidance phase, it is likely that the food or foods that were eliminated were in fact contributing to the symptoms. However, symptoms of many chronic conditions relapse and remit spontaneously, so it is important to reintroduce eliminated foods or food groups after symptoms are gone to see whether they recur. Because symptoms may take a few days to reappear, foods should be introduced back into the diet only every 3 or 4 days. It is best for a patient to use a small quantity of the reintroduced food at first, then to have a larger serving at subsequent meals on the same day (assuming no untoward effects are experienced with the first serving). In addition to chronic symptoms they have had previously, food-intolerant patients who reintroduce foods may experience lung congestion, increased mucus production, fatigue, concentration difficulties, digestive problems, constipation and diarrhea, bloating, fluid accumulation, mood swings, and drowsiness.[1,26]

During reintroduction, a previously eliminated food is eaten for only 1 day. It is then eliminated again if other foods have also been eliminated and need to be reintroduced. The Patient Handout contains a sample schedule for the elimination and reintroduction of foods in a moderate-intensity elimination diet.

Improvements in symptoms are readily apparent to the patient when they occur during an elimination diet. In fact, many patients are reluctant to attempt the challenge phase because their symptoms have improved so markedly.

Step 4: Creating a Long-Term Diet Plan

Once the initial three phases of the elimination diet are completed, long-term diet planning is necessary. Additional elimination diets may be needed at some point if symptoms are either unchanged or not fully resolved. Many recommendations exist regarding how long a food causing adverse reactions should be avoided. A reasonable approach is to continue the elimination for at least 3 to 6 months. After that, another challenge with the eliminated food or foods may be attempted. There is some evidence that when a food is reintroduced after a lengthy period, a food intolerance may no longer be found. In a study of 10 patients who had chronic urticaria or perennial rhinitis, 38% found their different food intolerances to be resolved at retesting a year or more after the initial evaluation.[27]

Risks of Elimination Diets

Although elimination diets are generally safe, particularly under the supervision of a health care professional, a few potential risks must be acknowledged, as follows:

- Elimination diets might activate "latent" eating disorders. The clinician should screen patients for anorexia and bulimia nervosa before initiating an elimination diet. Patients with irritable bowel syndrome may be especially vulnerable.[28]

- A food or food group that has led to an anaphylactic reaction should *never* be reintroduced without appropriate supervision by an allergist. In one small study, seven children with fish allergy eliminated it from there diets. When it was reintroduced, their hypersensitivity was more florid.[29]

- Malnutrition is a risk if a large number of food groups are eliminated. The clinician must ensure that dieters receive adequate fiber, nutrients (including vitamin D and calcium when dairy is restricted), and protein. Patients on gluten elimination diets often become deficient in zinc, selenium, copper, B_6, and B_{12} over time; gluten-free grains lack vitamins B_1, B_2, and B_3 as well as folate and iron. Special caution should be used in the treatment of autistic children, given that they tend to be limited in their diets at baseline.[30]

- The clinician must keep in mind the socioeconomic implications of prescribing an elimination diet: cost can become prohibitive—for example, various alternatives to gluten-containing grains can be costly or difficult to obtain; and patients following elimination diets have limited ability to eat at restaurants or other people's homes unless their dietary restrictions are clearly understood by those preparing their meals.[31]

- Enjoyment of eating, an important aspect of general health, may be diminished.

- A fear of food may be created. Some patients have significant symptom improvement with removal of a food. This success can lead to inappropriate association of symptoms with other foods that can snowball toward malnutrition. The goal should be temporary removal of a food, repair of the gastrointestinal ecosystem, and slow reintroduction of the food in the future if possible for non-IgE food intolerances.

- The likelihood of patient noncompliance with the diet must always be kept in mind; this can often be quite high, especially for diets prescribed for children.

> The clinician must be mindful of the potential pitfalls of prescribing elimination diets. Patient compliance, nutritional status, and the psychosocial impacts of such a diet must be given consideration. When judiciously used, elimination diets are associated with minimal risk.

References

References are available at expertconsult.com.

Patient Handout: Using an Elimination Diet

An elimination diet can be used to determine whether or not certain foods are contributing to your symptoms. If they are, the diet can also be used as a form of treatment.
There are four main steps to an elimination diet:

Step I: Planning
This step involves working with your provider to make a list of foods that might be causing problems. You may be asked to keep a diet journal for a week, listing the foods you eat and when you have symptoms. To decide what foods might be causing problems, ask yourself these questions:
   • What foods do I eat most often?
   • What foods do I crave?
   • What foods do I eat to "feel better" (comfort foods)?
   • What foods would be hard for me to stop eating?
The answers are foods you should try to eliminate. Other common problematic foods are listed below.

Step II: Avoiding the Foods on Your List
After you have made a list of foods to avoid, you start the elimination diet. You should stop eating the foods on your list for two weeks. If you make a mistake and eat something on the list, you should start over. The foods on the list should be avoided in their whole form and also when they are ingredients in other foods. For example, if you are avoiding all dairy products, you need to check labels for whey, casein, and lactose so you can avoid them as well. Elimination diets take a lot of willpower. You must pay close attention to food labels, and be careful if you are eating out, since you may not know all the ingredients of the foods you eat.

Many people notice that in the first week, especially in the first few days, their symptoms get worse before they get better. If your symptoms become severe or increase for more than a day or two, consult your healthcare provider.

Step III: Add the Foods Back
If your symptoms have not improved in two weeks, you will need to stop the diet and decide whether or not to try it again with a different list of foods. If you feel better after eliminating the foods, the next step is to see if your symptoms come back when you start eating the foods again. As you do this, keep a written record of your symptoms.

A new food or food group should be added every three days. It takes three days to see if your symptoms come back if they are going to. On the day you introduce an eliminated food back into your diet for the first time, start with just a small amount in the morning. If you don't notice any symptoms, eat a larger portion at lunch and dinner. After a day of eating the new food, wait for two days to see if you notice the symptoms. Then add back another eliminated food or food group. Follow the pattern until all foods are added back. If a food doesn't cause symptoms during a challenge, it is unlikely to be a problem food and can be added back into your diet for good. However, don't add the food back until you have tested ALL the other foods on your list.

Step IV: Create Your New, Long-Term Diet
Based on your results, you can plan how to change what you eat so that you'll be most likely to prevent your symptoms. Remember:
   • Some people have problems with more than one food.
   • Sometimes symptoms come and go for other reasons besides what foods we eat, so it can be confusing to tell for certain if a specific food is the cause.
   • Be sure that you are getting adequate nutrition during the elimination diet and as you change your diet for the long-term. For example, if you give up dairy, you must get calcium from other sources.
   • You may need to try several different elimination diets before you identify problematic foods.
   • If a food causes you to have an immediate allergic reaction, or causes you to have throat swelling, a severe rash, or other severe allergy symptoms, it is important to seek the care of an allergist before re-introducing foods that cause problems.

The elimination diet is not a perfect test. A lot of other factors could interfere with the results. Try and keep everything else (the other foods you eat, your stress level, etc.) as constant as possible while you are on the diet.

The Three Levels of Elimination Diets

Level 1: The Simple Diet
Eliminates milk, eggs, and wheat

	FOODS ALLOWED	FOODS ELIMINATED
Animal proteins	Beef, chicken, lamb, pork, turkey	Dairy products Chicken eggs
Grains and starches	Arrowroot, barley, buckwheat, corn, millet, oats, rice, rye, sweet potato, tapioca, white potatoes, yams	Wheat
Oils	Any non-dairy oils	Dairy-based butter and margarines
All fruits, vegetables, salt, spices, sweeteners, and vegetable proteins are allowed.		

Continued

Level 2: The Stricter Diet
The stricter diet eliminates several foods at once.

	FOODS ALLOWED	FOODS ELIMINATED
Animal proteins	Lamb	All others, including eggs and milk
Vegetable proteins	None	Beans, bean sprouts, lentils, peanuts, peas, soy, all other nuts
Grains and starches	Arrowroot, buckwheat, corn, rice, sweet potato, tapioca, white potato, yams	Barley, millet, oats, rye, wheat
Vegetables	Most allowed	Peas, tomatoes
Fruits	Most allowed	No citrus or strawberries
Sweeteners	Cane or beet sugar, maple syrup, corn syrup	Any others, including aspartame
Oils	Coconut, olive, safflower, sesame	Animal fats (lard), butter, corn, margarine, shortening, soy, peanut, other vegetable oils
Other	Salt, pepper, a minimal number of spices, vanilla, lemon extract	Chocolate, coffee, tea, colas and other soft drinks, alcohol

Level 3: A Few-Foods Diet
Only the foods listed below can be eaten. **All others** are avoided.
- Apples (juice okay)
- Apricots
- Asparagus
- Beets
- Cane or beet sugar
- Carrots
- Chicken
- Cranberries
- Honey
- Lamb
- Lettuce
- Olive oil
- Peaches
- Pears
- Pineapple
- Rice (including rice cakes and cereal)
- Safflower oil
- Salt
- Sweet potatoes
- White vinegar

Modified from Mahan LK, Escot-Stump S: *Krause's Food Nutrition and Diet Therapy*. 11th ed. Philadelphia: Saunders; 2004.

A Sample Elimination Diet Calendar

Day Number	Step
1	Begin Elimination Diet
2–7	You may notice symptoms worsen for a day or two
8–14	Symptoms should go away if the right foods have been removed
15	Re-introduce food #1 (for example, dairy)
16–17	Stop food #1 and watch for symptoms*
18	Re-introduce food #2 (for example, wheat)
19–20	Stop food #2 again and watch for symptoms
21	Re-introduce food #3
	...And so on, until all eliminated foods have been re-introduced

*You only re-introduce a new food for one day. Until the diet is over, it is not added back into the diet again.

Some Helpful Tips:
A number of foods can be 'disguised' when you look at food labels.

If You Are Avoiding	Also Avoid
Dairy	Caramel candy, carob candies, casein and caseinates, custard, curds, lactalbumin, goat's milk, milk chocolate, nougat, protein hydrolysate, semisweet chocolate, yogurt, pudding, whey. Also beware of brown sugar flavoring, butter flavoring, caramel flavoring, coconut cream flavoring, "natural flavoring," and Simplesse.
Peanuts	Egg rolls, "high-protein food," hydrolyzed plant protein, hydrolyzed vegetable protein, marzipan, nougat, candy, cheesecake crusts, chili, chocolates, pet feed, sauces.
Egg	Albumin, apovitellin, avidin, béarnaise sauce, eggnog, egg whites, flavoprotein, globulin, hollandaise sauce, imitation egg products, livetin, lysozyme, mayonnaise, meringue, ovalbumin, ovoglycoprotein, ovomucin, ovomucoid, ovomuxoid, Simplesse.
Soy	Chee-fan, ketjap, metiauza, miso, natto, soy flour, soy protein concentrates, soy protein shakes, soy sauce, soybean hydrolysates, soby sprouts, sufu, tao-cho, tao-si, taotjo, tempeh, textured soy protein, textured vegetable protein, tofu, whey-soy drink. Also beware of hydrolyzed plant protein, hydrolyzed soy protein, hydrolyzed vegetable protein, natural flavoring, vegetable broth, vegetable gum, vegetable starch.
Wheat	Atta, bal ahar, bread flour, bulgar, cake flour, cereal extract, couscous, cracked wheat, durum flour, farina, gluten, graham flour, high-gluten flour, high-protein flour, kamut flour, laubina, leche alim, malted cereals, minchin, multi-grain products, puffed wheat, red wheat flakes, rolled wheat, semolina, shredded wheat, soft wheat flour, spelt, superamine, triticale, vital gluten, vitalia macaroni, wheat protein powder, wheat starch, wheat tempeh, white flour, whole-wheat berries. Also beware of gelatinized starch, hydrolyzed vegetable protein, modified food starch, starch, vegetable gum, vegetable starch.

Data from Joneja JV. Dietary Management of Food Allergy and Intolerance. 2nd ed. Vancouver, BC: Hall Publishing Group, 1998; and Mahan LK, Escot-Stump S: *Krause's Food Nutrition and Diet Therapy*. 11th ed. Philadelphia: Saunders; 2004.

A One-Week Food Diary Chart
(Log in foods eaten and times. Note the symptoms you have and what times as well)

	Morning Foods	Morning Symptoms	Afternoon Foods	Afternoon Symptoms	Evening Foods	Evening Symptoms
Day 1						
Day 2						
Day 3						
Day 4						
Day 5						
Day 6						
Day 7						

Chapter 85

The Glycemic Index/Load

Sarah K. Khan, RD, MPH, PhD

At present, the American Diabetes Association (ADA)[1] does not recognize a role for the glycemic index in the prevention of disease. On the basis of its review, diets with a low glycemic index may reduce postprandial glycemia but may be difficult to maintain long term. The ADA holds that additional evidence to support the glycemic and lipid benefits of low–glycemic index diets is needed.[1,2] Data from a later review of the literature, however, suggest that glycemic index information should be incorporated into exchanges and teaching materials[3] specifically for disease prevention of diabetes, cardiovascular disease, inflammation, and, possibly, some cancers. In this chapter, the definitions of glycemic index and glycemic load are reviewed, and studies demonstrating their possible use in disease prevention are provided.

Glycemic Index

The glycemic index (GI) has proved to be a useful nutritional concept—the chemical classification of carbohydrate (simple or complex, sugars or starches, available or unavailable)—that fosters new insights into the relationship between the physiologic effects of carbohydrate-rich foods and health.[4] The GI measures how quickly a consumed carbohydrate affects postprandial serum glucose levels in a specified time. By definition, the GI compares equal quantities of available carbohydrate in foods and provides a measure of carbohydrate quality. Available carbohydrates can be calculated by summing the quantity of available sugars, starch, oligosaccharides, and maltodextrins.[5] In effect, the GI is an indicator of the relative glycemic response to dietary carbohydrates. Glucose and white bread are often used as the "gold standard" because they cause the fastest and most dramatic rise in glucose levels. In the evaluation of individual foods, either glucose or white bread is assigned a value of 100, the highest index possible. All other foods are then assigned proportionately lower values on the basis of how they affect serum glucose levels in comparison with glucose or white bread.[6] The GI is now widely recognized as a reliable, physiologically based classification of foods according to their postprandial

glycemic effects.[4] For example, in healthy individuals, stepwise increases in GI have been shown to predict stepwise elevations in postprandial blood glucose and insulin levels (Fig. 85-1).[5,7]

> The GI measures how quickly a consumed carbohydrate affects postprandial serum glucose levels in a specified time.

Glycemic Load

To provide a more accurate description of the quantity and quality of carbohydrate in a meal simultaneously, researchers developed the concept of the glycemic load (GL), which takes the concept of GI a step further, accounting not only for how rapidly a food's carbohydrates are converted to glucose but also the relative amounts of carbohydrate the food contains in an average serving. GL is generally held to be a more accurate measure of a food's overall effect on pancreatic insulin release and serum glucose levels. The GL of a food is calculated by multiplying the GI value by the amount of carbohydrates in grams provided by a serving of food and dividing the total by 100.[5] Therefore, the GL provides a summary measure of the relative glycemic impact of a "typical" serving of the food. In general, items with a low GI tend to have a correspondingly low GL. However, foods with a high GI may vary as to whether their GL is low or high. For example, the carbohydrates in watermelon are rapidly converted to glucose, so watermelon's GI is high at 72. However, because watermelon is made up primarily of water and contains little absolute carbohydrate content, its GL is relatively low at a value of 4.[4]

Several prospective observational studies have documented an independent association between a long-term consumption of a diet with a high GL and a higher risk for development of type 2 diabetes mellitus, cardiovascular disease, and certain cancers.[4] In another study, implementation of a low-GL diet was associated with substantial and sustained improvements in abdominal obesity, cholesterol concentration, and glycemic control.[8] A low-GL diet has been associated with more weight loss in young adults who are insulin resistant.[9] Use of GL to guide dietary choices has been found to have several benefits. High-GL foods can often lead to rapid release of large amounts of insulin, which can ultimately cause blood glucose levels to fall below fasting levels a few hours after eating. This rebound hypoglycemia can be characterized by fatigue, which decreases substantially when high-GL foods are removed from the diet. Interestingly, a low-GI meal leads to a lower glycemic response to subsequent meals as well.[10] On average, people who eat low-GL diets tend to eat smaller meals; their food cravings diminish. Diets of predominantly high-GI foods have been associated with a higher risk of insulin resistance syndrome and type 2 diabetes mellitus (Tables 85-1 and 85-2).[11]

FIGURE 85-1

Mean incremental blood glucose responses in healthy subjects 65 to 70 years of age. (Modified from Bjorck I, Granfeldt Y, Liljeberg H, et al. Food properties affecting the digestion and absorption of carbohydrates. *Am J Clin Nutr.* 59[suppl]:699S–705S, 1994.)

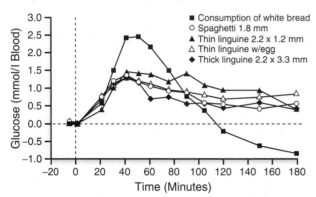

TABLE 85-1. Food Rating Values for Glycemic Index and Glycemic Load

VALUE	GLYCEMIC INDEX	GLYCEMIC LOAD
High	>70	>20
Medium	56-69	11-19
Low	<55	<10

TABLE 85-2. Calculating the Difference Between Glycemic Index and Glycemic Load

Example: Watermelon
Glycemic index: 72 (high)
Glycemic load: 4 (low)
Amount of carbohydrate per serving: 6 g (low)

Calculating Glycemic Load (GL)
GL = (Glycemic index)/100 × (carbohydrates per serving in grams)
or
72/100 (0.72) × 6 = 4

Note: Although the glycemic index of the sugar in watermelon is high, most of watermelon is water and the amount of carbohydrate per serving size is low (6 g), which results in a low glycemic load.

Disease Prevention

Diabetes

In sedentary middle-aged men with one or more traditional cardiac risk factors, a high-GI, high-carbohydrate diet was associated with the least favorable postprandial profile, whereas the low-GI, high-carbohydrate diet had the most favorable profile.[12] In another study, 4 weeks of a low-GI diet was shown to improve glycemic control, glucose use, some lipid profiles, and the capacity for fibrinolysis in type 2 diabetes mellitus.[13] Results of a 2004 meta-analysis support the use of the GI as a scientifically based tool to enable selection of carbohydrate-containing foods to reduce total cholesterol levels and to improve overall metabolic control of diabetes.[14]

In summary, a low-GI diet has been found to help with weight management, to improve insulin sensitivity and glycated hemoglobin level, and to reduce the overall risk of type 2 diabetes.[15]

> A low GI has correlated with a reduction in hemoglobin A1c, elevated high-density lipoprotein concentration, and lower levels of triglycerides.

Cardiovascular Diseases

In cardiovascular disease, dietary fats and lipids tend to receive the majority of attention. Carbohydrates with a high GI, however, may not be the ideal alternative when fats are restricted.[16]

Effects of a low-GI, low-GL diet on cholesterol appear to be most dramatic on triglycerides because there is less need for the liver to make this cholesterol to bind excessive glucose in the blood to be stored as fat. Mixed meals containing slowly digestible carbohydrate that induce low glycemic and insulinemic responses reduce the postprandial accumulation of both hepatically and intestinally derived triacylglycerol-rich lipoproteins in obese subjects with insulin resistance.[17] In a study comparing a low-GI diet with legumes and fiber to a healthy American diet with no legumes and less fiber, the GI diet was associated with lower fasting total cholesterol and low-density lipoprotein levels.[18] GL appears to be an important independent predictor of high-density lipoprotein cholesterol in youth.[19]

Findings suggest that high intake of refined carbohydrates is associated with risk for hemorrhagic stroke, particularly among overweight or obese women. In addition, high consumption of cereal fiber was associated with lower risk of total and hemorrhagic stroke.[20] An ad libitum low-GL diet may be more efficacious than a conventional, energy-restricted, low-fat diet in reducing cardiovascular disease risk.[21] When saturated fats were replaced with carbohydrates with a low GI, there was a lower risk of myocardial infarction in a prospective cohort of 53,644 men and women; but if saturated fat was replaced with carbohydrates with a high GI, the risk was increased.[22] A retrospective analysis of cardiovascular deaths in Denmark found that men who ate a high-GI diet were more likely to die of heart disease.[23] In an Italian cohort (The EPICOR study), a high-GL diet increased the overall risk of cardiovascular disease in women but not in men.[24]

Inflammation

The extent to which dietary GL can affect inflammation remains unclear, but a relationship does appear to exist. In both human and animal studies, hyperglycemia in the presence of diabetes has been linked to the production of reactive oxygen species, with consequent lipid peroxidation and resultant atherosclerosis. Hyperglycemia in nondiabetic subjects has similarly been found to increase the production of reactive oxygen species in vitro, with resultant oxidative cellular damage and the ultimate triggering of inflammatory responses. Leukocyte rolling, adherence, and movement from the bloodstream have also been noted in the presence of high glucose concentrations.[25] Subclinical inflammation, characterized by increased levels of interleukin (IL)-1beta and IL-6, has been noted to precede the development of type 2 diabetes mellitus in one large European study.[26]

The exact mechanisms by which elevated glucose values might be associated with inflammation are unclear, but increased production of tumor necrosis factor-alpha (TNF-alpha) may play a role. Production of acute-phase reactants rises in hyperglycemia, perhaps in response to TNF-alpha levels. Liu et al,[27] using prospective data from the Women's Health Study, found a statistically significant association between dietary GL and plasma levels of highly sensitive C-reactive protein (hs-CRP), a marker for systemic inflammation associated with an increased risk of coronary artery disease and other inflammatory disorders. The risk was higher in women who had an elevated body mass index.[27] This relationship may partially explain why it has been concluded, on the basis of epidemiologic data, that a diet with a high overall GL is associated with more coronary heart disease in women, independent of other known risk factors.[28]

Diets low in GL and high in fiber may increase plasma adiponectin concentrations in diabetic patients. Adiponectin may improve insulin sensitivity, reduce inflammation, and ameliorate glycemic control.[29] Higher adiponectin levels are associated with better glycemic control, more favorable lipid profile, and reduced inflammation in diabetic women.[30] A study of more than 3000 men and women in Greece found that those who most strictly followed the Mediterranean diet (rich in olive oil, fruits, vegetables, multigrain breads, fish, and lean meat) had, on average, 20% lower CRP levels, 17% lower IL-6 levels, 15% lower homocysteine levels, and 6% lower fibrinogen levels than those who did not follow the diet[31] (see Chapter 86, The Antiinflammatory Diet).

Additional research is needed to fully elucidate the relationship between GL and inflammation. However, given the relatively low risks associated with use of GL or GI to guide dietary carbohydrate choices, doing so may prove to be a useful part of an antiinflammatory diet.

Cancer

A number of case-control and cohort studies suggest a link between GL and various cancers. A positive association has been noted between GL and the risk for development of gastric,[32] colorectal,[33] and upper aerodigestive tract[34] cancers. Slightly higher risks of endometrial[35] and pancreatic cancers[36,37] have been suggested as well. A meta-analysis of 10 studies of 577,538 subjects showed that a high-GI diet is associated with a significantly increased risk of breast cancer, although this did not hold true for GL.[38]

Conclusion

The rate of carbohydrate absorption after a meal, as quantified by GI and GL, has a significant effect on postprandial hormonal and metabolic responses. A review of the literature demonstrates that the consumption of low-GI, low-GL foods may positively affect many parameters associated with diabetes, cardiovascular disease, inflammation parameters, and cancer progression.[11-37] Providing clinical guidelines for patients on how to benefit from a low-GI, low-GL food consumption is strongly encouraged. Table 85-3 lists GI and GL values for common foods.

Practical Clinical Guidelines

- Increase consumption of fruits, vegetables, and legumes.
- Consume fruits that are underripe instead of overripe (e.g., bananas).
- Consume grain products processed according to traditional rather than modern methods (e.g., al dente pasta, stone-ground breads, old-fashioned oatmeal).
- Avoid puffed grains and finely ground flour or grain products.
- Acid in food lowers GI (i.e., sourdough bread has a lower GI than non-sourdough bread).
- Limit intake of potatoes and concentrated sugars.
- Consume high glycemic foods with fat and protein to reduce their GI.[39]
- In general, reduce consumption of "white foods" (potatoes, breads, pasta) and increase consumption of multicolored whole, nonprocessed foods.

TABLE 85-3. Glycemic Index and Glycemic Load Values for Select Foods

FOOD ITEM	GLYCEMIC INDEX (glucose = 100)	SERVING SIZE (g)	AVAILABLE CARBOHYDRATE (g/serving)	GLYCEMIC LOAD (per serving)
Bakery Products				
Angel food cake	67	50	29	19
Pound cake	54	53	28	15
Apple muffin (no sugar)	48 ± 10	60	19	9
Bran muffin	60	57	24	15
Oatmeal	69	50	35	24
Pancakes	67 ± 5	80	58	39
Waffles	76	35	13	10

Continued

Table 85-3. Glycemic Index and Glycemic Load Values for Select Foods—cont'd

FOOD ITEM	GLYCEMIC INDEX (glucose = 100)	SERVING SIZE (g)	AVAILABLE CARBOHYDRATE (g/serving)	GLYCEMIC LOAD (per serving)
Beverages				
Coca-Cola	63	250 mL	26	16
Smoothie drink, soy, banana	30 ± 3	250 mL	22	7
Apple juice, pure, cloudy, unsweetened	37 ± 3	250 mL	28	10
Cranberry juice cocktail	68 ± 3	250 mL	36	24
Orange juice	50 ± 4	250 mL	26	13
Tomato juice, canned, no sugar	38 ± 4	250 mL	9	4
Gatorade	78 ± 13	250 mL	15	12
Breads				
Bagel (white)	72	70	35	25
Baguette (white)	95 ± 15	30	15	15
Oat-bran bread	44	30	18	8
Rye-kernel (whole-grain pumpernickel)	46	30	11	5
Wheat bread (80% intact kernels and 20% white-wheat flour)	52	30	20	10
Wonder enriched white bread	73 ± 2	30	14	10
Healthy Choice Hearty 7-Grain bread	55 ± 6	30	14	8
Breakfast Cereals and Related Products				
All-Bran	38	30	23	9
Cheerios	74	30	20	15
Cornflakes	92	30	26	24
Muesli	66 ± 9	30	24	17
Pop-Tarts, double chocolate	70 ± 2	50	36	25
Raisin Bran	61 ± 5	30	19	12
Special K	69 ± 5	30	21	14
Cereal Grains				
Sweet corn	60	150	33	20
Taco shells, cornmeal	68	20	12	8
White rice boiled	64 ± 7	150	36	23
Parboiled white rice (high amylose)	35 ± 4	150	39	14
Brown rice, steamed	50	150	33	16
Cracked wheat bulgur	48 ± 2	150	26	12
Semolina (roasted or steamed)	55 ± 1	150	11	6
Cookies				
Graham wafers	74	25	18	14
Vanilla wafers	77	25	18	14
Crackers				
Breton Crackers (wheat)	67	25	14	10
Corn Thins	87 ± 10	25	20	18
Rice cakes (low amylose)	91 ± 7	25	21	19
Rye Crisp bread	63	25	16	10
Stoned Wheat Thins	67	25	17	12
Dairy Products and Alternatives				
Milk	27 ± 4	250	12	3
Milk, condensed, sweetened	61 ± 6	250	136	83
Ice cream	61 ± 7	50	13	8
Yogurt	36 ± 4	200	9	3
Soy milk	44 ± 5	250	17	8
Tofu-based frozen dessert with high-fructose corn syrup	115 ± 14	50	9	10

TABLE 85-3. Glycemic Index and Glycemic Load Values for Select Foods—cont'd

FOOD ITEM	GLYCEMIC INDEX (glucose = 100)	SERVING SIZE (g)	AVAILABLE CARBOHYDRATE (g/serving)	GLYCEMIC LOAD (per serving)
Fruit and Fruit Products				
Apple (raw)	40	120	13	6
Apple juice (unsweetened)	40	250 mL	29	12
Banana (ripe)	51	120	25	13
Cranberry juice cocktail	68 ± 3	250 mL	35	24
Fruit cocktail (canned)	55	120	16	9
Grapes (raw)	43	120	17	7
Orange (raw)	48	120	11	5
Orange juice (reconstituted from frozen)	57 ± 6	250 mL	26	15
Pineapple (raw)	39 ± 15	120	12	5
Strawberry (raw)	40 ± 7	120	3	1
Strawberry jam	51 ± 10	30	20	10
Watermelon (raw)	72 ± 13	120	6	4
Legumes				
Black-eyed beans	42 ± 9	150	30	13
Chickpeas (garbanzo)	28 ± 6	150	30	8
Kidney beans	28 ± 4	150	25	7
Lentils (green)	22	150	18	4
Lentils (red)	26 ± 4	150	18	5
Mung beans	31	150	17	5
Pigeon peas	22	150	20	4
Pinto beans	39	150	26	10
Soya beans	18 ± 3	150	6	1
Pasta and Noodles				
Fettuccine (egg)	40 ± 8	180	46	18
Linguine (thick, durum wheat)	46 ± 3	180	48	22
Mung bean noodles (Lungkow)	26	180	45	12
Macaroni	47 ± 2	180	48	23
Rice noodles (dried)	61 ± 6	180	39	23
Rice noodles (fresh)	40 ± 4	180	39	15
Rice pasta (brown rice)	92 ± 8	180	38	35
Spaghetti (white)	32	180	48	15
Spaghetti (durum wheat)	64 ± 15	180	43	27
Spaghetti (whole meal)	32	180	44	14
Nuts				
Cashew nuts (salted)	22 ± 5	50	13	3
Peanuts	14 ± 8	50	6	1
Sport Bars				
Power bar (chocolate)	56 ± 3	65	42	24
Ironman PR Bar (chocolate)	39	65	26	10
Vegetables				
Beetroot	64 ± 16	80	7	5
Carrots (raw)	16	80	8	1
Corn (sweet, boiled)	60	80	18	11
Green peas	48 ± 5	80	7	3
Parsnips	97 ± 19	80	12	12
Baked potato (in skin)	60	150	30	18
Yam (peeled, boiled)	37 ± 8	150	36	13

Modified from Foster-Powell K, Holt SHA, Brand-Miller JC. International table of glycemic index and glycemic load values: 2002. *Am J Clin Nutr.* 2002;76:5–56.

http://www.glycemicindex.com	This is the official Web site for the Glycemic Index and International GI Database that is based in the Human Nutrition Unit, School of Molecular and Microbial Biosciences, University of Sydney. The Web site is updated and maintained by the University's GI Group, which includes research scientists and dietitians working in the area of glycemic index, health, and nutrition, including research into diet and weight loss, diabetes, cardiovascular disease, and polycystic ovary syndrome, headed by Professor Jennie Brand-Miller. Each month, the Group publishes a free e-newsletter, *GI News,* to bring consumers and health professionals up to date with the latest GI research from around the world.
http://www.fammed.wisc.edu/sites/default/files//webfm-uploads/documents/outreach/im/handout_glycemic_index_patient.pdf	Patient Handout on glycemic index/load from University of Wisconsin Integrative Medicine
http://www.ajcn.org/content/76/1/5/T1.expansion	International Table of Glycemic Index and Glycemic Load Values from the *American Journal of Clinical Nutrition*

References

References are available online at expertconsult.com.

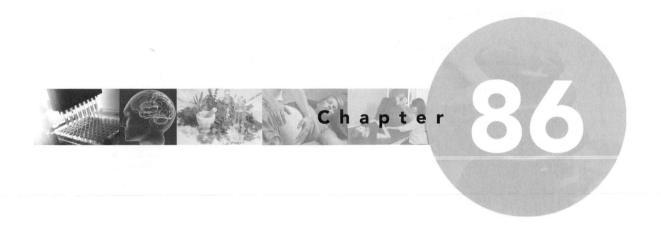

Chapter **86**

The Antiinflammatory Diet

Wendy Kohatsu, MD

Role of Inflammation in Disease

Chronic diseases affect more than 90 million Americans, accounting for 70% of all deaths[1] and about 75% of the nation's medical care costs.[2] In 2005, nearly one of every two American adults had at least one chronic illness.[3] It is now widely recognized that inflammation is the pathophysiologic mechanism underlying most chronic diseases—heart disease, diabetes, chronic pain, asthma, inflammatory gut disorders, degenerative diseases, obesity, cancer, and Alzheimer's disease. Inflammation is a natural response to acute injury; however, when it becomes chronic or systemic, the inflammatory process itself becomes a disease. A new term, *meta-inflammation,* has been coined to describe chronic, low-grade, metabolically induced inflammation that uses the same molecules and signaling pathways as classic inflammation.[4]

In allopathic medicine, medications are often prescribed to suppress the symptoms of inflammation, such as antipyretics for fever control, nonsteroidal antiinflammatory drugs (NSAIDs) for pain, and steroid inhalers for asthma. However, by the time the body signals the presence of inflammation, disease has already begun and medications may reduce symptoms but not necessarily address the root cause. To promote health and *prevent* inflammation, integrative physicians must promote lifestyle change and foremost learn to use food as medicine.

Markers of Inflammation

Markers of inflammation include C-reactive protein (CRP), interleukin-6 (IL-6), tumor necrosis factor (TNF), E-selectin, prostaglandin E_2 (PGE_2) and most of the even-series prostaglandins (series 2, series 4), adhesion molecules, and transcription factors; research is revealing many others. These factors play important roles in the balance between proinflammatory and antiinflammatory responses. CRP

is a commonly used marker of inflammation, and elevated CRP levels are a known independent risk factor for diabetes and cardiovascular disease.[5] (Low-risk level is 1.0 mg/dL.) Many studies on inflammation in humans also explore the role of the endothelium and genetic expression of inflammatory mediators and related markers. In general, free radicals (reactive oxygen species), often the byproduct of unhealthy intake and aberrant cell signaling, are considered markers of inflammation as well.[6]

What Role Does Diet Play in Inflammation?

It is estimated that at least 60% of chronic disease could be prevented by eating a healthy diet.[7]

Adherence to an antiinflammatory diet is critical if one expects to win the war on inflammation and chronic disease. On average, Americans ingest 4.7 pounds of food per day,[8] which the body burns as fuel, uses for cell synthesis, or, in the too-common case of excess, stores as fat deposits. We *can* take a more proactive, preventive approach by investing our 4+ pounds of daily food in healthy choices that decrease inflammation and thus chronic disease.

Of note, an antiinflammatory lifestyle also includes managing stress, limiting alcohol intake, smoking cessation, increasing exercise, and ensuring adequate sleep.[9]

How Do Foods Cause (or Inhibit) Inflammation?

Several mechanisms by which foods influence inflammation have been proposed.

• *Modulation of amount and types of eicosanoid activity.* Certain foods and spices contain compounds that, like medications, inhibit inflammation by acting on specific chemical pathways in the body. Our polyunsaturated fat intake profoundly affects the eicosanoid balance. Culinary spices such as turmeric contain compounds that suppress cyclooxygenase-2 expression, and nutmeg inhibits TNF-alpha release in animal studies.[10]

- *Pro-oxidant and antioxidant effects.* Some foods lead to the production of free radicals that help fight infection but in excess can also lead to significant inflammation and tissue damage. Whereas the use of high-dose, single antioxidant *supplements* has been called into question,[11] a healthy *diet* with a mix of antioxidant-rich foods can potentially protect against free radical–induced damage. Increased overall antioxidant capacity in the diet correlates with lower CRP levels,[12] and in one study, increased dietary intake of two antioxidant carotenoids correlated well with a lower incidence of joint inflammation.[13]

- *Effects of insulin and glucose levels.* Research has revealed links between elevated glucose and insulin levels with inflammation. Liu et al[14] found a strong link between high dietary glycemic load and elevated CRP concentrations in middle-aged women. CRP and nitrotyrosine (a marker of immediate antioxidant stress) double within 2 to 4 hours of a high-glucose, fatty beverage.[15] Type 2 diabetes seems to be preceded by elevations in inflammatory markers[16] (see Chapter 85, The Glycemic Index/Load).

- *Intracellular signaling, transcription factor activity, and gene signaling.* The food we eat can also alter gene signaling and influence the function of our cells. Omega-3 fats, in particular, can modulate gene expression related to inflammation.[17] Hypoxia, toxins, viruses, excessive calories, and oxidative stress can affect intracellular inflammatory responses.[4]

- *Gastrointestinal dysbiosis.* Another postulated mechanism for inflammation is alteration of gut bacterial flora[18] and disruption of the synergism with our commensal 10 trillion–plus gut microflora inhabitants.

What Is an Antiinflammatory Diet?

The antiinflammatory diet is founded on evidence-based principles of sound eating to promote health and to prevent and reduce inflammation in the body. There is no one antiinflammatory diet. Like other healthy plans, it emphasizes minimally processed whole foods; it is rich in beneficial fats, vegetables, and fruit, with appropriate amounts of whole grains and plant-based and healthy proteins.

Conversely, the standard American diet—higher in red meat, high-fat dairy, and refined carbohydrates and lower in magnesium—is more inflammatory, as measured by CRP levels.[19] The traditional Mediterranean and Okinawan diets are exemplary antiinflammatory diets built of many natural antiinflammatory foods and spices, with established track records of their health and longevity benefits.[20–22] The Mediterranean diet pyramid is presented as an example of a well-researched, healthy, and delicious diet with many antiinflammatory components that will be expounded on here (Fig. 86-1).

FIGURE 86-1
The Mediterranean diet pyramid.

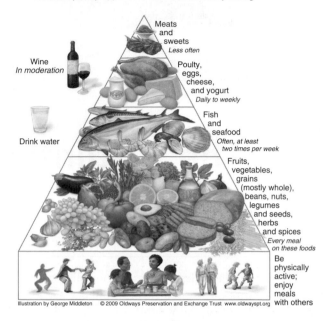

MEDITERRANEAN DIET PYRAMID
A contemporary approach to delicious, healthy eating

Illustration by George Middleton   © 2009 Oldways Preservation and Exchange Trust www.oldwayspt.org

Components of an Antiinflammatory Diet

Fats

Fats are the best-known component of the antiinflammatory diet because of their direct and powerful effects on inflammation and the eicosanoid cascades. Fats play many important roles in the human body. Every cell in the human body is surrounded by a phospholipid membrane composed of fatty acids. The fatty acid composition determines membrane fluidity and cellular transport, that is, what nutrients get in and what wastes get out of our cells. Fats are also involved in proper development of the central nervous system, energy production and storage, oxygen transport, and regulation of inflammation.

The Skinny on Fats

In nature, fats are usually a combination of the three basic fat classifications: saturated, monounsaturated, and polyunsaturated. Saturated fats are solid at room temperature, have hydrogen molecule saturation at every carbon, and have no double bonds. Lard, beef fat, butter, and coconut oil have high saturated fat percentages (41%, 44%, 66%, 92%, respectively).[23] High intake of animal sources of saturated fats has been associated with increased cholesterol and cardiovascular disease.[24,25] Monounsaturated fats are typically liquid at room temperature and have one double bond that imparts both chemical stability and fluidity. Food sources of monounsaturated fats include olive oil, nuts, avocado, and sunflower oil. As the nomenclature implies, polyunsaturated fats have more than one, usually multiple, double bonds that give this class the greatest nutritional benefits but on the other hand make these fats more susceptible to rancidity and chemical conversion to unhealthy fats.

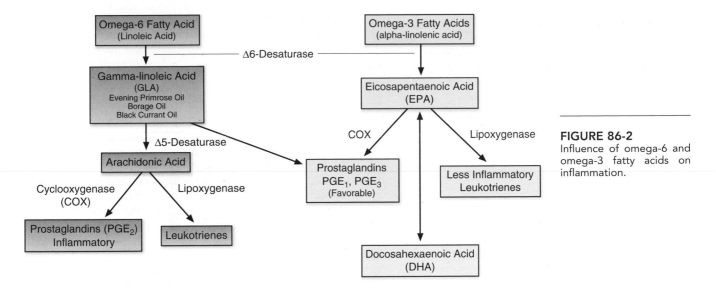

Essential fatty acids are fats that we must obtain from our diet because our bodies cannot synthesize them. The two essential fatty acid families, omega-6 and omega-3, are both polyunsaturated fats. However, they have opposing physiologic functions: omega-6 fats are proinflammatory, whereas omega-3 fats are antiinflammatory. On the omega-6 side, arachidonic acid leads to the production of the main proponents of the inflammatory cascade, the even-series prostaglandins (PGE_2) and leukotrienes (LTE_2). In contrast, omega-3 fatty acids have a more beneficial influence on inflammation. Omega-3 fatty acids lead to the production of antiinflammatory prostaglandins of the 1 and 3 series (PGE_1 and PGE_3) and fewer inflammatory leukotrienes. Because they compete for the same enzymes, the more omega-6 fatty acids we ingest, the less we are able to use the beneficial influences of the omega-3 fatty acids (Fig. 86-2).

Humans still require both omega-6 and omega-3 fats, but the optimal ratio is considered to be 2:1,[26] based on our Paleolithic-era genetics. The problem is that the standard American diet has a ratio of 10:1 to 25:1 omega-6 to omega-3, thus grossly tipping the dietary balance toward inflammation and chronic disease. Diets high in omega-6 fatty acids shift metabolism toward arachidonic acid and its subsequent metabolites that are prothrombotic and proaggregatory with increase in blood viscosity, vasospasm, and vasoconstriction.[27] This unfavorable shift toward the omega-6 cascade is also influenced by excessive alcohol consumption, diabetes, and stress, further exacerbating the risk for inflammatory complications in these diseases. Food sources high in omega-6 fats include corn oil, soy oil, and vegetable oil. The change from a farm-fed, free-range diet in the early 20th century to one of more processed convenience foods and saturated fats and *trans*-fats may play a role in the high incidence of chronic inflammatory conditions we now see in the 21st century.

Not All Omega-3 Fats Are Equally Effective

Another important concept to understand with omega-3 fats is that the end product, long-chain omega-3 fatty acids—eicosapentaenoic acid (EPA) and docosahexaenoic acid (DHA), are much more powerfully antiinflammatory than their precursor, alpha-linolenic acid (ALA). ALA is first converted into EPA, then into DHA. However, less than 1% of the original ALA is converted into the physiologically effective EPA and DHA.[28] For this reason, flax oil, which is rich in ALA, is not as effective as fish oil, which has higher amounts of preformed EPA and DHA (usually 18% and 12%, respectively), thus bypassing the rate-limiting conversion step. Higher dietary intake of EPA and DHA, but not of ALA, was associated with lower markers of inflammation.[29] EPA and DHA affect membrane composition and eicosanoid production far more effectively than ALA does. Omega-3 fats, especially EPA and DHA, have been shown in numerous studies to lower PGE_2, thromboxane A_2, and LTB_4 and to increase antiinflammatory PGI_3 and LTB_5.[30]

How Does One Get Omega-3 Fats?
▪ Animal Sources

Two servings of fatty, cold-water fish per week provide our minimal omega-3 needs. Eggs fortified with omega-3 are now sold with 100 to 225 mg DHA per egg, depending on whether the chicken feed was supplemented with flax or algae. Plant sources are flaxseed, hemp, chia seeds, and, to a smaller degree, walnuts, soy, and purslane. Plant-source omega-3 fats are largely in the form of ALA, which again must be converted to EPA and DHA to exert antiinflammatory effects.

A truly free-range egg has a favorably low omega-6/omega-3 ratio of only 1:3 compared with a conventionally raised egg with a ratio of 19:4.[27]

For the best sources of omega-3 EPA and DHA in cold-water fish, remember the acronym SMASH: salmon (wild Pacific), mackerel (Spanish), anchovies, sardines, and herring.

FIGURE 86-3
Hydrogenation of polyunsaturated fat.

cis and trans fatty acids

■ Supplements

The recommended minimum dose of purified fish oil is 0.5 to 1 g/day of combined EPA and DHA as adult maintenance. An average 1-g oblong-shaped fish oil capsule averages only 30% EPA and DHA; therefore, the correct dosing for 1 g of EPA and DHA is three or four capsules per day. A higher therapeutic dose may be needed (4 or 5 g/day) to treat inflammatory conditions. There are also vegan (non-fish) DHA supplements made from algae.

The Evil of trans–Fatty Acids

When a naturally liquid polyunsaturated fat is chemically converted by hydrogenation to a more solid fat, synthetic *trans*-fats are formed (Fig. 86-3). Although they are more shelf stable, these *trans*-fats (also known as hydrogenated fats or partially hydrogenated fats) wreak havoc in the body, disrupting the native *cis*-alignment of membrane fats[31] and increasing serum levels of lipoprotein(a) and triglycerides[32] as well as inflammatory mediators. Foods containing *trans*-fats should be eliminated from the diet altogether.[33]

A Word About Other Important Fats
■ Olive Oil

Olive oil, rich in monounsaturated fat, does not upset omega-6/omega-3 balance and has been shown to protect against inflammation.[34,35] Olive oil may also possess some NSAID-like activity.[36,37] A small study showed that extra virgin olive oil, but not regular olive oil or corn oil, reduces leukotrienes (LTB_4) and thromboxanes (TXB_2) in human subjects.[38] A healthy diet supplemented with virgin olive oil significantly lowered systolic blood pressure and fasting glucose concentration; CRP was lowered by 0.54 mg/L in this randomized trial.[39] Extra virgin olive oil is less refined and more healthy than regular olive oil because the natural polyphenols that also impart its characteristic color and "bite" remain intact. Extra virgin olive oil contains antioxidants and low-density lipoprotein (LDL)–lowering sterols and favorably affects antiinflammatory mediators.[40] Because of its high monounsaturated content, olive oil is less susceptible to *trans*–fatty acid conversion compared with other vegetable oils.

■ Coconut Oil

Currently, there is much interest in the use of coconut oil for health reasons. Whereas coconut fat is more than 90% saturated fat, 65% of this is specifically in the form of medium-chain fatty acids. Medium-chain fatty acids are readily metabolized in the liver to produce energy and therefore do not behave like other longer chain saturated fats with their adverse effects on cholesterol and fat accumulation.[31] The older scientific literature on coconut oil is mixed about its antiinflammatory effects; much of this is due to use of hydrogenated coconut fat and studies poorly designed to specifically measure the effect of coconut fat. Although it is not as powerful as fish oils, virgin (unprocessed) coconut oil may possess antiinflammatory effects[41] when it is taken in modest amounts; more studies need to be done to confirm its benefits.

Carbohydrates

A study from NHANES III concluded that grain consumption, especially whole grains, may reduce inflammation. Grain consumption was inversely correlated with elevated CRP levels.[42] Whole grains contain fiber, lignans, magnesium, zinc, B vitamins, and vitamin E that may help control inflammation. Dietary fiber, both soluble and insoluble, effectively slows digestion and reduces oxidant stress and inflammation. A study supports an inverse relationship between dietary fiber and risk of elevated CRP; greater protection was seen at a total fiber level above 22 g/day.[43] One study[44] of 522 diabetic patients showed that inclusion of 15 g of dietary fiber for every 1000 calories consumed daily with lifestyle changes (moderate exercise) significantly reduced CRP level by 27%.

Perhaps the single most important factor that determines the inflammatory potential of a carbohydrate-containing food is its glycemic load (GL; see Chapter 85, The Glycemic Index/Load). Excessive consumption of highly processed carbohydrates (e.g., white flour, refined sugars) with high GL causes abnormal surges in blood glucose and insulin levels and then overloads mitochondrial capacity to metabolize the excess, thus creating free radicals.[15] Immediate increases in CRP and inflammatory cytokines can be seen with a single meal.[45] One study found a strong link between high dietary GL and elevated CRP concentrations in women; CRP levels were more than doubled (3.7 mg/L) in the group consuming the highest GL compared with the lowest GL (1.6 mg/L).[14] Diabetics have elevated levels of glycation end products that have been associated with increased levels of inflammatory markers.[46]

Not surprisingly, diets rich in unprocessed, natural plant foods, such as the Okinawan and Mediterranean diets, have lower GL and substantially lower postprandial glucose levels and are associated with improved cardiovascular health and longevity.[47] Minimally processed low-GL foods (vegetables, fruit, nuts, seeds, whole grains) do not result in adverse postprandial inflammatory effects, but high-GL foods do.[9] Another reason to consume whole grains is that the active phytochemicals are concentrated in bran and the germ; refining wheat with removal of the fiber causes a 200-fold to 300-fold loss in phytochemicals![48]

Portion control is also important. Overconsumption of even healthy, low-GL foods can trigger a hyperglycemic response and inflammation. Excess calories regardless of source also contribute to obesity, which itself produces inflammation.[5]

Vegetables and Fruit

Vegetables and fruit, although often classified under the macronutrient carbohydrate, deserve their own stand-alone category because of their natural abundance of nutraceutical benefits. Vegetables contain the highest concentrations of vitamins, minerals, and other protective phytochemicals, with a lower calorie density compared with other foods. Rich in biochemical complexity, whole vegetables and fruit are superior to any single isolated nutrient. Citrus fruit, for example, contains not just vitamin C but some 60 flavonoids, 20 carotenoids, and limonoids. Higher intake of vitamin C from food sources has been associated with lower CRP and tissue plasminogen activator levels.[49]

The lack of adequate consumption of vegetables and fruit in the United States is appalling. It is estimated that Americans consume only 1.5 servings of vegetables per day and only one fruit per day.[50] Only 1 in 11 Americans consumes at least three servings of vegetables and two servings of fruit per day. Even sadder is that up to two thirds of this is fried potato products or iceberg lettuce.[51]

Studies support that people who consume more vegetables and fruit have lower rates of inflammatory disease, such as heart disease, stroke, and cancer.[52,53] High intake of vegetables and fruit, more than five servings per day, has a significant inverse dose-response association with inflammatory markers such as CRP, IL-6, and adhesion factors.[54–56] The more vegetables and fruit one eats, the less inflammation. Blueberries and cherries specifically showed reduced levels of inflammatory cytokines. Estimates from the U.S. Department of Agriculture flavonoid databases also show inverse association with high flavonoid intake (from fruit and vegetables) and lower CRP levels.[57] Flavonoids are responsible for the deep color of fruits and vegetables and often are a proxy marker for high nutritional quality. In epidemiologic studies, higher fruit and vegetable intake was shown to significantly decrease markers of inflammation in adolescents[58] and in adult women.[56]

> *Reminder:* steer patients away from fruit juice in your fruit recommendations because of its abnormally high sugar concentration and from French fries as a vegetable because of the high content of unhealthy fats and salt.

Avoid or minimize refined sugar. Sadly, more than 16% of daily calories of Americans comes from sucrose, corn syrup, and high-fructose corn syrup.[59] These empty calories from sugar-sweetened beverages and foods add minimal nutritional value and promote obesity. Do choose vegetables and fruits that are deeply colored throughout—carrots, spinach, broccoli, berries, peaches. Aim to eat at least five vegetable and fruit servings per day (Fig. 86-4).

Proteins

A large body of data supports the health benefits of plant-based proteins,[60–62] and they are a healthy alternative to animal sources of protein. Legumes are high in protein, fiber, iron, folic acid, and B vitamins. Most legumes are deficient in the essential amino acids methionine and tryptophan, but

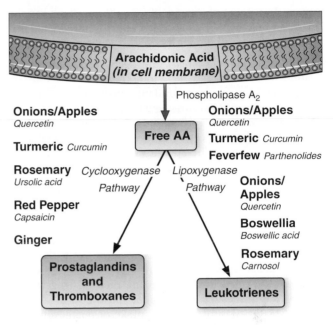

FIGURE 86-4
Food inhibitors of arachidonic acid (AA).

these are found in sufficient amounts in most grains; 80% of the protein in legumes is digestible, compared with about 90% from animal proteins.[63] Four servings of legumes per week in obese subjects resulted in significant decreases in CRP and complement C3 levels as well as in LDL cholesterol.[64] Nuts and seeds can also be added to an antiinflammatory diet for extra protein. Consumption of five or more servings of nuts and seeds per week was associated with lower levels of CRP, IL-6, and fibrinogen in a multiethnic study including more than 6000 patients.[65]

Meat

A handful of small studies show that lean, grass-fed, or wild sources of red meat may have less potential to trigger inflammation than does conventionally raised or processed red meat.[66–68] Larger and more conclusive studies need to be conducted to confirm these findings. Processed meats (bacon, hot dogs, salami, luncheon meats) are associated with 42% higher incidence of coronary heart disease and 19% greater incidence of diabetes.[69] For those who do eat meat, studies support trimming of visible fat[70] and avoidance of charring the food to lessen the inflammatory impact.[71]

Fish

Although it is a source of high-quality protein, fish often swim in waters contaminated with heavy metals, such as mercury, cadmium, and lead, and other pollutants, such as polychlorinated biphenyls. Even taking this into consideration, a review[72] reported that the benefits of fish intake outweigh the potential risks. Avoid those highest in methylmercury: shark, swordfish, golden bass (tilefish), and king mackerel. A serving of albacore tuna contains 0.35 ppm methylmercury; 1.0 ppm is the Environmental Protection Agency's "allowable" upper limit per day. Some of the safest fish are tilapia, anchovies, and wild salmon.

Other Antiinflammatory Foods, Spices, and Supplements

- *Wine:* A glass of red wine per day can lower plasma fibrinogen and factor VIIc levels.[73] Resveratrol in red wine may down-regulate inflammatory cyclooxygenase mediators.[74]

- Turmeric *(Curcuma longa),* the deep yellow spice commonly found in curries, has a long traditional use in Asian countries as a potent antiinflammatory agent. Turmeric has been shown to down-regulate cyclooxygenase-2 and lipoxygenase enzymes; to inhibit production of TNF, IL-6, and other inflammatory cytokines; and to modulate intercellular signaling.[75] Therapeutic doses ranged from 600 mg to more than 2 g/day.

- *Other spices:* Ginger, oregano, rosemary, clove, cumin, and cayenne also possess antiinflammatory properties[76] and add flavor to a wide variety of cuisines.

- Magnesium plays an important role in more than 200 critical enzyme reactions in the body, including mitochondrial energy production. Magnesium intake below the recommended dietary allowance (420 mg men, 320 mg women daily) was associated with higher likelihood of elevated CRP (≥3.0).[77] Ensure adequate intake of magnesium-rich green leafy vegetables, fruits, nuts, legumes, and whole grains or choose to supplement.

- Chocolate, one of nature's richest sources of dietary flavonols, has been shown to favorably affect antiinflammatory cytokines, to inhibit platelet aggregation, and to reduce lipoxygenase activity.[78,79] Dark chocolate (more than 70% cocoa mass) especially has been shown in human studies to modulate inflammation biomarkers,[80,81] to improve lipid profiles, and to decrease CRP in women.[82] A suggested antiinflammatory dose, based on research studies, is 2 to 3 ounces (or one quarter of a standard-sized bar) of dark chocolate per day.

Whole Fresh Food Nutrition

Many individual components of an antiinflammatory diet have been reviewed, but it would be an injustice to focus solely on the trees (nutrition components), lest we forget the forest of our entire dietary milieu. Maintaining an overall balanced diet with appropriate calorie intake is the key to long-term success. Whole diets, such as the traditional Mediterranean diet, have shown greater health benefits than relying on any single "magic bullet" component. In a study of more than 3000 men and women in Greece, it was found that those who most closely followed the Mediterranean diet had, on average, 20% lower CRP levels, 17% lower IL-6 levels, and 6% lower fibrinogen levels compared with those who did not follow the diet.[83,84] This healthy antiinflammatory diet pattern is characterized by high intakes of vegetables, fruit, legumes, fish, and whole grains; it is suitable for people from many ethnic backgrounds and is economically affordable.[15,85–87]

Medical Conditions That May Improve With the Antiinflammatory Diet

Table 86-1 provides a summary of some of the major diseases for which antiinflammatory diet modifications have shown therapeutic promise.

TABLE 86-1. Medical Conditions That May Improve With the Antiinflammatory Diet

CONDITION	COMMENTS
Coronary heart disease (CHD)	A review concluded that diets using healthy fats, whole grains, an abundance of fruit and vegetables, and adequate omega-3 fatty acids can offer significant protection against CHD.[88] The American Heart Association recommends the use of omega-3 fatty acids for cardiac risk reduction.[89] A study including more than 10,000 people found that in those consuming a Mediterranean diet, cardiac risk was reduced by half.[83]
Type 2 diabetes mellitus	A rise in inflammatory markers precedes type 2 diabetes.[14,16] Dietary patterns associated with type 2 diabetes also show higher levels of inflammation.[90]
Rheumatoid arthritis (RA)	Vegetarian diets and fish oil decrease numbers of tender and swollen joints.[91] One review noted average symptom scores to be decreased by roughly one third.[92] Patients with RA who consumed 1.8 g/day of EPA were found to have decreased morning stiffness and number of tender joints compared with controls.[93]
Chronic obstructive pulmonary disease (COPD)	There is a strong link between COPD and chronic systemic inflammation.[94] Omega-3 fats lower inflammatory cytokines in COPD patients.[95]
Alzheimer's disease (AD)	The cerebrospinal fluid in patients with AD was found to have four to five times higher levels of inflammatory markers.[96] High carbohydrate diets may correlate with increased Alzheimer's risk.[97] Fish, monounsaturated fats, cereal, and wine consumption seem to protect against cognitive decline.[98]
Inflammatory bowel disease	A supplement rich in vitamin C, vitamin E, selenium, and omega-3 fats improved clinical response and decreased steroid needs.[99] The Cochrane Collaboration found that omega-3 supplementation reduced the 1-year relapse rate from Crohn's disease by half with an absolute risk reduction of 31% and a number needed to treat (NNT) of only 3.[100]

TABLE 86-1. Medical Conditions That May Improve With the Antiinflammatory Diet—cont'd

CONDITION	COMMENTS
Atopic disease	Hempseed oil, with its high omega-3 content, decreases atopic dermatitis symptoms.[101] Supplementation with probiotics (*L. rhamnosus* GG) prenatally, during pregnancy, and in early infant life may prevent atopy in infants.[101] In a small trial, about half of asthma patients had decrease in airway hyperresponsiveness after consuming omega-3/omega-6 of 1:2 compared with a ratio of 1:10.[103]
Asthma	Hamburger consumption shows a dose-dependent relationship to asthma symptoms.[104] A diet high in polyunsaturated omega-6 fats doubled preschool children's risk for development of asthma.[105] There is promising epidemiologic evidence for omega-3 benefit, but study results have been equivocal.[106] In one study, fish oil supplements decreased symptoms, inflammation, and medication use in exercise-induced asthma.[107]
Cancer	One expert review estimated that 30% to 35% of cancer deaths are due to poor diet and thus preventable. Sulforaphane, carotenoids, and quercetin are fruit- and vegetable-derived chemopreventive compounds with some anticancer effects in vitro and in vivo.[108] Omega-3 fats have been linked in preclinical studies to decreases in inflammatory mediators involved in cancer cell growth, multiplication, and angiogenesis.[109] High meat and dairy consumption is linked to increased prostate cancer risk, and high tomato and fish consumption to less prostate cancer.[110] There may be a correlation between higher glycemic index diets and breast cancer risk[111] and colon cancer risk, at least in men.[112]
Fibromyalgia and low back pain	A small study showed that a vegan (no milk, meat, or eggs) diet improved fibromyalgia symptoms.[113] An intriguing hypothesis exists: phospholipase A_2 (PLA_2) is an enzyme that is at least 20 times more active in lumbar disk tissue. In persons who consume excessive omega-6 fats, PLA_2 may generate more proinflammatory eicosanoids.[6] Although it is difficult to assess because of the multifactorial nature of chronic pain, a diet that fights inflammation is likely one factor that may lessen its impact.
Depression	In a review and meta-analysis, greater positive effects of omega-3 fats were seen especially for the most depressed.[114] Two randomized pilot studies showed potential benefits for children with depression[115] and women with postpartum depression.[116]

Conclusion

Inflammation is the pathophysiologic mechanism underlying most chronic disease. The antiinflammatory diet is founded on evidence-based principles of sound eating to promote health and to prevent and reduce inflammation in the body. It is whole food–based nutrition that emphasizes omega-3 fats, vegetables and fruit, high fiber, whole grains, and healthy proteins. It can be recommended as "food as medicine" for a wide variety of common diseases including heart disease, diabetes, Alzheimer's disease, chronic obstructive pulmonary disease, inflammatory bowel disorders, cancer, depression, and pain.

KEY WEB RESOURCES

Anti-Inflammatory Food Pyramid: see http://www.drweil.com and search for "food pyramid"	Dr. Andrew Weil has published a patient-friendly and illustrative antiinflammatory food pyramid. This plan also features berries, Asian mushrooms, soy, tea, and dark chocolate.[116]
http://www.cfsan.fda.gov/~frf/sea-mehg.html	This helpful Web site provides information on mercury levels in fish from the Food and Drug Administration and the U.S. Environmental Protection Agency.
http://tcme.org/	The Center for Mindful Eating has information on eating mindfully.
http://www.amazon.com/Eat-Drink-Weigh-Less-Delicious/dp/1401302491	Great, patient-friendly book is *Eat, Drink, and Weigh Less* by Mollie Katzen and Walter Willett. Included are a Body Score tool and easy, inspiring recipes.
www.meatlessmonday.com	Check out the "Meatless Monday" campaign online. This Web site encourages all to explore healthy and tasty vegetarian alternatives to meat once a week and includes reader-inspired recipe contests.

References

References are available online at expertconsult.com.

Patient Handout: The Antiinflammatory Diet

Inflammation in the body is known to contribute to chronic disease such as diabetes, heart disease, asthma, inflammatory gut disorders, arthritis, obesity, cancer, and dementia. Eating an Antiinflammatory Diet may help to lessen inflammation and decrease chronic disease. Here are some simple guidelines:

Antiinflammatory diet guidelines:

1) Insure adequate omega-3 fat intake.
   - Eat two servings (4 ounces each) of fatty fish per week, or supplement with 1 gram (1000 mg) combined EPA + DHA daily. These will be listed on the supplement facts label.
   - Reduce use of omega-6 fats to keep ratio of omega-6:omega-3 in range of 2:1–4:1.

2) Choose healthy fats.
   - Substitute extra-virgin olive oil for other vegetable oils, trans-fats, or butter in your cooking for health benefits.

3) Increase vegetable and fruit intake (especially vegetables)
   - Eat 5–9 servings of vegetables and fruit per day, with more than half as vegetables.
   - Color your diet! – deeply colored fruits and vegetables contain higher amounts of protective phytochemicals.
   - Use the plate method – the biggest portion (half the plate) is where the vegetables go (excluding potatoes).

4) Choose whole grain carbohydrates and limit the portion sizes.
   - Choose carbs that are whole grain (requires chewing!), and aim for total of 25 grams of fiber per day.
   - Rx: Double your vegetable intake, and half your intake of refined carbohydrates (anything with flour and/or sugar)!

5) Get your protein from plant sources such as legumes, nuts and seeds, and/or choose lean, natural animal sources of protein in moderate amounts.

6) Spice it up! Include antiinflammatory herbs and spices such as garlic, turmeric, rosemary, ginger, oregano, cumin, and cayenne in your diet.

7) Eat mindfully
   - Be mindful of your food portions. Quality AND quantity matters. Regardless of how healthy your food choices are, excess calories from any source can increase inflammation and obesity.
   - Savor your food.

8) Adopt the Okinawan philosophy of "*hara hachi bu*" – stopping when nearly 8/10 full and paying attention to your hunger and satiety signals.[22] Remember to focus on the whole diet pattern, not just components. Choose food that is closest to its natural form (ie, less processed). Best dietary advice in 7 words: "Eat food. Not too much. Mostly plants." [116]

9) Adopt an antiinflammatory LIFESTYLE
   - Incorporate regular exercise that you enjoy into your life.
   - Keep weight under control. It is important to prevent and reduce obesity, especially abdominal obesity, as obesity itself sets up chronic inflammation in the body[117,118] Maintain body mass index (BMI) between 18.5–24.9.
   - Be aware of, and find healthy ways to reduce stress.

10) Enjoy 1–2 ounces of dark chocolate (at least 70%) as an occasional treat!

Eat More:	Eat Less:
Foods high in omega-3 fats • Cold water fish (Salmon, Spanish Mackerel, Anchovies, Sardines, Herring) • Ground flaxseeds or lignin rich flax oil • Walnuts	**Foods high in trans- and omega-6 fats** • Processed and red meats • Dairy products • Partially hydrogenated oils • Corn, cottonseed, grapeseed, peanut, soy oils
Vegetables • Yellow, orange, and red veggies (peppers, carrots, beets) • Dark leafy greens (spinach, kale, arugula, broccoli)	**Refined carbohydrates (with a high glycemic load)** • White breads or bagels • English muffins • Instant or white rice • Rice and corn cereals • Crackers, cookies, cakes
Deeply-colored fruit • Berries, melons, citrus fruit	**Sodas and juices** • Including "diet" drinks
Whole grains • Steel-cut or whole rolled oats • Sprouted-grain breads	
Antiinflammatory spices • Turmeric • Ginger • Rosemary • Oregano • Cayenne	

Information in this chart adapted from Rakel D and Rindfleisch A. *South Med J*. 98(3):302-10, 2005.

Chapter 87

The DASH Diet

David M. Lessens, MD, MPH, and David Rakel, MD

What Is the DASH Diet?

DASH stands for Dietary Approaches to Stop Hypertension. This eating plan was initially developed to lower blood pressure,[1] but it has since been found to modify several disease risk factors and outcomes, including improvements in cholesterol levels and insulin sensitivity. This diet favors meals that are low in animal and dairy fat and rich in fruits, vegetables, and whole grains. It is a well-balanced diet that can be followed by everyone, including those in low socioeconomic strata,[2] to help lead a healthy lifestyle (Table 87-1).

How Much Can I Expect My Blood Pressure to Come Down?

Two sentinel studies have investigated how adherence to the DASH diet can reduce blood pressure. The original study,[1] which took place among four academic health care centers, divided subjects into three groups; one ate a normal American diet, one ate an American diet but with more fruits and vegetables, and one ate the DASH diet. In those who did not have high blood pressure to begin with, the average systolic value (top number) dropped by 5.5 points and the diastolic value (bottom number) by 3 points for those eating the DASH diet. For those who already had high blood pressure, the systolic value dropped by 11.6 points and the diastolic value by 5.3 points. The blood pressure also dropped for group 2 (increase in fruits and vegetables) but not as much. Furthermore, these changes occurred after just 2 weeks on the diet.

The second DASH trial[3] examined the effect of a reduced dietary sodium intake (at three separate levels: 3300, 2300, or 1500 mg daily) as participants consumed a normal American diet or the DASH eating plan. Results showed that reducing dietary sodium lowered blood pressure for both eating plans (especially the group that consumed 1500 mg of daily sodium), but at each level, blood pressure was lower for those on the DASH eating plan. These studies emphasize the importance of dietary sodium on blood pressure but also highlight that other nutritional features of the DASH diet may play a role.

> In those with high blood pressure, the DASH diet on average lowers the systolic blood pressure 11.6 points and the diastolic blood pressure 5.3 points.

Besides Lowering of Sodium, by What Other Means Might the DASH Diet Benefit Our Health?

Oxidative stress represents an imbalance between the production and neutralization of reactive oxygen species or, more simply, one's ability to detoxify the products of cellular damage. Much of this damage is caused by inflammation, which plays a foundational role in many chronic diseases, including obesity. In a small study, investigators found that the DASH diet decreased blood pressure and enhanced antioxidant capacity, especially in obese individuals.[4] In addition, lower levels of proinflammatory markers, including C-reactive protein and interleukin-6, have been found in those consuming this diet.[5] These findings support the important role of inflammation in chronic diseases, including hypertension. More important, they illustrate another way that the DASH diet may lower blood pressure and other cardiovascular risks besides lower salt intake.

The importance of potassium, magnesium, and fiber in the DASH diet's role in lowering blood pressures has also been postulated. However, researchers have conducted a crossover study in which obese and lean individuals consumed a usual diet, the DASH diet, and the usual diet supplemented with specific amounts of potassium, magnesium, and fiber that match the DASH diet; each eating plan was also matched for calcium and sodium. After 3 weeks, only obese individuals adhering to the DASH diet showed an improvement in blood pressure and endothelial function. Nutritional factors other than these five must be contributing to the observed health benefits, and these remain a topic of further investigation.[6]

TABLE 87-1. The DASH Diet

FOOD GROUP	DAILY SERVINGS	SERVING SIZES	EXAMPLES AND NOTES	SIGNIFICANCE OF EACH FOOD GROUP TO THE DASH EATING PLAN
Grains and grain products	7-8	1 slice bread 1 oz dry cereal* ½ C cooked rice, pasta, or cereal	Whole wheat bread, English muffin, pita bread, bagel, cereals, grits, oatmeal, crackers, unsalted pretzels and popcorn	Major sources of energy and fiber
Vegetables	4-5	1 C raw leafy vegetable ½ C cooked vegetable 6 oz vegetable juice	Tomatoes, potatoes, carrots, green peas, squash, broccoli, turnip greens, collards, kale, spinach, artichokes, green beans, lima beans, sweet potatoes	Rich sources of potassium, magnesium, and fiber
Fruits	4-5	6 oz fruit juice 1 medium fruit ¼ C dried fruit ½ C fresh, frozen, or canned fruit	Apricots, bananas, dates, grapes, oranges, orange juice, grapefruit, grapefruit juice, mangoes, melons, peaches, pineapples, prunes, raisins, strawberries, tangerines	Important sources of potassium, magnesium, and fiber
Low-fat or fat-free dairy foods	2-3	8 oz milk 1 C yogurt 1.5 oz cheese	Fat-free (skim) or low-fat (1%) milk, fat-free or low-fat buttermilk, fat-free or low-fat regular or frozen yogurt, low-fat and fat-free cheese	Major sources of calcium and protein
Meats, poultry, and fish	2 or less	3 oz cooked meats, poultry, or fish	Select only lean; trim away visible fat; broil, roast, or boil instead of frying; remove skin from poultry	Rich sources of protein and magnesium
Nuts, seeds, and dry beans	4-5 per week	1.5 oz or ⅓ C nuts ½ oz or 2 Tbsp seeds ½ C cooked dry beans and peas	Almonds, filberts, mixed nuts, peanuts, walnuts, sunflower seeds, kidney beans, lentils	Rich sources of energy, magnesium, potassium, protein, and fiber
Fats and oils†	2-3	1 tsp soft margarine 1 Tbsp low-fat mayonnaise 2 Tbsp light salad dressing 1 tsp vegetable oil	Soft margarine, low-fat mayonnaise, light salad dressing, vegetable oil (such as olive, corn, canola, or safflower)	DASH has 27% of calories as fat, including that in or added to foods
Sweets	5 per week	1 Tbsp sugar I Tbsp jelly or jam ½ oz jelly beans 8 oz lemonade	Maple syrup, sugar, jelly, jam, fruit-flavored gelatin, jelly beans, hard candy, fruit punch, sorbet, ices	Sweets should be low in fat

From the Dietary Approaches to Stop Hypertension study, as published by the Joint National Committee on Prevention, Detection, Evaluation, and Treatment of High Blood Pressure and the National High Blood Pressure Education Program Coordination Committee. The sixth report of the Joint National Committee on prevention, detection, evaluation and treatment of high blood pressure. *Arch Intern Med.* 1997;157:2413–2446.
*Equals ½ to 1¼ C, depending on cereal type. Check the product's nutrition label.
†Fat content changes serving counts for fats and oils. For example, 1 Tbsp of regular salad dressing equals 1 serving; 1 Tbsp of a low-fat salad dressing equals ½ serving; 1 Tbsp of a fat-free dressing equals 0 servings.

Besides Lowering of Blood Pressure, How Else Does This Diet Affect Cardiovascular Health?

A study of 116 men and women with metabolic syndrome showed that consuming a DASH diet versus a control diet can reduce most of the metabolic risks, including total cholesterol, low-density lipoprotein, weight, triglycerides, and fasting blood glucose concentration while raising high-density lipoprotein. Although the magnitude of the effects varied by sex, they were positive for both groups.[7] An investigation of 31 type 2 diabetic individuals also found favorable changes in these parameters, including hemoglobin A1c (decrease of 1.7),[8] and adherence to this diet may actually have the potential to prevent type 2 diabetes.[9] Interestingly, the lipid- and glucose-lowering effect of the DASH diet seems to be independent of sodium intake, which again supports the notion that this eating plan works through several nutritional mechanisms.[10]

In a retrospective analysis using data from the Nurses' Health Study, a DASH score was composed on the basis of foods that individuals had consumed. In comparing the top and bottom 20% on the basis of this score, the investigators found a nearly 50% decrease in kidney stones, even in participants with lower calcium intake.[11]

As far as cardiovascular disease–oriented outcomes, the DASH eating plan has been shown to lower the rates of stroke,[5] heart failure events (including mortality),[12] and coronary artery disease by 10% to 20% during a 10-year period.[13]

Does This Diet Reduce the Risk of Cancer?

A prospective study assigning a DASH score to more than 100,000 participants showed an 80% reduction in colorectal cancer between the top and bottom 20% of scores during a 26-year period. Those following a Mediterranean diet had no such decrease in their risk.[14]

How Does This Diet Affect Bone Health?

Investigators at Duke University found that those who ate a DASH diet had evidence of less bone turnover that over time resulted in a stronger bone structure. This effect was enhanced when the DASH diet group further reduced their intake of sodium.[15]

What Foods Are Emphasized in This Diet, and How Do They Influence One's Health?

To summarize, the diet is

- High in fruits and vegetables
  These are rich in antioxidants (especially those with vibrant colors), are relatively low in calories, and contain significant fiber.

- Low in dairy, animal meat, and saturated fat
  These fats increase the risk of atherosclerosis.

- High in nuts, seeds, and beans
  These are high in protein and monounsaturated and polyunsaturated fats, which can decrease inflammation and cardiovascular disease.

- Low in snacks and sweets
  Many of these foods contain partially hydrogenated fats that act to preserve shelf life. These types of fats are sources of *trans*-fatty acids that play a significant role in increasing the risk of heart disease. Many common snacks are also composed of simple carbohydrates, which cause a rapid rise in insulin after they are consumed. Over time, elevations in insulin result in the body's becoming less responsive to its effect. In turn, the body will start to produce excessive amounts of insulin, which results in more inflammation and elevates the risk of cardiovascular disease.

- The diet is based on 2000 calories a day.
  Large portion sizes are a major contributor to rising obesity rates worldwide. Combining this diet with a regular exercise routine can lead to even more dramatic decreases in blood pressure and other chronic diseases.

Could the DASH Diet Be Improved?
Cooking Oils

The type of fat may prove to be more important than the amount of fat we eat. The DASH diet does not differentiate between the types of cooking oils. Many vegetable oils consist of partially hydrogenated oils that are a major source of *trans*-fatty acids. When possible, use monounsaturated oils such as olive or canola oil for cooking.

Types of Animal Protein

When eating meat, you may have greater benefit if you try to eat fish more than meat or poultry. Fish (particularly cold-water fish like salmon, herring, mackerel, and tuna) are rich in omega-3 fatty acids. These fats have been found to reduce the incidence of heart disease in part by reducing inflammation that can lead to atherosclerosis. Careful consideration of the sustainability of specific species and avoidance of mercury-containing products can also benefit our personal well-being.

How Can Someone Get More Information About the DASH Diet?

- The National Heart, Lung, and Blood Institute (NHLBI) is a part of the National Institutes of Health (NIH). You can get free information mailed to you or you may view it over the Internet by visiting http://www.nhlbi.nih.gov/health/public/heart/hbp/dash.

- Consulting with a nutritionist can provide valuable information on how to incorporate this diet into one's lifestyle.

References

References are available online at expertconsult.com.

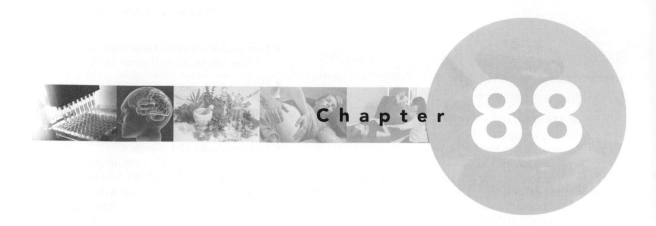

Chapter 88

Writing an Exercise Prescription

Michael J. Hewitt, PhD

Regular physical activity, whether it is accomplished through recreation, sport, labor, or participation in a structured exercise program, has been demonstrated to enhance function; to reduce, reverse and prevent age-related physiologic decline; and to lower the risks of a sedentary lifestyle.[1] Most physicians recognize the benefit of exercise, and most medical groups recommend regular physical activity.[2] However, because few medical training programs include even an overview of exercise physiology and few clinical rotations address exercise prescription, it is the rare physician who has experience in the decision-making process associated with recommending physical activity. Practically, prescribing exercise is no different from prescribing medication, surgery, or therapy; it is a thoughtful compromise between the potential benefits of the treatment and its potential adverse effects.[3]

Basic Principles

Two principles form the framework for making exercise recommendations; the overload principle and the concept of specificity of exercise. The overload principle, based on Hans Selye's general adaptation syndrome model, suggests that a body or physiologic system repeatedly exposed to a stressor of appropriate intensity ultimately adapts to that stressor. To scientists who specialize in exercise, this principle underlies the adaptations that occur after cardiorespiratory conditioning or strength training. In general, there is an inverted J-curve relationship between the volume or intensity of the stimulus and the physiologic adaptation. Infrequent strength training or work with light weights brings about modest increases in muscle strength, but consistent work with heavier loads results in greater strength gains. Too much load and consecutive lifting days, however, are often associated with injury. Cardiorespiratory adaptations follow a similar pattern.

> The challenge for physicians and their patients is to determine the appropriate exercise frequency and intensity for safe achievement of optimal functional enhancement.

Specificity of exercise refers to the relationship between the type of physiologic adaptation and the type of activity performed. It is widely accepted that strength training is beneficial, some say essential, to enhanced performance in sport. It is an unusual collegiate athletic team that does not have a strength coach. However, if one wishes to become a competitive swimmer or an Alpine skier, strength training alone is woefully inadequate. One must spend time in the pool or on the mountain. For similar reasons, sprinters train differently from middle- or long-distance runners. The implication for physicians is that cardiorespiratory health concerns, weight loss, and osteoporosis prevention all require different modes of exercise therapy.

The Five Components of Fitness

A useful model for exercise programming is one that addresses five components of fitness: cardiorespiratory or aerobic fitness, muscle strength and endurance, flexibility, body composition, and balance and agility. One could make an argument to include muscle power (i.e., the explosive application of strength), but lack of power is rarely a clinical limitation. Measurement of bone mineral content is another important component of body composition assessment. Balance and agility are the most commonly overlooked aspects of physical function, but they have significant implications for fall prevention and mobility and therefore are important to aging patients.[4]

There is typically an age-related decline in each of these components (with the exception of percentage of body fat, which rises with age) that can be attenuated or reversed by appropriate physical activity. In fact, much of the functional decline associated with aging can be more specifically called disuse atrophy.

> The five components of fitness are as follows:
> - Cardiorespiratory fitness (the ability of the heart, lungs, and vascular network to deliver oxygen to the working muscles)
> - Muscle strength (the maximal ability of the musculoskeletal system to move a heavy load) and muscle endurance (the ability to move that load repeatedly)
> - Flexibility (an index of joint range of motion)
> - Body composition (typically, the level of body fat, but a measure of fat-free body mass is of equal clinical significance)
> - Balance and agility

Body Composition

Body composition is the one component of fitness that does not require a specific exercise recommendation. Body composition changes as a consequence of cardiorespiratory exercise, strength training, and nutrient intake.[5] However, assessment of body composition is a highly useful tool to determine how patients should use their limited exercise time. For instance, a man with more than 25% body fat and a woman with more than 38% body fat are in a group with a statistically greater risk of heart disease, type 2 diabetes mellitus, hyperlipidemia, and hypertension.[6] Exercise programming should attempt to specifically address those risks as well as help reduce the level of body fat.

Quantification of fat-free body mass (FFB) further refines the exercise prescription. Many adults are at an appropriate weight on the weight-to-height scales or body mass index (BMI; weight in kg/height in m²) value but are underlean as indicated by a lower than optimal FFB. In general, cardiorespiratory exercise results in a reduction of percentage body fat but has a limited effect on FFB. In contrast, strength training increases FFB (as well as muscle strength) and can modestly raise metabolic rate, ultimately resulting in a reduction in percentage body fat. Most morbidly obese patients have developed adequate FFB simply to transport themselves and gain limited benefit from strength training, but their BMI and percentage of body fat respond favorably to cardiorespiratory activity. Smaller individuals who have acceptable weight-to-height values but who also have excess body fat benefit most from combining cardiorespiratory and strength programs.

The determination of bone mineral content (BMC, g) or bone mineral density (BMD, g/cm²) allows a superior level of exercise programming in terms of both efficacy and safety. Dual-energy x-ray absorptiometry (DEXA) is considered the new "gold standard" for simultaneous determination of percentage body fat, FFB, and BMC.[6] Its drawbacks are that the technique requires expensive equipment and patients experience a small radiation exposure. However, DEXA is fast, accurate, and reliable, and it does not depend on patient skill (as does underwater weighing) or measurer technique (as does anthropometry). If DEXA is not readily available or is cost-prohibitive and BMD data are not essential, bioelectric impedance analysis (BIA) is a practical alternative. As long as hydration status is controlled, BIA can rapidly and inexpensively provide accurate and repeatable measures of percentage fat and FFB. It eliminates measurement technique and patient cooperation errors and provides significantly more data, and a more meaningful assessment of health status, than does the ubiquitous determination of BMI. Several other field techniques can be effectively administered in a physician's office; these provide useful body composition data, but each method has limitations. A discussion of body composition assessment methodology is beyond the scope of this text, but interested readers are referred to three excellent summaries.[6-8]

> Dual-energy x-ray absorptiometry (DEXA) determines percentage of body fat, fat-free body mass (FFB), and bone mineral content (BMC).

The FITT Principle for Exercise Programming

For cardiorespiratory conditioning, strength training, flexibility, and balance-agility training, a simple exercise prescription tool is the FITT principle. FITT is an acronym for the following variables:

- Frequency
- Intensity
- Type
- Time (duration)

These are the four variables of physical activity that must be considered in exercise programming, and physicians should write a prescription specifically addressing each (Fig. 88-1). For example, individuals with elevated risk for heart disease should be encouraged to improve their cardiorespiratory condition. The type of exercise can be walking, jogging, or running, either outdoors or on a treadmill; bicycling, swimming, or hiking; aerobics and use of any of a variety of aerobic machines (stair climbers, rowing machines, cycle ergometers); or dancing, tennis, and many other possibilities. The choice is affected by geographic concerns (cycling in the Midwest United States during January is difficult) and economic limitations (some patients cannot afford a treadmill or the cost of participation in a fitness center), but the primary factor is patient preference. Exercise equipment manufacturers often promote their devices on the basis of efficiency and the effectiveness of the workout they provide. In reality, much of the inherent advantage of one type of exercise device over another is irrelevant when patients miss exercise sessions because they simply do not like the activity. The very best cardiorespiratory exercise is one that the patient will perform. Of course, a patient with knee limitations may not tolerate distance running, and a patient with severe osteoporosis should not be advised to take up ice skating.

FIGURE 88-1

Sample of an exercise prescription showing the first three components of fitness, with areas for the prescription to be individualized for the patient.

EXERCISE PRESCRIPTION

Name:_____   Date:_____

COMPONENT OF FITNESS	EXERCISE	FREQUENCY	DURATION	INTENSITY
Cardiorespiratory Fitness	_____ _____ _____	_____ days/week	_____ minutes	_____ beats/minute _____ beats/10 seconds
Strength	Free Weights Machines Elastic bands Floorwork	_____ days/week	_____ minutes _____ sets	_____ repetitions
Flexibility	Static	_____ days/week _____ repetitions	_____ seconds	Hold below pain threshold

Comments/Progression: _____

_____

_____

_____   By:_____
                                                         Exercise Physiologist

In 2011, the American College of Sports Medicine (ACSM) published a position stand on the recommended quantity and quality of exercise that is an excellent reference and should be in the library of any health professional who recommends physical activity.[9] In this position stand, quantity refers to the frequency and duration and quality to the intensity of physical activity.

Cardiorespiratory Training

The frequency of cardiorespiratory training is limited more often by patient compliance than by physiology. It is not inappropriate for one to exercise daily, but few people do. The ACSM recommends a frequency of 3 to 5 days per week for cardiorespiratory fitness and body composition enhancement and a duration of 20 to 60 minutes of continuous or intermittent exercise. Intermittent exercise is described as a minimum of 10-minute bouts accumulated throughout the day. The recommended intensity is 65% to 90% of maximum heart rate (HR_{max}) in healthy adults and 55% to 64% in very unfit individuals. The challenge, of course, is to know one's maximal heart rate. Graded exercise tests rarely continue to exhaustion; therefore, they do not provide a true HR_{max}, and prediction equations for HR_{max} (e.g., $220 - age$ in years) lack sufficient precision to be clinically useful. A maximal or submaximal exercise tolerance test performed by an exercise physiologist can provide a useful estimate of HR_{max} and a target heart range.

Graded exercise stress tests can identify hypertensive responses to activity and clinically significant electrocardiographic abnormalities with exercise and are thereby highly useful for providing a safe and effective cardiorespiratory exercise intensity range for at-risk patients. In healthy adults, heart rate is not essential for monitoring of exercise intensity. The Borg scale has been demonstrated to be an effective tool to assess cardiorespiratory exercise intensity (Table 88-1).[10] Healthy adults should maintain a subjective rating of perceived exertion (RPE) of "moderate" to "heavy," or about 13 to 15 on the scale. Beginners can improve compliance by limiting intensity to "light" to "moderate" (RPE 11 to 13). It is not uncommon for athletes to reach "very, very heavy" (RPE 19 to 20) for short bursts, particularly during interval training such as wind sprints and line drills, but there is little reason to recommend these levels for patients. The OMNI RPE scale, which provides illustrations representing exercise intensity as well as a 0 to 10 numerical rating scale, may be more appropriate for children as well as for adults for whom English is a second language.[11]

Another approach to recommendation of appropriate cardiorespiratory exercise intensity is based on the measured energy cost of the activity, reported in metabolic equivalents

TABLE 88-1. Borg Scale of Perceived Exertion

NUMBER	EXERTION LEVEL
6	
7	Very, very light
8	
9	Very light
10	
11	Light
12	
13	Moderate
14	
15	Heavy
16	
17	Very heavy
18	
19	Very, very heavy
20	

From Borg GA. Psychophysical bases of perceived exertion. *Med Sci Sports Exerc.* 1982;14:377–381.

(METs). One MET, defined as the energy expenditure of sitting quietly,[12] about 1 kcal • kg body weight^{-1} • hr^{-1}, requires about 3.5 mL of oxygen • kg body weight^{-1} • min^{-1}. Level walking on a firm surface at 3.5 mph is rated at 3.7 METs, and running at 7 mph (8.6 min • mile^{-1}) is 11.8 METs. A listing of the MET level of more than 400 recreational and occupational activities has been compiled.[12] This compendium provides a simple comparison of the energy costs of the activities, allowing physicians to suggest several equivalent options. Its utility is further enhanced if a graded exercise test has been performed to quantify the patient's sustainable and maximal MET capacities.

Because cardiorespiratory exercise is so critical to disease prevention and longevity, any program that increases participation should be welcomed. A 10,000-step program, *Walk to a Healthy Future*, has been endorsed by health providers and is promoted by the International Longevity Center.[13] Requiring only good walking shoes and an inexpensive digital pedometer, this program encourages participants to accumulate 10,000 steps daily, the equivalent of about 5 to 6 miles. The recommendations are based on research by a Japanese physician, Yoshiro Hatano, who reported that the typical (Japanese) adult takes between 3000 and 5000 steps per day.[14] In contrast, a 7-day study on the walking behavior of an Old Order Amish community in Ontario, Canada, whose members do not use electricity or motorized vehicles, found average daily step totals of 18,425 ± 4685 for adult men and 14,196 ± 4078 steps for adult women.[15] The highest recorded single-day total was 51,514 steps! It is not surprising that

rates of obesity (BMI ≥30) and overweight (BMI ≥25) among Amish adults average only 4% and 26%, respectively; in contrast, these rates are 30.9% and 64.5%, respectively, for the adult U.S. population.[16]

Resistance Training

A nearly universal physiologic change associated with aging is sarcopenia, the age- or disuse-related loss of muscle and FFB.[4,17–19] A reduction in FFB typically brings about a proportional drop in metabolic rate. In addition, the decline in FFB negatively influences strength, mobility, and balance, ultimately jeopardizing a person's independence.[19] Clinical rates for sarcopenia are 8% to 13% in persons younger than 70 years, about 17.5% in those aged 75 years, and more than 50% in the oldest old.[17,19] Subclinical levels of muscle loss are even more common. As prevalent and as significant as sarcopenia is, few physicians address it, and very few patients have heard the term. Fortunately, sarcopenia is highly preventable, and much of its effects can be reversed with resistance (strength) training. Although cardiorespiratory disease influences morbidity and mortality more than any other factor in our culture and appropriate preventive exercises should be prescribed for it, the prevention of sarcopenia and its long-term effects warrant nearly equivalent attention.

> Sarcopenia, the age- or disuse-related loss of muscle and fat-free body mass, reduces strength, mobility, metabolism, balance, and independence in older adults. Its effects can be attenuated or reversed by resistance training.

Resistance training has also been shown to be effective in combating osteopenia and osteoporosis, the bone loss analogues to sarcopenic loss of muscle. The Bone, Estrogen, Strength Training (BEST) study demonstrated that postmenopausal women, when exposed to a sufficient strength challenge with or without estrogen replacement therapy, could achieve small but significant increases in bone mineral density at the trochanter and lumbar spine (L2-4) sites.[20] Although the increases recorded during the 1-year study were modest (+0.77% to +2.00% for resistance training with estrogen; +0.02% to +1.13% for resistance training alone), they were in sharp contrast to the −0.13% and −0.57% losses recorded at the trochanter and L2-4 areas for women in the nonexercise, no-estrogen control group during the same period. The positive outcome in the BEST study can be attributed primarily to the significant and increasing weight challenge (intensity) participants faced during the study as well as to the frequency, time, and types of strength intervention imposed.

Thus, the FITT principle as suggested for cardiorespiratory programming can also be applied to resistance training. The ACSM suggests that one set of 8 to 10 weight exercises that work all major muscle groups be performed 2 or 3 days per week. A weight load that causes muscle fatigue in 8 to 12 repetitions is recommended. Older or frail individuals may find lighter weights that allow 10 to 15 repetitions before fatigue to be more appropriate.[9,19,21] A second or third set may be advantageous if time and patient interest permit, but the majority of the benefit is derived in the first set.[21] Although many physicians refer patients for an initial session with an exercise physiologist, physical therapist, or personal fitness trainer to learn the specifics of a strength training program, a program can be designed on the basis of general advice.[22] Flexibility and balance-agility recommendations should also follow the FITT principle.

Levels of Exercise Prescription

When prescribing exercise, the health care provider should determine the patient's desired outcome. Strategies exist to help patients overcome their physical and psychological barriers to exercise compliance.[23] Individuals hoping only to reduce disease risk may have a level of commitment different from that of others who seek true physical fitness or athletic performance. Table 88-2 summarizes exercise recommendations for several levels in the cardiorespiratory, strength, flexibility, body composition, and balance-agility areas. General recommendations for body fat and FFB at each level are also reported; however, body composition standards are subject to significant individual variation. A useful approach is to encourage patients to perform at least the recommended activity for the prevention of disease and to strive to consistently exercise at the "basic health" level. When these patterns become habitual, the health care provider can encourage physical activity at the level to achieve "enhanced fitness" (see Table 88-2).[3]

The most effective exercise prescriptions provide guidelines for variety and allow a progression of activity. The programs of long-term participants bear little resemblance to those of new exercisers. Compliance is enhanced if the initial program is broad enough and sufficiently challenging to effect measurable improvement but compact enough to fit into a patient's busy schedule. An experienced physician or exercise physiologist will develop a small starting program and suggest a progression during a specific time frame. One may start with a 10-minute walking or bicycle ergometer program three times weekly and progress to 20 minutes four times weekly within 2 or 3 months, ultimately striving for 40 minutes or longer on most days.

The Key Three Strength Program

In strength work, a simple starting program such as the Key Three[19,24] allows a basic whole-body strength workout to be completed in less than 10 minutes (Fig. 88-2). Few patients have an effective argument for why they cannot find 10 minutes for strength work twice a week. The Key Three can be performed with use of weight machines, inexpensive handheld dumbbells, or even elastic resistance bands, making

TABLE 88-2. Basics of Exercise Prescription

EXERCISE/FITNESS COMPONENT	FOR DISEASE PREVENTION	FOR BASIC HEALTH	FOR ENHANCED FITNESS	FOR PERFORMANCE-LEVEL FITNESS
Cardiovascular exercise	*Accumulate* 30-60 min of physical activity most days	Play or large muscle repetitive activity 20+ min* 3+ times/week	Play or aerobic exercise 40-60+ min* 4-6 times/week	*Add* interval training or competition
Strength training	Include weight-bearing activity most days	Key Three† or equivalent program 1-2 sets 2 times/week Lift to a "challenge" level in 8-12 or 12-15 repetitions	Balanced whole-body machine or free-weight program 2-3 sets 3 times/week. Reach "functional failure" in 8-12 repetitions	*Add* muscle endurance or power training *Add* Pilates work *Add* ascending or descending pyramids
Flexibility	Maintain range of motion by bending and stretching in daily activities	Perform 2-4 limitation-specific stretches after activity, 1 repetition Hold about 20-30 sec	Perform 6-10 whole-body stretches *after* activity and *before* competition, 1-2 repetitions	*Add* yoga, Pilates work, or facilitated stretches with a partner
Body composition	Men	≥ 5% ≤ 25% fat	12%-20% fat	8%-15% fat
		Maintain fat-free (lean) body mass at 125 to 150 lb. or more		
	Women	≥ 14% ≤ 38% fat	20%-30% fat	17%-25% fat
		Maintain fat-free (lean) body mass at 90 to 110 lb. or more		
Balance and agility	—	Act "like a child" Walk a balance line "Don't step on a crack ..." Brush teeth while standing on one foot	Recreational sports: tennis, bicycle, tai chi Social dancing Stability ball training	High-level sports: skiing, skating, surfing Yoga Martial arts Performance dancing Agility drills

Modified from Hewitt MJ. *Basics of Exercise Prescription.* Tucson, AZ: Canyon Ranch Health Resort; copyright © 2002.
*At a challenging intensity.
†Key Three consists of a double-leg press or squat, chest press, and lat pulldown or single-arm row.

FIGURE 88-2
Key Three exercises. **A,** Dumbbell squat (quadriceps, hamstrings, and gluteals). **B,** Supine bench press (pectoralis major and minor, anterior deltoid, and triceps). **C,** Single-arm dumbbell row (trapezius, latissimus dorsi, and biceps). (From Hewitt MJ. *The Key Three Strength Program.* Tucson, AZ: Canyon Ranch Health Resort; 2002. Illustration by Karen T. Wylie.)

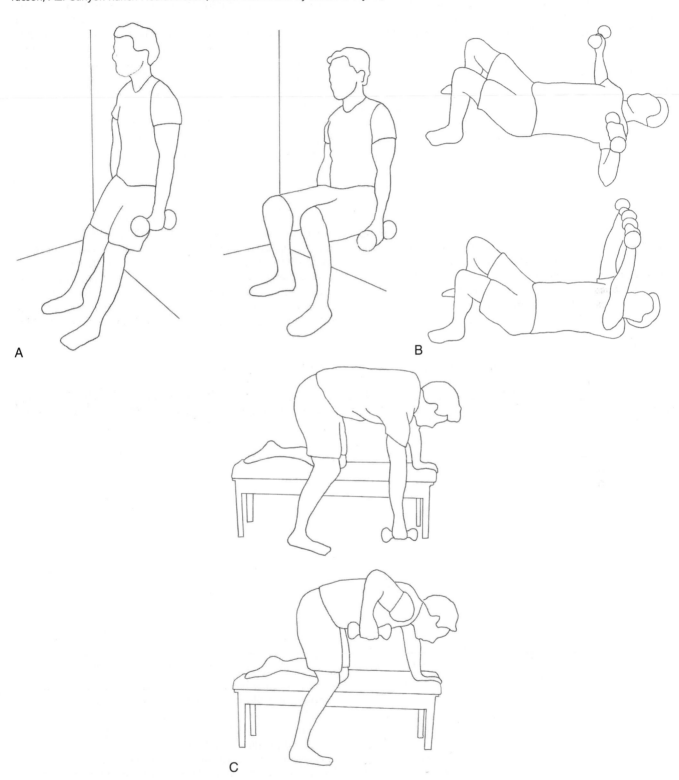

equipment and space limitations moot. The three exercises are the double-leg press machine or dumbbell squat, which can be performed against the wall for additional support (quadriceps, hamstrings, gluteals); the chest press machine or supine dumbbell bench press (pectoralis major and minor, anterior deltoid, triceps brachii); and either the lat pulldown or seated row machine or the single-arm dumbbell row (trapezius, latissimus dorsi, and biceps brachii). These three exercises challenge approximately 85% of the muscle system. Although bodybuilders might scoff at a basic program such as the Key Three, even smaller series of lifts have been demonstrated to rapidly improve strength, muscle mass, and mobility in older adults,[25-27] and these three core exercises can form the framework for more sophisticated lifting regimens.

Flexibility Versus Stability

Traditional thinking among exercise professionals and fitness enthusiasts is that more flexibility is preferable to less. Certainly this is true for dancers, gymnasts, and figure skaters, but it is not always the case for healthy adults. More modern thinking recognizes that optimal control of range of motion (ROM) requires an appropriate balance between limb flexibility and joint stability. Stretching programs have been demonstrated to effectively increase ROM, but physicians should use caution in recommending flexibility training regimens to patients exhibiting hypermobility tendencies (e.g., they can extend the thumb to touch the arm or can extend the elbows or knees significantly beyond 180 degrees). Hypermobile patients should be encouraged to preferentially participate in strength training to stabilize their joints. Most adults, however, will respond favorably to a modest flexibility program.

Static stretching, in which a joint is moved to a position eliciting mild tension and is held stationary, is the most commonly practiced method to improve joint ROM. There are places where ballistic stretching (incorporating bouncing movements), proprioceptive neuromuscular facilitation (hold-relax cycles with a partner or against an immobile object), and dynamic stretching (exaggerated movement mimicking sports-related activity) are indicated, but most patients will see safe and effective adaptations to a compact static stretching program.[28] The scientific evidence is equivocal in support for the common claim that improved

flexibility reduces the risk of injury, but enhanced and stable ROM is always desirable. Similarly, recommendations for the optimal time for holding a static stretch vary from as little as 2 or 3 seconds to well above 60 seconds, but most fitness professionals find that patients respond favorably to a hold period of 20 to 30 seconds.[28] Activities like yoga and Pilates also improve joint ROM, although a compact program of two or three static stretches performed daily is often preferable to a larger and more complex program performed only intermittently.

Balance and Agility

Balance and agility are the most often overlooked components of fitness, yet poor balance and its associated risk of falling are potentially the greatest health concerns for many older adults. Balance and agility require a rapid central nervous system (CNS) response to signals from the inner ears (vestibular signals), eyes (visual signals), postural muscles in the legs and back (proprioceptive signals), and touch (tactile signals). Although some deterioration in the quality of these signals occurs with age, it is primarily a slower rate of integration and response by the CNS that appears to cause the loss of function (disuse atrophy). Function loss is insidious and cyclical. Low function results in reduced confidence, which leads to avoidance of balance challenges; further reduction in function follows in a destructive cycle. Even highly skilled athletes lose function rapidly if they become injured or fail to practice.

Balance and agility can be restored by safe challenges to the system with appropriate exercises. Tai chi, dance, and simple balance exercises such as standing on one foot while brushing the teeth or hair provide effective signals to stimulate CNS adaptation.[29] In severe cases, ai chi, a form of tai chi performed in a swimming pool, provides a no-falling-risk stimulus to the balance control system. Sports such as tennis and bicycling are greater challenges and are associated with both higher risk and greater potential to achieve improvement. High-level activities, including skiing, skating, and martial arts, are appropriate for a select group of patients. Boating, whether on the gently rocking passageways of a ferry or cruise ship or on the heaving deck of an offshore sailboat, can provide a gentle to aggressive challenge to the balance centers.

THERAPEUTIC REVIEW

The ACSM[4,5,25,30] provides guidelines that illustrate the standard of care and prove invaluable for clinicians and physiologists who make exercise recommendations. This organization also offers a resource manual to support the guidelines, which includes background summaries in applied anatomy, exercise physiology, exercise testing and programming, emergency procedures, terminology, and more.[31]

A comprehensive exercise program has a synergistic effect. Improved strength in the postural muscles is reflected in better balance because those muscles can better respond to signals from the balance centers. Better cardiorespiratory conditioning allows a more challenging strength training program, and improved body composition allows greater range of motion for more effective stretching. Equally important, enhanced function allows greater participation, usually resulting in better compliance. Exercise prescription need not be complicated; virtually any activity has positive effects. The key is to gently challenge each of the physiologic systems in such a way to allow patients to experience enhanced function and then encourage them to modestly increase the stimulus.

KEY WEB RESOURCES

www.acefitness.org	The Web site for the American Council on Exercise, a not-for-profit organization that trains and certifies health and fitness professionals
www.ilcusa.org/pages/publications/healthy-aging/growing-older-staying-strong-preventing-sarcopenia-through-strength-training.php	An issue brief written by this author and published by the International Longevity Center on the basics of a small strength training program for the prevention of sarcopenia. All ILC-USA issue briefs can be reprinted for patients. Bulk orders can be obtained by contacting the ILC directly.
www.ilcusa.org/pages/publications/healthy-aging/walk-to-a-healthy-future.php	Another International Longevity Center issue brief, this one written by Robert N. Butler, MD, Founding Director of the National Institutes on Aging and late CEO and Founder of the ILC. *Walk to a Healthy Future* introduces the 10,000-step program and can be downloaded and reprinted for patients.
www.acsm.org	The American College of Sports Medicine is an international resource for information and certifications for exercise physiologists, sports medicine physicians, physical therapists, and other allied health professionals. The section on position stands provides downloadable documents illustrating the latest recommendations for exercise-based management of diabetes, weight control, and cardiorespiratory health.
www.canyonranch.com/connection	Canyon Ranch Health Resort's mission is "to inspire people to make a commitment to healthy living, turning hopes and intentions into the highest enjoyment of life." *Connection* is a periodic paper- and web-based publication featuring recommendations from their professional staff.
www.nsca-lift.org	Members of the National Strength and Conditioning Association earn certifications preparing them to be personal trainers and team strength coaches. The NSCA Web site's publications and education sections provide additional information for readers interested in a deeper understanding of this important component of physical activity.

References

References are available online at expertconsult.com.

Chapter 89

Breathing Exercises

Geeta Maker-Clark, MD

In ancient China, physicians were expected to keep themselves in excellent health and, by their example, to educate their patients in the correct way of living. It was thought that breath control was crucial to health—the physician learned how to control and regulate breath and was expected to teach patients these breathing techniques.

Jacqueline Young[1]

Breath as the Life Force

The breath is considered the basic force of life in many cultures. In India, the *prana* ("life," literally "breathing forth") of yogic tradition signifies the universal life force as well as the life force as it enlivens the individual being. In Zen tradition, the first 4 of the "112 ways" are instructions for breathing. In Chinese tradition, *qi* is the vital energy of life; a component of *qi* called natural air *qi* is absorbed by the lungs from the air we breathe. The Bible states that God "breathed into Adam's nostrils the breath of life," then later used a part of Adam's respiratory system, a rib, to give life to Eve. A rhythmic process of expansion and contraction, breathing is one example of the consistent polarity we see in nature—night and day, wake and sleep, seasonal growth and decay, and ultimately, life and death. As such, it is a powerful and necessary part of our daily life through which we can access improved mental and physical health.

Breathing as a Bridge to the Mind-Body Connection

In yoga, *prana* includes five aspects, or principle breaths, that are referred to as the gatekeepers of the heavenly world.[2] It was this understanding of the close relationship between breath and consciousness that led to the invention of the various techniques of breath control, or pranayama. Whereas

pranayama is also recognized as an essential means of rejuvenating the body, its ultimate purpose is to control the movement of the mind. In Ancient Tibet, it was said that the "breath is the horse and the mind is the rider."[3] A sigh during times of stress is an example of our mind-body "unconsciously" using the breath to stimulate relaxation. The breath can be considered a bridge to the mind-body connection; through regulation of our breathing, we can stabilize the nervous system, transcend the brain-dependent activities of the mind, and consciously stimulate relaxation and emotional harmony. In other words, we can use breathing exercises to achieve a balance between the mind-body, the conscious-unconscious, and the sympathetic-parasympathetic nervous system. One of the most beneficial things that can be done for both short-term and long-term physical and emotional health is to learn and to use proper breathing techniques.

An Example of How Life Affects Physiology

During times of emotional stress, our sympathetic nervous system is stimulated and affects a number of physical responses. During this fight-or-flight response, our heart rate rises, we perspire, our muscles tense, our digestion slows, and our breathing becomes rapid and shallow (as does our thinking, according to yogic tradition). Normally, this process is brought back into balance by the parasympathetic nervous system. With chronic stress, the sympathetic branch of the nervous system becomes overstimulated, leading to an imbalance of the autonomic nervous system that can result in inflammation, high blood pressure, muscle pain, and poor digestion, to name a few detrimental effects. Consciously slowing our heart rate, decreasing perspiration, and relaxing muscles is difficult to do voluntarily. Whereas breathing is one of our many involuntary body functions, it is the only one that we can easily influence voluntarily. Thus, the breath is an excellent tool to help facilitate a relaxation response. We can aid our body in regaining homeostasis by slowing and deepening our breathing.

Acknowledgment: This chapter was updated by the author from Rakel D, Mercado MA: Breathing Exercises. In: Rakel D, ed. *Integrative Medicine*, 2nd ed. Philadelphia: Saunders; 2007.

By simply changing the rate and volume of our inhalation and exhalation of air, we can directly stimulate the parasympathetic nervous system, resulting in relaxation and a reversal of the physical changes caused by the stimulation of the sympathetic nervous system during the stress response (Fig. 89-1).

The Breathing Process Can Be Trained

Our breathing can be trained to have both positive and negative influences on health. Chronic stress can cause us to breathe shallowly and erratically, leading to a restriction of the connective and muscular tissue of the thorax, resulting in a decreased range of motion of the chest wall. By causing decreased venous return to the heart during inspiration, this restrictive breathing pattern also decreases the variability of our heart rate.

During rapid, shallow breathing, the chest does not expand as much as it would during slower, deeper breaths, which causes the majority of the air exchange to occur at the top of the lung tissue, toward the head. This results in "chest breathing." Chest breathing is inefficient because the greatest amount of blood flow occurs in the lower lobes of the lungs, areas that have limited air expansion in chest breathers. Rapid, shallow chest breathing results in decreased gas exchange, causing less oxygen transfer to the blood and subsequent poor delivery of nutrients to the tissues as well as less removal of metabolic waste in the form of carbon dioxide from the body. The good news is that similar to learning to play an instrument or to ride a bike, we can train the body to improve the breathing technique. By focusing attention on the breath, we can move toward a sense of calm. It may take some practice and commitment, but long-term health benefits can be achieved. The relaxation response that is evoked can lead to a body and mind less susceptible to disease.

The Benefits of Abdominal Breathing

Abdominal breathing is also known as diaphragmatic breathing. The diaphragm is the biggest and most important muscle of respiration. When the diaphragm contracts, it is forced downward, causing the abdomen to expand. This produces a negative pressure within the thoracic cage, forcing air into the lungs. The negative pressure also pulls blood into the chest, increasing venous return to the heart. This leads to improved cardiac output, which results in improved stamina in both disease and athletic activity. Like blood flow, the flow of lymph, which is rich in immune cells, is also improved. By expanding the lungs' alveoli and improving the flow of blood and lymph, abdominal breathing helps prevent infection of the lungs and other tissues. Abdominal breathing can also decrease anxiety and depression by helping the mind-body to relax and reconnect. By practicing breathing exercises on a regular basis, we can improve our heart rate variability (which has been associated with increased longevity), blood pressure, digestion, sleep, and stability of our nervous system as well as stimulate a generalized relaxation response that results in emotional balance and an overall sense of well-being. Deep diaphragmatic breathing results in improved vital capacity by increased aeration of the alveoli. Refer to Table 89-1 for the scientific evidence supporting the physiologic benefits of breathing exercises on specific disease states.

FIGURE 89-1
Pathophysiologic effects of diaphragmatic breathing.

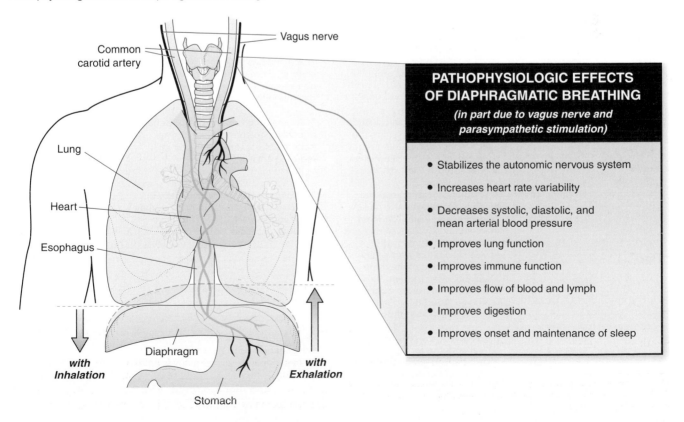

TABLE 89-1. A Review of the Literature on the Beneficial Effects of Breathing Exercises on Specific Disease States

DISEASE	STUDY	STUDY CHARACTERISTICS	RESULTS AND CONCLUSIONS	QUALITY*	GRADE†
Autonomic instability (e.g., poor heart rate variability)	Bernardi et al[4]	Italian study of 23 healthy adults comparing effects of recitation of the Ave Maria or a mantra on breathing rate, spontaneous oscillations in R-R interval, blood pressure, and cerebral circulation	"Baroreflex sensitivity . . . increased significantly. . . . Rhythm formulas that involve breathing at six breaths per minute induce favourable psychological and possibly physiological effects."	2	B⊘₁
	Pal et al[5]	Indian randomized controlled study of 60 men aged 17 to 19 years; either slow breathing or fast breathing exercises were practiced for 3 months	". . . regular practice of slow breathing exercise for three months improves autonomic functions [i.e., increased parasympathetic activity and decreased sympathetic activity], while practice of fast breathing exercise for the same duration does not affect the autonomic functions."	1	
	Sydorchuk and Tryniak[6]	Ukrainian study of 48 healthy adults; participants were observed to determine the influence of individually and differentially prescribed specific respiratory exercises on the vegetative nervous system state	". . . respiratory exercises . . . restore reliably a functional state of the vegetative nervous system [and] enable the sympathetic and parasympathetic nervous systems to regain the balance."	2	
	Oneda et al[7]	Brazilian study of 27 mild hypertensive patients; used slow breathing with interactive music (device-guided breathing) or listening to calm music to determine which decreased sympathetic nerve activity	"Only device-guided slow breathing was able to reduce peripheral sympathetic nerve activity" as measured by lowered blood pressure, decreased respirations and heart rate.	2	B⊘₁
Depression or anxiety	Han et al[8]	Chinese clinical study investigating the efficacy of breathing retraining on complaints, anxiety, and breath-holding in patients with medically unexplained dyspnea	"Breathing retraining profoundly improved . . . symptoms and decreased the level of state and trait anxiety. Breathing retraining turns out to be an effective therapy for those 'difficult to treat patients'."	2	B⊘₁
	Hibbert and Chan[3]	British controlled clinical study of patients who experienced panic attacks; the treatment group received training in controlled breathing, the control group received no training	"Observer ratings of anxiety showed a greater improvement for the group that received breathing training. . . . These findings suggest that training in controlled breathing . . . may have a non-specific effect in the treatment of patients with panic attacks."	2	
	Tweeddale et al[9]	Scottish controlled clinical study of 22 patients investigating the effectiveness of breathing retraining on hyperventilation, depression, and anxiety	". . . breathing retraining is of benefit, not only in restoring more normal patterns of breathing but also in reducing anxiety."	2	
	Feldman et al[10]	U.S. study comparing mindful breathing to progressive muscle relaxation and loving kindness meditation on negative reactions to repetitive thoughts; 190 novice meditators were assigned to complete one of the three 15-minute exercises and then completed measures of decentering, repetitive thought frequency, and negative reaction to thoughts	"Mindful breathing participants reported greater decentering . . . may help reduce reactivity to repetitive negative thoughts."	2	B⊘₁
	Brown and Gerbarg[11]	U.S. review article providing clinical evidence for the use of yoga breathing (pranayama) in the treatment of depression, anxiety, posttraumatic stress disorder, and victims of mass disasters	"By inducing stress resilience, breath work enables us to rapidly and compassionately relieve many forms of suffering."	2	B⊘₁

TABLE 89-1. A Review of the Literature on the Beneficial Effects of Breathing Exercises on Specific Disease States—cont'd

DISEASE	STUDY	STUDY CHARACTERISTICS	RESULTS AND CONCLUSIONS	QUALITY*	GRADE†
Hypertension	Grossman et al[12]	Israeli randomized controlled study of 33 adults aged 25 to 75 years; the effect of breathing exercises with interactive music on blood pressure was compared to control treatment (quiet music alone)	". . . average blood pressure [improved] by −5.0/−2.7 mm Hg in the active treatment group. Thus, breathing exercise . . . for 10 minutes daily is an effective non-pharmacological modality to reduce blood pressure."	1	A ① 1
	Schein et al[13]	Israeli randomized controlled study of 65 adults with hypertension; participants received self-treatment that guided slow and regular breathing using musical sound patterns or quiet music alone for 10 minutes daily for 8 weeks	". . . [slow, regular breathing] reduced systolic blood pressure, diastolic blood pressure, and mean arterial pressure by 15.2, 10.0 and 11.7 mm Hg respectively. Breathing pattern modification appears to be an important component in this reduction."	1	
	Viskoper et al[14]	Israeli multicenter clinical study of 17 patients with resistant hypertension; participants exercised device-guided slow breathing for 15 minutes daily for 8 weeks and self-monitored blood pressure	"Significant reductions in both office BP (−12.9/−6.9 mm Hg, P <.001) and home BP (−6.4/−2.6 mm Hg, P <.01/P <.05) [occurred] without side effects with 82% responders and good compliance. Resistant hypertensives can benefit from and are compliant with self-treatment by device-guided slow breathing."	2	
	Kaushik et al[15]	Indian clinical trial comparing mental relaxation to slow breathing (6 breaths/min) as adjunctive treatment of 100 patients with essential hypertension by observing effects on heart rate, respiratory rate, peripheral skin temperature, and electromyographic activity of frontalis muscle	"Even a single session of mental relaxation or slow breathing can result in temporary fall in blood pressure. Slow breathing caused a significantly higher fall in heart rate (p<0.05), respiratory rate (p<0.001), systolic blood pressure (p<0.05) and diastolic blood pressure (p<0.01)."	2	B ◯ 1
	Mourya et al[16]	Indian randomized controlled trial comparing slow breathing (5-6 /min) and fast breathing (30/min) in 60 patients with stage 1 essential hypertension. Outcomes on autonomic functions of blood pressure (BP), standing-to-lying ratio (S/L), Valsalva ratio, heart rate variation with respiration (E/I), hand-grip testing, and cold pressor response were then measured.	"Slow breathing had stronger effect than fast breathing. S/L ratio, E/I ratio, and BP response in hand grip and cold pressor test showed significant change only in patients practicing the slow breathing exercise. BP decreased longitudinally over a 3-month period with both interventions"	2	B ◯ 1
Insomnia	Choliz[17]	Spanish randomized controlled study of 46 patients with insomnia; participants were trained in the breathing process in the active group or received no breathing training in the control group.	"Increase in CO_2 has a sedative effect upon the central nervous system, and the beginning of sleep coincides with modifications in breathing. . . . Latencies to sleep for the insomniacs confirmed that the breathing process was useful in producing drowsiness."	1	A ① 1
	Manjunath and Telles[18]	Indian randomized controlled study of 69 nursing home residents; participants were randomly allocated to three groups: Yoga (including voluntarily regulated breathing), Ayurveda (an herbal preparation), and Wait-list control (no intervention).	"The Yoga group [whose practice included regulated breathing] showed a significant decrease in the time taken to fall asleep, an increase in the total number of hours slept, and in the feeling of being rested in the morning. The other groups showed no significant change."	1	
	Tsai[19]	Chinese controlled clinical study of 100 cardiology patients observed for 1 year; audiovisual relaxation training including deep breathing was compared with routine nursing care.	"Relaxation training [including deep breathing] significantly improved anxiety, sleep, and relaxation in the treatment group as compared to the control group."	2	

Continued

TABLE 89-1. A Review of the Literature on the Beneficial Effects of Breathing Exercises on Specific Disease States—cont'd

DISEASE	STUDY	STUDY CHARACTERISTICS	RESULTS AND CONCLUSIONS	QUALITY*	GRADE†
Pulmonary diseases (e.g., pneumonia, chronic obstructive pulmonary disease, asthma)	Chumillas et al[20]	Spanish randomized controlled study of 81 patients after upper abdominal surgery; the effectiveness of respiratory rehabilitation involving breathing exercises in preventing postoperative pulmonary complications was compared with no treatment.	"The incidence of postoperative pulmonary complications was 7.5% in the rehabilitation group [treated with breathing exercises] and 19.5% in the control group; the control group also had more radiologic alterations (p = .01)."	1	A↑₁
	Vraciu and Vraciu[21]	Clinical study of 40 patients undergoing open heart surgery; the effectiveness of breathing exercises in high-risk and low-risk patients in preventing pulmonary complications was compared with routine postoperative care.	"Breathing exercises reduced the incidence of pulmonary complications . . . in the high-risk group. These results justify the use of breathing exercises with the high-risk open-heart surgical patient [to prevent postoperative pulmonary complications]."	2	
	Yan et al[22]	Chinese multicenter, randomized controlled study of 324 patients with stable chronic obstructive pulmonary disease (COPD); the effectiveness of breathing exercises in preventing progression of COPD was compared with placebo medicine.	"It is shown preliminarily that breathing exercises had potent and lasting effect on respiratory muscle contraction [which is a key factor in preventing progression of COPD]."	1	
	Thomas et al[23]	U.K. multicenter randomized controlled trial comparing breathing training with asthma education; 94 subjects with asthma received three sessions of therapist-supervised breathing training, and 89 subjects received asthma nurse–delivered education. Outcome was measured by Asthma Quality of Life Questionnaire and secondary outcomes including spirometry, exhaled nitric oxide, and induced sputum eosinophil count.	"Breathing training resulted in improvements in asthma-specific health status and other patient-centered measures, but not in asthma pathophysiology."	1	B⊘₁
	Raupach et al[24]	European study investigating whether there is sympathetic activation in COPD patients in the absence of hypoxia and whether slow breathing has an impact on sympathoexcitation and baroreflex sensitivity, in 15 COPD patients and 15 controls	"Sympathovagal imbalance is present in normoxic COPD patients. Slow breathing significantly enhanced baroreflex sensitivity in both groups."	2	B⊘₁
	Genc et al[25]	Turkish study investigated respiratory and hemodynamic responses to deep breathing exercise (DBE) in the intensive care unit after major head and neck surgery; 35 patients were instructed to perform DBE every hour for 3 consecutive hours after surgery	"DBE improves oxygenation after major head and neck surgery, without causing additional harmful hemodynamic effects."	2	B⊘₁

*Quality: quality of study based on SORT criteria.
†Grade: evidence (letter) versus harm (number).

KEY WEB RESOURCES

http://www.holisticonline.com/yoga/hol_yoga_breath_home.htm	Sites that teach about breathing exercises and how to perform them
http://www.drweil.com/drw/u/ART00521/three-breathing-exercises.html	
http://www.fammed.wisc.edu/our-department/media/618/complete-breath	
http://www.fammed.wisc.edu/our-department/media/618/balanced-breathing	
http://www.fammed.wisc.edu/our-department/media/618/brief-introduction-yogic-breathing	Introduction to yogic breathing
http://www.fammed.wisc.edu/our-department/media/618/kapalabhati-breath	The energizing breath (Kapalabhati Breath)
http://www.yogajournal.com/practice/pranayama	Information on pranayama yoga breathing from *Yoga Journal*

References

References are available online at expertconsult.com.

Patient Handout: Breathing Exercises

Why is breathing well important?
Obviously, breathing is essential to life. However, breathing is even more important than you might think. How deeply you breathe, how rapidly you breathe, and whether you breathe from your chest or from your abdomen profoundly affect your body and mind. Learning and using proper breathing techniques is one of the most beneficial things that you can do for both your short-term and long-term physical and emotional health. Since breathing is something that we can control, it can be a very useful tool for achieving a relaxed state of mind and body. The regularity of practice is more important than the amount of time.

How does breathing affect health?
During times of emotional stress, our nervous system is stimulated and affects a number of physical responses. During this process our heart rate rises, our muscles tense, our digestion slows, we start to sweat, and our breathing becomes rapid and shallow. Normally, our nervous system is able to bring itself back into balance. However, with chronic stress, our nervous system becomes over-stimulated, leading to an imbalance of the system that can result in inflammation, high blood pressure, and muscle pain, to name a few detrimental effects.

We can aid our nervous system in regaining balance by voluntarily slowing and deepening our breathing. By simply changing our breathing, we can directly stimulate a reversal of the physical changes caused by our nervous system during the stress response. By practicing breathing exercises on a regular basis, we can improve our heart rate, blood pressure, digestion, sleep, and the stability of our nervous system, as well as stimulate a generalized relaxation response that results in less tension and an overall sense of well-being.

What are the side effects of breathing exercises?
Breathing exercises are easy, free, don't require any equipment, and can be done anywhere at any time. In general, breathing exercises are very safe. There is a risk of hyperventilation that can result in dizziness and/or loss of consciousness if breathing exercises are done too rapidly or if the Bellows Breathing Technique (see below) is done too much at the beginning of your breathing practice.

How are breathing exercises done?
There are many different breathing exercises. Listed here are two simple, yet very beneficial breathing techniques. To achieve the greatest benefit, breathing exercises should be practiced on a daily basis, preferably not immediately after eating or on an empty stomach.

Abdominal Breathing Technique

Breathing exercises such as this one should be done twice a day or whenever you find yourself under stress, your mind dwelling on upsetting thoughts, or when you are experiencing pain. Abdominal breathing is just one of the many breathing exercises, but it is the most important one to learn before exploring other techniques. The more it is practiced, the more natural it will become, improving your mind and body's internal balanced rhythm.

- Place one hand on your chest and the other hand on your abdomen. When you take a deep breath in, the hand on the abdomen should rise higher than the one on the chest. This ensures that the diaphragm is pulling air into the bases of the lungs.
- Place your tongue at the ridge of tissue behind your upper teeth, keeping it there through the entire exercise.
- After completely exhaling through your mouth, take a slow deep breath in quietly through your nose for a count of 4, imagining that you are sucking in all of the air in the room.
- Hold it for a count of 7 (or as long as you are able, not exceeding 7).
- Slowly exhale through your mouth for a count of 8. As all the air is released with exhalation, gently contract your abdominal muscles to completely evacuate the remaining air in your lungs. It is important to remember that we deepen respirations by completely exhaling air, rather than inhaling more of it.
- Repeat the cycle four more times for a total of five deep breaths. Do not do more than 5 at one time for the first few months of practice.

Tip
- In general, exhalation should be twice as long as inhalation.
- If you have trouble with the exercise, you can speed it up but maintain the 4:7:8 ratio. With practice you will be able to slow it down and breathe in and out more deeply.
- A rate of one full breath (inhalation and exhalation) every 10 seconds (for a total of 6 breaths per minute) has been found to have the most beneficial effect on stabilizing the nervous system and reducing blood pressure.
- The use of the hands on the chest and abdomen is needed only to help you train your breathing. Once you feel comfortable with your ability to breathe into your abdomen, you no longer need to do the hands placement of the exercise.
- Once you feel comfortable with this technique, you may want to incorporate words that can enhance the exercise. Examples are to say to yourself, "relaxation" (with inhalation) and "stress" or "anger" (with exhalation), so that you are breathing "in with the good and out with the bad." The idea is that you bring in the feeling/emotion that you want with inhalation and release those you do not want with exhalation.

The Bellows Breathing Technique (The Stimulating Breath)
If practiced over time, the abdominal breathing exercise can result in improved energy throughout the day, but sometimes we are in need of a quick "pickup." You can use the bellows breathing exercise (also called the stimulating breath or *kapalabhati*) during times of fatigue that may result from driving long distances or when you need to be revitalized at work. It should not be used in place of abdominal breathing, but in addition as a tool to increase energy when needed. It is a good thing to use instead of reaching for a cup of coffee.

The bellows breathing exercise is opposite to that of abdominal breathing. Short, fast rhythmic breaths, which are similar to the chest breathing we do when under stress, are used to increase energy. The bellows breath re-creates the nervous system's response to stress and results in release of energizing chemicals such as epinephrine. As with most bodily functions, this stimulation serves an active purpose, but overuse results in adverse effects, as discussed previously.

- Sit in a comfortable upright position with your spine straight, shoulders relaxed
- Place your hands at the base of the neck and the diaphragm to get a feel of where the breath should be
- With your mouth gently closed, breath in and out of your nose as fast as possible. To give an idea of how this is done, think of someone using a bicycle pump (a bellows) to quickly pump up a tire. The upstroke is the inspiration and the downstroke is exhalation, and both are equal in length.
- While doing the exercise, you should feel effort at the base of your neck, chest, and abdomen. The muscles in these areas will increase in strength the more this technique is practiced. This is truly an exercise!
- Do this breathing technique no more than 15 seconds when first starting. With practice, slowly increase the length of the exercise by 5 seconds each time. Do it as long as you are comfortably able, not exceeding 1 full minute.
- There is a risk for hyperventilation that can result in dizziness and/or a loss of consciousness if this exercise is done for too long or too much in the beginning. For this reason, it should be practiced in a safe place, such as a bed or a chair.
- This exercise can be used each morning on awakening or when needed for an energy boost.

HOW CAN I LEARN MORE?
The reader is encouraged to enroll in a yoga (particularly a hatha or pranayama yoga) class at a local community or fitness center. Most well-trained instructors will educate students about various breathing techniques and how the breath is used to enhance well-being with yoga practice.

An excellent book to help explore more advanced breathing techniques is *Conscious Breathing* by Gay Hendricks (New York, Bantam, 1995).

An excellent audiotape, *Breathing: The Master Key to Self Healing*, by Andrew Weil, discusses the health benefits of breathing and directs the listener through eight breathing exercises (Sounds True, 1999).

Chapter 90

Prescribing Movement Therapies

Patrick B. Massey, MD, PhD

The body of man is a machine which winds its own springs.

J. O. De La Mettrie, French physician, 1709-1751

Physical movement is crucial to ensure health as well as to treat disease. There are few illnesses that cannot be improved, and sometimes cured, with regular exercise. Indeed, exercise is the most effective health maintenance tool in the medical armamentarium, albeit underprescribed. In all of the programs described here, there is a recurrent motif of establishing and maintaining "balance." It seems to be a common theory that once the body is "in balance," good health is the result. Exercise, when it is done properly, may be the definition of "mind-body" medicine.

There are many exercise programs. However, the precise health benefits of most are unknown. For a small number of exercise programs, the growing data can steer us in the direction that could be, for the most part, beneficial to our patients. Some exercise approaches, like tai chi and yoga, for which there is more robust research, hold great potential as therapeutic tools and are increasingly incorporated into allopathic medicine (Table 90-1).

Not all exercise approaches may be appropriate for all patients. Some may be too demanding, whereas others may not be challenging enough. It is important to match the most appropriate movement therapy to the unique needs and beliefs of the individual patient. Regardless of the exercise therapy, movement is crucial to health.

Alexander Technique

History

Frederick Matthias Alexander (1869-1955), an actor and Shakespearean orator, at some point during his early career experienced chronic laryngitis. The traditional medical approaches proved to be insufficient, compelling him to develop a program that would enable him to regain his ability to speak loudly and clearly.

After exhaustive self-observations of his neck and facial muscles, he noted that greater tension with speaking resulted in laryngitis. He discovered that when he relaxed his neck muscles, his speech was better and he felt his spine "lengthen." Alexander hypothesized that there was a discrepancy between his kinesthetic senses of what he was doing and what he was actually doing. As a result, he sought to retrain his body and kinesthetic sense.

Theory

Alexander believed that tonic muscle activity, kinesthetic perception, and reactivity to contextual stimuli are interrelated fundamental aspects of an individual. He collectively referred to these as the "use of the self."[1] Alexander believed that automatic responses to stimuli could become habitual and lead to long-term adaptations of tonic muscle activity. Sometimes these adaptations are inefficient and may decrease the accuracy of kinesthetic self-perception. In other words, thought can set habitual patterns of action.

Alexander thought that these adaptations, in turn, reinforce excessive automatic responses and underlie numerous psychophysiologic conditions, such as anxiety disorders and back pain. Practicing specific postural adjustments of the head, spine, and other parts of the body, Alexander devised a method designed to readjust the kinesthetic sense and bring the body into balance. One of the benefits of the Alexander technique is that it may help uncover areas of imbalance, such as head position, spine movement, and arm and leg swing with walking.

Clinical Application

Although the Alexander technique does not specifically address pain, it does address underlying imbalances and disturbances in kinesthetic sense (Table 90-2).[2,3] A few clinical

TABLE 90-1. Quality of Evidence

GRADE	DEFINITION
A	Well-controlled and randomized studies showing benefit for specific medical conditions with statistical power
B	Clinical trials with statistical power to show benefit for specific medical conditions
C	Case studies and small clinical trials showing benefit or positive trend
D	Occasional case study, testimonial, and personal experience

TABLE 90-2. Summary of Alexander Technique

Evidence for effectiveness	C; limited studies or case reports and reported clinical experience
Risk of harm	Low
National licensure	No
State license	No
Alexander certification	Yes; Alexander
Continuing education	Yes, every 3 years; 24 hours of training in movement education, private practice, group presentation, group leadership
Medical conditions that Alexander technique may benefit	Limited movement Balance disorders Muscle spasms Parkinson's disease Sports injuries Back pain
Contact information	Society for Teachers of the Alexander Technique (STAT, United Kingdom): www.stat.org.uk/ American Society for the Alexander Technique (AmSAT): www.amsatonline.org/ Email: info@amsatonline.org PO Box 2307 Dayton, OH 45401-2307 Phone: 800-473-0620 or 937-586-3732 Fax: 937-586-3699

studies have demonstrated benefit of this technique in the gait and balance disturbances associated with Parkinson's disease and low back pain.[4-8] Interestingly, in a case study of low back pain, as the balance deficits improved, so did the pain.[7] These results were confirmed in a larger, randomized clinical trial comparing usual medical care, massage, and Alexander technique. At 1 year, Alexander technique was more effective for back pain than usual care and masssage.[9]

Quality of Medical Research: C

As with many nontraditional movement therapies, large, randomized clinical trials are rare even though personal experience and testimonials abound. The Alexander technique, however, is not specifically disease oriented and focuses on correction of underlying postural disturbances.

Feldenkrais Method

History

Moshe Pinhas Feldenkrais (1904-1984), an electrical engineer, was a recognized expert in the martial arts, judo, and jujitsu. As a result of his own injuries, he combined his training in martial arts with a number of relaxation techniques to devise his therapeutic approach, the Feldenkrais method. Like the Alexander technique, the Feldenkrais method is a learning process and not a specific medical or therapeutic technique.

Theory

Feldenkrais presumed that humans can learn at any age. He also presumed that the nervous system and musculoskeletal system are intertwined. Distortion or trauma in the development or function of the nervous system can have physical manifestations in the form of patterns of dysfunction. Over time, the result of this dysfunction may be pain and disability. Feldenkrais believed that this dysfunction can be unlearned through proper movement and education.

Therefore, the Feldenkrais method is a reeducation process using physical movement as the teaching tool. Increasing pain-free range of motion is the goal in the therapy, in addition to reeducating the interaction between the body and mind.

Clinical Application

The Feldenkrais method has been applied to a number of medical conditions, including chronic pain, gait disturbance, muscle spasm, and stress-related conditions (Table 90-3). It achieves its "reeducation" of the mind and body through two programs, Awareness Through Movement and Functional Integration.

Awareness Through Movement consists of verbally directing physical movement and is primarily offered to groups of people. Many sessions are available and are focused on specific physical functions or conditions. Each session may last between 30 and 60 minutes.

Functional Integration is a hands-on approach usually performed with the participant on a table. In this way, the practitioner can direct how the specific movements are done. This approach is done without the forceful techniques sometimes found in traditional physical therapy. The practitioner develops a tailored exercise program for the participant. Each session in this approach may also last between 30 and 60 minutes.

It is not unusual for licensed physical therapists to become qualified in these methods and to incorporate the Feldenkrais method into their clinical therapeutic approach to pain and dysfunction.

Quality of Research: C

As with many other movement therapy systems, the number of clinical studies of the Feldenkrais method published in the medical literature is limited. As a result, it is impossible to draw any firm conclusions as to its effectiveness.

TABLE 90-3. Summary of Feldenkrais Method

Evidence for effectiveness	C; limited studies or case reports and reported clinical experience
Risk of harm	Low
National licensure	No
State license	No
Feldenkrais certification	Yes; locations nationally and internationally
Training and continuing education	Yes; professional training program lasts 3 to 4 years All practitioners must complete 800 to 1000 hours of training; participate in Awareness Through Movement and Functional Integration lessons, lectures, discussions, group process, and videos of Dr. Feldenkrais' teaching Students are supervised for a period before receiving their certificate
Medical conditions that Feldenkrais method may benefit	Back and neck pain Stress Muscle spasms Pain Multiple sclerosis and Parkinson's disease (symptoms) Fibromyalgia
Contact information	Feldenkrais Educational Foundation of North America: www.feldenkrais.com/ 5436 N Albina Ave. Portland, OR 97217 Toll-free phone: 800-775-2118 Phone: 503-221-6612 Fax: 503-221-6616

One well-designed crossover study claimed no benefit for Feldenkrais method over a sham exercise for the symptoms of multiple sclerosis.[10] This study looked at the effects of the Feldenkrais method and sham exercise on a number of parameters, including hand dexterity, anxiety and depression, self-efficacy, symptoms, performance, and perceived stress. The Feldenkrais method seemed to improve stress and anxiety. Although both Feldenkrais and sham exercise improved self-efficacy, there were no significant improvements in function and performance. There were two drawbacks to this study, however. Only 20 people were enrolled, and each arm of the study lasted only 8 weeks.

In another study by James et al,[11] the Feldenkrais method was not found to be better than relaxation techniques and the control group's experience for improving hamstring flexibility. This study was flawed by the small number of sessions (14 total) and the fact that the Feldenkrais method is not specifically designed to increase flexibility, especially in otherwise healthy volunteers.

In a 2010 study, the use of Awareness Through Movement in an elderly population demonstrated significant improvements in balance and mobility and a decrease in the fear of falling compared with a wait-listed control.[12]

Given the international use of the Feldenkrais method, one would have to presume that there is some measurable benefit. Other published research suggests some potential for clinical benefit, but additional, well-planned studies are needed before firm conclusions can be reached and recommendations can be made.[13-16]

Martial Arts, Tai Chi, and Qi Gong

History

The basis of martial arts, be it tai chi, kung fu, or others, has always been development of the body, mind, and spirit. In Asia, martial arts and medicine have intertwined for thousands of years.[17] Unfortunately, in the United States, martial arts are commonly associated with pugilistic applications.

The histories of most martial arts are vague, given the tradition of passing knowledge orally from master to student.[17] According to these legends, however, martial arts have probably been practiced for thousands of years. A few, like tai chi, aikido, and tae kwon do, were systematized within the past few hundred years.[18] Although their lineage is clearer, it is likely that these disciplines may have developed as a synthesis from earlier martial art styles.

Some people believe that martial art movements originated from observation of the movements of animals, plants, and even water, focusing on the balance of flexibility, strength, and speed found in nature. Others believe that some martial arts, like kung fu, have their origins in yoga-type exercises.[17]

Although being flexible, strong, and fast has obvious benefits in self-defense, health has always been the driving force in martial arts. Throughout history in Asia, many famous physicians have also been experts in the martial arts, and martial art experts become physicians.[17]

Theory

Martial arts are commonly divided into two broad categories (with extensive overlap). "External" martial arts, like karate and tae kwon do, are those whose movements and exercises tend to be more ballistic and to use linear snapping motions. "Internal" martial arts, like tai chi, kung fu, and bagwa, emphasize circular movements, often at a slower pace. Qi gong (chee gong) breathing is a specific pattern of breathing and is often coupled with specific, repetitive movements. In Oriental medicine, the flow of qi (life energy) is believed to be vital for health. Qi gong is the foundation of most martial arts and, in this discussion, is considered to be part of the internal martial arts.

External martial arts primarily affect the muscles, creating strength and speed. As a therapeutic tool for the elderly and infirm, external martial arts may be limited.

The internal martial arts, it is believed, enhance the production and flow of qi. When the flow of energy is good, the body is healthy. Therefore, internal martial arts are effective not only for strength and speed but also for promoting health in the internal organs and joints, improving balance, and reducing stress.

Clinical Applications

Both categories of martial arts (internal and external) are exceptional sources of physical movement not commonly found in other types of exercise (Table 90-4). Tai chi has commanded the greatest amount of allopathic medical research. The exercises

TABLE 90-4. Summary of Martial Arts and Tai Chi

Evidence for effectiveness	A; randomized controlled clinical trials, meta-analysis, case studies, clinical trials
Risk of harm	Low
National licensure	No
State license	No
Martial arts and tai chi certification	Yes; locations nationally and internationally; however, no standardization of teaching
Continuing education	No; no set requirements for maintaining standards of training
Medical conditions that martial arts and tai chi may benefit	Balance, strength, fall prevention Stress relief Osteoporosis Cardiac disease, high blood pressure Parkinson's disease Back and neck pain
Contact information	No recognized, central governmental bodies for martial arts or tai chi Many hospitals, medical centers, and health clubs offer tai chi and other martial arts lessons and classes

or movements involved in tai chi encourage the body to move smoothly, without effort, through ranges of motion not commonly reached in activities of daily living.

Quality of Research: A

The majority of the medical research on the martial arts that has been published in the allopathic literature has focused on improved functioning in the elderly. Initial studies demonstrated improved balance and strength in the elderly who practiced tai chi.[19,20] These studies have been confirmed and expanded on to suggest an important role for tai chi in the prevention of falls in the elderly.[21,22] In these studies, the participants, elderly patients who were at substantial risk of falling, showed significant improvements in a number of balance and strength parameters as well as an increased feeling of security with daily activities. The potential benefits of tai chi and martial arts also include improvements in cardiovascular and pulmonary parameters, flexibility, immune function, osteoarthritis, arthritis pain, fibromyalgia, function, and strength as well as a better sense of well-being.[23–26] For more than a decade, a pioneer physical therapy program has been exclusively using martial art–based exercises to increase range of motion and strength in patients with therapy-resistant back and neck pain.[27]

A 2012 study of Tai chi for Parkinson disease showed that when compared with stretching and resistance exercise, tai chi was better for improving balance, control, walking and reducing falls after 6 months of training.[28,]

Tai chi and other martial arts are finding their way into traditional therapy programs,[29,30] cancer centers, and hospital-based fitness programs. The research for incorporation of tai chi into mainstream medicine is strong, and some have suggested that it be included in broader health strategies including diabetes, cancer, and even osteoarthritis.[31–34]

Pilates

History

Joseph Pilates (1880-1965) was the creator of the Pilates exercise method. As a child, Pilates had asthma and rickets and had survived rheumatic fever. By his mid-teens, however, through exercise, he was able to achieve good health. As a young athlete, he became accomplished in skiing, gymnastics, boxing, and other self-defense techniques.

During World War I, Pilates lived in England and was interned with other German nationals. It was during this time that he developed the foundations for Pilates training tables by using springs attached to hospital beds for the bedridden patients to perform resistance exercise.

In the 1980s, the Pilates method of exercise became popular in fitness studios. Today, it is not uncommon for Pilates methods to be offered in hospital-based fitness programs and health clubs.

Theory

Pilates believed that with conventional exercise, such as weightlifting, specific muscle groups are favored. As a result, the weak muscles tend to become weaker and the strong muscles to become stronger. In addition, weightlifting tends to create short, bulky muscles. This type of muscle, Pilates believed, results in an imbalance in the musculoskeletal system and raises the risk of injury and even of susceptibility to illness.

The Pilates approach emphasizes the core muscles in the abdomen and back. Breathing and body position are also important. Correct breathing and spinal-pelvic position enhance the mind-body connection and control of movement. The quality of movement is more important than adding weight or increasing the number of repetitions.

The Pilates method does not make any claims of treating specific pain conditions or illnesses. It emphasizes that a body in balance is resistant to injury and disease.

Clinical Applications

The Pilates method is taught in classes, small groups, or individually (Table 90-5). Its focus is not on treating a specific medical condition but on strengthening the body. There are no data to indicate the optimal amount of time for the lessons or the duration of training needed.

Specific apparatus may be used to help accelerate the strengthening and flexibility process. The apparatus can be expensive and is not always part of a health club Pilates program. In addition, use of the apparatus requires training and carries some risk if it is not done correctly.

Some physical therapists have incorporated the Pilates methods and apparatus into their own therapy programs. The effectiveness of this type of approach is unknown because there are no clinical trials comparing traditional physical therapy with Pilates methods.

Overall, however, like many other movement therapies, the Pilates method seems to be safe. There are no reports in the medical literature of adverse reactions to Pilates methods.

TABLE 90-5. Summary of Pilates Method

Evidence for effectiveness	C–; very limited studies or case reports and reported clinical experience
Risk of harm	Low; one case study of diaphragm rupture[64]
National licensure	No
State license	No
Pilates certification	Yes; no specific national or international governing body Certification requirements vary by location
Training and continuing education	Yes; Professional training programs vary significantly; some programs require >400 hours of training and supervision, and others confer a certification after 60 hours of training
Medical conditions that Pilates may benefit	Toning and strengthening Sports-related musculoskeletal injury
Contact information	The Pilates Method Alliance: www.pilatesmethodalliance.org/ Email: info@pilatesmethodalliance.com/ PO Box 370906 Miami, FL 33137-0906 Phone: 1-866-573-4945 Fax: 305-573-4461

TABLE 90-6. Summary of Trager Technique

Evidence for effectiveness	C; limited studies or case reports and reported clinical experience
Risk of harm	Low
National licensure	No
State license	No
International Trager certification	Yes; Trager International
Continuing education	Yes; four levels of training before practitioner certification, comprising 409 hours of supervised (226 hours) and unsupervised training Senior practitioner certification requires 500 supervised hours
Medical conditions that Trager technique may benefit	Back and neck pain[33] Stress[33] Muscle spasms Depression Multiple sclerosis, post-poliomyelitis status, cerebral palsy, Parkinson's disease (muscle tightness)[35] Tension headaches[36,37] Fibromyalgia
Contact information	United States Trager Association (USTA): www.trager-us.org/ 13801 W Center St, Suite C Burton OH 44021 Phone: 440-834-0308 Fax: 404-834-0365

Quality of Research: C–

Although the Pilates method is not considered a medical therapy, there is some limited information on its use for specific medical conditions. Mallery et al[35] evaluated the Pilates method as prevention of severe deconditioning in elderly, hospitalized patients. In a controlled study, these researchers randomly assigned 39 elderly (average age of 82 years), hospitalized patients to either a Pilates program with resistance exercises or a control group who experienced similar exercises done passively, with a physiotherapist moving their extremities. At the end of 4 weeks, the Pilates group seemed to have better endurance.

In a nonrandomized, noncontrolled study, health club participants performing Pilates exercises 1 hour per week for 24 weeks demonstrated improved flexibility.[36] In a similar type of study, trained gymnasts were able to increase their vertical leap by 16.2% and explosive power by 220% after 1 month of Pilates training.[37] Research has suggested that Pilates may be beneficial for chronic low back pain[38] and fibromyalgia.[39]

Trager Technique

History

The Trager approach was developed by Milton Trager, MD (1908-1997). As a young man, Dr. Trager became interested in how his body coordinated its physical movement while curing his chronic back pain. Dr. Trager held that physical restriction and stiffness, repeated over time, could become a habitual response. His belief was that the central nervous system is intimately involved with learned tautness and inflexibility, which over time results in pain.

Theory

Many movement therapies emphasize that misuse of soft tissues and improper function of joints result in inhibition of movement and, ultimately, inflammation and pain. Trager therapy focuses on reducing "un-natural" neuromuscular patterns of movement. It employs gentle, rhythmic movements to facilitate the release of mental and physical stress patterns manifested as tightness of muscles, ligaments, and other connective tissue. The aim is to achieve integration between the body and mind processes.

Clinical Application

A Trager work session takes between 1 and 1½ hours (Table 90-6). The patient usually lies on a massage table in loose-fitting clothes. The practitioner uses gentle rocking and vibrating movements to invoke a relaxed and supple feeling in the body.

Meditation can be incorporated and is referred to as a hook-up state. It is believed that in this increased state of relaxation, the results are more profound. After treatments, simple exercises, called Mentastics, are encouraged for home use.

The Trager technique has been recommended for back and neck pain as well as for pain in other joints and soft tissues. It may also have application in conditions such as fibromyalgia, chronic fatigue, and stress-related depression.

Quality of Medical Research: C

Trager therapy has been endorsed by leading practitioners in complementary and alternative medicine. However, vital medical research on the efficacy of the technique is lacking.[40] Although there is no paucity of case studies and reported clinical experiences, there are no quality studies in the allopathic literature.[41-45] Therefore, disproportionate claims of its effectiveness for specific diagnosis must be weighed against the available evidence.

The Trager technique appears to be safe as a therapeutic approach. No adverse results have been reported with the use of this therapy.

Yoga

History

Yoga, like martial arts, is not a therapy. It is a way to live one's life in harmony with nature, and good health is a result. Yoga may have been practiced for more than 5000 years. It was believed to be a path by which one could transcend the human. It later became a way to develop the self, mentally, physically, and spiritually, and thus through mental and physical discipline to achieve spiritual enlightenment. Yoga consists of the following five principles:

- Proper relaxation (savasana)
- Proper exercise (asanas)
- Proper breathing (pranayama)
- Proper diet (vegetarian)
- Meditation (dhyana)

In the United States, yoga is exemplified by the practice of postures (gentle stretching exercises), breathing exercises, and meditation. The body of research into the health benefits of yoga-based exercises and stress reduction is growing.

A number of different styles of yoga exist (Table 90-7). No style has been proved to have greater health benefits, and the style practiced may be personal preference or simply what is locally available.

Theory

Balance in all things leading to health is an idea common to many cultures. In allopathy, we know that excesses raise the risk for development of disease. Yoga emphasizes a three-pronged approach: practicing postures strengthens the body; controlling breathing creates a chemical and emotional balance; and meditation is a form of prayer. It is believed that the combination of these three aspects powerfully stimulates the inherent healing properties of each person.

Clinical Application

Despite its use for thousands of years, does yoga work? The medical literature contains hundreds of research and review articles debating yoga's benefits. As in much of the movement

TABLE 90-7. Styles of Yoga

STYLE	DESCRIPTION
Ananda	Classical style of hatha yoga that is gentle Not athletic or aerobic
Anusara	Spiritually oriented, using asanas with a mind-body emphasis
Ashtanga	Physically demanding, as participants jump from one posture to another Strength, flexibility, and stamina
Bikram	Practiced in a room at 100°F, performing a series of 26 asanas Cleansing the body and increasing flexibility
Kundalini	Believed to release Kundalini (serpent power) energy, at the base of the spine Involves asanas, but emphasis is on chanting and breathing
Iyengar	Strict attention to posture and alignment May use belts and blocks to help alignment

therapy research, there are more questions than answers. For yoga, however, a large body of evidence suggests benefit for a variety of chronic medical conditions (Table 90-8).

Solid medical research shows that exercise and stress reduction can reduce the risk of many diseases, including diabetes mellitus, heart disease, cancer, and even Alzheimer's disease.[46-50] Yoga may be a good way to modify some of the risk factors for a number of medical conditions.

Yoga and its rhythmic pranayama breathing techniques may help reduce the symptoms of asthma.[51-53] The exercise (asanas) and stress reduction techniques in yoga have also been shown to be beneficial in reducing medication use and improving nerve function.

Incorporation of yoga into a lifestyle can have almost immediate effect on reducing risk factors for heart disease and diabetes.[54,55] In one study, Bijlani et al[56] found that 9 days of exercise (asanas), stress reduction (including pranayama breathing), and proper nutrition resulted in significant reductions in low-density lipoprotein cholesterol, very-low-density lipoprotein cholesterol, and fasting serum glucose values as well as an increase in high-density lipoprotein cholesterol levels in patients with heart disease and diabetes.

The exercises and stress reduction techniques in yoga may also be effective for people with uncomplicated back and neck pain. Although high-quality studies have not yet been done, the available data do show that there is some benefit in the practice of yoga for chronic back pain.[57,58]

A number of studies suggest that yoga may be beneficial as an adjunctive therapy for cancer and the side effects of therapy (stress, pain, insomnia, and mood). Both exercise and meditation have been shown to be easily incorporated and beneficial.[59-61] Many cancer centers across the nation offer yoga to their patients for stress relief and mood enhancement and as a form of mild to moderate exercise.

The role of yoga in osteoarthritis, rheumatoid arthritis, and carpal tunnel syndrome is limited but promising. Use of yoga exercises has been shown to improve pain and function, with a decrease in the use of medications and other therapies.[62,63]

TABLE 90-8. Summary of Yoga

Evidence for effectiveness	B; large number of medical studies and clinical trials
Risk of harm	Low
National licensure	No
State license	No
Yoga certification	Yes and no; no specific national or international governing body Training from specific yogic masters a plus
Training and continuing education	Yes; professional training programs vary significantly Yoga is a process of continual learning but not structured; however, Iyengar yoga instructors must complete a 2- to 5-year training program
Medical conditions that yoga may benefit or prevent	Chronic disease Asthma Coronary artery disease Diabetes mellitus Stress-related disorders Menopause Cancer, side effects Musculoskeletal pain Carpal tunnel syndrome
Contact information	International Association of Yoga Therapists: www.iayt.org/ Email: mail@iayt.org 115 S McCormick St, Suite 3 Prescott, AZ 86303 Phone: 928-541-0004 Fax: 928-541-0182

Quality of Research: B

A search on the PubMed Web site using "yoga" yields more than 800 research and review articles on the use of yoga as a medical therapy. Not all of the medical study results are positive, but the majority of research shows benefits, especially in chronic disease.

The credibility of yoga as an important medical therapy suffers from a lack of high-quality, randomized, controlled studies. However, as the research continues to grow, it is certainly probable that those medical conditions improved by exercise, stress reduction, nutritional changes, and meditation will be shown also to benefit from yoga exercises and stress reduction techniques. Given the nature of chronic disease, yoga may play a role in treatment and, more important, prevention.

References

References are available online at expertconsult.com.

Chapter 91

Low Back Pain Exercises

Brian Degenhardt, DO and Coleen Smith, DO

The management of patients who seek treatment for low back pain can be difficult for any practitioner. The cause of low back pain can be the skin, soft tissue, or skeletal components. Low back pain can be referred from other sources, even visceral structures, or it can be secondary to postural decompensation.

History and physical findings should guide the practitioner to further evaluation and a treatment plan. Multidisciplinary treatment approaches are often necessary to facilitate healing for the patient with low back pain. Understanding of the patient's belief system about his or her low back pain may be an important component of recovery.[1] A treatment plan may include an exercise prescription. Movement, strengthening, and flexibility in patients with chronic lumbar back pain has demonstrated benefit.[2]

The traditional exercise prescription is a written description of the exercise, including the number of repetitions per set, number of sets per session, and frequency of sessions. This format is specific for strength exercises and has been applied to flexibility exercises. Many traditional exercise routines are assigned and performed too literally, without recognition of the subtle changes the patient experiences day to day in a healing exercise program. The goal of any complementary exercise recommendation is to encourage a dynamic interchange between the patient's awareness and the body. With appropriate education, the patient can become more sensitive to information being generated from the body and perform the exercise program in a much more precise, safe, and effective manner. Attention to the body's feedback mechanisms should be encouraged to allow the patient to modify any portion of the exercise prescription. This enables the patient to achieve optimal outcomes from the rehabilitation program. The outcomes of an exercise plan are to enhance flexibility, to minimize or to eliminate pain by reducing muscle tension, and to improve strength, thereby encouraging joint stability. A complementary exercise plan for a person with lumbar back pain should include the following approaches:

- Breathing and relaxation training
- Flexibility training
- Strength training
- Coordination training

The National Institute of Health and Clinical Excellence (NICE) has reviewed the evidence of therapies that have been found to be most useful for low back pain. Of all therapies used for low back pain, the evidence for benefit with least harm supported an exercise program, manual therapy, and acupuncture.[3]

The Patient Handout at the end of this chapter contains examples of the exercises and approaches discussed here.

Breathing and Relaxation Training

Flexibility and relaxation techniques are often great starting points in a patient's exercise prescription. They calm the patient and foster awareness of information from the body that helps guide and individualize the exercise prescription. These exercises enhance diaphragmatic function and improve oxygenation, lymphatic flow, and autonomic nervous system regulation. To begin this component of the exercise prescription, the patient should choose a comfortable position and minimize distraction, perhaps by listening to soothing background music. The patient must use the abdominal diaphragm while taking a slow, deep breath and both the diaphragm and the rib cage as inspiration continues (see Chapter 89, Breathing Exercises). The number of repetitions is likely to vary from day to day because stress and tightness also change daily. The patient needs to learn to recognize when the body is relaxed and ready to move on to other components of the exercise prescription. Once relaxation and focus have been obtained, participants should use deep breathing throughout all cycles of the exercise plan.

Flexibility Training

The flexibility portion of an exercise plan uses stretching to promote greater range of motion in all planes. Properly performed, stretching allows better neuromusculoskeletal function, promoting less pain and more motion. To stretch properly, the patient must move to the point of tension and then perform deep breaths to gently stretch the tight tissue. It is important to move slowly and gently in and out of stretches. Other models describe how to stretch, but this approach minimizes the chance of exacerbating a patient's back pain by overstretching. Although an outline of a stretch gives the patient a guide to promote flexibility of specific areas of the body, the patient listens each day to the information the body is generating to determine where the tightness is. This approach allows the patient to modify a stretch and to maximize its effectiveness each day. The stretch is considered complete only after the patient appreciates a change in the tension while holding the stretch. This change can occur after only one or two repetitions, or it may need more repetitions, as determined by the patient through attention to the body's feedback system. Patients must stay within their pain limitations to prevent reflex muscle tightening and injury.

In most patients with chronic low back pain, specific instruction is necessary for hip flexors and extensors. For recovery from muscle tightness and to decrease pain, it is also important to achieve greater flexibility as well as a balance of flexibility between the same muscles on the two sides of the body and between reciprocal muscles, particularly with the hamstring, iliopsoas, and piriformis muscles.

Strength Training

Strengthening exercises encourage active use of muscle groups, leading to better muscle tone and greater strength. It is important not to sacrifice flexibility for strength; the two are equally important for proper lumbar mechanics in patients with low back pain. The clinician can evaluate the patient's strength clinically by having the patient perform isometric contractions against the physician's resistance to determine whether there is gross asymmetry of strength. Asymmetry of strength may lead to or be secondary to hypertonicity in one muscle group and weakness in the opposing muscle groups. Once strength asymmetry or weakness has been diagnosed, specific instructions must be given first to stretch the hypertonic muscles and then to motivate the patient to exercise the weakened muscles. Patients are often unaware of this local muscle weakness. In many exercise programs, patients focus on rote repetition of exercises, strengthening hypertonic muscles rather than conditioning weakened muscle groups. It can be beneficial for the patient with hypertonic lumbar extensors to perform abdominal curl-ups to strengthen weakened antagonistic abdominal muscles after stretching the lumbar erector spinae muscles. Both exercises decrease hypertonicity in the lumbar extensor muscle group.

In many cases of lumbar back pain, strengthening activities must start out as isometric exercises instead of the typical isotonic exercises because isometric exercises are safer. Isometric exercises allow the origin and insertion of the involved muscle to remain in constant position while the patient presses against a resisting force that is equal to the patient's force.

> An example of an isometric exercise is pushing against a solid wall without moving. Isometric exercises are often useful for patients who have arthritis, in which joint movement causes pain and limitation.

Coordination Training

Differences in proprioception exist in individuals with and without back pain. Coordination training in patients with low back pain is based on the observation that the response of a patient's spine to stress causes the postural muscles to tighten and the antagonist muscles to react with inhibition, weakness, and atrophy.[4] Coordination training is imperative for improvement of overall postural balance in the patient with lumbar back pain. Proprioceptive education in patients with low back pain begins with improving ankle, knee, and pelvis coordination, perhaps through the use of a wobble board or fitness ball. The physician must remind the patient of safety precautions at the start of coordination training. Basic coordination exercises can usually be taught in the office and then performed by the patient independently. Advanced proprioceptive training usually requires supervision to ensure correct technique and safety.

KEY WEB RESOURCES

http://www.nlm.nih.gov/medlineplus/tutorials/backexercises/htm/_yes_50_no_0.htm	MedlinePlus slideshow on back exercises from The Patient Education Institute.
http://www.acatoday.org/pdf/BackPainExercise.pdf	Handout from the American Chiropractic Association on back pain exercises.
http://video.about.com/backandneck/Back-Stretches-for-Back-Pain.htm	Video of a back exercise and stretching routine to be done each day to prevent back pain from About.com.
http://www.egoscue.com/	The Egoscue technique addresses strengthening and balancing of the whole body unit to reduce back pain. A book that includes back stretching exercises from this method is Escogue P, Gitnes R: *Pain Free: A Revolutionary Method for Stopping Chronic Pain.* New York: Bantam Books; 2000.
http://www.fammed.wisc.edu/our-department/media/618/feldenkrais-low-back-pain	Video on how Feldenkrais therapy can be used for low back pain from the University of Wisconsin Integrative Medicine Program.

References

References are available online at expertconsult.com.

Patient Handout: Exercise Program for Low Back Pain

1. Listen to your body signals; the amount of exercise may vary from day to day. Always stay within pain limitations when performing any exercises.
2. It is important to breathe properly. While performing all aspects of your stretching program, breathe into your abdomen and feel the sides of your rib cage expand.
3. Move slowly and gently during stretching exercises. Do not bounce!
4. If you experience pain during or after a specific exercise, decrease the duration and intensity of the exercise. If the pain reoccurs, eliminate that exercise from your routine and consult with an exercise professional.

Breathing and Relaxation Exercises
Breathing and Body Stretch

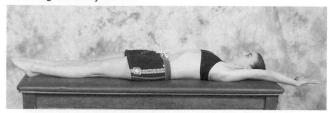

1. Lie on your back. Place your hands on your abdomen. Relax. This is your time to focus on yourself.
2. Breathe deeply into your abdomen so that your hands rise and fall with each breath. Feel the sides of your rib cage expand.
3. Hold your breath in for 3 to 5 seconds, and then exhale slowly.
4. Repeat steps 2 and 3 slowly and gently for 2 minutes.
5. Place your arms above your head and reach upward as you point your toes downward.
6. Hold the stretch for 5 slow, deep breaths.
7. Slowly return to the starting position, and repeat the stretch until the tissue tension experienced during the first stretch has resolved (often 2 times).

Stretching Exercises
Pelvic Tilt Exercise

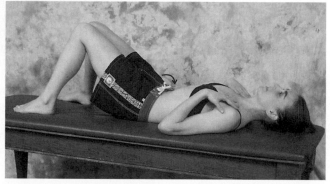

1. Lie on your back. Bend your knees, placing your feet flat on the floor and allowing your knees to touch.
2. Roll your pelvis backward by pushing your belly button toward your spine.
3. Hold this position for 20 to 40 seconds or until fatigued, while breathing slowly and deeply.
4. Release slowly. Repeat.

Low Back Flexion Exercise

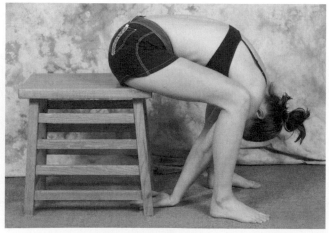

1. Sit. Curl your spine forward one vertebra at a time, from the head, to the neck, chest, and low back. Stop at and hold at any area of muscle tightness.
2. Hold position for 3 deep breaths or until the tissue relaxes.
3. Gently return to a sitting position.
4. Repeat at least 2 times, likely curling farther than the time before, until the tissue tension experienced along the spine has resolved, or if soreness has developed. Be patient with this stretch. It may take weeks before you can easily stretch all the way down the back.

Low Back Extension Exercise

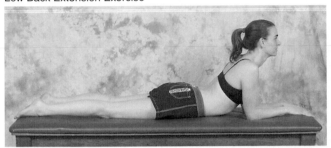

1. Lie on your stomach with your feet shoulder-width apart and your toes pointing downward.
2. Bring your elbows under your shoulders to support your weight.
3. Gently raise your head and slowly arch your back, letting your belly relax forward toward the floor. Go only as far as is painless until your muscles are more flexible.
4. Hold position and breathe into your abdomen for at least 3 deep breaths or until the tightness in your back releases.
5. Repeat until the tissue tension experienced during first stretch has resolved (often 2 times).

Cat/Dog Stretch Exercise

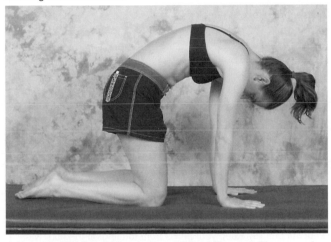

1. Kneel on the floor with your knees hip-width apart. Place your hands on the floor shoulder-width apart and palms down.
2. Slowly arch your back from your tailbone to your upper back like a cat stretches. Allow your head to lower comfortably. Hold position for 3 slow breaths.
3. Slowly release the stretch in the reverse order.
4. Once in the starting position, lift your buttocks upward, let your belly relax forward toward the floor, and slowly look toward the ceiling.
5. Hold this position for 3 breaths and gradually return to the starting position.
6. Repeat until the tissue tension experienced during the first stretch has resolved (often 2 times).

Hip Flexor Stretch Exercise

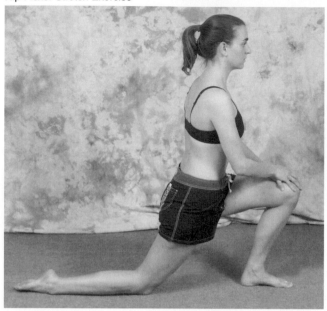

1. Kneel on one knee. Bend your other knee to 90 degrees and place your hands on it for balance.
2. Lean your trunk forward while keeping your low back straight.
3. Hold this position for 3 slow breaths, and then slowly return to the starting position.
4. Repeat until the tissue tension experienced during the first stretch has resolved (often 2 times).

Piriformis Exercise

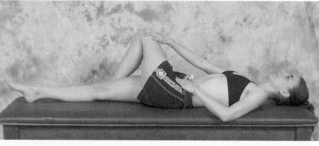

1. Lie on your back with your legs straight. To stretch the left side, bend your left knee and place your left ankle over your right knee with the left foot on floor.
2. Place your left hand on the left side of the pelvis and your right hand on your left knee.
3. Slowly pull your left knee across the right leg, feeling the stretch in your left buttock. Keep your pelvis from rotating off the floor with your left hand.
4. Hold this position for at least 3 slow deep breaths.
5. Slowly and gently return to the resting position.
6. Repeat steps 1 thru 6 until the tissue tension experienced during the first stretch has resolved (often 2 times).
7. Repeat with the right leg.

Hamstring Exercise

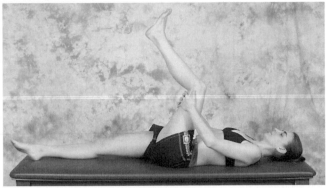

1. Lie on your back with your legs straight.
2. Gently bend one knee and grasp behind the thigh. Do not lift your pelvis or other knee off the floor during this exercise.
3. Straighten your knee. Go only as far as your flexibility will comfortably allow, and hold for 3 slow breaths.
4. Slowly lower your leg to the floor, and repeat for the other leg.
5. Repeat each side until the tissue tension experienced during the first stretch has resolved (often 2 times).

Strength Exercises
Abdominal Curl-Up Exercise

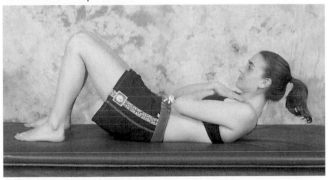

1. Lie on your back with your knees comfortably bent and your arms placed across your chest.
2. Keeping your neck and shoulders relaxed, lift your rib cage from the floor. Move only as far as your body will allow without pain. Hold position for 1 or 2 deep breaths.
3. Slowly and gently return to resting position.
4. Repeat until your abdominal muscles weaken or you notice that you are using your neck and shoulder muscles to perform the exercise.

Gluteus Maximus Exercise

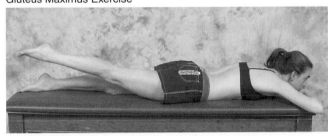

1. Lie on your stomach with your toes pointing downward and your legs straight.
2. Slowly raise one leg as far as is comfortable. Keep your pelvis flat on the floor and the buttock on that side tight.
3. Hold position for 3 deep breaths, or until muscles feel fatigued.
4. Gently return to the resting position. Repeat with the other leg.
5. Repeat with both legs until your muscles feel fatigued.

Gluteus Medius Exercise

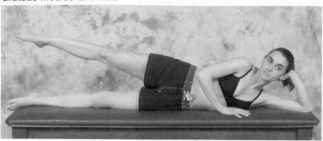

1. Lie on one side, keeping the leg that is on the floor straight or bent at the hip and knee and your top hand on the floor in front of you to maintain stability.
2. Raise your upper leg as far as is comfortable and painless, using your hip muscles only.
3. Hold this position for 3 slow breaths, and slowly return the leg to the resting position.
4. Repeat until fatigued or until you are using other than your hip muscles, and increase repetitions as tolerated.
5. Turn to your other side and repeat steps 1 through 4.

Coordination Exercises
Standing-on-One-Leg Exercise

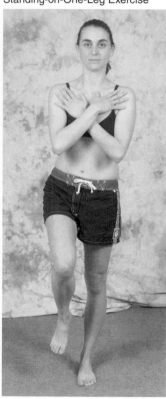

1. Stand on one leg and maintain your balance. Keep your back straight and your arms across your upper chest.
2. Hold this position for 1 minute while continuing slow, deep breaths.
3. Gently return to resting position and repeat 2 times on each leg.
4. After mastering this exercise, perform step 2 with your eyes closed.

Section II Mind-Body

Self-Hypnosis Techniques

Steven Gurgevich, PhD

Hypnosis is a system or collection of methods that allows us to enhance the communication and sharing of information between and within the mind-body. Because the body "hears" everything that enters the subconscious mind, these methods are a way of accessing and influencing subconscious effects on the body. We can do this entirely by ourselves, with the help of others, or by use of learning materials such as books, videos, and audio programs. Whether someone helps us (such as a trained therapist) or we do it by ourselves, all hypnosis is self-hypnosis.

One of these methods is trance. A hypnotic trance is a state of consciousness in which our focus of awareness allows us to become greatly absorbed in the experience and sensations of our ideas. A daydream is a good example of trance. In a daydream, we are aware of where we are and what we are doing, but at the same time, we are absorbed in the experience and sensations of the daydream—our thoughts, ideas, and images. In other words, a hypnotic trance and a daydream are very similar. Although most daydreams might occur spontaneously when we are bored or have too little to actively think about, a hypnotic trance is a state of consciousness we create deliberately. Learning to use this exquisite tool to enhance mind-body communication for healing, greater performance, comfort, and relaxation is easy and beneficial.

Hypnosis includes many different ways of creating that daydream-like state of mind. Among them are induction techniques, imagery methods, focusing concentration, and forms of passive relaxation and meditation. Once we learn them and discover how to achieve the desired results, we own those abilities for as long as we practice them.

What kinds of abilities might we learn this way? A very short list includes overcoming anxiety on an airplane, relaxing the smooth muscle of the intestines for more comfortable digestion, relieving pain, healing skin conditions, improving sleep patterns, changing habits, improving concentration skills, alleviating nausea associated with chemotherapy, improving surgical outcomes, and unlearning physiologic stress response systems. Andrew Weil, MD, says, "In general, I believe that no condition is out of bounds for trying hypnotherapy on."[1]

Although there are many different techniques to access subconscious influence on the body, for practicality this chapter focuses on one tool that primary care providers can easily use and teach their patients. This tool requires the following six main principles:

- Educate to remove preconceived fears and prevailing misconceptions.

- Tailor to match images, ideas, and hypnotic suggestions to the individual.

- Induce trance: thumb-and-finger release technique to trigger trance and staircase technique to help with progressive muscle relaxation and deepening of trance.

- Use trance for a specific purpose (headache, surgery).

- Re-alert to guide the patient out of trance.

- Debrief to develop insight into what worked and how to implement future techniques.

The Six Main Principles

Educate

To remove any fear and misunderstanding and to achieve a better clinical response, you must take time to educate your patient about hypnosis. Your first task is to dispel the myths and misconceptions. The most predominant misconceptions, and their corrections, are as follows.

- That hypnosis is "done to someone." Hypnosis is not done to anyone; it may be guided and taught, as all hypnosis is self-hypnosis.

- The subject loses consciousness and conscious control: At all times, the subject is consciously aware of where he is and what he is doing.

- The subject can be made to do things or to reveal things that she ordinarily would not do in a waking state: The subject is very much aware and is always in control of what she is choosing to experience.
- The subject must be gullible or weak-minded to be hypnotized: Again, this concept is false. Research has shown that some of the best subjects are those with greater intellectual capacity, open-mindedness, and creativity.

The next task is to define trance as a heightened state of conscious awareness in which an individual is more prone to suggestion. Emphasize that everyone has experienced trance many times. One example is daydreaming. Another is being absorbed in a good movie, when we are less aware of activities around us and more responsive to suggestions emanating from the screen. We might jump at the sudden appearance of the hideous alien monster, or we might cry at the plight of a character. At the same time, we are always in control and can go get popcorn if we want.

Like a good movie, hypnosis involves three factors: absorption, dissociation, and suggestibility. Through an induction technique, the subject becomes fully absorbed in the matter at hand, resulting in dissociation from various distractions. This creates a heightened state of awareness that allows the subject to be more receptive to suggestions that can influence physical and behavioral change. In addition to these factors, the vital ingredients[2] that enhance therapeutic effectiveness are the patient's motivation, belief, and expectations for success.

> Hypnosis requires three key factors: absorption, dissociation, and suggestibility.

Tailor

The talented therapist tailors the hypnotic technique to the subject's unique needs and beliefs. The more the technique relates to the subject, the more that person will accept hypnosis and find it useful. In contrast, if you use a technique that encourages an image associated with anger or fear or that is simply foreign to the patient, the process is counterproductive. Think of tailoring as your effort to make the hypnotic experience personally familiar to the subject.

Although there are more complex ways of performing this tailoring, here are a few easily remembered questions or suggestions you can use to help personalize the hypnosis to a patient's beliefs and interests:

- Imagine a favorite place, one that brings comfort and a sense of peace.
- What is your favorite color?
- What are some of your favorite activities and pastimes?
- What kinds of events and activities give you the greatest pleasure?

Testing Hypnotic Talent
In familiarizing yourself and your patients with their current level of hypnotic talent, inform them that you would like to explore their present ability for "mind-body communication" with one or both of these simple procedures.

▪ The Hand Clasp

- Clasp your hands together and interlace your fingers. Imagine that your hands are glued together. Feel how tight the glue holds them.
- Now imagine that the glue between your hands has grown even stronger, or you can imagine that your hands are in a vise that keeps them together.
- Continue to concentrate on how firmly your hands are stuck together. Perhaps you have felt how strong superglue is. Keeping the "stuckness" firmly in mind, try to pull your hands apart while focusing on the image or idea of your hands stuck together.
- If your hands remain stuck to one another, let yourself play with the idea and how well your body responded to your thoughts.
- Then imagine your hands free of each other and gently pull them apart.
- If your hands did not remain stuck together, even a little, play some more and see what happens. Sooner or later, your subconscious will accept the idea and image in your mind. The key is to make the image in your mind the dominant idea as you do this.

Ask your patient, Were you able to feel as if your hands were stuck together, even momentarily? The greater the ability, the more hypnotic talent.

▪ Ideosensory Experience
Ideosensory experience refers to the ability or capacity of the mind-body to respond to the idea or imagination of sensory stimuli (idea + sensory = ideosensory), that is, an idea in mind that produces a sensory response. Proceed speaking through each step as you help your patient develop the image as fully as possible in the imagination.

- Imagine that you have a freshly picked lemon in your hand. Imagine holding the lemon, feeling its weight, examining the texture of the skin, the color.
- Imagine scraping the skin enough to release some of the oil from the skin. If you are demonstrating this to your patient, squint or act as if lemon oil is squirting from the rind as you scrape it.
- Imagine the smell of the freshly released lemon scent.
- Now imagine that you are placing the lemon on a cutting board and slicing it slowly into two parts.
- See, in your imagination, the lemon juice released as the knife cuts through the lemon.
- Picture the lemon juice on the cutting board as you pick up one half of the freshly cut lemon.
- Imagine bringing the lemon half to your mouth and licking the juicy surface with your tongue.
- If needed or desired, have the patient close the eyes and repeat the instructions.

Ask the patient, Could you feel the weight of the lemon? Were you able to smell the lemon? Could you see the oil released when the rind was scraped or the juice released when you cut or squeezed it? Could you taste it? The stronger the sensation, the more hypnotic talent.

If the patient is not able to experience either of these sensations, that person may not be an ideal candidate for hypnotherapy.

Induce Trance

The practitioner performs trance induction for the first hypnosis session so that the patient can become familiar with it. It will be helpful if you can walk the patient through this so he or she feels comfortable doing it himself or herself. Children can do this easily, but adults often need a little practice.

In trance induction, it is helpful to use a trigger (i.e., a conditioned response) to tell the body it is time to relax and focus. Each time the individual uses or rehearses hypnosis with that particular method of induction, the procedure signals the associated responses, and the body "learns" and becomes conditioned. This creates a more automatic response to the trigger, and the more it is used, the easier it becomes to induce trance. It is important to use your voice to convey the message you intend. That is, use inflections, pauses, tone and volume, and accent to emphasize your message. It is also important to embed statements of positive reinforcement during the trance work so patients can develop the ability to do this on their own.

There are many different techniques for trance induction. Two examples are described here.

■ Thumb-and-Finger Technique

Instruct the patient to gently press the tips of the thumb and index finger together in the OK sign. Then tell him that when ready, he may close the eyes, take a deep breath, and hold that breath while you count to 5. With each increasing number, tell the patient that he is deliberately increasing some acceptable anxiety and to make it a physical experience by pressing his thumb and finger more tightly together. Let the patient know that he is in control of this form of tension and anxiety, and when you reach 5, he is to exhale the breath and release and relax the thumb and finger. Tell the patient to continue with the eyes closed and to permit the hand to relax and to allow breathing to become calm and regular. You may say that this acts as a cue or signal for him to relax and go into trance. This technique can be used at any time by the patient for self-hypnosis. Again, with repetition, it creates a conditioned response that facilitates a faster and easier induction.

■ Imagining a Relaxation Staircase

By imagining a beautiful staircase with 10 steps, the patient can use each step to focus on relaxing a different part of the body as she descends to her favorite place. In the brackets in the following passage, insert the patient's preferences that you learned during tailoring, such as favorite place or color. The relaxation staircase technique, which is also a technique for deepening of the trance, may go something like this:

Imagine a beautiful [favorite color] staircase that has 10 steps. These 10 steps lead to a peaceful and relaxing [favorite place]. In a moment, I am going to start counting backward from 10 to 1. With each step, you can notice your body relaxing more comfortably, allowing you to gently relax deeper and deeper with each step. It will be so very nice to discover which parts of your body relax more quickly and easily, as tension is automatically released.

As you start at the top of the staircase, allow each exhalation to release any tension or strain in your body. Let each breath now be a "relaxing breath."

10 . . . Relax your face and jaw, letting your tongue gently rest at the floor of your mouth.

9 . . . Relax your temples, eyes, and eyelids as we step down to . . .

8 . . . Relax the back of your neck and shoulders, simply letting go.

7 . . . Relax your arms, knowing that there is nothing for them to do.

And sometimes you will notice that your body is already getting ahead of my voice and the numbers, and sometimes it feels so comfortable when your body catches up to your relaxation.

6 . . . Relax your chest, with each rise and fall of the breath.

5 . . . Relax your abdomen, setting the muscles free.

4 . . . Relax your pelvis, allowing it to sink into the chair.

Sometimes your body may feel so "heavy" that it feels like you are sinking, and other times you feel so "light" that it may seem that you are floating. Whatever you experience is correct for you . . . let it happen.

3 . . . Relax your legs, giving them the day off with nothing to support.

2 . . . Relax your toes as we arrive at . . .

1 . . .

And continue past zero as you feel comfortable and at ease with this very relaxed form of concentration.

Hypnotic Strategies

We distinguish two hypnotic strategies or approaches in using clinical hypnosis in practice. One strategy is symptomatic, in which the emphasis of the hypnotic work is exclusively directed toward altering or removing symptoms. In most cases, the symptomatic approach is simple and effective. However, when symptoms do not respond to the symptomatic approach or when "symptom substitution" follows the removal of the original condition (when one symptom resolves but is replaced by another), then we look for a possible underlying or subconscious origin. That is, we look for underlying emotional conflicts that are being expressed by the body. This other strategy is called psychodynamic, and it more specifically addresses the origins or causes of the symptoms. The metaphor for exploring symptoms psychodynamically might best be thought of as the symptoms are "out of mind, but not out of body."

An example to illustrate the two strategies might involve a headache, for which the symptomatic approach relies on relaxation and imagery of comfort to relieve tension. The psychodynamic approach for a headache resilient to the symptomatic approach would address metaphorical questions, such as, Who is the pain in the neck? or What is the pain in the neck for you? In later examples, we are exploring the possibility of an underlying psychodynamic process in which emotional stresses are being expressed as physical symptoms. For our purposes in this chapter on self-hypnosis techniques, we will limit our examples and exercises to the symptomatic strategy or symptomatic approach.

Use

Use is the process of focused attention (trance) for a therapeutic purpose, such as symptom relief. This phase is what distinguishes hypnosis from meditation and relaxation exercises.

This section describes scenarios that may be used for some common problems seen in the primary care setting.

Gastrointestinal Disorders: Gentle Movement or Healing Color

Hypnosis is an excellent tool for unlearning and relieving gastrointestinal conditions such as irritable bowel syndrome, although the imagery you use can be modified to describe healing comfort from upper gastric distress, constipation, or other gastrointestinal symptoms.

One easy method to use with patients is to have them visualize a soothing color as it travels the entire alimentary canal from mouth to rectum, calming and healing as it goes. For example, you might speak as follows to your patient:

Recognize that your digestive system, your alimentary canal, from mouth to rectum is lined with smooth muscle that functions automatically. And throughout the alimentary canal, the smooth muscle produces a gentle wavelike motion, called peristalsis, which moves food through you in the proper direction from swallowing to elimination. Your thoughts and mental images are messages that slow or speed up this gentle wavelike motion so that you are comfortable and can enjoy natural, healthy, and comfortable digestion.

Now imagine that you are swallowing [patient's favorite color] in the form of a gentle light or a soothing liquid that will travel all the way through your digestive system in a comfortable, peaceful, healthy way. Follow that soothing [color] from your mouth and down your esophagus. As the [color] flows downward, let yourself feel a calm inner peace as your digestive tract begins to relax and restore itself, so that you can easily digest a wide variety of foods comfortably and easily and with peace of mind. As the soothing [color] gently moves down your esophagus, it comes to your stomach. Visualize the lining of your stomach as healthy and producing exactly the right amount of digestive juices to easily and comfortably digest your food. And as the soothing [color] begins to move into your intestine, you can know that it helps your food move through at the proper rate so your body absorbs all the nutrients from your food, to provide you with vitality, energy, and resources for healing.

The beautiful [color] continues to move through your intestines, easily guided by the gentle wavelike motion of peristalsis, as your body remains calm and relaxed and unaware of this motion. Your body is learning from this experience, and now you have the ability to choose a great comfort, a wonderful soothing comfort throughout your stomach and intestines and colon. Even when your body lets you know there are stresses around you, you can quickly override the bodily stress response by making a conscious decision to give your body the message for comfort as you are doing right now. You can now "let go" of stress. And "let go" is a phrase that will now provide a powerful and soothing message whenever you want to detach from stress around or within you. Let yourself "feel" the calm inner peace and comfort within your digestive tract, the healthy, gentle, calm process by which you easily digest and eliminate your food. Your body has just memorized this experience with you.

Headache: Cool Breeze Technique

The imagery of cooling the head helps facilitate vasoconstriction. Add the imagery of warming the hands to direct greater circulation to the extremities and to help reduce pressure and pain in the head, particularly for migraines.

This induction technique often also reduces pain by facilitating relaxation. Further time spent on relaxation of the head muscles is warranted because tension is often involved in the pathogenesis of headaches. You might say the following or something similar to your patient:

Feel the muscles in your temples relax, focus your attention on your eyes and forehead, and let them relax with each breath out. With each breath, let the muscles relax more and more. Now follow the muscles through the scalp to the base of the skull and relax this area, exhale, and feel the whole head relax. Imagine walking along a snowy path in the mountains with a cool breeze blowing across your face, cooling your head, your face, and your eyes. Imagine a cool and soothing sensation across your forehead and above each eye. Your hands are tucked in your pockets, so they are warming, and they are warm. Your hands are warm and comfortable, while a cool breeze and cold air make your head feel cooler, soothing and relaxing every muscle, releasing any tightness, any stress. Just feel a calm sensation flow through your eyes and forehead. You are calm and comfortable and relaxed. Just notice the cool breeze of each breath coming in your nose and softly blowing up and into your forehead, and the air warmed by your hands and body now being exhaled. Cool air in, soothing your head . . . warm air out, relaxing your body.

Repeat if needed.

Localized Pain From Injury or Preparation for Painful Procedure: Glove Anesthesia Technique

The glove anesthesia technique involves creating numbness in one of the patient's hands that then can be transferred from the hand to any part of the body for pain relief. Tailor the technique by asking the patient's favorite color and say something like the following:

Focus your attention on one of your hands. Direct all of your attention on that hand, and begin to imagine that hand becoming numb. Recall a time your hand fell asleep and how wooden your hand felt. As you numb your hand, imagine it gradually turning [insert favorite color]. Your hand is turning [favorite color], and as it does, there is a tingling in your fingertips, and warmth flows through your hand. Soon all the feeling will drain out of your hand as it turns a deeper [favorite color]. Let it go, let the feeling drain from your hand. That hand is feeling so numb, so very numb. That hand feels heavy, and it feels as if it were made of wood. Let all the feeling drain from your hand, so it now begins to glow a beautiful [favorite color]. Let your hand feel numb; let it feel numb as it glows brighter, glows like a beautiful [favorite color] light bulb. Your hand is now completely numb and filled with [favorite color] light.

Now place your numb [favorite color] hand on your [insert part of body . . . knee, jaw], place your hand on your [body part], and now let the numbness and the [favorite color] light drain into your [body part]. Feel your [body part] become numb and watch as the numbing [favorite color] light slowly leaves your hand and covers your [body part], making it numb, wooden-like, heavy, numb, numb, thick, as if it were made of wood. When all the [favorite color] light has left your hand numbing your [body part], place your hand back down into a comfortable position [pause]. You can keep your [body part] numb for as long as you need to, as long as you need to. When you have completed this process, just let go and feel the numbness and the [favorite color] light drain away, drain away, and your [body part] returns to normal. When you no longer need it to be numb, it returns to normal.

Warts: Hand Tracing Technique

This technique is best used for children with warts. Proceed as follows:

1. Have the patient trace both hands (or draw other parts of the body that may contain warts) on a piece of paper.
2. Have the patient draw where the warts are located on the tracing (Fig. 92-1).
3. Tailor the technique by asking about his or her favorite place and color.
4. Have the patient go to this favorite place (children are able to do this quickly and easily, but adults may have to use the induction technique discussed previously).

   Then say something like the following to the patient:

   Imagine that you are miniaturized. Small enough to get in a beautiful [favorite color] spaceship and travel through your body to where your warts are.

   Look at the roots of the wart and see what they are like. What would you like to do to prevent the roots from getting any nourishment from your body? Would you like to spray them or paint them with a powerful chemical that only warts can feel? Or would you like to cap them off with a plastic bubble, or cut them off and take them out of your body?

   As the patient invents a method to "treat" the roots of the warts, you might give some brief suggestions that reinforce the patient's power to do this from within himself or herself.

   Go ahead and do that now and make sure that you treat all your warts.

   Do you need more time to work on the warts?

   When the patient says that he or she has finished, ask him or her to do "one more thing" to ensure that these warts do not stand a chance.

   Your body will continue to work on these warts, even while you are sleeping.

   How long do you think it will take your body to remove these warts? I wonder how quickly your body will get the job done for you?

5. Then have the patient return to normal size and come out of the body. Offer encouragement on how well he or she did, how powerful his or her images seem, and how well his or her body heard everything it needed to do its part of the job.
6. After the patient comes out of trance, have him or her erase the warts on the tracing created previously. Have the patient use an eraser or paint the warts with white correction fluid.
7. Have the patient perform this technique one more time at home. Success with wart resolution has been found with two or three imagery sessions.

Improving Surgical Outcomes

Much evidence shows that patients can use hypnosis to make surgery a more comfortable experience by lessening pain, blood loss, and nausea and vomiting due to anesthesia and also by speeding up wound healing and overall recovery. Furthermore, studies have shown that hypnotic suggestions to these ends are equally effective if they are delivered by a person or by an audio program.

If at all possible, patients should practice this technique on their own for at least 3 days before surgery. Be sure to emphasize that they are preparing themselves very well for their healing experience by doing so. Postoperatively, they should begin the technique as soon as possible and continue for as long as needed. Overall, the suggestions should indicate that the surgical experience is comfortable and that recovery is rapid, effective, and easy for them.

Before surgery, the following suggestions will be effective:

You are preparing for a wonderful healing experience. Your body and mind are using only your positive words, images, and expectations for a comfortable and effective healing experience. Each time you practice or rehearse with your self-hypnosis, your body and mind are memorizing the positive messages as special instructions for comfortable healing. Any anxiety is easily replaced now by relaxing thoughts and feelings of comfort. You are in control of your inner comfort and can use any sounds or sensations from the environment around you to deepen your comfort.

Whenever you are distracted, you can quickly and easily return to your special place within you, your place of inner peace and confidence that reminds you that you are doing well, all is going well, and that you are preparing for a wonderfully comfortable and effective healing experience. Your body has begun performing its natural function of protecting you from any infection, managing blood flow, and using the procedure to enhance its inner-healing work. During and after the procedure, you will have all the "comfort control" [spoken with emphasis] you need to awaken feeling peacefully at ease with little or no discomfort.

The following postoperative suggestions will assist in rapid recovery:

You have done very well, and now your body is concentrating its powerful healing energy to mend the cells and tissues as your immune system maintains a peaceful balance of protection. Your body is releasing an abundance of the natural chemicals of comfort called endorphins, which circulate everywhere within you and concentrate themselves where you need the greatest comfort now. Immediately after the procedure, your body awakens each system and function

FIGURE 92-1
Patient's location of warts on a tracing of the hands.

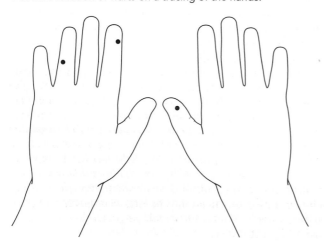

to continue the healing process. Your intestines and bowels awaken comfortably and gently begin their natural action. Sensations of hunger and thirst awaken gently, and you welcome the nourishment. Your body is healing rapidly and effectively, and you are feeling confidently in control through this rapid recovery time. You recognize how well you have done, and you deserve to take credit for how well you have done.

Re-Alert

Re-alerting the patient out of trance is simply the reversal of the induction technique, such as climbing the staircase with energy coming back into the relaxed muscles, with a suggestion to return to a fully alert, waking state feeling refreshed and at ease. The process of re-alerting involves not only speech but also tone of voice. As you come closer to having the patient open the eyes, the tone of your voice should reflect "refreshment" accordingly. You should reinforce the idea that the patient has done well and can comfortably use this technique as needed in the future.

For re-alerting, say the following or something like it to the patient:

It is now time to shift over and bring yourself to a fully alert, waking state. As we climb the staircase, counting each step, afterward you will be happy that you have done well with this method and proud because you realize that you can revisit this place whenever you need or desire.

As you proceed up the first step, feel the energy awakening your body, starting at your toes …

2 … And now allow it to flow up your legs …

3 … into your pelvis and lower back …

4 … traveling to your abdomen, as you feel your body refreshing itself.

5 … Take in this energy with each rise of your chest.

Your voice can become stronger as you return to a more normal pattern of speech.

6 … as you feel it travel into your arms …

7 … going up to your shoulders and neck …

8 … into your temples, eyes and eyelids.

Your voice should now be normal to waking state.

9 … Feel your tongue, jaw, and the muscles of your face energize, and allow your eyes to open when you are ready to feel wonderfully refreshed and energized.

You want to make sure that your patients are out of trance, and that can be done by taking time to engage in conversation, asking them how they are feeling and ensuring that they are fully reoriented to time, place, and person. The debriefing conversation that follows the trance work is also a good time to make sure that they are fully alert and oriented.

Debrief

After the procedure, when the patients are alert, engage them in a conversation that allows you to assess their experience during the self-hypnosis. You might ask about physical sensations, nature of any resistance, what they liked, what they did not like, and so on. The time to debrief after the hypnotic trance work lets you gain insight not only into what they experienced but also into what you want to remember to use with them in future sessions. The debriefing is an excellent opportunity to provide patients with encouragement about what they achieved and how they will continue to improve with these mind-body skills with practice.

Homework for the Patient

Your patients should first undergo induction, use, and re-alerting from trance with you as a learning experience in a clinical setting so they can see how to do it on their own. Think of it as a rehearsal for what you want your patients to practice by themselves. With the exception of removing warts (which requires only one or two sessions because further sessions may actually hinder the process), it is important to encourage your patients to practice or rehearse their self-hypnosis method to become more proficient with it. For conditions such as pain, there is no limit to the frequency of use.

Educate your patients to use this tool on their own by practicing at home what they experienced with you in the office. Review from beginning to end the steps the patients took with you; remind them that the body reacts to everything the patient may say, hear, think, and imagine and that it uses the patient's thoughts and ideas as instructions for the inner work to be achieved. Ask your patients to tell you where they plan to practice at home and what they are going to say or think to themselves to make it happen. Provide instructions as necessary to set them in motion for a positive experience at home. You might even give them a handout containing the words you spoke, along with instructions, or recommend an audio CD or audio program specific to them.

> Hypnotic induction and suggestion is an art that takes time and practice, yet simple techniques such as those discussed should be used to enhance care in the primary care setting. For more complicated cases, referral should be made to a licensed practitioner.

What to Look for in a Consultant

When referring your patient for hypnosis, be sure to review the therapist's qualifications to treat the underlying condition. A good rule of thumb: never refer a patient to a practitioner who does not have the qualifications to treat the specific condition without hypnosis.

There are many so-called certified hypnotherapists advertising their services. Frequently, their certification comes from a lay school of hypnosis that teaches them only the techniques of hypnosis, and they do not possess any education in medicine, psychology, social work, or dentistry. Choose a practitioner licensed in a clinical specialty who is certified by the American Society of Clinical Hypnosis (ASCH). This professional organization provides extensive, comprehensive training and requires supervised practice before granting certification. The American Society of clinical Hypnosis Web site (www.asch.net) provides referrals to qualified practitioners.

KEY WEB RESOURCES

www.cancer.gov/bcrisktool/Default.aspx	National Cancer Institute breast cancer risk calculator
www.asch.net	The American Society of Clinical Hypnosis offers excellent workshops that lead to certification and provides information for finding certified practitioners in clinical hypnosis. Their number is 630-980-4740.
http://www.sceh.us/	The Society for Clinical and Experimental Hypnosis offers professional training in clinical hypnosis for licensed physicians, psychologists, dentists, clinical social workers, nurses, and counselors. Ample resources are provided for professionals interested in clinical hypnosis.
http://erickson-foundation.org/	The Milton H. Erickson Foundation is dedicated to promoting and advancing the contributions made to the health sciences by the late Milton H. Erickson, MD, through training of mental health professionals and health professions worldwide.
http://www.ijceh.com	*International Journal of Clinical and Experimental Hypnosis*
http://www.apa.org/divisions/div30/	American Psychological Association, Society of Psychological Hypnosis, Division 30
www.HealingwithHypnosis.com	Steven Gurgevich, PhD, Healing with Hypnosis Web site with more than 50 audio, DVD, and book titles of therapeutic applications of clinical hypnosis, including *Surgery and Recovery, Cancer Support: Chemotherapy and Radiation Therapy, Immune Booster,* and *Healing Mind, Healing Body*
http://www.thehealingmind.org/	The Healing Mind, books and audios in guided imagery by Martin Rossman, MD
http://www.healthjourneys.com/	Health Journeys, guided imagery audios by Belleruth Naparstek

References

References available online at expertconsult.com.

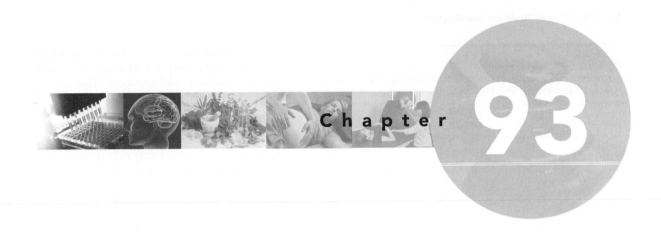

Relaxation Techniques

Michael Lumpkin, PhD, and David Rakel, MD

Historical Perspective

In the early twentieth century, the physiologist Walter Cannon discovered that when subjects were exposed to certain physical and mentally stressful events, they secreted a large amount of epinephrine that prepared them for action. Cannon later coined the term "fight-or-flight response" to describe this physical reaction to stress. In contrast, in the 1930s, the Nobel Prize–winning Swiss physiologist Walter Hess found that by stimulating certain areas of the brain of laboratory animals, he was able to induce a physical reaction opposite to that seen with the fight-or-flight response. Specific areas of the brain triggered signs of relaxation, such as reductions in muscle tone, breathing, and heart rate. Herbert Benson, working from the same laboratory as Cannon had years earlier, helped pioneer this field when he described the relaxation response and how meditation could be used to decrease the response of the sympathetic nervous system. Meditation was found to reduce heart rate, respiratory rate, plasma cortisol, and pulse rate and to increase electroencephalogram alpha waves, which are associated with relaxation.[1] Evidence accumulated to confirm that lifestyle practices can have a direct influence on disease and its prevention.

> Relaxation techniques are tools that will help balance the effects of stress but are not substitutes for exploring problems that may be causing the stress.

Pathophysiology

The Hypothalamus

That stress has damaging effects on health through dysregulation of the autonomic nervous system and the hypothalamic-pituitary-adrenal (HPA) axis is well established.[2]

As can be seen in Figure 93-1, stress triggers emotions that release chemicals through these sites to stimulate somatic changes that can lead to poor health. Chronic stress results in a continuous activation of cycle A in the figure, which helps explain the association between chronic stress and increased susceptibility to disease. To understand this link more clearly, it is helpful to outline the mechanisms by which stressors disrupt the mind-body balance, that is, how they perturb homeostasis. Stressors, whether physical, metabolic, psychological, or emotional, fall into one of two broad categories. They can be the acute, short-lived type or they can be chronic and unrelenting. When a person experiences acute stress, a rapid coordination of nervous, endocrine, and immune system responses occurs to promote the immediate survival of the individual. The brain's hypothalamus is the central element in these essential interactive responses. The hypothalamus is the integrative center of the central nervous system because it simultaneously monitors neural, hormonal, metabolic, and immune signals arising from inside the body and compares these inputs with information being sent to it from inside and outside the body by various receptor systems. Further, the state of mind—whether one is fearful, depressed, angry, or happy—is perceived by higher brain centers, and this information is also projected to the hypothalamus for processing and comparison with the baseline activities of the other organ systems as detected by the hypothalamus.

Specific information about the body's stress reactions is transmitted to the hypothalamus, in part, by bloodborne solutes such as glucose, electrolytes, fatty acids, amino acids, hormones, peptides, cytokines, and other compounds that serve as communication molecules. The hypothalamus also receives information through neural inputs from lower brain centers such as the midbrain and spinal cord and from the higher brain structures of the cerebral cortex, hippocampus, and amygdala. This makes the hypothalamus the conversion point for peripheral and central signals that can be integrated in such a way that proper

FIGURE 93-1
A simplified chart showing the cyclic mind-body and body-mind influences of stress (A) and relaxation (B) on health. As our body experiences the physical responses to stress and relaxation, our central nervous system remembers them, thus causing a continuation of the cycle, with long-term positive or negative physical consequences. HR, heart rate; Resp, respiratory.

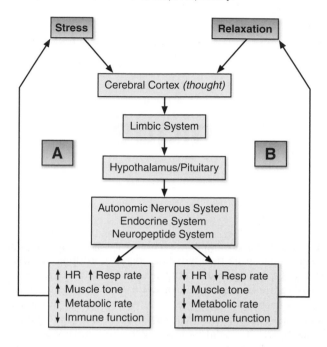

hormonal, autonomic, and behavioral changes are executed in the biologic defense of the individual.

Specifically, the hypothalamus responds to these signals by producing and releasing the "master" neurohormones known as the hypothalamic releasing factors that regulate anterior pituitary hormone secretion that, in turn, govern stress responses, reproductive activity, metabolism, growth, lactation, and fluid balance. To ensure a coordinated stress response, the hypothalamus also governs sympathetic and parasympathetic information flow to the visceral organs, tissues, and blood vessels of the body. The nervous connections of the cortical and limbic structures to the hypothalamus noted earlier form the anatomic basis for the transmission of conscious thoughts, emotions, and memories to the hypothalamus so that it can make appropriate adjustments in hormone secretion and autonomic outflow in an attempt to maintain homeostasis. On perceiving a stressor, the hypothalamus alters visceral organ activity to maximize the activation of critical functions such as increasing blood pressure and heart rate while reducing blood flow to tissues such as the gut and kidneys, where needs are less immediate.[3] This overall arrangement forms the very basis for the mind-body connection and can explain physiologically why relaxation techniques can reduce stress and favorably affect stress-related disorders.

Often, to be motivated to practice relaxation techniques, a person must first become aware that he or she is not at ease and is in need of stress reduction. Neurophysiologically, this may happen because the pathways of connectivity described earlier allow the factual information and conscious thoughts

of the cerebral cortex to arrive at the hippocampus and amygdala, where they are placed into a usable context by attaching memory and emotion. This consolidated information is then projected into the hypothalamus.[4] At this point, the hypothalamus and its various releasing hormone neurons elicit the specific hormonal, autonomic, metabolic, and behavioral changes that are appropriate for the physical or emotional stress being experienced. Most of the time, these autonomic alterations in the body's physiology are not consciously perceived. Because of projection pathways exiting from the hypothalamus that relay this information to the thalamus and from the thalamus back to the cerebral cortex, however, individuals can become aware of changes in their physiologic responses to stress. With this increased perception of stress and agitation, a person may choose to act on or moderate these responses. These neuronal pathways and their linkages to hypothalamic (autonomic) signaling provide the basis for the effectiveness of mind-body relaxation techniques such as biofeedback to address stress-related dysfunction.[5]

Hypothalamic-Pituitary-Adrenal Axis

Acute Stress Response
That most stressors stimulate the hypothalamic release of corticotropin-releasing hormone (CRH) and that CRH stimulates adrenocorticotropic hormone (ACTH) from the anterior pituitary gland are well known.[6] ACTH then increases the synthesis and release of the glucocorticoid hormone cortisol, as well as the androgens androstenedione and dehydroepiandrosterone from the adrenal cortex. The stress hormone cortisol is critical during an acute fight-or-flight challenge because it maintains blood glucose concentrations to fuel metabolic processes and supports sodium and water retention to maintain blood volume and perfusion pressures to activated organs. During the healthy and useful acute stress response, the blood concentrations of cortisol increase until they negatively feed back on the hypothalamic-pituitary unit to decrease the elevated levels of CRH and ACTH to their baselines.[7] This action prevents unnecessarily extended elevations in CRH, ACTH, and cortisol after acute stress.[8] In this acute situation, metabolic substrate mobilization, fluid retention, and increased blood volume occur only when a specific need exists.

Chronic Stress Response
In stark contrast, when an individual experiences chronic stress along with maladaptive responses or a lack of coping, cortisol levels may remain elevated because of ongoing activation of the CRH-ACTH-cortisol axis. The high concentrations of cortisol may cause glucocorticoid receptor desensitization in the hypothalamic-pituitary unit and may result in the loss of negative feedback restraint on CRH, ACTH, and cortisol. The subsequent elevations of cortisol may also damage hippocampal neurons (which also have glucocorticoid receptors) and thereby impair memory functions. Other pathophysiologic changes may include the following: the redistribution of fat from the buttocks to the abdominal and cervical regions ("buffalo hump") because of mobilization of free fatty acids; the development of insulin resistance from excessive glucose in the circulation; proteolysis in muscle, bone, and connective tissues; and the

inhibition of peptide and protein hormone formation, especially by the pituitary gland.[9] Ongoing high cortisol levels also suppress immune system function.[10] Rising cortisol levels decrease the proliferation and activity of blood lymphocytes, eosinophils, basophils, monocytes or macrophages, and neutrophils. Chronically elevated glucocorticoids can also decrease antibody and immunoglobulin production. At the same time, increased CRH acts in the brain to stimulate sympathetic outflow and inhibit parasympathetic activity. Because immune tissues such as the thymus gland, spleen, and bone marrow are innervated by sympathetic nerves, and because their immune cells have adrenergic receptors, they are subject to influence by stress-triggered sympathetic outflow.[10] The action of sympathetic catecholamines causes lymphopenia and suppression of natural killer cell activity.[11]

■ Chronic Stress and Gastrointestinal Function

Another organ system adversely affected by chronic stress is the gastrointestinal tract. Stress-induced elevations in hypothalamic CRH change the ratio of sympathetic to parasympathetic inputs to gastrointestinal components. The net outcomes for the stomach are inhibition of gastric contractility and decreased emptying that lead to sensations of fullness and bloating. Conversely, at the colon, the movement of material through the lumen is accelerated, and poor absorption of nutrients and water is the result. Diarrhea and inflammation of the bowel can occur if the stress is of sufficient intensity and length. Some investigators believe that this altered autonomic regulation of the gut resulting from persistent stress may account for the development of irritable bowel syndrome and the exacerbation of Crohn's disease.[12] These inflammatory conditions of the bowel may result in the leaky gut syndrome whereby poorly digested food antigens can provoke inappropriate immune responses that manifest as food allergies, as happens in the gluten sensitivity syndrome of celiac disease.

When one considers the impact of chronic stress on the many different organs and tissues discussed earlier, it is not surprising that poorly managed stress reactions may lead to greater susceptibility to chronic disease development, infectious conditions, and cancer cell proliferation.[13] However, the skillful use of relaxation techniques typical of mind-body medicine methods may be able to short-circuit the entire stress cascade that contributes to the development of disease.

Corticotropin-Releasing Hormone and Stress-Related Behaviors

CRH not only directs the neuroendocrine stress response but also acts directly in the brain as a neurotransmitter to drive stress behaviors that correspond to neuroendocrine events. For example, CRH acts in the brain to enhance locomotor activity, the startle response, and anxiogenic behaviors characteristic of the fight-or-flight response just as levels of stress hormones such as epinephrine and cortisol begin to rise to fuel the whole process.[14,15] CRH injected into the brains of experimental animals induces behaviors that closely mimic the signs and symptoms of major clinical depression in humans.[16] Investigators also know that CRH levels are elevated in the brains and cerebrospinal fluid of people with depression. Not surprisingly, these individuals also demonstrate chronic elevations in the diurnal pattern of cortisol secretion that would then account for some of the hormonal and physiologic disturbances they also endure. In fact, some of these patients may even develop features resembling those seen in Cushing syndrome.[17]

Stress Disorders: High Versus Low Hypothalamic-Pituitary-Adrenal Axis Activity

Whereas certain physical and behavioral disorders of chronic stress are associated with excessive HPA axis activity, some physical and behavioral dysfunctions result from an underfunctioning HPA axis following chronic stress. Clinical investigators Chrousos and Gold sorted out some of the disorders that fall between these two categories of HPA activity.[17]

In addition to chronic stress, long-term activation of the HPA axis is seen in melancholic depression, anorexia nervosa, obligate exercise, diabetes mellitus, metabolic syndrome, and premenstrual syndrome. Some stress-related conditions are so long lasting and severe that the adrenal glands cannot keep up with the added physiologic demands for cortisol. In these situations, a relative deficiency of cortisol (so-called adrenal exhaustion) may result even though the hypothalamus may continue to produce high levels of CRH (and thus may, in fact, drive more depressive behavior). Insufficient cortisol activity is seen in chronic fatigue, fibromyalgia, postpartum depression, posttraumatic stress disorder, and rheumatoid arthritis. Because most or all of these conditions have chronic stress and high states of CRH activation in common, perhaps all could be favorably affected by the use of relaxation techniques that lower stress and thereby lower CRH stimulation and the downstream stress responses it triggers.

In fact, by giving attention to lifestyle changes that reduce stressful triggers and by practicing techniques that activate the relaxation response (cycle B in Fig. 93-1), this approach can have significant health benefits. The relaxation response can be learned, but practice is required for the body to benefit from it. Regular use results in long-term physiologic changes that last throughout the day, not only during the specific time when the relaxation technique is practiced.[18]

> With chronic stress, corticotropin-releasing hormone (CRH) levels are elevated and can exacerbate depressed mood. Cortisol becomes less sensitive to CRH effects, and levels start to drop, resulting in more depression and fatigue. This condition is most effectively treated with a change in perception toward a more relaxed state.

The Evidence for Relaxation

More than 3000 studies show the beneficial effects of relaxation on health. To think that we could cover all of them here would be foolish. Many studies document the value of relaxation exercises such as meditation, breathing, and progressive muscle relaxation. Beneficial effects of relaxation have been shown in tension headaches,[19] anxiety,[20] insomnia,[21] psoriasis,[22] blood pressure,[23,24] cardiac ischemia and exercise tolerance,[25] cardiac arrhythmia,[26] premenstrual syndrome,[27] infertility,[28] longevity and cognitive function in older adults,[29] use of medical care,[30] medical costs in treating chronic pain,[31] smoking cessation,[32] and serum cholesterol levels.[33] Recommending relaxation therapy is very important in the primary care setting because more than 60% of all visits to physicians are stress related.

What Relaxation Exercises Have in Common

It is our mind's thoughts that trigger the physiologic changes that can result in poor health. Working to "get the mind off of it" involves focusing on something other than those thoughts that cause stress. Mental focus is what all relaxation techniques have in common. Meditation may focus on a mantra, yoga may focus on a body posture (asana) or the breath, guided imagery focuses on an image, and progressive muscle relaxation focuses on the muscles. Relaxation does not need to include these traditional mind-body therapies; it may simply involve focusing on a hobby such as painting, playing an instrument, or gardening. Whatever task is used, the mind has a tendency to wander. If this happens, we can simply accept it and bring our attention back to the activity at hand. Using a more structured technique will help stress the importance of this process. Focus frees the mind from its usual stressful thoughts, such as worry, planning, thinking, and reasoning, and dampens the production of adrenergic catecholamines that stimulate the hypothalamus, which in turn inhibits immune activity.

Relaxation and Aerobic Exercise

We usually do not associate relaxation with exercise, but Herbert Benson et al[34] found that the relaxation response could also be elicited during aerobic exercise. Compared with a control group, volunteers who focused their thoughts on a word or phrase while riding a stationary bicycle reduced both their oxygen consumption and their metabolic rate, resulting in better efficiency.[34]

Few people may have the time to meditate for 20 minutes twice a day, exercise for 30 minutes, spend good-quality time with their families, and make a living while getting 8 hours of sleep. Combining relaxation and exercise into one activity uses the time more efficiently.

Matching the Technique to the Individual

Relaxation techniques are similar to ice cream flavors. Someone who finds a flavor he or she likes thinks everyone else should try it. The important thing is not to have every patient meditate, but rather to match a technique to each patient's lifestyle. In fact, investigators have shown that various relaxation techniques, such as meditation, biofeedback, hypnosis, guided imagery, and progressive muscle relaxation, induce the same physiologic response.[35] Many different ways are available to arrive at the desired outcome. A technique that is matched to the individual is more successful in inducing relaxation and will be used more often. For example, a body-vigilant woman with breast cancer may not respond well to progressive muscle relaxation because this technique requires focus on specific parts of the body. An anxious, type A individual may do better with this technique because it gives an active mind a focal point. A relaxation exercise should be as individualized as prescribing a medication for hypertension.

Relaxation exercises are low-cost, well-tolerated therapies that can be recommended for many problems seen in the primary care setting. This approach may be most useful in patients suffering from anxiety, heart disease, recurring pain syndromes, and chronic illness, but it also is beneficial in helping patients find a balance, thus leading to the best medicine of all—prevention. Table 93-1 provides brief summaries of various relaxation exercises, as well as resources.

> The most important task is for the medical provider to match the relaxation technique to the patient's personality, beliefs, and lifestyle.

Growing Beyond the Relaxation Technique

Prescribing relaxation techniques can be a useful tool in helping improve health and reduce symptoms, but exploring our lives and making changes so we do not need to use these tools as often are also important. We are not facilitating deep healing if we maintain a stressful lifestyle and think that it will all be OK if we simply spend 20 minutes each day meditating or doing progressive muscle relaxation. We need to make choices that help us understand how we can live every minute in a more peaceful way. The goal is to require less of these techniques as we learn how to live in a way that resembles how our body feels when practicing one of them.

Peace

It does not mean to be in a place where there is no noise, trouble or hard work. It means to be in the midst of those things and still be calm in your heart.

Unknown

TABLE 93-1. Relaxation Techniques

RELAXATION TECHNIQUE	SUMMARY	FURTHER RESOURCES
Breathing Exercise (see Chapter 89, Breathing Exercises)	The foundation of most relaxation techniques. The subject places one hand on the chest and the other on the abdomen. He or she then takes a slow deep breath, as if sucking in all the air in the room. While doing this, the hand on the abdomen should rise higher than that on the chest. This exercise promotes diaphragmatic breathing, which increases alveolar expansion in the bases of the lungs. The subject holds the breath for a count of 7 and then exhales. Exhalation should take twice as long as inhalation. Repeat for a total of five breaths. Subjects should do this exercise three times a day.	Hendricks G. *Conscious Breathing: Breathwork for Health, Stress Release, and Personal Mastery.* New York: Bantam; 1995. Lewis D. *Free Your Breath, Free Your Life: How Conscious Breathing Can Relieve Stress, Increase Vitality, and Help You Live More Fully.* New York: Shambala; 2004. Weil A. *Breathing: The Master Key to Self Healing (The Self Healing Series)* (audio CD). Louisville, Colo: Sounds True; 2000. Instructional videos on breathing techniques can be found through the University of Wisconsin Integrative Medicine program: http://www.fammed.wisc.edu/our-department/media/integrative-medicine
Meditation (see Chapter 98, Recommending Meditation): Transcendental Meditation (TM) and the Relaxation Response	To prevent distracting thoughts, the subject repeats a mantra (a word or sound) over and over while sitting in a comfortable position. If a distracting thought comes to mind, it is accepted and let go, with the mind focusing again on the mantra.	For information on transcendental meditation: www.tm.org/
Mindfulness Meditation	Represents the philosophy of living in the present moment. The body scan is one technique whereby the subject uses breathing to obtain a relaxed state while lying or sitting. The mind progressively focuses on different parts of the body, where it feels any and all sensations intentionally but nonjudgmentally before moving on to another part of the body. A patient with back pain, for example, may focus on the quality and characteristics of the pain, to understand it better and bring it under control.	For full description of this technique, see Kabat-Zinn J. *Full Catastrophe Living: Using the Wisdom of Your Body and Mind to Face Stress, Pain, and Illness* (reprint). New York: Delta; 1990. Mindfulness stress reduction courses are offered throughout the United States. For more information on training programs, go to the Center for Mindfulness through the University of Massachusetts Medical School: http://www.umassmed.edu/cfm/home/index.aspx
Centering Prayer	A form similar to TM but with a more religious foundation. The subject repeats a "sacred word" similar to a mantra. As thoughts come to mind, they are accepted and let go, thus clearing the mind to become more centered on the spirit within. The subject regards the mind's preoccupied thoughts as the layers of an onion, which are peeled away to allow better understanding of the spirit at the core.	For a nondenominational discussion, go to the centering prayer Web site of Contemplative Outreach: www.centeringprayer.com/
Progressive Muscle Relaxation (PMR)	A form of relaxation in which the subject is attuned to the difference in feeling when the muscles are tensed and then relaxed. In a comfortable position, the subject starts by tensing the whole body from head to toe. While doing this, the subject notices the feelings of tightness. The subject takes a deep breath in and, while letting it out, lets the tension release and the muscles relax. This is then followed by progressive tension and relaxation throughout the body. One may start by clenching the fists, then tensing the arms, shoulders, chest, abdomen, hips, legs, and so on, with each step followed by relaxation.	Helpful Web sites for PMR include A Guide to Psychology and Its Practice (www.guidetopsychology.com/pmr.htm) and the American Medical Student Association (www.amsa.org/healingthehealer/musclerelaxation.cfm). Free guided body scans and relaxation exercises are offered by the University of Wisconsin School of Medicine: http://www.fammed.wisc.edu/our-department/media/mindfulness
Visualization/Self-Hypnosis (see Chapter 95, Guided Imagery, and Chapter 92, Self-Hypnosis Techniques)	The subject uses visualization to recruit images that create a relaxed state. For example, if a person is anxious, visualizing images of a place and time that was peaceful and comforting will help induce relaxation. This approach is best used in conjunction with a breathing exercise.	Many audio tapes and CDs are available that can guide people through a visualization "script" that results in relaxation. Belleruth Naparstek's Health Journeys are good audio guides: http://www.healthjourneys.com/index.asp Kaiser Permanente offers free downloadable guided relaxation audios through their Healthy Living Audio Library. Search: "Kaiser Permanente Audio Files"

Continued

TABLE 93-1. Relaxation Techniques—cont'd

RELAXATION TECHNIQUE	SUMMARY	FURTHER RESOURCES
Autogenic Training	Induces a physiologic response by using simple phrases. For example, "my legs are heavy and warm" is meant to increase the blood flow to this area, thus resulting in relaxation. The subject performs this process progressively from head to toe with the use of deep breathing and repetition of the phrase. After completion, the subject focuses attention on any body part that may still be tense and then focuses the breath and phrase to that area until the whole body is relaxed.	The British Autogenic Society is a good resource for more information: www.autogenic-therapy.org.uk/
Exercise and Movement: Aerobic	While performing an aerobic exercise, the subject focuses attention on a phrase, sound, word, or prayer and passively disregards other thoughts that may enter the mind. Some people focus on their breathing and say to themselves "in" with inhalation and "out" with exhalation. Or they repeat "one two, one two" with each step while jogging. Doing this helps the mind focus and prevents other thoughts that may cause tension.	Benson H, Klipper M. *Beyond the Relaxation Response* (reissued). New York: Harper/Torch; 1976. This book includes discussion of Benson's research on relaxation response while exercising.
Yoga	Has been practiced for thousands of years. To simplify, yoga is divided into three aspects: breathing (Pranayama yoga), body postures or asanas (Hatha yoga), and meditation to maintain balance and health. Regular practice induces relaxation.	For yoga, tai chi, and qi gong, it is best to encourage your patients to take a class at a local community center or gymnasium and to pick up an introductory book at a library or bookstore.
Tai Chi	This ancient Chinese martial art uses slow, graceful movements combined with inner mindfulness and breathing techniques to help bring balance between the mind and body.	As above
Qi Gong	This traditional Chinese practice uses movement, meditation, and controlled breathing to balance the body's vital energy force, qi (pronounced "chi").	As above

Adapted from Rakel DP, Shapiro DE. Mind-body medicine. In: Rakel RE, ed. *Textbook of Family Practice*. 6th ed. Philadelphia: Saunders; 2001.

References

References are available online at expertconsult.com

Chapter 94

Enhancing Heart Rate Variability

Malynn L. Utzinger-Wheeler, MD, MA

The human heart does not beat at a steady rate, but rather fluctuates from beat to beat, to create patterns that can be regular, as in respiratory sinus arrhythmia, or irregular, as in atrial fibrillation. These beat-to-beat changes and larger patterns collectively are called heart rate variability (HRV). In general, high HRV is an indicator of health, whereas too little variability is a predictor of disease, as exemplified by research showing that low baselines measures of HRV are predictive of all-cause mortality[1] and *independently* predict cardiovascular death.[2] HRV reflects sympathovagal balance, which, in turn, affects inflammatory pathways common to many illnesses.[3-9] Research reveals strong links between HRV and diseases in the cardiovascular,[10-21] neurologic,[22-28] psychological,[29-36] endocrine,[37-39] rheumatologic[40-42] pulmonary[43,44] gastroenterologic,[45,46] and dermatologic[47,48] systems. Even cognitive capacities[49-53] are associated with HRV. All these links will be explored in this chapter.

The ultimate aim of this chapter is to provide clinicians and patients with practical, meaningful, and effective tools to monitor and improve HRV. Preceding this is a review of basic physiology, followed by a discussion of the associations between HRV and health.

Background

HRV is driven by a highly dynamic, bidirectional interplay between the heart and the respiratory system, mediated by the two branches of the autonomic nervous system (ANS), the sympathetic and parasympathetic nervous systems.[54] A standard explanation for the association between disease states and lowered HRV is that neural damage from disease impairs vagus nerve functioning and thereby lowers parasympathetic tone. One of the most fascinating alternative considerations to emerge from research on inflammatory reflexes is that loss of normal vagal tone may lead to diminished functioning of the cholinergic antiinflammatory pathway that may result in downstream immune dysfunction and exaggerated cytokine release triggered by otherwise harmless stimuli.[7] In simple terms, loss of vagal function may *allow* inflammation and disease in the first place.[7] This means that clinicians have a potential opportunity to prevent or slow many conditions by helping people maintain sympathovagal balance.

> Down-regulation of vagal function can worsen chronic inflammation by reducing parasympathetic tone and the cholinergic antiinflammatory pathway.

Before exploring HRV physiology, we should look at the heart itself, which plays a more complex role in health than previously appreciated.[49,55-58] Not only does the heart have novel endocrine roles, such as those of the cardiac receptors for oxytocin, the bonding hormone normally associated with reproduction,[59] but also it has an extensive, intrinsic nervous system that allows it to process and respond to certain emotional and physiologic cues even before the brain does.[56,60,61] Moreover, the heart is the body's strongest generator of electric and magnetic signals, which are 60 times and 5000 times stronger, respectively, than those coming from the brain. These signals can be detected throughout the body by electrocardiography (ECG) or even several feet away by magnetocardiography.[62,63] A theory reviewed and developed by McCraty et al at the Institute of HeartMath is that the heart is not merely a pump. Rather, it provides an organizing force throughout the body, especially in the brain, where synchronization has been observed between R waves on the ECG and alpha waves on the electroencephalogram (EEG).[56,64] Pulsatile signals from the heart travel afferent vagal pathways and arrive in the brainstem and thalamus, where pacemaker cells appear to mediate synchronization of millions of incoming signals from the sensory cortex.[65] In other words, the heart itself may participate in interpreting our experience of the world by synchronizing cortical signals. The positive emotional states and biofeedback tools discussed later appear to increase this synchronization and improve cognitive performance.[29,34,49–51,56,66] In summary, the heart is a pump, a rhythm generator, a sensory organ, and a key node in body-wide communication.

> The heart itself may participate in interpreting our experience of the world by synchronizing cortical signals.

Physiology and Measurement of Heart Rate Variability

As stated earlier, HRV is driven by the ongoing interplay between the sympathetic and parasympathetic nervous systems to keep the body in a state of dynamic balance, or homeostasis.[54] Under conditions of rest, the healthy heart is largely under parasympathetic dominance. Vagal predominance exists during most of the sleep cycle, digestion, and times of quiet, focused attention, such as meditation or prayer. The arousal and erection stages of love-making are also driven by the parasympathetic system.

When a stressor, such as injury, acute illness, pain, or fear, is introduced, sympathetic drive kicks in, increasing catecholamine production necessary in the short run to increase heart rate, cardiac output, muscle strength, and vigilance and thus allowing the body to outrun a real or perceived threat.

In healthy people, sympathetic tone and parasympathetic tone are finely tuned, each rising and falling as demand changes. Unfortunately, daily stress, which can feel threatening, often erroneously triggers increased catecholamines. When this happens on a long-term basis, the body pumps out stress hormones more often than is healthy or necessary. The ANS may try to compensate by turning up parasympathetic control. Ultimately, sympathetic drive that simmers continuously can deplete the reserve needed to meet true challenges. This depletion usually translates into a feeling of being constantly "on edge" yet sluggish and lacking vitality.[56]

When the two systems compete inappropriately, the heart's electrical system can become unstable, causing arrhythmias, platelet aggregation, coronary artery constriction, increased stress on the left ventricular wall, and unhealthy remodeling. Reestablishing proper vagal input antagonizes these sympathetic overcompensations and rebalances the system. This

happens in part through cardiac baroreceptors, or mechanosensory receptors, which are sensitive to stretch and pressure changes and act centrally to restore proper vagal tone and blood pressure.

Baroreceptor sensitivity is a marker of the body's capacity to augment vagal tone reflexively and has a direct link to HRV, observed in respiratory sinus arrhythmia. During inspiration, intrathoracic pressure decreases, and the heart rate increases to compensate. During expiration, intrathoracic pressure rises, and the heart rate drops. In general, with faster breathing, sympathetic tone increases, and the heart rate climbs. With slower breathing, between six and four breaths/minute,[67,68] the balance shifts toward the parasympathetic system, and the heart rate slows.

Therefore, the healthy heart does not beat at a steady rate but rather varies in coordination with the breath and environmental cues. A well-known example of this phenomenon is in obstetrics, in which the fetus is assessed for adequate heart rate accelerations higher than baseline to ensure a favorable response to the challenges of labor (Fig. 94-1).

A flexible, well-coordinated ANS helps us respond appropriately to stress, and positive emotions seem to cultivate this dynamic synergy. In the state of appreciation, for example, parasympathetic and sympathetic systems both show moderate output, and they oscillate in relative regularity to produce what is known as a coherent HRV pattern, which is a smooth, sine wave–like curve and an overall shift toward parasympathetic dominance.[56] In contrast, during stress, anger, or chronic illness, the HRV curve becomes more erratic and shallow, thus reflecting the less-coordinated functioning between the two branches of the ANS and a shift toward sympathetic drive.[61]

Figures 94-2 and 94-3 are examples of graphed HRV plots. The tachogram in Figure 94-2, from the HeartMath Institute, demonstrates the use of a biofeedback technique to shift from frustration, shown with the erratic HRV curve, to appreciation, with a smooth curve. Although both graphs demonstrate similar peak-to-nadir differences in heart rate (reflecting the same absolute amount of variability), the patterns of the curves are quite different. Each segment of the frustration tachogram is erratic and shallow, reflecting low coherence. In contrast, the appreciation curve is both higher in amplitude, more regularly oscillating, and smoother. This *pattern* of variability, and not absolute amount of variability, determines coherence and optimal ANS output.[61]

In Figure 94-3, three emotional states are compared: anger, relaxation, and appreciation. Tachograms are displayed along with power spectra analyses, which plot power (variability) distributed as a function of frequency. Short-term power spectra analyses produce peaks or clusters of data points mostly within three main regions[69]:

FIGURE 94-1

Fetal heart tones. This fetal heart tone strip shows that the baby's heart regularly rises higher than the baseline of 130 beats/minute.

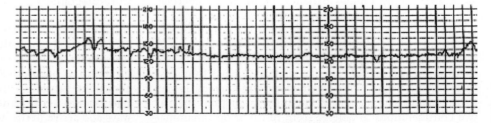

1. High frequency (HF), from 0.15 to 0.40 Hz, reflects the activity of the parasympathetic system and efferent vagal flow.
2. Low frequency (LF), from 0.04 to 0.15 Hz, most likely reflects both parasympathetic and sympathetic activity.
3. Very low frequency (VLF), from 0.003 to 0.04 Hz, reflects the sympathetic nervous system and factors possibly including input from chemoreceptors, thermoreceptors, and the renin-angiotensin system.

The Ultralow frequency region (ULF) is relevant for long-term measurements, such as 24-hour Holter monitor readings.

The *anger* curve demonstrates a disordered pattern with increasing heart rate. The spike in the VLF range demonstrates sympathetic dominance.

In *relaxation,* the tachogram shows a HF, low-amplitude pattern reflecting an overall *decrease* in ANS outflow. The spike in the HF range correlates with parasympathetic dominance.

In *appreciation,* a smooth, highly ordered (or coherent) sine wave is seen. The large, narrow spike in the LF band at 0.1 Hz is indicative of optimization between the sympathetic and parasympathetic branches of the ANS, as well as an entrainment among heart rate, respiration, and blood pressure.[56,70]

Although appreciation and relaxation share a shift toward parasympathetic dominance, appreciation has higher outflow of both parasympathetic and sympathetic drives (higher amplitude), and the two branches are more highly synchronized, shown by the smoothness of the curve and the spike seen at 0.1 Hz in the LF zone of the power spectrum. These qualities define coherence or resonance in HRV.[56,70] Several studies indicated that coherence leads to even greater improvements in health than does relaxation alone.[49,50,56,57,71,72]

In theory, coherence may be achieved at a higher average heart rate, (e.g., during light exercise), but obtaining accurate

---

FIGURE 94-2

Frustration to appreciation. Here a person's heart rate variability (HRV) goes from erratic and shallow during frustration to smooth with a more regularly oscillating HRV curve during appreciation. (From McCraty R, Childre D. *The Appreciative Heart: The Psychophysiology of Positive Emotions and Optimal Functioning.* Boulder Creek, CA; Institute of HeartMath; 2000. Copyright 2000, Institute of HeartMath.)

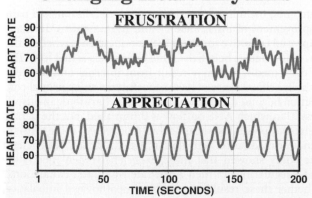

readings is difficult when a subject is moving. Novel technologies including sensors embedded in a T-shirt,[73] a mattress or pillow,[74,75] using wireless ECG,[76] in a Web cam,[77] or using microwave technology[78] soon will make it possible to track HRV coherence under dynamic conditions.

Advanced and Exploratory Concepts in Heart Rate Variability

In HRV dynamics, some physiologic relationships appear to be linear and predictable, whereas others require more complex, nonlinear modeling. Linear metrics, such as time and frequency domain analysis, have made useful predictions about risk stratification and mortality.[79-80] However, growing numbers of studies show that HRV is better described by nonlinear measures such as "sampling entropy," "detrended fluctuation analysis," and "fractal scaling."[81-83] Although a thorough discussion of this topic is beyond the scope of this chapter, a few key principles are useful in evaluating the literature.

In 2008, the editors of *Chaos* posed the question, "Is the normal heart rate chaotic?" Professor Leon Glass of McGill University in Montreal summarized the results of this ongoing discussion and stated that the dynamics of HRV technically are not chaotic, although they are *complex,* meaning the following: (1) the system is very sensitive to initial conditions or to small perturbations; (2) the number of independent, interacting components is large; and (3) the system's trajectory may evolve through multiple pathways. Ultimately, researchers have adopted the term multifractal to describe normal HRV. Turbulence, stock market trends, street riots, and embryogenesis are all described through multifractal models.[84]

Fractals are (1) self-similar, (2) generated through an iterative process, and (3) look the same at any scale. A good example is a tree or the bronchial tree of the lungs. The largest branches grow similar smaller branches, and so on. The formation of ice crystals, mountain ridges, and geothermal flows all illustrate fractal development. In multifractality, whole series of fractals cluster around one "singularity exponent," which contains an unknown or erratic variable. Therefore, the heart and respiratory systems are considered bidirectional, nonlinear oscillators.[54]

Researchers have made links between multifractality and human vitality.[55,85] Knowing that fixed, shallow patterns, such as the slow, periodic gasps of Cheyne-Stokes breathing in congestive heart failure, are signs of impending death (Fig. 94-4), researchers probed for patterns linked to vitality. Dr. Irving Dardik theorized that in optimum health, people's ultradian and circadian rhythms (e.g., hormonal cycles), as well as faster rhythms (e.g., respiration, heart rate, and brain waves), all align as nested or embedded waves, oscillating constructively, without destructive interference.[86] Limited, preliminary data show that heart rate and HRV themselves have both robust, endogenous circadian rhythms and faster, individual rhythms that synchronize with brain waves.[87,88]

An interesting paradox exists, however, in states of deep meditation when heart rate, breath rate, and HRV drop nearly to zero, thus making the meditator appear close to death. Because meditation is associated with several positive health

FIGURE 94-3

Anger, relaxation, and appreciation. In these three conditions, note the shift from the erratic heart rate variability curve of anger to the somewhat more regular, but low-amplitude curve of relaxation, and finally into the smooth, sine wave–like curve of appreciation, consistent with "coherence" or good synchronization between sympathetic and parasympathetic systems and the rest of the bodywide network of inputs. (From McCraty R, Childre D. *The Appreciative Heart: The Psychophysiology of Positive Emotions and Optimal Functioning.* Boulder Creek, CA; Institute of HeartMath; 2000. Copyright 2000, Institute of HeartMath.)

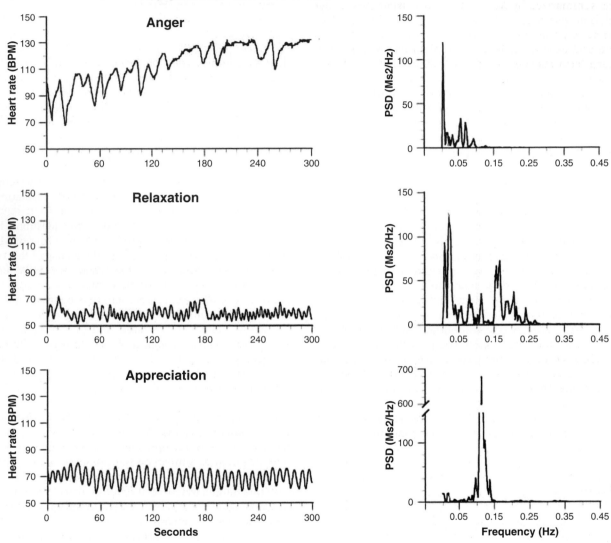

FIGURE 94-4

Cheyne-Stokes breathing in congestive heart failure (CHF). Here, the heart rate is regular, but dangerously so. Apparently, some ability to oscillate and respond to bodily cues has been lost in this end stage of CHF.

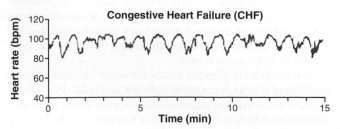

outcomes, including lower blood pressure, diminished pain, improvement of inflammatory and immune disorders, and improved cognitive function,[89-93] the question is whether this low-HRV state is beneficial. One hypothesis is that low HRV in deep meditation may result from internal quiescence, a "wholly selfless sense of love, peacefulness and spiritual connection beyond mere relaxation,"[56] or a "harmonic inclusiveness,"[94] in which ANS outflow is diminished, but the person feels alive, present, and connected. Conversely, some forms of dynamic meditation activate sympathetic drive,[95] and at least one study showed that more experienced Zen meditators had irregularities in their heart rate right after exhalation.[96] Whether these results represent sympathovagal imbalance, disease, or spiritual attunement is yet to be determined.

A parallel paradox is seen in high-intensity exercise, which temporarily elevates heart rate and *lowers HRV*, thus transiently placing high-risk populations, such as people who have experienced myocardial infarction, at greater risk for dangerous arrhythmias. Yet exercise is associated with *long-term improvements in HRV* and cardiovascular recovery, as summarized by Millar et al.[97] My hypothesis is that parallels in "psychological and emotional exercises," such as the mindful experience of anger or grief, may challenge the system and expand one's array of experience while building long-term resilience. For example, a study of bereavement showed that in the first week after loss of a loved one, multiple HRV-related measures worsened in the bereaved person. By 6 months, however, measures had recovered to values of nonbereaved controls.[98] Whether these and similar studies demonstrate psychological resilience[99] or a mere, expected return to baseline is unclear and thus bear greater exploration.

Heart Rate Variability and Health

Although HRV is linked to systemwide health, an important caveat to the following section is that normative data are still limited, and existing reviews show up to 260,000% individual variation, especially in spectral measures.[100] More research and experience are needed to contextualize test results for individual patients.

Many studies have found that HRV declines with age, potentially as one loses time in deep sleep.[101,102] However, the decline slows after the fifth decade. Parasympathetic function reaches its nadir in the eighth decade and increases in extreme old age, possibly aiding longevity.[103] HRV tends to be lower in postmenopausal women than in girls and younger women,[104] and it has not been shown to improve with hormone replacement therapy.[105] Men have higher sympathetic tone and lower parasympathetic tone than women in general; as women age, however, they appear to lose their parasympathetic dominance more markedly than do men.[101]

In cardiovascular health, low HRV is an independent predictor of future events and mortality, including cardiac-related sudden death from myocardial infarction, fatal arrhythmias, and all-cause mortality in certain populations.[5,8,10,14,16,106-108] HRV profile stratifies risk for worsening congestive heart failure,[109-111] coronary heart disease,[13] and atherosclerotic plaques, even in young, asymptomatic adults,[112-114] as well as elevated triglycerides.[115] Similarly, HRV correlates with early insulin resistance,[116] obesity in children and adults,[38,115,117,118] multiple metabolic syndrome,[119] and hypertension.[120-122] Hot flashes are associated with a significant decrease in vagal tone[39] and hence may be a cardiac risk.

Research has verified significant links between HRV and the following: neurologic disorders such as epilepsy, Parkinson disease, restless leg syndrome, migraine, and insomnia[22-28,123]; rheumatologic disorders including fibromyalgia, rheumatoid arthritis, and lupus[40-42]; gastroenterologic dysfunctions including functional dyspepsia and IBS[45,46]; and other inflammatory diseases such as asthma[43,44] and atopic dermatitis.[47,48] In addition, many studies tracked the effects of HRV on markers of inflammation and immunity.[3-9]

Innovative researchers are now using HRV to *predict* the onset of infection several days before symptoms and track its severity.[124-126] Similarly, low HRV can independently predict complicated recovery after abdominal surgery.[127] Conversely, working to improve HRV appears to reduce perception of pain.[128]

In mental health, low HRV is linked with depression, social isolation, bereavement, posttraumatic stress disorder, and suppressed anger,[29-36,129-131] and it may partially mediate the significantly increased risk of cardiac mortality in depressed individuals after myocardial infarction, although antidepressants do not always improve HRV.[33] Even in otherwise healthy individuals, stress has been demonstrated to change short-term HRV profiles, for example, in surgeons performing high-stress operations[127] and in physicians during and after a call.[132]

Environmental and work-related factors also affect HRV. Although results of studies are mixed, most suggest that pollution and tobacco smoke worsen HRV.[133-139] Exposure to factory toxicants, job stress, and shift work all diminished HRV,[140] whereas improving workspace and ambient light improved HRV and cortisol rhythms.[141] Disturbingly, a Japanese study showed that people who ate the provisional tolerable weekly intake (PTWI) of methylmercury (3.4 mcg/kg/week) from big eye tuna and swordfish for 14 weeks had significant increases in sympathovagal imbalance, which returned to normal 15 weeks later; controls showed no changes.

Factors That Improve Heart Rate Variability

Fortunately, many interventions improve HRV. In the case of lethal arrhythmias, cardiac resynchronization therapy (pacing) is sometimes necessary.[142] Other medical procedures, including spinal stimulation,[143] vagal nerve stimulation,[66,144,145] and acupuncture,[146] all show positive effects. Among pharmaceuticals and supplements, beta blockers and some calcium channel blockers appear to be useful.[147-150] In depressed individuals, selective serotonin receptor inhibitors (SSRIs) and cognitive-behavioral therapy improve HRV,[151,152] whereas tricyclic antidepressants and caffeine lower it.[153,154] St. John's wort was associated both with improvements and no change in two separate studies,[155,156] and gamma-aminobutyric acid (GABA)–covered chocolate boosted HRV recovery after stress.[157]

Foods, including green, leafy vegetables,[158] omega-3 polyunsaturated fatty acids in fish and fish oil,[159,160] and a Mediterranean diet[161] improve HRV. Wine paired with omega-3 fatty acid intake shows some benefit, but whether this benefit exists independently is unclear.[162] In fact, separate studies found that long-term moderate alcohol consumption and alcohol mixed with energy drinks both had deleterious effects on HRV.[163]

Lifestyle links with clear benefit include smoking cessation, which results in immediate improvements in HRV.[164,165] Although exercise showed no HRV benefit in one study,[106,166] most of the research demonstrated significant exercise-related benefit,[166-170] even including reversal of cardiac neural remodeling after myocardial infarction.[171] Entering a hotter or colder ambient temperature shifts HRV; cold environments acutely decrease heart rate and raise HRV. Whether these conditions, exemplified in the Polar Bear Plunge, result in lasting benefit is unclear.[172]

Simple mind-body techniques show much promise for improving HRV. Slow breathing or chanting a prayer or a mantra strongly affects HRV and baroreceptor sensitivity, even in people with advanced congestive heart failure.[68,173] Prayer in itself, especially centering prayer and prayers of gratitude, can produce high measures of HRV coherence,[57] as does expressive writing.[174] Listening to classical music or meditation music also significantly improves HRV.[175]

Biofeedback based on control of breath rate or focus on positive emotion is one of the most highly researched therapies to improve HRV.[176] Studies showed improvements in the following: cortisol and dehydroepiandrosterone levels; symptoms of depression, posttraumatic stress disorder, and mood regulation[35,57,177]; blood pressure[71,72]; cholesterol levels; aggression levels; and job satisfaction among correctional officers.[84] This same technique allowed high school students to perform better on standardized tests and function at a new, higher baseline of HRV coherence after training in biofeedback.[49,50] In summary, much evidence indicates that mind-body techniques have a positive effect not only on HRV itself, but also on health, emotions, and cognitive performance.

The Basics Matter

In keeping the heart rate variability profile healthy, the most powerful, safe, and reliable measures are the simple ones, namely, learning to develop a positive or appreciative view on life. Acting out these feelings daily in a healthy dose of fun or compassion makes a difference. So be sure to tell your patient that he or she will be practicing good medicine by evaluating life and priorities and maintaining gratitude and social connectedness.

Making Recommendations to the Patient

Given the foregoing data, you can develop an integrative plan to help patients maintain or enhance their HRV. In making an integrative treatment plan, you should ask the following questions: What are the known effects? What are the risks? What is the evidence? What is the cost or the availability? And, importantly, what does the patient believe or value? As a practitioner, your relationship with the patient and your own experience with a particular approach to healing strongly affect this last point. For that reason, you may want to experiment with several of these approaches yourself before talking to patients about them. Not only will you have the chance to improve your own health and well-being, but also you will have a personal experience that allows you to step on a common path with the patient. This kind of mutual and personal teaching honors the spirit of integrative medicine, in which the health and wisdom of both patient and health care practitioner are important, indeed critical, to healing! Luckily, many of the approaches listed here are fun. You may even want to try them with your office

staff or at home for your own learning. The Institute of HeartMath offers just such office-based trainings (see Key Web Resources).

Steps to Enhance Heart Rate Variability

Remember that patients do not need to attempt all or even most of these therapies immediately. A wise approach is to suggest that patients pick a few therapies that appeal to them first and then modify them as they come to know their own needs.

Step 1: Follow Good Preventive Measures

- Quit smoking.
- Maintain a healthy weight.
- Keep cholesterol levels in check.
- Eat a diet rich in omega-3 fatty acids, either from fish or from fish oils (see Chapter 86, The Antiinflammatory Diet).
- Keep alcohol consumption low to moderate.
- Exercise regularly but moderately, with guidance from a physician if heart disease or other significant illness is present.

Step 2: Maintain a Healthy State of Mind

- Keep up social connections or make new ones. Healthy relationships are powerful determinants of heart health.
- Obtain professional help for serious symptoms of depression or anxiety.
- Develop practices that help you feel calm, centered, present, and appreciative (see Chapter 93, Relaxation Techniques). Music often makes this easier.

Deep, Slow Breathing
This breathing exercise is cheap, safe, and easy to perform in just a few minutes. The best results come when people maintain six breaths/minute or simply focus on an appreciative or caring emotion that slows the breath and creates coherence automatically.

Meditation
Choose walking meditation, mindfulness meditation, chanting, or any other form that is appealing.

Prayer
Pray either on your own or in a group, for the social connection.

Journaling
Even writing down a few words and phrases per day can be healing.

A Simple Beginning

In the office, a simple way to help patients to begin enhancing heart rate variability is to teach them a deep-breathing technique.

1. Have the patient place a hand on his or her belly—while you demonstrate!
2. Make sure to have him or her "deep belly breathe" so that the stomach rises on the inbreath. On the outbreath, the belly falls.
3. In general, have the patient aim to breathe out for twice as long—or whatever he or she can sustain, as compared with the inbreath. A 4 to 8 count, for example, works well.
4. Have the patient repeat this twice a day, morning and night, or whenever stress arises, for 3 to 5 minutes to train the body-mind. If focusing on the breath per se is difficult, focusing on a positive feeling can work just as well.

Biofeedback

Several good computerized tools are on the market to help you learn to use biofeedback.

- www.wilddivine.com. This visually intriguing computerized adventure is driven as you learn skills to control your bodily rhythms through biofeedback.

- www.heartmath.com. This organization provides literature, handheld devices, and desktop biofeedback software, as well as thorough training for health care professionals and lay people. One limitation is that a person must be still to use these devices, but seeing live feedback is tremendously engaging to many who try it. Music can also be included in the program to assist you. Ultimately, the tools train you to function well without them.

Guided Imagery

Excellent resources for tapes or CDs are as follows:

- www.healthjourneys.com
- www.soundstrue.com

Step 3: Consider Medical Therapies and Supplements

- Beta blockers, verapamil (and possibly other calcium channel blockers), and antiarrhythmics may improve HRV, but their use must be guided by a physician.

- For depression, tricyclic antidepressants appear to worsen HRV, whereas SSRIs appear to improve it. St. John's wort may be beneficial. GABA appears to help HRV recovery from stress.

KEY WEB RESOURCES

HeartMath: www.heartmath.com	This organization provides literature, handheld devices, and desktop biofeedback software, as well as thorough training for health care professionals and lay people. They offer the emWave computer biofeedback system, which costs approximately $300.
Wild Divine: www.wilddivine.com	This visually intriguing computerized adventure teaches skills to control your bodily rhythms through biofeedback. The program costs approximately $300.
StressEraser: http://stresseraser.com/	The StressEraser is a small biofeedback device that monitors breathing and heart rate to enhance heart rate variability. It costs approximately $180.

References

References are available online at expertconsult.com.

Guided Imagery and Interactive Guided Imagery*

Martin L. Rossman, MD

Imagination is more important than knowledge.

Albert Einstein

As a physician treating primarily people with chronic and life-threatening illnesses for nearly 40 years, I have found working with mental imagery, especially in an interactive manner, one of the most useful approaches I have ever encountered.

As doctors, we are trained to diagnose and treat physically observable manifestations of disease and illness. In some instances, we can provide definitive, even lifesaving interventions, and both we and our patients are pleased and grateful. In many circumstances, however, our attempts to help do not result in a neat and acceptable result. We may not be able to diagnose the source of our patient's condition (84% of the 15 most common symptoms presented to a primary care doctor never come to be diagnosed as a disease state), or, alternatively, we can give the condition a name and perhaps provide some relief but can do little or nothing about much of the suffering that accompanies it. This is especially true for our patients with chronic illness, who often represent the most challenging and time-consuming aspects of our practices.

People with chronic illness need not only excellent medical care but also attention to what we may call the invisible yet important aspects of health care that are accessible only through their own awareness. A skilled clinician with sophisticated imagery skills can help such patients work effectively with their own strengths to help them fare better, whatever their medical condition may be.

What Is Guided Imagery?

Guided imagery is a term variously used to describe a range of techniques from simple visualization and direct imagery-based suggestion through metaphor and storytelling. Guided imagery is used to help teach psychophysiologic relaxation, to relieve pain and other symptoms, to stimulate healing responses in the body, and to help people tolerate procedures and treatments more easily.

Interactive Guided Imagery (IGI) is a service-marked term coined by the Academy for Guided Imagery for a process in which imagery is used in a highly interactive format to evoke a patient's autonomy. This technique gives patients ways to draw on their own inner resources to support healing, to make appropriate adaptations to changes in health, and to understand more clearly what their symptoms may be signaling.

Imagery is a natural way that the human nervous system stores, accesses, and processes information. It is the coding system in which memories, fantasies, dreams, daydreams, and expectations are stored. It is a way of thinking with sensory attributes, and in the absence of competing sensory cues, the body tends to respond to imagery as it would to a genuine external experience. The most common and familiar example of this phenomenon is sexual fantasy with its attendant physiologic responses.

Imagery has been shown in dozens of research studies to be able to affect almost all major physiologic control systems of the body—respiration, heart rate, blood pressure, metabolic rates in cells, gastrointestinal mobility and secretion, sexual function, and even immune responsiveness. Imagery is also a rapid way to access emotional and symbolic information that may affect both physiology and the way that patients care for themselves. For instance, a patient may talk at length about the nature of his or her back pain, yet the clinician may not appreciate it as much as when the patient uses imagery-laden language and says, "It feels like a knife twisting in my

---

* Interactive Guided Imagery is a particular approach taught by the Academy for Guided Imagery, in Malibu, California, of which Dr. Rossman is a founder and codirector.

back." Not only does this give a graphic, sensory description of the symptom, but also it may lead to important psychosocial information involved in the perception of the pain. In this case, respectful questioning about betrayals or related feelings would be appropriate (Box 95-1).

The following personal case history shows how imagery can help us become more aware of the interplay of feelings, physiology, and symptoms.

Case History (Headaches)

A 28-year-old woman with chronic mixed headaches came to my office with a severe migraine. We had worked together before, so I guided her through a simple progressive relaxation technique and asked her to focus directly on her pain and invite an image to come to mind that could tell her something useful about the pain. An image came of a large mynah bird, sitting on her head and pecking away in the area of her pain.

"Why's he doing that?" she asked, and I suggested that she ask him and imagine that he could answer in a way she could understand.

To her surprise, the bird answered, "Why not? You let everyone else pick on you!" She started crying and told me that the day before she had accidentally overheard a fellow employee making fun of her in the coffee room. She started to get angry, but then became nauseated and started to feel a migraine aura. She went home for the day, and the migraine developed into the headache that brought her in to see me. In her imagery dialogue, the bird agreed to work with her to understand and prevent her headaches more effectively. She left feeling 90% relieved without any other intervention.

The patient's continuing dialogues with the mynah revealed a long-standing pattern of low self-esteem and non-assertiveness. The bird told her that the result was holding anger and directing it toward herself, a process that ultimately led to her headaches. I referred her to a good therapist; after 18 months, she was not only relieved of headaches but also much happier and heading in a more successful direction in her life.

Applications in Medicine

Because imagery is a natural language of the unconscious and the human nervous system, its potential uses in the healing professions are protean. Guided imagery is essentially a way of working with the patient, rather than of treating particular disease entities, but it is especially effective in the following areas:

- Relaxation training and stress reduction
- Pain relief
- Management of chronic illness and prevention of acute exacerbations
- Preparation for surgery and medical procedures
- Medication compliance and adherence issues
- Cancer treatment and life-threatening illnesses
- Terminal illnesses and end-of-life care
- Fertility, birthing, and delivery
- Grief therapy
- Posttraumatic stress disorder
- Anxiety disorders
- Depression

Guided imagery is a broad term comprising techniques that are applicable in the course of brief medical office visits or in longer counseling or psychotherapy formats. Physicians may practice it themselves or may employ ancillary health professionals to offer longer sessions. Physicians may also teach their patients guided imagery skills for self-care by educating them about it and recommending or prescribing appropriate guided imagery books, compact discs (CDs), and audio downloads (see the later section on resources and the Key Web Resources box).

Is Research Literature Available on Guided Imagery?

A large body of clinical research supports the everyday use of imagery in medicine, and research in this area has significantly increased in the past few years. Of more than 1200 PubMed articles on guided imagery research since 1969, nearly 500 have appeared since 2005, and half of them have been published since 2009. More than 90% of the studies show positive benefits in clinical situations that include stroke rehabilitation, preparing for childbirth, treating anxiety disorders and posttraumatic stress disorder, relieving pain in both children and adults, preparing for surgery and medical procedures, changing eating habits, smoking and drug cessation, and supporting patients during cancer treatment. A summary of the evidence on guided imagery and visualization on immune function is summarized in Box 95-2.

How Does Imagery Work?

Research with functional magnetic resonance imaging indicates that when people visualize things or events, they activate the occipital cortex in the same way they do when

BOX 95-2. Guided Imagery Effects on Immune Function as Summarized by Trakhtenberg

- A relationship exists between immune system functioning and guided imagery and stress/relaxation.
- Guided imagery and relaxation interventions can reduce distress and allow the immune system to function more effectively.
- Changes in immune system functioning are correlated with either an increase or a decrease in white blood cell (WBC) count or with changes in neutrophil adherence.
- Stress/relaxation may account for qualitative (nature of neutrophil adherence) or quantitative (WBC count) changes in immune system functioning.
- Cell-specific imagery may predict in which WBC category (i.e., type of WBC—neutrophils or lymphocytes) changes in WBC count will occur.
- An active cognitive exercise or process involved in the initial stages of guided imagery is associated with decreases in neutrophil adherence. In contrast, relaxation without an active imagery exercise is associated with increases in neutrophil adherence.
- Decreases in WBC count occur only in the initial stages of exposure to guided imagery or relaxation interventions. After 4 to 5 weeks of training, however, WBC count increases.
- Increases in WBC count may be caused by an increase in WBC production as a result of enhanced relaxation ensuing from extensive visualization practice, and decreases in WBC count in the initial stage of visualization training are secondary to a decrease in WBC production as a result of possible pressure ensuing from an attempt to learn new training techniques.
- Decreases and increases in WBC count may be caused by the effect of margination. This means that imagery training may change the movement of WBCs and their location within the body, rather than decreasing or increasing production of WBCs.
- The change in WBC count may occur earlier in medical patients with a depressed WBC count and later in physiologically normal, healthy individuals.

Adapted from Trakhtenberg EC. The effects of guided imagery on the immune system: a critical review. *Int J Neurosci.* 2008;118:839–855.

they actually see the same things or events. Similarly, the temporal cortex is activated when music or speech is imagined, and the motor or premotor areas of the cortex are activated when a person imagines movement. We believe that this cortical activation sends neural and neurochemical messages to lower centers of the brain that can activate or deactivate stress responses. Neuropeptides can also affect physiology at a distance and can modify physiologic states, including blood pressure, clotting mechanisms, and immunity.

Clinically, we have known for many years that when people worry, which is an imaginative function, they can activate stress physiology, which over time can lead to physiologic exhaustion, maladaptive behavior, and vulnerability to illness. In the same way, when a patient imagines himself or herself in a beautiful, peaceful, safe place and concentrates on what he or she imagines seeing, hearing, and feeling there, the patient tends to induce a state of relaxation similar to what he or she would feel if actually in that place. The physiology of the "relaxation response," as described by Benson, takes over, thus allowing a break in the chronic stress state and facilitating certain reparative and restorative processes the body uses for healing. With regular practice, the creation of this state can help reverse some of the effects of chronic stress.

The creation of a relaxed state also allows the patient to experience that he or she has some choice in feelings about and response to stressors, which can lead to greater self-efficacy and change in lifestyle patterns that affect health. Finally, in a relaxed yet aware state, the body is more responsive to images and suggestions of pain relief, comfort, enhanced or reduced blood flow, and even up-regulation of immunity.

> Worry is an example of how negative images can trigger stress physiology. Imagery can also be directed toward positive physiologic responses.

Imagery is sometimes referred to as a "right brain" type of thinking because it tends to be synthetic, creative, and emotional. This type of thinking contrasts with the "left brain" form of linear, logical thinking with which we are all highly familiar.

These attributions are best considered a shorthand way of referring to modes of thinking that are associated with but not restricted to the respective hemispheres of the brain. They may be more accurately termed simultaneous versus sequential information processing. To illustrate the difference between these two types of thinking, let us imagine watching a train go by from two different perspectives. From the left brain or sequential processing perspective, one would observe the train from the level of the track. One would see the engine go by, then the first car, then the next, and the next, and so on—one car at a time, each following the one before. The right brain or simultaneous perspective would place one high above the train, where one could see not only the whole train, but also the tracks for miles ahead and behind, the countryside through which it travels, the place it started, and its next destination. Similarly, the holistic perspective of imagery shows one the forest, whereas the analytic perspective of linear thinking lets one more closely examine the trees. Both are useful.

Perhaps the reason that imagery seems so mysteriously powerful is that we have almost systematically ignored it in scientific culture and, as it is rediscovered, its many advantages in mind-body healing make us marvel at its utility. Imagery provides many advantages over analytic thinking when it is applied to personal healing. One is the big picture perspective that it offers. As the previous case history and the following example illustrate, imagery can often show how life events, emotions, and physical symptoms are connected.

Case History (Lumpy Breasts)

A patient with lumpy breasts was invited to allow an image to come that represented the lumps. She was surprised that she imagined them as pearls. On exploring the pearl image, she realized that pearls are formed in response to something irritating that could eventually turn harmful. Her orientation changed as she considered this idea. "Maybe the lumps are trying to protect me," she said. "They want me to reduce the stress I've been living with and the caffeine I've been using to try to keep up." This understanding led her to stop drinking coffee and change the way she was living to reduce her stress; her fibrocystic lumps soon disappeared.

Another advantage of imagery in mind-body healing is that it is closely related to emotion. Imagery is the basis of the arts, the essence of painting and sculpture, but also of poetry, storytelling, dance, drama, and even music. Imagery moves us and can represent what affects us emotionally. Because unexpressed emotions are often expressed in the body, many common and unexplainable symptoms that doctors see represent patients' feelings that are unrecognized and unattended. Imagery can bring these connections to light and make them available for expression and potential resolution (see Chapter 100, Emotional Awareness for Pain).

Imagery is also closely related to physiology. Imagining sucking on a lemon stimulates salivation in most people, whereas imagining frightening events elevates the heart rate and blood pressure. Imagining muscle relaxation produces muscle relaxation, and regular imagining of an activated immune system increases both the number and aggressiveness of natural killer cells. This psychophysiologic connection may account for the wide range of syndromes in which imagery has proved useful. These diagnoses include, but are not limited to, asthma, allergic rhinitis, tension and migraine headaches, neck and back pain, irritable bowel syndrome, premenstrual dysphoria, dysmenorrhea, Raynaud syndrome, anxiety, depression, hypertension, angina, and even diabetes. Imagery has also been shown to relieve anxiety and complications of invasive medical and surgical procedures, including endoscopy, colonoscopy, biopsy, and angiography, as well as childbirth.

> Guided imagery acts as a bridge of communication of information between the subconscious and conscious mind that the patient can use to find health.

Commonly Used Treatment Techniques

The list of techniques used in guided imagery is quite extensive, because this approach has been applied to problems ranging from chronic pain, to posttraumatic stress, to stimulating healing responses in the body, to enhancing mind-body awareness, and more. However, some of the more basic techniques are described here.

Mental and Physical Relaxation

Imagery is often the easiest way for many Western patients to learn to relax. Typically, patients are instructed in abdominal breathing and sequential or progressive relaxation suggestions and are then invited simply to daydream themselves to a place of great beauty, safety, or peacefulness or a place that they experience as healing. Patients are guided to notice what they see, hear, feel, and even smell as they imagine themselves in a relaxing place. As they immerse themselves in the imagery in this way, they tend to relax easily and deeply.

Symptom Relief Through Healing Imagery

Symptomatic imagery techniques reduce physical symptoms such as pain, anxiety, and insomnia without concern for the causes. Such techniques are useful alternatives or complements to medications and are particularly helpful when discomfort has a stress-related or functional basis. Many different situations and techniques are used, such as relaxation and then imagining how healing could happen in an area that is symptomatic. When patients are successful in relieving pain or other symptoms with imagery, they find the experience profoundly therapeutic and empowering.

Interactive Imagery Dialogue

Interactive imagery dialogue can be used with an image that represents anything the client or therapist wants to know more about; in many ways, it is the quintessential insight technique. This method is used to explore an image of a symptom (whether physical, emotional, or behavioral), an image that represents resistance arising anywhere in the process, an image of an inner resource that can help the client deal with the current problem, or an image of the solution.

With interactive imagery, the point is not to analyze the images but to communicate with them as if they are alive (which, of course, they are). This is not to say that the images have an existence apart from the client, but rather that they represent complexes of thoughts, beliefs, attitudes, feelings, body sensations, expectations, and values that at times can function as relatively autonomous aspects of the personality. These constellations were referred to as "subpersonalities" by Roberto Assagioli,[1] the originator of psychosynthesis, and as "ego states" by Watkins and Watkins.[2]

The Inner Advisor

The inner advisor is a specific type of IGI dialogue whereby clients are invited to converse with an imaginary figure that is specified to be both wise and loving or, as characterized in analytic terms, an "ego ideal." This figure can be referred to as the "inner guide," "inner healer," "inner wisdom," "inner helper," "inner physician," "higher self," or any other term that is meaningful to and comfortable for the client. Because the client is invited to imagine a figure that has these qualities, a dialogue with whatever figure arises is usually meaningful and helpful. Specifying the positive qualities offers some safety to clients if they find themselves exploring issues that may be emotionally difficult.

Evocative Imagery

The state-dependent technique called evocative imagery helps clients to shift moods and affective states at will, thus making new behaviors and insights more accessible to consciousness. Through the structured use of memory, fantasy, and sensory recruitment, the client is encouraged to identify a personal quality or qualities that would serve especially well in his or her current situation. For instance, a client may feel the need for more "calmness" or "peace of mind" to deal more effectively with a life issue or a medical illness. The guide then invites the client to relax and recall a time when peace of mind was actually experienced. Through the use of sensory recruitment and present-tense recall, the client is encouraged to imagine that he or she is in that time again now, feeling that peace of mind. Once this peaceful feeling state has been well established and amplified, the patient is invited to let the past images go, but to come back to the present, bringing along the feelings of peace of mind. As the client now becomes aware of the situation while strongly in touch with this feeling, he or she is usually able to tolerate it far more effectively.

Dr. Sheldon Cohen[3] at Carnegie-Mellon University in Pittsburgh researched evocative imagery and found it to be highly effective in shifting affective states. Research aimed at assessing the effects of those altered affective states on subsequent behavior, problem-solving, and self-efficacy remains to be done and offers a fertile field for future psychological and behavioral study.

Grounding: Moving From Insight to Action

Grounding is the process by which the insights evoked by imagery are turned into actions and greater awareness and motivation are focused into a specific plan for attitudinal, emotional, or behavioral change. This process of adding the will to the imagination involves clarification of insights, brainstorming, choosing the best option, affirmations, action planning, imagery rehearsal, and constant reformulation of the plan until it actually succeeds. It is often the missing link in insight-oriented therapies because it connects the new awareness to a specific action plan. Grounding is "where the rubber meets the road," and imagery can be used to enhance the process by providing creative options for action; the guide and client can use imagery rehearsal to troubleshoot and anticipate obstacles to success.

How to Get Started With Guided Imagery

The first thing the practitioner should do is notice how much imagery-laden language and suggestion are used in daily interactions with patients. Notice the terms patients use when they describe "knife-like" pains or the feeling of a "hot poker in my stomach." The practitioner should notice his or her own uses of imagery, too, such as in describing the mechanisms of a medication or intervention. Simple word pictures are commonly used when we prescribe and try to motivate patients to follow the regimen. Simple descriptions such as "This will relax the little muscles in your blood vessels, and that will lower your blood pressure" and "Acupuncture releases brain chemicals that relax your muscles and relieve pain" are very brief forms of what can be called guided imagery. Physicians can sometimes forget this effect when they become caught up in the necessities of informed consent, which tends to focus too much on the negative potential of treatments. Without "overpromising," physicians should accompany any prescription or recommendation with an expectation that it will be of help, and a brief word picture of how that can happen conveys a large amount of information in a concise way.

The practitioner should read books on guided imagery and experiment personally with guided imagery CDs or audios available through mp3 downloads (see later "Resources"). The more personal experience a practitioner has with guided imagery, the easier it will be to teach these skills to patients or simply to recommend or prescribe particular guided imagery exercises, lessons, or techniques. Some physicians set up their offices for guided imagery as follows: First the patient listens to guided imagery CDs; then the physician debriefs the experience with the patient, answers questions, and offers guidance on how to use the technique on a continuing basis.

The physician who wishes to guide patients through imagery experiences but has no experience or training in any form of relaxation, hypnosis, or meditation should pursue such training. Continuing medical education courses or local classes at community colleges or through other local sources are means of becoming familiar with mind-body approaches. Training that is specifically created for physicians or health professionals is more likely to be quickly usable with patients. For example, the Academy for Guided Imagery offers an excellent introductory course in a home study format, "The Fundamentals of Interactive Guided Imagery." This course provides rationale, references, and an introduction to clinical skills that can allow the physician to explore guided imagery safely in practice. I consider such a course the minimum a professional should study before using guided imagery in practice.

The Structure of a Typical Interactive Guided Imagery Session

At the Academy for Guided Imagery, we refer to the time spent before entering into a formal guided imagery exploration as the "foresight" part of the process. Along with evaluating the appropriateness of using imagery with the client or patient, the guide works with the client to establish the desired goals and objectives for their work together.

As with any medical or psychological situation, goals can be defined in physical, emotional, or behavioral terms, and a reasonable trial period of exploration is agreed on by the client and guide. We often ask patients to have three exploratory sessions and then decide whether this approach seems useful to them, whether they can best use guided imagery as self-care, in a brief, time-limited period of work (10 to 15 sessions), or whether longer-term work seems to be needed.

The typical processes involved are described here. Not every session uses the same approach; all sessions may use any of a wide variety of processes and methods of exploration drawn from the guide's training and experience (Boxes 95-3 and 95-4).

Precautions and Contraindications

Although directive guided imagery sessions are generally quite safe, receptive imagery, as used in IGI, can be a powerful tool that can connect people with emotional material very quickly. If patients are emotionally fragile, have a history of psychosis, or have repressed traumatic material, receptive imagery can reveal affective content that can be

BOX 95-3. A Typical Interactive Guided Imagery Session (see also Box 95-4)

1. Assessment (foresight):
   a. Ask what symptom, illness, or thoughts the patient would like to explore.
   b. Ask what the patient wants to get out of the session.
   c. Ask patient to narrow the problem to a short phrase or question.
   d. Formulate a one-sentence summary of goals.
   e. Obtain the patient's consent.
2. Imagery process (insight):
   a. Relaxation:
      (1) Ask how the patient best relaxes.
      (2) Use the patient's best method or teach him or her a method.
   b. Imagine a beautiful, safe place:
      (1) "Allow yourself to imagine a comfortable and peaceful place. It may be a place that you have been before or something that's just coming into your imagination now. If you imagine several places coming to mind, allow yourself to pick just one to explore now."
      (2) Ask the patient to describe the place in regard to sensations ("What do you see, hear, smell, feel, and taste? What makes you feel comfortable there?")
      (3) Invite the patient to find a comfortable place to settle down.
   c. Imagery dialogue:
      (1) Invite the patient to form an image that represents the illness, symptom, or issue.
      (2) Ask the patient to describe the image in detail. (Have him or her describe at least three things, such as appearance, character, and emotions of the image.)
      (3) Ask the patient to describe the qualities that the image portrays.
      (4) What feelings does the patient have about the image?
      (5) Invite the patient to express these feelings to the image, and allow the image to respond.
      (6) "Imagine that it can communicate with you in a way you can easily understand."
      (7) Facilitate the imaginary conversation as needed, using "content-free" questions and suggestions such as the following:
         (a) "Do you have any questions you would like to ask the image?"
         (b) "How does it respond?"
         (c) "Ask the image what it wants from you, and let it respond."
         (d) "What does it want you to know?"
         (e) "What does it need from you?"
         (f) "What does it have in common with you?"
         (g) "What does it have to offer you?"
         (h) "Ask the image what it can tell you about the problem so you can better understand."
         (i) "Ask the image what it can tell you about the solution so you can better understand."
         (j) "Go back to the safe place, and return from the inner place."
   d. When the image communicates, you may ask the patient how he or she feels about that or wants to respond, then encourage the patient to respond, and let the image respond to that. Your role is to facilitate the dialogue, not provide the answers.
   e. If the patient appears frightened, ask whether he or she feels safe; if not, have the patient go back to the safe place or ask what he or she needs to feel safe.
3. Evaluation (hindsight):
   a. Ask the patient what he or she felt was interesting or significant about the dialogue.
   b. Ask the patient whether he or she learned anything from or about the image or the symptom.
   c. Ask the patient whether the information changes his or her perspective or how he or she wants to respond.
   d. Ask the patient what he or she would do next with what was learned.

Many physicians, nurses, and therapists work for a defined period of time (6 to 20 sessions) with patients in a psychoeducational or counseling model, with well-defined symptomatic or behavioral goals, and they refer patients to mental health practitioners if their work becomes psychologically complex. At the same time, we urge mental health practitioners to take precautions to ascertain the medical status of any patient and to ensure that the patient is also aware of the medical options.

At the end of each session, and at the end of the agreed-on period, the goals of the work are reviewed, and progress is assessed. After this evaluation, an agreement is made to terminate treatment, to continue for another period, to refer the patient to another practitioner, or to define a period in which the patient will do "ownwork" and then return to report his or her progress.

---

overwhelming. The practitioner should be sufficiently trained in guided imagery skills to be able to recognize potentially problematic situations and to prevent or remedy them when encountered unexpectedly.

Although guided imagery can sometimes help shed light on a puzzling diagnostic situation, it should not be used in lieu of proper medical diagnosis, to avoid overlooking necessary medical treatment. With due attention to this issue and the precautions and contraindications listed in Boxes 95-5 and 95-6, the practitioner can practice guided imagery safely and help patients become more active participants in their own health.

BOX 95-4. Common Interactive Guided Imagery Suggestions and Questions

- Allow an image to form.
- What do you notice about it?
- What are you aware of?
- What are you experiencing?
- What would you like to notice yourself having?
- What would you like to say to it?
- What sensations are you aware of?
- Let me know when you are ready to move on.

BOX 95-5. Contraindications to Guided Imagery

- Strong religious beliefs proscribing the use of imagery
- Disorientation, dementia, or impaired cognition in response to pharmacologic or other agents
- Inability to hold a train of thought for at least 5 to 10 minutes
- Potential litigation (Guided imagery may be considered a form of hypnosis, which affects the legal status of information obtained with its use.)

BOX 95-6. Conditions in Which Guided Imagery Should Be Used With Caution*

- History of physical or sexual abuse
- Active psychosis or prepsychotic state
- Diffused dissociative disorders
- Posttraumatic stress disorder or anxiety disorders
- Personal history of suicide attempt or family history of suicide or suicide attempt
- Unstable medical problems, such as severe asthma, heart disease, and pain

*Practitioners treating people with these conditions/situations should be very well versed in both the treatment of the underlying disorder and the use of guided imagery.

Resources

Training

Simple guided imagery for relaxation and healing is generally safe if the guidelines provided are followed. IGI is a powerful proprietary method of personal and psychological inquiry that can rapidly expose high levels of affect that can be overwhelming to certain patients. Practitioners desiring to use IGI should have an appropriate level of training for the applications they choose. The "Fundamentals of Interactive Guided Imagery" is a 13-hour home study course that will give you a thorough and meaningful introduction to this form of treatment and its roles in medicine, along with several essential skills you can begin to use in your practice. The Academy for Guided Imagery (800-726-2070; see also Key Web Resources box) also offers in-depth training that leads to certification in IGI.

Guided Imagery Recordings and Self-Study Programs

Audio recordings and self-study programs can be helpful tools to facilitate healing. Some respected resources for imagery tapes and CDs are listed in the Key Web Resources box. These Web site listings offer disease-specific recordings, as well as recordings addressing general topics such as surgical preparation and recovery, immune support, and cancer therapy.

KEY WEB RESOURCES

The Healing Mind: www.thehealingmind.org	This Web site offers many guided imagery CDs and self-study programs by Dr. Martin Rossman and others, based on interactive imagery principles, as well as research, health tracker, interactive opportunities, and other material useful to patients and professionals.
The Source: www.drmiller.com	Dr. Emmett Miller has spent many years studying and practicing psychophysiologic medicine and offers a wide variety of excellent health-oriented guided imagery and hypnosis recordings.
Tranceformation: www.tranceformation.com	Dr. Steven Gurgevich, on the faculty of the Integrative Medicine program at the University of Arizona, uses the art of hypnotherapy and provides tapes for many medical conditions.
Health Journeys: www.healthjourneys.com	This large selection of excellent guided imagery CDs on many health topics is created by Belleruth Naparstek, LISW.
Academy for Guided Imagery (AGI).\: http://www.academyforguidedimagery.com/about/index.html	This Web site provides information, research, resources, and certification in guided imagery.
Kaiser Permanente audio library: https://members.kaiserpermanente.org/redirects/listen/?kp_shortcut_referrer=kp.org/listen	This audio library contains free downloadable guided visualizations for various health conditions including preparing for surgery.

References

References are available online at expertconsult.com.

Chapter 96

Journaling for Health

David Rakel, MD

I find, by experience, that the mind and the body are more than married, for they are most intimately united; and when one suffers, the other sympathizes.

Lord Chesterfield

The sorrow that hath no vent in tears may make other organs weep.

Henry Maudsley

Pathophysiology of Disclosure

The expression of emotionally upsetting experiences by writing or talking has been found to improve physical health, enhance immune function, and result in fewer visits to medical practitioners.[1]

In attempting to understand the pathophysiology behind the positive clinical effects of disclosure, we can review a study by James Pennebaker,[2] a pioneer in the field. He interviewed polygraphers (operators of lie detectors) who worked for the Federal Bureau of Investigation and Central Intelligence Agency. In performing these tests, the polygraphers would look for changes in parameters of the autonomic nervous system, such as heart rate, blood pressure, respiratory rate, and skin conductance, for clues of validity. Pennebaker described what was called the polygraph confession effect, in which readings in these areas significantly dropped after a person confessed. These changes were consistent with those seen with relaxation. Investigators believe that to inhibit actively one's thoughts, feelings, and behaviors requires physical work, work that can result in a chronic low-grade stress to the autonomic nervous system, which may, in turn, lead to disease. This inhibition can also lead to dysregulation of the hypothalamic-pituitary-adrenal axis and cause hypercortisolemia and immune suppression.[3]

Disclosing stressful events transfers repressed thoughts from the unconscious to the conscious level, at which they can be organized and controlled. This transfer removes the need for chronic low-grade stress to stimulate the autonomic nervous system and the hypothalamic-pituitary-adrenal axis

that can lead to disease and somatic symptoms. Disclosing allows the mind to interpret this new information from the subconscious and unlocks emotions that can stimulate positive physical results.

To illustrate how a stressor is stored in the mind, let us consider the money machine that is often an attraction at a county or state fair. The machine consists of an enclosed booth, a pile of paper money, and a fan. A lucky person wins the chance to enter the booth and grab as much money as possible while the fan blows it all around. When the human mind stores a stressful event, the event is not organized and stored as a concrete thought, but rather exists as a chaotic accumulation of a multitude of images, sensations, and emotions, like the money in the booth. Not until we grab the money, hold it in our hand, and count it are we aware of what we have. Disclosing is the process of organizing chaotic thoughts, thus allowing a person to interpret and evaluate the stressor. When this is done, the chronic somatic stress improves because the body no longer needs to sympathize.

When people put their emotional upheavals into words, either through expressive writing or talking, their physical and mental health improves.

Journaling After a Stressful Event

A review of online journal entries before and after the World Trade Center destruction in New York City on September 11, 2001 (9/11) offers insight into how a community discloses and communicates after a tragic event. If a community opens up and talks about the event, the health of the community improves. After 9/11, the city of New York had fewer visits to health care providers. It appears that this tragic event opened people up and stimulated communication that fostered relationships and a sense of community. The words they used in their writing switched to include less use of the ego-centered "I" to a more communal use of "we." This event brought the community together and reduced social isolation, in part by allowing its members to express their emotions (Box 96-1).[4]

BOX 96-1. How to Journal

1. Find a quiet place where you will not be disturbed.
2. Using pen, pencil, or computer, write about an upsetting or troubling experience in your life, something that has affected you deeply and that you have not discussed at length with others.
3. First describe the event in detail. Write about the situation, surroundings, and sensations that you remember.
4. Then describe your deepest feeling about the event. Let go and allow your emotions to run freely in your writing. Describe how you felt about the event then and how you feel now.
5. Write continuously. Do not worry about grammar, spelling, or sentence structure. If you come to a "block," simply repeat what you have already written.
6. Before finishing, write about what you may have learned or how you may have grown from the event.
7. Write for 20 minutes for at least 4 days. You can write about different events or reflect on the same one each day.
8. If the process proves helpful, consider keeping a journal regularly.

Adapted from Rakel DP, Shapiro D. Mind-body medicine. In: Rakel RE, ed. *Textbook of Family Practice.* 6th ed. Philadelphia: Saunders; 2001.

This process happens naturally in the first 2 to 3 weeks after a tragic event. This period is called the emergency phase, during which people and the media open up and discuss the event openly. Approximately 3 weeks after the event, the amount of discussion significantly declines, even though emotions and thoughts about it remain (Fig. 96-1). At this time, called the inhibition phase, when thoughts of the event remain but no one is talking about it, one may wish to encourage continued emotional expression.

Although seeing how this process unfolds in communities is interesting, how may this process of disclosure help us facilitate better health for individual patients? Let us first explore some key studies that show benefit.

Key Areas of Research

Asthma and Rheumatoid Arthritis

Smyth et al[5] asked 107 patients with asthma or rheumatoid arthritis to write either about the most stressful event of their lives (study group) or about daily events (control group) for just 20 minutes over 3 consecutive days. Four months after journaling, the asthmatic patients in the treatment group showed a 20% improvement in lung function, compared with no improvement in the control group. The patients with rheumatoid arthritis who wrote about stressful events showed a 28% reduction in disease severity, whereas the control group showed no change. These are excellent results requiring only paper, pencil, and 60 minutes of a patient's time.

Memory Function

Writing about emotional events may enhance cognitive function and memory. In one study, college freshmen at North Carolina State University who were assigned to write about

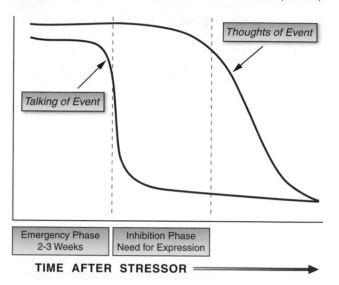

FIGURE 96-1
Pattern of talking compared with thinking about a traumatic event. Journaling is most beneficial during the inhibition phase, when talking decreases but thoughts remain. (Adapted from Rakel DP. Journaling: the effects of disclosure on health. *Altern Med Alert.* 2004;7:8–11.)

their thoughts and feelings about coming to school showed better working memory after 7 weeks compared with students who wrote about trivial topics.[6] Another group in the same study who wrote about their negative emotions had not only better memory but also less intrusive thinking; they were better able to focus on their studies. When students write about the stress of an upcoming test, they perform better on the examination.[7] Other research has linked such writing to higher grades among college students.[8,9]

Wound Healing

A study of similar design showed that writing about emotional events resulted in quicker wound healing than writing about trivial topics such as time management.[10] (No noticeable health benefit has been found in control groups who write about managing time in their lives.) In the second week, after writing for 20 minutes a day for 3 days, the subjects underwent a punch biopsy in the upper arm. Those who wrote about traumatic events had significantly smaller wounds 14 days after the puncture than did those who wrote about trivial topics.[10]

Irritable Bowel Syndrome

Of 103 study subjects with irritable bowel syndrome, 82 in the writing group were asked to write at an online portal for 30 minutes on 4 consecutive days about their deepest thoughts, emotions, and beliefs regarding the disease and their perception of its effects. Compared with the nonwriting control group, the expressive writing resulted in improved disease severity and fewer negative thoughts about their irritable bowel syndrome.[11]

Blood Pressure and Infectious Disease

Steffen et al[12] reported that African American subjects who had a higher level of perceived racism with the suppression of anger were also found to have higher blood pressure than subjects with lower levels of perceived racism. The first group also had higher blood pressure during sleep, a finding suggesting a baseline elevation in sympathetic tone.

Another study showed a higher incidence of infectious diseases and cancer in homosexual men who concealed their homosexual identity than in those who were open about their sexuality.[13]

Employment

In times of challenging economies and job layoffs, learning how the expression of emotions through writing can enhance the ability to obtain a job can be helpful. A group of senior-level engineers who wrote about the emotions of being laid off found new jobs more quickly than did those who did not write. The writing allowed the former group to address the anger, deal with it, and move on. The researchers of the study concluded that this work allowed the first group to have a more positive interview presence when they were looking for a job.[14]

Writing Characteristics Associated With Health

For therapeutic benefit, the health care practitioner does not need to read what is written. In fact, more harm can come from having patients read their writing to others. The therapeutic benefit comes from the expression of the emotions themselves. In evaluation of such writing, however, the following key characteristics have been most commonly associated with a shift toward improved health[15,16]:

- The writer constructed an evolving story. People who created a story with a beginning, middle, and end did better than those who wrote the same story day after day. Creating a story transforms the event into one that is easier to understand and learn from.

- The writer developed insight and used more causal words (realize, understand).

- The writer developed more optimism, with greater use of positive words and a moderate number of negative words.

- As the story evolved, pronouns changed from first person singular (I, me, my) to second person plural (we, us), suggesting that with writing, the person became less isolated and more connected to his or her community.

> The writing topic is less important than the exploration of emotions and thoughts of a topic.

Precautions

The process of disclosure may improve physical but not always mental health.[17] Our minds suppress traumatic events for a reason, and uncovering these events can be difficult for the conscious mind to handle, especially in children. In many cases, patients should work closely with a licensed therapist so they can continue to heal from this expression.

Timing of disclosure is also important. When the body-mind is ready to deal with repressed emotions, it generally has a way of letting us know. The danger comes in encouraging someone to write or express emotions when he or she is not ready to do so. This gives meaning to the old Zen saying, "Don't push the river." Do not encourage writing immediately after a stressful emotional event. Research suggests that this is not helpful and may be harmful.[18] A general recommendation on when to write is to consider expressive writing when the individual finds his or her mind focusing on an event repetitively or ruminating over something.

In helping others explore emotions of past events, one must avoid creating guilt. Little evidence shows that traumatic events in our lives can increase the risk of a disease such as cancer. We must not create this association but simply learn how these events can help us improve our current and future health.

Relationship-Centered Care

The primary care practitioner is in an ideal position to help patients heal through disclosure because people are more likely to discuss stressful events with someone who is accepting and whom they trust.[15] This relationship takes time to develop to a point at which a patient feels comfortable with disclosure. It takes an average of 1 month for children to discuss an abusive event with a psychotherapist.[19] The most important aspect of relationship-centered care is that we provide an environment in which the patient feels comfortable exploring issues that allow us to discover the root of what can influence long-term health. In doing this, whatever tool we use, be it journaling or counseling, will work better because our patients have a connection with someone with whom they feel comfortable sharing their deepest and most meaningful stories. Listening with intention and compassion may be our most valuable therapeutic tool.

The Patient Handout at the end of this chapter offers directions for patients on how to journal to improve health.

KEY WEB RESOURCES

James W. Pennebaker: http://homepage.psy.utexas.edu/homepage/Faculty/Pennebaker/Home2000/JWPhome.htm	This Web site of one of the key researchers in the field includes relevant publications, research tools, and links.
Dr. Howard Schubiner's Mind Body Program: http://www.unlearnyourpain.com/index.php	This program, offered by Howard Schubiner, MD, uses expressive writing to help provide healthy expression of emotions to reduce pain and tension.
Center for Journal Therapy: www.journaltherapy.com/	The Center for Journal Therapy offers classes and instruction on using journaling for health.
My Therapy Journal: https://www.mytherapyjournal.com/	This online journal with secure entries provides multiple ways to express oneself. A fee is required.

References

References are available online at expertconsult.com.

Patient Handout: Using Journaling to Aid Health

What Is Journaling?

Journaling is the process of writing about times in our lives that were stressful or traumatic. It provides an avenue for the expression of thoughts and memories that may have been internalized. These repressed emotions can often lead to a worsening of physical symptoms. William Boyd, a pathologist active in the early to mid-twentieth century, described this process well; he wrote, "The sorrow that hath no vent in tears, may make other organs weep." Journaling is one type of therapy that can be used to aid this process.

How Does It Work?

Studies have found that if we express feelings about a time in our lives that was very traumatic or stressful, our immune function strengthens, we become more relaxed, and our health may improve. Writing about these processes helps us organize our thoughts and create closure to an event that our minds have a tendency to want to suppress or hide. This can be done in the privacy of your home and requires only pen and paper.

Does Anybody Need to Read It?

No. No one needs to read what you write. The most benefit comes from writing the document, and the words can be thrown away if you desire. In fact, some people find that burning or destroying the document can add ceremony to the process. Letting the wind carry away the smoke can act as a positive metaphor that helps to let go, forgive, and heal. Others, however, prefer to keep their writings private, so they can look back on them and see how they have grown from the events. Be sure to keep the writing in a safe location to prevent others from reading it if there is information you want to keep private.

Are There Any Side Effects or Things I Should Be Aware of?

Recalling stressful memories can make you feel uncomfortable for a few days. If this were not the case, the body would not use so much energy trying to repress them. The benefits of journaling become most apparent weeks to months after writing. Do not feel the need to journal about every stressful event. The research shows that expressive writing provides the most benefit when used to express emotions of events that you find yourself ruminating about or that may come into your mind's thoughts time and time again.

This process can bring back into mind some frightening events for which you may need the help of a licensed counselor. Please notify your medical practitioner if you develop feelings that would benefit from further discussion. This is often the first step toward creating an environment that will promote healing from within that will have healthy effects long term.

How Is It Done?

Emotions can be expressed in many different ways. Journaling is simple and inexpensive and can be done independently. It would be beneficial to keep a regular journal to write about events that bring anger, grief, or joy. If that is unlikely and you just want to deal with a specific event or see whether this technique will help your condition, however, follow these steps:

1. Find a quiet place where you will not be disturbed.
2. Using pen, pencil, or computer, write about an upsetting or troubling experience in your life, something that has affected you deeply and that you have not discussed at length with others.
3. First describe the event in detail. Write about the situation, surroundings, and sensations that you remember.
4. Then describe your deepest feeling about the event. Let go and allow your emotions to run freely in your writing. Describe how you felt about the event then and how you feel now.
5. Write continuously. Do not worry about grammar, spelling, or sentence structure. If you come to a "block," simply repeat what you have already written.
6. Before finishing, write about what you may have learned or how you may have grown from the event.
7. Write for 20 minutes for at least 4 days. You can write about different events or reflect on the same one each day. The event is less important than the process of expressing emotions about an event.
8. If the process proves helpful, consider keeping a journal regularly.

How Can I Learn More?

An excellent resource for more information on this subject can be found through the following publications written by leading researchers in the field:

Opening Up: The Healing Power of Expressing Emotions by James W. Pennebaker (Guilford Press, 1997)

Writing to Heal: A Guided Journal for Recovering from Trauma and Emotional Upheaval by James W. Pennebaker (New Harbinger Press, 2004)

The Writing Cure: How Expressive Writing Promotes Health and Emotional Well-being by Stephen J. Lepore and Joshua M. Smyth (American Psychological Association, 2002)

The Center for Journal Therapy offers classes and instruction on using journaling for health. www.journaltherapy.com/

Howard Schubiner, MD, offers a program that uses expressive writing to help provide healthy expression of emotions to reduce pain and tension: http://www.unlearnyourpain.com/index.php

This online journal allows private journal entries that can be tracked and searched. It can be used for all types of journal entries. A fee is required: https://www.mytherapyjournal.com

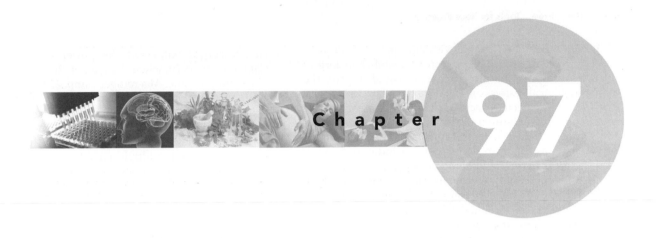

Healing Through Forgiveness

J. Adam Rindfleisch, MD, MPhil, and Gayle Reed, PhD, RN

> If you want to see the heroic, look at those who can love in return for hatred. If you want to see the brave, look for those who can forgive.
>
> *The Bhagavad-Gita*

Of central importance to the integrative approach to medicine is the creation of empathic, trusting relationships between caregivers and patients. If their caregivers provide them with a safe place to do so, patients often disclose traumatic experiences they may not feel comfortable discussing elsewhere. They may describe experiences of abuse—physical, emotional, or sexual. Pain inflicted by others, from minor slights and insults to the most horrifying experiences of brutality or betrayal, can significantly influence health at multiple levels; providers of integrative medicine must bear this in mind. For many people, being able to forgive others or themselves is an absolutely vital component of the process of reclaiming wholeness.

Some people freely recognize the role of forgiveness in healing the damage caused by traumatic experiences; others do not. How and when to address issues of forgiveness can be one of the most challenging aspects of caring for others. Addressing such issues can also be one of the most powerful and rewarding tools a patient is given.

This chapter explores the role that past traumas and forgiveness play in health. The process of forgiving is outlined, and methods for helping patients to forgive are suggested. Additional resources for further reading are also provided.

Traumatic Experiences and Health: The Need for Forgiveness

A strong relationship exists between traumatic experiences and the emergence of physical and mental health problems. In a 1999 study conducted at Harvard University in Massachusetts, 91 people with various chronic pain syndromes were asked to complete several measurement instruments. The researchers found that at least half the people in the study had strong histories of traumatic childhood events, a proportion much higher than that seen in the general population.[1] A 2001 Canadian study revealed that women with a history of childhood sexual abuse were much more likely to both use health care resources and have chronic pain symptoms than a group of matched controls.[2] A 2001 review in the *Annals of Internal Medicine* noted, "Both childhood maltreatment and psychological trauma in adulthood have been associated with increased vulnerability to psychiatric illness and more medical symptoms."[3] Research findings increasingly demonstrate that "...adverse personal, social, and interpersonal experiences, especially when they occur early in life, can result in physical and psychological difficulties in adulthood."[4]

How may an integrative provider help someone overcome the health effects of negative past experiences? Since the 1990s, a steadily growing body of research has emerged indicating what philosophical and spiritual traditions worldwide have acknowledged for some time: Forgiveness has the power to restore well-being. Simply imagining oneself granting forgiveness alters physiology. Blood pressure is lowered, heart rate decreases, and skin conductance changes.[5] Psychological measures of emotional state are also favorably affected.[6] People who are more inclined to forgive are less likely to experience symptoms of depression,[7] anxiety,[8,9] and posttraumatic stress.[10] Forgiveness of self is associated with less blood viscosity and better ratios of helper T to cytotoxic T white blood cells.[11]

Forgiveness clearly has the potential to serve as a powerful healing tool in multiple ways.

> A strong relationship exists between traumatic experiences and the emergence of physical and mental health problems.
> Strong evidence also indicates that forgiveness can improve health in individuals with various physical and psychological conditions.

A 2005 study of 61 people with chronic low back pain found a direct relationship between an inability to forgive and pain intensity; the more a person could forgive, the less psychological distress and pain he or she experienced.[12] Forgiveness has been associated with lower cardiovascular risk, possibly because it decreases anger and hostility; it has even been linked to improvements in lipid measures.[13] Forgiveness was found to decrease anger-induced myocardial ischemic events as well.[14] It decreased anger, depression, anxiety, and vulnerability to drug use in past substance abusers,[15] and a 4-week intervention helped terminally ill older patients with cancer to enhance levels of hope and quality of life.[16] Forgiveness therapy also lowered depression, anxiety, and posttraumatic stress and improved self-esteem, emotional mastery, and the ability to find meaning in suffering in women suffering from spousal emotional abuse.[17] It improves mental health by decreasing the tendency to ruminate, and it probably has secondary effects of improving social relationships as well.[11] Investigators have suggested that forgiveness therapy may hold great potential in the treatment of fibromyalgia and chronic fatigue,[18] and perhaps for any chronic health conditions.[4] Meta-analyses also pointed out the benefits of forgiveness for healing intergenerational pain, recovery from sexual abuse and incest, and abortion-related guilt.[19,20]

The Nature of Forgiveness

Several different measurement instruments are used to conduct research studies, and many have proven quite useful. Ultimately, however, each person must discern his or her own way of defining forgiveness and knowing when and how it has occurred. Even when people do not actually feel equipped to forgive, they are often able to recognize that forgiving is important. When patients are ready, integrative providers can guide them through the process.

As Jack Kornfield, a well-known writer and teacher of Buddhist meditation, noted, "We have all heard stories about the mysterious power of compassion and forgiveness in the lives of others. Each time we are inspired by these accounts, we remember that we, too, can forgive."[21]

Remarkable descriptions of forgiveness abound. Some examples are as follows:

- Forgiveness is an important teaching in the New Testament of the Bible. The Gospel of Matthew refers to the importance of "turning the other cheek," and Jesus asked for forgiveness for those who crucified him.

- The Dalai Lama continually reminds the Tibetan people to practice kindness and compassion toward the Chinese, despite the persecution his people have experienced under Chinese rule.

- Father William Meninger describes the tale of Sister Catherine, a 55-year-old nun who was informed that a physician had mistakenly injected a lethal medication into her during the brain operation she had just undergone. Her response was to call in her fellow church officials and declare, "There will be no repercussions. No one is to be held at fault. ... I forgive without reservation anyone who may have been in any way responsible for what has happened." She died 2 hours later.[22]

- Jack Kornfield witnessed the power of forgiveness in Cambodia in 1979, when the Khmer Rouge was committing mass genocide. At a refugee camp, 25,000 people gathered together despite knowing that they could be killed for doing so. The leader of the meditation recited one phrase from the time of the Buddha: "Hatred never ceases by hatred, but by love alone is healed. This is the ancient and eternal law." After multiple recitations, people began to chant with him, despite all the losses—of home, of freedom, of loved ones—that they had endured.[23]

- Bishop Desmond Tutu, during the era of apartheid in South Africa, was known to pray for the well-being of the white government officials despite their role in perpetuating the system that was so painful for his congregation, the country's black Africans.

- Multiple accounts exist of Jewish people's forgiving those who perpetrated the Holocaust during World War II. For instance, Rabbi Joseph Gelberman, whose family was exterminated by the Nazis, stated he was able to forgive because he "had to let go of what happened."[22]

Such accounts are powerful, but it is not to say that forgiving cannot occur on a personal level for "everyday" people as well as for religious leaders and spiritual communities. Giving and receiving pain are part of the human experience, and forgiving and being forgiven must therefore be part of it as well.

Guidelines for Helping People to Forgive

William Meninger defines the process of forgiveness as follows:

We begin to deal with our wounds by denying or minimizing them. When we finally do face them squarely and recognize the ones who inflicted them, we move on to the next step. This usually involves trying to excuse the perpetrator and blaming ourselves for causing or, at least, not stopping, the original wounds. When we are able to cease the self-blame, we begin to feel sorry for ourselves and to wallow in a mud hole of self-pity, bitterness, and recrimination. The next step is anger. We determine that we will do something about what happened to us and move forward with our lives. We stop rubbing salt in our wounds, and we actively seek healing. This leads us to the final stage, wholeness.[22]

Figure 97-1 illustrates some of the key steps that occur as a person goes through the forgiveness process. These steps need not always occur in a particular order, and not every person experiences every step before forgiveness occurs.

Stepwise approaches guiding forgiveness have been developed by several authorities, and suggestions derived from several of these are summarized in the Patient Handout at the end of this chapter. For further information, clinicians are referred to the work of Robert Enright[24,25] at the University of Wisconsin, Madison, and Frederic Luskin,[26,27] coordinator of the Stanford Forgiveness Project in Palo Alto, California. Additional recommended books and Web sites for both patients and providers are listed in the previously mentioned Patient Handout.[28-35]

FIGURE 97-1

The forgiveness process. General stages in the process are listed in the column on the *left*. Boxes overlying the *arrow* list major obstacles to forgiving. Specific actions are listed on the *right*. More detailed steps are outlined in the resource list in the Patient Handout at the end of this chapter. *Often the most difficult step.

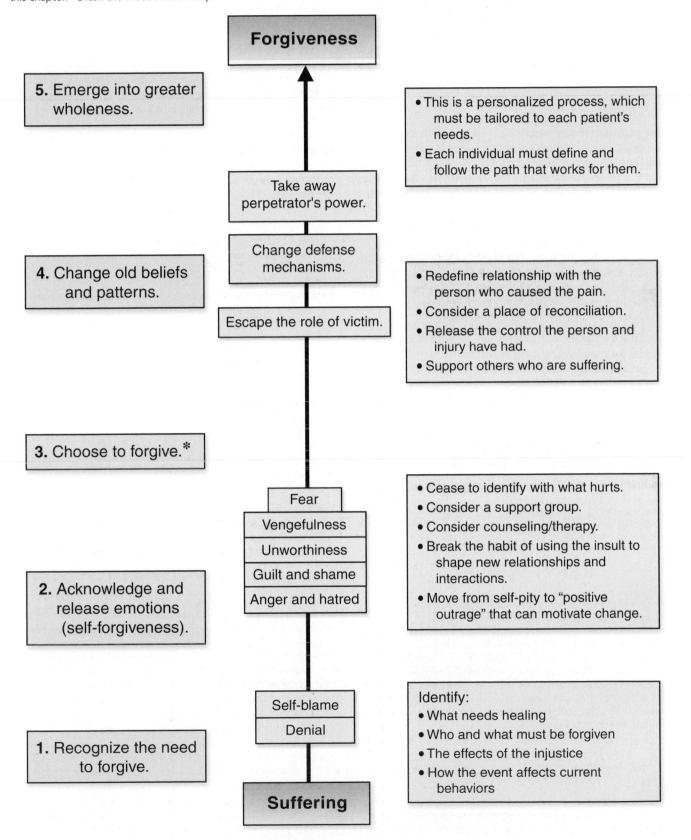

In discussing forgiveness with patients and using the Patient Handout, keep the following in mind:

- As with counseling for weight loss, substance abuse, or other types of behavioral change, suggesting that people cultivate forgiveness is only likely to be useful if people are "in a place" where they are willing and able to consider doing so. Some people may be offended if they are encouraged to forgive when they are not yet prepared to begin the process. As in motivational interviewing for substance use, the provider must assess readiness for change. Is the patient precontemplative, contemplative, or already taking steps toward forgiveness?

- The provider should emphasize, as noted in the Patient Handout, that forgiveness is not the same as tolerance, passivity, or forgetting what happened. No expectation exists that the patient must accept the perpetrator's behavior as acceptable or allowable. Forgiveness is done for the person doing the forgiving; the goal is to free him or her as much as possible from the negative consequences of a traumatic experience.

- Moving through the steps described in this chapter may be associated with an intense release of emotions. The provider must carefully assess whether mental health professionals are needed to assist a patient with the forgiveness process.

- Asking a person to forgive may be asking him or her to move away from a pattern of thoughts and feelings that has been present for many years. It is not a simple process for many people. Follow-up is important. The process takes time.

- A person's concept of forgiveness is based on his or her cultural and religious background. The provider should take a spiritual history and be aware of cultural beliefs, to suggest forgiveness as part of an individualized treatment plan that respects these beliefs and encourages appropriate social support.

- Meditation has shown promise in bringing about forgiveness and should be considered.[36]

- Forgiveness is not just a therapeutic intervention, it is an end point—a healthier state of being—unto itself.[4]

An integrative provider must carefully gauge whether a person is prepared to do forgiveness work. Readiness to change must be carefully assessed.

A spiritual history can be useful in guiding a discussion of forgiveness as a tool for improving health.

Forgiving can be a difficult, emotion-laden, and time-consuming process. Be certain someone has the support he or she needs before beginning the process. Strongly consider requesting assistance from mental health professionals.

Conclusion

Viktor E. Frankl, a psychiatrist and Holocaust survivor, summarizes the importance of how we deal with traumatic experiences in his work, *Man's Search for Meaning*:

> We must never forget that we may also find meaning in life even when confronted with a hopeless situation, when facing a fate that cannot be changed. For what then matters is to bear witness to the uniquely human potential at its best, which is to transform a personal tragedy into a triumph, to turn one's predicament into a human achievement.[37]

Patients continually seek the meaning underlying their illnesses, their suffering, and their terrible losses. As healers, we can help to guide this search. Forgiveness is one tool that may help us all move through tragedy and pain toward greater wholeness.

The Nature of Forgiveness

The following perspectives are based in part on the work of Enright and Luskin, as provided in Further Reading list.

- Forgiveness is a transformation. The key is to release suffering and thereby increase inner peace and understanding.
- Forgiveness is not forgetting. In fact, you have to remember and acknowledge negative emotions and events before forgiveness can occur.
- Forgiveness is not pardoning, excusing, or saying that something will be treated as acceptable behavior in the future.
- Forgiveness is, first and foremost, done for the person doing the forgiving. It is paradoxical in that when you forgive others, you heal yourself.
- Forgiveness is a path to freedom. It frees you from the control of the person who caused the harm. That person loses his or her power to cause you to feel negative emotions.
- Forgiveness can break old patterns that may otherwise interfere when you try to create new relationships.
- Forgiveness can take a long time and much hard work.
- Forgiveness need not require "making up" with the person who caused the harm. It is an internal process. It is primarily for you. The goal is to help you heal, to help you grow.
- Thinking about forgiveness may not be enough. For many, tapping into principles described in various spiritual traditions from around the world is necessary. Meditation, interpersonal dialogues, and intense emotional work may be essential parts of the forgiveness process for many people (see the Further Reading list and the Key Web Resources box).

References

References are available online at expertconsult.com.

Patient Handout: Healing Through Forgiveness

To err is human; to forgive, divine.
—*Alexander Pope*

Scientific research has indicated that forgiving past wrongs can be helpful for a variety of health problems, including anxiety, depression, substance abuse, and chronic pain. When we focus on forgiving, our blood pressure drops and our heart rate slows down. Our mood improves. Forgiveness can alter the state of our health.

What follows is a series of steps designed to help you forgive a past wrong. Follow each step, one at a time, and take a moment to write down your answers to each question. You need not share your answers with others. This process should be based on what feels best for you.

1. Think of a person who has wronged you, someone who you have not been able or willing to forgive thus far.
2. Describe the experience or experiences in which this "offender" harmed you or treated you unjustly. Does it help to have the pain and unfairness validated by a trusted person?
3. Describe the emotions you feel as you consider these events. Do you feel anger? Shame? Guilt? How much time do you spend thinking about or reliving what happened? Take as much time as you need to acknowledge your feelings and experiences and put them into words.
4. How has being unable to forgive affected your health? Has it affected your ability to relate to others? Did it change your view of the world? How has being hurt in the past caused you to protect yourself? Does how you defend yourself limit you in any way?
5. Consider what it means to forgive as well as the potential benefits of forgiving.
6. Are you ready and willing to forgive? When you feel that the answer is "yes," continue with the steps described below. Sometimes just deciding to forgive is the most difficult step of all! (Note: The following guidelines/suggestions are inspired by the works listed in the Further Reading section at the end of this chapter. Follow the steps in whatever order works best for you.)
7. Consider a situation in which another person had to forgive you for something. How did you feel? Recognize that everyone is involved in both forgiving and being forgiven. If you put yourself in the position of the person who hurt you, considering his or her life history and current circumstances, can you understand why he or she did this? (Again, understanding helps you to develop empathy for the person; it does not mean you are minimizing, condoning, or excusing what he or she did.)
8. Practice withholding resentment and developing goodwill toward the one who hurt you. You could consider performing an act of kindness toward the person who hurt you, if it is safe and possible to do so, but any attitude of goodwill that honors your decision to forgive is important. Do what respects your inherent worth as a human being as well as the inherent worth of the one who hurt you.
9. Consider that being realistic about the relationship with the person who hurt you can also be an aspect of goodwill. It can be helpful for both you and the person who hurt you to break any harmful patterns or connections.
10. Mourn and release the pain and emotions that the unjust event(s) caused you. Ask for support from friends or family members as you do this. In this way, you will no longer waste energy on this past injury, and you will be able to avoid passing the pain from the injury back to the person who hurt you and to other people around you.
11. Now that you are facing the pain in order to move through it, what virtues will you choose to follow to turn your suffering into triumph? Will you choose courage, compassion, kindness, love… forgiveness itself? What meaning will you discover? What kind of person are you becoming?
12. As you experience meaning and release, offer support to others who are experiencing similar difficulties. Helping others who have been suffering can help you find renewed purpose as a result of your own painful experiences.
13. For additional insight and assistance, consider discussing these issues with a health professional (counselor, psychologist, physician) or referring to the books mentioned in the Further Reading section of this chapter.

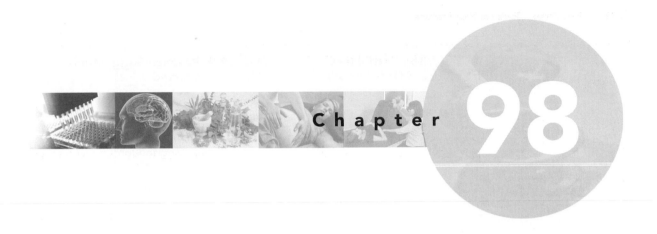

Chapter 98

Recommending Meditation

Luke Fortney, MD

What is Meditation?

Found in cultures, spiritual traditions, and healing systems throughout the world, meditation is a mind-body practice with many methods and variations, all of which are grounded in the silence and stillness of compassionate, nonjudgmental present-moment awareness. Although contemplative meditation practices are rooted largely in the world's spiritual traditions, the practice of meditation does not require belief in any particular religious or cultural system. In fact, public familiarization with meditation and increased research within the fields of neuroscience, psychology, and medicine have led to an increased understanding of consciousness and improved treatment for many health conditions.

Mindfulness is one aspect of the meditation experience that reflects the basic and fundamental human capacity to attend to relevant aspects of experience in a nonjudgmental and nonreactive way, which, in turn, cultivates clear thinking, equanimity, compassion, and open-heartedness. According to University of Massachusetts Center for Mindfulness founder Jon Kabat-Zinn, "Meditation is simplicity itself. It's about stopping and being present. That is all." Stated as simply as possible, *meditation means being present with what is.*

The goal of mindfulness is to maintain fluid awareness in a moment-by-moment experiential process that helps one disengage from strong attachment to beliefs, thoughts, or emotions in a way that generates greater sense of emotional balance and well-being.[1] This simple yet radical assertion holds the potential for wide-reaching therapeutic benefit for many current health care challenges such as rising health care costs,[2] chronic lifestyle-influenced illness,[3] practitioner burnout,[4] patient dissatisfaction,[5] and generalized stress for both practitioner[6] and patient.[7]

Meditation means being present with unmanipulated experience as it arises moment by moment.

Why Meditate?

Prescribed meditation practice can elicit physical ease and mental stability, which provide a foundation for health and wellness as it directly influences one's ability to meet the challenges resulting from stress, burnout, and illness for patient and practitioner alike. For most people, illness brings out feelings of confusion, anxiety, fear, and anger. Shock, isolation, depression, fear, and helplessness are some common experiences patients face in dealing with chronic disease.[8] Feeling out of control or losing one's grounding can give rise to reactivity of the mind and body that leads to increased pain and suffering. Applying the simple practice of nonjudgmental present-moment awareness and experiencing how this process influences one's relationship with life stressors are ways that meditation practice addresses the epidemic of mind-body afflictions that are expressed physically, such as acid reflux, migraine headache, low back pain, restless legs, fibromyalgia, chronic fatigue, irritable bowel, and many other conditions. These and other conditions disproportionately burden health care systems and often do not respond to conventional treatment alone.[2] Meditation is an inward-orienting, self-empowering practice that can stimulate the healing process and help patients and health care practitioners navigate unsettling and turbulent experiences. According to long-time meditation teacher Charlotte Joko Beck,[9] "The practice of meditation provides a skill that affords a greater sense of self determination—the ability to cultivate and draw upon inner resources to help meet all circumstances with equanimity and clarity." To learn the basic elements of meditation practice, see Boxes 98-1 through 98-4 and Figure 98-1.

The practice of meditation serves one's threefold physical, mental, and spiritual health.

BOX 98-1. Getting Started With Mindfulness Meditation Practice: SOLAR or SOL Acronym

Stop

- Find a quiet place where you will not be interrupted for the next several minutes.
- Set your cell phone alarm to vibrate in 5 or more minutes, and then forget about time altogether. You can adjust the length of your meditation time as you feel is appropriate.
- Sit comfortably in an alert position with a straight and relaxed back. With eyes open or closed, position your hands as you like.
- Allow an intention for this time, such as, "May I allow myself to be present to the simplicity of movements in the body as breathing, feeling, and sensing. May I enjoy the benefits of silence and stillness."

Observe

- Direct your attention into noticing sensations in the body and notice posture, feet on the floor, hips on the chair, or feeling a sense of being balanced and grounded.
- Allow the breath to flow in and out of the nose at a natural and unforced rate and depth. Avoid manipulating either a slower or faster rate. Just let the body breathe. In your own bodily experience, notice the sensations of simply breathing.
- Moment by moment, allow yourself to take *pause*, *breathe*, and *feel* just what arises in your experience.

Let it Be

- For this time now, *let everything be as it is* without reacting to or trying to change any of it. Like a watchful bystander, just witness your experience moment by moment as it happens right now, however it may be, pleasant or unpleasant.
- If you become caught up in any particular storyline, fantasy, daydream, rumination, compulsive thought, or distraction gently stop, drop into your body, and allow all experiences to roll on past the screen of your awareness like moving frames in a film.

And...
Return

- Let the breath be your anchor in the present moment. If you become distracted or caught up in any particular *thought, image, emotion*, or *sensation (TIES acronym)*, just bring your attention back to the breath, and *return again and again* to the experience of breathing in a nonjudgmental and self-forgiving way.
- At the end of your meditation period, remain still for a few more moments. Notice how you feel. Invite the intention to be mindfully present by taking a moment to *pause, breathe,* and *feel* whatever is happening in any experience throughout your day.

BOX 98-2. Practice Suggestions and Getting Started

- For "formal practice," find a quiet place to sit, with few distractions. In the beginning, it may be difficult to sit still for even 5 minutes. You may note restless or even disturbing thoughts. Over time with regular practice, the mind will become more stable and clear.
- Do not meditate too long in the beginning. It may be useful to start with short guided practices (http://www.fammed.wisc.edu/our-department/media/mindfulness).
- Commit to a set amount of time specifically for meditation. A good intention before you start is, "For this short time now, I have nowhere to go and nothing to do." Having a timer such as a smart phone application (e.g., Zen Timer) can ease any worry of having to keep track of time.
- Sit in a comfortable and alert position with an upright spine. For most people, sitting in a chair with feet flat on the floor is ideal. Other positions can include crossed legs, kneeling on a bench, or straddling a cushion.
- With eyes open or closed, allow the gaze to settle easily.
- Be persistent and regular with daily meditation. Progress comes by maintaining constant effort in daily practice. In time, try to meditate for 15 to 20 minutes in the morning just after rising and again before going to bed, but any duration and opportunity for meditation is beneficial, even if it is only one breath or 1 minute. The daily commitment of meditation requires a continual nonjudgmental return to the practice itself, over and over again every day. If you miss a day, or a week, or even years, simply return to the practice of meditation without judgment.
- For "informal practice," try to approach everyday activities with the same mindful intention, attitude, attention and presence as in "formal" meditation. While driving to work, focus on driving. When at work, concentrate on the performance of each task. At home, live and be completely present with others. Keep in mind that meditation is not about withdrawal from the world or responsibilities. It is about living with purpose, awareness, and kindness.
- A deepening of spiritual life and religious experience may occur. Although this can be pleasant, it can also be disconcerting early on and may require the reassurance and guidance of an understanding teacher.

Review of Meditation Research

Evidence pointing to the medical benefits of meditation is widely documented and continues to increase in quality and quantity. In 2007 alone, more than 70 scientific articles were published on mindfulness meditation practice. In particular, the biologic correlates of meditation experience have received the most attention in research, quite out of proportion to the complete meditative experience, which includes both objective external effects and subjective

BOX 98-3. Precautions and Recommendations for Meditation Practice

- Leg and back discomfort can be a common concern. Do not strain the body. Sit in an alert and comfortable position. Remember that meditation is about openness and not about contracting the body into discomfort.
- In the beginning, intrusive, repetitive, or disturbing thoughts may make it difficult to sit still for even 5 minutes. Keep in mind that meditation is not about making things go away. It is simply the nonjudgmental process of staying present with whatever is happening moment by moment, pleasant or unpleasant. However, over time and with regular practice, the mind will become more stable.
- In learning meditation, one should be guided by teachers and practice that resonate authentically, are nondivisive, and instill feelings of support. Do not forfeit personal boundaries and safety for any teacher or teaching. Listen to your intuition and reason, and trust that the experience you are having is exactly what you need in this moment.
- Meditation can at times uncover preexisting stressors or traumas, similar to peeling back the layers of an onion, thus revealing unpleasant underlying emotions. A professional counselor familiar with contemplative practice can help facilitate the healthy release of these emotions.
- Be attentive to and honest about your experience. In a compassionate way, attend to realizations and insights that arise from regular meditation practice. This may include journaling, creative expression, and talking with a skilled meditation teacher.
- Including a gentle form of movement is encouraged, such as contemplative or mindful walking, walking a labyrinth, hatha yoga, Pilates, nia, tai chi or qi gong, swimming, or biking. However, avoid striving and straining.

BOX 98-4. Summary of Mindfulness Meditation Practice

The Experience (TIES Mnemonic)
- **Talk/thoughts:** mental chatter, incessant thinking, storyline narratives
- **Images:** mental pictures, imagined scenes, visualized scenarios
- **Emotional feelings:** love, hate, fear, joy, sadness, anxiety, etc.
- **Physical Sensations:** sound, touch, sight, taste, smell

The Process (SOLAR or SOL Mnemonic)
- **Stop:** Pause and drop into this experience right now.
- **Observe** being aware of and noticing what is actually happening in this moment.
- **Let it be:** Acknowledge and allow this arising experience to be what it is, pleasant or unpleasant.
- **And...**
- **Returning** again and again to the present moment, remember to pause, breathe, and feel whatever is happening.

internal experience. However, research is only beginning to elucidate how the mind-body connection affects health in promoting wellness, as well as in managing and preventing disease.

The interplay between the mind and the body has been difficult to describe and operationalize from a scientific standpoint. However, many case examples reveal the potential value in developing clinically oriented mind-body therapies. As early as 1935, French cardiologist Brosse[10] studied Indian yogis capable of decreasing their heart rates to almost zero as shown on electrocardiography. In 1961, Bagchi and Wenger[11] found that some expert meditation subjects could produce bidirectional changes in every measurable autonomic variable. The *Lancet* published an account of the voluntary live burial of a yogi who sat cross-legged underground for 62 hours while continuous vital sign recordings revealed no distress.[12] In 1968, Hoenig[13] witnessed an experiment in which a yogi confined for 9 hours in a small enclosed pit and monitored with electroencephalography and ECG demonstrated a normal waking rhythm for the full 9 hours. This finding led Hoenig to conclude that the subject was awake and relaxed throughout the experiment. This researcher also observed a variable heart rate from 40 to 100 beats/minute in recurring cycles on ECG.[13] As in fetal heart monitoring, later research showed that synchronous increases in heart rate variability in adults predict a decrease in cardiovascular mortality,[14,15] which can be reproduced using meditation practices.[16,17]

Benson et al[18] helped pioneer academic interest in meditation through their research on the physiologic and neurochemical principles of *the relaxation response,* which is defined as a hypometabolic state of parasympathetic activation.[18] Further, many studies have demonstrated that meditation training reduces anxiety and increases positive affect,[19-21] whereas others have shown that mindfulness meditation prevents recurrence of depression.[22,23] In a 1985 study by Kabat-Zinn et al,[24] patients with chronic pain showed a statistically significant reduction in various measures of pain symptoms when they were trained in mindfulness-based stress reduction. Meditation practices have also shown beneficial effects on tension headaches,[25] psoriasis,[26] blood pressure,[27-29] serum cholesterol,[29] smoking cessation,[30,31] alcohol abuse,[32] carotid atherosclerosis,[33] coronary artery disease,[3,34,35] longevity and cognitive function in older adults,[36] psychiatric disorders,[18-23,37] excessive worry,[38] use of medical care,[39] and medical costs in treating chronic pain.[40] A 2004 meta-analysis found mindfulness-based stress reduction training useful for a broad range of chronic disorders that are difficult to treat, such as depression, anxiety, fibromyalgia, mixed cancer diagnoses, coronary artery disease, chronic pain, obesity, and eating disorders.[41] The investigators noted consistent and strong effect sizes across these very different situations, thus indicating a generalized application of meditation for both daily life distress and more extraordinary medical disorders.[41]

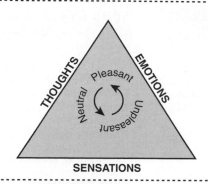

FIGURE 98-1
Mindfulness "practice as you go" cards (cut-out handout for patients).

Mindfulness practice (SOAP):

- **Stop:** Pause, notice your breathing, settle into the present moment just as it is...
- **Observe:** Drop into the body, being aware of and feeling whatever is happening in this moment (sensations/feelings/thinking)...
- **Assess:** Without judgment, recognize the pleasant/unpleasant/neutral nature of this experience and let it go...
- **Proceed:** Take a deep breath, and move on...

Triangle of mindful experience:

- **Mental thoughts:** Rumination, thinking, storylines, narratives, mental images,
- internal conversations, and so on...
 Emotional feelings: Love, hate, fear,
- guilt, anger, joy, sadness, anxiety, and so on...
- **Physical sensations:** Sound, touch, taste, smell, vibration, pressure, and so on...

Intentional kindness practice:

- May I/you/we be well
- May I/you/we be at ease
- May I/you/we be safe and protected
- May I/you/we understand and be understood

In a meta-analysis of brain imaging studies on various meditation styles, Newberg[42] suggested that the neurophysiologic effects derived from various meditation practices seem to outline a consistent and reproducible pattern of significant brain activity in key cerebral structures. Research focusing more specifically these physiologic effects of meditation by Davidson et al[43] described a positive correlation between meditation practice and left-sided prefrontal cortex activity, which is associated with positive affect. In this study, mindfulness meditation was associated with increases in antibody titers to influenza vaccine, a finding suggesting correlations among meditation, positive emotional states, localized brain activity, and improved immune function. Corroborating research demonstrated a direct link between immune function and mood, with positive affective states resulting in stronger immune function and decreased incidence of illness.[44-46] Lutz et al[47] observed increased left-sided prefrontal cortex gamma wave activity and synchronicity in expert Tibetan Buddhist meditators with more than 10,000 hours of meditation experience when compared with novice meditator controls, both at rest and during meditation. This finding suggests that attention and affective processes are flexible skills that can be learned.

Although ongoing research aims to elucidate the measurable biologic correlates of meditation and its significance with regard to health, the experiential knowledge that has arisen from time-tested practices of the great spiritual traditions should be acknowledged. Meditation practitioners within these spiritual systems continue to explore the subtle inner dimensions of meditative experience by using methods and perspectives that equally address the human condition in our search for healing and well-being.

Meditation is useful for any indication, including daily life and extraordinary medical disorders.

Mindfulness in Medical Practice

Practicing health-oriented medicine in dysfunctional health systems and institutions that do little to honor health is increasingly difficult.[48] As clinicians are asked to see more patients, they are forced to limit their focus to a physical process, laboratory test, imaging study, or quick prescription. For clinicians, maintaining a balance between personal needs and the demands of medical training and practice is often neglected at the cost of well-being and health. Sleep, exercise, relaxation, and personal interests take a back seat to long clinical hours and academic demands that contribute to burnout.[49] Research suggests that mindfulness meditation cultivates present-moment awareness that may reduce medical error and improve patient care. For example, faulty thinking, such as snap judgments, distracted attention, inadvertent stereotyping, and other cognitive traps, lead to critical mistakes in patient care.[50] Growing research also shows that practitioners who themselves exhibit healthy habits are more effective in motivating patients to make significant positive changes in their own lives.[51] This is also true of health practitioners who themselves practice meditation. In a randomized controlled trial of 124 psychiatric inpatients managed by 18 psychology residents, Grepmair et al[52] showed that patients of interns who received mindfulness training did significantly better than did patients treated by interns who did not receive mindfulness training.

To address these concerns, the University of Wisconsin Integrative Medicine Program created a collaborative online education module (http://www.fammed.wisc.edu/mindfulness; see Box 98-5 first item) to provide ongoing support for mindfulness practice and to help clinicians bring mindfulness into the clinical encounter by using a three step process: (1) pause, (2) presence, and (3) proceed[53] (see Chapter 3, The Healing Encounter). The first step, pause, encourages the user to stop, pause, and be present in the moment. The second step, presence, encourages the user to drop into the moment and become aware of sensations, emotions, and thoughts that arise without judgment or analysis. The third step, proceed, encourages health-oriented action that responds in a skillful and compassionate way by using insight from steps 1 and 2. For example, the disease- or symptom-focused visit would result in a medication to abort a migraine headache, but the mindful session could also address emotional stressors that are main migraine triggers. This approach focuses more on the underlying causes of suffering that may be exacerbating pain than on the symptoms of pain alone. The mindful clinical encounter encourages the clinician to pay attention to and illuminate key healing mechanisms that arise from the patient-clinician interaction.

Types of Meditation

Most types of meditation are embedded in a specific historical time period, based on the realizations of a particular teacher or group, and should be considered with their original cultural background in mind. Most techniques are best understood within the context of their particular spiritual traditions. The collection of information, teachings, and practices is massive, however, and selecting your own meditation practice can be challenging. One way to help is to read books, visit Web sites, attend local retreats and classes, and meet with teachers and groups to help discern what practices are a good fit for you. Keep in mind that *no one way is best*. Although insights and realizations from meditation practice have a universal quality, many practice styles exist. As the common saying goes, "all paths lead to Rome." After considerate searching, choose a practice that has personal resonance and meaning of some kind for you. For help with this process, see Boxes 98-5 and 98-6, and Table 98-1.

> "What joy awaits discovery in the silence behind the portals of your mind no human tongue can tell. But you must convince yourself; you must meditate and create that environment."
> Paramahansa Yogananda

Movement as Meditation

Often, we think of meditation as sitting on a cushion, folding your legs under you, closing the eyes, and focusing the attention on something such as a candle, a word, or a chant. These are just a few of the many varieties of meditation style, but this is not the only way meditation can be done. "Formal" meditation practice, however, typically involves being seated and still in certain comfortable and alert positions, generally on a firm chair or a floor cushion (Fig. 98-2, meditation postures). Most styles of meditation practice also recommend some form of movement practice such as yoga, contemplative or mindful walking, tai chi, labyrinth walking, dance, and so on. Being present and

---

BOX 98-5. Resources and Links to Learn Meditation

- http://www.fammed.wisc.edu/mindfulness (Online guided practices and resources for mindfulness in medicine from the University of Wisconsin)
- http://www.umassmed.edu/content.aspx?id=41252 (University of Massachusetts Center for Mindfulness)
- https://www.fammed.wisc.edu/aware-medicine/mindfulness (University of Wisconsin Aware Medicine Curriculum)
- http://eomega.org/ (New York/East Coast Omega Institute)
- http://nccam.nih.gov/ (National Center for Complementary and Alternative Medicine)
- http://diydharma.org/about-us (Do It Yourself Dharma)
- http://www.spiritrock.org/ (California/West Coast Spirit Rock Meditation Center)
- http://www.contemplativeoutreach.org/site/PageServer (Contemplative Outreach [Centering Prayer])
- http://www.christinecenter.org (Wisconsin/Midwest Christine Center)
- *Meditation for Beginners,* by Jack Kornfield, PhD (book and CD)
- *Guided Mindfulness Meditation,* by Jon Kabat-Zinn (CD)
- *Full Catastrophe Living,* by Jon Kabat Zinn (book)
- *Open Mind Open Heart,* by Fr. Thomas Keating, OCSO (book)
- *The Beginner's Guide to Contemplative Prayer,* by James Finley, PhD (CD)

BOX 98-6. Other Popular Meditation Styles, Teachers, and Spiritual Practices

- Ram Dass, formerly a Harvard University psychologist and researcher, learned Hindu meditation and chanting from his guru Maharaji. Books: *Be Here Now* and *Still Here.* Web site: www.ramdasstapes.org
- Eckhart Tolle, formerly an Oxford University research scholar, experienced a spiritual transformation and teaches contemporary spirituality. Book: *The Power of Now.* Web site: www.eckharttolle.com
- Tom Brown, Jr was mentored by "Grandfather," an Apache Medicine Man and Scout. Book: *The Vision.* School: Nature and Wilderness Survival Schools. Web site: www.trackerschool.com
- Ken Wilber, creator of the unified field theory of consciousness. Book: *A Brief History of Everything.* School: Integral Institute. Web sites: www.kenwilber.com, www.integralinstitute.org, http://wilber.shambhala.com
- John Main, a Catholic monk, founder of Christian Meditation inbreath mental mantra "MA-RA" and outbreath "NA-THA" Sanskrit for "Come Lord Jesus." Book: *Word into Silence.* Web site: www.wccm.org
- Neale Donald Walsch, author of *Conversations with God* and founder of Re-Creation retreats. Web site: www.nealedonaldwalsch.com

TABLE 98-1. Systems of Meditation Table*

	CENTERING PRAYER/ CONTEMPLATION	KABBALAH (QABALAH)	MINDFULNESS MEDITATION	RIDHWAN SCHOOL DIAMOND APPROACH	SELF-REALIZATION FELLOWSHIP (SRF)	TRANSCENDENTAL MEDITATION	TIBETAN BUDDHISM	ZEN BUDDHISM/ CH'AN
Traditional Background	Catholic/Christian (inclusive)	Jewish mystical (inclusive)	Vipassana/insight; mindfulness-based stress reduction medical (inclusive)	Sufi Islam, mystical psychology (inclusive)	Hindu Kriya yoga (inclusive)	Vedic Hindu (inclusive)	Various Tibetan lineages (inclusive)	Numerous Chinese and Japanese lineages (inclusive)
Teachers	Thomas Keating; Thomas Merton; Cynthia Bourgeault; M. Basil Pennington; William Meninger	Yehuda Ashlag; David Cooper; Michael Laitman	Jon Kabat-Zinn; Bhante Gunaratana; Sharon Salzberg; Jack Kornfield; Thich Nhat Hanh	A. H. Almaas (Hameed Ali)	Paramahansa Yogananda; Sri Daya Mata	Maharishi Mahesh Yogi (Various)	Fourteenth Dalai Lama; Panchen Lama; Chogyam Trungpa; seventeenth Karmapa	Bodhidharma; Eisai; Dogan; Huang Po; Charlotte Joko Beck; Claude A. Thomas
Technique	Sacred word; prayer; lectio divina	Kabbalah	Breath/body awareness	Inquiry	Kriya yoga; Hong-Sau; Aum	Personalized mantra	Mantra; visualization; chanting	Zazen
Body/Activity Focus	Contemplative walking	Self-directed	Mindful walking; Hatha yoga; body scan	Breathing exercises	Energization exercises	Self-directed	Rlung-sgom walking; mudras	Martial arts-Kungfu; Zen arts (ceramics, archery, calligraphy)
Readings/ Books	New Seeds of Contemplation (by Merton); Open Mind Open Heart (by Keating)	A Beginner's Guide to Kabbalah (CD); A Heart of Stillness (by Cooper)	Mindfulness in Plain English (by Gunaratana); Full Catastrophe Living (by Kabat-Zinn); A Path with Heart (by Kornfield)	Essence; The Diamond Heart Series I-IV; Inner Journey Home (by Almaas)	Autobiography of a Yogi; SRF Lessons (by Yogananda)	Science of Being and Art of Living: Transcendental Meditation (by Maharishi)	The World of Tibetan Buddhism; Path to Bliss (by Gyatso); Start Where You Are (by Chodron)	Zen Mind Beginner's Mind (by Suzuki); The Three Pillars of Zen (by Kapleau) Everyday Zen (by Beck)

	Coursework	Main Sites/Headquarters	Web Sites/Contact Information	Comments
	Teacher-student	Shaolin Temple, China (birthplace); multiple centers	www.dharmanet.org; www.tricycle.com	Chinese/Japanese tradition arrived in the United States after World War II; most Zen meditation research in Japanese
	Teacher-student; lineage directed	Lhasa, Tibet; Dharamsala, India; multiple	www.tibet.com; www.deerparkcenter.org; www.dawnmountain.org; www.drikungtmc.org	Model of nonviolence, loving compassion of sentient beings; ongoing dialogue with neuroscience researchers
	Seven-step coursework; interviews; personal mantra; retreats	Fairfield, Iowa; multiple; (Transcendental Meditation Independent UK)	www.tm.org; www.maharishipeacepalace.org; 1-888-learnTM; (www.tm-meditation.co.uk, independent, less expensive)	Popularized in 1960s, expanded meditation in the United States; large corpus of health research at Maharishi Vedic University
	Mailed lessons; Retreats; guru relationship; interviews with monks	Los Angeles; multiple (see also Yogoda Satsanga Society of India, sister organization to SRF)	www.srf-yogananda.org	Founded in 1920; popularized yoga-meditation in the United States; teaches direct path to self-realization through ancient Kriya yoga
	Diamond approach lessons; retreats	Berkeley, Calif; Boulder, Colo; multiple	www.ahalmaas.com; www.ridhwan.org	Founded in 1970s; called the Work; draws from psychology and integrates spiritual approach to self-liberation
	Mindfulness-based stress reduction / cognitive therapy	Insight Meditation Society, Mass; University of Massachusetts (for mindfulness-based stress reduction); Spirit Rock, Calif; Plum Village, France; multiple	www.dharma.org; www.umassmed.edu/cfm/mbsr; www.eomega.org; www.spiritrock.org; www.plumvillage.org	Popularized in 1980s; from an 8-wk course in a medical/research setting; many vipassana/insight sanghas or groups
	Tree of Life; Ten Sefirot; Devekut; teacher directed	Multiple	www.kabbalah.info; www.kabbalah.com; 1-800-kabbalah	Ancient oral tradition of wisdom and mystery; tells of Light of Creation; Jewish renewal movement
	Retreats; contemplative outreach	Abbey of Gethsemani, Trappist, Ky; Snowmass Colo; multiple/regional	www.centeringprayer.com (also see Christian Meditation: www.wccm.org)	Contemplation dates back to St. Anthony and the Desert Fathers; revived after Vatican II; in the tradition of Christian saints and mystics

*This table is representative and not exhaustive.

FIGURE 98-2
Meditation postures. **A,** Seated position with chair. Maintain a straight back. **B,** Full lotus position. Maintain a straight back. Use of a cushion, shawl, mat, or blanket for comfort may be helpful. **C,** Half-lotus position. Maintain a straight back. Use of a cushion, shawl, mat, or blanket for comfort may be helpful. **D,** Kneeling position with bench. Maintain a straight back. Use of a shawl, mat, or blanket for comfort may be helpful.

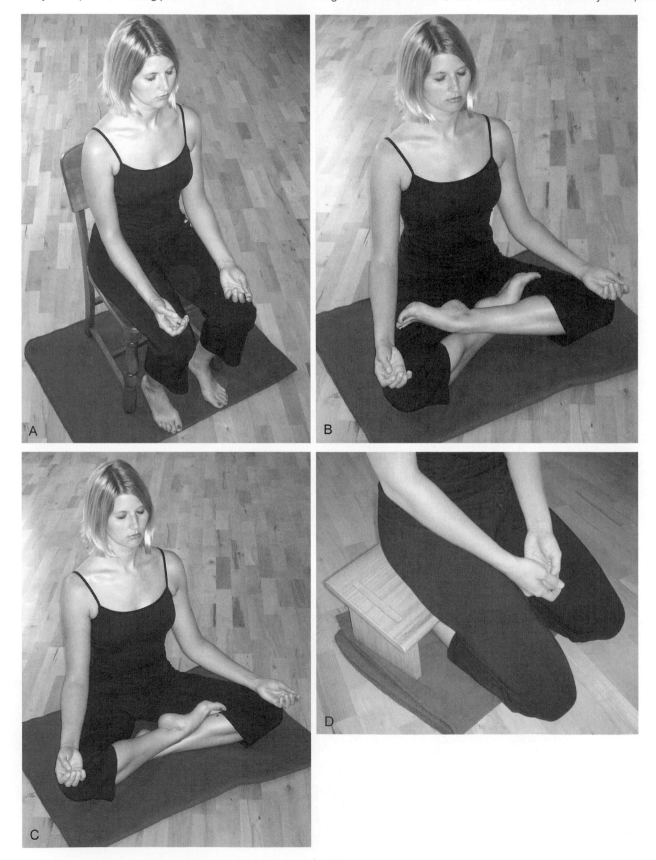

connected with the body and really noticing the qualities of the various physical sensations that arise with movement are important. Allowing the body to be your guide is a way of experiencing grounding and centering. Participating in activities that are safe and appropriate for each person is recommended.

Through meditation, one learns how to be present with and see through the obstacles of dissatisfaction, restlessness, and overidentification that imprison and obscure the mind.

References

References available online at expertconsult.com.

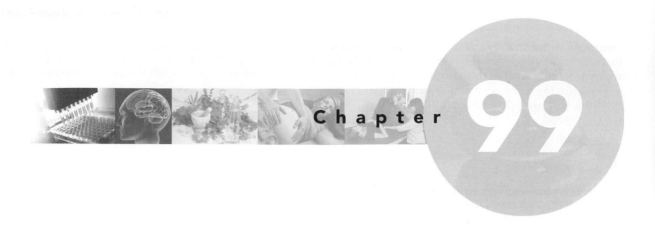

Motivational Interviewing

Robert Rhode, PhD

Health care providers often diagnose a patient's condition and recommend health-promoting behaviors (e.g., take this drug as prescribed, exercise, stop smoking, decrease substance use, make appointments for care, follow a diet). Integrative medicine is more than just recommending some alternative or nonallopathic health-promoting behaviors. It also involves the way in which those recommendations are made to the client.

Three Helping Styles

Directing

In most allopathic health care settings, the recommendation to the client is given in a directing helping style, which often includes identifying the health goal or destination and giving clear advice on how to reach that destination. The health care provider is using his or her expertise, identifying the problems to be addressed, and prescribing treatments or proscribing behaviors. The client would do well to heed and follow this well-intended advice. This style is initiated with medical students who are taught how to recognize symptoms and relevant treatments. Their excitement about their growing knowledge almost guarantees that when they start seeing clients, they will expound on their expertise and treatment recommendations with enthusiasm and direct the client on what to do. Medical students may be quite surprised and frustrated to find many of their clients explicitly rejecting this sound advice during the consultation (by responding with, "Yes, but…") or to have clients returning for a follow-up consultation with the same problem after ignoring the earlier proffered advice. Health care providers with years of experience are familiar with this dance and may have acquiesced to clients' not following treatment recommendations.

Although a directing helping style does not always facilitate the desired health improvement, it is necessary in health care, and some clients are responsive to it. Some clients prefer to be told what to do, and when their clinicians speak, they listen and implement the advice received. In some situations, the client's cooperation cannot be solicited, such as during an emergency or when the client is unconscious. At such times, the clinician takes charge, acts unilaterally, and institutes treatment.

Following

Another style often used in health care can be called a following helping style, which has no destination or goal other than developing rapport, or staying with the client. Health care providers offer healing by being genuinely present and attending to clients with heart and mind. In some situations, no obvious treatment or choice exists, and just being with the client is the medicine. This approach may be more valued in an integrative medicine setting than in one that emphasizes only allopathic approaches. A following helping style is also useful to clinicians in other situations, such as when the client is uncertain about changing jobs, relationships, donating an organ, or becoming pregnant. When one choice or another has no obvious risks or benefits, the clinician is very likely to use a following helping style to facilitate the client's talking about his or her choices and avoid advocating or directing toward either choice.

Guiding

A guiding helping style is a third way, and may be somewhere between a directing and a following helping style. This approach solicits the patient's experience and yet still moves toward a health goal. A clinician using a guiding helping style may be similar to a hiking guide. The hiking guide can be useful to point out the trail and warn about looming clouds and the need to pick up the pace before a storm arrives. The hiking guide is not going to carry the hiker to the top of the mountain, however. Motivational interviewing can be considered a specialized version of a guiding helping style that assists clients to access their own reasons and desires to engage in the health-promoting behavior. It may be a style that is most useful when the client must collaborate with the clinician to implement the health-promoting behavior.

Many lifestyle behaviors fall into this category because it is the client who has to exercise, eat more nutritiously, engage in meditation, or abstain from smoking.

> Motivational interviewing can be considered a specialized version of a guiding helping style that assists clients to access their own reasons and desires to implement the health-promoting behavior.

The proportions among communication skills used in these three helping styles have been depicted as in Figure 99-1.[1] With a directing helping style, the health care provider engages in extensive informing, teaching, advising, and passing on of expertise. He or she asks questions to learn about the client's experience and makes a diagnosis or determines which treatment may be best. He or she listens to the answers the client gives to those questions. With a following style, the clinician does much less informing and much more listening, facilitated perhaps by asking questions to help the client say more. With a guiding style, clients do some informing but less than in a directing style and more than in a following style. Questions are asked so the client learns (in that manner of "Now that I hear myself say it, I realize…") and not so the clinician can make a diagnosis or provide an answer or treatment. The clinician who uses a guiding style does more listening than when using a directing style but less than when using a following style. A guiding style involves going toward a destination, and in that way it resembles a directing helping style. It also is client centered, by collaborating with the client and recognizing the client as an expert and primary decision maker, and in that way it is similar to a following style.

A directing helping style has been called a "push technology."[2] The clinician is attempting to install knowledge or motivation as if the client is missing it. A guiding helping style is a "pull technology." The health care provider is attempting to pull the knowledge and motivation from the client's existing resources and experiences. A directing helping style is consistent with the clinician's role as healer, the one who cures, and the expert. A guiding helping style emphasizes healing rather than the healer, with two experts (the client and the clinician) in the consultation room. In settings where a directing helping style is common, the recipients of care are often called "patients." When a guiding or following helping style is more often used, the care recipients are often called "clients" or even "consumers." Figure 99-2 shows that the health care provider who uses a directing helping style does the most talking, whereas clients do very little. With a following helping style, the client does most of the talking, and the health care provider does much less. A guiding helping style is in between the two styles.

A health care provider who can use all three of these helping styles in response to different clients and situations likely sees more client improvement. All these styles are helpful. This chapter focuses on the guiding helping style and, in particular, on motivational interviewing, not because it is always better but because it is often underused, given the common reliance on a directing helping style in health care settings. A guiding helping style may also be more consistent with integrative medicine.

Foundation or Spirit of Motivational Interviewing

A motivational interviewing approach has three foundational values. Many clinicians, particularly integrative medicine clinicians, agree in principle on the first two, even if they are not always able to demonstrate them during their consultations or interactions.

1. Collaboration: The clinician comes alongside, joins up, looks at the client's life or situation together with the client, and partners with the client to consider a difficult situation.
2. Respecting the client's autonomy: The clinician respects that it is the client who has to engage in the health-promoting

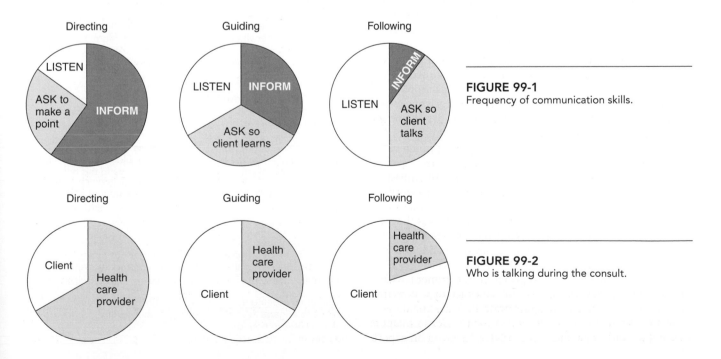

Directing   Guiding   Following

FIGURE 99-1
Frequency of communication skills.

Directing   Guiding   Following

FIGURE 99-2
Who is talking during the consult.

behavior. The clinician supports that the client can decide to change now, later, or not at all.

3. Curiosity: This leads to mining for, fishing for, and nurturing the client's reasons for engaging in the health-promoting behavior. Before giving any advice or teaching, the health care provider solicits what the client knows.

A directive helping style does not often involve collaboration with the client because the health care provider is adopting an expert role and is "driving the bus." Similarly, not much need exists to be curious about the client's experience because the clinician is deciding what needs to be done. An example of this is when the clinician tells the client that he or she is drinking too much, meets the criteria for alcoholism, needs to attend Alcoholics Anonymous meetings, and should abstain from drinking. The client's objection to the diagnosis and treatment recommendation does not change the clinician's conviction and is often labeled, very logically, by the clinician as an example of the client's denying reality or the truth ("The patient is in denial.").

When a motivational interviewing style is used, the clinician respects the client as capable and competent, and therefore it makes sense to collaborate with him or her. If the clinician intends to collaborate with the client, it makes sense to respect and support the client's autonomy. The client will literally be the one to implement (or not) the health-promoting behavior. During a stay in the hospital, health care providers may have more control over the patient's diet, activity, and medication. When the client is out of the hospital, the client decides what to eat, what to do, and what medication to take. Respecting that reality and explicitly recognizing that the client will make these decisions relieves the clinician of the frustrating task of trying to control the client. The clinician is no longer driving the bus but is "on the bus" with the client.

If the client is capable, competent, and believed to be the key person to implement any treatment, then it makes perfect sense to be curious about the client's experience and his or her reasons for embracing or rejecting the health-promoting behaviors. The client who is drinking too much is now approached differently. The clinician still maintains a focus on the destination of less drinking or abstaining. Instead of telling the client what the problem is, however, he or she now asks what the client thinks about the drinking and how it fits with other goal or values. Instead of pushing a treatment, the clinician explores what makes sense to the client to try. The client's objections to abstaining are not heard as denial but rather as the client's natural ambivalence to giving up something that he or she enjoys or to which he or she is attached. The clinician may help the client find his or her motivation to change this drinking by exploring which of the client's goals are hindered by the current drinking.

This collaborating with a capable client seems consistent with integrative medicine as described by Andrew Weil[3]: "There is this tremendous innate healing capacity that we all have. When I sit with a person who is sick, always at the back of my mind is the question, 'What is blocking healing here? What is preventing it? What can I do from outside that can facilitate that process?'"

Table 99-1 describes some ways to experiment with a motivational interviewing style, in contrast to a directing helping style. Another way to generate a motivational interviewing approach is for the health care provider to imagine quitting his or her job and envision that he is not an expert.

Suspending the expert role will very likely lead to joining with the client who is facing the challenge of improving well-being or managing a chronic condition. Although "care" today has the connotation of intervening in a beneficial way, another meaning is "to be with." Collaborating includes looking together at the situation, and from there, being curious about the client's motivation for the health-promoting behaviors is easy.

What Difference May It Make If a Motivational Interviewing Approach Is Used?

Meta-analysis and reviews of the effectiveness of motivational interviewing have been published.[4–8] Following the initial description of motivational interviewing in 1983, much of the research has related to health behaviors in the area of substance use. Over the years, more studies have focused on a broader range of health-promoting behaviors (Fig. 99-3). The effect sizes for various health behaviors 3 and 12 months after treatment are shown in Figure 99-4.

TABLE 99-1. Ways to Experiment With a Motivational Interviewing Style in Contrast to a Directing Helping Style

DIRECTING HELPING STYLE	MOTIVATIONAL INTERVIEWING STYLE
These may be methods a health care provider could use to help a client. These fit with a directing helping style.	Instead of using a directing helping style, a health care provider could use a motivational interviewing style, as follows:
Explaining why the client should engage in the health-promoting behavior.	Listening with the goal of understanding the client's dilemma concerning the health-promoting behavior.
Teaching the client, telling him or her what to do, or giving advice.	Asking what the client knows, then providing some information or advice, and finally asking how that fits with his or her life.
Describing specific benefits that would result from doing the health-promoting behavior.	Asking, "What benefits may there be for you if you engaged in this health-promoting behavior?"
Telling the client how to implement the health-promoting behavior.	Asking, "What are you already doing that would make it possible for you to engage in this health-promoting behavior?" Or, "How may you engage in this health-promoting behavior so it fits into your day?"
Emphasizing how important it is for the client to engage in the health-promoting behavior.	Asking, "Why is it important to you to think about or engage in this health-promoting behavior?"
Telling or inspiring the client to engage in the health-promoting behavior.	Asking, "Why would you want to enhance your health?"

Perhaps the Strength of Recommendation Taxonomy rating for the evidence would be grade A for health behaviors such as substance use and human immunodeficiency virus risk behaviors. For other health behaviors such as nutrition, exercise, and smoking, the rating may be grade B. The rating for potential harm may be grade 1 for all health behaviors.

Helping Clients Find and Use Their Motivation

Motivation is not binary, on or off, there or not there. Most clients are ambivalent about engaging in health-promoting behaviors, rather than either being motivated or not motivated. They have some reasons for the health-risky behavior and some reasons for the health-promoting behavior. They enjoy smoking but know they should quit. They want to lose

weight but have failed in the past. They want to reduce their blood pressure but have no time to meditate. When clinicians use a motivational interviewing approach, they respect that this ambivalence is a common human experience and does *not* indicate denial or resistance.

A client who is not engaging in some health-promoting behavior can be conceptualized by the health care provider as not having sufficient motivation to do what would be health promoting. Trying to instill more motivation either by inspiration or by threat can be seductive. That kind of directing helping style sometimes works. A health care provider who intends to use a motivational interviewing style similarly recognizes that the client does not have sufficient motivation to engage in the health-promoting behavior; in this case, however, the clinician goes looking for what motivation there is and ways that the client may find additional motivation.

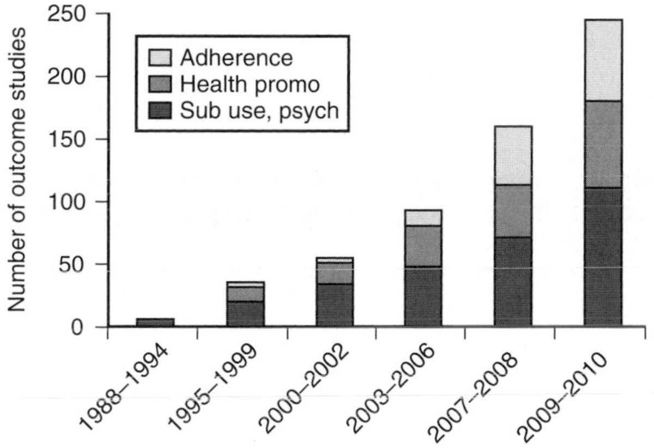

> Noncompliance can be defined as a situation in which two people (the clinician and the patient) work toward different goals.

Finding the client's motivation can be easier when the clinician thinks about various aspects of motivation. Researcher Paul Amrhein[9] identified that statements about desire, ability, reasons, and need often occur in conversations with a focus on changing a particular behavior (in motivational interviewing, this particular behavior or goal is called the target behavior). Statements the client makes in these categories probably indicate the client's movement toward taking action, and two additional categories related to the client's action can be observed: taking steps and commitment. Clients can make statements in any of these six categories in the direction of health (in which case it is referred to as change talk) or in the direction of not engaging in the health-promoting behavior (in which case it is referred to as sustain

FIGURE 99-3
Growth of motivational interviewing studies. promo, promotion; psych, psychological issues; sub use, substance use.

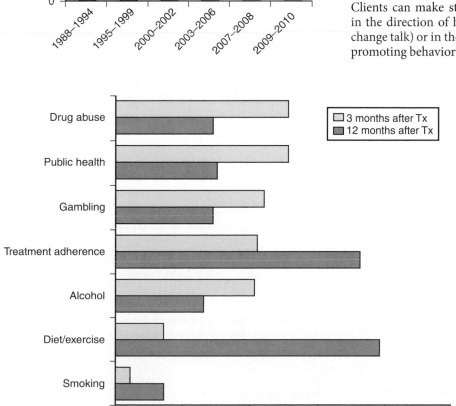

FIGURE 99-4
Effect size comparing motivational interviewing to no motivational interviewing at 3 and 12 months. (From Hettema J, Steele J, Miller W. A meta-analysis of research on motivational interviewing treatment effectiveness (MARMITE). *Annu Rev Clin Psychol.* 2005;1:91–111.)

talk, as in maintaining the status quo). Table 99-2 provides additional descriptions of each of these categories.

These categories provide the health care provider with guidance about where to go fishing for the client's motivation. A client who says "I don't have time to meditate" is describing something about ability. The clinician may then focus on a different category to try to solicit a motivation for meditating: "You don't have time to meditate, but it sounds like you wish you did." This statement involves recognizing ability in the sustain direction and fishing for desire in the change direction. If the client complains about following a new cholesterol-lowering diet, the clinician can respond: "You are not finding it fun to follow this diet, so why are you intending to do so?" This question involves recognizing desire in the sustain direction and fishing for reasons in the change direction. Table 99-3 provides examples of each category of motivation in both sustain and change directions for the target behavior of engaging in behaviors that would promote heart health after a heart attack.

These categories can be used by the health care provider to guide the interview. Several research studies found that the goals of the consult where change talk is elicited were associated with the desired behavior change. In one study of clients in treatment for alcohol problems, 16% of the days a client abstained 9 to 15 months after treatment could be predicted from how much the client was drinking at the start of treatment. A similar amount, 19% of the days a client abstained and 34% of the amount the client drank, could be predicted from how much change talk the client said in a single session 9 to 15 months earlier.[10] Change talk during today's consultation may be a good proxy for the actual behavior change in the future.

One way of understanding how motivational interviewing may be used by clients to implement change is also a way for the health care provider to guide verbal behaviors during the consultation. People tend to believe what they say more than what they hear. If the consultation is arranged so the client is describing out loud his or her desire to drink less, the ability to drink less, the need to drink less, the reasons for drinking less, steps to be taken to drink less, and ultimately the commitment to drink less, he or she may be talking himself or herself into the actual behavior of drinking less.

If a directing helping style is used, the health care provider is the one reinforcing the health-promoting behavior of drinking less. The client is passive and may or may not act on the health care provider's recommendations. The client may even be more able to propose objections to the change because the health care provider is inadvertently alleviating the client of having to identify the advantages of the change and thereby freeing the client to focus on the disadvantages of the change.

A second way of understanding how motivational interviewing may be used by clients to implement change is to recognize who must actually engage in the health-promoting behavior. During the consultation, the clinician or nurse who uses a directing helping style can check the client's blood glucose level, talk about the importance of lowering blood pressure, or underscore the need to exercise. The client, however, is the one who must engage in these same behaviors after the consultation is over and when the health care provider is no longer around. If the health care provider uses a motivational interviewing style and arranges the consultation so the *client* talks out loud about the reasons to check blood glucose levels, the way he or she will eat as to lower blood pressure, or what kind of exercise would be enjoyable, the client is rehearsing the very behavior needed to be implemented an hour, a day, a week, or a month after the consultation.

TABLE 99-2. Change Talk and Sustain Talk by the Client

CATEGORY	CLIENT TALKS ABOUT	WORDS THAT MAY BE CLUES		
Desire	What the client may enjoy or not enjoy, like or dislike, find as fun or not fun, want or not want.	I want I would like I enjoy	I don't want I hate I wouldn't enjoy	I wish
Ability	What the client perceives he or she is able or unable to do, what is possible or impossible, what he or she can or cannot do.	I can I'm unable I could	I can't I'm able I cannot	
Need	What the client thinks he or she should do, has to do, should not have to do, what is just or unjust, what the "right" or "wrong" thing is to do.	I need to I should I'd better	I have to I shouldn't have to I'd better not	I ought to
Reasons	The rationale, justification, or motive for doing or not doing the behavior.	Reasons are often preceded by "so," "because," or "so that," and they often follow statements in other categories, particularly need: "I don't need to because…"		
Steps	Behaviors the client has performed (in the recent past) that may be in the direction of change or in the direction of staying the same.	Steps are not the target behavior but are on the way toward or away from the target behavior.		
Commitment	What the client will or will not do in the future and intentions or agreements about the future. The strength of the commitment can vary, but they are commitment statements because they talk about the future.	I'll try I definitely will I promise	I may I won't I suppose	I will

TABLE 99-3. Categories of Motivation in Both Sustain and Change Directions for the Target Behavior of Engaging in Behaviors That Would Promote Heart Health After a Heart Attack

Target behavior is engaging in behavior that would reduce the risk of another heart attack. The client says this:	Is the client's statement in the direction of health (change talk) or in the direction of continuing the health risk (sustain talk)?	Within what category may the client's statement fit?	Possible response by the health care provider to manage the sustain talk or pull for or reinforce the change talk:
I don't like reduced-salt foods.	Sustain	Desire	"So using a salt substitute is going to be hard to do. Why were you thinking it may be a good idea?" (Recognize the desire in the sustain direction, and then pull for reasons in the change direction.)
I can't get to that evening Healthy Heart meeting.	Sustain	Ability	"You aren't able to get there, but it sounds like you have some recognition that it may be useful." (Recognize the sustain talk, and then pull for reasons or need in the change direction.)
The support from the Healthy Heart class would be helpful.	Change	Reason	"You may like the class." (Attempt to evoke change talk in an additional category of desire.) Or, "You can imagine some benefits from the class." (Reinforce the change talk in the reason category.)
I shouldn't need to do all this for my heart.	Sustain	Need	"It's not fair." (Acknowledge the sense of injustice and injury.) Or, "You would prefer that your heart just work." (Recognize how taking care of the heart is not enjoyable, but begin to call attention to the client's desire for the heart to work, which could lead to steps to take care of the heart.)
I think I may enjoy that support group.	Change	Desire	"You are looking forward to it." (Reinforce the enjoyment.) Or, "What are you hoping to get out of it?" (Attempt to evoke additional change talk in the reason category.)
I got a salt substitute.	Change	Step	"Good for you." (Affirm the client's action in the change direction.) Or, "What will you do next?" (Pull for more change talk in the step category.)
I'm not having any angina anymore, so I figure I don't need to take that medication.	Sustain	Reason	"You're glad your angina is gone." (Stay away from the reason category, go to another category, desire, and hope to find change talk there.)
I threw out those recipes with less salt.	Sustain	Step	"Something else makes more sense to you to try than reducing your salt." (Avoid trying to install reasons or motivation to reduce salt, and pull for other things the client may be willing to try.)
I could get a ride to the Heart Health class.	Change	Ability	"Sounds like it is important to you to try it out." (Pull for change talk in the need or reason category.)
I won't be weighing myself every day.	Sustain	Commitment	"If you thought that would make a difference, you could consider doing it." (Avoid arguing about what the client is going to do, and pull for reasons in the change direction.)
I probably need to go to a yoga class every day.	Change	Need	"It's something that you think would help." (Pull for change talk in the reasons category.)
I will be going to that exercise class tomorrow.	Change	Commitment	"You've made up your mind to try it out." (Reinforce the change talk in the commitment category.)

TABLE 99-4. Target Behavior Is to Engage in Those Behaviors That Would Manage a Diabetic Condition

SUSTAIN TALK	CHANGE TALK
I don't like sticking my finger.	I want to reduce my risk of losing my eyesight.
I can't take my meter with me during the day.	I could get that new, smaller meter.
I don't need to do all this checking and changing my diet.	I must learn more about the glycemic index.
I don't follow my diet sometimes because I don't want people to know I have diabetes and have to accommodate my dietary needs.	If I lower my sugars maybe I won't wind up like my mother, who had diabetes and lost her foot.

A client who says things such as those listed in the change talk column of Table 99-4 is rehearsing what he or she literally must think or say after the consultation is over to remind, justify, or motivate himself or herself to engage in behaviors related to managing diabetes. In addition, a client who is making statements such as those in the sustain talk column is probably reducing his or her motivation to engage in health-promoting behaviors after the consultation. One way that health care providers inadvertently arrange this is by saying the change talk. The client, who is ambivalent, then brings up the sustain talk, and that is what he or she may remember after the consultation. However, a health care provider who says the sustain talk before the client says it may be perceived as very empathic. The client experiences the clinician as someone who understands why it is so difficult to engage in the health-promoting behavior. By saying the sustain talk first, the health care provider alleviates the client from having to say it and decreases the client's reinforcement of the status quo. Having recognized the sustain talk, the health care provider has perhaps earned the client's cooperation and increased the probability that the client will shift to some change talk.

Helping the Client Say More Change Talk

Helping the client say more change talk can sometimes be as simple as asking the client to describe his or her desires, needs, or reasons for engaging in the health-promoting behavior:

"What would you *enjoy* about meditation?"

"How may you be *able* to arrange to take your medications reliably?"

"Why do you think you *need* to reduce the salt in your diet?"

"What *reasons* do you have for continuing with your exercises?"

"If you decided to eat less red meat, what *could you do* today or tomorrow?"

Open questions typically work better than closed questions. Open and closed questions have the typical definitions and perhaps also this aspect: the clinician may be surprised by the client's answer to an open question, whereas the clinician probably already has a very good guess about the client's answer to a closed question. Open questions ask the client to talk about what is important to him or her, whereas closed questions ask the client to talk about what is important to the health care provider. When the client says change talk, providing reinforcement and encouragement through affirmation, paraphrase, or summary can be useful.

Sometimes, change talk can be solicited by having the client envision the future. The health care provider can ask the client to talk about what he or she imagines in the future if changes are made or if changes are not made. Possible examples are as follows: "What do you imagine will happen in the future if you don't lower your blood pressure this year?" or "How do you think this _____ (health-risky behavior) might become worse?" Both these examples pull for reasons to engage in the health-promoting behavior.

Facilitating the client's talking about goals or values and how they fit or do not fit with health behaviors may also evoke change talk. This could sound like these examples: "How does the _____ (health-risky behavior) help or hurt your work?" or "How would taking care of your heart fit with what you want to do with your family?"

Sometimes, the health care provider hears a client's misconception, and providing accurate information is important. The health care provider may also have a recommendation or resource that he or she would like the client to consider. These concerns or snippets of advice can fit within a motivational interviewing style by respecting the client as competent. First, the health care provider elicits permission to provide the information, concern, or advice: "I have a concern about your situation. Would you like to hear it?" Or "I have an idea of something that may work for you if you would like to hear it." If the client agrees, which occurs most times, the health care provider then describes concisely the information or advice and returns the focus back to the client as ultimate decision maker with something such as this: "You are in the best position to decide whether this works for you." Or "How do you think that fits your situation?" Steve Rollnick,[1] one of the field's experts, has called this way of introducing advice or recommendations elicit-provide-elicit: elicit the client's permission, provide the information, and elicit the client's interpretation of the information. Another expert in the field, Terri Moyers,[11] has taught that if collaboration with the client is extensive, the client's change talk is actively solicited, and the client's autonomy is highly respected, some direct advice offered during the consultation is often heard and accepted by the client even when that same advice would be rejected by the client if given in the context of a directing helping style.

Because most clients are ambivalent about engaging in health-promoting behaviors, some sustain talk by the client is normal and expected. To help the client increase his or her motivation for the health-promoting behavior, however, the health care provider should be active in managing the sustain talk. Often, a first step is to demonstrate to the client that the sustain talk has been heard and understood. This is where the health care provider's skill in expressing empathy through paraphrasing or summarizing is necessary.

TABLE 99-5. Examples of Providing an Alternative Meaning for the Client's Observation in Sustain Talk

Observation the client has made	I've tried in the past and haven't succeeded in (stopping smoking, maintaining my exercise, improving my diet).
Meaning client may give this observation	I can't do this. Or I'm not successful. (Notice this statement is sustain talk in the ability category.)
Meaning you may want the client to have	This is important to you. You have tried out several ways that have not worked as well as you want. (The past failures are given a new meaning, and attention is called to desire, which is a different category than ability.)

Sometimes, the client will return to change talk if the health care provider overstates the sustain talk the client has just said. Possible examples are as follows:

Example 1: Client:"I don't really see the ankle swelling as a problem. They just hurt some."

Counselor: "You're not using the ankle swelling to think at all about your heart."

Example 2: Client:"I doubt if there is a problem. I don't have difficulties moving around."

Counselor: "As long as you can move, *everything* is OK."

The health care provider must say these kinds of amplified reflections (called amplified because the health care provider is increasing the emphasis or overstating the sustain talk) in a neutral voice tone. Sarcasm or criticism will very likely increase the client's sustain talk rather than decrease it.

Earlier in this chapter, examples were given of managing sustain talk by first paraphrasing the sustain talk and then focusing on a different category. These double-sided reflections will help manage sustain talk if the first side or phrase is the sustain side and the second side or phrase is the change side. The client is more likely to talk about the side (sustain or change) on which the health care provider finishes his or her statement. Another way to manage sustain talk is to provide an alternative meaning for the client's observation (Table 99-5).

Enhancing Your Motivational Interviewing Skills

Most health care providers use all three helping styles. Although the directing helping style is most frequently used, most health care providers occasionally use a guiding helping style and even the more specialized motivational interviewing style whether or not they have received formal training in it. Research has demonstrated that reading or attending workshops is probably not sufficient to enhance motivational interviewing skills. Listening to actual recordings of

BOX 99-1. A Way to Enhance Your Practice

Audiotape a session with a client. By yourself or with a colleague:

- Count the number of open questions and closed questions. You are more likely to be using a motivational interviewing style if at least 50% of your questions are open.
- Count the number of reflections you made. You are more likely to be using a motivational interviewing style if you have at least twice as many reflections as questions and you have at least one reflection every minute. Complex reflections often elicit more change talk than do simple reflections.
- Did you talk less than the client? You are more likely to be using a motivational interviewing style if the client talks approximately twice as much as you.
- Listen for where you did or could have solicited or reinforced any client statements about desire, ability, need, reasons, or steps statements toward the healthy alternative (change talk).
- Identify instances in which the client was engaging in sustain talk. Now that you have more time to think about your response, how else could you have demonstrated that you understood this sustain talk and called attention to possible change talk?
- Look at any instance where you gave the client advice. Did you use an elicit-provide-elicit format or in some other way ask for permission and ask the client to consider how well the advice fit?
- Did you warn the client of any possible consequences, confront the client regarding the behavior, or raise concerns without using elicit-provide-elicit? You are more likely to be using a motivational interviewing style if you avoid warning or confronting the client.

the clinician's consultations with clients is probably necessary. Whether alone, with one or several peers, or with an expert in motivational interviewing, the health care provider can listen for the characteristics listed in Box 99-1. A health care provider who practices with as few as 6 hours of recordings may significantly enhance his or her motivational interviewing skills.

One perhaps memorable way to remember the approach described here are these clinical pearls:

1. Quit your job. Do not be the only expert in the room. Imagine that you do not know, because it will make it easier for you to avoid adopting an expert role and easier for you to be curious about the client's experience.
2. Get on the bus. Be with the client, ride with him or her for a while, and look together at his or her life and dilemma of making this change. Respect that the client is going to get off the bus at whatever stop he or she chooses.
3. Go fishing. This is easier to do if you give up being the expert and the one who has to solve the problem. Treat the client as competent. Then it makes sense to go looking with the client for his or her motivation and the solutions he or she can create.

KEY WEB RESOURCES

Motivational Interviewing: http://www.motivationalinterviewing.org/	This central resource for trainers of motivational interviewing includes readings, links to other resources, and transcripts of some interviews focused on substance use problems.
MI Nordic: http://www.motiverandesamtal.org/ICMI	Videos show experts in the field presenting at an international conference on motivational interviewing held during the summer of 2010 in Stockholm.
Stephen Rollnick: http://www.stephenrollnick.com/	Stephen Rollnick provides resources and a discussion forum for motivational interviewing in medical (rather than substance use) health care settings.

References

References are available online at expertconsult.com.

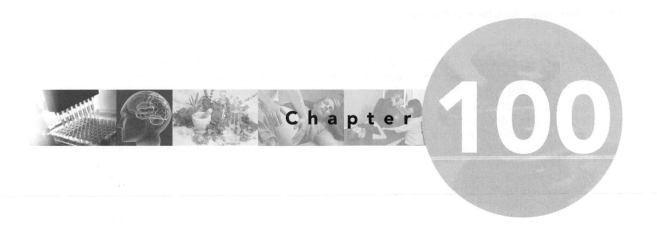

Emotional Awareness for Pain

Howard Schubiner, MD

An epidemic of chronic pain and related disorders is occurring in the United States and around the world.[1-3] Investigators estimate that 113 million individuals have chronic pain in the United States, and this number is increasing.[4-6] Back pain, neck pain, fibromyalgia, tension and migraine headaches, temporomandibular joint syndrome, and abdominal and pelvic pain syndromes are among the most common reasons for most primary care visits and consume a significant proportion of medical costs.[7] These disorders, along with various commonly associated disorders such as chronic fatigue, irritable bowel syndrome, interstitial cystitis, postural orthostatic tachycardia syndrome, and others, are among the most common concerns expressed to traditional and integrative practitioners.[8]

> Many pain syndromes seen in primary care practices are caused by psychophysiologic mechanisms.

The traditional biomedical model attempts to identify an underlying local and structural cause of pain. The efficacy of this approach has not been demonstrated for these chronic painful conditions[9,10] however, as is clear when one considers the number of people who suffer with these conditions on a regular basis. Chronic back pain is a good example of a disorder for which the purported causes of pain (herniated disks, spinal stenosis, spondylolisthesis, facet joint dysfunction, and other syndromes) have not been confirmed, nor have specific biomedical treatments been shown to be effective.[11,12] Whiplash is another example of a chronic pain syndrome shown to be unrelated to ongoing injury or a specific disease process in the neck.[13] The disorders considered in this chapter exclude those with objective evidence of structural disease, such as cancer, fractures, and inflammatory and infectious conditions.

Many central nervous system neurotransmitters have been found to be associated with fibromyalgia and migraine headaches.[14] Specific peripheral disease processes have not been identified, however. Little doubt exists that genetic predispositions occur with many conditions, such as migraine, anxiety, and depression.[15] However, studies have shown that life events are required to trigger these conditions, that is, to cause expression of underlying genetic predispositions.[16] In fact, one study showed that a particular genotype for depression can be activated by a stressful childhood (thus increasing risk for depression) and can be deactivated by a healthy childhood (thus decreasing depression risk).[17]

Because of the inability to identify and treat the underlying cause, attention has shifted to pain management. However, biomedical approaches to pain management, including pain medications (including opiates), injection techniques, and surgical and chemical ablations, have also not been shown to be efficacious.[9-13] Clearly, a new model for these disorders is needed. This chapter describes a mind-body model in which these disorders are considered to be related to individual reactions to stressful events and unresolved emotions.

Their Pain Is Real

Neuroscientists have identified areas of the brain that process pain, accentuate pain, and reduce pain.[18-21] We now recognize that all pain is real, no matter whether it is induced by a peripheral noxious event (e.g., bone fracture), by events in the nerve tissue (e.g., peripheral neuropathy), or in the brain (as in mind-body syndromes). In fact, clear evidence indicates that pain can originate in the absence of a tissue disorder in the area where pain is being felt, as seen in phantom limb syndrome.[22] A study by Derbyshire et al[23] confirmed that pain initiated by the brain is identical to pain originating in peripheral tissues.

> Learned nerve pathways and central sensitization often produce chronic pain.

The anterior cingulate cortex (ACC) is a key area within the brain that, when activated, augments pain.[19,21] Pain also activates the amygdala and the autonomic nervous system (ANS).[24,25] Emotional memories are stored in the amygdala, and people with adverse childhood experiences are known to be more likely to develop migraine, fibromyalgia, interstitial cystitis, irritable bowel syndrome, and chronic pelvic pain.[26-32] Evidence also indicates that the amygdala, the ACC, and the ANS are activated when emotions are experienced.[33,34] To summarize, these areas are involved in the activation of pain pathways, and these pathways are strongly influenced by thoughts and emotions.[19-21,35]

Learned pain pathways can develop after an injury (even a mild one) or can be created during times of significant stress and emotional reactions. Although most injuries heal within a reasonable amount of time, pain pathways can persist (become "wired"), thus creating chronic pain that is often refractory to medical therapies. These pain pathways are often very specific and can involve discrete or large areas of the body. Pain induced by psychophysiologic processes frequently moves or changes, as opposed to the pain caused by a specific injury or disease process.

Built-in central mechanisms for reducing pain exist. Notably, activation of the dorsolateral prefrontal cortex (DLPFC) area results in diminished pain.[18] Positive emotional states are correlated with activation of the DLPFC[36] (Fig. 100-1).

Psychology of Pain

The mind has two major components: conscious and subconscious. We are obviously aware of many of our actions, decisions, thoughts, and feelings. However, most of our thoughts and emotions are actually derived from subconscious processes.[37,38] In addition, these subconscious processes typically form the basis for most of our actions. Thus, many of our activities are routine and programmed by our subconscious minds, such as walking, talking, eating, and driving, as well as reactions to people, places, smells, and situations. These activities and reactions are carried out by sets of learned nerve pathways.

Another function of the subconscious mind is to protect us from physical threats. Therefore, we continuously monitor our environment for stimuli that could be "dangerous" in some way.[34] Innate pathways cause our bodies to react very quickly to a snake, a thrown object, or other physical threats. Our reactions to these threats are immediate, physical events and do not involve conscious processing (i.e., we are aware of them after they occur).[34,38] The subconscious mind also notices emotional threats and causes our bodies to react to them in a similar fashion. We are all aware that our bodies react to stress with various reactions, including facial flushing, tight stomach muscles, sweaty palms, voice changes, and others. Given the foregoing, we should not be surprised that during times of significant tension and stress, our bodies can develop physical reactions in a myriad of ways, such as the development of neck or back pain, headache, gastrointestinal or genitourinary symptoms, and many other symptoms.

> A detailed psychological history typically elicits the underlying psychological causes of psychophysiologic disorders.

People who were subjected to adverse childhood events develop a priming of the brain's emotional responses and a corresponding emotional memory for specific types of threats.[39] Often, these children suffer from stomach upsets, insomnia, anxiety, headaches, and other disorders.[26,27] Later in life, if new emotional or physical threats occur (especially if they are similar to those that occurred in childhood), brain pathways can be activated, and new symptoms often develop, including severe pain.[40] In a typical history, a girl who grows up with an emotionally abusive and controlling parent may develop migraine headaches as a teen when she is subjected to an emotionally abusive and controlling boyfriend.

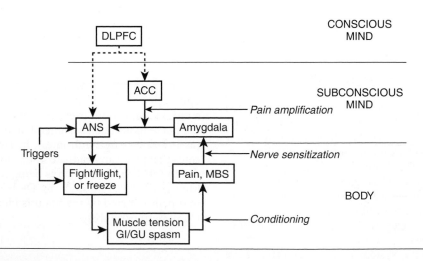

FIGURE 100-1

The neurology of psychophysiologic disorders (*thick solid line*, activating; *dashed line*, deactivating). ACC, anterior cingulate cortex; ANS, autonomic nervous system; DLPFC, dorsolateral prefrontal cortex; GI/GU, gastrointestinal/genitourinary; MBS, mind-body syndrome.

If she marries a controlling and abusive husband in her 20s, she may develop abdominal or pelvic pain. In her 30s, when subjected to a threatening work situation, she may develop widespread pain that is often diagnosed as fibromyalgia.

These physical reactions are real, and the pain they cause is real. However, they are physiologic, rather than pathologic, responses. In other words, they do not involve tissue destruction and can be reversed. They are responses created by the subconscious mind in an attempt to protect us from some threat (e.g., a controlling boss, an abusive husband, an overwhelming set of responsibilities). These threats activate fear and anger in the "internal child" portion of the mind. We currently use the term psychophysiologic disorders (PPDs) to describe them, but they have also been termed psychosomatic or functional disorders, tension myositis syndrome,[41] stress-related illness,[42] and mind-body syndrome.[40]

Another observation commonly made about persons who develop psychophysiologic reactions is that they tend to have a highly developed conscience, or "internal parent."[41] Those who exhibit certain characteristics—being selfless, highly responsible, or self-critical, feeling excessive guilt, lacking assertiveness, being perfectionists, holding themselves to very high standards, caring what others think of them, and holding emotions in—are commonly affected with this group of disorders. Large international studies have shown that women are more likely than men to display these characteristics, possibly because of higher rates of childhood and adult victimization and gender-based socialization.[43,44] These factors may play a role in the higher rates of chronic pain and other PPDs disorders among women (Fig. 100-2).

> Ruling out structural alterations is critical before the diagnosis of a psychophysiologic disorder is made.

Diagnosis of Psychophysiologic Disorders

PPDs should be suspected in patients who present with symptoms of one or more of the common PPD diagnoses (Box 100-1) and for whom a specific structural condition is not identified. PPD is therefore suspected in most patients presenting to a primary care physician or health care provider. A medical workup should be conducted to rule out any structural conditions such as tumors, fractures, infections, or inflammatory conditions. Conditions that are present in the asymptomatic population in equal proportions, such as bulging disks, mild spondylolisthesis, or spinal stenosis, do not exclude a diagnosis of PPD. A physical examination to rule out evidence of nerve root compression or signs of other disease processes is mandatory.

Once this is accomplished, the topic of PPDs should be broached with the patient. Talking with patients about PPDs should be done in a way that emphasizes that their symptoms are real and empathizes with their situation and their frustration with not achieving remission of symptoms. The clinician should explain that real symptoms, including severe and chronic pain, can frequently occur in the absence of structural disease processes, and one can use phantom limb syndrome as an example of this phenomenon.[22] Introducing the concept of learned nerve pathways helps patients to connect their

---

BOX 100-1. Syndromes Commonly Caused by Psychophysiologic Disorders

Chronic Pain Syndromes
- Tension headaches
- Migraine headaches
- Back pain
- Neck pain
- Whiplash
- Fibromyalgia
- Temporomandibular joint syndrome
- Chronic abdominal and pelvic pain syndromes
- Chronic tendinitis
- Vulvodynia
- Piriformis syndrome
- Sciatic pain syndrome
- Repetitive stress injury
- Foot pain syndromes
- Myofascial pain syndrome

Autonomic Nervous System–Related Disorders
- Irritable bowel syndrome
- Interstitial cystitis (irritable bladder syndrome)
- Postural orthostatic tachycardia syndrome
- Inappropriate sinus tachycardia
- Reflex sympathetic dystrophy (chronic regional pain disorder)
- Functional dyspepsia

Other Syndromes
- Insomnia
- Chronic fatigue syndrome
- Paresthesias (numbness, tingling, burning)
- Tinnitus
- Dizziness
- Spasmodic dysphonia
- Chronic hives
- Anxiety
- Depression
- Obsessive-compulsive disorder
- Posttraumatic stress disorder

FIGURE 100-2
The psychology of psychophysiologic disorders. MBS, mind-body syndrome.

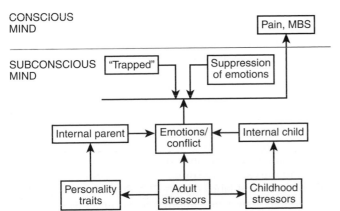

symptoms to central nervous system processes. The practitioner should state that learned nerve pathways are simply sets of nerve connections that have developed through experiences, such as the pathways that allow us to ride a bicycle, throw a ball, or walk and talk a certain way. Once these pathways are learned, they can continue for several years and can be reactivated after many years. Pain and other symptoms are easily learned and are the underlying cause of PPDs. Reassure the patient that no physical, structural disease process is present, and offer hope that the real condition that they suffer from can be reversed. Whether or not a physical injury occurs, stressful situations and powerful subconscious emotions are universal triggers of pain pathways in PPDs. These pathways become engrained in the presence of situations and emotions that remain unresolved. In addition, chronic pain frequently leads to frustration about ongoing pain and fear of an underlying physical disease. These reactions further activate pain pathways in the brain by activation of the amygdala, ANS, and ACC.[45,46] This educational process is extremely important to allay fears of a disease process, explain the reason for the symptoms, and offer hope and the expectation that these symptoms can be resolved. Treatment of PPDs in the absence of understanding and accepting these principles is typically not effective.

Diagnostic Interview

Many practitioners are not trained to conduct an in-depth psychological interview that begins with a patient's childhood history and attempts to elicit key psychological factors that have created psychophysiologic disorders. However, I have published a template for this type of assessment that can be used by patients or practitioners.[40] A brief description of this interview is provided here. As mentioned earlier, before diagnosing a form of PPD, the practitioner should rule out a pathologic medical condition, to ensure that the practitioner and patient are comfortable that they are dealing with a form of PPD. Before the interview, the patient should complete a checklist of symptoms and syndromes that are commonly caused by PPDs (Box 100-2).

Begin the interview by gathering data on the patient's family of origin, and ask probing questions about parents, siblings, and any other important individuals in childhood. Gently inquire about episodes or patterns of the following: emotional, physical, or sexual abuse; criticism, taunting, teasing, blame, humiliation, or judging; and overly high expectations or conditional love. Ask about parental relationships, alcohol or drug abuse, divorce or extramarital affairs, unequal treatment of siblings, and family psychological and physical illnesses. Ask about sibling relationships, with special regard to episodes of cruel behaviors, psychological or physical illness, or acting-out behaviors. Synthesize the patient's childhood experiences and reactions by the patient, in an attempt to understand the effects of upbringing on personality and development. Most people with PPDs have a set of personality traits that include an overly developed conscience (superego) and a deficiency of self-esteem, self-worth, and assertiveness (Box 100-3). Typically, one finds events and responses that prime the ANS and thereby set the stage for the development of PPDs later in life. Some of the common patterns are those of loss, abandonment, fear, guilt, resentment, and anger. In some instances, people with PPDs had very healthy childhoods, and when they are exposed

BOX 100-2. Common Symptoms of Psychophysiologic Disorders

- Heartburn, acid reflux
- Abdominal pains
- Irritable bowel syndrome
- Tension headaches
- Migraine headaches
- Unexplained rashes
- Anxiety or panic attacks
- Depression
- Obsessive-compulsive thought patterns
- Eating disorders
- Insomnia or trouble sleeping
- Fibromyalgia
- Back pain
- Neck pain
- Shoulder pain
- Repetitive stress injury
- Carpal tunnel syndrome
- Reflex sympathetic dystrophy (chronic regional pain disorder)
- Temporomandibular joint syndrome
- Chronic tendinitis
- Facial pain
- Numbness or tingling sensations
- Fatigue or chronic fatigue syndrome
- Palpitations
- Chest pain
- Hyperventilation
- Interstitial cystitis/spastic bladder (irritable bladder syndrome)
- Pelvic pain
- Muscle tenderness
- Postural orthostatic tachycardia syndrome
- Tinnitus
- Dizziness
- Posttraumatic stress disorder

to stressful situations later in life that contradict the values learned in childhood, PPD symptoms can develop.

The next phase of the interview consists of an evaluation of the events that trigger PPD syndromes. A simple approach is to inquire about the onset of each of the PPD symptoms from Box 100-2. Table 100-1 provides sample data filled in for a hypothetical patient. Although the onset may coincide with injury or a viral infection, these events create the nerve pathways that the body experiences on a temporary basis. The PPD symptoms become chronic by the development of learned nerve pathways only if the individual is in a situation in which several of the following circumstances are present: an inherently stressful situation; triggering by current events of emotional memories of priming events from childhood; experiences of guilt, self-criticism, a strong sense of responsibility, or other issues listed in Box 100-3; and an inability to express emotions of fear or anger or feeling trapped in the triggering situation. These situations trigger PPD symptoms that can easily become chronic once they are learned, especially if the symptoms are worrisome, seen as resulting from a disease process, and labeled by health practitioners as something other than a psychophysiologic process. Complete this process with each of the PPD symptoms that have occurred in the lifetime of the patient. Clear patterns frequently emerge that will help the patient understand that the symptoms are, in fact, caused by PPDs and that the patient is not crazy, incompetent, or disabled, but rather someone who has been exposed to series of events that have created physical or psychological symptoms in response to a particular combination of emotions developed in their life. When this understanding occurs, patients can be encouraged to see that they are not to blame for the symptoms, that they are not physically or psychologically damaged, and that they have the opportunity to overcome these symptoms.

> Stressful childhood events play powerful roles in the development of psychophysiologic and physical disorders.

If it is appropriate, the interview may be concluded with the following clear messages:

BOX 100-3. Personality Traits Common to Patients With Psychophysiologic Disorders

- Having low self-esteem
- Being perfectionists
- Having high expectations of themselves
- Wanting to be good or be liked
- Frequently feeling guilty
- Feeling dependent on others
- Being conscientious
- Being hard on themselves
- Being overly responsible
- Taking on responsibility for others
- Often worrying
- Having difficulty making decisions
- Following rules strictly
- Having difficulty letting go
- Feeling cautious, shy, or reserved
- Tending to hold thoughts and feelings in
- Tending to harbor rage or resentment
- Not standing up for themselves

"You have a form of PPD, rather than a structural disease process. PPD is caused by learned nerve pathways that have been triggered by the particular set of stressors that you have encountered. It is not your fault. Almost everyone gets PPD, and anyone would likely develop these symptoms given the events that occurred. You can get better because learned nerve pathways can be reversed. A path for unlearning your pain and other PPD symptoms exists if you are willing to do the work."

Treatment Approach

Because PPD is a disorder caused by stress and unresolved emotions, everyone with PPD can experience dramatic improvements or remissions. However, primarily patient-related factors determine successful treatment, rather than practitioner-related factors. In my clinical experience, successfully treated patients are those who are convinced that they have PPD rather than a structural disease process, are confident that they can address the issues that created PPD, are willing and able to devote a significant amount of time to psychological interventions, and have adequate resources as well as a lack of overwhelming obstacles in their lives. The practitioner's job is to help patients develop the first of these attributes; the rest of them are primarily up to the patient.

Two studies documented the efficacy of the therapeutic approach described in the next section. The first was a randomized controlled trial for individuals diagnosed with fibromyalgia.[47] In this small trial, at a 6-month follow-up, those who participated in a 3-week intervention had a mean decrease in pain of 2.5 on a 10-point Likert pain scale. In addition, 45% had a decreased pain level of at least 30%, and 25% had a decrease of at least 50%. A second study described the outcomes of patients with various musculoskeletal pain syndromes, including fibromyalgia, back and neck pain, headache, and other syndromes. Patients had a mean duration of pain of 8.8 years and had even better results. After the month-long intervention, 6-month follow-up pain scores showed that 67% had at least a 30% pain reduction, and 53% had at least a 50% reduction in pain.[48]

Therapeutic Program

Once a biomedical condition has been ruled out, the interview has demonstrated the linkages between priming and triggering events and the onset of PPD symptoms, and the

---

TABLE 100-1. Synthesis of the Diagnosis of Psychophysiologic Disorder Chart

AGE	PPD SYMPTOM	POTENTIAL TRIGGERING EVENTS	EMOTIONS THAT WERE TRIGGERED/CORE ISSUES
7	Stomach aches	Parents arguing	Fear of parents separating/loss
16	Irritable bowel syndrome	Parental divorce	Loss of father, mother depressed
28	Migraines	Husband "cheating"	Loss, anger, betrayal
38	Fibromyalgia/fatigue	Divorce/difficult boss	Loss, fear, powerlessness

PPD, psychophysiologic disorder.

BOX 100-4. Expressive and Therapeutic Writing Exercises

- Free writing: uncensored expressive writing about an emotionally charged topic
- Unsent letters: expressing thoughts and feelings fully in a letter format
- Dialogues: creating an imaginary conversation between two entities who discuss a relevant issue
- Gratitude: writing about things for which one is grateful
- Forgiveness: writing to express forgiveness toward oneself or others
- Barriers: writing about potential barriers, both internal and external, that may prevent healing
- Creating new responses: writing how one chooses to respond to potentially difficult situations
- Life narratives: creating an alternative life story that emphasizes overcoming obstacles rather than being victimized

---

BOX 100-5. Affirmative Script for Reducing Symptoms of Psychophysiologic Disorders

- When pain or other symptoms occur, stop and take a deep breath. Then take a moment to remind yourself that nothing is seriously wrong with your body. You are healthy, and the symptoms of mind-body syndrome will subside soon.
- Tell your mind that you realize that the symptoms are just a way of warning you about underlying feelings of fear, guilt, anger, anxiety, shame, inadequacy, or other emotions. Tell your mind to stop producing the symptoms immediately. Do this with force and conviction, either out loud or silently.
- Take a few deep breaths, and move on with what you were doing.

---

patient has been educated and accepts the diagnosis, then the intervention may proceed. There are resources and a comprehensive programs designed to empower the patient and guide him or her toward healing (see resources below).[40] These programs typically consist of a mixture of cognitive-behavioral, mindfulness, and emotional expressive techniques. The author's program has been shown to increase an internal locus of control (i.e., patients begin to believe that their thoughts and actions are capable of reversing their PPD symptoms).[47]

Several authors have developed various expressive and therapeutic writing techniques.[49,50] Research on many of these techniques conducted by James Pennebaker and others documented beneficial effects on health and well-being.[50-52] These techniques, along with others, are incorporated into programs designed to reverse PPDs.[40] These techniques are summarized in Box 100-4 and are discussed in Chapter 96, Journaling for Health.

Meditations and visualizations are used as part of healing in PPD. Mindfulness meditation has been shown to reduce reactivity to emotional issues and reduce pain,[53,54] and guided imagery is an effective tool to create the images of health and well-being that are essential to this therapeutic model.[55,56] Chapter 95, Guided Imagery and Interactive Guided Imagery, and Chapter 98, Recommending Meditation, provide practical advice on using these methods.

Affirmations are a key element of this program. The rationale for positive self-talk is the following. Pain resulting from PPDs is triggered by subconscious thoughts and emotions. Although one can often discern the origin of these subconscious processes, these processes can continue to create pain if they remain unchallenged. For example, a common thought of people with back pain is that they will hurt their back if they lift things or exercise. The conscious production of positive thoughts about one's health and well-being activates the DLPFC and deactivates the ACC. These processes, in turn, act to reduce pain. Remarkably, simple, strong assertions can often reverse pain within minutes when one is convinced of the diagnosis of PPD and of one's power in overcoming

it. Patients can "speak" to the pain on a consistent basis to reprogram learned pain pathways, particularly if they have been longs-standing. Box 100-5 offers an affirmation script for patients to use.

Another key component in healing is to challenge triggers that maintain symptoms. A trigger can be defined as a stimulus that leads to PPD symptoms, yet it would not typically cause a symptom in someone else. Typical examples are weather changes, bright lighting, foods, wine or other alcoholic drinks, family gatherings, visits to certain people, places, movements, driving, and many others. Triggers become activated by subconscious processes in a way similar to that by which pavlovian responses develop (i.e., operant conditioning). Therefore, triggers cause symptoms because they activate learned nerve pathways, rather than causing a physical reaction in the body. Triggers can be attenuated by understanding this process and by actively challenging them. One must be careful to rule out a structural relationship or a true allergic reaction before encouraging patients to challenge these triggers. Avoiding triggers allows them to exert even greater effects, so patients should be encouraged to seek out these triggers and expose themselves to them to overcome them. See Box 100-6 for a script regarding eliminating triggers.

As mentioned earlier, many patients with PPDs have personality traits of being overly responsible, self-critical, and unassertive. Individuals with PPDs often find themselves in situations in which they feel trapped or conflicted. They may be caring for an ailing parent who was abusive, work for a boss who is controlling and manipulative, or have a spouse or child who continually takes advantage of them. In these situations, taking action is often necessary. Pain is often dramatically reduced when a difficult situation is resolved or ameliorated to a significant degree. Clinicians must frequently encourage patients and help them find acceptable methods for dealing with these situations.

Finally, individuals who have endured significant childhood and adult stressors and who have suffered with chronic pain often have a negative view of themselves and low levels of self-esteem and self-efficacy. Therefore, an overarching theme for guiding individuals with PPDs to health is the development of love and kindness toward oneself. This can be accomplished in many ways, such as by positive affirmations, by

BOX 100-6. Affirmative Script for Reducing Triggers of Psychophysiologic Disorders

- When you notice you are encountering any symptom triggers or any stressful situations, immediately stop and take a deep breath. Then take a moment to remind your mind that this activity or trigger will *not* cause symptoms or problems any more. For example, when I lift heavy items, I always remind myself, "This will not cause any back problems. My back is healthy and strong, and I can do this without pain." Have a deep understanding of mind-body syndromes and the fact that your body is healthy and that you can get better by using these methods.
- Keep reminding yourself that you will not allow your mind to produce symptoms of a psychophysiologic disorder this time.
- Be firm and assertive.
- Repeat whatever positive phrases you choose every time you encounter any of your triggers until your brain unlearns the pathways of PPD.

meditations and visualizations, and by encouraging patients to stand up for themselves and take time to do things for themselves.

An empathic, insight-based treatment approach for psychophysiologic disorders has been demonstrated to be effective.

Conclusion

Most people with chronic pain do not have a structural cause for this pain and are actually suffering from PPDs. Biomedical approaches to PPDs often lead to an endless cycle of pain and interventions. When a biomedical condition is ruled out, a careful interview usually identifies the priming and triggering events leading to the onset of pain. Education about PPDs will help patients discard the biomedical explanation for their pain and empower the patient to take control of their symptoms and their lives. Even pain that has persisted for many years can be reversed or reduced by this relatively simple approach.

KEY WEB RESOURCES

Unlearn Your Pain: http://unlearnyourpain.com	The Web site of Dr. Howard Schubiner
Dr. John Sarno: http://johnesarnomd.com	The offical Web site of John Sarno, MD
Stress Illness: http//:www.stressillness.com	The Web site of Dr. David Clarke
Dr. David Schechter: http//:www.schechtermd.com	The Web site of Dr. David Schechter
PPD/TMS Peer Network: http://tmswiki.org	A participant-oriented information site on psychophysiologic disorders, including a list of practitioners who practice in this area and an active forum
RSI-Back Pain: http://rsi-backpain.co.uk/	A patient-run information site for people suffering with chronic painful conditions

References

References are available online at expertconsult.com.

Energy Psychology

Larry Stoler, PhD, MSSA

The cell is a machine driven by energy. It can thus be approached by studying matter, or by studying energy. In every culture and in every medical tradition before ours, healing was accomplished by moving energy.

Albert Szent-Gyorgyi, Nobel Laureate in Medicine

Case Study: Fear of a Flu Shot

A patient enters your office, and you recommend that she receive a flu shot. However, this patient is terrified of needles. You learn that because of this fear, the patient has never had a flu shot, despite being at risk. You explain to the patient that you can help her overcome this fear of needles by teaching her how to calm herself using a simple technique. You obtain her consent, and then you ask her to rate her fear of needles from 0 to 10, where 0 means she has no fear at all and 10 is the worst imaginable fear. She says that her fear at that moment, while just thinking about getting the flu shot, is a 9. This is her Subjective Units of Distress (SUDS) rating. Then you instruct her to tap on several acupuncture points on her hand, face, and chest. The procedure takes a couple of minutes. Immediately following this intervention, you observe that she has become calmer: her breathing has slowed down; she is smiling; her body posture is softer. You ask her how high her fear rating is now. She pauses briefly, has a somewhat confused expression on her face, and reports that the fear is hardly there. She reports that her SUDS rating is now 3. You ask her what the fear is based on now. She says that it is the image of the nurse preparing the needle. You ask her to focus on this image and you guide her in repeating the tapping on the same acupoints. When she completes the tapping sequence, you ask her to rate her fear level again, and she reports that she does not feel any fear. Her SUDS rating is 0. You then ask her to imagine receiving a flu shot in full detail. She does this imaginal exercise without any fear. You review with her the tapping sequence she just used and advise her that she can do this as a self-treatment any time she needs to and that she can use it to help her overcome any

fear or limiting beliefs that she encounters in her life. You can tell her in full confidence that because she reached a 0 in this brief treatment, the likelihood is great that she will have little or no fear when she receives her flu shot. You send her over to your nurse, who administers the flu shot. The patient has no adverse reactions. It took you 10 minutes to help this patient.

> The SUDS score stands for Subjective Units of Distress and is measured from 0 to 10, with 10 being the maximum amount of subjective feelings of distress and unrest.

Case Study: Neck Pain

You see another upset patient. He reports chronic neck and shoulder pain and insomnia. You note from the chart that these conditions were not reported in past annual physical examinations. Except for some mild hypertension, this patient has been in good health. Because you use energy psychology (EP) techniques, you have become more comfortable asking your patients about their emotional lives. When you ask about the origin of these symptoms, the patient becomes visibly more distressed and reports that 4 months ago, while on a road trip, he witnessed a fatal car accident. It was an icy winter day. The road appeared clear, but patches of black ice were present. He was driving cautiously. Suddenly, he had to stop his car to avoid hitting cars in front of him who were avoiding a car that had spun out of control and rolled over off to the side of the road. He was not directly injured in the accident, but he did see that the driver of the car that had rolled over was bleeding profusely from head injuries. He arrived safely to his destination, but heard on the news that that driver had died of his injuries. He did not think about the accident much at first. However, several days later, he began to have nightmares and difficulty sleeping through the night. Then he started to have neck

BOX 101-1. Overview of Energy Psychology

1. Uses meridian, chakra, or biofield interventions to treat the symptom
2. Provides rapid, gentle, nonretraumatizing treatment for a wide range of emotional and psychological conditions
3. Does not require deep emotional processing of the problem
4. Activates hope because long-standing problems can often be helped
5. Is easily taught as a self-help method

and shoulder pain. Over-the-counter pain remedies have not relieved his pain. You offer him the same treatment as in the previous case, after listening to a detailed account from him regarding precisely how he experienced this traumatic event. You then tailor the treatment to address the aspects of the traumatic event that are most upsetting and salient to him, including his image of the driver bleeding and his instinctive reaction to hold onto the steering wheel of his car very tightly while driving after seeing this accident. As a result of this treatment, the patient quickly calmed down, and his neck and shoulder pain dramatically improved at the same time. You also give him a handout with a self-treatment protocol to follow and ask him to call your office with an update the next day (see Patient Handout). The patient called and said that his neck and shoulder pain were 90% better and that he slept the entire night without any difficulties. Follow-up 3 months later revealed that his problems had completely resolved.

These two examples show how physicians, nurse practitioners, and other health care professionals can use EP methods to help patients overcome significant and debilitating problems (Box 101-1).

What Is Energy Psychology?

Energy psychology (EP) is the name of a family of treatment methods that address emotional, psychological, and behavioral problems by treating disturbances in the human energy field. These methods emerged in the early 1980s as an outgrowth of the continuing convergence of medical and healing systems of the West and the East that in modern times began with journalist James Reston's 1971 postsurgical treatment with acupuncture while he was accompanying President Nixon to China. EP also reflects profound shifts in scientific thinking as the implications of quantum theory are applied to healing practices.[1] Along with this is a renewed appreciation of the role of consciousness, intention, and energy in wellness and healing.[2] In current practice, the energy dimension of EP treatments focuses on making corrections in the acupuncture meridian system, the chakra system, and the more global human biofield. At the time of this writing, many EP treatment modalities are in use in the United States and increasingly throughout the world. Examples of popular modalities are the Emotional Freedom Techniques (EFT), Thought Field Therapy (TFT), Tapas Acupressure Technique (TAT), Energy Diagnostic and Treatment Methods (EDxTM), and Advanced Integrative Therapy (AIT), with EFT being the most commonly used method. These approaches are being used by a wide range of professionals and lay people. Psychologists, social workers, and other mental health practitioners—along with physicians, nurses, chiropractors, career coaches, educators, sports performance experts, yoga teachers, and lay people, among other groups—are integrating EP methods into their work (see Chapter 112, Human Energetic Therapies).

In the United States by the late 1990s, EP had gained the attention of increasing numbers of experienced psychologists and other mental health professionals because of its effectiveness as a rapid and comprehensive trauma treatment. These therapists who were already familiar with other effective trauma therapies, such as exposure therapies and Eye Movement Desensitization and Reprocessing (EMDR),[3] began to embrace EP because of the positive results they found in the treatment of patients who were traumatized by sexual abuse, violent attacks, car accidents, natural disasters, terror, and war. In clinical practice, as in the case studies at the beginning of this chapter, patients typically experience rapid and robust relief from trauma symptoms, usually after only a couple of sessions. Significantly, EP treatment is gentle and does not retraumatize the patient. EP treatment typically leads to nearly immediate and simultaneous positive changes in emotions, mind, body, and overall well-being. In practice, this means that upsetting emotions are calmed, disturbing thoughts are neutralized and positive ones spontaneously appear, and physical symptoms abate. Patients often report that they feel lighter, more optimistic, and reconnected to themselves.

Outside the clinic, trauma relief teams using EP interventions on site in trauma zones have obtained similar dramatic results. These trauma relief teams have had a significant impact by helping survivors of the following situations rapidly overcome posttraumatic reactions: the attacks of 9/11, the Indonesian tsunami, earthquakes in Guatemala and Pakistan, Hurricane Katrina in New Orleans, and the war in Serbia and Bosnia. EP is showing great promise as an effective treatment for U.S. military veterans stricken with posttraumatic stress disorder (PTSD). In each instance, EP treatment brought quick resolution of disturbing symptoms, such as nightmares, flashbacks, hypervigilance, and emotional numbness. As an empowerment strategy, patients were taught how to use EP for symptom maintenance and as an effective generalized self-help method. Because EP can be quickly taught to indigenous relief workers who are not mental health professionals, treatments can be locally administered while relying on only a few trained outside professionals. This method of treatment delivery was used successfully in Guatemala and Indonesia, as well as in Rwanda.

In the case of Rwanda, in 2006, members of the Trauma Relief Committee of the Association for Thought Field Therapy Foundation worked with children at the El Shadai orphanage. Many of the children there had witnessed the murder of their parents and other family members during the Rwandan genocide. The therapists worked with 50 children, ages 13 through 18 years. These children suffered typical PTSD symptoms including flashbacks, nightmares, bedwetting, depression, withdrawal, isolation, difficulty concentrating, and aggression. The children's level of PTSD was evaluated using standardized tests. The children's average scores exceeded the cutoffs for a diagnosis of PTSD as outlined in the fourth edition of the *Diagnostic and Statistical*

Manual of Mental Disorders. These 50 children were treated with 3 TFT sessions lasting 20 minutes each. After the TFT sessions were administered, most of the children experienced an immediate decrease in the frequency and intensity of flashbacks and other symptoms. The clinical improvement was matched by improvement in the children's test scores. At the conclusion of the 3 sessions, the tests were readministered, and the children's scores were found to be no longer in the PTSD range. These improvements continued to hold a year later when the children were retested.[4]

In general clinical practice, well-trained EP practitioners can help people rapidly recover from a broad range of problems, including the following: panic attacks, phobias, and generalized anxiety; traumatic reactions including PTSD; persistent negative emotional states such as sadness, grief, anger, and depression; and blocks to creative expression and peak performance. EP approaches can be helpful adjuncts to more severe problems such as bipolar disorder and personality disorders, including borderline personality disorder.

In 1999, the Association for Comprehensive Energy Psychology (ACEP) was founded (see the Key Web Resources box). The purpose of this nonprofit international professional organization, which is headquartered in the United States, is to promote the education, research, and professional practice of EP. In addition, ACEP is a leader in addressing the ethics and scope of practice issues that arise from the spread of this relatively new alternative and integrative therapy. ACEP offers education and certification in its own proprietary comprehensive EP model, and it offers training and certification programs in EFT. Recognizing that EP methods have an important role in mental health contexts, in broader health care settings, and in all areas in which people are working to help others advance themselves and overcome problems (e.g., education, corrections, coaching, sports performance), ACEP developed advanced training programs for both mental health professionals and allied health practitioners.

What Is the Evidence for Energy Psychology?

Although research is still at an early stage, evidence supporting EP is growing and echoes the positive anecdotal clinical reports. In any new field, research evidence accumulates in a hierarchic fashion from anecdotal reports to outcome studies without control groups to the gold standard randomized controlled trials. The preponderance of evidence across all these studies supports the efficacy of EP interventions. Positive findings have been obtained in studies examining the effectiveness of EP in patients with needle phobias, test anxiety, claustrophobia, public speaking anxiety, and trauma related to automobile accidents.[4]

EP methods show great promise in the treatment of returning veterans. In a randomized controlled trial of EP in combat veterans, 49 veterans had scores higher than the PTSD cutoff. After 6 treatment sessions, 42 of these veterans had scores that were no longer in the PTSD range. These gains were maintained at the 6-month follow-up.[5]

EP treatment often results in rapid and dramatic calming of the cognitive and emotional symptoms associated with distress. Some pilot data suggested that EP treatment produces rapid neurobiologic changes. As an example, Diepold

and Goldstein published a study in which they compared a patient's quantitative electroencephalography pattern before and after a single TFT session. The pattern was abnormal when the subject brought to mind a specific personal trauma, but it was normal when the subject thought about a neutral event. Following a single TFT treatment, no abnormalities were observed in either the traumatic or neutral condition. These positive changes in brain wave patterns remained at 18-month follow-up.[4]

In a health psychology application, TAT was shown to be an effective weight loss maintenance approach compared with a qi gong group and a no-treatment social support and education control. To be included, study participants had to have lost 3.5 kg during a 12-week weight loss program that focused on education and social support. Study subjects participated in a 12-week weight loss maintenance program. TAT was shown to be superior to the two other approaches at the end of the study.[6]

> Energy psychology, although a shift from the conventional Western medical belief, appears to be an easy to practice, low-cost with low-harm intervention that can empower patients to recruit internal resources that can resolve stressful emotions. Results have been shown to be sustained over time.

How Does Energy Psychology Work?

The debate on how EP modalities work is lively. Some investigators, such as Ruden,[7] argue that the clinical results seen in EP treatment can be explained by extending current neuroscience understanding of neuroplasticity in the brain. In a supportive line of inquiry, Kathleen Hui's work[8] at Harvard University demonstrated that stimulating acupoints can lead to modulation of the limbic system. Feinstein argued that EP is an accelerated exposure therapy. In other words, the somatic component of EP treatments, by stimulating the meridian system, accesses a much more rapid information processing system that turns off the body's alarm response and leads to repatterning of negative memory patterns. Presumably, Feinstein's argument could be expanded to include EP methods (e.g., TAT and AIT) that are somatically focused but do not employ percussive tapping on acupuncture points.

Roger Callahan,[9] the developer of TFT, proposed an informational and energetic model suggesting that stimulating meridian points helps to collapse perturbations in the patient's thought field. These energetic perturbations are presumed to be caused by some initial upsetting or traumatic incident. The notion of the existence of a thought field, which is a field of information fundamentally energetic and not localized in brain tissue, appears to be supported by Rupert Sheldrake's work on morphic resonance.[10] In addition, studies on mind effects at a distance offer further support for the possibility that our mind extends beyond the brain.[11] These latter energy- and consciousness-based explanations may better fit actual clinical experience, because many clinicians report positive EP clinical outcomes by activating body energy centers without touching the body or through intention only. Larry Dossey[12] argued that the evidence for nonlocal mind is compelling, and this nonmechanistic view points to new possibilities for healing. At the same time, it echoes ancient ideas about human interconnectedness.[13] The EP movement may well be one manifestation of this new view.

How Do I Get Started?

Because EP approaches can be used for self-help, one of the best ways to learn about EP is to begin by trying it out yourself. A basic tenet of EP treatment (similar to acupuncture) is that symptoms occur when we are in a state of energetic imbalance or disharmony. So, a good starting point for self-treatment is a comprehensive energy balancing practice.

A good option is the Four Energy Gates (Fig. 101-1 within the Patient Handout). According to Master Nan Lu, daily practice of these qi gong energy exercises drawn from traditional Chinese medicine can promote overall wellness and contribute to the improvement of emotional and physical symptoms.[14]

To work on a personal issue, follow these four basic steps: begin with a basic balancing practice (the Four Energy Gates); identify the problem; perform an energy clearing or balancing exercise (e.g., the EFT tapping sequence); and evaluate the results and repeat, if necessary (Box 101-2).

For example, let us say that you have an important speaking event coming up and you are experiencing apprehensions about presenting. As the day of the event approaches, you notice that you are avoiding preparing for the talk; you have an unsettled feeling in your belly when you think about it; when you respond to your colleagues' questions about it, your voice trembles; you worry that will embarrass yourself. Of course, these anxieties are common, but you feel your fears are excessive. You decide that you are going to help yourself overcome this problem by using an EP approach. You have already noted the behavioral (avoidance), physical (distress in your belly and shaky voice), emotional (anxiety), and cognitive (worry about embarrassment) components of your anxious reaction. Considering these symptoms, you identify your worry that you will embarrass yourself as the most salient aspect. You establish that your SUDS rating when you think about these worries is a 9. Many EP options are available for addressing this problem. Here is one that is easy to do and is generally very effective. It is based on the EFT, the most popular EP method. If you choose the more comprehensive of the self-treatment protocols, you would begin with the Four Energy Gates practice. This takes approximately 15 to 20 minutes. The acupuncture points used in the Four Energy Gates improve the flow and distribution of your body's Qi. The first three open up the energy flow to the head, middle of your body, and lower body, respectively.

BOX 101-2. Steps for Energy Psychology Self-Treatment

1. Begin with a balancing practice (four energy gates).
2. Identify the issue (cognitive, emotional, behavioral aspects).
3. Hold the problem in mind while doing the Emotional Freedom Techniques tapping sequence.
4. Evaluate the results and repeat, if necessary.
For a shortcut, do only steps 2 to 4.

The last one helps to integrate and harmonize the Qi flow in the body. Many times, just doing the Four Energy Gates can lead to a significant improvement in the problem.

If, after completing the Four Energy Gates, your anxiety remains (you still feel distress when you think about embarrassing yourself when you give the speech) and your SUDS level is not 0, you can then proceed to treat your worry of embarrassing yourself by using the following energy tapping protocol (Fig. 101-2 within the Patient Handout):

1. While tapping firmly and steadily on the side of the hand (sh on the chart), say out loud:
   "Even though I have this worry that I'll embarrass myself, I deeply love and accept myself." Another version you can use is this: "Even though I have this worry that I'll embarrass myself, I'm attracting love and compassion into my heart." Repeat these statements three times.
2. Next, tap approximately seven to nine times on each of these acupoints while repeating at each point this phrase, which serves to keep you attuned to the problem: "this worry." Again, steady and firm tapping works best.
3. Move from one point to the next until you have tapped on all seven points:
   Eyebrow: eb
   Side of the eye: oe
   Under the eye: e
   Under the nose: un
   Under the lower lip: ul
   Under the collarbone: c
   Under the arm: ua
   (Note: You can tap on all the points on the chart, but usually tapping on these seven points is sufficient. Also, do your best to tap on the location shown in the chart. If you are not sure whether you are doing it correctly, do your best and continue with the procedure.)
4. After you have tapped on these points, stop and reevaluate the intensity of the problem. What is the SUDS level now? How much distress remains? To what extent are you able to imagine yourself in the situation and be free from worry and distress? If any upset remains, repeat these steps. However, this time adjust the first statement to this: "Even though I still have some of this worry, I deeply love and accept myself." The reminder phrase could be " the remaining worry" or "still have some worry." Complete the tapping sequence and reevaluate. Sometimes, you need to shift the focus of the treatment to a different facet or aspect of the problem, say from the worry of embarrassment to the queasy feeling in your belly. By doing this, usually the problem significantly subsides or disappears after a few rounds of tapping. In some instances, more persistence is required. If you do not experience immediate improvement, keep at it.
5. Usually, when your SUDS reaches 0, and you have no distress when you imagine experiencing the situation, the likelihood is high that you will be able to go through the actual event with little or no distress. However, because the tapping is easy to do, you can always use it as a self-help booster whenever you feel the need. You should test out the treatment as much as possible to be sure that you are completely free of the negative reactions. As you start to notice improvements, push yourself to imagine the target situation at its worst to see whether you experience any distress. If you do, repeat the tapping, targeting those specific reactions.

How Do I Get Trained?

EP appears simple, and for many issues it can be. Using EP clinically to treat a diverse clinical population with a range of problems requires advanced training, however. Furthermore, knowledge of various ways of working energetically allows you to individualize treatment. EP training for professionals is becoming more rigorous. ACEP sponsors several training programs, and you can also go to the Web sites of other methods to discover ways to learn and become certified in those approaches (see the Key Web Resources box).

Importance of Personal Practice and Development

As you use EP methods more frequently, an important shift occurs. You internalize your experience that entrenched and difficult to treat problems can often be transformed quickly. Contrary to the generally held idea that you must work through the deep psychological roots of problems, you can reliably facilitate deep and enduring personal change by addressing the energetic foundations of problems.

In all energy work, indeed in all healing, the practitioner's personal development is critical. Caring, compassion, and technical skill are essential to the healing encounter. So, however, is the internal energetic level of the practitioner. Practitioners should establish a personal practice that can increase their energy level. For example, performing the Four Energy Gates everyday gradually improves your internal energy and helps you to be more effective. Other examples could include a regular meditation practice, doing yoga, or taking daily walks in nature. Time devoted to your personal practice has many visible and invisible benefits.

> As with any healing-oriented practice, work on yourself first by grounding and balancing your own energy. This can be done in various ways, including the four energy gates technique, meditation, breath work, and others.

Energy Psychology as a First-Line Treatment

Patients come to see their doctors and health care practitioners to seek treatment for disturbing symptoms. That many of these symptoms are not based on any significant disorder is well known. Often, these symptoms are somatic messages related to ongoing stress and disharmony in the patient's life. Having EP as part of your tool set will enable you to alleviate your patients' symptoms by helping them deal with the underlying stress that is at the root of their distress. An added benefit is that by offering EP treatment, you can help patients leave your office feeling better. In addition, they will have an effective, inexpensive, and safe self-help tool that they will be able to use forever.

KEY WEB RESOURCES

Association for Comprehensive Energy Psychology: www.energypsych.org

The Association for Comprehensive Energy Psychology is an international nonprofit professional organization whose goals are to promote the education, training, research, and ethical practice of comprehensive energy psychology.

EFT Universe: www.eftuniverse.com

This Web site contains many articles and case examples of the application of The Emotional Freedom Techniques (EFT).

http://video.google.com/googleplayer.swf?docid=6887426238803490578&hl=en&fs=true&autoplay=1

Of particular interest is a short video showing the before and after results of EFT treatment of four severely traumatized veterans.

TATLife: www.tatlife.com

This is the home site for the Tapas Acupressure Technique.

Energy Psychology: www.energypsych.com

This is the Web site for Dr. Fred Gallo, who is credited with coining the term energy psychology and who wrote the first textbook on it *(Energy Psychology)*. He has developed numerous methods, including Energy Diagnosis and Treatment Methods (EDxTM).

Innersource: www.innersource.net

This is Dr. David Feinstein's and Donna Eden's Web site, which includes links to many of Dr. Feinstein's articles, as well as information about Donna Eden's energy medicine workshops and trainings.

Traditional Chinese Medicine World Foundation: www.tcmworld.org

This Web site describes the many programs offered by Master Nan Lu. Energy psychology has direct links to traditional Chinese medicine. Master Lu's programs and training are a natural way to deepen your grasp and appreciation of the healing principles behind energy psychology.

Patient Handout: Energy Psychology Self-Care Patient Handout

Use the 4 Energy Gates (Figure 101-1) for daily self-care. Also, use this practice when dealing with an emotional, personal, or physical problem that is not passing on its own. You can do one or more of the 4 Energy Gates throughout the day, whenever you need a pick-me-up. *(Remember to consult with your physician if you have any serious health concerns.)*

Use the tapping method (Figure 101-2) to address a particular distressing emotional or personal issue.

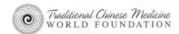
Traditional Chinese Medicine
WORLD FOUNDATION

The Four Energy Healing Gates: Universal Pathways to Health

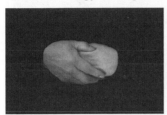

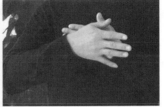

On the web between the thumb and index finger: With firm pressure, make small circles for 4 to 5 minuts. Note: the outside, active hand supports and protects.

On the center line of the body between the breasts: Place one palm over the other, and using light pressure only, circle in a clockwise direction at least 200 times (can also be done counter-clockwise).

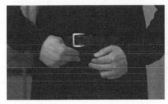

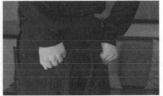

Just to each side of the center line, four fingers below the navel: Tap this area with two fingers of each hand for 4 to 5 minutes.

In the center "dimple" of the main muscle of the buttocks: Keeping arms, shoulders and hips relaxed, hold a loose fist and alternately punch this area for 4 to 5 minutes.

Traditional Chinese Medicine World Foundation
34 West 27th St, Site 1212, New York, NY 10001
212-274-1079 • fax: 212-274-9879 • www.tcmconference.org

Fig 101-1. Energy Psychology Meridian Tapping Protocol
From: Traditional Chinese Medicine World Foundation. http://www.tcmworld.org/_downloads/FourEnergyGates_FullPage.pdf
Accessed June 20, 2011.

1. Identify the problem that is blocking you. Is it primarily an emotional, cognitive, or behavioral issue? Is it physical (e.g., shoulder pain)? Rate it from 0–10 (10 is the most distress).

2. Then while tapping firmly and steadily on the side of the hand (sh on the chart) say outloud (to yourself):
*"Even though I have this **[insert your problem]**, I deeply love and accept myself."* Or, use this:
*"Even though I have this **[insert your problem]**, I attract love and compassion into my heart."*
Repeat 3 times.

3. Next, tap steadily and firmly about 7–9 times on each of the following acupoints, while saying at least once at each point, a brief reminder of the issue you are working on. (See Fig. 101-2.)
        Eyebrow – eb
        Side of the eye – oe
        Under the eye – e
        Under the nose – un
        Under the lower lip – ul
        Under the collarbone – c
        Under the arm – ua
(Note: You can tap on all of the points on the chart, but usually tapping on these 7 points is sufficient. Also, do your best to tap on the location shown in the chart. If you are not sure if you are doing it correctly, do your best and continue with the procedure.)

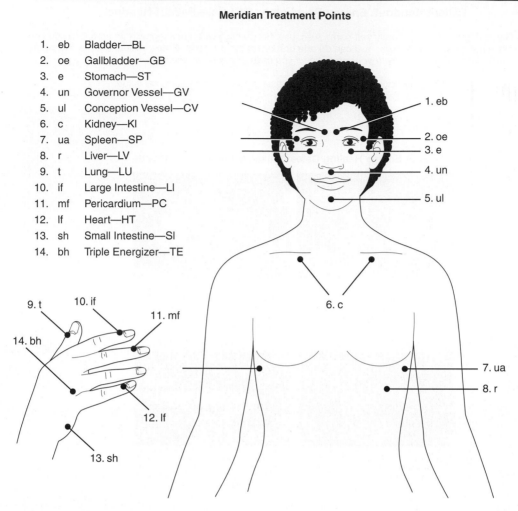

Meridian Treatment Points

1. eb   Bladder—BL
2. oe   Gallbladder—GB
3. e   Stomach—ST
4. un   Governor Vessel—GV
5. ul   Conception Vessel—CV
6. c   Kidney—KI
7. ua   Spleen—SP
8. r   Liver—LV
9. t   Lung—LU
10. if   Large Intestine—LI
11. mf   Pericardium—PC
12. lf   Heart—HT
13. sh   Small Intestine—SI
14. bh   Triple Energizer—TE

Figure 101-2. Energy tapping protocol.

4. Reevaluate the problem. How is it now? Repeat steps 2 and 3 if the problem still bothers you. Target the aspect of the problem that it is most distressing. For example, it may have started as a physical discomfort and has become more clearly emotional. Be persistent and repeat as necessary.

5. Usually, when your SUDS reaches 0, and you have no distress when you imagine experiencing the situation, the high likelihood is that you will be able to go through the actual event with little or no distress. However, because the tapping is easy to do, you can always use it as a self-help booster whenever you feel the need. Note: it is important to test out the treatment as much as possible to be sure that you are completely free of the negative reactions. As you start to notice improvements, push yourself to imagine the target situation at its worst to see whether you experience any distress. If you do, repeat the tapping targeting those specific reactions.

References

References are available online at expertconsult.com.

Section III Biochemical

Chapter 102

Prescribing Probiotics

J. Adam Rindfleisch, MD, MPhil

What Is a Probiotic?

Our intestines harbor trillions of organisms; in fact, they constitute 95% of the cells in our bodies.[1] Metagenomics and DNA studies indicate that the human gut houses somewhere on the order of 30,000 to 40,000 different organisms,[2] and with each passing year, new physiologic roles for these organisms have been discovered. Some investigators have gone so far as to refer to the enteric flora as "the forgotten organ" of the body.[3]

Since the 1980s, tremendous interest has developed in ways the ecosystem of the gut may be altered, not only to decrease pathogen numbers but also to promote overall health. Many different foods and supplements that contain microbes—namely, species of bacteria or yeasts—are now available over the counter. These products are widely known as probiotics, a hybrid word created by combining the Latin *pro-* ("for") with the Greek adjective *-biotic* ("life").[4] For all the commercial and scientific attention these supplements currently receive, only in the 1990s did the word probiotic enter both medical and general lexicons on a regular basis. The word was first put into play in 1965,[5] but its very definition remained elusive for many years. Most experts would now agree that a probiotic is a preparation or product containing a defined single or mixed culture of live microbes that, when ingested in sufficient numbers, will exert beneficial effects on health beyond basic nutrition by altering the gastrointestinal microbiota.[5-8]

For a food or supplement to be considered a probiotic by most definitions, it must meet several criteria, including the following[9]:

1. It must contain live organisms capable of colonizing the gastrointestinal tract, meaning that, among other things, it should be acid and bile tolerant.
2. It should improve the health and well-being of the host.
3. Its organisms should be generally recognized as safe (GRAS) and not pathogenic. (In the case of some *Enterobacter* species that have been used, this may not be the case.)
4. Host-specific strains of organisms should be used; humans should receive strains specific to humans and not to animals.

Increasing evidence indicates that many (but by no means all) products meet these specifications. Thirty to 40 species account for 99% of the bacteria present in the gut and often inform the selection of strains used therapeutically. The two most common genera of bacteria used in probiotics are *Bifidobacterium* (e.g., *Bifidobacterium bifidus*) and *Lactobacillus* (e.g., *Lactobacillus reuteri*). Strains of *Streptococcus* and Enterobacteriaceae are less commonly included.[10] *Saccharomyces boulardii*, a probiotic yeast, has been found to have a wide array of benefits and is gaining popularity.[10,11] *Escherichia coli* Nissle 1917 (the last part of the name is the subspecies designation) was discovered in the feces of World War I soldiers who were resistant to salmonellosis and shigellosis and is widely used in Europe. Products may contain just one species, or they may contain a mixture of different organisms.

> The most common probiotic species used are *Lactobacillus* and *Bifidobacterium*. *Saccharomyces boulardii*, a probiotic yeast, has also shown promise for many indications.

Why Are Probiotics Used to Promote Health?

Probiotic therapy is not a new idea; in fact, its genesis can be traced to ancient times. Reference to such therapy was made in the Persian version of Genesis (18:8), which states, "Abraham owed his longevity to the consumption of sour milk."[12] The Roman historian Plinius noted that fermented foods could be of benefit to persons with signs and symptoms compatible with what would now be termed gastroenteritis.[7]

The modern use of microbial interference therapy, or probiotics, is tied to the late nineteenth century observation by microbiologists that the resident bacterial flora of people who were healthy was different from that of people who were symptomatically ill.[13] In the early twentieth century, the Russian scientist and Nobel laureate Elie Metchnikoff posited that ingestion of lactobacilli in fermented foods contributed to the longevity of Bulgarian peasants by optimizing the balance between gastrointestinal pathogens and nonpathogens.[14,15] Researchers theorized over the years that the microbiota of the gut somehow influenced health and illness. It stood to reason that changing the microbial mix could lead to health benefits.

Most people in the general population consider the gastrointestinal tract a closed tube through which foodstuffs and then waste products pass, but this is an oversimplification. To explain why probiotics may be used to promote health, a review of some important gut functions is worthwhile. Some of these functions include the following:

1. Permeability (and screening what moves into and out of the bloodstream). The intestinal mucosa has a very large surface area, and it serves as an important interface with "the outside world," constantly exposed to foreign molecules, bacteria, fungi, and viruses.[8] The mucosal system that begins in the mouth and ends at the anus is, in fact, a permeable system that leaches microbes (translocation) and dietary antigens into the systemic circulation and tissues. Probiotics influence this permeability in many ways.[1,11]
2. Motility (peristalsis), as directed by the enteric nervous system. The gut flora influences chemical mediators that affect the physiology of the elaborate enteric nervous system and ultimately influence the body's nervous system as a whole.[16] Research shows that gut microbiota may even influence brain development and subsequent adult behavior in mammals.[17]
3. Immune function. At any given time, most immune system activity occurs within the gastrointestinal tract. Gut-associated lymphoid tissue is influenced by the types of bacteria that are present in the gut and the signaling mechanisms they trigger.[18]

Clearly, intraspecies and interspecies communication between gut microbes occurs (this is known as quorum sensing),[19] and a dialogue between bacteria and host is ongoing as well.[20] In fact, human evolution and the evolution of gut microflora are so intimately interconnected that it is easy to imagine the degree of complexity that now characterizes this commensal relationship.

Although gastrointestinal physiology and the composition of the microbiota are likely highly individualized, some common factors can have a negative effect on them, including the following:

- Poor eating habits
- Chronic physical and emotional stress
- Lack of exercise
- Insufficient rest
- Frequent exposure to antibiotics
- Geographic factors

How Do Probiotics Work?

Probiotics have been found to improve health through numerous different mechanisms, many of which may be specific to individual species. Different species predominate, based on the location along the gastrointestinal tract, in part because the rate of gut motility varies greatly from one part of the gut to another. In healthy persons, the transit time from mouth to anus is between 55 and 72 hours, of which 4 to 6 hours comprise the transfer time from the mouth to the cecum, and the remaining time reflects transit through the colon. Some species live close to the gut lining, whereas others live in the center of the lumen.[3,21] Some of the key mechanisms of action of probiotics, as described in the literature, include the following:[1,3,10,11,22]

1. Blockade of toxin receptor sites
2. Inhibition of the growth of pathogenic microbes
3. Inhibition of pathogen attachment to receptor sites
4. Engagement in cross-talk with other flora to enhance resistance to colonization. Biofilms, which are aggregations of ordered and often specialized groups of microorganisms that often perform complex functions, seem to play a role
5. Enhancement of tight junction bonding and prevention of impaired barrier function
6. Production of cytochrome P-450–like enzymes and facilitation of detoxification
7. Exertion of trophic effects by influencing transport pathways and the production of energy and protein, as well as by releasing enzymes that facilitate the maturation of enterocytes
8. Production of B vitamins and vitamin K
9. Interaction with the immune system. Potential mechanisms include altering secretory immunoglobulin A levels, decreasing inflammatory effects of natural killer cells, and trapping helper T cells in mesenteric lymph nodes to decrease the inflammatory response
10. Creation of a physiologically challenging environment (low pH, production of toxic byproducts)
11. Competitive consumption of nutrients
12. Reduction of concentrations of oncogenic enzymes in the gut
13. Direct DNA signaling. Even dead probiotic organisms can exert an influence on some (but not all) aspects of gut physiology; this has been referred to as the probiotic paradox.[23] One study examining the effect of probiotic organisms on a murine model of colitis found that nonviable organisms were just as effective as live microbes. In this study, the beneficial effects of probiotics were attributable not to microbial colonization and generation of metabolic byproducts, but rather to Toll-like receptor signaling mediated by microbial DNA (Fig. 102-1).[24]

The gut microbiota may actually help shape individual human physiology by influencing expression of genes critical to proper development of the intestines and functions, including nutrient absorption and metabolism, metabolism of toxins, gut maturation, and angiogenesis.[25]

Probiotics have multiple potential mechanisms of action. Different species have very different degrees of efficacy in clinical trials.

FIGURE 102-1
Schematic summary of some of the mechanisms of action of probiotics in the bowel. Probiotics can alter pathogenic bacterial adherence to the bowel wall through (1) a physical barrier, (2) an altered epithelial surface glycosylation pattern, and (3) increased mucin production. Other modes of action include (4) secretion of antimicrobial peptides and (5) modulation of the immune system. IFN, interferon; IL, interleukin; TNF, tumor necrosis factor. (Redrawn from Borowiec AM, Fedorak RN. The role of probiotics in management of irritable bowel syndrome. *Curr Gastroenterol Rep.* 2007;9:393–400.)

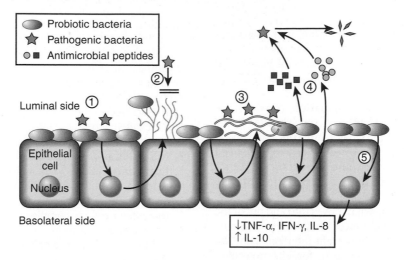

What Are Prebiotics, Synbiotics, and Postbiotics?

Prebiotics

Also known as probiotic enhancers or colon food, prebiotics are nondigestible nutrients that selectively stimulate the growth and activity of one or more colonic microorganisms that act to promote the health and well-being of the host.[26] The prebiotics developed thus far are mainly nondigestible oligosaccharides, which have traditionally been used to add fiber to foods without adding bulk. Prototypes include inulin (a chicory fructan) and fructooligosaccharides, which occur naturally in garlic, onion, leeks, asparagus, chicory, bananas, wheat, oats, soybeans, and artichokes.[27] Inulin and oligofructose stimulate the growth of bifidobacteria at the expense of *Bacteroides, Clostridium,* and coliform bacteria.[26] Chicory fructans have also been shown to enhance the absorption and balance of dietary calcium.[28,29] Other oligosaccharides, such as xylose, maltose, and mannose, also show promise as prebiotics. Lactulose is perhaps one of the prebiotics most familiar to medical practitioners.

> Common prebiotic foods include garlic, onion, leeks, asparagus, chicory, banana, wheat, oats, soybeans, and artichoke.

Synbiotics

Synbiotics are products that contain both prebiotic and probiotic ingredients. The thinking is that consuming both at once, instead of just the probiotic alone, may enhance microbe survival during transit through the upper gastrointestinal tract and lead to greater positive effects on the beneficial microbes already established in the intestines. Although most studies have focused exclusively on probiotics, a growing body of synbiotics research now exists. For example, one trial confirmed that a synbiotic of *Lactobacillus casei* and inulin reduced toxic protein fermentation metabolites in the gut.[30]

Synbiotics have been found to decrease levels of proinflammatory cytokines as well.[31] In vitro studies suggested that prebiotics and synbiotics could play a role in colon cancer chemoprevention by reducing the incidence of aberrant crypt foci, as was shown in rat studies in which intestinal changes were induced by known carcinogens.[32,33] Synbiotics were also found to be effective in improving clinical symptoms of active Crohn's disease.[34] In addition, synbiotics containing *Lactobacillus helveticus, Bifidobacterium infantis* and *Bifidobacterium bifidum,* and fructooligosaccharide were found to limit common winter infections in schoolchildren.[35,36]

Postbiotics

Postbiotics, which have received less overall clinical research thus far, are metabolic byproducts, generated by probiotics, that influence host physiology.[37]

How Does the Human Microbiota Become Established?

Every person's microbiota is initially determined at birth, specifically by the mode of delivery. A newborn's gut is sterile. When a baby is delivered vaginally, his or her gastrointestinal tract is seeded with organisms from the mother's vagina, whereas the gastrointestinal tract of a baby delivered by cesarean section is largely populated by organisms from the surrounding environment.[38–40] The following factors in the neonatal period also play a role in composition of the ultimate gut microbiota in a child:

- Breast-feeding versus bottle-feeding (higher concentrations of potentially beneficial bifidobacteria are found in the gut when babies are breast-fed, as are fewer potential pathogens[41])

- Term versus preterm birth

- Administration of antibiotics

- Surrounding environment (level of sanitation)

TABLE 102-1. Therapeutic Benefits of Probiotic Therapy*

Conditions for Which Probiotics Are of Proven Benefit	Diarrheal illness (viral): • Treatment and prevention of viral diarrhea[44,47] • Prevention of antibiotic-associated diarrhea[48] • Traveler's diarrhea prevention[49] Eczema (particularly when given prenatally)[50,51] Flatulence[52] Hepatic encephalopathy (minimal severity)[53] Irritable bowel syndrome (number needed to treat of 4 with bifidobacteria)[54] Necrotizing enterocolitis prevention in preterm infants[55] Prevention[45] • Colds in older adults[56] • Infections in daycare facilities (gastrointestinal) • Potentiation of response to influenza vaccine
Conditions for Which Data Suggest Probiotics Have Benefit	Acute diarrhea prevention[44,58] Bacterial vaginosis[59,60] (combination of *L. rhamnosus* GR-1 and *L. reuteri* RC-14 showed most promise in restoring vaginal microbiota) *Clostridium difficile* infection (namely, recurrences)[11] Diarrhea, persistent (more than 14 days)[61] *Helicobacter pylori* treatment enhancement[62] Inflammatory bowel disease[63,64] Infant growth (especially children of mothers with HIV infection)[65] Postoperative infections after abdominal surgery[45] Radiation-induced diarrhea[66] Respiratory tract infection (seems mainly to decrease severity, not duration)[67] Ventilator-associated pneumonia[68]
Conditions for Which Probiotic Therapy Holds Promise	Allergic rhinitis[69] Asthma[70] Attention deficit disorder and attention deficit hyperactivity disorder[71] Autism[72] Chemotherapy-induced diarrhea[73] Chronic fatigue–related cognitive function[74] Colic[43] Cancer prevention[45] Colon cancer recurrence[46] Cystic fibrosis[75] Dental diseases, including caries, gingivitis, halitosis[45,46] Diabetes (type 1)[76] Diverticular disese[77] Dyslipidemia[45,78] Food allergies[46,79] HIV-related diarrhea[11] Liver disease[45] Rheumatoid arthritis[45] Genitourinary tract infections[80,81] (especially insertion of *Escherichia coli* probiotics through a bladder catheter). Nephrolithiasis[82]
Conditions for Which Probiotic Therapy Has Not Proven Beneficial	Lactose intolerance[83] Otitis media[45] Pancreatitis[84] Spondyloarthropathies[85]

Data from references 10, 11, 21, and 43 to 85.
HIV, human immunodeficiency virus.
*Remember that benefits are strain specific. This list focuses on many of the conditions that have been studied, primarily using meta-analysis and systematic reviews, but it is by no means comprehensive.

• Socioeconomic status

• Geographic factors

> Positive effects on colonization of the gut with healthy flora can be listed as yet another clinically proven benefit of breast-feeding.

Investigators have found that supplementation of formula with probiotics can have several benefits for infants, including reducing Enterobacteriaceae and *Clostridium* counts, favorably altering stool pH, altering fecal immunoglobulin A and short-chain fatty acid concentrations (the latter connected to resistance to pathogen colonization), and decreasing intestinal permeability.[42] Once established, the intestinal microbiota is relatively constant and difficult to alter over the long term.

What Are Clinical Indications for Prebiotic and Probiotic Use?

Probiotics are intended to be used for prevention and, in some instances, treatment of many different specific maladies, as listed in Table 102-1, which summarizes key findings of numerous probiotic-focused systematic reviews and meta-analyses.[43-85] Different probiotics are used for different conditions; the reader should keep in mind which species were used in any given study.

How Should Probiotic Supplements Be Taken?

A simplistic view of probiotic therapy ("Just take any probiotic and follow the label instructions," or "Simply take acidophilus") does a disservice to published research in this field and also may not serve the best interests of patients. Clinicians must remember that therapeutic benefits ascribed to probiotic therapy are strain specific.[86] Numerous microbes are promoted as probiotics, and data comparing strains with one another in terms of clinical efficacy for specific maladies are largely lacking. With various studies using different strains in varying doses for numerous illnesses in dissimilar populations over disparate time courses and using different experimental models, one can see how generalizations about administration of probiotic therapy must be avoided and how urgently additional study is needed.

Daily dosages given for prebiotics and probiotics range widely, anywhere from 1 million to 20 billion colony-forming units (CFUs), but recommendations tend toward 1 to 10 billion CFUs for infants and 10 to 20 billion CFUs for older children and adults. A 2008 review of probiotics for diarrhea in children found that doses of at least 10 billion CFUs/day were necessary for effect.[47] To achieve and maintain a therapeutic effect, probiotics must be administered repeatedly to ensure a sufficient and consistent population level over time. Available data regarding the appropriate duration of therapy for various clinical conditions are limited, however.

Table 102-2 lists some of the key probiotics, the doses in which they are administered, and the indications for which they have been found to be effective.[87]

Some manufacturers beg to differ, but to minimize exposure to gastric acid, most experts recommend taking probiotics on an empty stomach. When taken during a course of antibiotic therapy, probiotics should be started as soon as possible and continued for 7 to 14 days after completion of therapy. Some authorities recommend separating antibiotics and bacteria-derived probiotics by 2 hours.[86] The body's microflora typically takes 6 to 8 weeks to recover after exposure to an antibiotic.

TABLE 102-2. Commonly Studied Organisms With Significant Probiotic Potential

PROBIOTIC SPECIES NAME	EXAMPLES OF CONDITIONS WHERE BENEFIT HAS BEEN FOUND	DOSE (COLONY-FORMING UNITS)
Lactobacillus		
• *Lactobacillus acidophilus*	Vulvovaginal candidiasis	8 oz yogurt with at least 10^8 CFU/mL daily for 6 mo
• *Lactobacillus reuteri*	Acute infectious diarrhea in children	10^{10}–10^{11} twice daily for up to 5 days
• *Lactobacillus rhamnosus* GG	Acute infectious diarrhea in children	10^{10} in 250 mL oral rehydration solution (infants); 10^{10}–10^{11} twice daily for 2–5 days (older children)
	Antibiotic-associated diarrhea	6×10^9–4×10^{10} daily for 1–2 wk
	Traveler's diarrhea prevention	2×10^9 daily from 2 days before leaving and throughout trip
	Irritable bowel syndrome (combined with other lactobacilli)	8–9×10^9 daily for 6 mo
	Atopic disease prevention	10^{10} daily for 2–4 wk before due date for pregnant women; then infant administration for 6 mo
	Vulvovaginal candidiasis	10^9 per suppository, inserted twice daily for 7 days
• *Lactobacillus salivarius*		
Bifidobacterium	Overall better scores for irritable bowel syndrome treatment	
	Necrotizing enterocolitis	
• *Bifidobacterium bifidum*		
• *Bifidobacterium infantis*	Irritable bowel syndrome	10^6–10^{10} daily for 4 wk
• *Bifidobacterium longum*	Combined with fructooligosaccharides, improvement in some outcomes in ulcerative colitis	
Other Forms		
• *Escherichia coli* 1917 Nissle	Ulcerative colitis	Acute flares: 5×10^{10} twice daily until remission, maximum of 12 wk, followed by once daily for maximum of 12 mo
		Flare prevention: 5×10^{10} daily
• *Streptococcus thermophilus*		
• *Saccharomyces boulardii* (yeast)	Antibiotic-associated diarrhea	4×10^9-2×10^{10} daily for 1–4 wk
	Clostridium difficile infection	2×10^{10} daily for 4 wk plus vancomycin and/or metronidazole
	Traveler's diarrhea prevention	5×10^9-2×10^{10} daily from 5 days before leaving and throughout trip
	Ulcerative colitis	Flares: 250 mg three times daily for 4 wk, plus mesalamine
	Crohn's disease	Maintenance: 1 g daily for 6 mo, plus mesalamine

TABLE 102-2. Commonly Studied Organisms With Significant Probiotic Potential—cont'd

PROBIOTIC SPECIES NAME	EXAMPLES OF CONDITIONS WHERE BENEFIT HAS BEEN FOUND	DOSE (COLONY-FORMING UNITS)
Combinations		
• L. acidophilus and B. delbrueckii subspecies bulgaricus	Antibiotic-associated diarrhea	2×10^9 daily for 5–10 days
• L. acidophilus and B. longum	Antibiotic-associated diarrhea	5×10^9 daily for 7 days
• L. rhamnosus GR-1 and L. fermentum RC-14	Vulvovaginal candidiasis	10^9 bacteria in skim milk, twice daily (taken orally) for 14 days
• VSL#3*	Irritable bowel syndrome	9×10^{11} daily for 8 wk
	Ulcerative colitis	Active flares: 1.8×10^{12} twice daily for 6 wk plus conventional therapy
	Pouchitis	1.8×10^{12} bacteria twice daily

From Williams NT. Probiotics. *Am J Health Syst Pharm.* 2010;67:449–458.
*A cocktail of eight different species: *S. thermophilus, B. breve, B. longum, B. infantis, L. acidophilus, L. plantarum, L. casei,* and *L. delbrueckii* subspecies *bulgaricus*).

This recovery period is decreased to just a few days with probiotic use.[88] Most studies of antibiotic-associated diarrhea have subjects take the probiotic for as long as they take the antibiotic therapy, and continuing for a few weeks after antibiotics are completed is a reasonable recommendation.

Treatment is typically well tolerated, and palatability is an uncommon issue because the capsules can be opened and mixed into drinks or soft foods. Sometimes, the agents are available as powders. If effective, treatment can continue indefinitely. Precautions do exist, however (see later). If a patient has not noticed a benefit after 6 weeks or more of use, a trial of a different species or another approach altogether is worth considering. Often, a trial of *Saccharomyces boulardii* may be merited if bacterial probiotics are not found to be helpful.[11]

Refrigeration is recommended for products that have been heat-dried, because they are more likely to die off with temperature extremes and need refrigeration. Lyophilized preparations (as noted on the bottle) do not need refrigeration and tend to have good overall long-term survival.

Brand choice is important. One study of 14 commercial probiotics sold in the United States found that 93% were incorrectly labeled; nearly 36% did not list strains on the label at all, and nearly 60% had contaminants.[89,90] Another study that tested 58 products from around the world found that only 38% contained the dose stated on the label, and 29% did not contain strains listed on the label.

How may one select a reliable probiotic brand? Consider the following:

• Use products from companies that have actively sponsored probiotics research.

• Consider using a Web site such as www.consumerlab.com (a subscription currently costs approximately $30/year). The laboratory tests different brands of supplements to verify whether they contain what they claim on their labels. Products that are of good quality are listed.

• Make certain products have a Good Manufacturing Practices (GMP) seal.

• Ensure that the product specifies which species it contains and in what quantities.

Although many companies manufacture probiotic cocktails (mixes of several different species), few studies have not reviewed the efficacy of combinations. Benefits vary by microorganism. For example, different bifidobacteria tolerate different pH levels and vary in terms of fecal recovery rates after they have been consumed.[91]

> General guidelines for taking probiotics:
> • Take 2 hours before or after antibiotics.
> • Take on an empty stomach.
> • Heat-dried formulations should be kept in the refrigerator; lyophilized ones can handle room temperature.
> • Most doses range from 1 to 10 billion colony-forming units once or twice daily.

Do Natural Food Sources Provide Probiotic Exposure?

Yes, but not without a few caveats. European, African, and Asian consumers have long been exposed to probiotics as found in functional foods, typically fermented and nonfermented dairy products such as yogurt, buttermilk, sauerkraut, kefir, and kimchi. However, the organisms typically found within these foods are often not the same microbes for which significant supportive research data exist regarding health benefits. For example, the live cultures in yogurt products frequently emphasize *Lactobacillus delbrueckii* subspecies *bulgaricus* and *Streptococcus thermophilus,* two organisms that may not survive passage through gastric acid and bile to colonize the gut mucosa.

Consumers should be sure to purchase products in which the probiotic organisms are added after pasteurization; otherwise, the bacteria are killed during that process.

Using products that clearly state "contains active cultures" or "living yogurt cultures" is best.[92]

Typically, frozen foods do not contain live cultures, and foods such as frozen yogurt likely do not constitute a good probiotic source. However, work is progressing in the development of probiotic ice creams.[93]

How Safe Are Probiotics?

Today, diets high in fermented foods remain popular worldwide. They have been used for decades, and little, if any, risk has been identified with them. Probiotic therapy, obtained through supplements or by dietary means, appears to be extremely safe.[10,11,43,45,46,94,95] Many of the safety concerns raised are linked to case reports only, and when compared with many commonly used medications (including antibiotics), probiotics and prebiotics fare much better in terms of adverse effects.

Bacteria do translocate, however, and case reports of bacteremia and liver abscess exist.[96,97] Case reports have been published documenting rare infectious complications with *Saccharomyces boulardii* in nonimmunocompromised patients who were nonetheless ill.[98,99] Caution is advised regarding the use of probiotics in the following settings[100]:

- Immunocompromised patients

- Premature infants. Studies of the use of probiotics for prevention of necrotizing enterocolitis demonstrated minimal risk, however. A 2010 study pooling side effects data for more than 1100 infants found probiotic use to be quite safe.[101]

- Patients with central venous access or other indwelling medical devices in place

- Use of an untested probiotic strain

- Pancreatitis. A 2008 study found increased mortality (relative risk, 2.53; 95% confidence interval, 1.22 to 5.25) in a group of 152 inpatients with severe acute pancreatitis.[102,103] Although systematic reviews have not reported mortality increases with probiotic use in patients with pancreatitis in general, they have not found that using probiotics for treating pancreatitis is beneficial. Avoidance of probiotic use, especially in patients with severe cases of pancreatitis, may be prudent.[84]

> As a general rule, most good-quality probiotics are quite safe with few side effects, but use caution in patients with severe pancreatitis, immunocompromised people, and those with indwelling medical equipment.

- Lactose hypersensitivity and yeast allergy. Some authorities recommend that *Lactobacillus* preparations be avoided in persons with hypersensitivity to lactose or milk, and yeasts should not be used in anyone with a yeast allergy. Bifidobacteria have no contraindications listed.[87] Probiotics should be used cautiously in people taking immunosuppressive therapies. The use of *Enterobacter* species is controversial, given the risk of pathogenicity.

A 2011 review concluded that prebiotics and probiotics are, based on the available data, safe to use in infant formula, with no adverse effects or negative impacts on growth.[103] A 2009 review of 11 studies of probiotic use during pregnancy found no adverse outcomes on gestational age, malformation frequency, cesarian section outcomes, or miscarriages, but the investigators cautioned that further research is needed.[104]

KEY WEB RESOURCES

International Scientific Association for Probiotics and Prebiotics: http://www.isapp.net/	This organization's mission is to disseminate reliable information about these substances.
Usprobiotics: http://www.usprobiotics.org/	This Web site has some nice summaries of the literature, as well as a useful resource page that includes Web casts.
Food Insight: http://www.foodinsight.org/	This well-done educational site involves food and nutrition. Users can click "Search" in the upper right corner of screen and gather probiotics information. It also has premade PowerPoint presentations on nutrition in the "For Professionals" section, as well as many resources on various food components, food safety, and weight management.
University of Wisconsin Integrative Medicine: http://www.fammed.wisc.edu/sites/default/files//webfm-uploads/documents/outreach/im/handout_probiotics_patient.pdf	This is a patient handout on probiotics.
American Gastroenterological Association: http://www.gastro.org/patient-center/diet-medications/probiotics	This is another patient handout on probiotics.

Acknowledgment

The author and editor would like to thank Russell Greenfield, MD for his help in preparing this manuscript.

References

References available online at expertconsult.com.

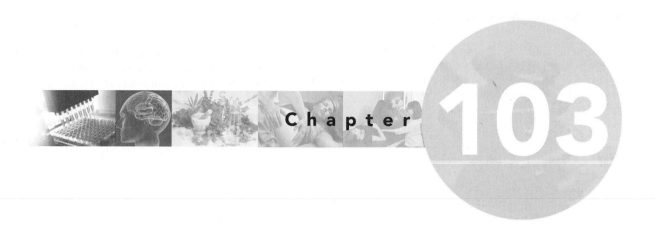

Chapter 103

Prescribing Botanicals

Paula Gardiner, MD, MPH, and Tieraona Low Dog, MD

A careful examination of the evidence regarding the safety and efficacy of herbal medicines should guide clinicians as they partner with their patients in creating optimal health care. In 1997, 42% of the U.S. population used some form of complementary and alternative medicine (CAM), and 12% of the population used herbal medicine.[1] In 2007, 18% of the U.S. population used herbs for health conditions, and annual expenditures for herbal supplements exceeded $25 billion.[2,3] Clearly, many of our patients are regularly using herbs and dietary supplements.

Who Uses Herbs?

Rates of herbal product use vary by age, gender, race, and ethnicity, but substantial numbers of all patient groups report using herbs and dietary supplements, particularly women and people with chronic or recurrent illnesses who also receive care from conventional health care professionals. In national studies, the medical conditions for which herb use is most commonly reported have been upper respiratory infections, arthritis, depression, musculoskeletal pain, memory improvement, and menopausal symptoms.[4,5]

What Else Are They Taking?

Additionally, more than 27 million people living in the United States may be taking an over-the-counter medication and an herb or a prescription medication and an herb concurrently.[6] Different patient populations are at high risk for drug-herb interactions and include human immunodeficiency virus–positive patients, chronically ill patients, patients with cancer, and older Medicare patients.[7–10]

No universally accepted guideline exists for managing a patient's prescription medication and herbal medicine in the outpatient or inpatient setting.[11] However, the Joint Commission (formerly the Joint Commission on Accreditation of Healthcare Organizations) requires that dietary supplements (herbs, vitamins, minerals) conform to the same hospital standards as prescription medications.[12]

Despite the documented high prevalence of patient use of herbal products, fewer than half of patients who use herbs typically discuss it with their clinicians.[9,13] Therefore, clinicians must have an approach to discussing herb use with patients.

Talking About Herbs With Patients

Health care providers must be able to talk with patients about many different treatment options, including those that fall outside what the health care provider learned in formal training. Because the use of herbs has the potential for both benefit and harm, providers must approach the topic of herb use in an open and nonjudgmental way. Many cultures have a rich history of using botanical medicines; indeed, herbal medicine is the most common form of traditional medicine in the world. Because so many different herbal practices and products are available in the United States, generalizations are difficult. Nevertheless, by asking a few open-ended questions, the physician should be able to assess the patient's beliefs and cultural practices regarding his or her use of herbal medicines. Examples of such questions are as follows:

- When you were growing up, did you or your family ever use any medicinal plants or herbal remedies to improve your health or treat an illness?

- If I were to walk around your house and look for containers of herbs, vitamins, or dietary supplements, what would I find?

- How do you use herbs or herbal remedies in your home?

- Are you taking any herbs or herbal medicines now? If so, what are you trying to treat, and do you think the herbs are working?

Using herbs in practice is a holistic process. Besides the patient's cultural and social background, the physician should take into account the patient's symptoms, any chronic or acute illness, any prescribed medications, and any non-prescribed medications, as well as judging how adherent the patient will be to the regimen the physician recommends.

Efficacy

How does the physician know whether an herb actually works for a patient's condition? Does strong historical evidence exist? Does the herb have a biologically plausible mechanism of action based on in vitro or animal research? Has the herb undergone controlled clinical trials? If so, which type of product was studied and at what dose? These are important questions to ask when trying to determine efficacy. First, here is a summary of the strengths and weaknesses of different types of evidence used to assess the efficacy of botanical medicines.

In vitro studies—objective measurements using isolated tissue or cell culture—are a well-accepted first step for understanding the physiologic or pharmacologic activity of a particular substance. Animal studies are often used in pharmacologic studies because they permit control over certain variables and can help explain potential mechanisms of action. The strengths of in vitro and animal studies are the following:

- They allow control over certain variables.
- They generate and test hypotheses for mechanism of action.
- They help determine safety at varying doses and duration.

These studies do have limitations, as follows:

- Results may not accurately predict physiologic effects in humans.
- Parenteral administration may give differing results from oral administration.
- Study of isolated constituents may not reflect use of the whole plant.
- Ethical issues surround the use of animals in medical research.

A long history of use is an important source of information regarding the safe and effective use of plant medicines. These historical data are almost exclusively based on observational data, and even today, a clinician's observations remain an important tool for assessing efficacy and adverse effects in the office. One strength of observational data is that they can provide useful insight when a therapy has been used by multiple cultures, over time, for similar purposes. In addition, the astute clinician may detect a therapeutic effect, or an adverse effect, that is not well known or recognized. An important limitation is the risk of bias if the observers are not studying a defined cohort of patients.

Nonrandomized and nonblinded, or uncontrolled, studies are valuable for generating hypotheses and assisting in the identification of adverse events, although they are best regarded as yielding supportive evidence. Strengths of uncontrolled studies are as follows:

- They are valuable for generating hypotheses.
- They are useful for identifying adverse events.

The limitation is that the presence of multiple uncontrolled variables increases the risk of bias in the results.

Outcomes research generally involves a cohort of patients with the same diagnosis (e.g., diabetes, heart disease) that relates their clinical and health outcomes (e.g., death, events, improvement) to the care they received (e.g., physical therapy, medication). The strengths of outcomes research are as follows:

- It reflects more closely the actual day-to-day practice of clinical medicine.
- It is well suited for whole systems approaches (e.g., traditional Chinese medicine, Ayurveda, naturopathy).

The limitation is that it is difficult to establish efficacy for any particular aspect of treatment.

In randomized double-blind clinical trials, patients are randomly allocated to different treatment groups, and neither the researchers nor the participants know who is receiving the experimental protocol. Considered the gold standard for pharmaceutical research, this type of study can greatly reduce bias. It has the following strengths:

- It provides safeguards against numerous forms of bias.
- The model is applicable for the study of many botanical interventions.

Limitations of randomized double-blind trials are as follows:

- The average randomly allocated patient may not adequately reflect the clinical subgroups seen in clinical medicine.
- This model may not be applicable for answering some clinical questions, such as individualization of therapy.
- The lack of a randomized controlled trial is often interpreted as lack of efficacy; this is a problem in botanical medicine, in which treatments may have been used for centuries but lack current gold standard evidence.

In addition to understanding the limitations of different research methods clearly, the physician must understand exactly what type of product is actually being tested. The complex nature of botanicals—the variations in constituents among species, plant parts, and preparation—makes it essential that authors of research articles provide an adequate description of the product used in the clinical trial. Descriptions should include identification (Latin binomial and authority), plant part (e.g., root, leaf, seed), and type of preparation (e.g., tea, tincture, extract, oil).

Tincture and extract description should include the identity of the solvent and the ratio of solvent to plant material. If the preparation is standardized to a chemical constituent, then that information should also be included. Precise and clear dose and dosage form should be provided.[14] These are critically important issues to consider when conducting and publishing research on botanical medicines. Thus, we must ask the question "Is the product my patient is taking for a particular condition similar to what was clinically tested?" In 2006, the Consolidated Standards of Reporting Trials (CONSORT) developed guidelines in reporting clinical trials of herbal medicine in the peer-reviewed literature that have been adopted by many journals.[15,16]

Increasing numbers of systematic reviews and meta-analyses are now available for busy clinicians to evaluate the evidence of efficacy for numerous botanicals including echinacea,[17] garlic,[18-21] kava,[22] ginkgo,[23,24] horse chestnut,[25] saw palmetto,[26] and St. John's wort.[27] While recognizing the value of meta-analyses in the medical literature, one potential problem exists with this approach in the field of herbal medicine: the pooling of different products to reach a specific conclusion about a particular plant. For example, a review of garlic pooled results from clinical trials using raw garlic, aged garlic extracts, dehydrated garlic, and garlic oil macerates to reach a specific conclusion regarding the benefit of garlic to cardiovascular health.[28] When one evaluates these products from an analytical perspective, the marked chemical differences among them make any general conclusion about the efficacy of garlic (or lack thereof) questionable.

Finally, we must consider what level of evidence of efficacy is acceptable to support the use of a medicinal plant by our patients. This must take into consideration the relative safety of the product, the medical condition being treated, and patients' personal beliefs and preferences.

Safety Considerations

As with any drug or chemically active constituent, whether an herb is toxic depends on its dose, form of product, what it is taken with, and the underlying condition of the patient. Overall, most herbs commonly used in the United States have a relatively good safety profile, and the incidences of herbal adverse events are low. From 2007 to 2009, the Food and Drug Administration (FDA) received more than 700 adverse event reports about dietary supplements.[29] In general, many case reports are of poor quality or are anecdotal, and frequently the adverse effects are caused not by the supplements themselves, but rather by contaminants.[30]

> Adverse effects of botanicals commonly arise not from the supplement itself but from contaminants within it.

Modern use of an herbal product may not reflect the use of herbal preparations in traditional medicine. For example, an excellent safety record of a traditional oral preparation may well have limited relevance to use of the same herb in a concentrated product at a high dose. Moreover, herbs that are apparently safe under normal conditions may be more hazardous in specific conditions (e.g., pregnancy, impairment of renal or liver function), under special circumstances (e.g., during the perioperative period), or when combined with certain conventional drugs.

When considering the safety of botanicals, one must look at the framework for regulating the sale of dietary supplements in the United States. The Dietary Supplement and Health Education Act (DSHEA), which was enacted in 1994, has had a profound influence on how herbal products are sold and marketed to the consumer. To discuss herbal products with patients, physicians must understand this Act.[31] The following points are important:

- The DSHEA allows dietary supplements to be marketed without prior approval of their efficacy and safety by the FDA.

- The manufacturer of an herbal product is responsible for the truthfulness of claims made on the label and must have evidence that the claims are supported; nevertheless, the DSHEA neither provides a standard for the evidence needed nor requires submission of the evidence to the FDA.

- Manufacturers are permitted to claim that the product affects the structure or function of the body, as long as (1) no claim of effectiveness is made for the prevention or treatment of a specific disease, and (2) a disclaimer appears on the container informing the user that the FDA has not evaluated the product for any claim.

- The manufacturer is responsible for controlling the quality and safety of the product, but if a concern about safety arises, the burden of proof lies not with the manufacturer but with the FDA, which has to prove that the product is unsafe.

- The FDA has released good manufacturing practices (GMPs) for herbal products. GMPs set standards for purity, strength, and potency of the supplements to reflect what is stated on the label.[32]

Even if we physicians are able to identify an herbal product that shows strong efficacy, the concern about the safety of herbal products overshadows our discussions with patients. These concerns include contamination with other products such as heavy metals, pesticides, microorganisms, or misidentified herbal ingredients and adulteration with a prescription drug.[33] The quality of plant material varies considerably, depending on where it is cultivated or gathered, the times and methods of harvest and drying, and environmental conditions such as climate and soil type. The composition of an herbal product may vary considerably among manufacturers, and discrepancies between label information and actual content may occur. Clinicians should be cognizant of potential adverse events from food or drug interactions. For instance, sufficient evidence from interaction studies and case reports demonstrated that St. John's wort (*Hypericum perforatum*) induces the cytochrome P-450 (CYP) 3A4 enzyme system and the P-glycoprotein drug transporter in a clinically relevant manner, thus reducing the efficacy of comedications.[34-36]

In December of 2006, the Dietary Supplement and Nonprescription Drug Consumer Protection Act was passed. It requires the reporting of a serious adverse event as a result of a dietary supplement and labeling of the manufacturer's address and phone number. The manufacturer is required to forward information on serious adverse events to the FDA within 15 days. The health care professional can also report a drug-herb interaction or an adverse effect to MedWatch, a program administered by the FDA. Another excellent resource is to contact the local poison control center; the current nationwide toll-free number for poison control is 800-222-1222.

Choosing a Brand or Product: A Question of Quality

Once the clinician has determined that an herb is efficacious and safe for a particular patient, he or she must advise the patient on choosing high-quality products. The quality of an herbal preparation partly determines its efficacy, as well as its safety. Even with the DSHEA, loopholes in the regulatory system have allowed poor-quality products to be introduced into the marketplace. The FDA is addressing some of the problems associated with manufacturing herbal products with its new GMPs.[32] Nonprofit and for-profit organizations have taken on the task of certifying manufacturers that are following good manufacturing practices and testing to see that what is on a label is in the bottle (Table 103-1). Guiding patients toward purchasing the best-quality herbal product is critical; high quality generally translates to better safety and efficacy.

TABLE 103-1. Information on Testing Dietary Supplement and Herbal Products

ORGANIZATION	WHAT TO LOOK FOR ON THE LABEL	WEB ADDRESS
The Natural Products Association (formerly the National Nutritional Foods Association) is a trade group that has a Good Manufacturing Practices (GMP) certification process and a Natural Seal certification process that tests for ingredient quality and contaminants.	NPA 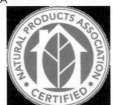	http://www.npainfo.org
NSF International is a nonprofit public health organization. NSF's certification service includes product testing, Good Manufacturing Practices (GMP) inspections, ongoing monitoring, and use of the NSF mark.	NSF 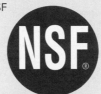	http://www.nsf.org
The United States Pharmacopeia (USP) tests for contamination, adulteration, and good manufacturing processes. The USP also examines products for pharmacologic properties.	USP 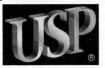	www.uspverified.org http://www.usp.org/USPVerified/ dietarySupplements/supplements. html
ConsumerLab evaluates commercially available dietary supplement products for composition, potency, purity, bioavailability, and consistency of products.	CL 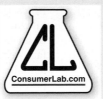	www.consumerlab.com
The U.S. government GRAS acronym stands for the phrase Generally Recognized as Safe. Under sections 201(s) and 409 of the Federal Food, Drug, and Cosmetic Act, any substance that is intentionally added to food is a food additive that is subject to premarket review and approval by U.S. Food and Drug Administration, unless the substance is generally recognized, among qualified experts, as having been adequately shown to be safe under the conditions of its intended use, or unless the use of the substance is otherwise excluded from the definition of a food additive.	GRAS	http://www.cfsan.fda.gov/~dms/ grasguid.html
Health Canada In Canada, dietary supplements are regulated by the government in a natural health products category ensuring the safety and efficacy of these products. This link includes all dietary supplements that are licensed for sale in Canada.		http://www.hc-sc.gc.ca

Dosing

Once the correct herb has been chosen for the correct patient's diagnosis, the clinician confronts confusing questions of dosing. Where is the dosing information on the label of the bottle? How much herb should the patient take and for how long? Is the dose different for a child?

Patients can prepare and use herbal medicines in many ways (Table 103-2). A traditional herbalist individualizes every treatment protocol on the basis of the patient's unique situation and often uses more than one herb or type of preparation. However, tailoring the herbal treatment to the patient can be difficult for the conventional provider in this age of uncertainty about the safety of all herbal products. Traditionally, most herbalists administered crude herbs in the form of teas, decoctions, tinctures, poultices, or compresses. These preparations are relatively inexpensive and easy to use. We encourage our patients to become involved with creating self-care routines (cooking with herbs, making a cup of tea, taking an herbal bath). Most commercial herbal products are sold in solid dosage forms, such as tablets and capsules, although teas, tinctures, and liquid extracts remain popular. Teas (water extracts) have a long history of use but are often limited by taste and rapid spoilage (they have to be made fresh). Hydroethanolic extracts, such as tinctures and fluid extracts, are more concentrated and easier to administer, although the alcohol content can be a problem for some patients.

Growing numbers of herbal preparations are now standardized to a specific constituent, or group of compounds, thus helping to ensure batch-to-batch consistency of the product. The standardizing compound may or may not be one of the "active" ingredients in the product. Most clinical trials are conducted on standardized products. A table from *The ABC Clinical Guide to Herbs* that lists commercial products used in clinical studies is adapted for this chapter (Table 103-3).[37]

The type of herbal preparation a clinician chooses to use depends on various considerations, including the patient, whether the medical problem is acute or chronic, personal preferences, and medicinal properties of the herb. For example, many people find valerian tea unpleasant tasting; recommending a tincture or capsule may improve the chance that the patient will adhere to therapy. Chamomile tea is quite appropriate for people of all ages. If using garlic for cardiovascular health, the patient could simply add garlic to the daily diet or choose a standardized extract.

For dose, the clinician can start by looking at the clinical trials—the product studied, the dose used, and side effects reported. Most herbal clinical trials have been conducted on standardized extracts in solid dosage forms (capsules and tablets). Excellent resources about correct dosages are also available on the Internet (Table 103-4). The clinician should nevertheless be aware that products in the marketplace vary widely in dose

TABLE 103-2. Preparation of Herbal Products

Balm or salve	A soothing, lipid-based topical preparation containing beeswax, vegetable, or mineral oil
Bath	An herbal preparation placed in a soaking bath; transdermal absorption extremely limited and mostly relevant to herbs with high volatile oil content. Herbal baths can be useful for skin irritation or enjoyed simply for their pleasant aroma.
Decoction	An extraction of the soluble compounds from hard plant material (e.g., bark or roots) in boiling water. Herbs are generally simmered for at least 10 min.
Essential oil	Volatile oils extracted from a plant, often through distillation. Essential oils are often many times more potent that the plant itself, which also means an increased risk of potentially adverse effects when used internally. Some popular essential oils include eucalyptus, peppermint, and tea tree oil.
Fluid extract	A hydroethanol solution with the strength of one part solvent to one part herb (more concentrated than a tincture; alcohol content can vary)
Glycerite	An herbal compound infused in a solution of glycerin (no alcohol)
Infusion	An extraction of soluble compounds from fresh or dried flowers, leaves, or seeds in hot water. Infusions are generally steeped for a minimum of 5–10 min (a tea).
Maceration	An herbal infusion made with cold or room temperature water
Pills, capsules, or tablets	May contain the whole herb (or particular plant part such as leaf, root, or seed) or the dried extract of a herb
Poultice	An herbal preparation wrapped in cloth and applied to the skin
Powders	An herbal preparation applied in a powder form (talc)
Syrup	Herbs infused in a syrup product
Tincture	A hydroethanolic solution of active plant constituents with a strength of greater than one part herb per one part solvent (alcoholic content can vary)
Tonic	A preparation used to invigorate and restore the body and generally taken on a daily basis (e.g., nettles)

TABLE 103-3. Commercial Products Used in Clinical Studies Listed in Single Herb Monographs

HERB	PRODUCTS USED IN CLINICAL STUDIES (MANUFACTURER)	OTHER NAMES (MANUFACTURER/DISTRIBUTOR)
Black Cohosh	Remifemin tablet (Schaper & Brümmer GmbH & Co. KG) CR BNO 1055, an aqueous/ethanolic extract Klimadynon/Menofen (Bionorica AG, Neumarket, Germany)	Remifemin (originally manufactured by Schaper & Brümmer; now manufactured and distributed by GlaxoSmithKline) Menofen (Vitamin Plus Company)
Echinacea	Echinacea Plus (Traditional Medicinals, Inc.) Echinacin (Madaus AG) Echinaforce (Bioforce AG)	Formerly imported by EchinaGuard (Nature's Way Products, Inc.); no longer in the United States Echinaforce (United States: Bioforce)
Garlic	Aged Garlic Extract (Wakunaga of America Co., Ltd.) Kwai forte 300 mg LI 111 (Lichtwer Pharma AG) KwaiN LI 111 (Lichtwer Pharma AG) Sapec (Lichtwer Pharma AG)	Aged Garlic Extract (extract used in Kyolic product line) Kwai HeartFit Garlic (United States: Abkit, Inc.) Kwai Garlic Supplement (United States: Abkit, Inc.)
Ginger	EV. Ext 77 (extract used in retail products) (Ferrosan A/S) Zintona (Herbalist & Doc)	FlexAgility (United States: Enzymatic Therapy) Zinaxin (Ferrosan A/S) Zincosamine (United States: FreeLife International LLC)
Ginkgo	Bio-Biloba (Pharma Nord ApS) EGb-761 (extract used in retail products) (Dr. Willmar Schwabe Pharmaceuticals) Geriaforce (Bioforce AG) LI-1370 (extract used in retail products) (Lichtwer Pharma AG)	Ginkgold (United States: Nature's Way Products, Inc.) Ginkoba (Pharmaton Natural Health Products) Tanakan (Beaufour-Ipsen) Tebonin (Dr. Willmar Schwabe Pharmaceuticals) Ginkai (United States: Abkit, Inc.) Ginkyo (Lichtwer Pharma AG) Kaveri (Lichtwer Pharma AG)
Ginseng, Asian	G115 (extract used in retail products) Gerimax Ginseng extract (Dansk Droge A/S) Pharmaton capsules (Pharmaton Natural Health Products)	Ginsana (Pharmaton Natural Health Products)
Saw Palmetto	IDS 89 (extract used in retail products) (Strathmann AG & Co.) Nutrilite Saw Palmetto with Nettle Root (Nutrilite) Permixon (Pierre Fabre Médicament) PRO 160/120 (Dr. Willmar Schwabe Pharmaceuticals) Prostagutt (Dr. Willmar Schwabe Pharmaceuticals) Prostaserene (Therabel Research)	Strogen 160-mg caps (Strathmann AG & Co.) Strogen forte (Strathmann AG & Co.) Strogen S (Strathmann AG & Co.) Strogen UN (Strathmann AG & Co.) WS 1473 (Dr. Willmar Schwabe Pharmaceuticals) Prostol (United States: Nature's Way Products, Inc.) SabalSelect (United States: Indena USA, Inc.)
St. John's Wort	Hyperiforce (Bioforce AG) Kira (Jarsin 300) (Lichtwer Pharma AG) Remotiv (Bayer Vital GmbH & Co.) WS 5572 (extract used in retail products) (Dr. Willmar Schwabe Pharmaceuticals)	Kira (United States: Abkit, Inc.) Ze 117 (extract used in retail products) Neuroplant (Dr. Willmar Schwabe Pharmaceuticals) Perika (United States: Nature's Way Products, Inc.)

Adapted with permission from the table "Commercial Products Used in Clinical Studies Listed in Single Herb Monographs." In: Blumenthal M, Hall T, Goldberg A, et al, eds. *The ABC Clinical Guide to Herbs*. Austin, TX: 2003:398-404. Copyright © American Botanical Council 2003. The 8 common herbs here were among 29 in the book, and the brands listed were used in the clinical studies that were reviewed in *The ABC Clinical Guide to Herbs*. Go to www.herbalgram.org for more information.

and may not accurately represent either what was historically used or the dose typically seen in clinical trials.

We recommend asking patients to bring to the office all their dietary supplement bottles, teas, tinctures, and so on. This can be a fruitful exercise in starting an open discussion, teaching the patient how to read supplement labels, and catching potential drug-herb interactions and adverse effects. Table 103-5 contains explanations of the elements of a label on a botanical product bottle.

Always document in the chart any dietary supplement or herbal product your patients are using.

TABLE 103-4. Evidence-Based Resources for Dietary Supplements

RESOURCE	DESCRIPTION	WEB SITE
Government Web Sites		
National Center for Complementary and Alternative Medicine (NCCAM)	The NCCAM provides helpful herbal summaries called Herbs at a Glance. CAM on PubMed is the product of a collaboration between the National Library of Medicine and the NCCAM to facilitate literature searches on various complementary and alternative medicine therapies, approaches, and systems. It contains citations, has links to full text, and allows searchers to limit retrievals by publication type. Look for the Alerts and Advisories, treatment information, resources, links to other organizations (e.g., Food and Drug Administration, Agency for Healthcare Research and Quality, Office of Dietary Supplements). (Free)	www.nccam.nih.gov http://nccam.nih.gov/research/camonpubmed/
MedlinePlus: Dietary Supplements	This consumer health database from the National Library of Medicine offers extensive information on dietary supplements. Links are organized using the same alternative medicine medical subject headings used by the National Library of Medicine. Some of the Natural Medicine Comprehensive Database abridged monographs are available under the dietary supplements link.	http://medlineplus.gov http://www.nlm.nih.gov/medlineplus/druginformation.html
Office of Dietary Supplements (ODS)	Under Health Information in this very helpful site are excellent dietary supplement fact sheets. (Free)	ods.od.nih.gov/index.aspx
Health Canada	The Canadian government regulates natural health products in Canada and licenses products with proof of safety and efficacy. This very helpful site lists products licensed in Canada and has useful monographs.	http://www.hc-sc.gc.ca
Additional Web Sites		
American Botanical Council	This nonprofit organization has helpful information and continuing medical education resources.	www.herbalgram.org
AltMedDex	Several hundred excellent monographs and patient information sheets on dietary supplements and medical conditions are updated semiannually. This site is a component of the larger Micromedex product, published by Thomson. A handheld version available. (Subscription required)	www.micromedex.com/products/altmeddex
Cochrane Collaboration Complementary Medicine	The Cochrane Library is an electronic resource produced by the Cochrane Collaboration to supply high-quality, comprehensive systematic reviews of research literature from throughout the world. (Subscription required)	http://www.compmed.umm.edu/cochrane_about.asp
Natural Medicines Comprehensive Database	This database was created by the publishers of the *Pharmacist's Letter.* You can search by dietary supplement or commercial product name. Monographs include extensive information about common uses, evidence of efficacy and safety, mechanisms, interactions, and dosage. It is extensively referenced and updated daily. In addition, continuing medical education, listserv, and interactions information are available. (Individual subscriber: $92/yr)	www.naturaldatabase.com
Natural Standard	This is an independent collaboration of international clinicians and researchers who created a database that can be searched by complementary and alternative medicine subject or by medical condition. The quality of evidence is graded for each supplement. A Palm version will soon be available. (Individual subscriber: $199.00/yr)	www.naturalstandard.com
Longwood Herbal Task Force	This site provides peer-reviewed monographs, clinician summaries, and patient information, as well as carefully evaluated links to other sites. (Free)	www.longwoodherbal.org
HerbMed	HerbMed is an herbal database that provides scientific data underlying the use of herbs for health. HerbMedPro, an enhanced version of HerbMed, is available for subscription, licensing, and data streaming. The public site has 20 herbs; HerbMedPro has an additional 233 herbs and continuous updating. (Individual subscriber: $45.00/yr or 48 hr for $9.95)	www.herbmed.org

TABLE 103-5. Interpreting Product Labels

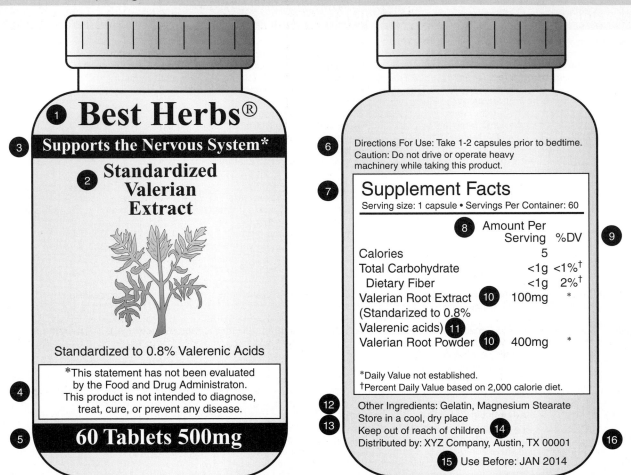

NUMBER	EXPLANATION
1.	Brand name
2.	Product/herb name
3.	Herbal products and other "dietary supplements" may make "statements of nutritional support," often referred to as "structure/function claims," as long as they are truthful and not misleading, are documentable by scientific data, do not claim to diagnose, cure, treat, or prevent any disease, and carry a disclaimer on the product label to this effect. The disclaimer must also note that FDA has not evaluated the claim. The product manufacturer must also notify the FDA of the structure/function claim within 30 days of bringing the product to market. According to current FDA regulations, examples of acceptable structure/function claims include "supports the immune system" and "supports a healthy heart," whereas claims such as "helps treat the common cold" and "helps prevent heart disease" are considered unacceptable because these are considered drug claims. Thus, "helps maintain urinary tract health" is acceptable, whereas "helps prevent urinary tract infections" is not.
4.	A structure/function claim requires this disclaimer when it appears on the label of a dietary supplement, as well as in any brochures or advertising. The disclaimer must be in bold type and in a box.
5.	Number of tablets, capsules, and net weight of each in package
6.	Directions for Use and Cautions
Items 7–10 are part of the "Supplement Facts Panel"	
7.*	"Serving Size" is the suggested number of tablets, capsules, softgels, tea bags, liquid extract, or tincture to take at one time.

TABLE 103-5. Interpreting Product Labels—cont'd

NUMBER	EXPLANATION
8.*	"Amount per Serving" first indicates the nutrients present in the herb and then specifies the quantity. The following items must be declared if in excess of what can legally be declared as zero: calories, fat, carbohydrates, sodium, and protein. In addition, the following nutrients must also be declared if present in quantities exceeding what can legally be declared as zero: vitamins A, C, D, E, K, B_1, B_2, B_3, B_6, B_{12}, folic acid, biotin, calcium, iron, phosphorus, iodine, magnesium, zinc, selenium, copper, manganese, chromium, molybdenum, chloride, and potassium. Most herbal products contain negligible amounts of these nutrients.
9.*	"Percent Daily Value" (%DV) indicates the percentage of daily intake provided by the herb. An asterisk under the "Percent Daily Value" heading indicates that a Daily Value is not established for that dietary ingredient.
10.*	Herbs should be designated by their standardized common names as listed in the book *Herbs of Commerce*, published in 1992 by the American Herbal Products Association. If the common name is not listed in *Herbs of Commerce*, then the common name must be followed by the herb's Latin name. The plant part must be listed for each herb. The amount in milligrams of each herb must be listed unless the herbs are grouped as a proprietary blend—then only the total amount of the blend need be listed. For herbal extracts, the following information must be disclosed: (1) the ratio of the weight of the starting material to the volume of the solvent (even for dried extracts in which the solvent has been removed, the solvent used to extract the herb must be listed), (2) whether the starting material is fresh or dry, and (3) the concentration of the botanical in the solvent.
11.	Standardization. If a product is chemically standardized, the product label may list the component used to measure standardization (e.g., ginsenosides in Asian ginseng, valerenic acids in valerian) and the level to which the product is standardized (e.g., 4% ginsenosides). Therefore, if a product contained 100 mg of Asian ginseng extract per capsule and the extract was standardized to 4% ginsenosides, one capsule would contain 4 mg of ginsenosides. In most, but not all, cases, the component used to measure standardization is bioactive, although the standardization component may not be responsible for the intended primary activity of the herbal supplement; other active compounds may be responsible. Products can also be standardized to "marker compounds" for purposes of quality control. Those markers may or may not be active.
12.	A list of all other ingredients, in decreasing order by weight, must appear outside the Supplement Facts box. In herb formulas containing multiple herbal ingredients, the herbs must be listed in descending order of predominance.
13.	The proper location for storage of herbal products is typically labeled as a cool, dry place.
14.	All herbal products and other dietary supplements should be kept out of the reach of children.
15.	The herb should be used before the expiration date for maximum potency and effectiveness. Expiration dates are often arbitrarily established by the manufacturer, regardless of the ingredients and their relative stability. Such dates are routinely set at 2 years from the date of manufacture of the finished dietary supplement, although this period may be longer or shorter, depending on the manufacturer's policies, stability testing, dosage form, and other variables.
16.	The product must list the manufacturer or distributor's name, city, state, and zip code.

*Data from the table "Interpreting Product Labels." In: Blumenthal M, Hall T, Goldberg A, et al, eds. *The ABC Clinical Guide to Herbs*. Austin, TX: American Botanical Council; 2003:xxiv. Copyright © American Botanical Council 2003. Go to www.herbalgram.org for more information on additional resources and continuing medical education for health care providers.
FDA, Food and Drug Administration.

Conclusion

In conclusion, the clinician should remember the following:[38]

- Ask all patients about botanicals and the supplements they use. (Offer examples of types of products meant in the question.)

- Record the responses in the patient's record so anyone consulting it can check for possible safety concerns such as herb-drug interactions.

- Advise patients about the safety and effectiveness of the products they are or are considering using.

- If unable to answer all the patient's questions about some botanicals, be prepared to refer the patient to evidence-based sources of information (see Table 103-4).

- Report a possible adverse effect to MedWatch, as previously discussed.

References

References are available online at expertconsult.com.

Detoxification

Luke Fortney, MD

What Is Detoxification and Why Do It?

Detoxification, as reviewed here, is the constellation of physiologic and psychological processes by which the body identifies, neutralizes, and eliminates toxic substances, metabolic byproducts, habits, and patterns. Alcohol and other narcotic withdrawal therapies are serious medical conditions requiring close supervision and are not discussed here.

For an increasing number of people living in a more polluted and stressful world, body systems can become overburdened and strained by various contaminants that may lead to health problems.[1] In general, these toxins can be identified within the following general categories[2]:

- *Antinutrients* such as high-fructose corn syrup, trans fats, caffeine, alcohol, and processed foods

- *Internal metabolic toxins* such as nitrogen, carbon dioxide, bile, urea, and stool

- *Medications* used improperly, inappropriately, or too often

- *Heavy metals* such as mercury, arsenic, lead, cadmium, tin, and aluminum

- *Chemicals* such as pesticides, herbicides, cleaning products, solvents, and glues

- *Allergens* such as food, mold, dust, pollen, and chemicals

- *Infectious organisms* such as bacteria, viruses, yeast, and parasites

Further, the following social, emotional, and spiritual challenges affect health and well-being[3,4]:

- *Stress,* such as lack of personal time, too much work, excessive worry, too little rest, and financial strain

- *Unhealthy mental states,* such as addictions, overeating, and destructive mental patterns

- *Ambient distractions,* such as pervasive noises, smells, lights, and images

- *Overstimulation* from advertisements, radio, computers, television, smart phones, and pagers

- *Lack of spiritual connection,* a loss of meaning and purpose

- *Isolation,* the lack of social support and community

- *Nature deprivation,* being disconnected from natural environments

- *Negative emotions* and persistent self-defeating thoughts, such as anger, fear, guilt, and hopelessness

Although too infrequently acknowledged, the body and mind already possess the capacity to handle these challenges. This process of maintaining biologic and mental balance is called homeostasis. The major systems that work together synchronously to maintain health and balance include the following:

- Liver and gallbladder (Figs. 104-1 to 104-3)

- Kidneys

- Gut

- Skin

- Lungs

- Lymphatics and circulation

- Mind and brain

Symptoms that may reflect an overtaxed or dysfunctional detoxification system are vague and nonspecific, but when seen in constellation they suggest a problem with the body's ability to restore itself. When potentially serious medical conditions have been ruled out by a reasonable allopathic workup, symptoms that may be attributed to a detoxification problem with the body often include the following[1,5,6]:

- Fatigue with sleep disruption and brain fog

- Mood disturbance, especially depression, anxiety, fear, and anger

FIGURE 104-1
Liver detoxification. OTCs, over-the-counter (drugs); vit., vitamin.

Endotoxins
 * end products of metabolism
 * bacterial endotoxins

Exotoxins
 * drugs (prescription, OTCs,
       recreational, etc.)
 * chemicals
      - agricultural
      - food additives
      - household
      - pollutants/contaminants
 * microbial

PHASE I
[cytochrome P-450 enzymes]

PHASE II
[conjugation pathw ays]

* **toxins**

(nonpolar ∴
  lipid-soluble)

Reactions
oxidation
reduction
hydrolysis
hydration
dehalogenation

**Enzymes, Cofactors
& Other Nutrients
Used**

riboflavin (vit. B_2)
niacin (vit. B_3)
pyridoxine (vit. B_6)
folic acid
vitamin B_{12}
glutathione
branched-chain
   amino acids
flavonoids
phospholipids

**intermediary
metabolites**

(more polar ∴
  more water-soluble)

**Reactive Oxygen
Intermediates**

sulfation
glucuronidation
glutathione conjugation *
acetylation
amino acid conjugation
   glycine
   taurine
   glutamine
   ornithine
   arginine
methylation

* N-acetylcysteine, cysteine,
methionine are precursors

**excretory
derivatives**

(polar ∴
  water-soluble)

Serum

Kidneys

Urine

Bile

Feces/stools

lipid-soluble (nonpolar)
toxins stored in adipose
(fat) tissue contribute to
increased/mobilized toxin
load with weight loss.

Superoxide

**Antioxidant/Protective
Nutrients/Plant
Derivatives**

carotenes (vit. A)
ascorbic acid (vit. C)
tocopherols (vit. E)
selenium
copper
zinc
manganese
coenzyme Q10
thiols (found in garlic, onions
            & cruciferous vegetables)
bioflavonoids
silymarin
pycnogenol

Free Radicals

**Secondary
tissue damage**

FIGURE 104-3
Phase 2 detoxification. CoA, coenzyme A; SAMe, S-adenosylmethionine. (From Bland JS, Costarella L, Levin B, et al. Environment and toxicity. In: *Clinical Nutrition: A Functional Approach.* Gig Harbor, WA: Institute for Functional Medicine; 1999:261.)

FIGURE 104-2
Phase 1 detoxification. P-450, cytochrome P-450.

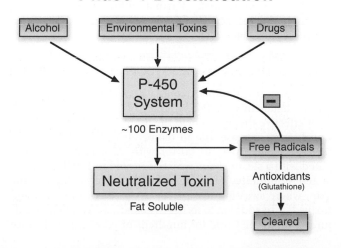

Phase 1 Detoxification

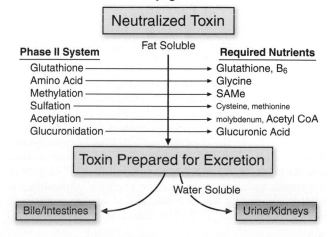

Phase 2 Detoxification
Conjugation

Phase II System		Required Nutrients
Glutathione		Glutathione, B_6
Amino Acid		Glycine
Methylation		SAMe
Sulfation		Cysteine, methionine
Acetylation		molybdenum, Acetyl CoA
Glucuronidation		Glucuronic Acid

Neutralized Toxin — Fat Soluble

Toxin Prepared for Excretion — Water Soluble

Bile/Intestines ← → Urine/Kidneys

- Muscle aches and joint pain
- Sinus congestion, dark circles under the eyes, and postnasal drip
- Headaches with neck and shoulder pain
- Bloating and gas
- Irritable bowel, foul-smelling stools, and dark urine
- Weight changes and loss of muscle tone
- Heartburn, recurrent colds, and persistent infections
- Infertility and low libido
- Premature aging and weakness
- Fluid retention and excess weight
- Rashes and canker sores
- Bad breath and adverse body odor

Although convincing scientific data supporting detoxification therapies are lacking, the question for a patient suffering from any of these symptoms remains this: "*What can I do to find relief?*" Unfortunately, many gimmicky, expensive, unnecessary, and potentially harmful products, programs, and practitioners exaggerate their detoxification claims. In general, patients should avoid dramatic and extreme approaches in favor of reasonable, safe, and health-promoting lifestyle changes that empower patients and avoid dependency and unrealistic expectations. The five basic components of any detoxification program should include the following:

- Exercise every day, such as yoga and walking (especially in natural environments)
- Regular sweating, through exercise, a sauna, a steam room, or a hot room yoga class
- Healthy nutrition, rich in organic fruits and vegetables and filtered water (see Figs. 104-1 to 104-3)
- Self-reflection, such as meditation and breathing-focused relaxation techniques
- Body work, such as massage and acupuncture

Testing for Toxins

Although testing the body for various chemicals has the appeal of suggesting certainty in naming alleged culprits to explain various symptoms, random testing for toxins remains largely unfounded with few exceptions, and evidence does not support regular or widespread use. The Centers for Disease Control and Prevention (CDC) conduct a biomonitoring program that tests random sample populations for environmental toxins, or body burden. Results continue to demonstrate the ubiquitous nature of toxic body burden across all demographic groups.[7-10] These findings indicate the widespread presence of societal chemicals and suggest that chemical body burden can be presumed for any presenting patient.[11-16] Given the expense, variable quality, questionable validity, and unknown significance of body burden, routine testing is not recommended at this time.[10,17,18] Moreover, the health significance of specific chemical exposures—at what levels, during which times, and at what frequency—is poorly understood.[19] Indiscriminate and unfounded causal

statements about exposure, harm, and treatment efficacy should be approached cautiously and skeptically. The focus should be on reducing the amount of toxicity we place in our living environments (see Chapter 105, Integrative Strategies for Planetary Health).

Chelation Therapy

Using safe and effective methods to prevent disease, treat symptoms, and achieve homeostasis is the primary goal of a good detoxification regimen. Appropriately, well-placed controversy and concern exists over many detoxification therapies, including chelation for the removal of various heavy metals from the body.[20] The safety of widespread chelation therapy remains in question. A study from the Emergency Department at Emory University in Atlanta found common adverse effects associated with intravenous chelation that included diaphoresis, hypotension, tachycardia, leukopenia, thrombocytopenia, electrocardiographic abnormalities, and increased serum creatinine.[21] The clinical significance of chelation therapy is also uncertain. A review by the Cochrane Database concluded that, at present, evidence of the effectiveness or ineffectiveness of chelation therapy in improving clinical outcomes of patients with atherosclerotic cardiovascular disease is insufficient.[22] However, the CDC did recommend that the calcium disodium edetate ($CaNa_2EDTA$) challenge test be considered for children who have blood lead levels of 1.21 to 2.12 mcmol/L (25 to 44 mcg/dL) to determine whether chelation is indicated.[23] Another option could include use of modified citrus pectin such as Pectasol, which may also have benefit in children whose test results are higher than acceptable levels for lead and other heavy metals.[24-28] The dose in one study was 5 g three times daily for 4 weeks.

> Unfortunately, pectin is a viscous fiber that is not absorbed into the bloodstream, and food sources (citrus, apples, legumes, cabbage) do not help chelate heavy metals. Modified citrus pectin is absorbed and does help reduce this burden.

In general, what can or should be done to address the ubiquitous nature of chemical body burden is uncertain. Caution and skepticism in the use of chelation therapy are therefore recommended. Further information regarding chelation therapy can be found online (see the Key Web Resources box, later).

Sauna Therapy

The body stores lipophilic toxins such as pesticides in adipose and subcutaneous fat. Taking a relaxing sauna or steam bath is an effective therapy to help the body detoxify.[29] The traditional sauna increases the air temperature to 160°F to 200°F (approximately 70°C to 90°C) with 25% humidity, compared with a steam room, which is heated to 120°F to 130°F at 100% humidity. The exogenous heat diverts blood to the skin, where sweating releases excess sodium, nitrogen, and toxins.[30-32] In addition to its use in Scandinavia and many cultures around the world for hundreds of years, research since the 1960s has demonstrated the health-promoting effects of regular sauna use including stress reduction, detoxification, lower blood pressure, and decreased pain.[33] Appropriate sauna use is safe for most people of all ages, although caution should be used in people who have undergone recent surgery, who have unstable cardiovascular conditions such as recent myocardial infarction or cerebrovascular accident, or who have multiple sclerosis, acute lung infections, or pregnancy complications.[34] Further, some evidence indicates that a lower-temperature infrared sauna may offer similar health benefits. Lower-temperature infrared saunas are typically heated to 120 °F and are a good option for those who cannot tolerate the higher temperatures of a traditional sauna or steam room. For further reading on the many health effects of sauna therapy, please refer to an excellent book entitled *The Holistic Handbook of Sauna Therapy*, by Nenah Sylver.[35]

Exercise

Reasonable and safe approaches to body burden detoxification include increasing awareness and adherence to healthy lifestyle behaviors such as regular exercise, healthy nutrition, stress reduction, mind-body practices, spiritual connection, and avoidance of harmful behaviors such as smoking. Exercise has been shown to enhance adipose tissue circulation and therefore increases the release of stored toxins.[36] Cardiovascular exercise also supports detoxification through sweating. Starting with gentle but regular forms of exercise, such as walking or bicycling for 30 or more minutes a day, is best. Ideally, a person should set a goal of 60 or more minutes of vigorous movement of any kind on a daily basis. Hot room yoga is particularly beneficial for detoxification, but any and all forms of movement are encouraged.

Nutrition

Nutrition is arguably the first and most important step in promoting health and supporting the body's efforts to remove harmful substances. What a person avoids eating is equally important as what is included in a healthy diet. By avoiding artificial additives and unhealthy fats, reducing excess calories (including less salt, saturated fat, and sugars), and adhering to a diverse whole food organic diet, a person will be better able to support the body's detoxification process, in large part by avoiding further environmental pollution[37-39] (see Chapter 86, The Antiinflammatory Diet).

Safe and Environmentally Friendly Fish and Seafood Choices

Consuming fish and seafood a few times per week has many benefits, but concerns also exist about contaminants that may affect our health and the environmental impact of fishing practices. Resources that you can use to help guide your choices in safe fish and environmentally sustainable seafood choices are provided in the Key Web Resources box.

TABLE 104-1. The Environmental Working Group's List of the "Dirty Dozen" (Foods Highest in Pesticides Used) and the "Clean 15" (Foods Lowest in Pesticides Used)

DIRTY DOZEN (BETTER TO BUY ORGANIC)	CLEAN 15 (LESS IMPORTANT TO BUY ORGANIC)
1. Celery	1. Onions
2. Peaches	2. Avocado
3. Strawberries	3. Sweet corn
4. Apples	4. Pineapple
5. Blueberries	5. Mangoes
6. Nectarines	6. Sweet peas
7. Bell peppers	7. Asparagus
8. Spinach	8. Kiwi
9. Cherries	9. Cabbage
10. Kale and collard greens	10. Eggplant
11. Potatoes	11. Cantaloupe
12. Grapes (imported)	12. Watermelon
	13. Grapefruit
	14. Sweet potato
	15. Honeydew melon

Data from the Environmental Working Group: http://www.ewg.org.

Pesticides in Produce

When deciding whether to invest in organic produce, it can be helpful to understand which conventional fruits and vegetables are highest and lowest in pesticide content. The Environmental Working Group puts out a guide that lists the "Dirty Dozen" (foods highest in pesticides used) and the "Clean 15" (foods lowest in pesticides used), as shown in Table 104-1 (see also the Key Web Resources box).

Fasting

Occasional and sensible fasting may be helpful as well. Several variations of fasting exist, some involving drinking only water or juices or other nonsolid foods. During fasting, the main source of energy used by the body comes from hydrolyzing fatty acids from triglycerides stored in adipose tissue.[40-43] Because many toxins are sequestered in fat, fasting may be helpful in releasing these toxins from the body. Initially, a person may feel worse during a fast because of the mobilization of toxins. Resting and drinking plenty of fluids are therefore helpful during a fast.

Manual Therapies

Manual therapies such as massage may be helpful in mobilizing and eliminating toxins from the body by stimulating the lymphatic system, among other possible benefits. Together with exercise and sauna therapy, massage can greatly enhance the ability of the lymphatic, cardiopulmonary, and hepatorenal circulatory systems to mobilize and eliminate toxins. For example, massage has been shown to reduce excessive fluid volume by 65% in patients with lymphedema.[44,45] Other forms of body work such as acupuncture may be helpful as well, in part by increasing the relaxation response, as well as treating Qi stagnation and myofascial restrictions.

Mind-Body Connection

Finally, any detoxification review or program that ignores the mind-body connection is remiss. Stress is arguably the most significant toxin confronting patients on a daily and long-term basis. As measures of happiness decline in the United States (Fig. 104-4), various mind-body syndromes such as fibromyalgia, migraine headache, chronic fatigue, irritable bowel, multiple chemical sensitivities, and others continue to affect more people.[46,47] Unfortunately, support and awareness are lacking for mind-body interventions that cultivate understanding, behavior changes, insight, and accountability for patients and health care workers.[48] Various chapters in this text offer helpful tools to support a healthy mind and heart.

FIGURE 104-4
U.S. Department of Commerce, Bureau of the Census.

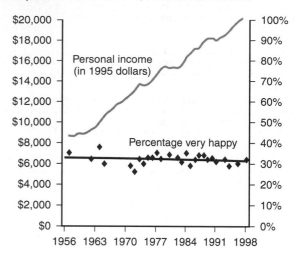

THERAPEUTIC REVIEW

See the Patient Handout at the end of this chapter.[49]

KEY WEB RESOURCES

University of Wisconsin Department of Family Medicine: www.fammed.wisc.edu/integrative/modules	This Web site provides a regularly updated, self-guided 7-day detoxification plan.
Environmental Working Group: www.ewg.org; http://www.ewg.org/safefishlist	This group offers excellent resources regarding information on harmful toxins in the environment with recommendations on how to avoid them, including information on toxins in fish and pesticides in produce.
Environmental Defense Fund seafood selector: http://www.edf.org/page.cfm?tagID=1521	This organization offers ratings of the best (least contamination) and worst (most contamination) for seafood consumption, as well as a pocket guide for selecting seafood.
Centers for Disease Control chemical exposure report: http://www.cdc.gov/exposurereport/	This national report details the health effects of human exposure to environmental chemicals.
Doctor's Data, Inc.: www.doctorsdata.com	This laboratory offers toxicology testing, as well as drinking water analysis. It also contains information on chelation therapy.
Bioneers: www.bioneers.org	This organization offers advice on sustainable living that supports nature's resources.
National Center for Complementary and Alternative Medicine: www.nccam.nih.gov	This National Institutes of Health Web site provides information on many topics, including chelation therapy.

Acknowledgments

I would like to thank Rian Podein, Mario Salguero, and David Rakel for their contributions to this chapter.

References

References are available online at expertconsult.com.

Patient Handout: Seven Day Detoxification Program Patient Handout

Many detox approaches are available, and very little evidence suggests that one is superior to the next. However, a 7-day commitment to healthy activities can relieve many symptoms by helping the body find balance. Most importantly, be creative and adapt to your needs. The following plan (found online at www.fammed.wisc.edu/integrative/modules) offers general guidelines for self-guided detoxification.

Getting Started

- This regimen is not intended to be an exhaustive resource, nor is it a test of will and endurance. It is designed to be a safe, easeful, useful, empowering, and accessible health guide taking into account personal variability and preference *with individual adaptations made as necessary.* However, *this process does require planning and preparation, so read through it and make preparations ahead of time.*
- In addition to physiologic approaches, this plan equally emphasizes mind-body approaches that can aid the relaxation response and unravel negative and unconscious mental patterns that often result in pain and discomfort.
- The most important part of going through a detox program is to first ask why you are doing it. Being clear about your intentions helps avoid inflated expectations and disappointment. Write down your reasons for going through a detoxifying program in language that is meaningful to you.
- The five basic ingredients of this detox regimen are self-reflection, exercise, sauna, nutrition, and manual therapy. The program offered here is designed to support and enhance your own ability to heal and experience well-being. It is intended for most people with few exceptions and is self-directed.
- The program has a strong emphasis on using organic, sustainable, local, responsible, gentle, natural, whole, balanced, and easeful products and methods that honor the global and spiritual aspect of health.

Precautions and Expectations

- **Healing crises** commonly occur during a detoxification regimen. Common and temporary symptoms of detoxification include feeling lousy, headache, lightheadedness, diarrhea, cramps, bloating, body aches, fatigue, mood changes, and weakness. These crises are caused by a combination of factors including the mobilization of toxins, low blood sugar, low fluids, electrolyte imbalance, withdrawal from various substances (such as alcohol, caffeine, sugar, nicotine), and even changes in your daily routine.
- Most often the best approach is to **continue with the detox**. However, you may need to stop or alter the detox if you experience ongoing distressing symptoms.
- **Dehydration** is common during a detox. Make sure that you drink a lot of fluids.
- **Address your particular needs** as you go along, such as more frequent snacks, larger meals, increase protein and healthy fats, less work, more rest, and less striving.
- In general, continued use of **prescribed daily medications** is recommended. If needed, use as needed medications sparingly for headaches or other problems you encounter.
- **Communicate with your health care provider**, therapist, or other healing practitioners about any concerns that arise during the detox as needed.

In the end, you will likely find that you feel better, have more energy, and may require less medication.

Below are three examples of 7-day detoxification programs. You can choose the one that best matches your needs and lifestyle. They progress from simple (#1) to more involved (#3).

Version #1 (short)
For 7 or more days:
- ☐ Eat only fruits and vegetables in any combination, amount, and preparation using healthy oils and spices as needed.
- ☐ Drink plenty of filtered water, juice, tea, and broth.
- ☐ Move and exercise the body in any variety, intensity, and duration.
- ☐ Keep a journal and practice any variety of self-reflection.

Version #2 (short)
- ☐ **Days 1 and 2:** Eliminate meat, eggs, dairy, wheat, alcohol, caffeine, chocolate, and sugar. Eat only organic vegan foods in any arrangement, preparation, and amount using cooking oils and seasonings.
- ☐ **Day 3:** In addition, eliminate grains, nuts, beans, and legumes. Eat only fruits and vegetables in any combination, amount, and preparation using oils and spices as needed.
- ☐ **Day 4:** Avoid eating any solid food. Drink plenty of water, broth, juice, and tea.
- ☐ **Day 5:** (same as Day 3)
- ☐ **Days 6 and 7:** (same as Days 1 and 2)

Version #3 (Long version. Supplements and bowel regimen are optional.)

Days 1 and 2

For the entire detox week, eliminate flesh foods/meat (e.g., fish, beef, pork, lamb, poultry), refined sugars (white/brown sugar and especially high-fructose corn syrup), and especially artificial sweeteners such as *saccharine, aspartame, and Splenda* (natural sweeteners such as honey, maple syrup, and molasses are okay to use in small amounts). Also avoid alcohol, tobacco, caffeine, cigarettes, chocolate, and recreational drugs for the entire week. It is advised to avoid dairy, wheat, and eggs during the detox week as well (instead try soy/almond/rice milk, soy cheese, soy yogurt, stanol/sterol spreads). Cooking preferences are guided by recipes that include soups, steaming, sautéing, etc.

Encouraged foods for days 1 and 2 include fresh/frozen/dried vegetables, fruit, and mushrooms (maitake, shiitake, oyster, and/or enoki, etc). Healthy grains are also recommended for days 1 and 2 (brown/wild rice, quinoa, buckwheat, oatmeal, millet, seeds, nuts, legumes, and flaxseed).

In addition, the following suggestions are encouraged:

- ☐ Use cold-pressed organic extra virgin olive oil as guided by your recipes and meals.
- ☐ Use spices and healthy seasonings as guided by your recipes.
- ☐ Drink 8–10 glasses of filtered water, including vitalizing beverage, detox broth, smoothies, and diluted juices.
- ☐ Drink tea throughout the day, such as peppermint, decaf green, chamomile, licorice, ginger, rooibos, and digestive tea.
- ☐ For snacks eat mixed nuts, dried and fresh fruit, vegetables, and detox broth (see Table 104-1).
- ☐ Consider using the optional herbs and supplements at recommended dosages.
- ☐ Consider 15–30 minutes of sauna or steam room therapy.

Continued

☐ Consider 30–60 minutes of light exercise such as walking, running, biking, skiing, jump rope, stretching, yoga, pilates.
☐ Practice any variety of self-reflection, including meditation and breathing exercises.
☐ Journaling is encouraged to reflect on the detox process.

Day 3
For day 3 also eliminate grains, nuts, seeds, legumes, beans, and mushrooms. *Eat only fruit and vegetables* fresh/frozen/dried in any combination and amount using healthy recipes. Just like days 1, 2, 6, and 7, the following items are suggested:

☐ Olive oil
☐ Spices and seasonings
☐ Filtered water, tea, vitalizing-beverage, detox broth, smoothies, and diluted juice
☐ Optional herbs and supplements at recommended dosages
☐ Sauna or steam room heat therapy
☐ Light exercise
☐ Journaling, self-reflection, or meditation

A new suggestion to add on day 3 is massage therapy to help mobilize toxins and stimulate the lymphatic circulation.

Day 4 (Modified Fasting)
Eliminate all solid food (i.e., using only water, tea, juices, and broth with modifications as needed). Most importantly, PAY ATTENTION TO THE NEEDS OF YOUR BODY! *Sensitive, ill, weak, and thin people should avoid or modify this day of fasting if needed, such as drinking more juice and broth as needed.*

Other suggestions include:

☐ Rest and relaxation; avoid exercise and sauna use today.
☐ Do minimal or no work today and avoid being overly active.
☐ **Stop all previous supplements for today.**
☐ Drink plenty of fluids and keep up with bowel and bladder fluid losses (tea with honey, vitalizing beverage, diluted fruit/vegetable juice, and detox broth).
☐ Use journaling, self-reflection, or meditation.

Optional bowel cleansing regimen (One at a time):

☐ Take 500–1000 mg of bentonite clay or activated charcoal capsules by mouth three times per day with water, **only for the day of fasting today** (*toxin binder for the gut*)
☐ Drink 300 mL of **magnesium citrate** (one bottle) in the morning for bowel elimination
☐ Use 1–2 saline **Fleet Enemas** in the afternoon or evening

Day 5 (Same as Day 3 except for Energy Work)
For day 5, add back *fruit and vegetables* in any combination, preparation, and amount using healthy recipes. Again, encouraged foods include fresh/frozen/dried vegetables and fruit (*but no mushrooms, grains, seeds, beans, legumes, or nuts*). Just like days 1–3, the following items are suggested:

☐ Olive oil
☐ Spices and seasonings
☐ Filtered water, tea, vitalizing-beverage, detox broth, smoothies, and diluted juice
☐ Optional herbs and supplements restarted at recommended dosages
☐ Sauna or steam room heat therapy
☐ Light exercise
☐ Journaling, and self-reflection, or meditation

A new suggestion to add on day 5 is an **energy work session** *such as acupuncture or Reiki to help balance your system.*

Days 6 and 7 (Same as Days 1 and 2)
In addition to fruits and vegetables, **add back** mushrooms, beans, legumes, seeds, nuts, and healthy grains. The following suggestions continue to be encouraged:

☐ Olive oil
☐ Spices and seasonings
☐ Filtered water, tea, vitalizing-beverage, detox broth, smoothies, and diluted juice
☐ Optional herbs and supplements at recommended dosages
☐ Sauna or steam room heat therapy
☐ Light exercise
☐ Journaling, self-reflection, or meditation

Detox broth recipe
Use fresh organic ingredients if possible. This is an excellent aid for fasting on Day 4. Ingredients can be varied according to taste and availability.

☐ 1 large soup pot or kettle
☐ 1 strainer
☐ 1 large bowl or container for straining the soup
☐ 3–4 quarts of filtered water (fill pot after all ingredients are in)
☐ 1 large chopped onion (white or yellow)
☐ 3–5 small bunches of various chopped greens (kale, parsley, cilantro, chard, or dandelion)
☐ 2 stalks of sliced celery
☐ 1 cup of fresh or dried seaweed (nori, dulse, wakame, kelp, or kombu)
☐ 1/2 small-medium head of chopped cabbage (any variety)
☐ 2 peeled carrots
☐ 2 stalks of peeled burdock root
☐ 1 large peeled daikon root
☐ 1 cup of squash (any variety) chopped into cubes
☐ 3 chopped root vegetables (turnip, parsnip, or rutabaga)

☐ 2–3 cups fresh/dried mushrooms (maitake, shiitake, oyster, or enoki)

Add all ingredients to the large pot at once and bring to a low boil for 40–60 minutes (add water to fill). Strain the stock to remove the solid material (keep the liquid broth and dispose the left over solid parts). Salt to taste. Store in the original soup pot or a tightly sealed container for use all week. Keep the remaining broth cooled in the refrigerator, and reheat for use. Enjoy as a sipping broth throughout the detox week, especially during the day of fasting on day 4.
Recipe Courtesy of Mark Hyman, MD

Smoothie recipe with supplements
Use organic ingredients when possible. This makes about 1 liter which is divided into 4 servings, or 2 days worth, a glass in the AM and PM.

☐ About 2 tablespoons (20 mL) of organic cold pressed extra virgin olive oil
☐ 1/2 avocado
☐ *About 4 tablespoons (20 g) of* **whey protein powder** *(optional)*
☐ *About 4 tablespoons (20 g) of* **modified citrus pectin** *(Pectasol, optional)*
☐ 1/2 cup of orange juice (or 100% organic juice of choice)
☐ 1/2 cup of vanilla flavored soy milk, rice milk, or almond milk
☐ About 4 tablespoons (40 g) of flaxseed (or psyllium)
☐ 8–10 ice cubes (or 1/2 cup of filtered water)
☐ 1 organic banana (sliced)
☐ 1 organic apple or pear with peel (sliced)
☐ 1/2 cup organic frozen or fresh blueberries (and/or seasonal berries of choice)

Place ingredients in a blender and grind up until smooth, adding more water as needed. Store remaining mix in the refrigerator. *Be creative; this can be varied according to taste and availability of various fruit.* Enjoy 1 tall glass twice a day with or between meals.

Digestive tea recipe
☐ 1/2 teaspoon (t) of whole fennel seeds
☐ 1/2 t of whole coriander seeds
☐ 1/2 t of whole cumin seeds

Add seeds to about one quart boiling water. Let the seeds steep for about 10 minutes. Enjoy after meals throughout the detox week. Other recommended teas include ginger, licorice, peppermint, chamomile, rooibos, and decaf green teas.
Recipe Courtesy of Kris Helgeson, FNP

Vitalizing beverage
This is an excellent aid for fasting on day 4.

☐ 1–2 tablespoons fresh lemon and/or lime juice (about 1/2 crushed or squeezed lemon/lime)
☐ 1–2 tablespoons of real maple syrup
☐ 1/10 teaspoon cayenne pepper (a small pinch)
☐ Purified, spring, or mineral water (carbonated water can also be used)

In a tall glass combine the juice, syrup, and cayenne. Fill the glass with water and stir well. Add crushed ice as desired. Enjoy throughout the detox, especially during fasting on day 4. Diluted fruit juice of any variety (1/2 real juice and 1/2 water) is also recommended.
Recipe Courtesy of Paramahansa Yogananda (adapted)

- *Hydrolyzed whey protein powder* 10 g powder two times per day mixed in smoothies or juice. Whey protein contains bonded cysteine that increases glutathione, a potent antioxidant, immune modulator, and detoxifier.
- *Pectasol powder (modified citrus pectin-MCP,* **NOT pectin fiber**) 10 g powder two times per day mixed in smoothies. MCP is absorbed in the gut and chelates heavy metals in the body that flow to the kidneys and liver where they are eliminated. It is easier to find online.
- *Milk thistle crude extract capsules* about 500–1000 mg three times per day with meals. This is a safe and beneficial herb used for 7 days for liver support.
- *Dandelion root capsules,* about 500–1000 mg three times per day with meals. This is a safe and beneficial herb for kidney and gallbladder support. It may increase urination.
- *Multivitamin tablet,* one daily with a meal.
- *Turmeric capsules,* about 500–1000 mg three times per day with meals. This is a safe and beneficial herb used for 7 days for inflammation and gut support.
- *Probiotics (Includes both lactobacillus and bifidobacteria),* one capsule three times per day. This is a safe and beneficial supplement used for 7 days to colonize the gut with healthy supportive bacteria.
- *Fish Oil omega-3 essential fatty acids,* 1000 mg total of EPA and DHA daily in liquid or capsule form. Vegetarian options include 2 tablespoons (T) daily of ground flaxseed or flax oil mixed in with smoothies. This supplement is used to reduce inflammation in the body.
- *Extra virgin, cold-pressed, organic olive oil,* 2 tablespoons in smoothies twice a day (and used in any amount in food for cooking). This healthy oil is rich in essential fatty acids.

DAY OF FASTING ONLY: *Activated charcoal or bentonite clay capsules, about* 500–1000 mg three times per day to bind gut toxins, but only taken during fasting. Always take about 1 hour *before* or *after* anything else by mouth.

From University of Wisconsin Integrative Medicine. *Detoxification Handouts.* www.fammed.wisc.edu/integrative/modules.

Integrative Strategies for Planetary Health

Nancy L. Sudak, MD, and James Harvie, PEng

Awareness of the ecologic impact of modern human activities necessitates urgent action on the part of governmental officials, public interest groups, and individuals. Integrative holistic practitioners intuitively understand that partitioning body from mind and spirit is unnatural; the separation of human health from the health of communities and the planet is similarly shortsighted. Holistic integrative practitioners, who are uniquely oriented toward an expansive worldview, are ideal educators for patients and colleagues about the steps that can be taken to mitigate ecologic health impacts and advocate for policies and practices that promote resilience at individual, community, and planetary levels. Understanding some general concepts is helpful, but extensive scientific knowledge is not required to implement ecologic preventive health strategies. Once individuals become aware of the enormity of environmental degradation, they may feel a call to action to protect humans and the planet from further harm (see Chapter 113, Creating a Greener Clinic: The Impact of Global Warming on Health).

This chapter provides a practical overview of some of the major issues eroding global ecologic services and of preventive strategies through a lens of climate change, the food system, and toxic chemicals.

Although acute toxicity is problematic, this chapter focuses on the long term. The chapter does not address the myriad established environmentally related occupational exposures, and it assumes an everyday workplace that is not dissimilar from our homes with respect to use of products, technologies, and consumption of foods and water. The important social health impact of our current materials economy is similarly beyond the scope of this chapter.

A Systems Approach

Human populations are tied to ecologic functions, and from a wellness perspective, differentiating between human and environmental effects is not useful. What food we grow, and how we grow it, has consequences with respect to nutrition, greenhouse gas emissions, water and air quality, and socioeconomic health.[1] Similarly, the toxic persistent cycle demonstrates the potential for distant releases to cause local exposures and the role of prevention at the local level in promoting global restoration. Figure 105-1 helps illustrate that when we pour something undesired down the drain, our action has multiple unseen effects, and although a burden may have been relieved on the home front, another burden occurs elsewhere. We must therefore understand that being healthy when living on an unhealthy planet is impossible.

The Precautionary Principle

An important concept that has evolved from the study of environmental health is the precautionary principle, a decision-making tool used if an activity raises the threat of harm, but cause and effect are not definite. The precautionary principle proposes that the burden of proof that an activity or product is *not* harmful should fall on the purveyors of a potentially harmful activity. This principle embodies the Hippocratic premise, "First do no harm," and is gaining widespread acceptance because it eliminates the barrier of uncertainty to allow for protective action. Rather than asking how much toxic damage is acceptable in a baby or an ecosystem, a precautionary approach asks how much exposure can be avoided.[2] For example, although we know that many industrial chemicals have adverse health effects and that our body burdens are noteworthy, we may not fully understand whether safe threshold limits exist or have the benefit of studies that demonstrate synergism among various chemical combinations. It is also reasonable to consider the biochemical diversity among detoxification mechanisms in human beings[3] and to acknowledge that what may be tolerated in one individual may have a devastating health impact on another. When consequences are not known with certainty,

FIGURE 105-1
Toxic persistent cycle. (From Western Lake Superior Sanitary District. *Safe Solutions to Toxic Problems: A Guide to Eliminating Persistent Toxic Substances from the Lake Superior Basin.* Duluth, MN: Western Lake Superior Sanitary District; 2007. <http://www.wlssd.com/Safe_Solutions_Toxic_Problems.pdf.pdf>.)

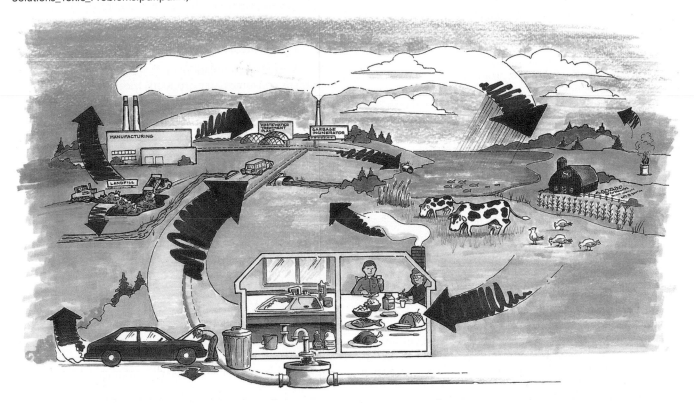

but are judged from available evidence to pose significant risk, avoidance is the most prudent course of action.

> The precautionary principle proposes that the burden of proof that an activity or product is *not* harmful should fall on the purveyors of a potentially harmful activity. When consequences are not known with certainty, but are judged from available evidence to pose significant risk, avoidance is the most prudent course of action.

The burden of scientific proof has become an obstruction to protecting health and the environment, because many people will be irreversibly sickened during the lengthy process required to prove that a substance is harmful. In fact, under current regulatory practice, proponents of harmful activities are served by investment in research that prolongs uncertainty. Many smokers died of lung cancer before cause and effect were definitively established between cigarette smoking and lung cancer. Application of the precautionary principle has become a critical component of environmental agreements throughout the world because it proactively combines scientific rigor from all current available evidence with the primary concern of protecting public health. When human health and environmental health are at stake, protective action is the most ethical course of action, even when it precedes scientific certainty. The challenge is that application of the precautionary approach is still limited in

scope. The following two examples demonstrate the importance of these considerations:

Nanotechnology

Nanomaterials are engineered particles made to have extremely small dimensions to take advantage of unique physical and chemical properties that exist at the nanoscale. As a result of their unique size, the physical and chemical properties of nanomaterials differ from their larger-scale particles and may act unpredictably and in ways that are currently not understood. For example, evidence indicates that nanomaterials can pass through skin and blood-brain barriers.[4] Scientific bodies have recommended that nanomaterials be treated and regulated as new chemicals[5] and that the precautionary principle be applied.[6] Nonetheless, hundreds of consumer products and food additives already on the marketplace contain nanomaterials. These products are typically undisclosed and untested for their impacts on human and environmental health.

Genetically Engineered Foods

Genetically engineered (GE) foods were first introduced to the marketplace in 1994, when producers in the United States brought out the Flavr Savr tomato. In 1996, GE soy became the first GE crop to be widely grown. GE technologies incorporate genetic material into the food supply and result in foods that would not otherwise occur in nature. Up to 70% of packaged foods in U.S. supermarkets may contain ingredients from GE corn,[7] soy, canola,[8] or sugar.[9] In 2009, GE beets were introduced to the U.S. market. U.S. residents have therefore been consuming GE foods without benefit of adequate studies to ensure that these foods will have no adverse impacts on human or animal health or on the environment. Health concerns associated with GE foods include both potential human and ecologic impacts. These include allergies,[10] antibiotic resistance,[11-18] food toxicity,[19-23] threats to nontarget species by contamination,[24-27] and gene dispersal.[28-34] Moreover, GE crop use promotes the increased use and toxicity of pesticides.[35-38]

In 1992, the U.S. Food and Drug Administration declared that GM crops are generally regarded as safe (GRAS) and therefore do not require any safety evaluations or labeling of GMOs.[39] Problematically, technology stewardship agreements state that the purchase of genetically modified seeds from patent owners (such as Monsanto) for purposes of research is explicitly prohibited unless that research is approved by the technology proponents. Leading researchers released a statement concluding that "as a result of restricted access, no truly independent research can be legally conducted on many critical questions regarding the technology, its performance, its management implications,… and its interactions with insect biology."[40] We continue to face a paucity of studies specifically designed to assess the potential for health effects from GE foods or feed. In 2005, a Parliamentary Assembly of the Council of Europe noted the health and safety issues around GE crops and the lack of studies assessing these threats by stating that "the health risks to humans (allergies, nutritional effects, etc.) so far have hardly been examined… [and] there is as yet no reliable information concerning their medium- and long-term environmental effects."[41]

In 2011, the Parliamentary Assembly adopted a resolution[42] that highlights the contrast between the U.S. approach to GMOs, which assumes safety without research, to the European approach, which hinges on the precautionary principle. Moreover, the resolution recommended that member countries "take the necessary steps to label products containing GMOs or derived from animals fed with GMOs" and "that the European Union guarantee the right of its member states to decide whether or not to cultivate genetically modified plants and, if such cultivations exist, to establish GMO-free zones." In 2009, a leading U.S. Catholic health system introduced a policy aimed at preferentially purchasing GE-free foods.[43] By 2011 the American Academy of Environmental Medicine (AAEM),[44] the American Nurses Association, the Illinois Public Health Association,[44a] and the American Public Health Association[44b] endorsed resolutions calling, in part, for the labeling of GMO foods. Specifically, the AAEM stated, "with the precautionary principle in mind, because GM foods have not been properly tested for human consumption and because there is ample evidence of probable harm, the AAEM asks, in part, that physicians educate their patients, the medical community, and the public to avoid GM foods when possible and provide educational materials concerning GM foods and health risks."[44]

Concepts in Ecotoxicology

Persistence

- Persistence is the tendency of a substance to resist degradation.

Bioconcentration

- Persistent chemicals accumulate in an organism and at higher levels of the food chain.

- Substances dispersed into air or water reappear in higher concentrations in foods derived from animals that are long-lived (dairy products and meats) or high on the food chain (large predatory fish).

- Accelerated accumulation of toxic burden occurs when humans consume dairy products, meat, and fish.

- Bioconcentrated substances may readily pass from mother to fetus and nursing infant at vulnerable periods of development.

Transient Exposures

- Chemicals that are not persistent or bioaccumulative can also be a threat if they are encountered in sufficient concentrations, particularly during windows of vulnerability.

- Epigenetic programming is commonly disrupted by environmental exposures, particularly during sensitive windows of development.[45]

Endocrine Disruption

- Endocrine disruption occurs when a substance acts as a hormone agonist or antagonist and thereby interferes with the body's normal hormonal functions.

- Malformed reproductive organs, endometriosis, and cancer are examples of associated conditions.

- A few known human endocrine disruptors include diethylstilbestrol (DES), dioxin, polychlorinated biphenyls (PCBs), dichlorodiphenyl trichloroethane (DDT) and other pesticides, bisphenol A (BPA), and phthalates.

- Unlike some chemicals, these disruptors have no threshold of toxicity, and their effects do not correlate linearly with magnitude of exposure; thus, miniscule exposures can result in dramatic modulation of function.

- A newly recognized class of compounds called obesogens interferes with the body's adipose tissue biology, endocrine hormone systems, or central hypothalamic-pituitary-adrenal axis. Obesogens are suspects in derailing the homeostatic mechanisms important to weight control.[46]

Effects of Chemical Mixtures

- No animal or individual experiences one toxin at a time, but toxicity studies are conducted individually.

- Although chemical mixtures represent a huge unknown area in toxicology, chemicals interact with one another to produce effects that may be inhibitory, additive, or synergistic.

Body Burden

- The body burden is the total amount of toxic chemicals, both naturally occurring and human made, carried in the body at a given point in time.

- This term may refer to single or multiple chemicals.

Highest Risk in Children[47]

- Children have higher consumption of air, food, and water per body weight.

- Their breathing zones are closer to the ground, where toxic residues settle in dust.

- Children have higher gastrointestinal absorption of heavy metals and other toxicants.

- They have immature glomerular and hepatic function.

Pressing Ecologic Problems in Today's World: Three Examples

Exploring ecologic health can feel daunting when we begin to comprehend the profound impact of modern life on the planet and its inhabitants. Remaining ignorant with respect to ecologic issues or adopting a mindset that an individual has little power to influence the solution is not uncommon. Patients have questions about these issues and look for answers and understanding about how to process these concerns, become empowered, and feel hopeful. However, until health care practitioners engage populations, we will continue to harm ourselves and all life on Earth. The following three issues are critically important to understand as we engage with our patients and the broader community.

Chemical Exposures and Associated Policies

Since 2000, studies conducted by the U.S. Centers for Disease Control and Prevention (CDC)[48] have begun to document the scale of our toxic body burden, as measured in human blood and urine. Many toxic chemicals have also been identified in umbilical cord blood, thereby demonstrating in utero exposure. Substances for use outside of the food and drug industries may be introduced into the marketplace without assessment for toxicity. Thus, the burden of harm is on consumers, rather than on product purveyors. Of the more than 80,000 chemicals in use today, approximately 5000 are used pervasively.

At the heart of many of the issues associated with toxic chemicals is the Toxic Substances Control Act of 1976 (TSCA), which was created with the intent to identify and regulate dangerous chemicals. A 2009 report by the U.S. Government Accountability Office (GAO) included the TSCA on its "High Risk" areas of government needing immediate reform. The GAO concluded that the Environmental Protection Agency (EPA) "does not have sufficient chemical assessment information to determine whether it should establish controls to limit public exposure to many chemicals that may pose substantial health risks."[49]

Food and Water Concerns

Since the early twentieth century, we have radically altered the way we produce and distribute food. The industrialization of our food system is fundamentally affecting the health of individuals and the planet. Not only are the foods we promote misaligned with dietary guidelines, but also methods of production and distribution divorced from natural ecologic processes are helping promote increased antibiotic-resistant bacteria, poisoned air and water, foodborne pathogens, and collapsing rural communities. Because poor nutrition is a risk factor for four of the six leading causes of death in the United States (i.e., heart disease, stroke, diabetes, and cancer), the public health, medical, nursing, and hospital communities have recognized the need to address the food system by promoting nutritious foods from sustainable food systems[50-53] (Boxes 105-1 and 105-2).

Like food, water is essential for life and good health. A lack of water to meet daily needs is a reality today for one in three people around the world.[54] Although most of the U.S. population has access to fresh treated water, increasing concerns are associated with contaminated water[55-57] and with water scarcity resulting from drought or resource depletion as agriculture, industry, and households become increasingly affected by climate change. Adding to the complexity is the role of water privatization in which water companies are purchasing aquifers, water supplies, and watersheds that had previously been held in the common domain.

Climate Change

According to the Intergovernmental Panel on Climate Change, warming of the climate system is now unequivocal, and evidence from all continents and most oceans shows that many natural systems are being affected by regional climate changes, particularly temperature increases.[58] The direct and indirect impacts on human health are not inconsequential and include asthma, loss of life, the range of

---

BOX 105-1. Key Principles of Chemical Policy

Key Principles of a Health-Oriented Chemicals Policy
- Immediately initiate action on the worst chemicals. Persistent bioaccumulative toxins are uniquely hazardous.
- Require basic information for all chemicals. Manufacturers should be required to provide basic information on the health hazards associated with their chemicals, how they are used, and the ways that the public or workers could be exposed.
- Protect the most vulnerable.
- Hold industry responsible for demonstrating chemical safety.
- Promote safer alternatives.
- Ensure the right to know.

Adapted from the Safer Chemicals, Healthy Families Coalition: <www.saferchemicals.org>.

BOX 105-2. Sustainable or Healthy Food System Characteristics

- Proximate (obtained close to home)
- Healthy, as part of a balanced diet
- Fairly traded
- Nonexploitive
- Environmentally beneficial
- Accessible and affordable
- Meeting animal welfare standards
- Socially inclusive
- Encouraging knowledge of food and food culture

infectious disease vectors, respiratory diseases, allergies, and childhood development problems.[59,60] In 2003, more than 35,000 people died in Europe as a result of heat stress. Clearly, the health care system will be required to carry a significant burden in treating climate-related health care costs. Approximately 30% of global emissions leading to climate change are attributable to agricultural activities, including land use changes such as deforestation.[61,62]

We must recognize that health care itself has a sizable greenhouse gas footprint. The National Health System (NHS) of the United Kingdom is a global health care climate mitigation leader through its comprehensive assessment of its climate footprint and the development of a climate mitigation and adaptation strategy.[63] The 2004 NHS greenhouse gas footprint was calculated as representing 3% of the total U.K. greenhouse gas footprint. In a similar, albeit less comprehensive, analysis, investigators estimated that U.S. health care greenhouse gas emissions in 2007 represented 8% of total U.S. emmissons.[64] Consistent with the U.K. calculations, prescription drugs represented a significant contribution to the U.S. health care footprint: 14% of total health care greenhouse gas emissions.

Because pharmaceutical interventions are used extensively for nutrition-related diseases such as stroke, heart disease, and diabetes, and given that our food system is a significant climate emissions contributor, we suggest that a dietary-focused primary prevention strategy would have health and climate benefits (see Chapter 113, Creating a Greener Clinic: The Impact of Global Warming on Health). Research indicates that we must increase the resilience of our social and ecologic systems considerably to cope with future climate change and other components of global change.[65]

Personal and Planetary Health in Everyday Life

Aside from specific occupations and their own unique set of environmental exposures, relative commonality exists in the nature of the foods we eat, the water we drink, and the products we use on our bodies and in our homes. Moreover, because white collar employment now comprises approximately 50% of the workplace, from an environmental health perspective, our workplaces may be almost indistinguishable from our homes.

Household Products

Many people are unaware of the magnitude of toxic exposure they receive through ordinary household products. Nearly every type of common household cleaner, deodorizer, drain clog substance, and laundry product has been identified as having some toxic properties.[66] Health effects associated with indoor cleaners include cancer, reproductive disorders, and respiratory or skin damage. Cleaning chemicals eventually enter the environment and may have deleterious effects, such as depletion of the ozone layer, diminution of drinking water quality, and accumulation in aquatic life. Some of the less safe chemicals are persistent and remain in the environment for many years or even indefinitely. Many cleaning chemicals are considered hazardous materials owing to their flammability, corrosivity, or toxicity, and they present safety and cost concerns in their handling, storage, and disposal.[67]

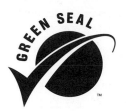

FIGURE 105-2
Green Seal Standard logo. (Courtesy of Green Seal, Inc., Washington, D.C.)

Almost all home cleaning products can be effectively replaced by common household ingredients. Recipes for specific uses are abundant on the Internet and are available in most public libraries. Typical suggested alternative ingredients are vinegar, baking soda, corn starch, salt, borax (toxic if ingested), lemon juice, olive oil, essential oils, mild liquid nondetergent soaps, reusable nonimpregnated steel wool, and nonchorine, non–sodium hypochlorite scouring powder. For people less interested in making their own products, many "green" cleaning products are available in the marketplace.[68] Environmentally preferable products (EPPs) have been designated by the Green Seal Standard for Industrial and Institutional Cleaners (GS-37)[69] (Fig. 105-2). Patients should be informed that the safety of a product is not guaranteed even when products are found on the shelves of their trusted stores. Learning to avoid toxic substances does require concern, the ability to read labels, and some scientific literacy. Physicians can help patients by compiling recipes for effective nontoxic cleaning solutions or lists of preferred commercial home cleaners. Hosting demonstrations and lectures in the clinic or hospital setting also sends an important message of public health to patients.

Because of the toxic persistent cycle, discarding toxic household products can be complicated. As a rule, these substances should not be poured down the drain, flushed down the toilet, or thrown in the trash. Because many common household products are considered hazardous waste, local environmental agencies, university extension services, or public works departments should be contacted for instructions on proper disposal. Some waste facilities have specialized departments that accept and properly manage toxic substances.

Personal Care Products

Most consumers would be surprised to learn that the government does not require health studies or premarket testing for cosmetics and other personal care products. Personal care products include soaps, hair dyes, body lotions, perfumes, cosmetics, and other similar products. Teenage girls use an average of 17 personal care products per day (compared with adult women, who use an average of 12 products per day).[70]

Serious health effects associated with personal care products include carcinogenicity and reproductive or developmental toxicity. Manufacturers are currently reformulating products in Europe to comply with an amendment to the European Union's Cosmetics Directive to ban the use of chemicals that are known or strongly suspected of causing cancer, mutation, or birth defects, but this effort was voluntary within the United States as of 2011. Patients should be counseled to reduce their use of personal care products and to avoid products with heavy fragrance, aerosols, and dark hair dyes (which may contain lead acetate).

Use of milder soaps and avoidance of nail polish, hairspray, and other phthalate-containing substances (known endocrine disruptors) should be encouraged. Despite the apparent confidence they engender in consumers, commonly used antibacterial soaps are harmful to our ecologic system, and they provide no added protection to household consumers. Triclosan is a bactericide used in a growing number of consumer products, including antibacterial soaps, toothpaste, shampoos, lotions, and deodorants. Even at low levels, it is acutely toxic to some aquatic organisms, particularly certain algae species, and it has been detected in surface waters.[12,71,72] Triclosan and tricarban are good examples of avoidable toxic substances with pervasive impacts and little to no consumer benefit. Triclosan is problematic for its persistence, its activity as an endocrine disruptor, and its potential to promote antibiotic-resistant organisms. As a protective measure to the people and aquatic species exposed, an informed consumer may simply learn to avoid the purchase and use of antibacterial (or antimicrobial) personal care products such as soaps, gels, cleansers, toothpaste, cosmetics, or other "antibacterial" or "antimicrobial" items such as cutting boards, towels, shoes, clothing, and bedding.

Cellular and Cordless Phones

In 1900, our experience of electromagnetic radiation was limited to natural sources. Since 1950, however, we have become increasingly reliant on electric technologies involving various electromagnetic frequencies. Accordingly, concern about health hazards (most notably cancer) has escalated. Conflicting results have emerged with respect to health risks and electromagnetic radiation exposure through microwaves, computers, and televisions. However, a study released in April 2007 revealed an increased risk of ipsilateral acoustic neuroma and high-grade glioma in long-term users (more than 10 years) of cell phones.[73] These same concerns have also been generated by cordless phones.[74] A large subsequent study was performed in 2010 by the Interphone Study Group and concluded that there is no increased risk of cancer in long term cell phone user. However, this study has been criticized for design flaws generated by selection bias, exposure bias, and age-range bias.[74a] In 2011 the World Health Organization (WHO) issued a press release stating that the International Agency for Research on Cancer and the WHO classified radiofrequency electromagnetic fields as possibly carcinogenic to humans, based on an increased risk for glioma associated with wireless phone use.[74b]

Based on the foregoing studies and the pervasive nature of cell phone and cordless phone use, the University of Pittsburgh (Pennsylvania) Cancer Institute issued practical recommendations regarding cell phone and cordless phone use,[75] including avoiding the use by children (whose brains absorb cell phone radiation more readily than those of adults), keeping the phone as far away from the body as possible, avoiding use when the signal is weak, purchasing phones with the lowest possible specific absorption rate (SAR), and other important suggestions.

Household Pesticides

The use of pesticides is widespread, and homeowners use substantially more per acre than does the agriculture sector. House dust typically contains 10 to 100 times the pesticide content of outdoor air. In the Nonoccupational Pesticide Exposure Study, a cross-section of homes was found to contain pesticide residues, including residues of substances banned years earlier.[76] The Ontario College of Family Physicians completed an extensive literature review of pesticides and determined that, "Exposure to all the commonly used pesticides … has shown positive associations with adverse health effects. The literature does not support the concept that some pesticides are safer than others; it simply points to different health effects with different latency periods for the different classes."[77] The College urged a focus on reducing exposure to all pesticides rather than targeting specific pesticides or classes. The investigators encouraged family doctors to learn about high-risk groups (women of childbearing age, occupationally exposed patients, children) and to teach methods of reducing pesticide exposures. Physicians are ideally suited to bringing these issues to the grounds of hospitals, schools, and government facilities and to suggest safer yet effective alternatives for landscaping and lawn care. Finally, the College suggested that physicians convey health concerns to politicians who make regulatory decisions about pesticide use and public health. As of 2010, every province and territory in Canada has pesticide-related legislation in place to protect its citizens from unnecessary exposure.

Various reduction strategies exist through application of integrated pest management (IPM), an approach to pest management that focuses on preventing and managing pest problems through nontoxic methods by using a hierarchy of strategies, with chemical controls as a last resort. Homeowners who use a pest control or lawn maintenance company should clearly communicate an IPM plan to the contractor. Many contractors now employ IPM, but homeowners are encouraged to request a thorough explanation of individual company IPM policies.

Furnishings

That furnishings of the typical U.S. home contain toxins is not intuitively obvious. However, substances such as wrinkle-resistant fabrics, permanent press sheets, curtains, and clothing, as well as modern furniture made from pressed composite wood, contain and emit formaldehyde and other substances. Carpeting is usually made of synthetic fibers that have been treated with pesticides, fungicides, and adhesives. Many office carpets emit a chemical called 4-phenylcyclohexene, an additive to the latex backing used in more commercial and home carpets, which is thought to be one of the chemicals responsible for "sick" office buildings.[78] Modern furniture also contains a significant amount of plastics and foam, which are highly flammable petroleum-based products requiring chemical flame retardants (polybrominated diphenyl ethers [PBDEs]). This is a topic of growing concern in environmental health. Perfluorinated compounds (PFCs), associated with fabric protectors and stain guards, constitute another type of persistent bioaccumulative toxin (PBT) of increasing concern. Vinyl (polyvinylchloride [PVC]) plastic coverings contain phthalates and release dioxin and furans during manufacture and breakdown.

Patients, let alone design professionals, may have trouble discerning the differences among various product components. As a general rule, products constructed from solid wood, metal, and natural fibers such as cotton and wool tend to be safe alternatives.

Meat, Poultry, and Seafood

Confined (or concentrated) Animal Feedlot Operations (CAFOs) epitomize the extreme of our industrialized food system. These operations confine large quantities of livestock to a closed area where all food and water inputs are carefully controlled. CAFOs are defined as more than 1000 beef cattle, 2500 hogs, or 100,000 broiler hens; they generate an estimated 575 billion pounds of manure annually.[79] The largest 2% of U.S. livestock farms now produces 40% of all animals in the United States.[80] In 2002, half of all hogs in the United States were raised on large-scale farms that managed more than 5000 hogs.[81] Ten companies produce 92% of the nation's poultry.[82] Although not exclusive to CAFOs, many different feed additives are provided, including growth hormones, antibiotics in feed and water, and arsenic. Public health and medical associations have called for a moratorium on CAFO construction because of concerns that include runoff, community impacts, air quality, worker health and safety, and issues of antibiotic resistance.[83-85] The Food and Agriculture Organization identified meat production alone as responsible for 18% of global greenhouse gas emissions.[86] The wide variety of public health and infectious disease has called attention to increasing concerns with antibiotic resistance.[87-91] The CDC noted that 90,000 patients died as a result of hospital-acquired infections, and more than 70% of the bacteria that cause hospital-acquired infections were resistant to at least one of the drugs most commonly used to treat them. Investigators estimated that more than 70% of all antibiotics consumed in the United States are used as feed additives for poultry, swine, and beef cattle for nontherapeutic purposes.[92] The strong consensus is that agricultural antibiotic use contributes to antibiotic resistance in humans, and more than 300 organizations, including the American Medical Association, have advised that restrictions on agricultural use of antibiotics are necessary.[93] Investigators have recommended that health professionals become aware of these trends as they promote healthier sustainable diets.[94]

Although fish is a good source of protein and omega-3 fatty acids, some species should be avoided because of PBT content. Mercury is the PBT most commonly associated with fish contamination; others are PBDEs, dioxin, furans, and PCBs. Mercury is bound to the protein component and cannot be removed. Most other PBTs accumulate in fat, which should be removed. Most fish advisories are based on federal guidelines developed to protect the average 160-lb man; patients should be advised to recognize this fact. Many Web sites have developed "fish calculators" that allow users to determine "allowable" fish intake on the basis of individualized weight, age, and sex. Patients who catch and eat their own fish should be advised to become familiar with local fish consumption advisories, which are typically developed for specific inland lakes. Many fish stocks are in serious decline as a result of overfishing. In addition, evidence indicates that salmon produced from the aquaculture industry has higher levels of PCBs than does wild-caught fish.[95,96] Table 105-1 lists fish choices that are of concern with respect to both overfishing and contamination. Fish listed in boldface in the table are contaminated with mercury, dioxin, PCBs, or pesticides,[97] or they are high on the food chain.

Organic Food Considerations

Conscientious health care practitioners are well aware of the challenges involved in encouraging patients to consume healthy foods. Warning patients about food contaminants adds a layer of complexity to the discussion. However, the issue of contaminated food is particularly relevant during vulnerable periods of life and should not be overlooked. This information can be introduced in the clinic setting and followed up with handouts, community presentations, and resource lists for patients (see the Key Web Resources box). Practitioners need not feel the burden of expressing every pertinent aspect of this problem to the patient. They should enlist the expertise of community professionals.

Growing children consume far more food and water per body weight than adults, and their biologic detoxification mechanisms are not fully developed. As a result of these differences and the qualities of foods eaten in high amounts by typical children, a child experiences a substantial burden of pesticide exposure in the first decade.[98] Consequently, elimination of pesticide residues is a sensible precautionary strategy. Although families may have budgetary challenges that do not allow for a complete transition to an organic diet, avoidance of the most contaminated foods is a useful approach. Table 105-2 lists types of produce that have been found to

TABLE 105-1. Fish Choices of Environmental Concern*

- Caviar: wild paddlefish and sturgeon eggs
- Chilean sea bass/toothfish
- Cod: Atlantic
- **Grouper**
- Halibut: Atlantic
- **Marlin**
- Monkfish/goosefish
- **Orange roughy**
- **Rock cod/boccacio/Pacific rockfish**
- **Salmon: farmed or Atlantic**
- **Shark**
- Shrimp/prawns: imported
- Skate
- Snapper
- **Sturgeon: wild**
- **Swordfish**
- **Tilefish**
- Tuna: blue-fin

*__Bold type__ indicates contamination with mercury, dioxin, polychlorinated biphenyls, or pesticides.[98] These fish are high on the food chain.

TABLE 105-2. Foods With High Pesticide Content

- Apples
- Bell peppers
- Celery
- Cherries
- Imported grapes
- Nectarines
- Peaches
- Pears
- Potatoes
- Red raspberries
- Spinach
- Strawberries

be highest in tested pesticide residues and are best to avoid when substitutes are available.[99]

Drinking Water

According to the EPA, the United States has one of the safest water supplies in the world.[100] We are fortunate that public regulation of drinking water has provided a public health benefit, but this relativistic assessment does not address potential exposure to unregulated contaminants found in the drinking water supplies or the relative safety of existing standards. The EPA has drinking water regulations for more than 90 contaminants. The Safe Drinking Water Act (SDWA) set up a process for identification of new contaminants that may require regulation in the future.

The EPA must periodically release a Contaminant Candidate List (CCL).[101] The contaminants on the list are known or anticipated to occur in public water systems. However, they are currently unregulated by existing national primary drinking water regulations. The most current list, published in 2011, contains many different industrial chemicals such as perchlorate (used in the manufacture of rocket fuel) and toluene, as well as a long list of pesticides, and even the pharmaceutical hormone estrogen. The water supply for approximately 15% of the U.S. population derives from sources separate from public supplies, such as wells, cisterns, and springs.[102] These sources are unregulated and require the homeowner to test the water for safety.

Many patients interested in a precautionary approach install water filters or treatment systems. Numerous systems are commercially available. Ideal water filtration devices are certified to remove specified contaminants. NSF International, an independent standard-setting organization, certifies water treatment systems.[103] Water filtration is especially advisable for patients who have private wells in proximity to industrial sites, landfills, combined annual feedlot operations, contaminated soils, or agricultural areas.

Patients may be under the misguided impression that bottled water is purer than tap water. A 1999 report, however, found that some bottled water contained bacterial contaminants and that several brands contained synthetic organic chemicals or inorganic contaminants.[104] The report also noted that bottled water regulations have gaping holes, and both state and federal bottled water regulatory programs are severely underfunded. Bottled water costs up to 10,000 times more than tap water (notwithstanding the energy use and pollution costs associated with transport across the country). Bottled water produces up to 1.5 million tons of plastic waste per year. In 2006, the U.S. population consumed more than 30 billion bottles of water, of which more than 80% went to a landfill or were incinerated. According to the Ocean Conservancy Institute, more than 6% of marine debris consists of plastic bottles. Water is essential to human life and is an inherent right, but access to affordable safe and sustainable water is becoming increasingly difficult around the world. By supporting and promoting publicly owned water infrastructures, the health care community can provide the moral voice for the right to affordable, safe, and sustainable drinking water. Drinking water concerns represent a challenging issue that jeopardizes our planetary health.

Conclusion

Rachel Carson was one of the first scientists to raise an alarm about the unconditional belief in "better living through chemistry" and reminded us of humans' intimate relationship with the environment. Clearly, many modern chemicals provide humans with products that are extraordinarily effective and convenient. We are beginning to realize, however, that despite the short-term benefits, these products have a host of recognized long-term impacts that have been either purposely or inadvertently ignored. This lesson parallels what we have learned about our unfettered use of energy and the industrialization of our food system. We are reminded

---

BOX 105-3. Key Advocacy Strategies

Develop and Adopt an Ecologic Health Mission Statement and Plan
Work with your clinic or institution to develop or tailor an existing ecologic health mission statement and plan. Use the plan meaningfully to guide purchasing and other practices.

Model Behavior in Home and Practice
Adopt policies and practices within your clinic and institution consistent with your ecologic health mission. As products and services become obsolete, change to those that are more ecologically benign. Consider the Green Guide for Health Care (see Key Web Resources box).

Educate
Provide resources and information to patients and colleagues within clinic or institution as hard copies or on website.

Meet With Your Hospital CEO
Numerous hospitals and clinics are adopting ecologically sustainable practices and policies. One physician's voice is important support for new or existing "green" or environmental teams; many physicians' voices add potency to the message.

Meet With Elected Officials
Elected officials and their staff are interested in meeting with constituents to hear their views. A physician's voice brings considerable moral authority. Most visitors are paid lobbyists representing industry and corporations, not typically the voice of community and health. Call and make appointments, and if that is not possible, speak to senior staff. Elected officials are busy; stay on point to keep your message relevant and concise. Ask for their specific position and try to gain a commitment. Follow up with a letter, and keep the ball rolling.

Continued

BOX 105-3. Key Advocacy Strategies—cont'd

Offer Your Voice to a Community Organization
Most community-based organizations have limited resources and welcome occasional help. Offer to write an article for their newsletter, be a spokesperson at media events, or meet with them and an elected official.

Media
Although media are changing, sharing your views on issues with the public is important. We need more health advocates. Letters to the editor and opinion editorials are widely read and shared. Call your newspaper to learn about word length and other submission guidelines.

Host Community Events: Book Signing, Movie Viewing
Many ecologic health multimedia resources are available. Host a community movie viewing or book reading and help integrate an ecologic health message.

Grand Rounds
Grand rounds are an important way to bring the latest science to your colleagues.

that we are part of a system with intricate feedback loops, and as we interfere with these relationships, we may create unintended consequences. These relationships suggest the necessity for an important global shift in our consciousness from one that has been oriented toward an efficient, linear, Western scientific model to one with greater appreciation of an interconnected resilient systems model.

As integrative physicians, this thinking is not new. We have recognized the value of pharmaceutical interventions, but we have worked first to explore primary prevention interventions and naturally sustainable treatment options.

Reports by the United Nations Millennium Assessment, the Intergovernmental Panel on Climate Change, and global governmental scientific bodies add a layer of urgency to holistic thinking and provide clarity that human activities are affecting ecologic systems. Our action today is imperative and requires an approach that moves from a model of disease treatment to one of ecologic prevention (Box 105-3).

PREVENTION PRESCRIPTION

- Substitute nontoxic alternatives for chemical pesticides for home and garden.
- Choose organically grown, locally raised produce and animal products.
- Eat low on the food chain
- Select "green cleaners."
- Purchase bath and beauty products that are free of phthalates and other toxic compounds.
- Purchase furniture and building materials that are produced from simple components (wood, metal, cotton materials).
- Avoid polyvinylchloride (vinyl) products.
- Purchase "green" computers and home electronics with a priority for those that may be returned to the manufacturer for recycling at the end of the product's life.
- Avoid polytetrafluoroethylene (Teflon) and stain treatment products.
- Avoid plastic bottles made of polycarbonate number 7.
- Avoid antimicrobials.
- Prefer metal, ceramic, or glass containers, especially for hot and acidic foods.
- Conserve energy and consume less.

KEY WEB RESOURCES

Cell Risk (list of cell phones with the lowest and highest specific absorption rate or radiation): http://www.cellrisk.com/
HealthCare Without Harm: The Campaign for Environmentally Responsible HealthCare: www.noharm.org
Practice Greenhealth: www.practicegreenhealth.org
Green Guide for Health Care (offers tools for creating healthy, healing environments): www.gghc.org
Pesticide Action Network pesticide guide (What's on My Food): www.whatsonmyfood.org
Pesticide Action Network physician network: www.panna.org/healthnetwork
Safer Chemicals Safer Families: www.saferchemicals.org
Monterey Bay Aquarium Seafood Watch: www.montereybayaquarium.org/cr/seafoodwatch.aspx
Our Stolen Future (database with focus on endocrine disruption): www.ourstolenfuture.org
The Collaborative on Health and the Environment: www.healthandenvironment.org
Science and Environmental Health Network: www.sehn.org
Physicians for Social Responsibility: www.psr.org
Environmental Working Group: Skin Deep (a safety assessment of reports and ingredients in personal care products; includes searchable database): http://www.ewg.org/skindeep/
Campaign for Safe Cosmetics: www.safecosmetics.org
The Story of Stuff (includes videos on the negative effects of overconsumption): www.thestoryofstuff.com
Council of Canadians: Water: http://www.canadians.org/water/index.html

References

References are available online at expertconsult.com.

Section IV Biomechanical

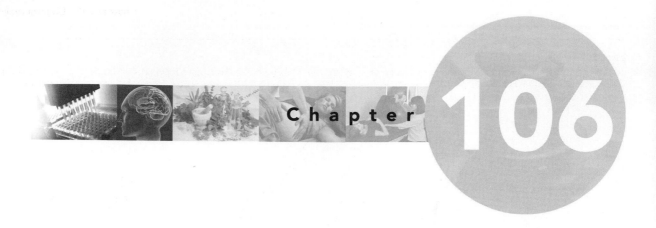

Chapter

106

Counterstrain

Harmon Myers, DO, and Julia Jernberg, MD

History and Theory of Counterstrain Therapy

In the 1950s, Lawrence Jones, an osteopathic physician in rural Oregon, discovered a novel, highly effective, low-risk form of manipulation that, 6 decades later, has become an internationally taught technique. In an attempt to ameliorate a farmer's severe back pain, Dr. Jones noted that the passive positioning of this index patient into a position of comfort and the holding of that position resulted in the complete resolution of the patient's back pain. Jones followed up this serendipitous discovery with the meticulous cataloging of hundreds of points that could be relieved by precisely positioning the patient.[1] The position needed to treat the patient's pain effectively could be determined by finding specific points of disease that Jones termed "tender points." Tender points were areas that, when palpated, caused the patient to experience discomfort at that site and that felt more taut to the examiner or were of a firmer consistency than the surrounding tissue. Jones believed that the cause—and subsequently the treatment—centered on the pathologic features of agonist and antagonist muscles of specific joints.

Jones (and subsequent theorists) ascribed the pathologic features of a tender point and the associated pain to the inappropriate and ceaseless firing of muscle proprioceptors and nociceptors that were, as a result, constantly "turned on" without any relaxation. Jones termed his treatment of the pain associated with these tender points, "strain-counterstrain" because he hypothesized that a rapid attempt to return a strained agonist muscle back to its neutral position would excessively accelerate the lengthening of the antagonist muscle. Because the antagonist was short while the agonist was stretched out (the strain), the proprioceptors within the shortened antagonist were hypervigilant for signs of stretch (i.e., the "gain" was increased to enhance the sensitivity to subsequent stretch). Thus, when the antagonist was rapidly lengthened (the counterstrain) as the agonist raced back to its neutral position, the antagonist's highly attuned proprioceptors could "see"

the prompt lengthening as a signal that the antagonist was being stretched beyond neutral, even though it was not actually longer than its neutral length. This false sensation that the antagonist was being stretched then led to chronic overfiring of the antagonist's proprioceptors. Because the muscle was signaling "stretch" when it was not actually lengthened, it had no opportunity to turn down the neural discharge. The muscle therefore continually tried to shorten (i.e., was chronically constricted) in its attempt to alleviate the false sensation of stretch (Fig. 106-1).

Strain-counterstrain, Jones reasoned, was effective because it enabled the cessation of the inappropriate firing of the proprioceptors in the antagonist muscle. If the muscle were shortened while it was not contracted, the perpetual firing that relayed the false sensation of stretch could be shut down, and the proprioceptors could be "reset" with the normal length of the muscle as the baseline. Thus, Jones' therapy is based on the *passive* shortening of the afflicted muscle into an optimum relaxed position that allows the afferent nerve impulses to dampen. As a result, the muscle can escape from signals to contract on a long-term basis.

While Jones was beginning to appreciate the therapeutic potential of strain-counterstrain manipulations, Janet Travell, MD, John F. Kennedy's physician, was embarking on what was to become an exhaustive study of myofascial trigger points and their pain referral patterns. Travell's trigger points were similar to Jones' tender points—in that they were nodular, taut areas in muscle that were tender to palpation. Travell noted that trigger points could refer pain to areas beyond the region of the trigger point, and she extensively mapped out both mundane and unexpected referred sites. For instance, Travell noted that a trigger point in the soleus muscle in the leg could cause pain in the leg, the sacral area and, surprisingly, in the jaw. Travell's therapy of the trigger points differed markedly from Jones' counterstrain manipulations. Travell's preferred method of treating trigger points was to anesthetize the skin topically with a cold spray and then to stretch out the muscle containing the trigger point. In addition, injection into a trigger point was also noted to relieve associated pain (Box 106-1).

FIGURE 106-1
Jones' neuromuscular model. EMG, electromyography. (From D'Ambrogio KJ, Roth GB. *Positional Release Therapy: Assessment and Treatment of Musculoskeletal Dysfunction*. St. Louis: Mosby, 1997; modified from Jones LH. *Strain and Counterstrain*. Newark, OH: American Academy of Osteopathy, 1981.)

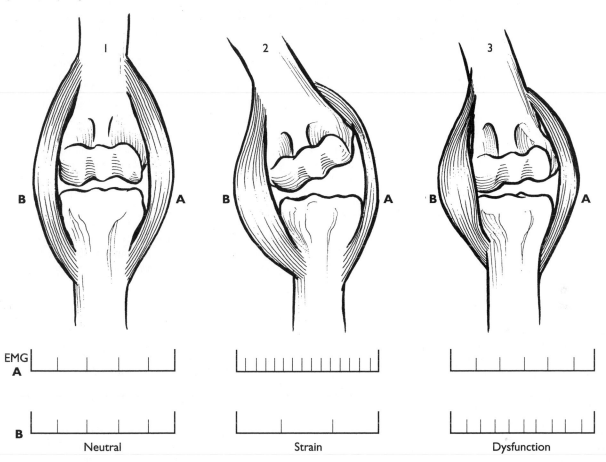

Harmon Myers, DO, was an early student and a subsequent teacher of Jones' technique. Myers synthesized the joint-centered tender points and manipulations of Jones with Travell's myofascial referral patterns of pain stemming from muscular trigger points. Myers realized that Jones' tender points and counterstrain treatment positions actually were locating and shortening Travell's myofascial trigger points and associated muscles. In counterstrain, the passively and optimally shortened position (held for 90 seconds) allowed the inappropriate firing of the proprioceptors located in the muscle containing Travell's trigger point to abate. When the chronically contracted muscle finally relaxed, Travell's trigger point palpably dissolved, and the myofascial pattern of pain ceased.

Often, complete symptom resolution was obtained with just a few counterstrain sessions. This was true not for just muscular pain, but also for other symptoms noted by Travell or Jones. Not uncommonly, patients with complaints of dizziness (sternocleidomastoid muscle), cough (pretracheal fascia and sternocleidomastoid muscle), gastric reflux, and bowel symptoms (rectus abdominis, external abdominal oblique, and longissimus thoracis muscles) dramatically improved with the application of Jones' positioning applied to Travell's myofascial patterns of pain.

The seemingly remarkable efficacy of this therapy, when administered in a finite number of sessions, along with the relatively benign nature of the treatment led to its appeal for patients and therapists alike. Without further provocation, a few sessions of counterstrain are often curative, even for long-standing pain problems. If continuing reasons for exacerbation exist (e.g., Crohn's disease–induced abdominal pain and back pain in a patient with chronic inflammatory bowel disease, lupus-associated recurrent headaches associated with disease severity, or back pain in a patient with leg-length discrepancy), then recurring treatments may need to be allotted based on activity of the underlying disease.

Practical Applications of Counterstrain Therapy

Evaluating the Patient for Therapy

To determine whether a patient might be helped by counterstrain, the practitioner must know the myofascial pain referral patterns, as well as the associated visceral and autonomic symptoms. Once the clinician is familiar with the referral patterns, especially for the more common muscles, then a search for tender points within those muscles can ascertain whether counterstrain is likely to be an effective therapy for that particular patient.

To help guide the search for culprit muscles further, ask yourself what muscles are stretched when the pain worsens, and then look for tender points within those muscles. If a patient complains of back pain and enters the office hunched over (back in flexion), then an examination of the anterior muscles (rectus abdominis, external abdominal oblique, and iliacus) may very well yield significant tender points. The back pain in this patient would worsen when the patient is standing straight, which stretches the anterior (abdominal) thoracic and lumbar muscles.

Myofascial pain is not limited solely to the somatic realm. Multiple examples of muscular pain stemming from the stomach and intestines exist, and ample evidence indicates

neural feedback between the viscera and the muscles and vice versa. A thorough understanding of the somatovisceral relationships, followed by subsequent treatment of identified muscular disorders, can prove invaluable in patients who have failed to attain relief by pharmaceutical and other conventional methods (e.g., for gastroesophageal reflux disease, inflammatory bowel disease, irritable bowel syndrome, and the associated back pain).

Some ailments associated with the more common myofascial pain patterns are listed in Table 106-1. More detailed lists can be found in the references.[1-3] Successful treatment of muscle disorders implicated in myofascial pain referral patterns can frequently spare patients unnecessary consumption of pain medications, can sometimes prevent surgery (e.g., appendectomy for a tender point in the right lower external abdominal oblique muscle), and, of course, can often provide pain relief.

Even if you should decide to refer patients elsewhere for treatment instead of endeavoring to treat them yourself, you must appreciate the contributions of myofascial patterns of pain. A clinician who is adept—or at least competent—in diagnosing myofascial contributions to pain and other dysfunctions will cultivate appreciative patients.

BOX 106-1. Pathophysiology of a Tender Point

Awareness of tender points in the myofascial system dates back to the Chinese Tang Dynasty (AD 618), when these areas were called Ah Shi points. Descriptions of these points in Western medicine have included terms such as trigger points, fibrositis, muscle callus, chronic myositis, and muscular nodules. The underlying mechanisms of pain and inflammation appear to share common origins. Tender points result from the following three mechanisms:

- A proprioceptive neural response to acute muscular strain that registers the rate of stretch of the muscle spindle fibers
- A nociceptive neural response to visceral disease, muscle strain, or injury that persists because of a lack of response to treatment
- An autonomic-somatic neural response to increased tone of the sympathetic nervous system that can result from anxiety and pain

   Within the area of the tender point, proinflammatory and vasoconstrictive chemical mediators, including histamine, prostaglandins, bradykinin, products of anaerobic metabolism, and potassium, accumulate. These mediators team with an influx of calcium ions and lead to chronic hyperstimulation of the associated muscle, thereby causing a neurologic reflex arc that further exacerbates and "tightens" the painful muscle. The underlying trigger of this phenomenon can be an acute injury, repetitive strain, imbalance of muscle use, visceral disease, or chronic stress and tension.

History and Examination
■ Clues From History
Determine the probable initial or continuing source of pain or dysfunction. This can lead to a directed search for related myofascial referral. For example, a patient with upper back pain who has a history of chronic gastroesophageal reflux disease would prompt evaluation of upper tender points in the anterior rectus abdominis and external abdominal oblique muscles, in addition to posterior tender points, whereas a patient who has headaches and dizziness that began after she ran into a truck's side mirror, with resultant forceful turning of her head, may well have tender points in the sternocleidomastoid muscle.

■ Exacerbating and Alleviating Factors
Assess what positions the patient naturally assumes to alleviate the discomfort and what movements make it worse. Realize that shortening of the culprit muscle lessens pain and stretching of that muscle worsens it. In addition, active use of an afflicted muscle worsens the pain. For example, low back pain that worsens with lumbar extension could implicate the anterior abdominal muscles, whereas pain in the knee on rising from a sitting position would prompt an examination of the groin for a tender point in the rectus femoris muscle.

TABLE 106-1. Myofascial Pain Patterns Associated With Common Ailments

HEADACHE AND NECK PAIN	BOWEL PROBLEMS	BACK PAIN
Sternocleidomastoid	External abdominal oblique	Quadratus lumborum
Trapezius	Rectus abdominis	Longissimus thoracis
Levator scapulae	Iliacus	Multifidus
	Longissimus thoracis	Rectus abdominis

Feel the Tender Point

Attentively "listen" to the patient's muscles with your fingers as you search for tender points. Closing your eyes and directing your full attention to the symphony of textures that your fingers encounter will markedly enhance your ability to appreciate tender points.

Treatment Logistics

Once the tender points have been discerned, treatment consists of *shortening* the affected muscles while they are in a *relaxed* state. This passively shortened position enables the constantly firing proprioceptors and nociceptors to sense that continual stretching is no longer occurring; thus, they can finally turn down their signal intensity to a normal level. For this to happen, the treatment position must be precisely determined so that the muscle is optimally shortened. A solid knowledge of anatomy helps the counterstrain practitioner envision the correct position, and the palpable softening of the previously taut tender point confirms the optimum treatment position. Subjective input from the patient is also very helpful in finding the correct position. Palpation of the tender point initially elicits a painful sensation in the patient. When the patient is perfectly positioned for optimal shortening of the muscle, however, the patient will experience at least 70% improvement in the level of pain with palpation of the tender point. Often, complete amelioration of the pain with palpation at the tender point coincides with ideal muscle shortening, and the patient is incredulous that the palpating finger is still on the same tender point (as it should be throughout the treatment and after returning the patient to neutral position while the practitioner checks periodically for the texture and the subjective sensitivity of the tender point). Especially when a practitioner is first learning counterstrain, the patient's subjective input regarding tenderness from firm palpation of the tender point can be very helpful in guiding the proper positioning of the patient.

The final test for the efficacy of that position is to check for the disappearance of the tender point on returning the patient to a neutral position. Because the practitioner's finger remains on the tender point during the entire treatment, it is possible to reevaluate the consistency and sensitivity of the tender point after holding the optimum position for 90 seconds. If the maneuver is done correctly, the posttreatment tender point should no longer be tender (or should be at least 70% improved) and should no longer feel taut or ropey in the neutral position.

During counterstrain treatments, the patient is moved into and out of positions very slowly, so as not to reset the inappropriate receptor firing with any rapid stretching. The optimal position must be held for 90 seconds to turn off the inappropriately firing neurons effectively. Counterstrain should not be painful, and the patient should not experience any discomfort (except the occasional gentle stretching sensation in muscles opposite to those being shortened). The patient must be instructed to alert the practitioner if any pain or discomfort is experienced, and the practitioner should adjust the position accordingly to ensure that the position is comfortable.

Precautions

Although this technique can be powerfully beneficial, a few potential warnings are in order. Occasionally, the patient will feel sore or have flulike symptoms for 24 to 48 hours after a treatment, as the inflammatory mediators and byproducts of anaerobic metabolism are released into the circulatory system. This phase typically does not last more than 48 hours, and the patient is usually markedly improved thereafter. A more serious caveat of treatment applies to patients with severe posttraumatic stress disorder (PTSD). Relief of chronic and debilitating pain may destabilize the psychological state of a tenuous patient with PTSD who has come to rely on pain as a distraction from mental trauma. Other than these precautions, if a patient is treated in a position of comfort, then counterstrain can be an astonishingly effective, yet reassuringly benign, manual therapy to incorporate in your arsenal.

General Guidelines

Treat Referral Points First

Before you attempt to treat the tender points at the site of pain, search for the important and common myofascial pain referral areas and treat those first. If a patient has a headache, first examine and treat the neck referral muscles (sternocleidomastoid, trapezius, and levator scapulae) before you begin to treat any tender points in the head itself. Approximately half the time, abolition of tender points in these referral muscles alone will resolve the head pain. Similarly, if a patient has sacral or buttock pain, you must evaluate and alleviate any tender points in the quadratus lumborum or longissimus thoracis muscles that refer pain to this area before trying to remedy any points in the piriformis or gluteus muscles themselves. If you fail to remove disorders in the offending *referral* muscles before addressing the tender points within the area itself, therapy will often be ineffective because the major culprit of the pain—anatomically removed from the site of the discomfort—will continue to cause symptoms until it is treated.

Order of Treatment

Once you have located the tender points, treat the most severe or the middle of a chain of tender points first. Sometimes, this approach can "turn off" adjacent or milder tender points.

Be Slow and Gentle

Move the patient into and out of position very slowly and gently. Ask the patient to tell you if he or she has any discomfort beyond the mild stretching of muscles on the side opposite the one being treated.

Listen to Your Fingers and the Patient

As you strive to position the patient so that the afflicted muscle is at its shortest length, the palpable softening of the texture of the tender point combined with the patient's subjective assessment of the resolution of the discomfort noted during application of pressure to the tender point will guide you to the optimal position.

Hold

Hold the position for 90 seconds. This is how long it takes to reset the inappropriately firing nerves. If pain is long standing, you may need to hold the position for a minute or two more. Use the sensation that the tender point is dissolving to know when the patient can be returned to neutral position.

Check Response

Keep your fingers on the tender point during treatment, and occasionally check back to make sure the tender point is soft and painless. When you return the patient to neutral position after treating that particular muscle, recheck the tender point. It should be at least 70% improved for lasting therapeutic efficacy.

Variations in Position

Although each particular muscle has general guidelines to direct you to the correct position, each patient will differ in the extent needed to achieve ideal resolution of the tender point. Often, younger, more limber patients need more flexing, bending, or rotating, whereas older, stiffer patients experience complete tender point and pain relief with much less dramatic contortion of the body.

> Anterior tender points tend to be treated with flexion, whereas posterior tender points tend to be treated in extension. The more lateral tender points tend to need more side-bending or rotation, whereas the more midline tender points tend to evoke more flexion or extension in their resolution.

Comfort Is Paramount

Always treat the patient while he or she is in a position of comfort. Counterstrain is an inherently low-risk therapy as long as the patient is comfortable during treatment. Obviously, extreme extension of the cervical spine (rarely used in counterstrain) should be undertaken with a degree of caution in the older adults or in young women and others more prone to vertebral artery issues.

Sequelae

Discuss with the patient that he or she may feel sore or have flulike symptoms for 24 to 48 hours after treatment. Most ailments need three or fewer treatments to resolve. If the pain persists beyond three sessions, then the source of the pain needs to be reevaluated.

Examples of the Technique

This section contains illustrations of referral patterns, tender points, and treatment positions for several muscle groups that are commonly involved in pain. This discussion provides just a short sample, and the reader should refer to referenced resources or continuing medical education for more information.[2,3]

Headache, a common and frequently debilitating complaint, aptly illustrates the need for a clinician to be familiar with the myofascial pain patterns and also provides an example of the ease and efficacy of using counterstrain in clinical practice. Many headaches are associated with tender points in three noncranial muscles: sternocleidomastoid, trapezius, and levator scapulae. These tender points are relatively easy to locate, and the positions of treatment are readily learned. Because the neck is not extended, the risk of vertebral artery dissection is not a concern. Thus, this is a rewarding set of muscles on which to learn the counterstrain technique. Consider checking to see whether these muscles are implicated in patients with migraines, stress headaches, or other head or neck pain complaints.

Trapezius Muscle

The trapezius muscle, an expansive muscle in the upper back, can have various trigger point locations. The trapezius muscle can refer pain from the posterior neck into the head and sometimes causes discomfort in the frontal sinus area. The two most common tender points (medial and lateral) that refer pain to the head and neck are found by pinching the uppermost area between the shoulder and the neck and are depicted by the Xs in Figure 106-2A.

Tender Points

Tender points are located in the fibers of the upper part of the muscle at the junction of the neck and shoulder and are found by pinching the muscle between finger and thumb.

- Medial point: The medial point is found in the webbing at the junction of the neck and thorax (a gentle version of the Star Trek "Vulcan death grip").
- Lateral point: The lateral point is found a centimeter or two more lateral than the medial point as you pinch out toward the shoulder.

Referral Pattern

- Medial point: Pain can be located at the angle of the jaw, behind the eye, and through the temporal region into the lateral neck.
- Lateral point: Pain is found in the suboccipital area through the posterior neck (see Fig. 106-2B).

Treatment Position

With patient lying on back:

- Medial points: Side-bend the patient's cervical spine toward the side of pain so the ear is moved toward the shoulder.
- Lateral points: Flex the patient's shoulders so that the arms are approximately 150 to 170 degrees overhead (so that the humerus is though the plane of the eyes), as shown in Figure 106-2C, and apply steady, gentle cephalic traction (in effect, moving the scapular attachments closer to the vertebral origins of the muscle).

Levator Scapulae Muscle

Chronic contraction within the levator scapulae muscle can be a frequent source of pain in the shoulders and the posterior neck, with radiation of pain into the occipital area. This condition is seen in people with tension and anxiety (chronic shoulder shrug), those who work extensively with a keyboard, or those who regularly hold a telephone between the ear and the shoulder. A hint that the levator scapulae is in need of treatment comes when a patient holds his or her contralateral hand over the area between the shoulder and neck and rubs the upper back with his or her fingers.

- Tender point: This point is located at the superomedial border of the scapula between the scapula and the nape of the neck (Fig. 106-3A). Slide your fingers medially over the scapular spine and move laterally to medially. When the spine of the scapula ends, hook your fingers up and onto

FIGURE 106-2
The counterstrain technique applied to the trapezius muscle. See text for details. **A,** Tender points. **B,** Pain referral pattern. **C,** Treatment position for lateral trapezius points.

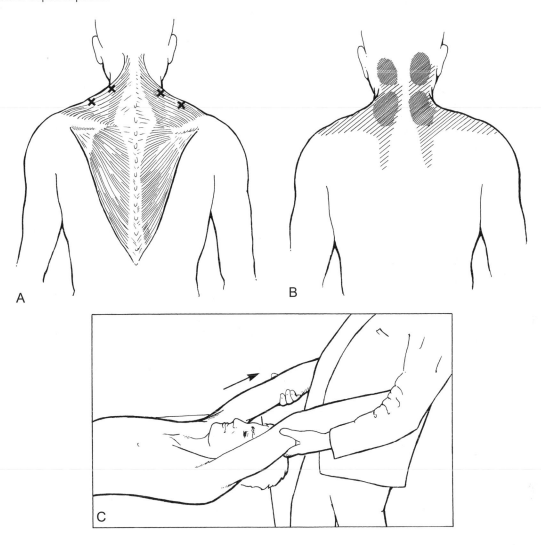

the superior medial border of the scapula, and press posterior to anterior and medial to lateral against the medial edge of the scapula.

- Referral pattern: Pain is felt in the posterior neck through the shoulder, with referral pain in the occipital area (see Fig. 106-3B).

- Treatment position: With the patient supine, side-bend the neck toward the side of the tender point. Flex the patient's shoulder to approximately 30 to 45 degrees with the elbow flexed. Abduct the shoulder slightly and apply a cephalic force through the shaft of the humerus to elevate the scapula. It feels as though you are shoving the shoulder toward the ear (see Fig. 106-3C).

Sternocleidomastoid Muscle

This muscle is a myofascial culprit often implicated in headache, ear pain, or sinus symptoms. Additionally, the sternal branch attachment can be associated with dry cough, whereas disorders of the clavicular belly of the muscle can be associated with postural dizziness and a sense of imbalance. Generally, patients do not actually complain of any discomfort in the anterior neck, and thus awareness of Travell's myofascial patterns of pain can be important in resolving the many headaches and other symptoms originating from dysfunction in the sternocleidomastoid muscle.

- Tender point: This is located anywhere in the body of either the sternal or the clavicular division of the muscle (or the sternal attachment in the case of cough). Pinch the belly of the muscle with your thumb and index finger to help find the tender point. Obviously, care should be taken to avoid carotid massage (Fig. 106-4A).

- Referral pattern: Pain is referred to the suboccipital, frontal, maxillary, or other areas of the head. Further symptoms stemming from the sternocleidomastoid muscle include ear, eye, or temporomandibular joint symptoms, dizziness or imbalance, and dry cough (see Fig. 106-4B).

FIGURE 106-3
The manipulation technique applied to the levator scapulae muscle. See text for details. **A,** Tender point. **B,** Pain referral pattern. **C,** Treatment position.

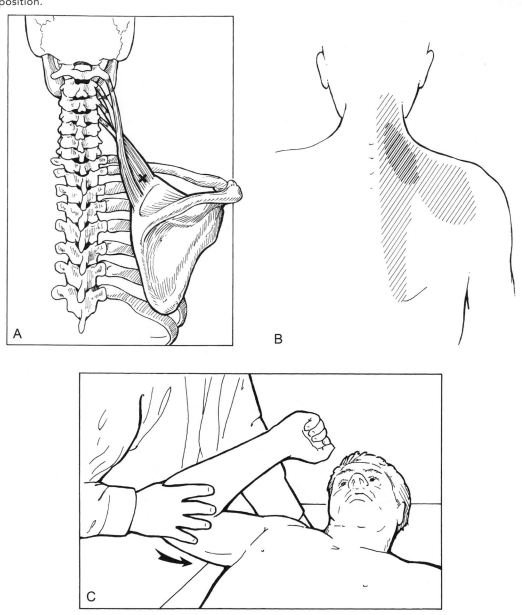

- Treatment position: With the patient supine, support the head as you gently but markedly flex the neck, rotate the head away from the tender point, and side-bend it toward the tender point. Imagine coaxing the patient's ear toward either the sternum (for the sternal branch) or the clavicular insertion (for the clavicular branch). Sometimes, using a pillow helps the patient relax enough to soften the sternocleidomastoid muscle while the patient's head is elevated off the table (see Fig. 106-4C).

Piriformis Muscle

The sciatic nerve and the piriformis muscle are in close proximity (Fig. 106-5). In fact, in 5% of the population, the nerve runs through or over the muscle, thus making irritation of the nerve much more likely when the muscle is inflamed. This condition, called piriformis syndrome, is a common cause of buttock pain with radiation of pain down the back of the thigh. Before treating the piriformis muscle, be sure to assess for and treat any tender points in the quadratus lumborum and longissimus thoracis muscles because both these muscles can radiate to the sacral or buttocks area. The rectus abdominis and external abdominal oblique muscles can also be involved anteriorly.

- Tender point: This point is located within the piriformis muscle, which is 3 inches medial and slightly cephalad to the greater trochanter. Tender points can occur anywhere within muscle, which runs between

FIGURE 106-4
The manipulation technique applied to the sternocleidomastoid muscle. See text for details. **A,** Tender point. **B,** Pain referral pattern. **C,** Treatment position.

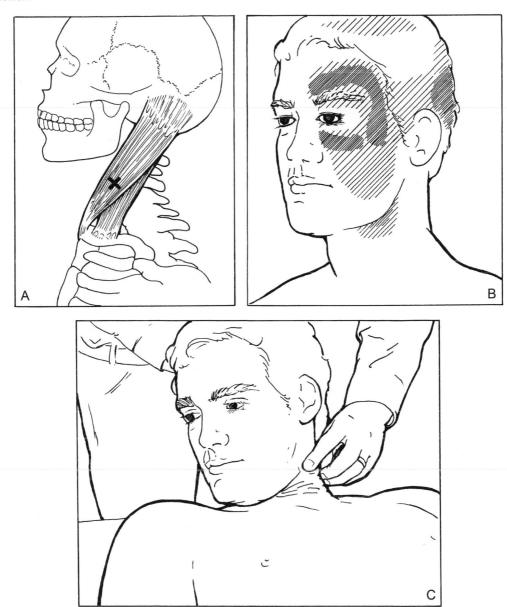

the midsacrum and the greater trochanter of the proximal femur (see Fig. 106-5A).

- Referral pattern: Pain may occur in the buttock and the back of the thigh (see Fig. 106-5B).

- Treatment position: The patient is prone. The therapist sits on the same side as the tender point. The patient's leg on the tender point side is suspended off the table with the patient's anterior ankle resting on the therapist's thigh. Flex the patient's hip 120 to 130 degrees, adduct the hip to tolerance, and slightly rotate the hip internally by gently pulling outward on the foot (see Fig. 106-5C).

Benefits

The counterstrain technique is beneficial for the following reasons:

- It often provides immediate relief of discomfort. The benefits are frequently long lasting or even permanent, and they can usually be achieved in a few sessions.

- It readily and efficiently helps the body regain normal function and range of motion that may have been severely and chronically limited by a remote injury that led to continual myofascial dysfunction.

FIGURE 106-5
The manipulation technique applied to the piriformis muscle. See text for details. **A,** Tender point. **B,** Pain referral pattern. **C,** Treatment position.

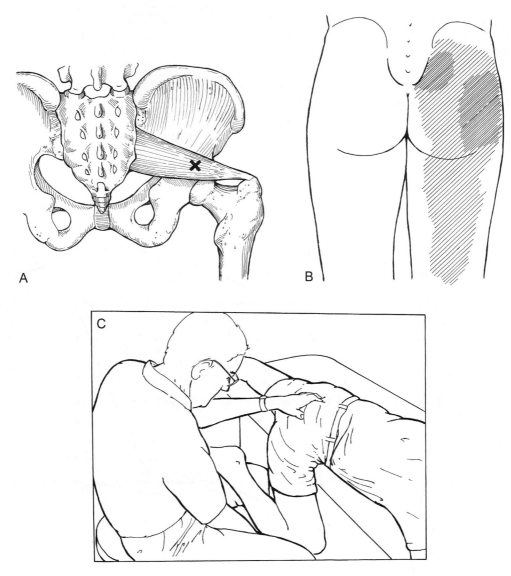

- Not only is it comfortable for the patient to experience, but also counterstrain can be highly rewarding for the practitioner to perform. Counterstrain is easy to learn (especially using Myers' method of combining Travell's myofascial trigger point and Jones' positioning) and not difficult to master at an advanced level.

- It enables you to touch the patient and thereby increase a sense of caring and rapport in a time when technology is creating barriers between practitioner and patient.

- In addition to treating pure somatic pain, counterstrain can help relieve visceral symptoms and the associated somatic pain resulting from somatovisceral or viscerosomatic neural feedback loops.

- It uses a position of comfort, with almost negligible inherent risk to the patient.

- The acquisition of this technique can be readily accomplished by most medical practitioners who have a fundamental medical or anatomic knowledge base.

Limitations

The limitations of counterstrain therapy are as follows:

- Although pain relief is usually permanent, in some cases pain can recur. Recurrence is more likely when the initial source of injury is not adequately addressed.

- A somewhat localized technique such as this may not be the most effective approach for treating a patient with diffuse and disseminated tender points (e.g., fibromyalgia). In addition, it may not be as rewarding when treating someone with frequent or continuous recurrent reinjury (e.g., as seen in untreated Crohn's disease or gastroesophageal reflux disease in which the visceral problem restimulates the somatic disorder).

- The technique is conceptually easy to learn but takes practice to become thoroughly adept at it. The practitioner should start by becoming familiar with the common and important muscle groups and then progress from there.

- When able, one should begin the counterstrain technique by practicing on children because their limited soft tissue

mass allows for easy identification of tender points, and their small frames enable ready maneuverability into treatment positions.

- If psychological problems are not addressed, a patient who "needs" somatic pain to maintain equilibrium can become destabilized. Close coordination with a mental health professional is recommended in patients with a history of severe psychological issues or with significant PTSD before attempts are made to relieve the somatic pain.

KEY WEB RESOURCES

American Academy of Osteopathy: http://www.academyofosteopathy.org/	Many courses in manual medicine, including counterstrain, are offered annually.
Jones Institute: http://www.jiscs.com/Article.aspx?a=0	This organization coordinates counterstrain workshops in the United States and internationally.
Tucson Osteopathic Medical Foundation: www.tomf.org/	This group offers hands-on classes in strain/counterstrain, taught by Myers twice a year.

KEY EDUCATIONAL TEXTS

Travell J, Simons D. *Travell and Simons' Myofascial Pain and Dysfunction: The Trigger Point Manual.* Philadelphia: Lippincott; 1998.	Travell and Simons' two-volume text documenting the myofascial pain and dysfunction referral patterns encompasses an amazingly thorough life's work, replete with interesting observations of common and unique myopathic associations.
Travell J, Simons D. *Travell and Simons' Trigger Point Flip Charts.* Baltimore: Williams & Wilkins; 1996.	This useful trigger point flip chart is based on Travell's work.
Myers H. *Clinical Ap plication of Counterstrain.* Tucson: Osteopathic Press; 2006.	Myers' counterstrain manual combines Travell's findings with Jones' work to provide a succinct, visual, and hands-on approach to learning and applying counterstrain.

References

References are available online at expertconsult.com.

Acupuncture for Headache

Aaron J. Michelfelder, MD

Overview

Acupuncture is the technique of piercing the skin with needles in specific points on the body to treat or prevent various conditions. Acupuncture has been used for thousands of years by practitioners in many different cultures and societies around the world. Because acupuncture has become more popular, physicians must have at least a basic working knowledge of the technique. The best physicians use all their knowledge of integrative medicine to provide the most comprehensive care available for patients.

Acupuncture points are not random. They are palpable, and points often correspond to depressions in muscles or bones or to neural foramina. An acupuncture point usually has its own neurovascular bundle, which distinguishes it from surrounding tissue, and is sometimes quite tender to palpation. In traditional Chinese medicine, these points connect to energy (qi) channels within the body called meridians. Fourteen principal meridians (6 bilateral [total of 12] and 2 central) are recognized, typically named after organs of the body: kidney (KI), heart (HT), small intestine (SI), bladder (BL), liver (LV), master of the heart, also called pericardium (MH), triple heater (TH), gallbladder (GB), spleen (SP), lung (LU), large intestine (LI), stomach (ST), conception vessel (CV), and governor vessel (GV).

Mechanism of Action

The exact mechanism of action of acupuncture is unclear. However, significant evidence indicates that acupuncture effects changes in the muscles where the needle is inserted, changes starting at nerves near the needle and passing all the way up to the higher cortex, as well as changes in circulating and local hormones, cytokines, neurotransmitters, and other body chemicals.[1]

Safety of Acupuncture

Despite the use of sterile needles to pierce unsterilized skin, serious adverse reactions to acupuncture are very rare. A systematic review of the world literature on prospective studies of the safety of acupuncture revealed that in 9 trials involving tens of thousands of treatments, pneumothorax was the only life-threatening complication, and it occurred twice; infections did not occur at all.[2] A prospective survey of 34,000 treatments by traditional acupuncturists in the United Kingdom found no serious adverse events.[3] In the largest prospective trial to date, involving 97,733 patients and more than 760,000 treatments performed by 7050 physicians in Germany, pneumothorax occurred twice, as well as one occurrence each of exacerbation of depression, acute hypertensive crisis, vasovagal reaction, and asthma attack with hypertension and angina.[4] The reactions most commonly reported were needling pain in 3.28%, hematoma in 3.19%, bleeding in 1.38%, and orthostasis in 0.46% of patients. Overall, nonserious adverse events were reported to occur in 7.1% of patients.[4]

Training in Acupuncture

Laws concerning the practice of acupuncture are defined by each state. Practitioners include the following: licensed acupuncturists, who have completed at least 3 years of training at a college of Oriental medicine; chiropractors, who receive variable amounts of training in chiropractic school but may have additional training after school; and physicians and dentists who have completed acupuncture training courses outside their regular professional training. For physicians to practice acupuncture, some states require no training at all, others require 200 hours, and some mandate 300 hours of acupuncture training. Board certification is available to physicians through the American Board of Medical Acupuncture. Details on physician training and licensure can be found on the Web site of the American Academy of Medical Acupuncture (see the Key Web Resources box, later).

Techniques

Technique for Acupressure

Acupressure is essentially massage, but with the purpose of stimulating an acupuncture point for a desired effect. Acupressure can also be used to relax trigger points, as well as other areas of spasm within muscles that may or may not be acupuncture points.

The purpose of the technique is to find the point or area to be stimulated, as follows:

1. With your index finger or thumb, start superficially and apply just enough pressure to move the skin.
2. Move the finger or thumb in gentle, slow circles.
3. With every few circles, apply more and more pressure until you feel the muscle fibers beginning to relax beneath your fingers. If you are stimulating an area without a muscle, such as over the supraorbital foramen, just keep applying slow, steady downward, circular pressure over the foramen.
4. With stimulation of an acupuncture point, the patient should eventually feel a dull, aching sensation. Stimulation of the point should last at least several minutes past which the patient feels this aching sensation. You may have to apply acupressure intermittently, such as for a few minutes, several times an hour.

This technique is a good one to teach patients to perform on themselves for problems such as sinus headaches and pressure.

Technique for Acupuncture

Acupuncture needles come in all sizes, from very small (approximately 40 gauge) to much larger (up to 20 gauge). An acupuncture needle comes to a very sharp point and has a plastic or wrapped metal handle. Because acupuncture needles are not hollow like phlebotomy needles, they are believed to separate tissue more than to cut it (Fig. 107-1).

1. After the desired acupuncture point is found, palpation of the point is important to prepare the body for the needle (Fig. 107-2).
2. A very small needle may need an introducer, which is included with most needles. The introducer is a plastic tube a few millimeters shorter than the needle. Place the introducer on top of the acupuncture point, and then drop the needle into the introducer (Figs. 107-3 and 107-4). The handle of the needle will protrude a few millimeters from the top of the introducer.
3. Holding the introducer between the thumb and third finger of your dominant hand, tap the needle into the skin using your index finger (Figs. 107-5 and 107-6). With practice, the right amount of force needed to pierce the skin is simple to recognize.
4. After the initial tap of the needle into the skin, carefully remove the introducer. Then, the needle may be pushed in deeper and angled to wherever you would like it to go. Typically, the needle enters the body of a muscle, but the depth depends on the acupuncture point. A point on the back of the neck may be 2 to 3 cm deep, but a point on the forehead may only be a few millimeters deep.

Inserting the needles without the plastic introducer requires some training and supervision and is beyond the scope of this chapter.

FIGURE 107-1
Package of acupuncture needles.

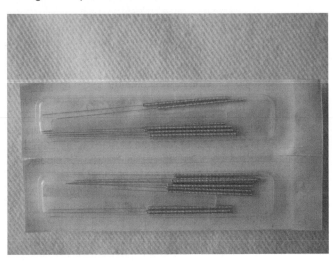

FIGURE 107-2
Palpation.

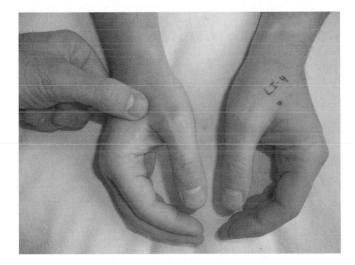

Once a needle has been inserted, it can either be stimulated or left alone. If it is left alone, the coiled handle and temperature difference between the needle tip in the body and the needle handle at room temperature will cause electrons to move from inside the body into the needle. Inserting a needle and then leaving it alone is called *needle in dispersion*. The needle becomes a capacitor removing electrons from the body. In traditional Chinese medicine, this action is believed to be calming, cooling, and depleting.

To add electrons to the body, the needle can be stimulated by a back-and-forth twirling action, which the acupuncturist achieves by rotating the needle approximately 180 degrees alternately clockwise and counterclockwise. The needle can also be stimulated by warming with something like Chinese moxa, an herb pressed into an incense-like stick that, when lit, smolders and emits a steady stream of heat. Electrical stimulators are very popular and may be connected to the

FIGURE 107-3
Positioning the introducer.

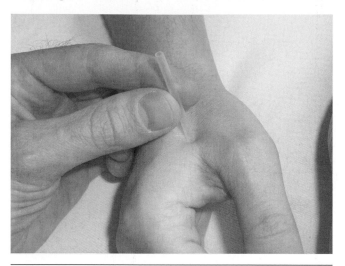

FIGURE 107-4
Needle in introducer.

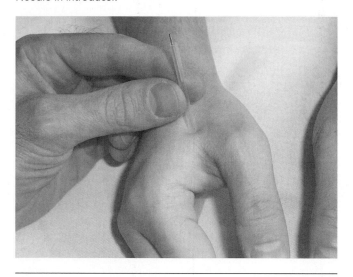

FIGURE 107-5
Tapping needle into place.

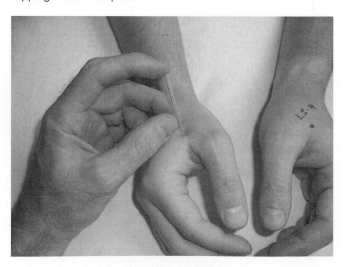

FIGURE 107-6
Needle in place.

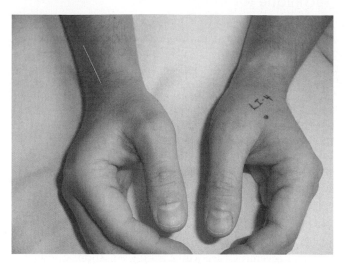

needles in a circuit to add electron flow from one needle to another. This is the process for percutaneous electrical nerve stimulation, the acupuncture version of transcutaneous electrical nerve stimulation. Lasers can also be used to stimulate acupuncture points with or without needles.

> Both acupuncture and acupressure can be used to stimulate acupuncture points. Patients can be taught to perform their own acupressure, thus empowering them to help themselves.

Evidence for Acupuncture in Headache

The allopathic tradition of the randomized placebo-controlled clinical trial is very difficult to apply to acupuncture. Defining placebo acupuncture is challenging because many people argue that any needle piercing the skin is acupuncture. Many studies use no acupuncture as the control intervention, or they use sham acupuncture, which usually means inserting needles into places that are not acupuncture points. Some studies have tried to use acupressure as the control. In any case, many studies have been unsuccessful in blinding patients or their physicians regarding whether they had acupuncture, and the acupuncturist is certainly not blinded regarding whether traditional or sham acupuncture is being used on the patient. Many studies also use protocols whereby every patient receives the same treatment. Most acupuncturists individualize the acupuncture treatment to each patient and modify treatments based on response to earlier treatments.

To put acupuncture studies into context, the U.S. Food and Drug Administration requires only two studies of a drug to show that the drug is better than placebo before the agent can be approved. A drug could show neutral results in many studies, but as long as two studies have positive results, the drug can be approved for use. Possibly because of the difficulties in experimental design, many studies of acupuncture have had positive results, and many have had neutral results.

In 1999, Melchart et al[5] performed a review of 22 randomized controlled trials of acupuncture for headache involving 1042 patients from European countries. These reviewers concluded that the trials tended to be small and had methodologic problems; however, the evidence suggested a role for acupuncture in headache treatment.[5] In a newer, well-designed trial reported in 2004, Vickers et al[6] studied acupuncture in 401 patients with chronic headaches in the United Kingdom. Subjects underwent either acupuncture treatments once a week for 3 months or no acupuncture. Over 1 year, the treatment group had a 34% decrease in headache score, versus 16% in the control group. In addition, the treatment group was found to have 20 fewer days of headache per year, 15% less medication use, 25% fewer visits to the general practitioner, and 15% fewer days off work. Wonderling et al,[7] examining the cost effectiveness of acupuncture for headaches in the United Kingdom, found that acupuncture improved health-related quality of life at a small additional cost and was relatively cost effective.

Two Cochrane Collaboration reviews of acupuncture performed meta-analyses of available acupuncture trials for headache. The first meta-analysis of acupuncture trials included 22 studies with a total of 4419 patients in whom acupuncture was used for migraine prophylaxis. The reviewers concluded that these "studies suggest that acupuncture is at least as effective as, and possibly more effective than, prophylactic drug treatment, and has fewer side effects." They recommended acupuncture as a treatment option for patients with migraines.[8] The second meta-analysis concerned acupuncture for tension headaches and included 11 trials with a total of 2317 participants. The reviewers found that patients had a statistically significant reduction in the number, frequency, and intensity of tension headaches over 3 months, but none had studied effects beyond 3 months. The reviewers concluded that "acupuncture could be a valuable non-pharmacologic tool in patients with frequent episodic or chronic tension-type headaches."[9]

> The latest evidence shows that acupuncture is helpful in treating headaches.

Selecting Acupuncture and Acupressure Points

Selection of acupuncture or acupressure points for treatment of headaches should proceed as follows:
1. Start with general relaxation or calming points.
2. Release trigger points in the posterior cervical region.
3. Depending on the type of headache, use local points.

General Relaxation and Calming Points

Governor Vessel 20
The GV20 point is at the top of the head, over the sagittal suture, which is created by the closure of the posterior fontanelle. Often, a bony ridge is present at this point. Visually, GV20 can be found by tracing an imaginary line from the ear lobes up through the middle of the top of the ears (the helix) and up to the midline. Where that line crosses the sagittal

suture (midline) is the GV20 point. The patient can apply acupressure to this point, or a needle can be inserted here and left in dispersion (Fig. 107-7).

Large Intestine 4
The LI4 point is located in the body of the first interosseus muscle in the hand, between the first and second metacarpal bones. This point is usually tender, and patients can easily perform acupressure to this point bilaterally on themselves (Fig. 107-8).

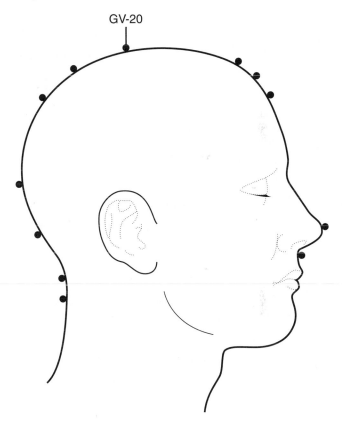

FIGURE 107-7
The governor vessel 20 (GV20) acupuncture point.

GV-20

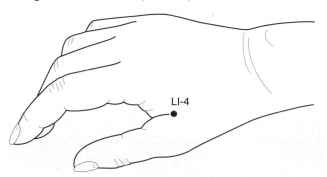

FIGURE 107-8
The large intestine 4 (LI4) acupuncture point.

LI-4

FIGURE 107-9
The gallbladder 20 (GB20) acupuncture point.

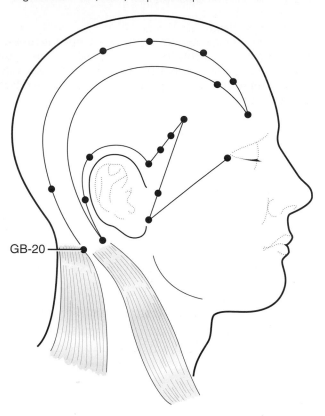

GB-20

Trigger Points in the Cervical Region

People with headaches tend to have stiff posterior cervical muscles. Massage, heat, chiropractic and osteopathic manipulation, acupressure, trigger point injections, and acupuncture can all help release the muscle spasm.

Gallbladder 20

The GB20 point is located at the base of the skull, posteriorly, between the insertions of the sternocleidomastoid and the trapezius muscles. Start by placing the thumb and index finger of one hand on the mastoid processes and then slide them posteriorly. Your fingertips will "fall into" two depressions at the base of the skull. Superiorly, you will feel the skull. On either side of your fingers, you will feel the sternocleidomastoid or trapezius muscles (Fig. 107-9).

> Palpate all the muscles of the posterior neck from the base of the skull down to the shoulders. Any tender points or areas of spasm should be addressed with massage, acupuncture, or acupressure.

Local Points

Frontal Headaches

For frontal headaches, including sinus, tension, and migraine, the GV24.5 may be used. GV24.5 is located on the glabella, between the eyebrows (Fig. 107-10).

FIGURE 107-10
Acupuncture points governor vessel 24.5 (GV24.5), bladder 2 (BL2), and stomach 2 (ST2).

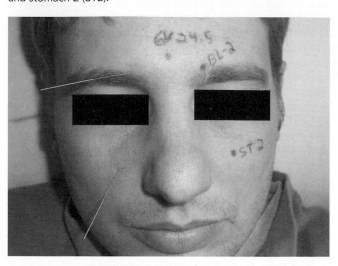

Sinus Headaches

- *Bladder 2:* The BL2 point is located at the frontal notch, just medial to the supraorbital foramen (see Fig. 107-10). Insert the needle from above.

- *Stomach 2:* The ST2 point is located lateral to the nose in a depression where the infraorbital foramen is found. Needle this point starting laterally, aim toward the medial canthus of the eye, and insert the needle subcutaneously (see Fig. 107-10).

Tension Headaches

- *Temporal muscle tender points:* Palpate the muscles of the scalp carefully, and perform acupressure or acupuncture at any tender areas or regions of spasm found, especially in the temporal region.

Migraines and Cluster Headaches

Migraines and cluster headaches are complicated to treat with acupuncture. Follow the same principles of general relaxation points, then cervical points, then GV24.5. After those procedures, search for any tender points on the scalp. If needling tender points on the scalp does not provide satisfactory relief, a more systemic approach with acupuncture may be more successful. Such an in-depth approach is beyond the scope of this chapter.

During an Acupuncture Treatment

Needles stay in place for approximately 30 minutes. Patients should be relaxing in a comfortable room with the lights low and perhaps some calming music in the background. Distractions should be minimized.
Remove acupuncture needles as follows:
1. Place one finger on the skin next to the needle.
2. While holding your finger in place, use the other hand to pull the needle out gently.

3. Sometimes a drop of blood may be released. Applying pressure is not necessary; simply dab the blood away with sterile gauze.

Posttreatment Home Program

Patients are instructed to moderate their activity for 24 hours after a treatment. They should avoid very hot or very cold foods, consumption of alcohol, sexual activity, and other physically demanding activities. They should also drink plenty of water and get lots of sleep.

Patients can continue to perform acupressure on themselves starting 24 hours after the treatment. A good approach is to stimulate GV20, LI4, and local neck and head points twice a day and as needed.

Ideally, acupuncture is integrated into a regimen of headache trigger avoidance, healthful diet, exercise, and stress reduction, as well as possible medication therapy. Acupressure is a great way to empower patients to take control of their own symptoms.

What to Look for in an Acupuncturist

A physician acupuncturist should have completed training in one of the programs approved by the American Board of Medical Acupuncture. Board certification in medical acupuncture identifies individuals who have completed at least 200 hours of training, passed a board examination, practiced at least 2 years, and performed at least 500 acupuncture treatments.

A nonphysician acupuncturist should be licensed. The letters "L.Ac." should follow a licensed acupuncturist's name. In addition, the National Certification Commission for Acupuncture and Oriental Medicine has a database of certified acupuncturists (see the Key Web Resources box).

Conclusion

- Training for physicians to learn acupuncture is available through several continuing medical education programs.

- Acupuncture is useful for treating headaches, and patients can be taught acupressure to empower them to take control of their own health.

- In treating headaches: (1) start with general relaxation points (GV20, LI4), (2) release trigger points in the posterior cervical region (GB20 and any tender points), and (3) depending on the type of headache, use local points.

- For referral, look for a physician acupuncturist, licensed acupuncturist, or chiropractor with documented training and, ideally, certification in acupuncture.

KEY WEB RESOURCES

American Academy of Medical Acupuncture: http://www.medicalacupuncture.org/index.html	The main certifying group of physician acupuncturists
National Certification Commission for Acupuncture and Oriental Medicine (NCCAOM): www.nccaom.org	Certifying group maintaining a database of certified acupuncturists
National Center for Complementary and Alternative Medicine (NCCAM): http://nccam.nih.gov	Part of the National Institutes of Health
Acumedico: http://www.acumedico.com/acupoints.htm	A list of acupuncture sites with illustrations
Acupuncture Today: http://www.acupuncturetoday.com/mpacms/at/home.php	Acupuncture news source with information on clinicians and acupuncture research

References

References are available online at expertconsult.com

Acupuncture for Nausea and Vomiting

Aaron J. Michelfelder, MD

Overview

For an overview of acupuncture, its mechanism of action, safety, training for, and techniques for performing acupuncture and acupressure, please see Chapter 107, Acupuncture for Headache.

Extensive data are available concerning acupuncture and acupressure for nausea and vomiting, especially with regard to the following causes or types of these disorders:

- Postoperative status
- Chemotherapy
- Pregnancy
- Motion sickness

Postoperative Nausea and Vomiting

In 1997, the National Institutes of Health (NIH) convened a panel of nonadvocate scientists to assess the current evidence concerning acupuncture and its efficacy. At that time, the panel concluded that clear evidence indicated that acupuncture was effective for adult postoperative and chemotherapy-induced nausea and vomiting.[1] Since then, six studies have also demonstrated efficacy for preventing postoperative nausea and vomiting in children.[2-4] A 2004 Cochrane Review of 26 trials involving 3347 children and adults showed that acupuncture, with and without electrical stimulation, and acupressure were effective in decreasing the incidence of postoperative nausea and vomiting in comparison with controls.[5] When compared, acupuncture and acupressure were equivalent to antiemetic drugs for preventing vomiting but were actually better for preventing nausea.[5] A Cochrane meta-analysis including 40 trials with a total of 4858 participants looked specifically at stimulation of the wrist acupuncture point pericardium 6 (PC6) for preventing postoperative nausea and vomiting.[6] The reviewers found that acupuncture and acupressure at the PC6 acupoint significantly reduced the risk of postoperative nausea and vomiting when compared with sham in both children and adults. The reviewers also found that PC6 stimulation was equivalent to antiemetic drugs.[6]

Chemotherapy-Induced Nausea and Vomiting

As previously stated, the 1997 NIH Acupuncture Consensus Panel concluded that acupuncture was effective for chemotherapy-induced nausea and vomiting. Dundee and Yang[7] found that acupressure was effective for decreasing nausea in hospitalized patients but worked much better when the acupressure bands were stimulated every hour. In an attempt to make this effect stronger, these investigators gave acupuncture with electrical stimulation to 105 patients, all of whom had had sickness after an earlier chemotherapy treatment. This treatment prevented sickness in 66% of patients, and only 6% did not have some benefit from the acupuncture.[7] A meta-analysis of 11 studies including 1247 patients found that self-administered acupressure prevented chemotherapy-induced nausea and vomiting, and electroacupuncture also had a positive effect.[8] The reviewers concluded that these studies suggested a biologic effect of acupuncture in preventing and treating chemotherapy-induced nausea and vomiting.[8]

Pregnancy-Related Nausea and Vomiting

The data for use of acupuncture in pregnancy-related nausea and vomiting are equivocal.[9] A Cochrane Review of available studies found limited evidence to support the use of wrist and ear acupressure or acustimulation to treat pregnancy-related nausea and vomiting and cited the need for higher-quality, more focused studies in this area.[10]

Motion Sickness

Several devices, including acupressure and electrical stimulation devices, are approved by the U.S. Food and Drug Administration for the prevention of motion sickness. Hu et al[11] reported that acupressure reduced the symptoms of motion sickness and decreased abnormal gastric myoelectric activity and tachyarrhythmia. However, Miller and Muth,[12] who tested two available acupressure and acustimulation bands for the prevention of motion sickness, found that the devices delayed the onset of, but did not prevent, the sickness.[9]

> Acupuncture and acupressure are effective for postoperative and chemotherapy-induced nausea and vomiting, but data are equivocal for pregnancy-induced nausea and vomiting, as well as for motion sickness. Acupuncture, with or without electrical stimulation, and acupressure appear to be equivalent to antiemetic drugs for the prevention of nausea and vomiting.

Acupuncture Points for Nausea and Vomiting

Naming of acupuncture points and techniques for performing acupuncture and acupressure are discussed in Chapter 107, Acupuncture for Headache.

Three main points are relevant to this discussion: (1) master of the heart 6, also called pericardium 6 (MH6, PC6, or P6), (2) stomach 36 (ST36), and (3) liver 3 (LV3).

Master of the Heart 6

MH6 is located on the anterior surface of the wrist, approximately three fingerbreadths proximal to the distal wrist crease. It lies between the tendons of the flexor carpi radialis and palmaris longus muscles. Because the median nerve can be very superficial, insert the needle only a few millimeters under the skin starting proximally and direct it very superficially toward the hand. Warn the patient that if he or she feels a shooting or shocklike sensation into the hand, it is nothing harmful, and then redirect the needle more superficially (Fig. 108-1).

Stomach 36

ST36 is a depression in the anterolateral aspect of the shin, between the tibialis anterior muscle and the extensor digitorum longus muscle. You can find this point by placing your thumb on the anterior border of the tibia and sliding superiorly. Where the tibia starts to fan out near the patella (tibial tuberosity), allow your thumb to travel laterally until it encounters a depression approximately six fingerbreadths below the patella and one fingerbreadth lateral to the tibial tuberosity. The needle is inserted perpendicular to the skin, approximately 1 to 2 cm deep, and is stimulated with clockwise and counterclockwise twisting (Fig. 108-2).

FIGURE 108-1
The master of the heart (MH6; also called pericardium [PC6 or P6]) acupuncture point.

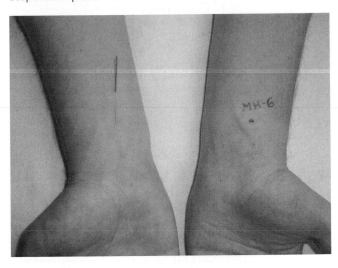

FIGURE 108-2
The stomach 36 (ST36) acupuncture point.

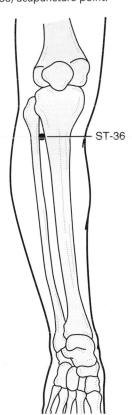

Liver 3

LV3, also a very important point for the treatment of nausea and vomiting, is located on the dorsum of the foot between the first and second metatarsal bones. If you place a finger between the first and second toes and slide it up the foot

FIGURE 108-3
The liver 3 (LV3) acupuncture point.

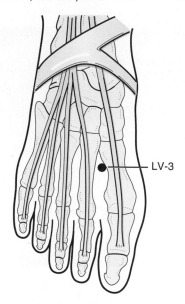

between the first two metatarsal bones, LV3 is the last place where you can access the underlying muscle between those two bones. The needle is directed toward the tip of the calcaneus and is inserted to a depth of approximately 1 cm (Fig. 108-3).

Practical Use of These Points

To prevent nausea, stimulate the MH6 point, either with acupressure with a finger, a commercially available acupressure band, an acustimulator or with acupuncture. To treat nausea and vomiting, start with MH6, and then add ST36 with stimulation and LV3 in dispersion (see Chapter 107, Acupuncture for Headache, for the distinction between stimulation and dispersion).

During an Acupuncture Treatment

For the prevention of nausea, needles should be placed at least 30 minutes before the antiemetic effect is needed and continued for as long as required. For the treatment of nausea and vomiting, needles stay in for as long as needed. Patients should be relaxing in a comfortable room with the lights low and perhaps some calming music in the background. Distractions should be minimized.

Remove acupuncture needles as follows:
1. Place one finger on the skin next to the needle.

2. While holding your finger in place, use the other hand to pull the needle out gently.
3. Sometimes a drop of blood may be released. Applying pressure is not necessary; simply dab the blood away with sterile gauze.

Posttreatment Home Program

Patients are instructed to moderate their activity for 24 hours after a treatment. They should avoid very hot or very cold foods, consumption of alcohol, sexual activity, and other physically demanding activities. They should also drink plenty of water and get lots of sleep.

Patients can continue to perform acupressure on themselves whenever needed. Acupressure is a great way to empower patients to take control of their own symptoms.

What to Look for in an Acupuncturist

A physician acupuncturist should have completed training in one of the programs approved by the American Board of Medical Acupuncture. Board certification in medical acupuncture identifies individuals who have completed at least 200 hours of training, passed a board examination, practiced at least 2 years, and performed at least 500 acupuncture treatments.

A nonphysician acupuncturist should be licensed. The letters "L.Ac." should follow a licensed acupuncturist's name. In addition, the National Certification Commission for Acupuncture and Oriental Medicine has a database of certified acupuncturists (see the Key Web Resources box).

Conclusion

- Acupuncture has been shown to be effective for the prevention and treatment of postoperative and chemotherapy-induced nausea and vomiting. Acupuncture may be helpful for the prevention of pregnancy-induced nausea and vomiting, as well as motion sickness.

- For prevention of nausea, stimulate the MH6 point with acupuncture, acupressure, or electrical stimulation.

- To treat nausea and vomiting, use MH6, but also add ST36 with stimulation (clockwise and counterclockwise twisting action) and LV3 in dispersion (needle left alone).

- For more information about learning acupuncture, visit the American Academy of Medical Acupuncture Web site (see the Key Web Resources box).

KEY WEB RESOURCES

American Academy of Medical Acupuncture: http://www.medicalacupuncture.org/index.html

The main certifying group of physician acupuncturists

Acumedico: http://www.acumedico.com/acupoints.htm

A list of acupuncture sites with illustrations

National Certification Commission for Acupuncture and Oriental Medicine (NCCAOM): www.nccaom.org

Certifying group maintaining a database of certified acupuncturists

Acupuncture Today: http://www.acupuncturetoday.com/mpacms/at/home.php	Acupuncture news source with information on clinicians and acupuncture research
Sea-Band: http://www.sea-band.com/	A commercial product that stimulates PC6 for nausea and vomiting
Mayo Clinic: http://www.youtube.com/watch?v=XWdDMrS8WlA	You Tube video on acupuncture for nausea

References

References are available online at expertconsult.com.

109

Saline Nasal Irrigation

David Rabago, MD, and
Aleksandra Zgierska, MD, PhD

Saline nasal irrigation (SNI) is an adjunctive therapy for upper respiratory conditions that bathes the nasal cavity with saline delivered as a spray or liquid.[1,2] SNI likely originated centuries ago in the Ayurvedic medical tradition.[3] In the West, several administration devices, indications, and solutions for SNI were described in the *Lancet* in 1902.[4] Although the exact use prevalence is not known, the popularity of SNI has increased over time, in context of studies reporting positive effects in several upper respiratory conditions, as well as publicity in news and popular media outlets, including the Oprah Winfrey Show on television (May, 2007) and National Public Radio.[5] The most common method of liquid SNI is the so-called neti pot, which uses a gravity-based administration. Endorsement of SNI by physicians is common; in a survey of 330 family physicians, 87% reported recommending SNI to their patients for one or more conditions.[6]

Mechanism and Indications

The exact mechanism of SNI action is not known.[2] SNI may improve the nasal mucosa's immune response to infectious agents, inflammatory mediators, and irritants through several reported physiologic effects including direct cleansing by irrigation,[7-9] removal of inflammatory mediators,[10,11] and improved mucociliary function as demonstrated by increased ciliary beat frequency.[12,13] Chronic sinus symptoms (lasting more than 12 weeks) are the most common indications for SNI.[6] Based on positive results in clinical and functional outcomes, the Cochrane Collaboration concluded that SNI is appropriate adjunctive therapy for the symptoms of chronic rhinosinusitis.[2,14,15] Users of liquid SNI also reported significantly decreased antibiotic and nasal spray use.[1] These results were corroborated for liquid SNI, but not for nasal spray SNI.[15] Data for other indications are less rigorous, including irritant rhinitis,[16,17] viral upper respiratory infection,[18-20] allergic rhinitis,[21-23] and postoperative care after endoscopic sinus surgery,[24] although positive study results exist for each indication. SNI has been recommended by content experts for mild to moderate rhinitis of pregnancy,[25] acute rhinosinusitis,[26] sinonasal sarcoid,[27] and Wegener granulomatosis[28] (Table 109-1).

> Gravity liquid irrigation using a neti pot appears to be more effective than nasal spray irrigation for reducing antibiotic use in patients with recurring sinus infections.

Technique Variations

SNI can be performed using positive-pressure (spray or squirt bottle) or gravity-based pressure (a vessel with a nasal spout) devices (Fig. 109-1 in the Patient Handout). Each type of device is available over the counter. Saline is instilled in one nostril and is allowed to drain out the other.[2] Although liquid and spray SNI have both been assessed, liquid SNI is reported to be significantly more effective than spray SNI for chronic sinus symptoms[15] and allergic rhinitis.[11,21] Uniform recommendations regarding liquid versus spray SNI and other use-related variables are less evidence based for other indications. Ideal salinity of SNI for any given condition is not known; 0.9% to 3% saline solutions have been most often used. Similarly, optimal pH and temperature are not known.[2] Each may be patient specific,[22] and SNI has been reported

TABLE 109-1. Recommended Indications for Saline Nasal Irrigation

KEY CLINICAL RECOMMENDATIONS	EVIDENCE RATINGS*	REFERENCES
Nasal irrigation is effective adjunctive treatment for symptoms of chronic rhinosinusitis.	A	14 and 15
Nasal irrigation may be effective adjunctive treatment for symptoms of several other conditions based on limited trial evidence: irritant rhinitis or congestion, allergic rhinitis, viral upper respiratory congestion, and postoperative care after endoscopic sinus surgery.	B	16–24
Nasal irrigation has been recommended by content experts for mild to moderate rhinitis of pregnancy, acute rhinosinusitis, sinonasal sarcoid, and Wegener granulomatosis.	C	25–28

Adapted from Rabago D, Zgierska A. Saline nasal Irrigation for upper respiratory conditions. *Am Fam Physician.* 2009;80:1117–1119.
*A, consistent, good-quality patient-oriented evidence; B, inconsistent or limited-quality patient-oriented evidence; C, consensus, disease-oriented evidence, usual practice, expert opinion, or case series.

to be safe within the pH and temperature ranges used in the cited studies. In the United States, lukewarm tap water from municipal water systems or intact wells deeper than 40 feet seems safe for saline preparation; surface water should not be used for nasal irrigation. If these criteria are not met, or if potability is otherwise in doubt, boiled water cooled to room temperature, or distilled water, is recommended for saline preparation.

Recommended Dose for Treatment and for Prevention

The effective dose of SNI for treatment of chronic sinus symptoms in randomized controlled settings has been reported to be once[1] or twice[15] daily. Long-term use is less well known, but subjects with chronic sinus symptoms in one study stabilized their use of liquid SNI at approximately three times weekly for prevention of symptoms.[29] Recommendations for acute rhinosinusitis, upper respiratory infection, and rhinitis are more difficult to make. NSI once daily or spray saline up to three times daily has been reported to be safe.[20,30]

Safety

SNI appears safe. No study assessing SNI has reported any adverse events.[2] SNI is associated with frequent, minor side effects that are self-limited or resolve with practice or adjustment of the procedure.[1,15,22,31] Minor side effects include a sense of discomfort and nervousness with the first use of liquid SNI.[22] Side effects noted by fewer than 10% of SNI users include self-limited ear fullness, stinging of the nasal mucosa, and epistaxis (rare)[1,15,31]; these side effects were ameliorated by technique modification and salinity adjustment,[22] and they did not cause subjects to discontinue SNI.[1,15]

Practical Uses

SNI has been identified as "an important component in the management of most sinonasal conditions [that is] effective and underutilized."[32] Most interested patients with appropriate conditions would be considered appropriate for a trial of SNI. Examples of inappropriate patients include those with the potential to leak saline into unwanted tissue planes or spaces (e.g., incompletely healed facial trauma), patients with neurologic or musculoskeletal problems that could facilitate aspiration, or patients who otherwise cannot perform the procedure.

References

References are available online at expertconsult.com.

KEY WEB RESOURCES

University of Wisconsin Department of Family Medicine: http://www.fammed.wisc.edu/research/past-projects/nasal-irrigation

Guidelines on how to perform saline nasal irrigation and prepare saline solution, with directions available in English and Spanish

Patient Handout: Using Saline Nasal Irrigation for Upper Respiratory Conditions

Chronic sinus symptoms (nasal congestion, runny nose, or postnasal drip) are very common and have several potential causes and treatments. Saline nasal irrigation is a therapy you can do at home in addition to your current care plan for sinus symptoms. This technique improves symptoms by rinsing the area behind the nose with salt water. This handout describes how to perform saline nasal irrigation using a nasal cup, also known as a neti pot.
What you will need: A nasal cup and prepackaged salt are commercially available at many pharmacies.

Saline nasal irrigation has three steps.

Step 1: Mix the solution
- If you are using prepackaged salt, simply prepare the salt water as directed on the package. To make your own salt solution, measure 1 tsp of salt and 1/2 tsp of baking soda and stir into a pint (16 oz) of lukewarm water. Place 4 fluid oz (100 mL) in the nasal cup.

Step 2: Position the nasal cup (Fig. 109-1)
- Lean over a sink so you are looking directly into the basin.
- Rotate your head slightly and gently insert the spout of the nasal irrigation pot into the upper nostril so that it forms a comfortable seal. Do not press the spout against the "middle," or septum, of the nose.

Step 3: Irrigate the nose
- *Breathing through your mouth*, raise the nasal irrigation pot so that the solution enters the upper nostril. The solution will soon drain from the lower nostril.
- When the nasal pot is empty, gently exhale through both nostrils to clear them of excess solution and mucus. Gently blow your nose into a tissue.
- Repeat the procedure for the other nostril.

Nasal cup care: Mix new solution when you plan to irrigate your nose, and discard extra salt water immediately. Wash the nasal pot after irrigation.
Troubleshooting: You may notice some drainage of salt water up to 30 minutes after nasal irrigation; this is normal. Many users of nasal irrigation carry tissues. If stinging or burning occurs, try decreasing the salt content by half; you may also adjust the temperature of the water slightly. Do not use very hot or very cold water. Nasal irrigation can also be done in the shower.
Want more information? A more detailed patient handout (including a version in Spanish), instructions for making and adjusting salt water using bulk ingredients, instructional videos and links, scientific reports, and a radio story by National Public Radio (NPR) are at http://www.fammed.wisc.edu/research/past-projects/nasal-irrigation

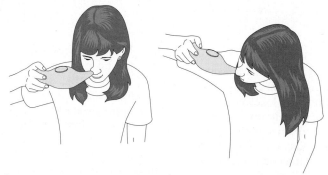

FIGURE 109-1
A common nasal irrigation technique using a nasal cup, or neti pot. Liquid saline is instilled in one nostril and is allowed to drain out the other. (From Rabago D, Zgierska A, Mundt M, et al. Efficacy of daily hypertonic saline nasal irrigation among patients with sinusitis: a randomized controlled trial. *J Fam Pract*. 2002;51:1049-1055.)

Redrawn from University of Wisconsin Department of Family Medicine *: Nasal irrigation instructions.* <http://www.fammed.wisc.edu/research/past-projects/nasal-irrigation>; Accessed 15.02.12.

Section V Bioenergetics

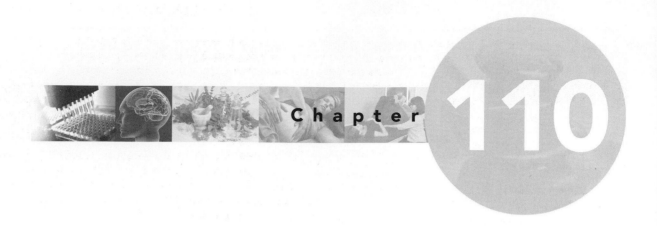

Chapter 110

Integrating Spiritual Assessment and Care

Gregory A. Plotnikoff, MD, MTS,
and Douglas E. Dandurand, PhD, MDiv

Spiritual and religious practices such as prayer represent the most prevalent complementary therapies in the United States. More than twice as many U.S. adults use prayer for health and healing than use herbal medicines.[1] Nearly 80% of U.S. adults believe that religion, to a large extent, helps patients and families cope with illness.[2] Nearly 75% of the public believes that praying for someone else can help cure his or her illness, and 56% of adults state that faith has helped them recover from illness, injury, or disease.[3] By definition, whole person medical care integrates the spiritual dimensions of the patient and the family.

Spirituality may or may not involve formal religion. Spirituality is subjective, complex, and fluid and therefore difficult to define or measure. Anandarajah[4] advanced our cognitive understanding of spirituality in his description of its three dimensions, based on answers from more than 800 health professionals to the question, "What does the word *spirituality* mean?" (Table 110-1). As a more formal definition, spirituality is a journey toward, or experience of, connection with the source of ultimate meaning. Spirituality includes connection with oneself, with others, with nature, and with a higher power. This connection is often with a greater story that makes sense of one's life.

In clinical settings, both spiritual support and spiritual distress demand professional attention. Spiritual beliefs are frequently important in medical decisions.[5] Spiritual well-being is closely linked to successful coping,[6] faster recovery,[7] and higher quality of life.[8] Many patients may want help with meaning, hope, or overcoming fears.[9] Unmet spiritual needs are associated with despair,[10] increased mortality,[11] and unnecessarily increased use of health care resources.[12] This last point is crucial for both primary and subspecialty care because it expands the differential diagnosis to consider in patients requiring frequent encounters with the health care system for ambiguous or nonspecific symptoms (Fig. 110-1).

U.S. adults consistently report that it is good for doctors to talk with patients about spirituality.[13,14] In 2004, 83% of 921 primary care patients surveyed in Ohio reported that they wanted physicians to ask about spiritual beliefs in certain circumstances, such as serious illness or loss of loved ones.[15] In response to the accumulating data on the importance of spirituality and health, the Joint Commission (formerly the Joint Commission for the Accreditation of Healthcare Organizations [JCAHO]) now requires that patients' spirituality be addressed as part of routine inpatient care.[16] Despite patients' interest and needs, however, a nationwide survey of 1,732,562 patients reported very low ratings of satisfaction with the emotional and spiritual aspects of care received.[17]

Integrative clinicians should be prepared to inquire about and engage patients in discussions of spirituality. To ignore the patient's source of meaning, purpose, richness, and direction places the physician at risk for providing inefficient, ineffective, and unsatisfactory care.[18] The challenge is to identify the best means of doing so.

Multiple mnemonics exist to guide physicians in their interviews. These include FICA,[19] HOPE,[20] and SPIRIT,[21] which are outlined in Box 110-1. These mnemonics highlight content and provide questions that may lead to important insights on care for the patient and family. For appropriate integration of spiritual assessment and care into clinical settings, this chapter identifies five practical goals. When these goals are addressed, three practical outcomes result: (1) improved diagnostic accuracy, (2) appropriately focused and directed resources, and (3) a strengthened therapeutic alliance.

TABLE 110-1. Three Dimensions of Spirituality: Head, Heart, and Hand

COGNITIVE	EXPERIENTIAL	BEHAVIORAL
Beliefs	Love, compassion, altruism, forgiveness	Duties: daily behavior, moral obligations
Values	Connection, relationship with: self, others, community, environment, nature, the transcendent	Choices: life choices, medical choices
Ideals	Inner energy, strength, resilience	Specific practices: prayer, meditation, yoga, chanting, rituals, diet, nature walks, etc.
Meaning	Inner peace, comfort, support	Participation in religious community
Purpose	Hope	
Truth	Faith (trust)	
Wisdom	Transcendence	
Faith (belief)		

From Anandarajah G. The 3 H and BMSEST models for spirituality in multicultural whole-person medicine. *Ann Fam Med.* 2008;6:448–458.

The Five Clinical Goals of Spiritual Assessment and Care

Clinical Goal 1: Anticipate the Presence of Religious and Spiritual Concerns in Both Adult and Pediatric Care

Spiritual and religious concerns in clinical care range from rituals or practices such as prayer to complex crises such as despair. Every illness is a potential spiritual crisis. This is true for the patient and family, as well as for the care team. These crises can be found in both acute care and chronic care, but they may be most easily seen in end-of-life care. For example, common spiritual or religious concerns at the end of life include the following:

- Not being forgiven by God

- Not reconciling with others

- Dying alone or cut off from God

- Not having a blessing from a family member or clergy person

- Wondering whether anyone will miss you or remember you over time[22]

Spiritual concerns can arise at any time. To recognize religious and spiritual concerns in others, one should be able to recognize them in oneself. Whole person health care

FIGURE 110-1

Unmet spiritual need cycle may result in increased demand and service use. (Redrawn from Grant L, Murray SA, Sheikh A. Spiritual dimensions of dying in pluralist societies. *BMJ.* 2010;341:c4859.)

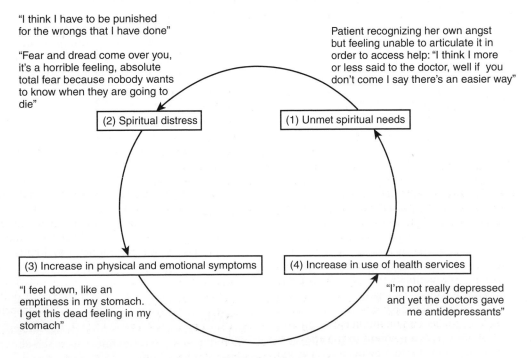

"I think I have to be punished for the wrongs that I have done"

"Fear and dread come over you, it's a horrible feeling, absolute total fear because nobody wants to know when they are going to die"

Patient recognizing her own angst but feeling unable to articulate it in order to access help: "I think I more or less said to the doctor, well if you don't come I say there's an easier way"

(2) Spiritual distress

(1) Unmet spiritual needs

(3) Increase in physical and emotional symptoms

(4) Increase in use of health services

"I feel down, like an emptiness in my stomach. I get this dead feeling in my stomach"

"I'm not really depressed and yet the doctors gave me antidepressants"

BOX 110-1. Spiritual Assessment Tools

FICA (Pulchaski et al*)
F: *Faith or belief:* What is your faith or belief?
I: *Importance and influence:* Is it important in your life? How?
C: *Community:* Are you part of a religious community?
A: *Awareness and addressing:* What would you want me as your physician to be aware of? How would you like me to address these issues in your care?

HOPE (Anandarajah and Hight†)
H: *Hope:* What are your sources of hope, meaning, strength, peace, love, and connectedness?
O: *Organization:* Do you consider yourself part of an organized religion?
P: *Personal spirituality and practices:* What aspects of your spirituality or spiritual practices do you find most helpful?
E: *Effects:* How do your beliefs affect the kind of medical care you would like me to provide?

SPIRIT (Maugans‡)
S: *Spiritual belief system:* What is your formal religious affiliation?
P: *Personal spirituality:* Describe the beliefs and practices of your religion or spiritual system that you personally accept or do not accept.
I: *Integration within a spiritual community:* Do you belong to a spiritual or religious group or community? What importance does this group have for you?
R: *Ritualized practices and restrictions:* Do you carry out specific practices as part of your religion or spirituality (e.g., prayer and meditation)? What significance do these practices or restrictions have to you?
I: *Implications for medical care:* What aspects of your religion or spirituality would you like me to keep in mind as I care for you?
T: *Terminal events planning:* As we plan for your care near the end of life, how does your faith affect your decisions?

*Data from Puchalski CM, Larson DB, Post SG. Physicians and patient spirituality. *Ann Intern Med.* 2000;133:748–749.
†Data from Anandarajah G, Hight E. Spirituality and medical practice: using the HOPE questions as a practical tool for spiritual assessment. *Am Fam Physician.* 2001;63:81–88.
‡Data from Maugans TA. The SPIRITual history. *Arch Fam Med.* 1996;5:11–16.

means proactively engaging the spiritual life, as opposed to waiting for a crisis to bring that awareness to light. Hence, all clinicians are challenged to develop self-awareness of their own spiritual history and perspectives.[23] In clinical care, the goal is to not to react to one's own spiritual needs or beliefs, but rather to acknowledge and bracket them and then respond to the patient's spiritual concerns. This occurrence of responding to the patient rather than to one's own emotional responses is termed being present.

Both culture and spirituality can be implicit and unconscious. Patients and physicians can be blind to the effects of their own perspectives in clinical interviewing and decision making. For this reason, health care professionals should begin by conducting cultural and spiritual assessments of themselves before they complete such assessments on patients. The most effective interviewing allows the patient's deeply held implicit and unconscious beliefs to be understood, acknowledged, and affirmed by the clinician. The clinical challenge is to create a safe and conducive setting in which spiritual concerns can be recognized and shared.

> Spirituality is about questions, not answers. The challenge is for health care professionals to step out of their role as answer givers and into their role as listeners.

When patients believe that they will not be judged, that someone will listen and not try to fix, dismiss, or deny their concerns, they often freely share their most private concerns. The sense of being heard is itself frequently therapeutic.

From an ethical viewpoint, physicians should maintain respect for their patients' beliefs and recognize patients' vulnerability to their own attitudes. No practitioner should impose his or her own religious, or antireligious, beliefs on patients.[24,25] All practitioners need to recognize that their answers are their answers only.

To address spiritual and religious concerns does not require specifically religious or spiritual questions. Good open-ended questions include the following:

- How else do you hurt?

- Serious illness can affect lives in many unexpected ways. How has this illness affected your life?

- What do you miss most or fear most as a result of this illness?

- What are some of the things you wish you could talk about? Is there anyone you wish you could talk to?

- What's most important to you right now?

The answers to such questions frequently reflect the patient's spiritual values and worldview, in addition to identifying important connections that have been disrupted.

Clinical Goal 2: Comprehend How Patients Want Their Religious or Spiritual Beliefs and Community to be Seen as Resources for Strength and Recovery

Faith and related religious worldviews may be considered medically relevant only when they obstruct implementation of scientifically sound biomedical care.[26] However, this attitude is profoundly naive. Every religion and cultural tradition has teachings, practices, and rituals that facilitate spiritual healing.[27]

> The challenge is not to seek omnicultural and spiritual competency, but rather to develop a humility that allows patients to teach about what is important to them.

Patients often display many clues that can be keys to the beginning of a conversation. For example, "Mrs. Xiong, I see that you have white and red strings tied around your wrist. Could you share with me their importance to you?" Such questioning would lead the health care professional into a deeper understanding of the patient's worldview and sources of strength. Such questioning would also prevent profound patient harm by accidental cutting and removal of sacred objects to make way for an intravenous placement or other biomedical intervention.

Related questions include the following:

- In the past, from where have you drawn the strength to cope with difficult situations?

- How can I be helpful regarding your spiritual concerns and practices?

- With regard to your care, what is most important to you?

The principal guideline in any such questioning is to listen for understanding, rather than to express agreement or disagreement.

Clinical Goal 3: Understand Better Your Patients' Subjective Experiences and Subjective Understanding of (Ultimate) Reality

Every effective health care professional is broadly familiar with the religious worldviews of the cultural groups within his or her patient population. Patients and their families can teach health care practitioners about the specifics. This is important because significant danger exists in extrapolating the truth for one patient of one cultural group and making it the truth for all such patients. This approach constitutes practice by stereotype (e.g., this patient is Hmong; therefore….). The challenge is to understand what *this* illness means for *this* particular patient.[28]

The following seven concepts and questions help guide the clinician's understanding:

1. How is ultimate health understood?
2. How are affliction and suffering understood?
3. What are the different parts of a person?
4. How is the patient's illness, sickness, or disease understood?
5. What intervention or care is believed necessary by the patient?
6. Who is seen as qualified to address the different parts that need healing?
7. What do the patient and family mean by efficacy or healing?

Given the frequently implicit and unconscious nature of the answers to these questions, these questions should be seen only as prompts or guides. Health care professionals should ask themselves whether they could answer these questions for their patients based on their interviews. Doing so directs interviewing toward the clinically relevant meaning of the illness for the patient. The response to an open-ended question such as "What do you fear most about surgery?" often leads to a dialogue that may help answer these questions. Should this information reveal a spiritual concern that cannot be addressed medically, further questioning can help identify the interventions that are needed and the persons who should perform them.

Clinical Goal 4: Determine What Impact, Positive or Negative, Your Patients' Spiritual Orientation Has on Their Health Problems and Perceived Needs

Although spirituality is frequently seen in a positive light, it also has a shadow side. The fourth edition of the *Diagnostic and Statistical Manual of Mental Disorders* (DSM-IV) added an axis IV concern: a religious or spiritual problem.[29] Examples cited include distressing experiences that involve loss or questioning of faith, problems associated with conversion to a new faith, or questioning of other spiritual values that may not necessarily be related to an organized church or religious institution.

When patients are asked about their sources of support, what worked previously may not be not perceived to be working at present. Spiritual distress is often exacerbated when a patient's understanding of his or her spiritual life and spiritual support conflicts with the religious beliefs of his or her faith tradition. For example, if the Source of Life (God) is feared or is understood as punishing, the person in distress has nowhere to turn and thus is at high risk for panic and despair. This situation often surfaces when patients hear a diagnosis of a life-threatening or life-changing illness.

In such cases, traditional spiritual sources of support, such as teachings, practices, and rituals, may paradoxically be barriers to spiritual well-being. For this reason, health care professionals are at risk for creating a sense of shame or guilt by denying, dismissing, or silencing doubts or theologic challenges. Examples of valid spiritual suffering include the following:

Spiritual Alienation
"Where is God now when I need Him most?"
"Why isn't He listening?"

Spiritual Anxiety
"Will I ever be forgiven?"
"Am I going to die a horrible death?"

Spiritual Guilt
"I deserve this."
"I am being punished by God."
"I didn't pray hard enough."

Spiritual Anger
"I'm mad at God."
"I blame God for this."
"I hate God."

Spiritual Loss
"I feel empty."
"I don't care anymore."

Spiritual Despair
"There's no way God could ever care for me."
"I'm just a corpse waiting to happen."[16]

When spirituality is understood as including connections with oneself, with others, with nature, and with God or a higher power, then spiritual suffering can be seen as resulting from the loss of such connections: betrayal by one's body, loss of social roles, dependence on technology, and theologic doubt or loss of faith. Healing therefore is the process of resolving such broken connections and recovering one's wholeness. The focus of healing is the human experience of illness. Healing can occur in any dimension: physical, emotional, social, and spiritual. Healing as the resolution of brokenness may or may not include curing disease. Healing is never quick or easy.

Frequently, when patients are diagnosed with a life-threatening or life-changing illness, they turn toward their God and pray for healing. Healing, in its truest sense of making whole, means personal (spiritual) growth and development through embracing the illness (or any other presenting issue) and discovering their God as a source of love in it.

"Healing" and "cure" are terms and intentions that, for many, if not most, people are used interchangeably and synonymously. Therefore, when one prays for healing, one may more truly be praying for cure. This lack of distinction between healing and curing is crucial for clinicians to understand because it addresses the patient's understanding of his or her relationship with their God or Source of Life. A person who prays for cure, which is not always possible, sets himself or herself up for an experience of disconnection with his or her God and may perceive that God as an abandoning God. This experience needs to be considered in the differential diagnosis of spiritual distress or despair.

Spiritual healing begins with recognition and acknowledgment of spiritual pain. For this reason, the American Academy of Hospice and Palliative Medicine's mnemonic LET GO can be quite helpful (Box 110-2).[30] The challenge here is to respond not as an expert with answers, but as a fellow human being also struggling to make sense of tragedy. Listening, acknowledging, and validating are means of connecting at a deep level and are the most profound means of strengthening the therapeutic alliance. This connection between clinician and patient is the foundation for healing. Without this connection, without listening to the patient at a deep level, referral of patients to professionals with expertise in pastoral care and counseling may be perceived as abandonment by these patients.

BOX 110-2. Spiritual Suffering Response Mnemonic

LET GO: American Academy of Hospice and Palliative Medicine
L: Listen to the patient's story.
E: Encourage the search for meaning.
T: Tell of your concern and acknowledge the pain of loss.
G: Generate hope whenever possible.
O: Own your own limitations, seek competence, and refer when appropriate

---

Generating hope whenever possible does not mean creating fake scenarios or deceiving patients. Generating hope means identifying what is important to the patient and working to achieve that. What constitutes hope and its shadow side, despair, changes throughout the course of an illness.

As with any medical referral, pastoral experts are available for assistance in understanding complex or difficult cases. Referrals can enhance the quality of care and, frequently, the patient's quality of life.

Clinical Goal 5: Determine Appropriate Referrals to Chaplains, Clergy, or Traditional Healers for Spiritual Care

Many spiritual concerns are addressed as a variation on the following questions: "Why? Why me? Why now?" Clearly, multiple members of the health care team can recognize the many varieties of such spiritual concerns in clinical settings. Even if time allows, however, these are not questions that should be answered by health care professionals. To do so is to risk harming patients. For every such question, the best answers are found, rather than given. The health care professional's role is to help give voice to such questions and to support the patient's search for answers.

Today, no member of a health care team needs to be a self-sufficient virtuoso. This is especially true when Clinical Pastoral Education (CPE)–trained chaplains are available in hospital settings. Chaplains offer well-tuned skills in listening for, and responding to, spiritual concerns in acute care settings. Furthermore, they can help identify when a spiritual guide (director) or a culture's spiritual healer (e.g., priest, pipe holder, or shaman) may be the most appropriate professional for a patient's spiritual concerns.

Professionally trained spiritual directors (guides) serve in outpatient settings. This setting allows the spiritual director to enter a long-term or more expansive relationship with the patient. Spiritual direction is emphatically not about giving preformed or formulaic answers. Spiritual directors are trained in the art of meeting the person where he or she is experiencing life. Spiritual direction ideally addresses integration of the *all* of life without judgment.

Care plans should identify a patient's spiritual resources, spiritual needs, and preferred spiritual care provider. Truly integrative medicine requires that a relationship be built between the physician and available chaplain services, thus leading to establishment of a network of local consultants and patient- or family-preferred spiritual care providers who can offer assistance.

THERAPEUTIC REVIEW

When spiritual assessment and care are integrated into clinical settings, three practical outcomes result: (1) improved diagnostic accuracy, (2) appropriately focused and directed resources, and (3) a strengthened therapeutic alliance. To achieve these outcomes, clinicians should consider integrating these eight summary points:

1. Mnemonics exist to guide inclusion of spirituality in clinical care. Expand the social history.
2. Spiritual needs can arise at any time or place. Anticipate them.
3. Spiritual healing begins with recognition and acknowledgment of spiritual pain. Listen intentionally.
4. Spirituality is about questions, not answers. Help voice the questions.
5. The best answers are found, rather than given. Support the search.
6. Care plans should include patients' spiritual needs, resources, and preferred spiritual care providers. Identify them.
7. Every religious tradition has teachings, practices, and rituals that are potential resources for strength and recovery. Integrate these into the care plan when appropriate.
8. Every illness is a potential spiritual crisis. Refer to pastoral care specialists (chaplains, clergy, spiritual directors) for assistance.

KEY WEB RESOURCES

Duke University Center for Spirituality, Theology and Health: http://www.spiritualityandhealth.duke.edu/

The center is focused on conducting research, training others to conduct research, and field-building activities related to religion, spirituality, and health.

George Washington Institute for Spirituality and Health (GWish): http://www.gwish.org/

GWish is working toward a more compassionate system of health care by restoring the heart and humanity of medicine through research, education, and policy work focused on bringing increased attention to the spiritual needs of patients, families, and health care professionals.

HealthCare Chaplaincy: http://www.healthcarechaplaincy.org

The multifaith HealthCare Chaplaincy is a national leader in the research, education, and practice of spirit-centered palliative care, which helps people with life-altering illness to live well and live fully.

References

References are available online at expertconsult.com.

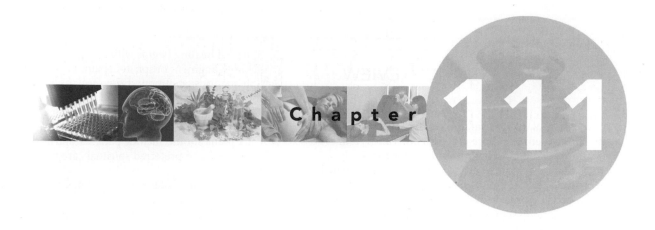

Chapter

111

Therapeutic Homeopathy

Paul E. Bergquist, MD

Why Homeopathy?

"When I was a medical student I felt sure that any one of us would have been ashamed to be caught looking into a homeopathic book by a professor. We had to sneer at homeopathy by word of command. Such was the school opinion then, and I imagine similar [sentiments]… exist in the medical schools today."[1]

So spoke William James, philosopher and physician, in 1898, when he made a plea to the Massachusetts legislature to support homeopathy. Medical practitioners today are no less skeptical about homeopathy than they were a century ago. Homeopathy is just as implausible, irrational, and misunderstood today as it was then.

How is it possible that homeopathic remedies containing infinitesimal amounts of active substance can cure illness? Proponents of homeopathy believe that the use of microdoses stimulates human defense and homeostatic self-regulatory mechanisms to resolve illness. Cure is possible in many acute and chronic diseases, some of which have little or no chance of cure in regular medicine. Despite a relative lack of scientific data to support its theory, homeopathy has been used safely and effectively by millions of people worldwide for more than 2 centuries.

What is Homeopathy?

Homeopathy is derived from the Greek words for "like" and "suffering." The guiding principle "likes cure likes" has its origins in ancient Egyptian medicine, as well as in Hippocratic medicine of the ancient Greeks, but the practice of homeopathy was codified by Samuel Hahnemann, a seventeenth-century German medical doctor. Disillusioned with the medical practices of his day, which included bloodletting, purging, cathartics, and cupping, Hahnemann decided to experiment with medicinal substances on himself.

He started with quinine, an herbal medicine known at the time to cure malaria:

"I took by way of experiment … four drams of good China (quinine). My feet, fingers, at first became cold; I grew languid and drowsy; then my heart began to palpitate, and my pulse grew hard and small; intolerable anxiety, trembling, prostration throughout all my limbs; then pulsation, in the head, redness of my cheeks, thirst, and, in short, all those symptoms which are ordinarily characteristic of intermittent fever, make their appearance. This paroxysm lasted two or three hours each time, and recurred if I repeated this dose, not otherwise; I discontinued it and was in good health again."[2]

This was the first proving of a homeopathic medicine, and it led Hahnemann to formulate the Law of Similars, which states that a remedy can cure a disease if it produces similar symptoms in a healthy person. Hahnemann also found that symptoms of poisoning by a drug were often the same as the symptoms of the disease cured by the drug. Hahnemann and his followers went on to prove hundreds of plant, mineral, animal, and disease substances. These symptoms were collected and catalogued in the Homeopathic Materia Medica, which today includes more than 2000 remedies. Each remedy has a full profile of mental, emotional, and physical pathologic symptoms. Homeopathic remedies are compiled in the Homeopathic Pharmacopeia of the United States, which is recognized by the U.S. Food and Drug Administration.

How Are Homeopathic Remedies Prepared?

Because many remedies are toxic in their crude form, Hahnemann attenuated the remedies by serial dilution and succussion, a process whereby the solution is struck on a pad a given number of times between dilutions. This process eliminated almost all the side effects of the crude substance. A 12 C potency, for example, is prepared by diluting 1 drop of the crude tincture in 99 drops of an alcohol-water solution, succussing it, and then taking a drop of that diluted solution and diluting it in another 99 drops of alcohol-water solution; this process is repeated 12 times to reach the 12 C, or 12 centesimal, potency. The decimal (X or D) potencies are diluted 1:9 and are considered less potent. Beyond a 12 C or 24X dilution, Avogadro's rule designates that not a single molecule of the original substance should remain in solution.[3] Paradoxically, however, in clinical practice, the higher the number of dilutions and succussions, the more potent the remedy. French scientists Jacques Benveniste et al[4] were able to demonstrate mast cell degranulation by a homeopathic dilution of immunoglobulin E antibodies in a laboratory setting, even at very high dilutions in which not a single molecule of immunoglobulin E remained in the solution. Because of its implausibility, their study, published in the scientific journal *Nature,* was rejected by the scientific community. However, the study was repeated 10 years later in a rigorous pan-European trial published in 1999. Again, the investigators demonstrated statistically significant results showing activity of hyperdilute solutions.[5]

Table 111-1 lists the common homeopathic potencies and their usual dosing methods.

How Do Homeopathic Remedies Work?

The exact mechanism by which homeopathic remedies work is unknown. The clinical success of homeopathy is often attributed to the placebo effect. Reilly and Taylor et al[6-9] conducted four double-blind placebo-controlled trials of homeopathy in the treatment of allergies and found that homeopathy was significantly more effective than placebo. These researchers concluded that either homeopathy works or the clinical trial was flawed. Since 1980, more than 190 controlled and 115 randomized trials of homeopathy have been performed. Several groups have conducted comprehensive meta-analyses of the entire body of data, results of which again suggest that homeopathy is more than a placebo-based approach.[10-12]

Transfer of bioelectric wave signatures from medicinal substances to water in hyperdilute solutions has been posited as a possible mechanism of the action of homeopathic remedies.[13] French virologist and Nobel Laureate Luc Montagnier et al[14] published a study showing that dilute solutions containing the DNA of pathogenic bacteria and viruses (including human immunodeficiency virus [HIV]), "could emit low frequency radio waves" that induced surrounding water molecules to become arranged into nanostructures. Once induced, these water molecules could then also emit radio waves. These investigators suggested that water could retain these properties even after the original DNA-containing solutions were ultradiluted to the point where no molecules of the original DNA remained (much like a diluted and potentized homeopathic remedy).[14]

TABLE 111-1. Common Homeopathic Potencies

COMMON POTENCIES	SERIAL CYCLES (OF DILUTION AND SUCCUSSION)	USUAL DOSING METHOD
6X	1:10 dilution 6 cycles	3–5 pellets every 5 min–every hr for acute illness
12X	1:10 dilution 12 cycles	3–5 pellets every 15 min–every 2 hr for acute illness
30X	1:10 dilution 30 cycles	3–5 pellets every 1–8 hr for subacute illness
6C	1:100 dilution 6 cycles	3–5 pellets every 5 min–every hr for acute illness
12C	1:100 dilution 12 cycles	3–5 pellets four times daily in acute case, or 5 pellets daily in chronic case
30C	1:100 dilution 30 cycles	3–5 pellets three times daily in acute case, or daily for 10 days in subacute case
200C	1:100 dilution 200 cycles	5 pellets every hr or daily in very acute case, 10 pellets once in chronic case
1M	1:100 dilution 1000 cycles	5 pellets every hr in severe acute case, 10 pellets once in chronic case
10M	1:100 dilution 10,000 cycles	5 pellets every hr in severe acute case, 10 pellets once in chronic case
50M	1:100 dilution 50,000 cycles	5 pellets daily in severe acute case, 10 pellets once in chronic case
CM	1:100 dilution 100,000 cycles	5 pellets daily in severe acute case, 10 pellets once in chronic case

How Are Homeopathic Medicines Prescribed?

When the body is threatened by harmful external forces, such as trauma, bacteria, and viruses, it produces symptoms such as fever, cough, and pain. These symptoms often reflect certain innate purposes: to inactivate bacteria or viruses, to carry off irritating byproducts of disease, and to force the individual to rest and recuperate. Although these symptoms may be uncomfortable for the patient, they represent a healthy reaction of the body's defense mechanisms. They are also the only true guides to individual manifestations of disease.

The homeopath, recognizing the individual as body, mind, and spirit, takes an extensive history of all physical, mental, and emotional symptoms. The location, quality, severity, frequency, and time of aggravation of symptoms are discovered. Underlying causes such as trauma, bereavement, change of job, abuse, and physical changes (pregnancy, teething, menarche, menopause) are important.

Amelioration or aggravation of symptoms, fears and phobias, food cravings and aversions, sex drive, and energy level are all considered. Body habitus, physiognomy, mannerisms, behavior, and psychological symptoms are examined. The homeopath is especially interested in unusual symptoms, or strange, rare, and peculiar symptoms.

The homeopath builds a complete picture of the pathologic features of the person in the course of taking the history and then attempts to find a remedy that most closely matches the whole picture of symptoms. In an acute case, the acute symptoms are primarily taken into account. In a chronic case, in what is often called constitutional prescribing, all symptoms, past and present, may help the homeopath find the right remedy.

The process of finding the correct remedy can be the most challenging aspect of the clinical practice of homeopathy. A homeopathic repertory of symptoms and a homeopathic materia medica are the two essential references for practicing homeopaths (Boxes 111-1 and 111-2). After the most important symptoms are elicited, a repertory of symptoms is consulted to see which remedies cover all or most of the important symptoms in the case. Those remedies are studied more closely in one or more of the materia medicas, which are encyclopedias of remedy characteristics and symptoms. The remedy that appears to match the pathologic features and essential nature of the case most accurately is given to the patient. Several remedies may match the case closely enough to stimulate the natural homeostatic mechanisms of the body to move toward cure. If the remedy chosen is not a close match to the case, it will do nothing for the symptoms.

Remedy Prescription

In acute illnesses, the remedy is usually given in lower potencies, such as 12 C or 30 C, three to five pellets by mouth every 5 to 60 minutes. If the remedy does not help the symptoms after four or five doses, a different remedy should be chosen.

In less acute illnesses, the remedy can be given three or four times a day for 1 to 2 days. If no improvement is noted, a different remedy is chosen.

Once improvement is noted, the remedy is given only when symptoms recur. In chronic illnesses, a higher potency, such as 200 C, is used once at the beginning of treatment. Symptoms are monitored over the next 1 to 2 months. If improvement is followed by relapse, the remedy is repeated once. If no improvement is noted, a different remedy is chosen. A patient who is taking other medications may need a daily dose of a lower potency (e.g., 12 C) after the initial 200 C to counter the interfering effects of the other medications.

Box 111-3 contains a list of several reputable homeopathic pharmacies.

For Which Conditions Can Homeopathic Treatments be Used?

Many conditions, chronic and acute, can be effectively treated with a homeopathic approach. They include pediatric problems, such as recurrent otitis media,[15–17] pharyngitis,

BOX 111-3. Small Sample of Reputable Homeopathic Pharmacies

Boericke & Tafel, Inc.: 2381 Circadian Way, Santa Rosa, CA 95407; telephone: 707-571-8202; fax: 707-571-8237

Boiron-Bornemann, Inc.: Box 449, 6 Campus Avenue, Building A, Newtown Square, PA, 19073; telephone: 800-BLU-TUBE

Hahnemann Laboratories, Inc.: San Rafael, CA 94901; telephone: 888-4-ARNICA; fax, 415-451-6981

Helios Homeopathic Pharmacy: 97 Camden Road, Tunbridge Wells, Kent, TN1 2QR, United Kingdom; telephone 01892-537 254

Homeopathic Educational Services: 2124 Kittredge Street, Berkeley, CA 94704; telephone: 510-649-0294; fax: 510-649-1955

Standard Homeopathic Company: Box 61067; 204-210 West 131st Street, Los Angeles, CA 90061; telephone: 800-624-9659

Washington Homeopathic Products: 260 Hawvermale Way, Berkeley Springs, WV 25411; telephone 800-336-1695

TABLE 111-2. Remedies for Teething

REMEDY*	INDICATION	BETTER FROM/IN	WORSE FROM/IN
Calcarea Carbonica	Constipation, delayed teething, milk intolerance	Heat	Cold, wet, dairy products
Chamomile	Irritability, screaming, capriciousness	Being carried, rocked hard, car ride	Night, heat, being held still
Pulsatilla	Weepiness, whining	Gentle rocking, being held	Overheated, stuffy room
Nux Vomica	Irritability, burping, gas	Nap, evening	Morning

*All doses 12C to 30C; three pellets given every hour as needed in the cheek. If no improvement is seen after four to five doses, choose another remedy.

TABLE 111-3. Remedies for Colic

REMEDY*	INDICATION	BETTER FROM/IN	WORSE FROM/IN
Chamomile	Irritability, being cross	Being carried, being rocked hard	Open air, night
Calcarea Carbonica	Sweaty head, plumpness	Dry, warm	Cold, wet
Colocynthis	Doubling up, distended abdomen	Firm pressure, heat, bending legs up	Anger, eating, drinking

*All doses 12C to 30C; three pellets given every hour as needed in the cheek. If no improvement is seen after four to five doses, choose another remedy.

attention deficit hyperactivity disorder,[18] enuresis,[19] constipation, diarrhea,[20] asthma, allergic rhinitis, eczema,[7,21,22] juvenile arthritis, chronic bronchitis, and recurrent pneumonia. Adult problems well treated by homeopathy include anxiety,[23] bruising and ecchymosis from trauma and surgery,[24-26] poisonings,[27] anemia,[28] acquired immunodeficiency syndrome/HIV infection,[29,30] insomnia,[31,32] vertigo,[33] tinnitus,[34] depression,[23,35,36] bipolar disorder, headaches,[37] gastroesophageal reflux disease, colitis, Sjögren syndrome,[38] rheumatoid arthritis,[39,40] heart disease,[41] multiple sclerosis (management and arrest of progression), perimenopausal symptoms,[42,43] fibromyalgia,[44] chronic fatigue syndrome,[45] infertility,[46] dysmenorrhea,[47,48] postoperative ileus,[49] chronic or recurrent urinary tract infection, trigeminal neuralgia,[50] psoriasis,[51] numerous other dermatologic conditions,[52,53] influenza,[54,55] snoring,[56] and chronic cough. Traditionally, homeopathy has been used effectively for the treatment of epidemics; during certain cholera epidemics and severe influenza epidemics, homeopathy was significantly more effective than any of the allopathic approaches to management.

In a study funded by the Cuban government, Bracho et al[57] created a homeopathic preparation of four strains of *Leptospira* and administered it to 2.3 million people at high risk during an epidemic of leptospirosis in Cuba. A significant decrease in the disease incidence was observed in the intervention regions. No decrease was noted in the regions where no remedy was administered. The epidemic was controlled, and the incidence of leptospirosis fell below the usual levels.[57]

Classical homeopaths use constitutional prescribing for chronic disease and complicated cases. Although most health care practitioners will probably not want to prescribe constitutionally, homeopathy may be used in a cookbook fashion to achieve results in many acute illnesses and some chronic illnesses. Tables 111-2 through 111-5 list some of the commonly used remedies for various problems.[58]

Otitis Media

Acute and chronic recurrent otitis media responds well to homeopathic remedies.[17] Acute otitis media often improves without treatment over 3 to 5 days. Antibiotics can often be avoided, and the appropriate homeopathic remedy will sometimes speed healing and prevent recurrence (Table 111-6).

Sinusitis

Several remedies are appropriate for acute sinusitis[59] (Table 111-7). Chronic or recurrent sinusitis can be treated by referral to a classical homeopath for constitutional treatment. Referral to an ear, nose, and throat consultant may be helpful to rule out more serious disorders.

Allergies, Asthma, and Atopic Eczema

Allergic rhinitis, asthma, and atopic eczema can be cured over several years with a constitutional classical homeopathic approach. Referral of a patient with such a problem to

TABLE 111-4. Remedies for Severe Brain Injury and Mild Traumatic Brain Injury*

Severe acute head trauma[†]	Arnica	10 M–100 M (CM)	5 pellets (oral/axilla/buccal mucosa), every 15 min in the first 12–24 hours, then every day for 10–30 days Decrease frequency of dose as patient improves Continue through rehabilitation
Chronic effects of head trauma (posttraumatic brain injury)	Suggest constitutional homeopathic therapy (e.g., Arnica, Calcarea Carbonica, Cicuta, Helleborus, Natrum Sulphuricum, Opium Silica)	200 C–1 M	5 pellets once; repeated as necessary if improvement is followed by relapse

*Homeopathic remedies have been used for acute severe concussion and intracranial hemorrhage as adjunctive therapy to neurosurgical approaches and in posttraumatic brain injury for speeding rehabilitation.[58]
[†]Homeopathic treatment would be adjunctive therapy to a hospital intensive care unit protocol for treatment of head injury.

TABLE 111-5. Remedies for Acute Injury and Emergencies

INDICATIONS	REMEDY	POTENCY	DOSE
Shock	Arnica	200 C or up to 50 M	5 pellets PO every 5 min–every day
Shock with fear	Aconite	200 C or up to 50 M	5 pellets PO every 5 min–every day
Head injury	Arnica	200 C or up to 50 M	As above; the more severe the trauma, the more frequently repeated and the higher the potency
Blow to spine or whiplash	Hypericum	200 C or up to 50 M	5 pellets PO every 5 min–every day
Trauma with bleeding, bruising, contusion, laceration	Arnica Hypericum	30 C or up to 200 C 30 C or up to 200 C	As above; remedies may be given concurrently
Eye injury	Aconite	30 C–200 C	5 pellets PO every 5 min–every day
Black eye	Ledum	30 C–200 C	As above
Cut nerves, crush injuries	Hypericum, Arnica	30 C–200 C	As above; may give concurrently
Fractures	Arnica, Symphytum, Ledum	200 C	5 pellets of each daily for 10–14 days
Puncture wounds	Ledum	30 C–200 C	5 pellets PO every 5 min–every day, depending on severity
Bites, bee stings	Apis, Ledum	As above	As above
Muscle, ligament, and joint sprains and strains	Arnica, Ruta	30 C-200 C	5 pellets PO three times daily for 10–14 days
Chronic sprains or strains	Rhus Toxicodendron	30 C or 200 C	5 pellets daily for 7–10 days or 10 pellets one dose once
Burns First-degree Second-degree Third-degree Sunburn	Calendula Urtica Urens Causticum Urtica Urens Hypericum Cantharis, Hypericum Belladonna	Topical oil, lotion 30 C 30 C 30 C–200 C 30 C–200 C, topical 30 C–200 C 30 C	Apply to burn 5 pellets PO every 5 min prn 5 pellets PO every 5 min prn 5 pellets PO every 5 min prn Tincture dilute 1:3 in water 5 pellets PO every 5 min prn 5 pellets PO every 5 min prn
Heatstroke: hot, red, dry	Antimonium Crudum, Belladonna,	30 C–200 C	5 pellets every 15 min prn
Throbbing headache	Glonoine	30 C–200 C	As above
Electrical burns	Phosphorus	30 C–200 C	5 pellets PO three times daily prn

TABLE 111-5. Remedies for Acute Injury and Emergencies—cont'd

INDICATIONS	REMEDY	POTENCY	DOSE
Epistaxis	Phosphorus	30 C–200 C	5 pellets PO every 5 min prn
Blood, fluid loss	China Officinalis	30 C–200 C	As above
Dental extraction with blood loss	Phosphorus	30 C–200 C	As above
Syncope, collapse	Carbo Vegetabilis	30 C–200 C	5 pellets PO every 5 min prn
Food poisoning	Arsenicum Album	30 C	5 pellets PO every 5 min prn
Mucus, vomiting	Ipecac	30 C	5 pellets PO every 5 min prn

PO, orally; prn, as needed.

TABLE 111-6. Remedies for Otitis Media

REMEDY*	INDICATIONS	BETTER FROM/IN	WORSE FROM/IN
Aconite	Sudden onset, high fever, restlessness, being hot, dry, thirsty, or fearful	Open air, rest	Night, warm room, noise, cold wind, teething, touch
Belladonna	Red face, being hot, right ear, throbbing pains, high fever	Sitting up, wrapping up in warm room	Light, getting head wet or cold, teething, 3 AM–3 PM
Calcarea Carbonica	Thick discharge from ear, decreased hearing	Warmth, dryness, lying, massage	Cold, wet, exertion, teething, milk
Chamomile	Being cross, screaming in pain, pushing people away	Being carried rapidly, warm weather	Wind, 10 PM–10 AM, teething, cold, being looked at
Ferrum Phosphoricum	Early stages, gradual onset, pallor	Cold applications, touch, cold drinks	Night, motion, noise, right side, warm drinks
Hepar Sulphuris	Great sensitivity to pain, fits of screaming	Warmth, warm applications	Hating to be examined, cold, drafts of air
Lachesis	Rare, extreme pain, left ear, pharyngitis	Open air, discharge, loosening clothes	After birth of second child/ jealousy, wind, tight clothes
Mercurius Vivus	Sickly child status, precociousness, foul discharge, salivation at night, pus in ears	Rest, morning	Night, warmth of bed, being too hot or too cold, being held
Pulsatilla	Weepiness, sensitivity, thick yellow discharge, left ear	Wanting to be held, carried, or comforted; open air, lying on painful side	Twilight, after eating, warm stuffy room, left side, fat-rich food
Silica	Constipation, being chilly, ruptured eardrum with watery or cheesy discharge, sweaty feet	Rest (fatiguing easily), warmth, covering up	Milk, teething, cold air, night, combing hair, touch

*All remedies are 12C or 30C; three pellets are given every 5 minutes to every hour as needed until better. If no improvement is seen after four to five doses, choose another remedy.

a classical homeopath is recommended. Asthma and eczema symptoms are not always easily palliated, and the constitutional homeopathic approach, combined with steroid and bronchodilator inhalers and minimal use of steroid creams, is recommended. Allergic rhinitis symptoms, conversely, can be alleviated in a palliative manner.[9] Table 111-8 lists some of the more common remedies for palliation of these problems.[60,61]

Chronic Bronchitis

For cough that persists after all other causes—infections, asthma, allergies, neoplasms, chronic obstructive pulmonary disease, and gastroesophageal reflux disease—have been ruled out and empirical therapy has failed, the homeopath can prescribe Ignatia 200 C once or Ignatia 30 C daily for 7 days. If emotional trauma or loss precedes the cough, this remedy is especially indicated.

TABLE 111-7. Remedies for Sinusitis

REMEDY*	INDICATIONS†	BETTER FROM/IN	WORSE FROM/IN
Arsenicum Album	Burning nasal discharge, restlessness, anxiety	Warm drinks, hot applications, food, lying head up	Midnight or after, cold, exertion, ice, draft, tobacco
Hepar Sulphuris	Pain at root of nose, sensitivity, irritability, stuffy nose, later stage	Warmth, wrapping up, eating	Cold draft of air, touch, lying on painful side
Hydrastis	Thick, yellow discharge from posterior nares, nose sores, bloody crusts	Pressure, warm wraps, dry weather, rest	Inhaling cold air, night, open air, motion
Kali Bichromicum	Most common sinus remedy, pain in maxillae and bridge of nose, thick stringy discharge, stuffy nose	Heat, pressure, motion	Cold, damp air, undressing, 2–3 AM, alcohol, after sleep
Mercurius Vivus	Raw nostrils, ulcers, bloody discharge, hurried, bad breath	Moderate temperatures, rest, morning	Night, extremes of temperature, heat, drafts, lying on right side
Natrum Muriaticum	Fluent white nasal discharge, violent sneezing	Rest, open air, lying on right side, massage	Heat of sun, morning, emotions, exertion, consolation, touch
Nux Vomica	Snuffling, stuffiness, impatience, anger, feeling chilly, sneezing on waking	Rest, allowing discharge freely, hot drinks, evenings	Uncovering, coffee, alcohol, drugs, morning, overeating, pressure of clothes
Pulsatilla	Ripe cold with yellow mucus, loss of smell, weepiness, clinginess	Gentle exercise, open air, weeping, massage	Warm and stuffy room, beds, rich fatty food, time before or during menses
Silicea	Dry nose crusts, sensitive nasal bones	Warmth, warm wraps, summer, wet weather	Cold air, noise, light, confrontation, talking, mental exertion

*All remedies are three pellets, 12C or 30C, given every 2 to 4 hours as needed until better. If no improvement is seen after four to five doses, choose another remedy

TABLE 111-8. Remedies for Allergic Rhinitis

REMEDY*	INDICATIONS†	BETTER FROM/IN	WORSE FROM/IN
Allium Cepa	Bland eye tearing, sneezing, excoriating nasal discharge	Open air, cold room, cold water, motion	Warm room, wet feet, evening, spring, damp weather
Arsenicum Album	Burning eye and nasal discharge, thin mucus, feeling chilly, restlessness	Heat, hot applications, hot drinks, motion, lying with head elevated	Midnight or after, sight or smell of food, cold drinks, alcohol
Arundo	Itching inside nose, palate, or ear canals; salivation with runny nose	Desire for sour foods, drinking	Urination
Arum Triphyllum	Raw sores in nostrils, excoriating discharge, stuffy nose, mouth breathing	Warmth	Talking, overuse of voice, cold wet wind
Euphrasia	Profuse burning tears, bland nasal discharge, eyes filled with tears, red eyes	Winking, wiping eyes, dark, open air, coffee	Night, lying down, wind, sunlight, warmth, indoors
Galphimia Glauca[13]	Sneezing, hives, cold sores, skin allergy, eyelid edema		Weather changes
Natrum Muriaticum	Watery white nasal discharge, cold sores, sneezing, cracked lip, headache	Fresh air, cool bath, thirst, sweating, skipping meals	Heat, sun, light, 9–11 AM, time after menses, warm room, consolation, grief, loss
Nux Vomica	Violent sneezing in spells, daytime runny nose with nighttime stuffiness	Indoors, warmth, hot drinks	Outside, cold air, drafts, coffee, stimulants, alcohol, overwork

TABLE 111-8. Remedies for Allergic Rhinitis—cont'd

REMEDY*	INDICATIONS†	BETTER FROM/IN	WORSE FROM/IN
Sabadilla	Sneezing in spells, exhaustion, tickling in nose, red burning eyelids, dry mouth	Warmth, warm drinks, open air, eating	Cold air, cold drinks, odors (especially flowers), sneezing
Wyethia	Tremendous itching of upper palate, dry mouth	Clucking palate, swallowing saliva	Afternoon, eating, exercise, motion
Homeopathic combination remedies	Many over-the-counter preparations available; can be used for generic rhinitis symptoms		
House dust mite remedy†	Used if dust mite allergy is known		

*All remedies are three pellets, 12 C to 30 C, every 2 to 4 hours as needed until better.
†Data from Lewith GT, Watkins AD, Hyland ME, et al. Use of ultramolecular potencies of allergen to treat asthmatic people allergic to house dust mite: double blind randomized controlled clinical trial. *BMJ*. 2002;324:520–523.

Cancer

Homeopathic remedies are used in cancer to stimulate the immune system and for palliation of symptoms.[62-64] They can also be used to reduce the side effects of cancer treatment.

Calendula 30 C or Fluoric Acid 30 C at a dose of five pellets every 4 hours daily or Calendula ointment applied two times a day after radiation treatment has been found to be highly effective for prevention of grade 2 or higher acute dermatitis in patients with breast cancer.[65] Radiation-induced itching in such patients can also be treated with several other remedies, including Causticum, Ignatia, Kali Bichromicum, Psorinum, Rhus Toxicodendron, and Gamma Ray.[66]

Radium Bromatum 30 C, five pellets once or three times daily, can be used for other side effects of radiation therapy, such as Lhermitte sign, nonhealing burns or ulcers, postradiation pain and myalgias, fatigue, and other skin problems.

Gastrointestinal Disorders

Table 111-9 lists common remedies for gastrointestinal disorders.[20,67]

Obstetrics

Homeopathic remedies are well suited to pregnancy. The remedies have no side effects and can be safely prescribed for various prenatal difficulties, including miscarriage, morning sickness, heartburn, headaches, constipation, induction of labor[68] and preeclampsia, as well as postpartum problems such as hemorrhage,[69] mastitis, depression, and newborn nursing difficulties[70] (Table 111-10).

TABLE 111-9. Remedies for Acute Gastrointestinal Disorders

REMEDY*	INDICATIONS†	BETTER FROM/IN	WORSE FROM/IN
Arsenicum Album	Diarrhea, vomiting, thirst for small sips, cramping, blood in stool or emesis	Heat, warm drinks, lying with head up, company, rest	Eating, spoiled food, cold drinks, spicy food, right side, cold
Cantharis	Burning stool, burning pains, blood in stools or emesis	Belching, flatus, warmth, rest, rubbing	Drinking liquids, coffee
Croton Tiglium	Gushing watery diarrhea, vesicular rash, loud gurgling, sloshing intestines	Time after sleep, gentle rubbing	Drinking or eating least amount, touch, motion, summer, washing
Carbo Vegetabilis	Feeling chilly, indigestion, gas, bloating, belching	Belching, fanning, cold, bending over double	Eating, evening, lying down, wine, warmth, rich food
China	Gas that will not come up or down, belching that gives no relief, indigestion	Bending double, hard pressure, open air, warmth	Light touch, night, eating, drafts, every other day
Colocynthis	Vomiting, diarrhea, with severe cramps, doubling up with pain	Warmth, pressure, rest, after stool	Anger, indignation, drafts, taking cold

Continued

TABLE 111-9. Remedies for Acute Gastrointestinal Disorders—cont'd

REMEDY*	INDICATIONS†	BETTER FROM/IN	WORSE FROM/IN
Gelsemium	Green or white diarrhea, heaviness of limbs and eyelids, tremor	Motion, profuse urination, bending forward, sweating	10 AM, anticipation, thinking of ailment, emotion, shock, humid weather
Ipecac	Continuous nausea and vomiting, increased salivation	Rest, open air, pressure, cold drinks, motion	Food smells, vomiting, warmth of room, overeating
Lycopodium	Indigestion, bloating, rumbling gas, heartburn, craving for sweets	After midnight, warm food and drink, uncovering, getting cool	Lying on right side, 4–8 AM, cold drinks, warm room, pressure of clothes
Nux Vomica	Constipation, vomiting, nausea	Evening, nap, warmth, wrapping head, hot drinks	Overindulgence, morning, spicy food, stimulants, narcotics, cold open air
Phosphorus	Vomiting, hematemesis, thirst for cold water	Cold, eating, sleep, cold food and water, dark	Warm food and drink, touch, evening, light, wind, odors, emotion
Podophyllum	Painless gushing diarrhea, colic, flatus, offensive odor	Massage over liver, lying on abdomen	Morning, teething, hot weather, eating, drinking, milk
Pulsatilla	Indigestion, heartburn, weepiness	Open air, motion, cold applications	Rich fatty food, time after eating, warm room
Sulfur	Constipation, diarrhea, burning anus with itching, large hard stools	Open air, lying on right side, dry heat, walking, drawing up limbs	Bathing, standing, warmth of bed, being overheated, suppressed symptoms

*All remedies are three pellets, 12C to 30C, every 2-4 hours as needed until better.
†Data from Jacobs J, Jonas WB, Jimenez-Perez M, Crothers D. Homeopathy for childhood diarrhea: combined and metaanalysis from three randomized, controlled clinical trials. *Pediatr Infect Dis J.* 2003;22:229–234.

TABLE 111-10. Remedies for Obstetrics

INDICATION	REMEDY	POTENCY	DOSE
Induction of labor	Caulophyllum with Blue Cohosh tincture or capsules	30C–200C One dropperful or one capsule alternating with Caulophyllum every 2 hr	5 pellets every 2 hr for five doses. Repeat next day if no labor. If no labor after 2 days, wait for several days before repeating
Turning a breech baby	Pulsatilla	30C–CM	5 pellets one dose
Weak, exhausted labor, rigid os, poor contractions	Gelsemium	30C	5 pellets every 5–10 min for four doses
Ineffectual labor, lack of dilation, no progress	Caulophyllum	30C	5 pellets every 5–10 min for four doses
Arrested labor with shooting pains and cramps in thighs	Cimicifuga	30C	5 pellets every 5–10 min for four doses
Back labor, occiput posterior position	Kali Carbonicum	30C	5 pellets every 5–10 min for four doses
Fainting, desire for cool air, labor with poor progress, weepiness	Pulsatilla	30C	5 pellets every 5–10 min for four doses
Fear, anxiety during labor	Aconite	30C	5 pellets every 5–10 min as needed
Retained placenta	Cantharis, Sepia	30C	5 pellets every 5–10 min for two doses of one remedy. If no results, try the other remedy
Completion of a miscarriage	Cimicifuga. Take with tinctures of Blue and Black Cohosh	200C–1M 1 dropperful of each	5 pellets once, with tinctures orally every 2–4 hr until bleeding slows and tissue passes

Conclusion

Homeopathy is a safe and effective tool that can be integrated into a practicing clinician's armamentarium as either first-line therapy or adjunctive treatment. It is relatively free of adverse side effects, enhances the body's ability to restore balance, is curative in some diseases that would otherwise be managed only with allopathic medicine, speeds healing in adjunctive approaches, and is inexpensive. Homeopathy has survived the ultimate test of any medical therapy—the test of time in the field of clinical practice. Perhaps elucidation of an underlying mechanism of action that can be understood in scientific terms will return homeopathy to a more prominent role in common clinical practice in the future.

KEY WEB RESOURCES

American Institute of Homeopathy (AIH): www.homeopathyusa.org	This is the principal professional organization of licensed medical practitioners who are practicing homeopaths. The Institute publishes a quarterly journal for practitioner members.
National Center for Homeopathy (NCH): www.nationalcenterforhomeopathy.org	This national organization of lay and professional homeopaths is one of the primary homeopathic associations in the United States. It is dedicated to providing information on postgraduate training in homeopathy and dissemination of homeopathic educational materials and resources.
Homeopathic Educational Services: www.homeopathic.com	Homeopathic Educational Services is a retail outlet for homeopathic books, tapes, remedies, software, and educational materials. This site also includes the *Homeopathic Family Medicine eBook,* by Dana Ullman, MPH, a review of homeopathic treatment for numerous clinical problems with associated footnoted references.
Whole Health Now homeopathy software: www.wholehealthnow.com/homeopathy_software/index.html; and Kent Homeopathic Associates: www.kenthomeopathic.com/referenceworks.html	These computer programs contain materia medica designed to help match a remedy to specific symptoms from the entire homeopathic database.

KEY RESOURCES FOR FURTHER STUDY

Coulter H. *Divided Legacy.* Washington, DC: McGrath; 1973.	A comprehensive history of homeopathy
Dean ME. *The Trials of Homeopathy.* York, UK: University of York; 2001.	A review of all the clinical research conducted on homeopathy from the early 1800s to the present
Herscu P. *The Homeopathic Treatment of Children.* Berkeley, CA: North Atlantic Books; 1991.	A review of some of the most often used remedies for a variety of common pediatric illnesses
Morrison R. *Desktop Companion to Physical Pathology.* Nevada City, CA: Hahnemann Clinic Publishing; 1998.	A concise desk reference written for physicians to aid in remedy selection for a group of common disorders
Panos M, Heimlich J. *Homeopathic Medicine at Home: Natural Remedies for Everyday Ailments and Minor Injuries.* Los Angeles: Jeremy P. Tarcher; 1990.	A resource for patients and practitioners in choosing remedies for common acute ailments at home
Perko S. *Homeopathy for the Modern Pregnant Woman and Her Infant.* Berkeley, CA: Benchmark Homeopathic; 1997.	A practical guide for using homeopathy in obstetrics and neonatal care
Ramakrishnan AU, Coulter C. *A Homeopathic Approach to Cancer.* St. Louis: Quality Medical; 2001.	A homeopathic adjunctive approach to the treatment of cancer
Sankaran R. *Soul of Remedies.* Mumbai: Homeopathic Medicals; 1997.	A description of the constitutional nature of a selected group of remedies by an experienced homeopath
Ullman D. *Homeopathic Family Medicine eBook.* Homeopathic Educational Services: www.homeopathic.com; 2010.	A review of homeopathic treatment for a wide variety of clinical problems with associated footnoted references

References

References are available online at expertconsult.com.

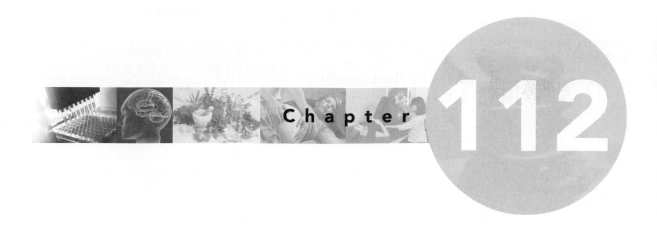

Chapter 112

Human Energetic Therapies

J. Adam Rindfleisch, MD, MPhil

We are surrounded by energy and vibration, and in truth, physics informs us that we ourselves *are* energy and vibration. One of the best-known of all physics equations, e = mc², defines a link, albeit challenging to describe without the use of mathematics, between energy and matter. We perceive photons, which behave as both particles and waves, as our sense of sight. We are aware of vibrations in the air as sound. Even our most basic sense, touch, is fundamentally based in the interactions among fields. Matter is mostly space that contains (or perhaps gives rise to) a smattering of subatomic particles that influence one another through mysterious forces of attraction and repulsion. The nature of the links among energy, physical reality, and consciousness is one of the great mysteries of our times.

How may these concepts of physics—vibrations, fields, and energy—inform healing? Dozens, if not hundreds, of different cultures and traditions have words referring to a life force that animates living things. Examples include chi, prana, pneuma, fohat, mana, and orgone. Many people within these cultures have suggested the possibility both to perceive and to manipulate this life force. Human energetic therapies have been practiced for millennia.

In the first section of this chapter, key concepts of energy medicine are introduced, and some of the most commonly used human energetic therapies are described. Research related to human energetic therapies is then summarized, and suggestions are offered on how health care providers can work collaboratively with energy medicine practitioners.

The final section is for those practitioners who are interested in exploring energy medicine in greater depth through their own experience. Exercises that can be incorporated into any form of integrative practice are described, and the reader is offered additional resources for further exploration.

One caveat: Energy medicine is perhaps one of the most mysterious and controversial of all forms of therapy. At the time of this chapter's writing, whether the National Institutes of Health will continue to fund research in this area is unclear. Even for some of the most objective of scientists, the topic of energy medicine strikes a highly emotional chord.

As integrative medicine providers explore the use of these therapies, the concept of "scope of practice" takes on a new meaning. At some point, every integrative provider will be required to determine his or her stance regarding the validity and utility of these approaches.

Of course, a textbook chapter can offer only a taste of this varied and complex array of therapies. Trying to understand energy medicine solely by reading about it is akin to trying to appreciate a Beethoven symphony without ever having heard it. The reader is strongly encouraged to learn and explore through direct experience.

> Truly learning about human energetic therapies requires one to experience them firsthand.

Defining Energy Medicine

The National Center for Complementary and Alternative Medicine classifies human energetic therapies according to whether the energy they profess to manipulate is (1) veritable (dealing with forms of energy that can be measured in a laboratory) or (2) putative (held by most, although not all, researchers as not being measurable with current technology).[1] The approaches described in this chapter are typically classified as putative—or subtle—energy therapies, but many practitioners claim to have measured these energies through different means.[2]

According to the 2007 National Health Information Survey, at least 0.5% of the U.S. population had used some form of energy medicine in the past year.[3] A 2002 study by the Centers for Disease Control and Prevention found that 0.5% of respondents had used qi gong and 1% had used Reiki.[4] Surveys may underestimate energy medicine's use because practitioners of other modalities, such as massage therapists, chiropractors, and naturopathic doctors, commonly blend energy medicine into their practices without labeling what they are doing as energy medicine per se. More than 50 hospitals and clinics in the United States offer some form of biofield therapy to their patients.[5]

Many different schools, or styles, of human energetic therapies exist, especially if one includes the various shamanic techniques that have arisen in many of the world's indigenous cultures. *The Encyclopedia of Energy Medicine* identifies nearly 50 popular approaches used in the United States.[6]

Although various approaches to energy medicine may work with different aspects, or parts, of the energy field or enlist different techniques for manipulating or maneuvering energy, most share some common elements[7]:

- They assume the presence of an energetic anatomy, or pattern, that has an influence on health. Common examples include the chakra system, the aura, and the meridian system used in acupuncture. Some schools of thought propose the existence of several different layers, or levels, of the energy body, each with unique characteristics. Because the chakra system is intrinsic to most techniques, and because it is often referenced by integrative medicine patients, it is described in more detail, in Table 112-1.

- Patterns in the energy body may precede or cause physical problems. They may also be linked to emotional, mental, social, or spiritual issues.

- Most energy practitioners enlist one or more methods of perceiving the energy field. For example, some practitioners claim to see it, some feel it through touch, some

enlist the use of pendulums or other dowsing techniques to assess it, and some report being guided by intuition or direct knowing. Many enlist the assistance of "helper" energies in their work.

- Many healers have experienced a health crisis (taken the healer's journey) themselves that precipitated their foray into energy healing.

- Energy is said to respond to intention. Practitioners may manipulate energy through any number of means, which may include healing rituals, hands-on techniques, visualization exercises, or nonlocal (distant) healing practices.

Table 112-2 lists various forms of human energetic therapies, with key Web sites for each.

> Although styles and forms of biofield therapies are myriad, many of them share common elements.

Energy Medicine Research

Through technology, we routinely perceive and manipulate various forms of energy. Our cellular phones and televisions can pick up precise frequencies from among thousands that bounce through the atmosphere. Western medicine relies on energetic properties of the body to obtain electrocardiograms

TABLE 112-1. The Chakras

CHAKRA NAME(S)*	LOCATION IN THE BODY	COLOR	ASSOCIATED ISSUES
First (root)	Base of spine	Red	Physical health and security, materialism, body awareness
Second	Lower abdomen, just below umbilicus	Orange	Emotions, especially toward oneself, reproduction, creativity (in some traditions)
Third	Solar plexus (just below xyphoid)	Yellow	Mental well-being, logic, will, sense of control
Fourth	Heart area, but in midline rather than to the left	Green (sometimes rose)	Connections to others, relationships, forgiveness, compassion
Fifth	Throat	Blue (sometimes turquoise)	Self-expression, creative pursuits, speaking one's truth
Sixth (third eye)	Center of forehead	Indigo or violet	Vision, perception, intuition, dreams
Seventh (crown)	Top and center of scalp	Purple or white	Spirituality, connection with a higher power, unity
Eighth and higher	Vary greatly among traditions; some describe an eighth chakra 6–12 inches over the seventh chakra and a ninth chakra 6–12 inches below the feet	Varies (the one below the feet is said to be brown)	Variable; eighth chakra sometimes described as a point where the boundaries of an individual begin to disappear; in some traditions, linked to the collective consciousness or past lives; ninth chakra may be tied to grounding, connection with the earth

For more information on how energetic anatomy is conceptualized in different traditions, see the various Web sites listed in Table 112-2.
*Names, numbers of chakras, and locations vary among different traditions. In Indian traditions, each chakra 1 to 7 has an associated sound (lam, vam, ram, yam, ham, am, om, respectively), as well as a musical key (the first starts with C and the others follow up the scale). Each chakra is linked to different glands as well; this often guides how energy medicine practitioners work with different conditions. In some traditions, the glands are, from chakras 1 to 7, the adrenals, gonads, pancreas, thymus, thyroid, pituitary, and pineal, respectively. Some traditions ascribe adrenals to the third, and some link the prostate to the first.

TABLE 112-2. Energy Healing Modalities: Descriptions and Key Web Sites*

ENERGY MODALITY	DESCRIPTION AND RELATED WEB SITE*
Acupuncture and acupressure	Needles are inserted into points said to be located along different meridians, or energy channels, within the body. In electroacupuncture, electricity is passed through the needles. http://www.yinyanghouse.com/
Barbara Brennan School of Healing	This approach focuses on energy healing according to detailed descriptions of energy anatomy and flow. Many schools of healing are based on the experiences or techniques of a specific individual, and this is one example. http://www.barbarabrennan.com/
Crystal therapy and Gem therapy	Minerals are used to influence the energy field. Different stones are believed to have specific vibrational properties. http://healing.about.com/od/crystaltherapy/Crystal_Therapy.htm
Emotional Freedom Techniques and Thought Field Therapy	These methods were created by Gary Craig and Roger Callahan, respectively. Tapping of various meridian points is said to release stored negative emotional energy. http://www.emofree.com/ and http://www.rogercallahan.com/index.php
Eye Movement Desensitization and Reprocessing (EMDR)	Rapid alternation of eye movements from left to right and tapping of specific groups of points on the body are used in various patterns to release energy-based problems. http://www.emdr.com/
Flower essences	Various flower extracts are said to influence people according to the nature or energy of the extracts' plants of origin. http://www.bachcentre.com/
Healing Touch	Developed in the 1980s by Janet Mentgen, RN, this method is based on principles used in therapeutic touch and other such techniques. Extensive instruction and training are required for certification. http://www.healingtouchinternational.org/
Homeopathy	Created by Samuel Hahnemann in 1796, this approach uses highly diluted solutions said to hold the vibrational principle of a given remedy, which is carefully tailored after a detailed evaluation of a person's symptoms. http://www.homeopathic.org/
Jin Shin Jyutsu	Developed by Jiru Murai in the early 1900s and brought to the West by Mary Burmeister in the 1960s, this method focuses on the use of 26 safety energy locks to unlock energy flow. http://www.jsjinc.net/
Johrei	Founded by Mokichi Okada, who envisioned a "paradise on earth" brought about through energetic detoxification and adherence to seven key principles, this method does not involve direct physical touch. http://www.johreifoundation.org
Matrix Energetics	This system of "consciousness technology" was created by Richard Bartlett DC, ND. It holds that anyone can be a healer through manipulating the matrix of information that is the foundation on which a person's reality is built. http://www.matrixenergetics.com/
Polarity Therapy	Based on the work of Randolph Stone, this approach combines diet, exercise, and other techniques to optimize the health of the energy field. http://www.polaritytherapy.org/
Pranic Healing	Systematized by Choa Kok Sui and tied to Arhatic yoga, this method involves visualizing colors and directing them through different techniques. http://www.pranichealing.org/
Qi gong	This technique enlists various precise body movements to alter one's capacity to store and manipulate qi, or energy. http://www.qigonginstitute.org/main_page/main_page.php
Quantum-Touch	In this system created by Richard Gordon, energy is directed through intention, breathwork, and other techniques, with a strong focus on musculoskeletal issues, among others. http://www.quantumtouch.com/
Reflexology	Certain parts of the feet, believed to be correlated with various body parts, are massaged or treated with essential oils. http://www.reflexology-usa.org/
Reiki	This technique originated in Japan with Mikao Usui. Trainees are given attunements said to allow them to pass universal healing energy through them to others. Many different schools exist. http://www.reiki.com/
Shamanic healing	This modality is often classed as spiritual, rather than energetic. The healer intuitively determines the source of a health problem and enlists ritual, helpful spirits, journeys to the spirit world, or other techniques to bring about healing. Hundreds of shamanic traditions exist. http://www.shamanresource.com/
Therapeutic Touch	This technique was developed in the 1970s by Dolores Krieger, a nurse, and Dora Kunz. Gentle touch is used to influence the biofield. http://www.therapeutictouch.org/
Zero Balancing	Created by Fritz Smith, MD, in the 1970s, this method holds that gentle touch and traction can balance energy at a "zero point," a place where the energetic and physical bodies are aligned. http://www.zerobalancing.com

This list is by no means comprehensive. For instance, prayer and spiritual healing are also classified by some investigators as human energetic therapies. All Web sites accessed 11.11.11.
*Table based in part on data from Rindfleisch JA. Biofield therapies: energy medicine and primary care. *Prim Care*. 2010;27:165–179.

(ECGs), electroencephalograms (EEGs), magnetic resonance imaging (MRI) scans, computed tomography (CT) scans, x-ray studies, and many other tests. All these devices are powered by electricity, another form of energy.

> Research has shown that human energetic therapies can positively influence outcomes in numerous circumstances, but much remains to be learned about the mechanism of action, the differences in effect among different energy modalities, and the best ways to integrate these approaches into other types of healing practices.

We know that individuals' energy fields interact. When people are near one another, one person's pattern on an EEG will reflect another's pattern on an EEG, and vice versa.[8] A 1994 study reported that one person's brain could share information with another's.[9] This was the case even when the people were in different rooms and one of those rooms was an electromagnetically impenetrable (Faraday) chamber. In some instances, after pairs of subjects meditated together and established a rapport (found they liked each other), investigators reported that flashing lights viewed by one subject influenced the EEG for the ophthalmic region of the brain of his or her partner in the sealed room.[9] A 2004 study found similar results.[10]

What is the status of energy medicine research? The current body of research on human energetic therapies is relatively small, but some fascinating discoveries have been made.

Three important suppositions related to energetic therapies require validation for energy medicine to be considered plausible from a scientific standpoint. The following must be established:

1. Subtle energy exists, and it has explicable mechanisms of action through which it influences biologic systems.
2. People can perceive and manipulate this energy.
3. Manipulating this energy has clinically important effects on human health.

As far as suppositions 1 and 2 are concerned, suffice it that fascinating studies have been conducted, many with remarkable findings, but much remains to be learned. Quantum theory, biophoton emissions, and an array of novel measurement devices have offered insights into the mechanism of action of energy therapies. Other research indicates that test subjects can influence random number generators and gather information about distant, unseen objects better than would be predicted by chance alone. The following books, which summarize this research in detail, are recommended:

- Jonas WB, Crawford CC, eds. *Healing, Intention and Energy Medicine: Science, Research Methods, and Clinical Implications.* New York: Churchill Livingstone; 2003.

- Laszlo E. *Science and the Akashic Field: An Integral Theory of Everything.* Rochester, VT: Inner Traditions; 2007.

- McTaggart L. *The Field: The Quest for the Secret Force of the Universe.* New York: Harper; 2008.

- Oschman J. *Energy Medicine: The Scientific Basis.* New York: Churchill Livingstone; 2002.

- Oschman J. *Energy Medicine in Therapeutics and Human Performance.* Edinburgh: Butterworth Heinemann; 2003.

- Schwartz GE, Simon WL. *The Energy Healing Experiments: Science Reveals Our Natural Power to Heal.* New York: Atria Books; 2007.

As for the third supposition, that energy therapies have clinically meaningful effects, the body of research is slowly growing. Many studies have raised the possibility that human energetic therapies may influence patients. For instance, a study conducted in Hawaii found that 11 healers, from various traditions, affected the brain activity on functional MRI scans of people with whom they felt a close connection. This result occurred even with the healers and their partners separated by hundreds of miles. The healers were asked to send "distant intentionality" at random 2-minute intervals; the recipients were unaware of the timing of this transmission. Functional MRI findings indicated that activity levels in several areas of the brain changed at precisely the time the healers were sending their intentions ($P = .0000127$).[11]

Table 112-3 summarizes some of the key clinical studies of the effectiveness of human energetic therapies and focuses primarily on meta-analyses and systematic reviews.[12-33] The most commonly studied therapies are healing touch, Reiki, qi gong (which is also, to some degree, a movement-based therapy), and therapeutic touch.

Guidelines for Making an Energy Medicine Referral

The keys to making an appropriate referral to an energy medicine practitioner are in many ways the same as when one refers to any sort of nonbiomedical practitioner:

1. Know the practice and the practitioner. This not only includes knowing in general about the nature of the modality practiced, but it also means being aware of the practitioner's qualifications and training. How willing is the practitioner to work collaboratively with Western medicine practitioners? Both innate talent and amount of experience influence a given healer's effectiveness.[8] The best way to get to know providers is to experience their practice as a client.

2. Know when to refer. Many energy medicine practitioners suggest that any patient-related concern is "fair game" when someone is referred for energy work. However, keep in mind that not all providers work according to Western medicine diagnostic categories. Trust your instincts as the referring provider. In my experience, energy medicine is especially worthy of consideration for the following:

- People with generally heightened sensitivity. These people are often uncomfortable with crowds, highly intuitive, finely attuned to the feelings of others, or very sensitive to foods, medications, or environmental pathogens.

- People with a history of severe emotional traumas

- People with pain (physical or otherwise)

- People with fatigue or a sense that they can never "keep their energy in." This can include those who are constantly giving to or supporting others and not taking time for their own needs.

- Those who seem "starved for energy." This group includes those patients who leave a provider completely drained at the end of a visit.

TABLE 112-3. Summary of Key Systematic Reviews, Meta-Analyses, and Randomized Controlled Trials Relating to Clinical Efficacy of Human Energetic Therapies

FOCUS OF STUDIES	FINDINGS

General Reviews	• A 2010 systematic review of 67 biofield therapy studies concluded that biofield therapies "…are promising complementary interventions for reducing pain intensity in numerous populations, reducing anxiety for hospitalized populations, and reducing agitated behaviors in dementia, beyond what may be expected from standard treatment or nonspecific effects. Effects on longer term clinical outcomes are less clear, and more systematic research is needed."[12]
	• A 2008 Cochrane Review evaluated findings for 1153 patients in 5 Healing Touch, 15 Therapeutic Touch, and 5 Reiki trials to determine whether touch therapies were helpful for pain. Pain was reduced an average of 0.83 points on the 10-point pain rating scale, with a 95% confidence interval of −1.16 to −0.5. The investigators concluded "touch therapies may have a modest effect on pain relief."[13]
	• A 2003 research survey reviewed 2200 published reports related to spiritual healing, energy, medicine, and the effects of mental intention. Findings were summarized as follows[14,15]:
	    • 75% of 130 studies on the link between religious/spiritual practices and health showed positive findings, but overall study quality was poor. Nearly all the research was observational.
	    • 11 out of 19 trials of energy healing involving 1122 people reported positive effects (Cohen's D effect of 0.6). Overall research quality was judged as fair (Jadad score, 3–4 out of 5). Most trials involved Therapeutic Touch.

Healing Touch	• A 2004 review concluded that although 30 available studies of Healing Touch did not allow for generalized conclusions, the technique holds promise.[16] • A 2010 pilot study found that Healing Touch lowered stress and improved heart rate variability in 9 pediatric oncology patients.[17] • Vitality, pain, and physical functioning was improved in a group of 78 women with gynecologic cancers who were undergoing radiation therapy.[18] • Healing Touch decreased anxiety and length of stay in patients recovering from coronary bypass surgery, but it led to no change in pain medication or antiemetic use or atrial fibrillation incidence.[19]
Qi Gong	• A 2010 study of 162 oncology patients found that medical qi gong improved quality of life, reduced treatment side effects, and reduced inflammation with no adverse effects.[20] • Of 58 studies of qi gong's in vitro effects reviewed in 2003, most showed positive effects, but trial quality was poor. The same was true for 33 clinical studies.[15] • Qi gong training for 5 weeks decreased tinnitus in 80 patients for more than 3 months.[21] • A small noncontrolled trial involving 18 patients with chronic fatigue found that qi gong training significantly improved pain, sleep, mental attitude, and general mobility.[22]
Reiki	• A 2009 review that included 12 studies found that 9 of 12 of them reported significant therapeutic effects of Reiki, but 11 of the 12 were ranked as poor quality based on the Jadad score.[23] • A 2010 study conducted in a Yale University cardiology ward found that heart rate variability and positive emotional status improved markedly with the provision of Reiki to patients, as compared with patients in the control group or those who listened to meditative music.[24] • Review of study data through 2007 concluded that the benefit of Reiki "remains unproven."[25] • A review by Vitale in 2007 held that the Reiki literature includes 1 of 4 studies with significant findings for stress and depression, 1 study with significant findings for acute pain, and 1 of 3 studies that showed benefit for chronic pain.[26]
Therapeutic Touch	• A 2010 study found that Therapeutic Touch improved pain and fatigue in a study of 90 patients undergoing chemotherapy.[27] • A 2010 study of 21 postoperative patients found that Therapeutic Touch significantly decreased pain, cortisol, and natural killer cell levels.[28] • A 2010 Cochrane Review found Therapeutic Touch not helpful for acute wound healing, given that 2 trials showed improvement and 1 trial showed slowed healing.[29] • A 2007 Cochrane Review did not find any good-quality studies to assess the general effect of Therapeutic Touch on anxiety.[30] • A 2008 review concluded that Therapeutic Touch does reduce pain and anxiety in patients with cancer.[31] • Therapeutic Touch was found to decrease behavioral symptoms in people with dementia.[32] In a subsequent study of a group of 64 residential patients, this technique was found to decrease restlessness and cortisol variability significantly.[33]

• Anyone who lacks focus or seems "ungrounded"

• Patients suffering from an array of nonspecific or unrelated complaints or whose symptoms are not easily explained from a biomedical perspective

• Patients whose chief complaints have something of a supernatural or paranormal bent. Again, the integrative providers' belief system will guide how they approach such concerns.

3. Be aware of safety concerns. Energy medicine has a very low risk of negative effects or outcomes, although one must use caution about relying on human energetic therapies to the exclusion of conventional, potentially lifesaving interventions, especially during life-threatening emergencies or when dealing with severe physical trauma. In addition, patients with psychosis may not do well with energetic approaches.

Energy medicine can be considered for use to maintain health or to treat practically any condition, with minimal adverse effects. Caution is recommended with use in people with a history of psychosis or when use could lead to a delay in potentially life-saving allopathic interventions.

4. Obtain feedback from the recipients of the care. Are people getting better after you refer them? Is healing occurring?

Incorporating Energy Medicine Approaches Into One's Own Practice

As with any approach to healing, practitioners must find appropriate mentorship when adopting new techniques. However, energy medicine is something that anyone can try. Many practitioners teach the family members or friends of an ill person techniques they can practice with their loved ones themselves.

The exercises in this chapter are starting points. As you gain experience, create your own, tailoring to the needs of your specific practice.

As you experiment with these exercises, keep in mind that a health care provider should not "take on" the energy of others, nor is it appropriate for him or her to feel that personal energy is lost during energy work with another person. Always ask for permission before doing one of these exercises with someone. Be sure to allow the recipient of the practice to have sufficient time to recover afterward; some people move into a trancelike state as they work with these techniques. Persons familiar with Interactive Guided Imagery and mindfulness practices will note that many energy exercises contain elements of both.

The following four practices can be readily incorporated into a patient encounter:
1. Grounding
2. Charging up your energy
3. Setting appropriate boundaries
4. Draining away a symptom

Grounding

This exercise can be used when people seem overly distracted by their emotions or too much "in their head," thinking about an issue but not remaining aware in other ways. Grounding can be helpful for bringing someone into the present moment or into a more enhanced awareness of their physical state. It is also good for people who tend to go off on tangents in conversation. This exercise can be useful for providers before, between, or following encounters with patients. Caution: Some people cope with pain or suffering by not being grounded; this exercise may be stressful to them.

- Remove your footwear as able. Socks are permissible.
- Sit up or lie straight. If possible, the soles of your feet should be kept in contact with the floor.
- Keep your legs and arms uncrossed, if possible.

- After a few slow, deep breaths, bring all your attention to the soles of the feet. Imagine the breath moving in and out through them. Continue until this feels comfortable. If you feel any resistance, simply note it and continue to breathe.
- Feel, visualize, or imagine on the outward breath that the feet are extending into the ground like the roots of the tree, slowly spreading through the soil. Sense how these roots add stability and a sense of connection with the earth.
- With each inward breath, feel, visualize, or imagine energy flowing into the feet through those roots, the way that nutrients and water flow into a tree. Let the energy move into the body up through the feet and to wherever it is needed.
- Continue this exercise for at least 20 breaths.
- It may be helpful to follow this exercise with an overall body scan, in which a person is asked to tune in sequentially, without judging or analyzing, to various parts of the body. (e.g., "Focus on your left toes…then your left foot…then the ankle…knee…thigh")

Charging Up Your Energy

Many variations of this exercise exist. It can be done by anyone who is feeling fatigued or weary, as well as by someone intending to share energy with another person. The best approach always is to maintain your own energy level and allow additional energy to flow through to others without ever feeling that you are losing your own energy in the process.

- In a place that feels safe, assume a comfortable position and close your eyes. You may find it helpful to place your hands on your lap, with the palms facing upward.
- Bring your awareness to the breath, and take several deep breaths.
- When you inhale, begin by imagining white light moving in through the soles of the feet and up through the body to the heart.
- After the flow from the feet to the heart can be perceived, do the same with the top of the head, and imagine white light moving in, down through the center of the head, neck, and chest, to the heart.
- Continue this process, and allow the heart to fill to overflowing with the white light. Thinking about whatever fills your heart with the strongest sense of joy, compassion, love, or enthusiasm is often helpful.
- Once the heart feels full, it should remain so through the rest of the exercise. Repeat the previous steps if the heart does not continue to feel full.
- As the heart overflows, send the white light (or, if preferred, the feeling of love or compassion) from the heart and down the arms into the hands. This energy is ready to be shared with another part of your own body by placing the palms over wherever extra energy is desired. It may also be shared with another person, with permission.

Setting Appropriate Boundaries

This exercise is especially helpful to people who feel overwhelmed by the energy, emotions, or simply the physical presence of others. It may be useful for people with fibromyalgia, whose senses are heightened to a point of causing dysfunction, or for people with chronic fatigue, whose energy seems to leak out of them in a way they cannot control. This practice also may be useful for people who feel as though others are somehow draining their energy. It can help a person feel less defensive or adversarial.

- Ideally, this exercise should be done at a time and place where you feel safe enough to close your eyes.

- Take a moment to tune in to how you feel, right now. Do you feel drained? Tired? Overwhelmed? Where in the body do you have these feelings? Where do you feel vulnerable?

- After several deep breaths, imagine yourself surrounded by a clear, bright, white, force field. This force field surrounds you like a protective bubble that allows in only what you choose and deflects anything that is unnecessary or harmful away from you.

- Strengthen the force field in any places where you feel vulnerable.

- If desired, you can choose to maintain knowledge of whatever bounces off the force field; understand that you can do this without its affecting you emotionally or energetically.

- Imagine white light radiating from a point at the exact center of the bubble of force that clears out anything that does not belong inside the bubble.

- Enhance the force field further by using additional imagery, sounds, or feelings that you associate with strength and well-being. Pause after adding each extra layer, and focus on the breath.

- With practice, a person can rapidly move through this exercise before entering an uncomfortable environment or facing a challenging interpersonal encounter. This exercise can also be good to use on first awakening or when retiring for the night.

Draining Away a Symptom

Healing touch and other human energetic therapies often use this technique in various forms. This exercise can be helpful when a symptom can be localized to a specific area of the body. For example, a pain drain can be used for headaches or joint pain. Practitioners can also ask those experiencing emotional pain where in their body they feel it the most.

- Close your eyes and focus on the part of the body where you feel the pain, discomfort, or imbalance most strongly.

- Describe what you notice there. Does it have a color? Is it an image? A memory? What sound do you hear when you tune into this area? What temperature is it, and how does it feel compared with the rest of your body?

- Take some time to focus your awareness on the discomfort. This can be distressing, given that we may spend time trying to avoid, ignore, or control our symptoms. Just observe. Stay as neutral as possible.

- Now, focus on how the area should be. At its healthiest, how does it look, sound, and feel? Take time to develop a strong sense of this. Again, stay objective.

- With each exhalation, envision the symptom—all that you noticed about it—being exhaled. Some people let it leave with the breath, and others release it into the ground through the bottoms of their feet. Some people release it in the form of emotions that arise. For others, it just seems to fade away.

- With each inhalation, breathe in your sense of how the part of your body receiving your attention can feel at its healthiest, at its most whole. Draw in the imagery you generated around health for this location. This can come in with the breath, through the top of the head, through the bottoms of the feet, or in any other way that seems appropriate.

As a provider present with someone doing this exercise, you can often enhance the experience by placing your hand on or near the part of the patient's body that is receiving attention. If it seems appropriate, you may envision sending what is required through yourself. Use the steps outlined in the grounding exercise to ensure that you are not giving your own energy, but rather letting it flow into and through you, as though you are an antenna. Similarly, if you the provider feel comfortable doing so, you may feel or see the symptom being released from the person being healed into your hands. If this occurs, simply intend that whatever is released be deflected away from both the patient and you into the ground.

> If you choose to try energy medicine exercises with those who seek your care, feel free to experiment. Shape these or other exercises as you find appropriate, and develop some of your own.

If you find the foregoing exercises helpful, you may want to consider some of the following resources, which offer other useful exercises and ways of conceptualizing human energetic therapies:

- Brennan BA. *Hands of Light: A Guide to Healing Through the Human Energy Field.* New York: Bantam Dell; 1993.

- Brennan BA. *Light Emerging: The Journey of Personal Healing.* New York: Bantam Dell; 1993.

- Bruyere RL. *Wheels of Light: Chakras, Auras, and the Healing Energy of the Body.* New York: Fireside; 1994.

- Dale C. *The Subtle Body: An Encyclopedia of Your Energetic Anatomy.* Boulder, CO: Sounds True; 2009.

- Eden D. *Energy Medicine for Women: Aligning Your Body's Energies to Boost Your Health and Vitality.* New York: Tarcher Penguin; 2008.

- Eden D. *Energy Medicine: Balancing Your Body's Energies for Optimal Health, Joy, and Vitality.* New York: Tarcher Penguin; 2008.

- Gordon R. *Quantum Touch: The Power to Heal.* 3rd ed. Berkeley, CA: North Atlantic Books; 2006.

- Ingerman S. *Shamanic Journeying: A Beginner's Guide.* Boulder, CO: Sounds True; 2008.

- Myss CM. *Anatomy of the Spirit: The Seven Stages of Power and Healing.* New York: Random House; 1996.

- Weil A, Chiasson AM. *Self-Healing with Energy Medicine* (Self Healing CD Series). Boulder, CO: Sounds True; 2009.

KEY WEB RESOURCES*

Alternative Medicine Foundation resource guide on energy work: http://amfoundation.org/energywork.htm	Provides descriptions, links, and introductory readings for a number of different energy medicine modalities.
Association for the Scientific Study of Consciousness: http://assc.caltech.edu/	Organization dedicated to the study of consciousness, with regular international conferences
Institute of Noetic Sciences: http://www.noetic.org/	Group dedicated to the study of consciousness and energetic, founded by astronaut Edgar Mitchell
International Society for the Study of Subtle Energies and Energy Medicine: http://www.issseem.org/	Group devoted to the study of energy medicine that publishes a newsletter and hosts annual conferences focused on energy medicine

*See also the Web sites listed in Table 112-2.

References

References are available online at expertconsult.com.

Section VI Other Therapeutic Considerations

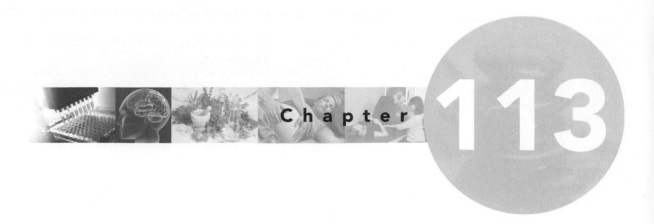

Chapter

113

Creating a Greener Clinic: The Impact of Global Warming on Health

Rian J. Podein, MD, and Michael T. Hernke, PhD

Global warming and climate change are transforming ecosystems on an extraordinary scale and at an extraordinary pace, resulting in what some consider to be the greatest public health disaster facing us today.[1,2] The etiology of climate change has been identified and reported by the Intergovernmental Panel on Climate Change, concluding with strong evidence that most of the global warming that has occurred during the past 50 years is attributable to human activities and specifically the consumption of fossil fuels producing carbon dioxide and other greenhouse gases (GHGs).[3] Because of the familiarity and predominance of carbon dioxide among the greenhouse gases, it is often used as a representative, or surrogate, for estimating, monitoring, and reporting of GHG emissions. Reporting of carbon dioxide emissions can be expressed as the specific carbon dioxide quantity (e.g., tons per year) if this is the only GHG emission measured. When other GHG emissions are taken into account, the result may be expressed in terms of global warming potential (GWP). GWP is a measure of how much a given mass of greenhouse gas is estimated to contribute to global warming relative to the same mass of carbon dioxide over a given time, facilitating measurements in units of carbon dioxide equivalents.[4] All sectors of society, including health care, contribute to the increasing accumulation of atmospheric GHG. For many countries, the health care sector is responsible for consuming significant amounts of goods and services and is an important contributor to gross domestic products. In general, the more that a health care system consumes, the greater the amount of carbon emissions associated with the consumption, and the greater the size of its carbon footprint. Carbon emission estimates have been completed for the United States and the National Health System (NHS) in England. The U.S. health care system emits more than 434 million tons of carbon dioxide annually, which represents 7% of total annual U.S. carbon emissions; and the NHS England carbon emissions total 18 million tons per year, which represents 3.2% of total carbon emissions in England.[5,6]

> Greenhouse gas emissions are represented by the quantity of carbon dioxide measured in tons. Global warming potential incorporates all gases and is a measure of how much a given mass of greenhouse gas is estimated to contribute to global warming relative to the same mass of carbon dioxide over time.

The public health consequences of GHG accumulation and climate change are already present, and future projections are alarming. The direct human health effects as a result of climate change have been reported through a multitude of pathways, including temperature-related illnesses and deaths, extreme weather, air pollution, allergic diseases, infectious diseases, malnutrition, and displaced populations.[7] The global burden of disease morbidity and mortality attributable to the human-caused portion of climate change is significant, with approximately 5 million disability-adjusted life years per year and more than 150,000 lives annually, with projections to more than double by 2030.[8]

Whereas the health care sector can play a key role in helping societies adapt to the effects of climate change and the risk it poses to human health, the role of mitigation has more recently emerged. This was demonstrated by a World Health Organization mandate for member states to develop "programs for health systems that will contribute to reducing their own greenhouse gas emissions."[9] Individual, organizational, and national motivations for reducing green-house gas emissions may vary, but health care practitioners and health care organizations must be motivated to do no harm, and it is therefore incumbent on us to reduce, with the goal to eliminate, the carbon footprint of medicine and health care.

> The U.S. health care system emits more than 434 million tons of carbon dioxide annually, which represents 7% of total annual U.S. carbon emissions. The NHS England carbon emissions total 18 million tons per year, which represents 3.2% of total carbon emissions in England.

A Primer on Life Cycle Assessment

Quantification of the carbon emissions of a health system, hospital, or clinic is important to approximate the overall impact toward climate change, to identify strategies for carbon reduction, and to clarify the potential value of mitigation efforts. Life cycle assessment (LCA) is a technique that can be used for this process. LCA evaluates the environmental impacts precipitated by a product or a service (i.e., health care) from sourcing materials through end of life. LCA is composed of three stages:

1. Identify and quantify environmental loads—energy and materials usage, emissions, and waste.
2. Assess and evaluate potential environmental impacts associated with the loads.
3. Assess the opportunities for improvement.

LCA considers all processes over the life cycle—extraction and processing, manufacturing, transport and distribution, use, reuse, maintenance, recycling, and final disposal.[10,11]

A product life cycle can be seen as a linear progression that starts with extraction of raw materials, such as ore and oil, which are processed into basic materials, such as aluminum and plastics. Finished materials then compose parts and components, such as a car body, which along with other components are assembled into final products. A life cycle also includes the use phase and the end-of-life activities, such as disassembly and recycling. Transportation and distribution between life cycle phases are also considered.

Activities across a life cycle require material and energy resources and generate wastes and emissions, including GHG. LCA gathers information about the quantity of these resources and wastes at each life cycle stage. Thus, the effect of producing an automobile would include not only the impacts at the final assembly facility but also the impact from mining metal ores, making electronic parts, forming windows and parts that are needed to build the car, and of course the emissions precipitated from driving.

LCA provides a fairly complete picture within the scope of investigation of a product's or service's known environmental impacts. It lets you see which parts of a product or facility life cycle most negatively affect the environment and helps prioritize improvements or select alternative products and services to achieve safer and more efficient energy and materials use (Fig. 113-1). LCA approaches alone do not

FIGURE 113-1
Improving the environmental profile of health care. (Originally presented by Hernke MT. Customer-focus across the lifecycle. *10th International Greening of Industry Network Conference: Corporate Social Responsibility—Governance for Sustainability.* Göteborg, Sweden; June 23-26, 2002.)

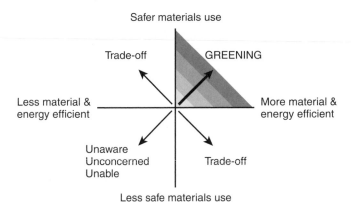

Improving the Environmental Profile of Health Care

provide a vision of health care in a sustainable society, a task for which broader science-based principles are useful and have been described elsewhere.[12]

The U.S. and England health sector carbon footprint estimates, mentioned previously, were calculated by use of the LCA technique. Their findings identified not only the total GHG emissions but also that the three greatest areas of carbon emissions within health care are attributed to building energy use, pharmaceuticals, and travel, each of which accounted for about 22% of emissions in the England study (Fig. 113-2).[6] In the United States, building energy use and prescription drugs accounted for about 20% and 15% of emissions, respectively; emissions attributable to travel were not considered.[5,13]

Energy Use

Energy use to heat, to cool, and to power medical facilities is highly intensive and expensive, and it is one of the largest contributors to health care's carbon footprint by the use of non-renewable fossil energy sources. Fortunately, this area offers many opportunities for improving efficiency.

A variety of calculator tools use energy consumption information to enable health care facilities to estimate their GHG (including carbon dioxide) emissions, to compare energy use with similar buildings nationwide, to estimate the health impacts and medical costs due to power plant emissions from the consumed energy, and to obtain third-party recognition and verification for energy consumption benchmarks (see Key Web Resources).

Energy consumption and carbon tracking tools can help people and organizations monitor efforts to reduce energy consumption and resultant carbon emissions. Major targets for energy use mitigation include conserving energy, making operations more energy efficient, and purchasing renewable energy or installing renewable energy infrastructure (Box 113-1).

New health care facilities can reduce their energy use and subsequent carbon emissions by incorporating energy efficiency and renewable energy into their design

FIGURE 113-2
The three greatest areas of carbon emissions within health care.

Top Three Sources of Carbon Emissions in Health Care

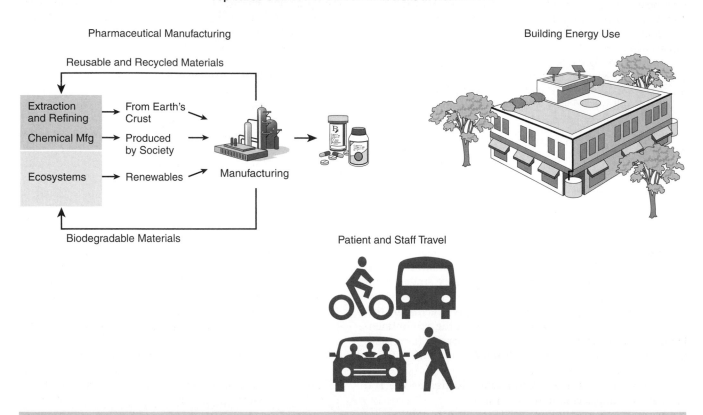

and construction. To facilitate this goal, the U.S. Green Building Council has created the Leadership in Energy and Environmental Design (LEED) program for the health care industry, a best practices guide for more sustainable building design, construction, and operations.[14] LEED is a certification system providing third-party verification that a building was designed and built with a focus on energy savings, water efficiency, carbon dioxide emissions reduction, improved indoor environmental quality, and stewardship of resources and sensitivity to their impacts.

LEED is perhaps the most well known green building standard but certainly not the only one worth considering. Retzlaff[15] and Haapio and Viitaniemi[16] reviewed LEED and other green building standards to help users understand their substantial differences and merits with respect to various sustainability dimensions, such as the relative emphasis on energy use and indoor air quality and other facility goals, such as community or civic use.

When health care facilities, organizations, and national systems reduce their energy use or increase the contribution of renewable energies, co-benefits in addition to carbon reduction and climate change mitigation are realized through direct public health benefits and economic savings. For example, the health effects due to pollution from the emissions of fossil fuels, especially from coal combustion, include cardiovascular disease, cancer, stroke, and respiratory disease as well as asthma and delayed neurologic development in children.[17-19] In addition, the cost of fossil fuels promises to increase over time as supply decreases, thereby positioning energy conservation, efficiency, and alternative energy measures to provide for long-term financial benefits.

Health systems have been encouraged to respond to the challenge of climate change by addressing our own energy consumption and to lead by example: "The health sector is one of the most trusted and respected sections of society, and it is also one of the largest employers and consumers of energy. This presents both a responsibility and an opportunity to be an 'early mover' to achieve climate-neutrality in its own operations, and to demonstrate that this can go hand-in-hand with improved effectiveness and cost savings."[20]

Pharmaceuticals

Pharmaceutical medications are also one of the largest contributors to health care's carbon footprint; most of their emissions result directly from the energy used in pharmaceutical production in the manufacturing plants.[6] There has been a steady increase in the demand for pharmaceutical interventions and the use of prescription medications within modern medicine. Globally, pharmaceutical sales are expected to reach $880 billion in 2011, with the United States as the single largest market with sales of more than $300 billion.[21]

If health care continues to increase its reliance on and use of pharmaceutical medications, its contribution to the carbon footprint will also continue to increase in addition to significant public health and ecologic consequences. Medication-related errors at all points of care, including prescribing of medications, dispensing by pharmacists, and unintentional nonadherence on the part of patients, are a major contributor to avoidable morbidity, mortality, and cost.[22] Ecologically, pharmaceutical medications are being excreted and discarded into the environment at a rate faster than they can be degraded,

causing them to accumulate in waterways and drinking water. The majority of waterways tested in the United States now show traces of common medications such as acetaminophen, hormones, blood pressure medicine, codeine, and antibiotics, with mounting concerns regarding their deleterious effects on aquatic organisms.[23] Strikingly, a vast array of these pharmaceuticals, including antibiotics, anticonvulsants, mood stabilizers, and sex hormones, have found their way into the drinking water supplies throughout the United States.[24] Because of multiple concerns, including pharmaceutical use in large ongoing amounts, environmental accumulation, resistance of some pharmaceutical parent compounds or active metabolites to biodegradation, newer drugs with poorly understood modes of biochemical actions, potential for ecologic harm, and potential for unknown subtle effects from long-term exposures to low concentrations of bioactive compounds, pharmaceuticals have been named by the Environmental Protection Agency as one of the top five "emerging" contaminants affecting human and ecologic health.[25]

Integrative medicine, with its incorporation of nonpharmaceutical complementary and alternative medicine interventions, is a proven approach that can reduce health care's reliance on pharmaceuticals.[26, 27] Compared with pharmaceutical interventions alone, an integrative medicine approach often holds the potential to be as effective or even better, to be less expensive, and to pose more limited or even positive side effects. One such example is the treatment and prevention of migraine headaches. Acupuncture has demonstrated benefit for the acute treatment of migraine headaches and could therefore be considered in association with or instead of pharmaceuticals.[28] For migraine headache prophylaxis, acupuncture is at least as effective as or possibly more effective than pharmaceutical drug treatment, has fewer adverse effects, and can be cost-effective.[28-30] In addition, another nonpharmaceutical intervention, biofeedback, has been shown to be equally efficacious compared with the commonly used pharmaceutical propranolol for migraine headache prevention.[31]

Efforts within the practice of medicine and health care to facilitate pharmaceutical reductions are crucial for the goal of reducing carbon emissions and for providing optimal quality patient care. A couple of areas warrant an increased focus for change. First, providers, organizations, and health systems would benefit by addressing the great imbalance of resources currently provided for disease treatment and away from wellness promotion and disease prevention. The benefits of this would reduce the need for pharmaceutical and nonpharmaceutical interventions alike. Second, support for the education of health professional students and providers regarding the role of an integrative medicine approach is already under way, with an increasing presence of complementary and alternative medicine electives in medical schools, integrative medicine curriculum within medical residency programs, integrative medicine fellowships, and continuing medical education programs, all of which will contribute to an increasing base of providers who will have the knowledge and training to consider nonpharmacologic interventions when appropriate.

Procurement and Transportation

Other noteworthy areas for carbon mitigation efforts within health care include food procurement and on-road transportation. According to the National Academy of Sciences, outside of direct energy use, these have been identified as the two biggest lifestyle factors when it comes to the net contribution to climate change.[32]

Environmentally preferable purchasing (EPP) is the act of purchasing products and services whose environmental impacts have been considered and found to be less damaging to the environment and human health compared with competing products or services that serve the same purpose. Although EPP can be used for all products and services, one emerging example within health care is the purchase of more local, healthy, and sustainable foods. Most foods travel an average of 1500 miles from "farm to plate," with significant GHG emissions as a result of transportation and fossil fuel use.[33] More locally produced foods reduce the "food miles" of a product, with a resultant reduction in the amount of carbon and GHG emissions. In addition are the co-benefits of reduced air and water pollution associated with long-distance transport. More specifically, one of the leading contributors to food system climate change is recognized to be meat consumption and production, responsible for nearly a fifth of total global GHG emissions.[34] Some health care organizations have acted by significantly reducing their meat offerings. Notably, the British NHS has instituted vegetarian menus and reduced meat offerings in all of the nation's public hospitals to reduce its carbon footprint.[35] Inspired by the Meatless Monday project, a nonprofit initiative in association with the Johns Hopkins Bloomberg School of Public Health, numerous health care organizations within the United States have endorsed a voluntary one-day per week meatless menu (to learn more, visit www.meatlessmonday.com). The United Nations climate chief has validated the utility of these efforts, stating that having a meat-free day every week is the biggest single contribution people could make to curbing climate change in their personal lives.[36]

> *People should have one meat-free day a week if they want to make a personal and effective sacrifice that would help tackle climate change.*
> Rajendra Pachauri, Chair of the United Nations Intergovernmental Panel on Climate Change
> (Originally published in *The Guardian*, September 7, 2008.)

Supporting more sustainable food procurement products, including reduced meat consumption, provides health care organizations an opportunity to model healthy eating patterns for patients, reduces carbon and GHG emissions, and offers health benefits too. The regular consumption of meat products increases the risk of chronic diseases, especially some of the leading causes of death, such as cardiovascular disease, stroke, diabetes, and some cancers.

Road transportation in the form of staff and patients driving automobiles plays a significant role in health care's carbon footprint. Health care organizations have the opportunity to encourage staff and patients to shift from sedentary automobile travel to more active and healthy travel, such as walking, cycling, and public transport. In addition to reducing carbon and GHG emissions, these more active transportation methods provide exercise, reduce fatal accidents, increase social contact, and reduce air pollution.[37]

FIGURE 113-3
Virtuous cycle for transportation. (From *Saving Carbon, Improving Health*. NHS Carbon Reduction Strategy for England, January 2009.)

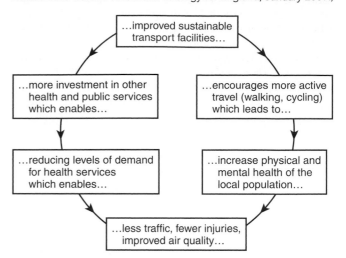

Consideration should be given to senior-level creation of an active travel plan for the organization, incentives for staff and patients for active travel, establishment of monitoring metrics for monitoring, routine review of organizational travel needs and alternatives (e.g., teleconferencing), and moving health care delivery closer to the home. Efforts to reduce carbon emissions, including for transportation, have the potential to save money, to benefit population health, and to reduce health inequalities. In fact, many efforts that improve health also contribute to more sustainable development and vice versa. This may be illustrated as a virtuous cycle, a condition in which a favorable circumstance or result gives rise to another that subsequently supports the first, as demonstrated for transportation (Fig. 113-3).

Conclusion

In 1987, the United Nations published a report that provided guiding principles for sustainable development.

> *Sustainable development is development that meets the needs of the present without compromising the ability of future generations to meet their own needs.*
> World Commission on Environment and Development
> (Originally published in *Our Common Future.*
> New York: Oxford University Press; 1987.)

The more recent Millennium Ecosystem Assessment, an extensive assessment of the consequences of ecosystem change for human well-being, has highlighted our global unsustainability according to this principle, concluding that human actions are depleting Earth's natural capital, putting such strain on the environment that the ability of the planet's ecosystems to sustain future generations can no longer be taken for granted.[38] Reducing carbon and GHG emissions is a critical component in mitigating the consequences of global climate change and for moving toward a more sustainable society. The common mission of health care professionals and their institutions to facilitate health and to reduce suffering along with good societal standing positions them well to model carbon reduction practices. To transition toward a reduced carbon medical practice and health care system, we may look to prior successes, such as addressing global health interdependence by promoting peace and nuclear disarmament and antismoking advocacy. With climate change, the stakes are high for global catastrophe, as they are with nuclear weapons. In addition, the scientific evidence supports the risks of exposure to secondhand smoke, and the evidence for global warming and climate change is unequivocal that secondhand carbon is harmful too.

KEY WEB RESOURCES

Energy and Greenhouse Gas Emission Calculator Tools

Practice Greenhealth (membership organization for health care institutions): http://practicegreenhealth.org/tools-resources/energy-impact-calculator

Energy Impact Calculator
Calculates carbon dioxide emissions on the basis of the amount of energy consumed by the building; estimates health impacts and medical costs due to power plant emissions

Energy Star (a joint program of the U.S. Environmental Protection Agency and the U.S. Department of Energy): www.energystar.gov/index.cfm?c=healthcare.bus_healthcare

Portfolio Manager
Calculates greenhouse gas emissions (including carbon dioxide, methane, and nitrous oxide) on the basis of the amount of energy consumed by the building; allows comparison of energy use to similar buildings nationwide; potential to earn Energy Star recognition

World Resources Institute and World Business Council for Sustainable Development (a joint project of a global business association and an environmental think tank): www.ghgprotocol.org/

Greenhouse Gas Protocol
Provides a comprehensive accounting framework and extensive suite of tools and guidance for emissions accounting for standards and programs around the world, including tools for "office-based and service sector organizations," suitable for health care

Climate Registry (a membership organization for North American organizations): www.theclimateregistry.org/

Climate Registry Information System (CRIS)
Online tool for greenhouse gas calculation, reporting, and third-party verification; emissions can be estimated on the basis of sources and fuel type or directly reported

References

References available online at expertconsult.com.

Patient Handout: Steps You Can Take to Improve Your Health and Reduce Your Carbon Footprint

1. Nutrition: Eat more plants and less meat!

> "People should have one meat-free day a week if they want to make a personal and effective sacrifice that would help tackle climate change."
> Dr Rajendra Pachauri, chair of the United Nations Intergovernmental Panel on Climate

Fruits and vegetables play a significant role in preventing certain chronic diseases. When compared to people who eat only small amounts of fruits and vegetables, those who eat more generous amounts, as part of a healthy diet, tend to have reduced risk of chronic diseases. To learn more about how many fruits and vegetables you need each day, how to include fruits and vegetables in your daily diet, delicious recipes, and much more, visit: www.fruitsandveggiesmatter.gov.

"Meatless Monday" is a movement with the goal to help reduce meat consumption which is a significant contributor to climate change and chronic diseases. To learn more and join the growing number of individuals, families and institutions pledging to improve their health and the health of our planet go to www.meatlessmonday.com.

2. Walk more, drive less.

> "The true miracle is not walking on water or walking in air, but simply walking on this earth."
> Thich Nhat Hanh Buddhist monk

Automobile use is a significant contributor to climate change, local air pollution, pedestrian injuries, and obesity. Active travel modes such as walking, cycling and using public transport offer great benefits for your health and the environment. One fun way to set goals and increase your motivation is to measure the number of steps you take during the day with a pedometer, a step counter that you wear on your waist. To learn more about how to start a walking program, the benefits of physical activity and how to use a pedometer see: www.aafp.org/online/etc/medialib/aafp_org/documents/clinical/pub_health/aim/onestep.Par.0 001.File.tmp/OneStepAtATime.pdf

3. Healthy habits, less pharmaceuticals

> "One of the first duties of the physician is to educate the masses not to take medicine."
> Sir William Osler, MD, "Father of modern medicine"

Pharmaceutical medications are one of the largest contributors to health care's carbon footprint due to the increased energy it takes to make and transport them. We are using so many pharmaceutical medications that they are even starting to show up in our drinking water. Often times wellness can be maintained and medical conditions can be treated with the use of lifestyle modifications such as physical activity, nutrition, and stress reduction. Discuss with your health care provider how lifestyle approaches can prevent, reduce, or eliminate the need for pharmaceutical medications.

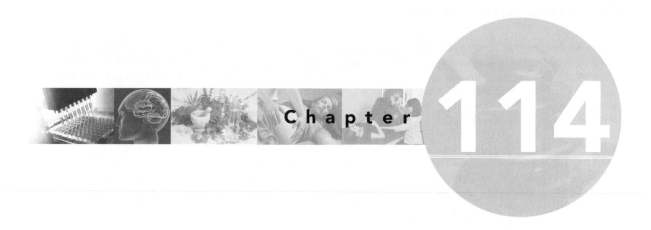

114

Creating Ceremony and Ritual in the Medical Encounter

Howard Silverman, MD

Philosophy

The use of ceremony and ritual has been connected to health and healing across time and cultures. When the scientific revolution began in earnest, the ceremonial roots of the healers' art began to separate from the specific techniques and approaches used by scientifically based clinicians. Increasingly, clinical interventions are focused almost exclusively on the physical aspects of disease. The impact of this approach has been amazing, yet patients and families are left to make sense of the meaning aspects of illness privately. Clinicians face many of the same issues as the amount of time they spend with patients diminishes and administrative, financial, and legal pressures mount.[1] The growth of interest in complementary and alternative therapies during the past 20 years[2,3] reflects, in part, a compensatory movement; that is, patients are seeking ways to recover the sacred as it relates to health and disease. They are eager for better communication with their clinicians, active participation in their treatment, and approaches that value an emphasis on the whole person.[4]

Few conventionally trained clinicians feel comfortable working on this level with patients and families, although notable exceptions can be found in geriatrics and hospice settings.[5,6] Complementary and alternative medicine (CAM) practitioners vary widely as well, although many of the modalities lend themselves to a more ceremonial application. Consider, for example, the scents and ritual involved in massage or acupuncture. Furthermore, CAM practitioners frequently spend more time with their patients, thereby facilitating this level of interaction.

This chapter discusses what is meant by ceremony and ritual; explores the importance of ceremonies and ritual; discusses the underlying structure of ceremonies and rituals,

including examples; and offers specific suggestions for incorporation of ceremony and ritual appropriately into clinical practice.

What Do We Mean by Ceremony and Ritual?

It is helpful to define what we mean by the terms *ceremony* and *ritual*.[7,8] They can be defined as follows:

> The words "ritual" and "ceremony" are so widely used that they mean many things to different people. Generally, both words refer to processes that separate the ordinary from the extraordinary. Some of these processes are repetitive ("rituals") and others may be performed only on special occasions ("ceremonies").[7]

We all perform various rituals many times per day—brushing our teeth or driving to work. Often, we perform these activities on "autopilot." For example, we may arrive home and not even remember specific locations or turns along the way. Some might call this daydreaming, but it is associated with an altered mental state that may be accompanied by time distortion and amnesia, common counterparts of hypnotic states. Most rituals offer a limited opportunity to suspend the pressures of the day and allow some "downtime." Activities such as meals are often mere rituals, but they can also be valuable family ceremonies with some minor alterations.[9]

Ceremonies, on the other hand, generally occur only on special occasions, have a specific purpose, and are consciously designed to have beneficial effects. In the space that is created, extraordinary things are allowed to happen, at least for a while. Things can be safely said that might not otherwise be comfortable to share. Connections can be made that might not occur in day-to-day life. Powerful insight may come in the twinkling of an eye. Yet the paradox is that one can never predict whether such a thing will happen, when it will happen, or how. We offer our intention to forces beyond our understanding but cannot control the outcome. Ceremonies may be derived from family or religious traditions. With the increasingly mobile nature of our culture and resulting disruptions in stable communal life, ceremonies are increasingly becoming lost or fractured. In addition, it is often challenging or inhibiting to find common ground with regard to ceremony, particularly if the participants come from different cultures or religions. Sadly, we increasingly see negative ceremonies, such as gang initiations, replacing functional ceremonies that are rooted in communal life.

> Ceremonies provide the opportunity to reframe, reformat, reinvent, and retell the stories through which we orient and explain our lives and are healing not only for patients but for clinicians as well.

The good news is that the human need for ceremony in connection with healing is so strong that ceremonies persist even in conventional medicine. As discussed in more detail later, this statement applies to medical procedures such as surgery and office visits as well as to medical education (e.g., grand rounds or ward rounds). The difficulty, however, is that the meaning and connection have been lost, and therefore these ceremonies no longer retain their full vibrancy and healing potential.

The Importance of Ceremonies

One view of what is really happening within a ceremony is that first we suspend our ordinary time-space relationships in a safe place. When we do so, the way is opened for extraordinary things to happen. In this protected time-space, we can revitalize our sustaining connections to the truth within ourselves and to things other than ourselves: to people, forests, animals, land, and some things we believe in. Ceremonies provide the opportunity to reframe, reformat, reinvent, and retell the stories through which we orient and explain our lives.

> A ceremony usually occurs on a special occasion and has a specific purpose to beneficial effects. During this time, things can be safely discussed that may not be comfortable to share outside the ceremony.

What is ultimately possible is rarely achieved through certainty; more often it takes a "leap of faith." Ceremonies provide a lens through which we can see things in a new light. They provide the structure by which we can lift our hearts from self-doubt. They provide an access into the world of faith and the human spirit. Ceremonies help provide roadmaps that restore our dreams, express our visions, and give us hope. They give us a time to experience awe, a state in which we lift ourselves out of the ordinary into a different level of consciousness. Awe is the ultimate reminder that we are small and the universe is large. Awe helps us find the faith to move forward.

Two powerful effects of ceremonies are (1) offering an opportunity to exert control over situations and (2) linking members of a community to provide mutual support.

Control

Individuals who are diagnosed with serious or life-threatening illness face an enormous loss of control in their lives. They lose a sense of predictability over their futures and frequently perceive no choice other than to simply defer to their clinicians' recommendations for diagnosis and treatment. In some cases, they may experience significant loss of function, dignity, or body parts. In wishing to re-exert control over their situation, some may inappropriately reject conventional interventions, often to their detriment. Another option to regain control over a situation like this is to reframe the significance and meaning related to it. For example, a parent may feel helpless to affect the outcome of a disabled child, but even in the face of this situation, he or she can choose to accept the loss and seek whatever good might arise from this situation. This approach advocates not denial of the reality of the situation but, rather, transcendence of the perception that it is hopeless or all bad. Ceremonial interventions can offer a powerful tool to help patients and families cross the chasm from denial toward acceptance while alleviating undue fear, suffering, depression, and dysfunction.

Black Elk, a legendary Oglala Sioux medicine man, lived in the early part of the twentieth century. In his biography of this remarkable man, John Neihardt[10] quotes Black Elk as saying, "A [person] who has a vision is not able to use the power of it until after he has performed the vision on earth for the people to see." That is, it is not enough to try to think differently about your situation; at some point, you need to act out a new vision before other people. Ceremony is one technique that allows this revisioning to happen. This is not a new concept, as reflected in our legal traditions, such as witnessing or notarizing the signing of important documents. One could argue that witnessing and notarizing are simply legal requirements to prevent fraud, but they nonetheless retain a vestigial ceremonial aspect. Ceremonies are an important tool to reestablish control over difficult situations, and studies support the positive health effects of perceiving that one has control over one's situation. An example is that people in assisted living and care center settings live longer when they have a choice about their food, furniture arrangement, plants, and pets.[11,12]

Community

Human beings rely on one another for support and interaction. If we were to remove ourselves entirely from contact with others, we would likely die. As mentioned previously, increasing mobility exerts a significant disruptive effect on our communal connections. Paradoxically, we most need community when facing a serious illness, but illness can disrupt a person's communal fabric in many ways:

1. One often experiences a significant diversion of time for medical diagnosis and treatments.
2. The stigma of disease may cause friends and family members to limit or avoid contact.
3. Impairments from acute or chronic conditions may limit one's ability to participate in meaningful communal life.

The second major benefit of ceremonies is that they can act as powerful glue to initiate, renew, and sustain functional communities. The presence of friends and family during a ceremony serves the purpose of witnessing, but there is more to it. Everyone can remember a time when they participated in a ceremony and felt strongly connected to the other participants. It might have been a reunion, a wedding, or participation in team sports. Whatever the circumstance, most people report a strong sense of connection and bonding that persists long after the event is over. The social networks established and maintained in this way are important in maintaining health and even more so in addressing the logistical, emotional, and spiritual effects of illness.

Structure of Ceremonies

Some ceremonies derive from ancient or family traditions, and others are created to serve a specific purpose. Before the exploration of how ceremonies are put together, it is important to note a few caveats:

- Ceremonies are best used to bring meaning, control, and connection into patients' lives. Under no circumstances should one think of them as inviting some kind of "magical" cure.

- From an ethical and effectiveness perspective, it is crucial that ceremonies remain entirely patient centered, particularly with respect to purpose, process, and symbols.

Components

One useful way to think about the inner structure of ceremonies is listed in Box 114-1.

Shared Purpose

It is important that all of the participants of the ceremony understand and share the purpose for the event. This idea should be clarified and communicated clearly and should be realistic. For example, parents of a disabled child may state that they wish to let go of their grief about the disability and move into the future. This is a suitable, clear, and realistic purpose. Saying they want to hold a ceremony to "cure" the child, however, is neither suitable nor realistic.

BOX 114-1. Components of a Ceremony

Shared purpose
Shared preparation
Community and facilitator
Opening
Materials
   Sacraments
   Ceremonial objects
   Ceremonial dress
Process
   Sharing
   Metaphor and symbols
   Trance
   Ceremonial language
Closure

Shared Preparation

There is a practical element to preparation, in that the materials and processes for the ceremony need to be assembled during the preparation phase. Preparation is a time laden with possibility. Relationships can be forged or strengthened as participants work together toward a common purpose. It is also a wonderful opportunity for reflection and introspection. For example, the preparation involved for a wedding is a time for the two families to get to know each other and (it is hoped) work in unison toward a common goal.

Community and Facilitator

For the ceremony to proceed smoothly, it must have a clearly designated facilitator who keeps people and processes on track. This is usually a person who has experience in such facilitation work and knows how to balance structuring of the unfolding events with being open to new possibilities that might arise. Ideally designated as the purpose is being defined, the facilitator also supervises planning and preparation. The community also must be defined, invited, and, when appropriate, prepared for or involved in the preparation phase. Ceremonies that people drift in and out of are generally not nearly as effective.

Opening

Because the ceremonial "bubble" is one in which extraordinary things can occur and a different quality of attention is invited from the facilitator and community, it is important to clarify when the ceremony has begun and when it has ended. This clarification can be made in a variety of ways—a reading, a song, lighting of a candle, or greeting the patient as one enters the examination or operating room.

Materials
Sacraments

The word *sacraments* has a special meaning in some religious contexts, but here it is used in a more general way to denote anything that affects the senses. Thus, sacraments can be ingested, felt, heard, or smelled. Of these, olfactory sacraments seem to be the most powerful, an observation that is consistent with the fact that our sense of smell is connected into our limbic systems and bypasses cortical areas. In some cultures, hallucinogens are ingested, and religious ceremonies may involve wine or special foods.

Another manifestation of the erosion of communal ceremonies in modern culture is the widespread abuse of sacraments, particularly tobacco, food, and alcohol. When sacraments are used outside a proper ceremony, their effect is lessened. This process leads to a kind of "sacramental tachyphylaxis," that is, more and more of the substance must be used to achieve the desired effect, in contrast to a small amount of the substance typically used in a ceremony. Thus, part of the effectiveness of addiction treatment programs such as Alcoholics Anonymous is related to the introduction of functional ceremony in the context of a supportive community.

Ceremonial Objects

Ceremonial objects are items usually only used during the ceremony; they may be created during the preparation phase or may be objects used over time for similar purposes. They should be chosen in service of the purpose and process and with sensitivity to the beliefs of the participants. Ceremonial objects that

TABLE 114-1. Examples of Nonclinical Ceremonies

COMPONENT	MARRIAGE	SUPER BOWL SUNDAY
Shared purpose	Forge a union between two individuals and two families	Go, team, go!
Shared preparation	Invitations, planning ceremony, food	Inviting friends and assembling food and drink
Community and facilitator	Minister, invited family members	Party host, family, and friends
Opening	Opening processional	Opening kickoff (for some, it's the pregame show)
Materials 　Sacraments 　Ceremonial objects 　Ceremonial dress	 Wine, candles, incense, flowers Family bible Wedding dress, tuxedos	 Beer A special football Team shirts, hats
Process 　Sharing 　Metaphor and symbols 　Trance 　Ceremonial language	 Vows Best man, bridesmaids, processional, rings Sense of a "cocoon" Blessings	 Screaming and shouting The forces of good versus evil Frequent as a result of beer and evidenced by football "widows/widowers" Technical football jargon and stats
Closure	Recessional and reception	Closing gun

have been used over time or have a strong connection to the past are particularly powerful. Some people might believe that surgeons who become upset if their special instruments are not available are acting "childish"; however, if they are seen as ceremonial objects, the reaction is much more understandable.

◼ Ceremonial Dress
Although it is not universal, the facilitator and participants may create or require various types of clothing that serve the purpose and process of the ceremony. Like ceremonial objects, ceremonial dress in most cases is used uniquely in the context of ceremony and may be assembled during the preparation phase. A wedding gown is a good example; imagine the power of wearing one's grandmother's gown or one handmade by a favorite relative. The white coat in medical care is another that is now used in ceremonies "welcoming entering medical students and [which] helps establish a psychological contract for the practice of medicine."[13]

Process
◼ Sharing
All ceremony involves some kind of sharing, usually in words although not exclusively so. A skilled facilitator will find ways to make sharing happen in a meaningful yet safe way and will give participants multiple options to share. For example, in a traditional Native American talking circle, an eagle feather (= ceremonial object) is passed around the circle of participants, and each is invited to talk if he or she wishes to. One participant in such a circle asked, "What was put in that feather? I fondly remembered things I haven't thought about in years!"

◼ Metaphor and Symbols
Humans respond strongly to metaphor and symbols, and a skilled facilitator makes use of this response during the ceremony. For example, in a ceremony to release unrealistic hopes and dreams for a disabled child, the hopes and dreams could be written on paper and burned. This is an area in which knowledge of the patient coupled with creativity and sensitivity can produce significant breakthroughs.

◼ Trance
Trance states are frequently involved in ceremonies. In some cultures, trance states may be intentionally induced through the use of hallucinogenic sacraments, drumming, or chanting. These states are frequently associated with a sense of time distortion, focal attention to the events of the ceremony, or amnesia. Trance states often happen in the operating room when excellent surgeons are at work and completely focused on the task at hand.

◼ Ceremonial Language
Specialized language that is common to the participants is often used during ceremonies. For example, in traditional religious ceremonies, Latin or Hebrew may be spoken. Interestingly, medical ceremonies have a highly specialized language or jargon, although it is usually not well understood by patients or family members.

Closure
See earlier discussion of opening. It is often desirable for the closure to be done in some way that connects with the opening, for example, blowing out a candle lit during the opening for closure with a patient in the examination room.

Examples

Examples of how these components apply to common nonclinical and clinical ceremonies are described in Tables 114-1 and 114-2. This type of analysis could be applied to a wide variety of clinical procedures and encounters. Observations over time indicate the following:

- There are very few widely shared ceremonies within the United States, with the possible exception of the Super Bowl.

- The common feature of medical ceremonies is the relative lack of sharing with regard to purpose and preparation. This generally results in an unsatisfying and sometimes unproductive experience for both the clinician and the patient.

TABLE 114-2. Clinical Ceremonial Examples

COMPONENT	CHILDBIRTH	SURGERY
Shared purpose	Have a healthy baby, decrease pain, and minimize morbidity	Patient and surgeon may have varying understandings of the purpose of the surgery
Shared preparation	Extensive—prenatal care	Usually separate—patient is in preoperative area and surgeon is elsewhere
Community and facilitator	Obstetrician usually facilitates; patient, coach, family, and labor and delivery staff	Family and operating room crew Facilitator may be surgeon, anesthesiologist, or scrub nurse, depending on who you ask
Opening	Variable—onset of contractions, admission to labor and delivery unit	Surgical incision
Materials Sacraments	Pain medications, music	Preoperative and intraoperative medications Coffee for operating room staff
Ceremonial objects Ceremonial dress	Forceps when necessary Special gowns	Surgeon's special instruments, other Scrubs, hospital gowns
Process Sharing	Entire delivery process is a team effort Many times, there is sharing of support, hopes, excitement	Very little
Metaphor and symbols	Many possibilities, e.g., asking father to cut umbilical cord	Very little
Trance	Definitely on the part of mother	Focused awareness, particularly noted in experienced surgeons
Ceremonial language	Medical jargon, but language often learned in prenatal visits and delivery training courses	Technical jargon
Closure	Crying of baby	Suture of incision

- Childbirth and a hospice death are two of the few medical ceremonies that continue to involve extensive sharing of purpose and preparation, and they remain a revitalizing and meaningful experience for both patient and clinicians.

- Almost any ceremony, medical or otherwise, can be renovated to make it more meaningful and effective (see next section).

Incorporating Ceremony and Ritual in Your Practice

Some clinicians may wish to engage their patients in the planning, preparation, and execution of formal ceremonies. Although most do not prefer to be in a position to do so, some lessons can be learned from ceremonial practice. These lessons can be easily and innocuously incorporated into clinical practice as follows.

1. Clinical scenarios in which these techniques are most applicable include
   a. The diagnosis of a life-threatening illness, such as cancer, heart disease, or multiple sclerosis
      (1) It is critical to assist the patient in gaining a sense of control over the situation and to prepare him or her for the road ahead.
      (2) Even without a ceremony, it is helpful to help the patient identify the major things he or she has lost as a result of this diagnosis and, for each of these, what he or she might gain as a result.
   b. Preparation for a significant surgical or diagnostic procedure
2. Reflect on what you do with patients every day, and consider how you might use this information to enliven these interactions. Small things can make a big difference.
   a. For procedures, enquire whether the patient has some special music he or she would like played or an article of clothing he or she would like to wear that would not interfere with the procedure.
   b. During office visits, have your staff allow the patient to sit in a chair while waiting for you, and take each history eye to eye with the patient. When examination time comes, moving the patient onto and then off of the table invites a sense of opening and closing. See Table 114-3 for a more detailed set of suggestions regarding office visits.
   c. Take a few deep breaths before entering the examination room, while reviewing the chart, or while washing your hands before an examination or procedure.
   d. Empower patients and staff to create appropriate rituals and ceremonies when it feels appropriate to do so.
3. Ceremonies are by definition healing not only for patients but for clinicians as well.
   a. Some medical clinics and offices have chosen to create and hold periodic office healing ceremonies focused on the well-being of clinicians and staff.
   b. When appropriate, attending patient life cycle rituals (weddings, births, funerals) can be healing for both the clinician and the family.
4. Experiment in your personal and professional arenas, and invite in the extraordinary and unexpected!

TABLE 114-3. Creating Ceremony Around the Healing-Oriented Office Visit

COMPONENT	OFFICE VISIT AS IT NOW IS	HEALING-ORIENTED OFFICE VISIT
Shared purpose	May or may not be mutually reviewed and fixed at the beginning of the office visit Often, nurse writes chief complaint on chart	Create the intention that this visit will focus on getting at the root of the problem
Shared preparation	Initial or interval history	Encourage the patient to tell "your story"
Community and facilitator	Clinician usually acts as facilitator; community is patient and anybody else in examination room	Encourage patient to invite key family and friends, and greet and acknowledge them individually
Opening	Door opening and initial greeting	Offer a moment of silence, reflection Reinforce the purpose by indicating that this is a visit to heal rather than to cure
Materials Sacraments	Smells of examination room, cold stethoscope, funky paper gowns	Create a warm and welcoming environment to facilitate introspection (indirect lighting, soft warm colors, comfortable seating)
Ceremonial objects	Otoscope, stethoscope, prescription pad	Encourage the patient, family, and friends to bring objects that are healing symbols for them Use a candle in a talking circle if appropriate
Ceremonial dress	Funky paper gown, white coat	The white coat still holds great power, but avoid the paper gowns

Process
  Sharing
  Metaphor and symbols
  Trance
 	
  Ceremonial language
	Interactivity during visit
	Limited—kind touch, language
	Limited
	
	Medical jargon, dosing
		Discussion of what really matters to the patient
		Variable—see ceremonial objects
		Encourage with periods of silence; these do not have to be long or uncomfortable but should be long enough to allow some reflection and "settling" of thoughts and feelings
		Consider inviting affirmations or prayer if appropriate and comfortable

Closure	Leaving examination room	Handshakes, but hugs preferred if appropriate and comfortable

References

References are available online at expertconsult.com.

Appendix Laboratory Testing Resources in Integrative Medicine

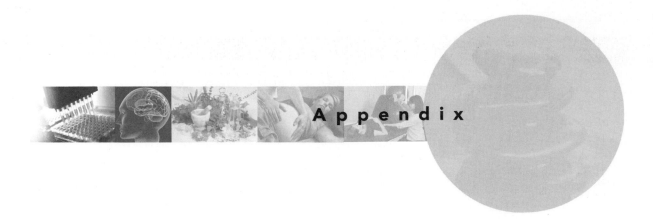

Laboratory Testing Resources in Integrative Medicine

David Rakel, MD

TEST	EXPLANATION	LABORATORY
Aging/Resiliency Markers Telomere length	Telomere length is given in relation to age group averages.	SpectraCell Laboratories
Digestion/Nutrition Stool culture and analysis	Digestive stool analysis includes a number of stool markers to assess digestion, absorption, metabolism, pancreatic function, inflammation, and fecal flora.	Doctors Data, Inc. Genova Diagnostics MetaMetrix
Intestinal permeability	This double sugar test measures the variable absorption of lactulose and mannitol after a challenge drink to measure permeability and absorption.	Doctor's Data, Inc. Genova Diagnostics
Small bowel bacterial overgrowth	A lactulose challenge test measures gas production (hydrogen and methane) during 2 hours to determine the level of bacterial fermentation in the distal small intestine.	Genova Diagnostics
Lactose intolerance	A lactose challenge test measures gas production to determine if lactose is digested properly.	EnteroLab
Micronutrient testing	Assesses the level and function of specific nutrients in blood	Doctor's Data, Inc. SpectraCell Laboratories
Essential Fatty Acids Plasma fatty acids	Rapid turnover will be an indication of current fatty acid intake; also allows assessment of triene/tetraene ratio.	MetaMetrix Nutrasource Diagnostics
Red blood cell fatty acids	Measure of erythrocyte cell membrane fatty acids will assess fatty acid intake in the past 2 to 4 months. Correlated with cardiovascular disease risk	Doctor's Data, Inc. Genova Diagnostics
Environmental Testing Drinking water	Evaluates water for heavy metals, fluoride, and pH	Doctor's Data, Inc.
Environmental pollutants	Tests urine for levels of common environmental pollutants, such as xylene, styrene, paraben, and phthalates	US BioTek
Heavy Metals Hair	Although considered of unknown value, these tests have been used for the past 25 years by the Environmental Protection Agency to monitor environmental changes in toxic metals.	Doctors Data, Inc. Genova Diagnostics MetaMetrix

TEST	EXPLANATION	LABORATORY
Urine	Random and timed urine tests can also provide another indication of exposure. This test is particularly important as a baseline evaluation before a chelating agent is given to determine total body burden.	Doctors Data, Inc. Genova Diagnostics MetaMetrix
Post-provocation urine	Chelating agents, including EDTA (to bind lead) and DMSA or DMPS (to bind mercury), are given before a timed urine test to assess total body burden of a given heavy metal. This is useful to monitor treatment in an individual, but post-provocation reference ranges are not available.	Doctors Data, Inc. Genova Diagnostics MetaMetrix
Hormones Salivary/adrenal	Salivary hormone levels of DHEA and cortisol measure free hormone availability and have been demonstrated to correspond with adrenal function	Diagnos-Techs Genova Diagnostics MetaMetrix ZRT Laboratory
Salivary/female	Salivary hormone levels of progesterone, testosterone, and estradiol have been normalized and correlate with free hormone availability. Data on changes in salivary levels in the setting of hormone therapy make it unclear as a tool for monitoring treatment levels.	Diagnos-Techs Genova Diagnostics ZRT Laboratory
Serum/hormone metabolites	Ratio of 2-hydroxyestrone/16-hydroxyestrone in blood has been demonstrated in the Women's Health Initiative cohort to be predictive of recurrence of breast cancer.	Genova Diagnostics
Urine/hormone metabolites	Ratio of 2-hydroxyestrone/16-hydroxyestrone in urine has been correlated with risk of breast cancer (low) and risk of osteoporosis (high).	Genova Diagnostics Meridian Valley Laboratory MetaMetrix Rocky Mountain Analytical US BioTek
Immunology Immune function	Flow cytometry evaluation of NK-cell function as well as presence/activity of immune cells and cytokines	ImmunoSciences Lab
Food allergies	Measures of IgE and IgG activation in the presence of various food antigens; IgE = allergic reaction, IgG = intolerance	ALCAT Elisa/ACT Genova Diagnostics Immuno Laboratories ImmunoSciences Lab Meridian Valley Laboratory MetaMetrix Rocky Mountain Analytical US BioTek
NutriGenomics	Broad-based term to represent genomic testing performed that highlights individual biochemical needs for particular macronutrients, micronutrients, and medications. It is experimental at this point because no outcome studies have demonstrated clinical validity.	Genova Diagnostics SpectraCell Laboratories
Oxidative Stress Markers Lipid peroxides, isoprostane, 8-hydroxydeoxyguanosine	Markers of oxidative end-tissue damage to fats, proteins, and DNA	Brunswick Laboratories Genox Corporation Genova Diagnostics MetaMetrix
Glutathione, total antioxidant capacity (TAC)/ total reactive antioxidant potential (TRAP), superoxide dismutase	Markers of capacity to deal with oxidative stress	Brunswick Laboratories Genox Corporation Genova Diagnostics

Laboratory Contact Information

ALCAT
Cell Science Systems
852 South Military Trail
Deerfield Beach, FL 33442
800-872-5228
www.alcat.com/

Brunswick Laboratories
6 Thacher Lane
Wareham, MA 02571
508-291-1830
www.brunswicklabs.com

Diagnos-Techs
6620 S 192nd Place, Bldg J
Kent, WA 98032
800-878-3787
www.diagnostechs.com

Doctor's Data, Inc.
3755 Illinois Avenue
St. Charles, IL 60174-2420
800-323-2784
www.doctorsdata.com

ELISA/ACT Biotechnologies
14 Pidgeon Hill Drive
Suite 180
Sterling, VA 20165
800-553-5472
www.elisaact.com

EnteroLab
10851 Ferguson Rd, Suite B
Dallas, TX 75228
972-686-6869
www.enterolab.com

Genova Diagnostics
63 Zillicoa Street
Asheville, NC 28801
800-522-4762
www.gdx.net

Genox Corporation
1414 Key Highway
Baltimore, MD 21230
800-810-5450
www.genox.com

Immuno Laboratories
6801 Powerline Road
Fort Lauderdale, FL 33309
800-231-9197
www.immunolabs.com

ImmunoSciences Lab
8693 Wilshire Blvd, Suite 200
Beverly Hills, CA 90211
800-950-4686
www.immuno-sci-lab.com

Meridian Valley Laboratory
801 SW 16th Suite 126
Renton, WA 98055
425-271-8689
www.meridianvalleylab.com

MetaMetrix Clinical Laboratory
4855 Peachtree Industrial Blvd, Suite 201
Norcross, GA 30092
800-221-4640
www.metametrix.com

Nutrasource Diagnostics
519-824-4120 x 58817
www.omega3testing.com

Rocky Mountain Analytical
Unit A, 253147 Bearspaw Road NW
Calgary, Alberta
Canada T3L 2P5
403-241-4513
www.rmalab.com/

SpectraCell Laboratories
10401 Town Park Drive
Houston, TX 77072
800-227-5227
www.spectracell.com/

US BioTek
13500 Linden Ave North
Seattle, WA 98133
877-318-8728
www.usbiotek.com

ZRT Laboratory
1815 NW 169th Pl, Suite 5050
Beaverton, OR 97006
503-466-2445
www.salivatest.com

Index

Page numbers followed by *f* refer to figures;
page numbers followed by *t* refer to tables; page
numbers followed by *b* refer to boxes; page
numbers with *e* refer to online-only material.

1007